MANUAL FOR Clinical Trials Nursing

THIRD EDITION

Edited by
Angela D. Klimaszewski, RN, MSN
Monica Bacon, RN
Julia A. Eggert, PhD, GNP-BC, AGN-BC, AOCN®
Elizabeth Ness, RN, MS
Joan G. Westendorp, RN, MSN, OCN®, CCRP, CIM
Kelly Willenberg, MBA, BSN, CCRP, CHRC

Oncology Nursing Society
Pittsburgh, Pennsylvania

ONS Publications Department
Publisher and Director of Publications: William A. Tony, BA, CQIA
Managing Editor: Lisa M. George, BA
Assistant Managing Editor: Amy Nicoletti, BA, JD
Acquisitions Editor: John Zaphyr, BA, MEd
Copy Editors: Vanessa Kattouf, BA, Andrew Petyak, BA, Laura Pinchot, BA
Graphic Designer: Dany Sjoen
Editorial Assistant: Judy Holmes

Copyright © 2016 by the Oncology Nursing Society. All rights reserved. No part of the material protected by this copyright may be reproduced or utilized in any form, electronic or mechanical, including photocopying, recording, or by an information storage and retrieval system, without written permission from the copyright owner. For information, visit www.ons.org/sites/default/files/Publication%20Permissions.pdf, or send an email to pubpermissions@ons.org.

Library of Congress Cataloging-in-Publication Data

Manual for clinical trials nursing / editors, Angela D. Klimaszewski [and 5 others]. – Third edition.
    p. ; cm.
  Includes bibliographical references and index.
  ISBN 978-1-935864-37-0
  I. Klimaszewski, Angela D., editor. II. Oncology Nursing Society, issuing body.
  [DNLM: 1. Clinical Trials as Topic–nursing. 2. Neoplasms–nursing. 3. Clinical Nursing Research. WY 156]
  RC267
  362.19699'40072–dc23

2015021838

Publisher's Note

This book is published by the Oncology Nursing Society (ONS). ONS neither represents nor guarantees that the practices described herein will, if followed, ensure safe and effective patient care. The recommendations contained in this book reflect ONS's judgment regarding the state of general knowledge and practice in the field as of the date of publication. The recommendations may not be appropriate for use in all circumstances. Those who use this book should make their own determinations regarding specific safe and appropriate patient care practices, taking into account the personnel, equipment, and practices available at the hospital or other facility at which they are located. The editors and publisher cannot be held responsible for any liability incurred as a consequence from the use or application of any of the contents of this book. Figures and tables are used as examples only. They are not meant to be all-inclusive, nor do they represent endorsement of any particular institution by ONS. Mention of specific products and opinions related to those products do not indicate or imply endorsement by ONS. Websites mentioned are provided for information only; the hosts are responsible for their own content and availability. Unless otherwise indicated, dollar amounts reflect U.S. dollars.

ONS publications are originally published in English. Publishers wishing to translate ONS publications must contact ONS about licensing arrangements. ONS publications cannot be translated without obtaining written permission from ONS. (Individual tables and figures that are reprinted or adapted require additional permission from the original source.) Because translations from English may not always be accurate or precise, ONS disclaims any responsibility for inaccuracies in words or meaning that may occur as a result of the translation. Readers relying on precise information should check the original English version.

Printed in the United States of America

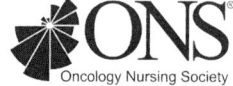

Integrity • Innovation • Stewardship • Advocacy • Excellence • Inclusiveness

For Joe, my love, my best friend and best time;
For Michael, my pride, inspiration, and role model
Always reach for the stars.

For my coeditors and authors, and the clinical trial nurses worldwide who contribute daily to improving the human condition while advocating for clinical trial participants and maintaining protocol integrity—thank you.

—Angela Klimaszewski

As with the second edition of this manual, I dedicate my contribution to oncology nurses worldwide. But I also wish to gratefully acknowledge two of the many unsung heroines of research—Henrietta Lacks and Rosalind Franklin.

—Monica Bacon

To the nurses working in clinical trials who offer opportunities for the newest state-of-the-art treatments (including the newest genetic technologies) and care to patients with cancer.

—Julia Eggert

Special thanks to my family for their continued love and support; to my authors and fellow coauthors for their expertise and patience; and to my colleagues for inspiring me to present clinical trial content in ways that the novice or expert clinical trial nurse will continue to learn.

—Elizabeth Ness

To the courageous patients who participate in clinical trials, whom I consider to be heroes. For all of the oncology nurses caring to make a difference in a patient's life—thank you.

—Joan Westendorp

For my husband, Dale, for always believing in me; to my twin daughters, Mariel and Brandy, who have proven to me that my greatest accomplishment in life is being a mom; to Dr. Eduardo R. Pajon, who introduced me to clinical trials nursing; and to Ryan D. Meade, Esq., who picked me up when I was down and opened the door to research compliance consulting.

—Kelly Willenberg

Contributors

Editors

Angela D. Klimaszewski, RN, MSN
Consultant
Port Monmouth, New Jersey
Chapter 14. Informed Consent; Chapter 44. Publishing Guidance for Clinical Trial Nurses

Monica Bacon, RN
Oncology Nurse and Researcher
Operations Manager, Gynecologic Cancer InterGroup
Kingston, Ontario, Canada

Julia A. Eggert, PhD, GNP-BC, AGN-BC, AOCN®
Doctoral Program Coordinator
School of Nursing
College of Health and Human Development
Clemson University
Clemson, South Carolina
Chapter 31. Pharmacogenetics and Pharmacogenomics; Chapter 33. Cytogenetics; Chapter 34. Tumor Profiling; Chapter 35. Storage of Genetic Material

Elizabeth Ness, RN, MS
Nurse Consultant, Education
Center for Cancer Research
National Cancer Institute
National Institutes of Health
Bethesda, Maryland
Chapter 4. Types of Clinical Research: Experimental; Chapter 10. The Research Team; Chapter 15. Protocol Development and Response Assessment; Chapter 28. Adverse Events; Chapter 42. Clinical Trial Nurse Education

Joan G. Westendorp, RN, MSN, OCN®, CCRP, CIM
Chief Nursing Officer
West Michigan Cancer Center
Kalamazoo, Michigan
Chapter 2. Drug Development; Chapter 3. Types of Clinical Research: Background; Chapter 7. Sponsoring Agencies; Chapter 27. Investigational Agents: Procurement, Accountability, and Administration of Research Study Drugs

Kelly Willenberg, MBA, BSN, CCRP, CHRC
Manager/Owner
Kelly Willenberg, LLC
Chesnee, South Carolina
Chapter 18. Billing, Budgets, and Funding; Chapter 19. Agreements and Contracts

Authors

Gloria Adams, RN, CCRP, OCN®
Clinical Monitoring Project Lead
inVentiv Health Clinical
Blue Bell, Pennsylvania
Chapter 40. Data and Safety Monitoring Plans

Kim Adler, RN
Clinical Trials Nurse Consultant
Calvary Mater Newcastle, Medical Oncology Clinical Trial Unit
Newcastle, New South Wales, Australia
Chapter 45. Australia

Sviatlana Alimpiyeva, MD
Chief Specialist, Republican Clinical and Pharmacological Laboratory
Republican Unitary Enterprise Centre for Expertise and Testing in Health Care
Minsk, Belarus
Chapter 47. Belarus

Rosa Maria Álvarez-Gómez, MD
Medical Researcher
Genomics and Massive Sequencing Unit
Instituto Nacional de Cancerología
Mexico City, Mexico
Chapter 57. Mexico

Eriko Aotani, RN, MSN, CCRP
Director
Global Health Research Coordinating Center
Kanagawa Academy of Science and Technology
Kanagawa, Japan
Chapter 56. Japan

Tammie L. Bain, BS, JD
Independent Consultant
Tacoma, Washington
Chapter 22. Financial Conflict of Interest

Carol Anne Bales, RN, MSN, CCRP
Retired RN
Wilmington, North Carolina
Chapter 8. Legal, Regulatory, and Legislative Issues; Chapter 27. Investigational Agents: Procurement, Accountability, and Administration of Research Study Drugs; Chapter 40. Data and Safety Monitoring Plans

Heather Benzel, BSN, RN, CCRP
Quality Management RN
VA Nebraska-Western Iowa Health Care System
Grand Island, Nebraska
Chapter 1. History and Background of Oncology Clinical Trials

Regina Berger, PhD, SC
Head of AGO Austria Clinical Trial Office
Department for Gynecology and Obstetrics, AGO-Studienzentrale
Medical University of Innsbruck
Innsbruck, Austria
Chapter 46. Austria

Lora Black, RN, MPH, OCN®, CCRP
Director of Clinical Research—Oncology
Sanford Research
Sioux Falls, South Dakota
Chapter 18. Billing, Budgets, and Funding

Chantale Blattler, HonBSc, CCRP
Program Manager
Princess Margaret Cancer Centre
Toronto, Ontario, Canada
Chapter 48. Canada

Belinda Chung Yee Borrmann, RN
Study Coordinator/RN
Kliniken Essen Mitte
Essen, Germany
Chapter 52. Germany

Valerie Bowering, RN, CONC
Clinical Research Coordinator III
Princess Margaret Cancer Centre
Toronto, Ontario, Canada
Chapter 48. Canada

Sally Brown, RN, BSN, MGA, OCN®, CBCN®, CCRP
Coordinator, Research Protocols
MedStar Franklin Square Medical Center
Baltimore, Maryland
Chapter 8. Legal, Regulatory, and Legislative Issues

Jane Bryce, MSN, AOCNS®
Researcher Nurse
National Cancer Institute
Napoli, Italy
Chapter 50. European Union Directives; Chapter 55. Italy

Pamela Carney, MSN, RN, OCN®
Manager, Vanderbilt-Ingram Service for Timely Access
Vanderbilt-Ingram Cancer Center
Nashville, Tennessee
Chapter 3. Types of Clinical Research: Background

Karen Carty, CCR
Project Manager
Cancer Research UK Clinical Trials Unit, Glasgow
Glasgow, Scotland, United Kingdom
Chapter 62. United Kingdom

Ting Chang, MN
Associate Director of Site Management Organization
SMO ClinPlus Co., LTD
Shanghai, China
Chapter 49. China

Adriana Chávez-Blanco, DVM
Clinical Trials and Harmonisation Operations Manager
Grupo de Investigación en Cáncer de Ovario y Tumores Ginecológicos de México
Mexico City, Mexico
Chapter 57. Mexico

Ann M. Lau Clark, RN, MSN, CCRC, CCRP
Clinical Research Nurse Team Leader
Loyola University Cardinal Bernardin Cancer Center
Maywood, Illinois
Chapter 28. Adverse Events

Wendy Cooper, RN, BSN, OCN®, CCRP
Manager of Outpatient Oncology
Sarah Cannon Cancer Center
Nashville, Tennessee
Chapter 17. Workload Determination and Resource Allocation

Patricia Cortés-Esteban, MD
Assigned Physician at the Medical Oncology Service
Gynaecologic Tumours Clinic
Instituto de Seguridad y Servicios Sociales para los Trabajadores del Estado
Mexico City, Mexico
Chapter 57. Mexico

Georgia Cusack, MS, RN, AOCNS®
Director of Research Nursing and Education
Office of the Clinical Director
National Heart, Lung, and Blood Institute
National Institutes of Health
Bethesda, Maryland
Chapter 4. Types of Clinical Research: Experimental

Kathy Czaplicki, RN, MSN, CCRC
Clinical Research Nurse Team Leader
Loyola University Cardinal Bernardin Cancer Center
Maywood, Illinois
Chapter 30. Psychosocial Distress

Sourat Darabi, PhD(c)
Graduate Research Assistant
Clemson University
Clemson, South Carolina
Chapter 33. Cytogenetics

Irene Fernández-Bravo Del Olmo, CTN
Clinical Trial Nurse
MD Anderson Cancer Center Madrid
Madrid, Spain
Chapter 60. Spain

Karri Donahue, MSN, RN, CCRP
Clinical Research Coordinator
Catholic Health Initiatives
CHI Health St. Elizabeth
Lincoln, Nebraska
Chapter 1. History and Background of Oncology Clinical Trials

Belinda Egan, RN Dip Cert.
Research Nurse Coordinator
Christchurch Hospital
Christchurch, New Zealand
Chapter 58. New Zealand

Gabriele Elser, RN
Head of AGO Study Office
AGO Research GmbH
Wiesbaden, Germany
Chapter 50. European Union Directives; Chapter 52. Germany

Rose Ermete, RN, BSN, OCN®, CCRP
Quality Assurance Nurse Auditor
SWOG
San Antonio, Texas
Chapter 43. Mentorship

Lyndon Vestal Evans, RN, BS
Manager, Oncology Clinical Research
NCORP of the Carolinas
Greenville Health System Cancer Institute
Greenville, South Carolina
Chapter 20. Financial Risk Assessment and Monitoring

Kelly Filchner, MSN, RN, OCN®, CCRC
Director, Clinical Operations
Fox Chase Cancer Center Partners
Fox Chase Cancer Center
Philadelphia, Pennsylvania
Chapter 16. Protocol Review and Approval Process

Lisa Francisco, BSN, RN, OCN®
Oncology Clinical Nurse Educator
Ipsen Biopharmaceuticals
Basking Ridge, New Jersey
Chapter 25. Adherence and Retention in Clinical Trials

Dolores Gallardo-Rincón, MD
Ovarian Cancer Program
Instituto Nacional de Cancerología
Mexico City, Mexico
Chapter 57. Mexico

David Gillogly, BS, MBA
Senior Director, Clinical Management
Otsuka Pharmaceutical Development and Commercialization
Princeton, New Jersey
Chapter 2. Drug Development

Contributors vii

Marjorie J. Good, RN, BSN, MPH, OCN®
Nurse Consultant
Division of Cancer Prevention
National Cancer Institute
National Institutes of Health
Bethesda, Maryland
Chapter 24. Accrual Base, Recruitment, and Promotion Strategies

Nicole Grant, RN, BSN, MPH
Director, Regulatory Affairs Office
Center for Cancer Research
National Cancer Institute
National Institutes of Health
Bethesda, Maryland
Chapter 39. Creating and Maintaining a Regulatory File

Daniela Grosso, MSN
Research Nurse
Assistant Director, Service Health Professionals
Istituto Oncologico Veneto IRCSS
Padua, Italy
Chapter 55. Italy

Clement K. Gwede, PhD, MPH, RN
Associate Member/Professor
H. Lee Moffitt Cancer Center and Research Institute
University of South Florida
Tampa, Florida
Chapter 17. Workload Determination and Resource Allocation

Jacqueline M. Hale, MSN, APNC, APNG-BC, AOCN®
Coordinator, Family Risk Assessment Program
Hunterdon Regional Cancer Center
Flemington, New Jersey
Chapter 32. Genetic Testing

Tasha D. Hall, PhD, RN
Associate Director, Medical Scientist
Gilead Sciences, Inc.
Foster City, California
Chapter 37. Documentation

Andrea Harkin, BA, CCR
Operations Director
Cancer Research UK Clinical Trials Unit, Glasgow
Glasgow, Scotland, United Kingdom
Chapter 62. United Kingdom

Elizabeth Hassen, MSN, OCN®
Lecturer, Adjunct Faculty
Doctoral Student in Interdisciplinary Healthcare Genetics
Clemson University
Clemson, South Carolina
Chapter 34. Tumor Profiling

Kathleen R. Hurtado, RPh
Independent Consultant
Nine 7 Consulting
Houston, Texas
Chapter 27. Investigational Agents: Procurement, Accountability, and Administration of Research Study Drugs

D. Marie Jackson, PhD, MBA
Director of Research Services and Finance
Office of Research Administration
Parkland Health and Hospital System
Dallas, Texas
Chapter 21. Internal Financial Audit and Quality Assurance

Annamalar Jeyasehar, PhD(c), MSN, RN
Graduate Student, Healthcare Genetics
Graduate Teaching Assistant, Healthcare Genetics Undergraduate Curriculum
School of Nursing, College of Health Education and Human Development
Clemson University
Clemson, South Carolina
Chapter 31. Pharmacogenetics and Pharmacogenomics

Manmana Jirajarus, MSN, APN
Advanced Practice Nurse (Oncology)
Ramathibodi Hospital, Mahidol University
Rachathewi, Bangkok, Thailand
Chapter 61. Thailand

Catherine Johnson, RN
Clinical Research Nurse and Gastrointestinal Cancer Care Coordinator
Department of Medical Oncology, Calvary Mater Newcastle
Waratah, New South Wales, Australia
Chapter 45. Australia

Satya Pal Kataria, MD, DM
Consultant and Head of Department of Medical Oncology
Vardhman Mahavir Medical College and Safdarjung Hospital
New Delhi, India
Chapter 53. India

Teresa Knoop, MSN, RN, AOCN®
Assistant Director, Clinical Trials Shared Resource
Vanderbilt-Ingram Cancer Center
Nashville, Tennessee
Chapter 3. Types of Clinical Research: Background

Bhavesh Kumari, MSc, MA
Vice Principal, College of Nursing
Vardhman Mahavir Medical College and Safdarjung Hospital
New Delhi, India
Chapter 53. India

Nathalie Le Fur, PhD
Clinical Project Manager
ARCAGY-GINECO
Hôpital Hôtel Dieu
Paris, France
Chapter 51. France

David Leos, MBA, RN, OCN®
Clinical Protocol Manager
Department of Plastic Surgery
University of Texas MD Anderson Cancer Center
Houston, Texas
Chapter 23. Public and Patient Education

Yanfei Liu, MN
Research Nurse, Administrator of Cancer Clinical Trials Office
Fudan University Shanghai Cancer Center
Shanghai, China
Chapter 49. China

Marisa Teruel López, CTN
Nurse and Clinical Trial Coordinator (Phases I–IV)
FINCIVO (Fundación de Investigación Instituto Valenciano de Oncología)
Valencia, Spain
Chapter 60. Spain

Yuting Luan, RN
Research Nurse
Fudan University Shanghai Cancer Center
Shanghai, China
Chapter 49. China

Lydia T. Madsen, RN, PhD, OCN®, AOCNS®
Advanced Practice Nurse
University of Texas MD Anderson Cancer Center
Houston, Texas
Chapter 15. Protocol Development and Response Assessment

Susan Markus, RN, BSN, MS, OCN®
Senior Research Nurse
Johns Hopkins University
Baltimore, Maryland
Chapter 8. Legal, Regulatory, and Legislative Issues

Volha Matylevich, MD, PhD
Leading Research Scientist
Gynecologic Oncology Department
N.N. Alexandrov National Cancer Center of Belarus
Minsk, Belarus
Chapter 47. Belarus

Sergey Mavrichev, MD, PhD
Head of Gynecologic Oncology Department
N.N. Alexandrov National Cancer Center of Belarus
Minsk, Belarus
Chapter 47. Belarus

Deirdre McDonnell, RN, RM
Clinical Research Coordinator
St. Vincent's University Hospital
Dublin, Ireland
Chapter 54. Ireland

Sandra A. Meadows, MPH, CIP
Senior Quality Improvement Specialist
The Ohio State University
Columbus, Ohio
Chapter 41. Preparing for Audits, Inspections, and Monitoring Visits

Abelardo Meneses-García, MD
General Director
Instituto Nacional de Cancerología
Mexico City, Mexico
Chapter 57. Mexico

Wendi Mitchell, RN, OCN®
Clinical Trials Coordinator
West Michigan Cancer Center
Kalamazoo, Michigan
Chapter 13. Elements of a Protocol

Anita Cizek Moore, MS, RN, CCRP
Director, Clinical Research Office
University of Maryland
Baltimore, Maryland
Chapter 9. Good Clinical Practice

Mariel D. Norton, JD
Baker, Ravenel, & Bender, LLP
Columbia, South Carolina
Chapter 19. Agreements and Contracts

Tanya O'Shea, MSc Oncology
European Clinical Operations Lead
Prothena Biosciences Limited
Alexandra House, The Sweepstakes Ballsbridge
Dublin, Ireland
Chapter 54. Ireland

Ellen A. Patricia, MS, CIP
Program Director, HRPP Quality Improvement
Office of Responsible Research Practices
The Ohio State University
Columbus, Ohio
Chapter 41. Preparing for Audits, Inspections, and Monitoring Visits

Pamela Perry, MS
Director, Clinical Management
Otsuka Pharmaceutical Development and Commercialization
Princeton, New Jersey
Chapter 2. Drug Development

Cecilia Petrowsky, RN, MSN, CCRC, OCN®
Manager, Cancer Clinical Trials Office
Loyola University Cardinal Bernardin Cancer Center
Maywood, Illinois
Chapter 11. Standard Operating Procedures

Adriana Placintar, RN
Nurse
Institute of Oncology—Day Hospital Unit
Cluj, Romania
Chapter 59. Romania

Dianne M. Reeves, RN, MSN
Associate Director for Biomedical Data Standards
National Cancer Institute
National Institutes of Health
Rockville, Maryland
Chapter 38. Data Management and Electronic Data Management Systems

Susana Baviera Rincón, CTN
Clinical Trial Nurse/Data Manager
FINCIVO (Fundación de Investigación Instituto Valenciano de Oncología)
Valencia, Spain
Chapter 60. Spain

Yuko Saito, MS, RN, CCRP
Clinical Trial Head/Clinical Leader
Novartis Pharma KK
Tokyo, Japan
Chapter 56. Japan

Geri L. Schmotzer, RN, MSN, MPH, PhD
Assistant Adjunct Professor
University of San Francisco
San Francisco, California
Chapter 5. Types of Clinical Research: Observational; Chapter 10. The Research Team; Chapter 29. Patient and Family Education

Kathleen Scott, PhD
Clinical Project Manager
ICORG—All-Ireland Cooperative Oncology Research Group
Dublin, Ireland
Chapter 54. Ireland

Saritha Shamsunder, MD, FRCOG
Senior Specialist OB/GYN
Vardhman Mahavir Medical College and Safdarjung Hospital
New Delhi, India
Chapter 53. India

Norma Sheridan-Leos, RN, MSN, AOCN®, CPHQ, CPPS
Performance Improvement Specialist
Houston Methodist Hospital
Houston, Texas
Chapter 23. Public and Patient Education

Suwannee Sirilerttrakul, MEd, APN
Advanced Practice Nurse (Oncology)
Ramathibodi Hospital, Mahidol University
Rachathewi, Bangkok, Thailand
Chapter 61. Thailand

Zelda Smith, RN, CBCN®, OCN®
Clinical Trials Coordinator
West Michigan Cancer Center
Kalamazoo, Michigan
Chapter 13. Elements of a Protocol

Douglas C. Stahl, PhD, MBA
VP of Enterprise Business Intelligence
City of Hope
Duarte, California
Chapter 21. Internal Financial Audit and Quality Assurance

Deborah A. (Lindberg) Standafer, RN-C, BSN, MBA, CCRC
Clinical Research Administrator
TriHealth Hatton Research Institute
Cincinnati, Ohio
Chapter 6. Expanded Access to Investigational Drugs

Connie M. Szczepanek, RN, BSN
Director
Cancer Research Consortium of West Michigan (CRCWM NCORP)
Grand Rapids Clinical Oncology Program
Grand Rapids, Michigan
Chapter 20. Financial Risk Assessment and Monitoring

Ashish Thakkar, MS
Clinical Protocol Coordinator
Loyola University Cardinal Bernardin Cancer Center
Maywood, Illinois
Chapter 36. Pharmacokinetic Trials

Lisa Tinker, RN, BScN, MHM
Nurse Manager—Ambulatory Care
Solid Tumor Oncology
Princess Margaret Cancer Centre
Toronto, Ontario, Canada
Chapter 48. Canada

Nina M. Trocky, DNP, RN, NE-BC, CCRA
RN to BSN Program Director
Assistant Professor
University of Maryland School of Nursing
Baltimore, Maryland
Chapter 26. Clinical Trial Registries

Brandy Troisi, BA, RN
Registered Nurse
Carolina Center for Behavioral Health
Moore, South Carolina
Chapter 18. Billing, Budgets, and Funding

Connie M. Ulrich, PhD, RN, FAAN
Associate Professor of Bioethics and Nursing
University of Pennsylvania School of Nursing
NewCourtland Center for Transitions and Health
Secondary Appointment, Department of Medical Ethics and Health Policy
University of Pennsylvania Perelman School of Medicine
Philadelphia, Pennsylvania
Chapter 12. Ethics of Clinical Research

Bénédicte Votan, MSc, Post Graduate
General Manager
ARCAGY-GINECO
Hôpital Hôtel Dieu
Paris, France
Chapter 51. France

Anita Walden, BS, CHI
Manager, Informatics Project Leader
Duke University Medical Center
Durham, North Carolina
Chapter 38. Data Management and Electronic Data Management Systems

Gwenyth R. Wallen, PhD, RN
Deputy Chief Nurse, Research and Practice Department
National Institutes of Health Clinical Center
Bethesda, Maryland
Chapter 12. Ethics of Clinical Research

Therese White, RN, MSN
Regulatory Affairs Specialist
National Cancer Institute
National Institutes of Health
Bethesda, Maryland
Chapter 39. Creating and Maintaining a Regulatory File

Kathy Wilkinson, RN, BSN, OCN®
Manager, Cancer Research and Registry
Billings Clinic Cancer Center
Billings, Montana
Chapter 35. Storage of Genetic Material

Patricia C. Woltz, PhD, RN
Director, Nursing Research
University of Maryland Medical Center
Baltimore, Maryland
Chapter 9. Good Clinical Practice

Siu-Fun Wong, PharmD, FASHP, FCSHP
Professor, Oncology
Associate Dean of Assessment and Scholarship
School of Pharmacy
Harry and Diane Rinker Health Science Campus, Irvine
Chapman University
Irvine, California
Chapter 27. Investigational Agents: Procurement, Accountability, and Administration of Research Study Drugs

Gema Piqueres Zafra, CTN
Clinical Trial Nurse
FINCIVO (Fundación de Investigación Instituto Valenciano de Oncología)
Valencia, Spain
Chapter 60. Spain

Vijay Zutshi, MD, FICOG
Consultant, OB/GYN
Vardhman Mahavir Medical College and Safdarjung Hospital
New Delhi, India
Chapter 53. India

Field Reviewers

Damiana M. Maloof, MSN, RN, OCN®
Oncology Research Nurse Program Supervisor, Office of Research
Newton-Wellesley Hospital
Newton, Massachusetts

Camille A. Servodidio, RN, MPH, OCN®, CCRP, CBCN®
Clinical Manager, Comprehensive Breast Center
Middlesex Hospital
Middletown, Connecticut

Janet F. Zimmerman, MS, RN
Assistant Clinical Professor
Drexel University
Philadelphia, Pennsylvania

Disclosure

Editors and authors of books and guidelines provided by the Oncology Nursing Society are expected to disclose to the readers any significant financial interest or other relationships with the manufacturer(s) of any commercial products.

A vested interest may be considered to exist if a contributor is affiliated with or has a financial interest in commercial organizations that may have a direct or indirect interest in the subject matter. A "financial interest" may include, but is not limited to, being a shareholder in the organization; being an employee of the commercial organization; serving on an organization's speakers bureau; or receiving research funding from the organization. An "affiliation" may be holding a position on an advisory board or some other role of benefit to the commercial organization. Vested interest statements appear in the front matter for each publication.

Contributors are expected to disclose any unlabeled or investigational use of products discussed in their content. This information is acknowledged solely for the information of the readers.

The contributors provided the following disclosure and vested interest information:

Kelly Willenberg, MBA, BSN, CCRP, CHRC: Kelly Willenberg, LLC, employment or leadership position, and consultant or advisory role; SWOG, honoraria
Lora Black, RN, MPH, OCN®, CCRP: Sanford Research, employment or leadership position, and research funding
Rose Ermete, RN, BSN, OCN®, CCRP: National Cancer Institute, research funding
Jacqueline M. Hale, MSN, APNC, APNG-BC, AOCN®: American Nurses Credentialing Center, employment or leadership position; Advanced Practitioner Society for Hematology/Oncology, Scripps Health, honoraria
Tasha D. Hall, PhD, RN: Gilead Sciences, employment or leadership position, and stock ownership
Catherine Johnson, RN: International Society of Nurses in Cancer Care, leadership position
David Leos, MBA, RN, OCN®: Oncology Nursing Society, honoraria
Connie M. Szczepanek, RN, BSN: National Cancer Institute NCORP Grant, employment or leadership position
Lisa Tinker, RN, BScN, MHM: AstraZeneca International National Ovarian Cancer Advisory Board, AstraZeneca International Saracatinib Nursing Advisory Board, AstraZeneca International Olaparib Nursing Advisory Board, consultant or advisory role
Siu-Fun Wong, PharmD, FASHP, FCSHP: SWOG, leadership position

Contents

Preface xvii

Acknowledgments xix

SECTION I. History and Foundation

Chapter 1. History and Background of Oncology Clinical Trials 3
   Introduction 3
   History 3
   Growth of International Guidelines and U.S. Regulations 5
   Treatment of Minorities and Women 6
   Treatment of Children and Older Adults 7
   Evolution of National Healthcare Reform 8
   Summary 8
   References 10

Chapter 2. Drug Development 13
   Introduction 13
   Where Does It All Begin? 13
   The Investigational New Drug Application 14
   Naming of Drugs 16
   Summary 16
   References 16

Chapter 3. Types of Clinical Research: Background 17
   Introduction 17
   Experimental Versus Observational Clinical Research 17
   Comparative Effectiveness Research 17
   Nursing Companion Studies 19
   Institute of Medicine Reports: Efforts to Improve the Clinical Trials
      Enterprise 20
   Summary 21
   References 21

Chapter 4. Types of Clinical Research: Experimental 23
   Introduction 23
   Key Concepts to Understanding Clinical Trial Designs 23
   Clinical Trial Designs 25
   Phases of Clinical Trials 27
   Summary 33
   References 33

Chapter 5. Types of Clinical Research: Observational 35
   Introduction 35
   Study Types 35
   Summary 38
   References 39

Chapter 6. Expanded Access to Investigational Drugs 41
   Introduction 41
   Expanded Access Programs 41
   Individual Patients, Including Emergency Use 42
   Intermediate-Sized Patient Populations 42
   Treatment Investigational New Drug Application or Treatment
      Protocol 43
   Charging Rules 43
   Availability in Community Health Organizations 43
   Implications for Clinical Trial Nurses 44
   Summary 44
   References 44

Chapter 7. Sponsoring Agencies 45
   Introduction 45
   Types of Sponsors 45
   Summary 48
   References 48

SECTION II. Clinical Trials: Fundamental Information

Chapter 8. Legal, Regulatory, and Legislative Issues 51
   Introduction 51
   Selected Historical Events 51
   U.S. Regulatory Authority 53
   International Conference on Harmonisation 57
   International Standards, Laws, and Guidelines 57
   Clinical Trials Registration and Patient Open Access 59
   Federal Clinical Trial Legislation 60
   State Clinical Trial Legislation 60
   Compliance Issues 61
   Summary 64
   References 64

Chapter 9. Good Clinical Practice 67
   Introduction 67
   Background 67
   Good Clinical Practice in a Global Economy 68
   U.S. Food and Drug Administration Good Clinical Practice 69
   Good Clinical Practice in Practice 69
   Summary 70
   References 71

Chapter 10. The Research Team 77
   Introduction 77
   Investigator 77
   Subinvestigator 80
   Research Participant 80
   The Nurse's Role 81
   Clinical Research Coordinator 84
   Clinical Data Manager 84
   The Interdisciplinary Team 84
   Summary 85
   References 86

Chapter 11. Standard Operating Procedures **89**
    Introduction 89
    Standard Operating Procedures and Quality Management 89
    Summary 92
    References 94

Chapter 12. Ethics of Clinical Research **97**
    Introduction 97
    Social and Scientific Value 97
    Informed Consent 99
    Therapeutic Misconception 99
    Institutional Review Boards 101
    Scientific Integrity 101
    Research Misconduct 102
    Conflict of Interest 102
    Ethics Consultation 103
    Summary 103
    References 104

SECTION III. Protocol Development, Review, and Approval Process

Chapter 13. Elements of a Protocol **109**
    Introduction 109
    Protocol Elements 109
    Summary 111
    References 111

Chapter 14. Informed Consent **113**
    Introduction 113
    Guiding Principles 113
    The Process of Informed Consent 115
    Required Elements of the Consent Form 115
    Assessing Comprehension and Improving Readability 117
    Special Populations 120
    Genetic Testing and Genomic Research 122
    Exemptions and Waivers 123
    Role of Clinical Trial Nurses 123
    Summary 123
    References 124

Chapter 15. Protocol Development and Response Assessment **127**
    Introduction 127
    Determining Primary and Secondary Objectives 127
    Selecting a Study Design 128
    Study Intervention and Required Procedures 129
    Oncology Trial Endpoints 131
    Statistical Considerations 134
    Analysis Plan 137
    Monitoring 137
    Summary 138
    References 139
    Additional Resources 140

Chapter 16. Protocol Review and Approval Process **141**
    Introduction 141
    Pre–Institutional Review Board Reviews and Approvals 141
    Institutional Review Board Ethical Review 143
    Types of Institutional Review Board Reviews 146
    Institutional Review Board Review Outcomes 150
    Additional Institutional Review Board Oversight Requirements 152
    Accreditation of Human Subject Protection Programs 153
    Summary 153
    References 154

SECTION IV. Financial Factors

Chapter 17. Workload Determination and Resource Allocation **157**
    Introduction 157
    Factors Affecting Workload Determination and Resource Allocation ... 157
    Promise of a Prospective Comprehensive Workload Tool 158
    Key Lessons Learned About Workload Measurement 160
    Protocol-Directed Resource Planning 163
    Graphics Used for Resource Planning and Allocation 164
    Summary 169
    References 170

Chapter 18. Billing, Budgets, and Funding **171**
    Introduction 171
    Administrative Components 171
    Estimating Accrual 176
    Nonrefundable Fees 176
    Billing Compliance for Medicare and Third-Party Payers 177
    Device Trials 178
    Patient Care Costs 178
    Laboratory Fees 178
    Pharmacy Costs 179
    Pharmacokinetic Sampling 179
    Staff Effort and Budgeting 179
    Hidden Costs 181
    Summary 182
    References 182
    Additional Resource 183

Chapter 19. Agreements and Contracts **185**
    Introduction 185
    The Agreement 185
    Implications for Clinical Trial Nurses 188
    Summary 188
    References 189

Chapter 20. Financial Risk Assessment and Monitoring **191**
    Introduction 191
    Areas of Potential Financial Risks and Risk Reduction Strategies 191
    Strategies to Reduce Risk 192
    Summary 197
    References 198

Chapter 21. Internal Financial Audit and Quality Assurance **199**
    Introduction 199
    Definitions of Terms 199
    Background 199
    The Financial Audit Process 200
    Failure Mode and Effects Analysis as a Quality System
        Framework 201
    Summary 201
    References 204

Chapter 22. Financial Conflict of Interest **205**
    Introduction 205
    Background 205
    Identifying Conflicts of Interest 206
    Definition of Financial Conflict of Interest 207
    Office of Management and Budget Requirements for Researchers 208
    U.S. Food and Drug Administration Requirements for Researchers 209
    U.S. Public Health Service Requirements for Researchers 209
    Grants and Cooperative Agreements Issued by Public Health
        Service Agencies 209
    Contracts Issued by Public Health Service Agencies 210
    Centers for Medicare and Medicaid Services Requirements 212
    Consequences of Noncompliance 213
    Summary 215
    References 215

SECTION V. Recruitment and Retention

Chapter 23. Public and Patient Education **219**
    Introduction 219
    Clinical Trial Nurses' Role in Education 219
    Effect of Education on Accrual 220
    Individual, Group, and Public Education 220

Opportunities and Preparation for Speaking to the Public 221
Credibility 222
Explain the Importance of Eligibility Criteria 222
Informational Materials 223
Underrepresented Populations 224
Summary 225
References 226

Chapter 24. Accrual Base, Recruitment, and Promotion Strategies 229
Introduction 229
Recruitment Considerations 229
The Recruitment Process 235
Recruitment Strategies 235
Summary 238
References 238

Chapter 25. Adherence and Retention in Clinical Trials 241
Introduction 241
Definitions of Adherence 241
Factors Affecting Adherence 242
Adverse Effects 243
Impact of Nonadherence 243
Assessment for Adherence 243
Determining Patient Adherence 244
Why Are Patients Nonadherent? 244
Interventions to Promote Adherence 244
Physician/Nurse Adherence Issues 245
Summary 245
References 246

Chapter 26. Clinical Trial Registries 247
Introduction 247
Purpose 247
Evolution of Registries 247
Other Registries 251
Current Trends 252
Implications for Clinical Trial Nurses 253
Summary 253
References 254

SECTION VI. Clinical Trial Participants

Chapter 27. Investigational Agents: Procurement, Accountability, and Administration of Research Study Drugs 259
Introduction 259
Procurement of Research Study Drugs 259
Accountability for Research Study Drugs 260
Documentation of Returned Drugs by Patients 263
Return of Research Drugs to the Supplier 263
Transfer of Research Drugs 263
Compassionate Use, Special Exceptions, or Emergency Use of an
    Investigational Agent for a Patient 264
Administration of Research Drugs 264
Role of Clinical Trial Nurses 267
Summary 267
References 268

Chapter 28. Adverse Events 271
Introduction 271
Definitions 271
Adverse Event Assessment 271
Event Terminology 271
Severity Rating Scales 274
Determining Attribution 276
Adverse Event Collection 278
Adverse Event Documentation 279
Adverse Event Recording 279
Adverse Event Reporting 279
National Cancer Institute–Sponsored Clinical Trials and Adverse
    Events 284

Unanticipated Problems 284
Summary 286
References 288

Chapter 29. Patient and Family Education 291
Introduction 291
Effective Patient Education Messages 292
Specific Informational Needs for Study Phases 294
Providing Clear and Effective Patient Education 298
Challenges to Learning 299
Summary 301
References 301

Chapter 30. Psychosocial Distress 303
Introduction 303
Background 303
Patient Motivation for Clinical Trial Participation 303
Physician Factors 304
Patient Factors 304
Phase I Trial Participation 304
Protocol Factors 305
Distress 305
Nursing Implications 309
Summary 310
References 310

SECTION VII. Genetics and Genomics

Chapter 31. Pharmacogenetics and Pharmacogenomics 315
Introduction 315
Drug Development Process 315
Review of Basic Genetics 316
Basic Pharmacogenomics for Clinical Trial Nurses 317
Pharmacogenetics and Common Anticancer Drugs 318
Pharmacogenetic Testing 320
Role of Clinical Trial Nurses 322
Summary 322
References 323

Chapter 32. Genetic Testing 327
Introduction 327
Hereditary Cancer Predisposition Testing 327
Informed Consent 331
Protection Against Discrimination 333
Hereditary Cancer Predisposition Testing in Clinical Trials 334
Commercial DNA Banking 335
Implications for Clinical Trial Nurses 335
Summary 335
References 336

Chapter 33. Cytogenetics 339
Introduction 339
Chromosome Banding Techniques 339
Cancer Genetics 339
Chromosome Alterations in Cancers 340
Leukemia 340
Summary 341
References 342

Chapter 34. Tumor Profiling 343
Introduction 343
Tumor Profiling 343
Kaplan-Meier Survival Curve 344
Biomarkers in Specific Cancers 344
Summary 347
References 347

Chapter 35. Storage of Genetic Material 351
Introduction 351
Informed Consent 351

    Human Specimen Collection..352
    Genetic Information Nondiscrimination Act Protection..............354
    Implications for Clinical Trial Nurses 354
    Summary..354
    References...355

Chapter 36. Pharmacokinetic Trials 357
    Introduction...357
    Role of Pharmacokinetic Trials in Oncology Drug Development..........357
    Pharmacokinetic Parameters..358
    Pharmacokinetic Clinical Trials Setting................................358
    Pharmacokinetic Models 358
    Summary..361
    References...362

SECTION VIII. Documentation and Data Management

Chapter 37. Documentation 365
    Introduction...365
    Basic Rules of Documentation in a Medical Record 365
    Source Documents 365
    ALCOA 366
    Research-Specific Documentation......................................366
    Challenges..368
    Summary..368
    References...368

Chapter 38. Data Management and Electronic Data Management Systems 369
    Introduction...369
    Clinical Data Management Practices..................................369
    Clinical Data Management Plans.......................................369
    Definition and Purpose..370
    Data Management Processes...371
    Clinical Research Standards..375
    Future Considerations..376
    Electronic Data Management System Implications in Clinical Trials....377
    Summary..380
    References...382

SECTION IX. Quality Assurance

Chapter 39. Creating and Maintaining a Regulatory File................... 387
    Introduction...387
    Overview..387
    Contents of the Regulatory File...387
    Format...393
    Centralizing Essential Documents......................................394
    Maintenance of the Regulatory File....................................394
    Summary..394
    References...395

Chapter 40. Data and Safety Monitoring Plans 397
    Introduction...397
    Background..397
    Data and Safety Monitoring Plans.....................................399
    Summary..401
    References...402

Chapter 41. Preparing for Audits, Inspections, and Monitoring Visits ... 403
    Introduction...403
    Purpose of an Audit...403
    U.S. Food and Drug Administration Inspections: Routine and For-Cause..404
    Investigational New Drug Application and Investigational Device Exemption Sponsors...405
    How to Prepare for an Audit 408
    Close-Out Meeting..410
    Summary..410
    References...410

SECTION X. Professional Development of Clinical Trial Nurses

Chapter 42. Clinical Trial Nurse Education 415
    Introduction...415
    Professional Development Activities..................................415
    Professional Development Log..418
    Professional Portfolio...418
    Summary..418
    References...418

Chapter 43. Mentorship 421
    Introduction...421
    Background..421
    Mentorship Defined...422
    Theoretical Frameworks for Mentoring...............................422
    Mentoring Competencies..423
    The Mentoring Relationship..424
    Communication..426
    E-Mentoring...426
    Mentorship and the Future...427
    Summary..427
    References...427
    Additional Resources...428

Chapter 44. Publishing Guidance for Clinical Trial Nurses................. 429
    Introduction...429
    Why Publish?..429
    Article, Abstract, or Poster 429
    Authorship...433
    Acknowledgments...435
    Medical Writers...435
    Writing With Integrity..435
    Summary..437
    References...437

SECTION XI. International Clinical Trials Research

Introduction to International Section 441

Chapter 45. Australia... 443
    Introduction...443
    History and Foundation 443
    Clinical Trials: Fundamental Information............................444
    Sponsoring Agencies..445
    Protocol Development, Review, and Approval 445
    Financial Factors...447
    Recruitment and Retention...449
    Clinical Trial Participants..450
    Genetics and Genomics..451
    Correlative Trials...451
    Documentation and Data Management..............................452
    Professional Development..452
    Summary..452
    References...453

Chapter 46. Austria... 455
    Introduction...455
    History and Foundation 455
    Clinical Trials: Fundamental Information............................455
    Protocol Development, Review, and Approval 456
    Approval Processes..456
    Financial Factors...457
    Recruitment and Retention...457
    Clinical Trial Participants..458
    Genetics and Genomics..458
    Correlative Trials...458
    Documentation and Data Management..............................459
    Quality Assurance...459
    Professional Development..460
    International Clinical Trials Research 460
    Summary..460
    References...461

Chapter 47. Belarus 463
- Introduction 463
- History and Foundation 463
- Clinical Trials: Fundamental Information 463
- Protocol Development, Review, and Approval 467
- Financial Factors 468
- Recruitment and Retention 468
- Clinical Trial Participants 469
- Genetics and Genomics 469
- Correlative Trials 469
- Documentation and Data Management 469
- Quality Assurance 470
- Professional Development 470
- Summary 470
- References 470

Chapter 48. Canada 473
- Introduction 473
- History and Foundation 473
- Clinical Trials: Fundamental Information 474
- Protocol Development, Review, and Approval 476
- Financial Factors 477
- Recruitment and Retention 478
- Clinical Trial Participants 479
- Genetics and Genomics 479
- Correlative Trials 480
- Documentation and Data Management 480
- Quality Assurance 481
- Professional Development 482
- Summary 482
- References 483

Chapter 49. China 485
- Introduction 485
- History and Foundation 485
- Clinical Trial Procedures in China 485
- Ethics Committees 486
- Protocol Development, Review, and Approval 486
- Informed Consent 486
- Financial Factors 486
- Recruitment and Retention 486
- Clinical Trial Participants 487
- Genetics and Genomics 487
- Correlative Trials 488
- Documentation and Data Management 488
- Quality Assurance 488
- Professional Development 488
- Summary 488
- References 488

Chapter 50. European Union Directives 491
- Introduction 491
- Proposed Clinical Trials Regulation 493
- Resources for European Clinical Trial Nurses 493
- Summary 494
- References 494

Chapter 51. France 497
- Introduction 497
- History and Foundation 497
- Clinical Trials: Fundamental Information 497
- Financial Factors 499
- Recruitment and Retention 499
- Clinical Trial Participants 499
- Genetics and Genomics 499
- Correlative Trials and Ancillary Studies 499
- Documentation and Data Management 500
- Quality Assurance 500
- Professional Development 500
- Summary 500
- References 500

Chapter 52. Germany 503
- Introduction 503
- History and Foundation 503
- Clinical Trials: Fundamental Information 504
- Protocol Development, Review, and Approval 504
- Financial Factors 505
- Recruitment and Retention 506
- Clinical Trial Participants 506
- Genetics and Genomics 508
- Correlative Trials 508
- Documentation and Data Management 509
- Quality Assurance 509
- Professional Development and Clinical Trials Nursing Education 510
- Summary 510
- References 510

Chapter 53. India 513
- Introduction 513
- History and Foundation 513
- Cancer Scenario in India 513
- Clinical Trials: Fundamental Information 514
- Protocol Development, Review, and Approval 514
- Financial Factors 515
- Recruitment and Retention 516
- Genetics and Genomics 516
- Correlative Trials 516
- Documentation and Data Management 517
- Quality Assurance 517
- Professional Development 517
- Summary 517
- References 517

Chapter 54. Ireland 519
- Introduction 519
- History and Foundation 519
- Clinical Trials: Fundamental Information 521
- Protocol Development, Review, and Approval 524
- Financial Factors and Trial Site Budgets 524
- Recruitment and Retention 526
- Clinical Trial Participants 526
- Genetics and Genomics 528
- Correlative Trials 528
- Documentation and Data Management 528
- Quality Assurance 529
- Professional Development 530
- Summary 531
- References 532

Chapter 55. Italy 535
- Introduction 535
- History and Foundation 535
- Clinical Trials: Fundamental Information 535
- Protocol Development, Review, and Approval 536
- Financial Factors 537
- Recruitment and Retention 537
- Clinical Trial Participants 538
- Genetics and Genomics 539
- Correlative Trials 539
- Documentation and Data Management 539
- Quality Assurance 540
- Professional Development 540
- Summary 541
- References 542

Chapter 56. Japan 545
- Introduction 545
- History and Foundation 545

Clinical Trials: Fundamental Information 546
Protocol Development, Review, and Approval 548
Financial Factors 549
Recruitment and Retention 550
Clinical Trial Participants and Nursing Components 551
Genetics and Genomics 553
Correlative Trials 554
Documentation and Data Management 555
Quality Assurance 556
Professional Development 556
Implications for Nurses 557
Summary 557
References 557

Chapter 57. Mexico 559
Introduction 559
History and Foundation 559
Clinical Trials: Fundamental Information 560
Protocol Development, Review, and Approval 560
Financial Factors 562
Recruitment and Retention 562
Clinical Trial Participants 562
Genetics and Genomics 563
Correlative Trials 564
Documentation and Data Management 564
Information System Resources and Patient Support 564
Quality Assurance 564
Professional Development 565
Summary 565
References 566

Chapter 58. New Zealand 567
Introduction 567
History and Foundation 567
Clinical Trials: Fundamental Information 567
Protocol Development, Review, and Approval 568
Financial Factors 568
Clinical Trial Participants 569
Genetics and Genomics 570
Ancillary Studies 570
Documentation and Data Management 570
Quality Assurance 570
Professional Development 571
Summary 571
References 571

Chapter 59. Romania 573
Introduction 573
History and Foundation 573
Clinical Trials: Fundamental Information 574
Protocol Development, Review, and Approval 575
Financial Factors 576
Recruitment and Retention 576
Clinical Trial Participants 576
Genetics and Genomics 577
Correlative Trials 577
Documentation and Data Management 577
Quality Assurance 577
Professional Development 578
Summary 578

Chapter 60. Spain 579
Introduction 579
History and Foundation 579
Clinical Trials: Fundamental Information 579
Protocol Development, Review, and Approval 580
Financial Factors 582
Recruitment and Retention 582
Clinical Trial Participants 582
Genetics and Genomics 583
Correlative Trials 583
Documentation and Data Management 583
Quality Assurance 583
Professional Development 583
Summary 584
References 584

Chapter 61. Thailand 585
Introduction 585
History and Foundation 585
International Clinical Trials Research 585
Clinical Trials: Fundamental Information 586
Protocol Development, Review, and Approval 586
Financial Factors and Budget 587
Recruitment and Retention 587
Clinical Trial Participants 587
Genetics and Genomics 588
Correlative Trials 588
Documentation and Data Management 588
Quality Assurance 588
Professional Development 589
Cultural Aspects 589
Summary 590
References 590

Chapter 62. United Kingdom 591
Introduction 591
History and Foundation 591
Clinical Trials: Fundamental Information 593
Safe Handling and Workplace Safety 594
Protocol Development, Review, and Approval 595
Financial Factors 597
Recruitment and Retention 597
Off-Treatment Follow-Up 597
Clinical Trial Participants 598
Genetics and Genomics 599
Correlative Trials 599
Documentation and Data Management 600
Quality Assurance 600
Professional Development 601
Summary 601
References 602

Appendices 603
Appendix 1. Terms of the Federalwide Assurance for the
   Protection of Human Subjects 605
Appendix 2. Oncology Nursing Society Oncology Clinical Trials
   Nurse Competencies 607
Appendix 3. National Cancer Institute Consent Form Template for
   Adult Cancer Trials 609

Index 627

Preface

Fifteen years have passed since the Oncology Nursing Society (ONS) Clinical Trial Nurses (CTNs) Special Interest Group developed the first edition of the *Manual for Clinical Trials Nursing*. At that time, clinical trials were increasing in number, and there was a shortage of experienced CTNs. Oncology nurses were recruited from medical-surgical settings, but they lacked the background and fundamental information about clinical trials and the know-how of trials regulation. The purpose of the manual was to introduce novice CTNs to clinical trials research and to act as a "how-to" resource for CTNs who needed a fast introduction to the research and regulations of the time. It was also the first comprehensive nursing work that contained chapters about clinical trials nursing outside of the United States, something the editors felt strongly about including. This third edition has expanded to become a guide for CTNs of all levels of experience in all practice settings, as well as a reference for advanced practice nurses, research scientists, and students of nursing and research.

This edition is the result of an extensive revision. New section editors Julia A. Eggert, PhD, GNP-BC, AGN-BC, AOCN®, Elizabeth Ness, RN, MS, and Kelly Willenberg, MBA, BSN, CCRP, CHRC, joined seasoned editors Joan G. Westendorp, RN, MSN, OCN®, CCRP, CIM, Monica Bacon, RN, and myself to present content in a logical format. The chapters have been reorganized to add clarity and facilitate location of desired content. Topics range from history and fundamental information through protocol development and financial factors, recruitment and retention, clinical trial participants, and genetics and genomics to correlative trials, quality assurance, professional development, and international research efforts. Implications for CTNs are incorporated throughout. The key points of each chapter are listed at the end of the chapter to highlight the primary content elements. However, clinical trials research is dynamic, and the reader is directed to specific websites throughout the manual to access the most current information available.

Two new sections were added based on feedback to editors. A section addressing financial factors of clinical research, including workload determination, billing and budgets, contracts, financial risk assessment and monitoring, internal financial audit and quality assurance, contracts, and conflict of interest, was added to help CTNs evaluate the financial impact of a protocol in their work setting and to aid in the preparation of protocol budgets. The second new section explores genetics and genomics. The editors recognize that the number of studies pertaining to genetics and genomics has increased over the last decade and is expected to continue to rise. Therefore, information addressing pharmacogenetics and pharmacogenomics, genetic testing, cytogenetics, tumor profiling, and storage of genetic material was included.

The international section has expanded to include Belarus, China, India, Ireland, Mexico, Romania, Spain, and Thailand, in addition to most of the countries represented in the second edition. This reflects the emerging international markets for clinical trials research, especially in the area of oncology, and delineates the emerging role of CTNs around the globe.

The appendices, which were expanded in the second edition, have been limited to three: federalwide assurances, oncology CTN competencies, and an informed consent document template. Again, as much as possible, the reader is referred to specific websites that are included in the text. This will ensure that the most current version of the document being discussed is presented to the reader.

The *Manual for Clinical Trials Nursing* is made possible through the support of ONS, and we are grateful for its continued backing. Most of all, our thanks go to the authors for sharing their expertise and experiences with clinical trials for the benefit of CTNs worldwide. It is the continued development of the *Manual for Clinical Trials Nursing* that makes it a valuable resource in today's clinical research environment.

Angela D. Klimaszewski, RN, MSN
Lead Editor

Acknowledgments

Special thanks to Lisa George, Amy Nicoletti, Judy Holmes, Dany Sjoen, and Laura Pinchot for their guidance and expertise in the production of this work. Your efforts are truly appreciated.

Special thanks also to Barb Sigler, who guided the production of books like this for 17 years at ONS and championed all three editions of the *Manual for Clinical Trials Nursing*.

SECTION I.

History and Foundation

Chapter 1

History and Background of Oncology Clinical Trials

Karri Donahue, MSN, RN, CCRP, and Heather Benzel, BSN, RN, CCRP

Introduction

The field of oncology has been extremely fortunate to experience the advancement of treatment from preliminary cancer surgeries offering limited results to in-depth, targeted therapies increasing the overall survival and quality of life for many patients with cancer. Because less than 5% of new patients with cancer participate in clinical trials, many resources are being developed in an effort to increase trial participation as well as quality and patient safety (American Society of Clinical Oncology, n.d.).

Understanding the history of clinical trials, including successes, failures, and the risk for patient endangerment, is paramount in establishing and maintaining a quality environment for clinical trial patient care. Through an elaborate sequence of events, clinical trials have developed layers of federal and international policies and procedures to help safeguard the patient experience, encourage increased participation, and facilitate the trajectory of oncology research.

History

Experimental research studies on human subjects can be traced to ancient times. Early clinical trials often were comparative studies (see Chapter 3) that focused on the prevention of communicable diseases and on nutritional disorders, which were prevalent until the latter half of the 20th century (Lilienfeld, 1982). As early as 1863, Rudolf Virchow deduced cancer to its cellular origin by using a microscope (DeVita & Rosenberg, 2012). In an effort to promote public health in the United States, a one-room laboratory was created in 1887 within the Marine Hospital Service (predecessor to the U.S. Public Health Service). The Hygienic Laboratory was established to provide funding for research on the prevention, detection, and treatment of disease. The Ransdell Act of 1930 was enacted to legislate public funding of medical research and changed the name of the Hygienic Laboratory to the National Institute of Health (Harden, n.d.). The name was later changed to the National Institutes of Health (NIH) to reflect the addition of new institutes.

The first documented clinical trial in the United States using a matched control group, random assignment, and single-blinding (see Chapter 4) was reported in 1931 by J. Burns Amberson and colleagues. The trial evaluated the use of sanocrysin, a gold compound, in the treatment of patients with pulmonary tuberculosis treated at the W.H. Maybury Sanatorium in Northville, Michigan. Twenty-four patients were matched and then randomized to either group I (sanocrysin-treated) or group II (control). As a result of substandard and often absent informed consent processes, subjects were not aware of the differences in the treatment regimens between the groups (Lilienfeld, 1982).

In 1937, President Franklin D. Roosevelt signed the National Cancer Institute Act, which established the National Cancer Institute (NCI) as a division of NIH. NCI was the first disease-oriented institute of NIH, now totaling 27 institutes (DeVita & Rosenberg, 2012). The act mandated funding to support cancer research and training (Jenkins & Lake, 1988; White-Hershey & Nevidjon, 1990). The Federal Food, Drug, and Cosmetic Act was passed the following year to ensure that a drug demonstrated safety in humans before it could be marketed to the public (Swann, 1998).

The authors would like to acknowledge Sheila Breslin, RN, MS, for her contribution to this chapter that remains unchanged from the previous edition of this book.

In 1944, scientist Oswald Avery discovered that cellular information was not transmitted by proteins but rather by DNA (DeVita & Rosenberg, 2012). With this discovery, the door to biotechnology research and sequencing of the genome was opened. Later, it would lead to developing the bench-to-bedside therapies concept of translating what works in the laboratory and applying this to the patient treatment level.

NCI began to fund cooperative oncology groups in an effort to expand enrollment in clinical trials in the mid-1950s. Cooperative oncology groups are composed of groups of physicians at institutions nationally who collaboratively design and implement clinical trials. The Clinical Trials Cooperative Group Program was originally composed of four pediatric and nine adult groups (Children's Oncology Group, n.d.; NCI, n.d., 2005) (see Figure 1-1). The initial consolidation occurred in 2000, when the four pediatric groups became one group, known as the Children's Oncology Group. The next consolidation occurred in 2014, when the nine adult groups were merged into four adult groups. The Cancer Therapy Evaluation Program, a branch of NCI's Division of Cancer Treatment, oversees the cooperative oncology groups (Cheson, 1991).

During the 1950s, there were great advancements in treatment with radiation and chemotherapy. Cobalt teletherapy was introduced to treat patients with radiation, along with the advancement in technology that allowed the beams to be delivered more accurately to the tumor and minimized exposure to normal tissue (DeVita & Rosenberg, 2012). In the mid-1970s, two breakthrough studies evaluated the use of single-agent and combination therapy in adjuvant breast cancer. Although NCI (2007) developed the combination regimen consisting of cyclophosphamide, methotrexate, and fluorouracil, the study was performed in conjunction with the Milan Cancer Institute in Italy because no major U.S. institution was willing to test combination therapy. Both studies had positive outcomes, and as a result of increased availability of treatments, including hormone and chemotherapeutic agents, as well as clinical trials and increasing diagnostic tools, the rate of cancer deaths began to decline by 1991. The war on cancer mandated the support of research as well as the reduction of incidence, morbidity, and mortality from cancer; these advancements assisted in fulfilling that directive (DeVita & Rosenberg, 2012).

The National Cancer Act of 1971 resulted in a large increase in NCI funding. NCI was charged with the responsibility of conducting basic scientific research in oncology and applying the results to clinical practice. The National Cancer Act also promoted the development of oncology training programs, facilities, and public education services (Jenkins & Hubbard, 1991; Jenkins & Lake, 1988).

By 1973, most oncology clinical trials were conducted at NCI-designated comprehensive cancer centers that received core grants from NCI to fund operations. Community oncologists, however, still were treating patients with cancer who might be eligible for enrollment in a clinical trial. In response, NCI developed outreach programs

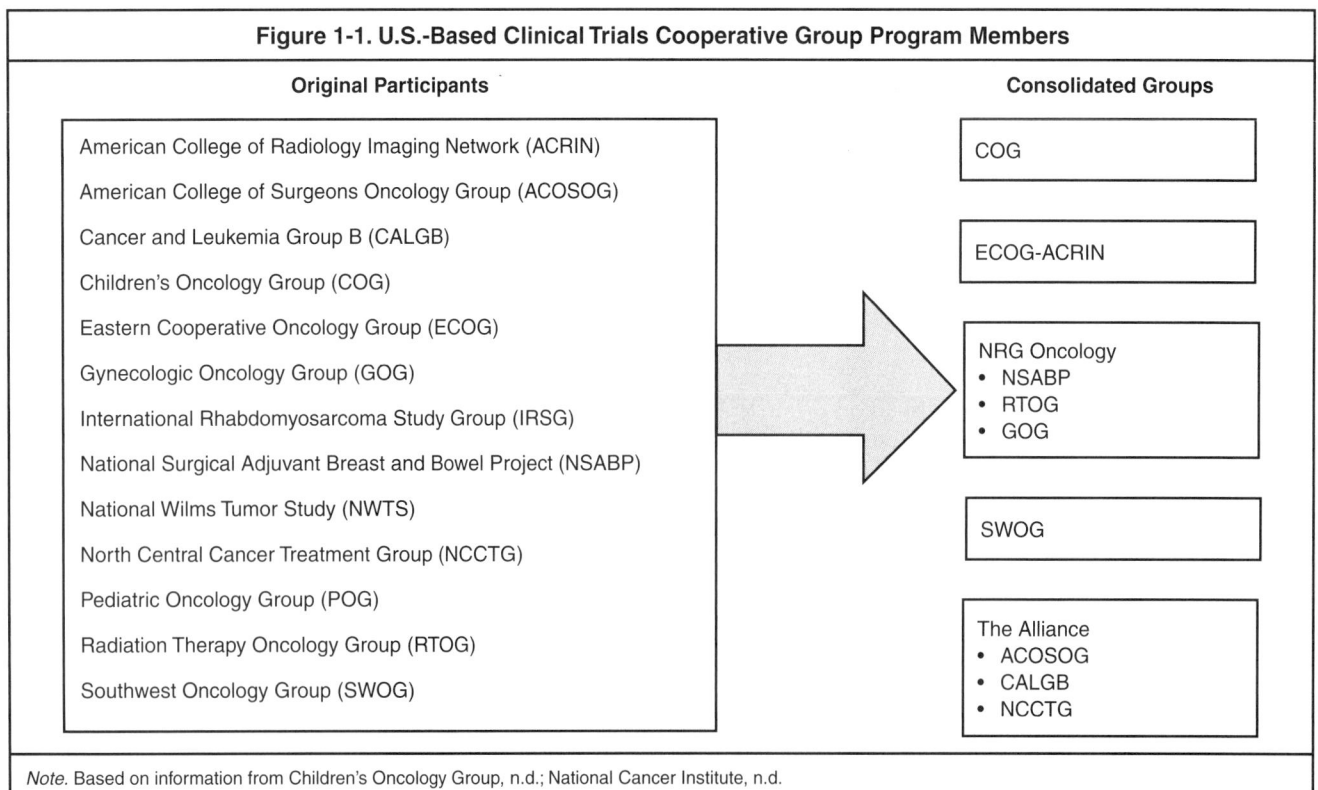

Figure 1-1. U.S.-Based Clinical Trials Cooperative Group Program Members

Original Participants
- American College of Radiology Imaging Network (ACRIN)
- American College of Surgeons Oncology Group (ACOSOG)
- Cancer and Leukemia Group B (CALGB)
- Children's Oncology Group (COG)
- Eastern Cooperative Oncology Group (ECOG)
- Gynecologic Oncology Group (GOG)
- International Rhabdomyosarcoma Study Group (IRSG)
- National Surgical Adjuvant Breast and Bowel Project (NSABP)
- National Wilms Tumor Study (NWTS)
- North Central Cancer Treatment Group (NCCTG)
- Pediatric Oncology Group (POG)
- Radiation Therapy Oncology Group (RTOG)
- Southwest Oncology Group (SWOG)

Consolidated Groups
- COG
- ECOG-ACRIN
- NRG Oncology
  - NSABP
  - RTOG
  - GOG
- SWOG
- The Alliance
  - ACOSOG
  - CALGB
  - NCCTG

Note. Based on information from Children's Oncology Group, n.d.; National Cancer Institute, n.d.

in an attempt to make clinical trials available to larger numbers of patients with cancer and to improve patient accrual into the trials. These programs provided funding for community physicians to participate in NCI-sponsored clinical trials (Cheson, 1991; Jenkins & Hubbard, 1991). Currently, approximately 85% of patients with cancer are seen and treated at community cancer centers or hospitals near their home communities with access to a wide array of clinical trial opportunities (NCI, 2014b).

The Cooperative Group Outreach Program, established in 1976 by the NCI Division of Cancer Treatment, allowed community physicians to affiliate with a cooperative group to offer their patients access to cooperative group trials. The Community Clinical Oncology Program, instituted in 1983, differed from the Cooperative Group Outreach Program in its funding source, research focus, accrual requirements, and affiliation policies. The NCI Division of Cancer Prevention and Control (DCPC) funded the Cooperative Group Outreach Program. Community physicians affiliated with cancer centers and cooperative groups to form a research base. In addition to cancer treatment, DCPC-sponsored clinical trials focused on prevention and early detection of cancer. The High-Priority Clinical Trials Program, established in 1988, targeted phase III cooperative group trials as high priority, thus increasing accrual (Cheson, 1991).

Transition took place among the cooperative groups, and NCI wanted to take the program a step further. NCI asked the Institute of Medicine (IOM) in 2009 to review the Clinical Trials Cooperative Group Program. In 2010, IOM recommended to consolidate the Clinical Trials Cooperative Group Program and fund no more than five groups (four adult groups and one pediatric group) (NCI, 2011) (see Figure 1-1). Grants were scheduled to be awarded to the five groups in spring 2014. The purpose of the consolidation was to (a) develop the competence of operations and data management centers so that more integration takes place, (b) enhance the ability to function together on a larger scale, and (c) prevent redundant studies that require large sample sizes to answer clinical questions among cooperative groups (NCI, 2012).

The NCI Board of Scientific Advisors approved the creation of the NCI Community Oncology Research Program (NCORP) on June 24, 2013. NCORP's purpose is to bring state-of-the-art cancer prevention, control, treatment, and imaging clinical trials; cancer care delivery research; and disparities studies to individuals in their own communities. NCORP is based at the Division of Cancer Prevention and replaced both the Community Clinical Oncology Program Network and the NCI Community Cancer Centers Program in 2014. To participate, institutions must apply within one of three NCORP components: research bases, community sites, and minority/underserved community sites. NCI aimed to provide an estimated $40.8 million and up to 40 awards for fiscal year 2014. Future amounts will be determined based on annual appropriations (NCI, 2013).

NIH released its NIH Roadmap in the early part of the 2000s, which enhanced the bench-to-bedside process by combining basic science and clinical medicine from clinical researchers to medical practitioner to patient (Kaitlin & DiMasi, 2011). With this came the push for bio-innovation. In 2004, the U.S. Food and Drug Administration (FDA) introduced the Critical Path Initiative with a goal of improving translation of basic research to safe and effective medicine and treatment options for patients (Kaitlin & DiMasi, 2011). This fostered identification of various biomarkers and other tools used to improve patient outcomes and survivorship rates and uncovered the potential to treat patients with targeted therapy, based on biomarkers and molecular abnormalities.

Growth of International Guidelines and U.S. Regulations

Fraudulent claims of safety and efficacy, as well as abuses in drug and device manufacturing, were rampant in the United States in the late 1800s, leading to untold numbers of serious injuries and deaths. As a result of these abuses, the 1906 Food and Drug Act was signed into law, establishing the first federal regulatory standards to ensure food and drug purity and truth in labeling. The Bureau of Chemistry, whose name was changed in 1930 to the U.S. Food and Drug Administration, implemented these laws. In 1938, a new, more stringent law was enacted that mandated drug safety testing and, for the first time, FDA approval prior to marketing. This legislation also brought the marketing of medical devices under the FDA's regulatory purview. The Kefauver-Harris Amendments to the Food and Drug Act were passed in 1962 after the discovery that thalidomide could cause fetal abnormalities. The amendment required preclinical testing of drugs, as well as proof of efficacy and safety, before use in humans. It also required that research subjects provide informed consent before participating in clinical trials (Swann, 1998) (see Chapter 14).

Research on vulnerable populations, such as slaves, prison inmates, people with mental illness and cognitive disabilities, the poor, children, and minority groups, was conducted in the United States from the mid-1800s to the mid-1900s without participants' informed consent (Allen, 1994; Merkatz & Junod, 1994). However, it was not until the exposure of medical atrocities performed on prisoners during World War II that a code of ethics for human experimentation was developed. The resulting Nuremberg Code of 1947 serves as the foundation for the ethical principles governing clinical research today (McCarthy, 1994; Merkatz & Junod, 1994; Nuremberg Code, 1949).

In 1964, the World Medical Association developed the Declaration of Helsinki, a set of international ethical guidelines for physicians involved in biomedical research.

These guidelines recommended preclinical studies before the implementation of human clinical trials, scientific justification for experimentation in humans, and a written protocol document with review by an independent committee. The declaration posited that research be conducted only by qualified medical personnel and offered guidelines for the provision of informed consent from human participants. The Declaration of Helsinki has been updated periodically since 1964, with the most recent update approved in 2013 (World Medical Association, n.d., 1996).

After the passage of the National Research Act (1974), the National Commission for the Protection of Human Subjects of Biomedical and Behavioral Research was created to develop written policies for the protection of human subjects. Published in 1979, the resulting Belmont Report led to the establishment of institutional review boards (IRBs), outlined protocol design criteria, and recommended that written informed consent be obtained from all research subjects (Jenkins & Hubbard, 1991; National Commission for the Protection of Human Subjects of Biomedical and Behavioral Research, 1979). These policies were codified in 1981 in the *Code of Federal Regulations* (National Commission for the Protection of Human Subjects of Biomedical and Behavioral Research, 1979; Sparks, 2002).

One of the most important of these regulations, known as the "Common Rule" (Basic HHS Policy for Protection of Human Research Subjects, 2009), outlined specific measures that investigators and institutions must follow to protect subjects who participate in federally funded research. The Common Rule included criteria for the provision of informed consent, guidelines for the conduct of IRBs, and requirements for the protection of vulnerable populations, as well as other subject protections such as the mandate for data and safety monitoring boards, regulations regarding investigator conflict of interest, and training of clinical research personnel (NCI, 2005).

In 1996, members of the International Conference on Harmonisation of Technical Requirements for Registration of Pharmaceuticals for Human Use (ICH) finalized a set of good clinical practice (GCP) standards for the conduct of clinical trials. Officially known as the *ICH Harmonised Tripartite Guideline for Good Clinical Practice* (ICH, 1996), its 13 principles (not regulations) were adopted by the United States, the European Union, Japan, Australia, Canada, and a number of other countries, as well as the World Health Organization. In addition to establishing consistent principles for the protection of human subjects, the goal of the ICH GCP guidelines is to streamline regulatory approvals of new drugs by developing consistent recommendations for the design, implementation, reporting, and interpretation of clinical trials worldwide (Dixon, 1999; U.S. FDA, 1996). (See Chapter 9: Good Clinical Practice for additional information.)

Passed by Congress in 1996 and implemented by the U.S. Department of Health and Human Services (DHHS) in 2003, the Health Insurance Portability and Accountability Act (HIPAA) influenced the conduct of clinical trials, mandating specific privacy protections for trial participants. For a detailed examination of the impact of HIPAA on clinical trials, the reader is referred to NIH Publication Number 04-5495 (U.S. DHHS, 2004).

Federalwide Assurance for the Protection of Human Subjects (FWA) (see Appendix 1) was passed in 2005 with the intent of enforcing that all research involving human study participants is subject to federal regulations and must be guided by ethical principles. The ethical principles specifically cited include the Belmont Report in addition to other appropriate ethical standards recognized by federal departments and agencies that have adopted the Common Rule (U.S. DHHS, 2014a).

The Office for Human Research Protections (OHRP) oversees the safety of participants in federally funded clinical trials. FWA is the only type of assurance of compliance currently accepted and approved by OHRP for institutions engaged in nonexempt human subject research conducted or supported by DHHS (U.S. DHHS, 2014b).

Treatment of Minorities and Women

Despite the increasing incidence of and mortality from cancer in the African American community, this group has been underrepresented in clinical trials (George, Duran, & Norris, 2014). Lack of participation by minorities in general and specifically African Americans largely had been attributed to fears of exploitation generated by the Tuskegee syphilis experiment conducted by the U.S. Public Health Service from the 1930s to the 1970s. This study allowed African American men with syphilis to go untreated, even after curative treatment was available, in order to study the natural progression of the disease. Therefore, there is a mistrust, feeling of fear, and lack of confidence regarding medical establishments and research among minorities, which continues to be a barrier for many researchers (Allen, 1994; George et al., 2014; McCarthy, 1994).

Lack of access to state-of-the-art health care; cultural or ethnic factors; economic status; language or literacy barriers; and long-standing fear, apprehension, and skepticism have been identified as obstacles to minority participation in clinical trials (George et al., 2014; NCI, 2005). However, because 40% of Community Clinical Oncology Program annual referrals are from minority populations, NCI provides funding to institutions that serve a high percentage of minority groups through its Minority-Based Community Clinical Oncology Program (MBCCOP), which was established in 1990 (NCI, 2005).

According to George and colleagues (2014), more than 30% of the U.S. population is of racial or ethnic minority; however, racial and ethnic minorities represent less than 18% of the participants in clinical trials. Causes of low participation in clinical trials by minority groups are complex. Reasons for low accrual may be due in part to a deficiency of available trials in communities with high disparate populations as well as the study design. Often disparate populations lack sufficient health care, resulting in an increase of disease processes. Clinical trial eligibility is often rigid and exclusionary of many of these comorbidities. MBCCOP accrued 10% of all ethnic minorities participating in NCI-approved clinical trials (NCI, 2005).

In 1977, women were excluded from participation in clinical trials because of concerns about the potential teratogenic effects of untested drugs on a developing fetus, partially as a result of severe birth defects caused by the drug thalidomide (effective in preventing nausea in pregnant women). This FDA-mandated exclusion applied to phase I clinical trials involving the use of untested drugs in pregnant women or women of childbearing potential. However, in practice, the exclusion was extended to all women in all phases of clinical trials (McCarthy, 1994).

These policies severely limited knowledge about gender- and race-related differences in drug safety and efficacy (Allen, 1994; McCarthy, 1994; Merkatz & Junod, 1994; Millon-Underwood et al., 1993). The AIDS epidemic highlighted the potentially discriminatory nature of these exclusionary practices (Kelly & Cordell, 1996; McCarthy, 1994). Between 1992 and 1993, 15% of all new AIDS cases reported were in women, and almost 75% of these women were either African American or Hispanic (Allen, 1994).

In 1986, NIH drafted its first policy promoting the inclusion of women in clinical trials (La Rosa, 1994). Since implementation of this policy, women of childbearing potential have been allowed to participate in phase I clinical trials as long as they are not pregnant. They must be advised of the potential for fetal damage if they become pregnant and must agree to use effective contraception while participating in a study (Merkatz & Junod, 1994). In 1990, NCI created the Office of Research on Women's Health to promote research on women's health issues and the participation of women in clinical trials (Pinn, 1994). The NIH Revitalization Act, passed by Congress in 1993, mandated the inclusion of women and minorities in all NIH-sponsored clinical trials (Pinn, 1994). As a result, participation of women in clinical trials is growing. Study data show women comprised 49% of NCI cooperative study enrollments between 1996 and 2002 for breast, colorectal, lung, and prostate therapeutic trials (Murthy, Krumholz, & Gross, 2004).

In 2010, the book *The Immortal Life of Henrietta Lacks*, written by Rebecca Skloot, was published. This story exposed the public to the struggle between ethics, race, and medicine. The book is based on the true story of Henrietta Lacks, better known as HeLa in the scientific world, who was diagnosed with cervical cancer in 1951. Cells were retrieved for the purpose of diagnosing her cancer; however, additional cells were taken without her knowledge or consent to contribute to research and are still being used in research today. The family was aware of the use of their mother's cells but was unaware of the full impact those cells have made in laboratories across the world until Skloot started communicating with them. With the use of Henrietta Lacks' cells and the publication of Skloot's book, bioethics began evolving, and the public became aware of the triumphs and tribulations of research today.

Treatment of Children and Older Adults

Historically, participation of children in cancer clinical trials has far exceeded adult participation. This is, in part, because childhood cancers are rare, and most children with cancer are treated at major academic institutions with access to clinical trials (Sateren et al., 2002). However, because children represent a vulnerable population, special protections have been implemented to safeguard their treatment. In 1983, laws to protect children in clinical trials were added to the *Code of Federal Regulations* (Burns, 2003; Hirtz & Fitzsimmons, 2002; Sparks, 2002).

Concerns have been raised that drugs used to treat adults were being administered without adequate testing in children (Hutchins et al., 1999; Sateren et al., 2002). In 1998, NIH issued a policy mandating the inclusion of children in clinical trials unless scientifically or ethically contraindicated (NIH, 1998). Then in 2002, the Best Pharmaceuticals for Children Act was passed, amending the Federal Food, Drug, and Cosmetic Act to improve drug safety and efficacy testing prior to use in children (Burns, 2003). Until recently, parental consent alone was sufficient for children younger than 18 years old to participate in clinical trials. Now, children younger than 18 years old are asked for their assent if they are mature enough to understand the trial and the expectations of the study. Although assent, unlike informed consent, is not required by law, many IRBs require it (NCI, 2014) (see Chapter 14: Informed Consent).

Underrepresentation of the older adult population has been another concern in clinical trials. In 1989, FDA published recommended guidelines for inclusion of older adults in clinical trials. However, they continue to be proportionally underrepresented in clinical trials, despite cancer incidence and mortality rates being highest in this population. Suggested reasons for underrepresentation include concerns about toxicities, the presence of comorbid conditions, perceived lack of benefit, advanced stage of disease at diagnosis, lack of awareness, quality-of-life concerns, and a variety of socioeconomic barriers (Hutchins, Unger, Crowley, Coltman, & Albain, 1999; Lewis et al., 2003; Talarico, Chen, & Pazdur, 2004).

Older adults' lack of participation in clinical trials may not only limit the generalizability of results to older patients, but actually may result in less aggressive approaches to treatment because of misconceptions about tolerability, thereby compromising survival outcomes (Hutchins et al., 1999; Talarico et al., 2004). Excluding the older population is problematic because it is the greatest burden to healthcare costs in the United States (Herrera et al., 2010). Herrera and colleagues (2010) noted that 36% of personal healthcare dollars are spent on older adults, and older adults spend 42% of all prescription drug dollars. Increased representation of older adults in clinical trials, therefore, is critically important. Today, cooperative group trials, such as treatment (e.g., chemotherapy), quality-of-life trials, and registries, are designed specifically to include older adults.

Table 1-1 summarizes the significant events in the history of clinical trials development.

Evolution of National Healthcare Reform

In 2007, Medicare's Clinical Trial Policy (Centers for Medicare and Medicaid Services, 2007) revised the coverage for Medicare patients who participate in clinical trials. This revision helped to cover expenses accrued during participation in qualified clinical trials. While many states have adopted a variety of state-specific agreements to cover varying aspects of clinical trial participation, very little consistency exists among insurance carriers across the nation. In March 2010, the enactment of the Patient Protection and Affordable Care Act introduced requirements for insurance companies to provide coverage for routine costs associated with clinical trial participation (Phillips, 2010). With this in place, patients are able to choose the best option for treatment without worrying that certain tests or procedures will not be covered based on their participation in a clinical trial (Repucci, 2012). The new requirements went into full effect in 2014. The federal law will address coverage in all 50 states as well as the District of Columbia and includes Employee Retirement Income Security Act (known commonly as ERISA) plans, "self-insured" plans that are not mandated by state regulations (Phillips, 2010).

Summary

The evolution of clinical trials has resulted in dramatic improvements in the prevention and treatment of many diseases, including cancer. Advances in medicine, improved surgical techniques, the development of new drugs and devices, the application of statistical techniques to research studies, recognition of the need for regulation, and the development of ethical codes all have influenced how clinical trials are now conducted both in the United States and internationally. The focus today is not only the treatment and prevention of cancer, but also patients' symptom management and qual-

Table 1-1. Selected Events in the History of U.S. Oncology Clinical Trials Development	
Year	Event
1747	Lind conducts the first documented comparative study on patients with scurvy.
1800s	Drugs and vaccines to treat smallpox, diphtheria, and cholera are developed and tested.
1887	The National Institutes of Health (NIH) is founded.
1900s	Research on prevention and treatment of infectious diseases begins.
1906	The Food and Drug Act, regulating drug purity, safety, and labeling, is signed into law.
1937	The National Cancer Institute Act establishes the National Cancer Institute (NCI).
1938	The Federal Food, Drug, and Cosmetic Act replaces the 1906 Food and Drug Act and requires that drugs be tested for safety before marketing.
1947	The Nuremberg Code establishes a basic code of ethics for experimentation on human subjects.
1962	The Kefauver-Harris Amendments to the Federal Food, Drug, and Cosmetic Act mandate preclinical testing and the provision of informed consent.
1964	The Declaration of Helsinki establishes specific guidelines for physicians conducting human research.

(Continued on next page)

Table 1-1. Selected Events in the History of U.S. Oncology Clinical Trials Development *(Continued)*	
Year	Event
1966	U.S. Surgeon General policy mandates independent review of all research on human subjects, proposing the establishment of institutional review boards.
1971	The National Cancer Act mandates NCI to conduct and apply basic cancer research.
1974	The National Research Act establishes the National Commission for the Protection of Human Subjects of Biomedical and Behavioral Research.
1976	NCI initiates the Cooperative Group Outreach Program.
1979	The Belmont Report outlines ethical principles and guidelines for protection of human subjects.
1981	Laws governing the protection of human subjects in research funded by the U.S. Department of Health and Human Services (DHHS) are added to the *Code of Federal Regulations*.
1983	NCI funds Community Cancer Outreach Programs.
1986	NIH establishes policies for the inclusion of women in clinical trials.
1988	NCI establishes the High-Priority Clinical Trials Program.
1989	The U.S. Food and Drug Administration publishes guidelines for the inclusion of older adult patients in clinical trials.
1990	The Office of Research on Women's Health is created.
1991	Sixteen federal agencies adopt the federal policy for the protection of human subjects, known as the "Common Rule."
1993	The NIH Revitalization Act mandates the inclusion of women and minorities in NIH-sponsored clinical trials.
1996	The International Conference on Harmonisation establishes good clinical practice guidelines for human subject research. Congress passes the Health Insurance Portability and Accountability Act (HIPAA).
1997	The Food and Drug Modernization Act mandates establishment of a public resource for information on clinical trials.
1998	NIH Policy and Guidelines on the Inclusion of Children as Participants in Research Involving Human Subjects mandates that children must be included in all NIH-sponsored research except under certain circumstances.
2000	The World Health Organization establishes international guidelines for ethics committees involved in the review of biomedical research.
2002	The Best Pharmaceuticals Act for Children amends the Federal Food, Drug, and Cosmetic Act to improve drug safety and efficacy testing for children.
2003	DHHS implements HIPAA.
2004	The International Committee of Medical Journal Editors issues a statement mandating public registration of clinical trials, including a description of informed consent and ethics committee approval as prerequisites for manuscript publication.
2005	Federalwide Assurance for the Protection of Human Subjects is required for all studies funded or conducted by DHHS that involve human subjects.
2006	NCI initiates phase 0 clinical trials to study the pharmacokinetics and pharmacodynamics of molecular-targeted drugs.
2007	Medicare's Clinical Trials Policy is revised with updated coverage rules for Medicare.
2007	Pilot program of NCI Community Cancer Centers Program (NCCCP) is launched and focuses efforts on cancer research, improving quality cancer care, and survivorship for patients who are treated at community hospitals.
2010	Enactment of the Patient Protection and Affordable Care Act requires insurers to cover routine costs of participation in clinical trials.
2012	Clinical Trials Cooperative Groups are consolidated from 13 groups to 5 (4 adult and 1 pediatric).
2013	NCI Community Oncology Research Program (NCORP) is created to bring state-of-the-art cancer prevention, control, treatment, and imaging clinical trials, cancer care delivery research, and disparities studies to individuals in their own communities. NCORP replaces the Community Clinical Oncology Program and the NCI Community Cancer Centers Program.
2014	Insurance coverage requirements for clinical trial participation go into effect as mandated by the Patient Protection and Affordable Care Act.

ity of life. Developments have been made to include more of the disparate populations and increase outreach activities within communities. Patients are more educated about their diagnosis and potential clinical trials and frequently seek out participation in research activities.

Key Points

- The progress made in clinical trials has positively affected the prevention and treatment of many diseases, including cancer.
- Factors that have influenced the way in which clinical trials are conducted include medical and surgical advances, development of new drugs and devices, application of statistical techniques to research studies, recognition of the need for regulation, and development of ethical codes.
- The focus today is not only the treatment and prevention of cancer but also symptom management and quality of life, genomics, personalized medicine, and biospecimens.

References

Allen, M. (1994). The dilemma for women of color in clinical trials. *Journal of the American Medical Women's Association, 49*, 105–109.

American Society of Clinical Oncology. (n.d.). About clinical trials. Retrieved from http://www.cancer.net/navigating-cancer-care/how-cancer-treated/clinical-trials/about-clinical-trials

Basic HHS Policy for Protection of Human Research Subjects, 45 C.F.R. 46 (2009). Retrieved from http://www.hhs.gov/ohrp/humansubjects/guidance/45cfr46.html

Burns, J.P. (2003). Research in children. *Critical Care Medicine, 31*, S131–S136.

Centers for Medicare and Medicaid Services. (2007, October 9). National coverage determination (NCD) for routine costs in clinical trials. Retrieved from http://www.cms.gov/medicare-coverage-database/details/ncd-details.aspx?NCDId=1&ncdver=2&bc

Cheson, B.D. (1991). Cancer clinical trials: Clinical trials programs. *Seminars in Oncology Nursing, 7*, 235–242.

Children's Oncology Group. (n.d.). Our history. Retrieved from https://childrensoncologygroup.org/index.php/history

DeVita, V.T., & Rosenberg, S.A. (2012). Two hundred years of cancer research. *New England Journal of Medicine, 366*, 2207–2214. doi:10.1056/NEJMra1204479

Dixon, J.R., Jr. (1999). The International Conference on Harmonization good clinical practice guideline. *Quality Assurance, 6*, 65–74.

George, S., Duran, N., & Norris, K. (2014). A systematic review of barriers and facilitators to minority research participation among African Americans, Latinos, Asian Americans, and Pacific Islanders. *American Journal of Public Health, 104*, e16–e28.

Harden, V.A. (n.d.). A short history of the National Institutes of Health. Retrieved from http://history.nih.gov/exhibits/history/index.html

Herrera, A.P., Snipes, S.A., King, D.W., Torres-Vigil, I., Goldberg, D.S., & Weinberg, A.D. (2010). Disparate inclusion of older adults in clinical trials: Priorities and opportunities for policy and practice changes. *American Journal of Public Health, 100*(Suppl. 1), S105–S112.

Hirtz, D.G., & Fitzsimmons, L.G. (2002). Regulatory and ethical issues in the conduct of clinical research involving children. *Current Opinion in Pediatrics, 14*, 669–675.

Hutchins, L.F., Unger, J.M., Crowley, J.J., Coltman, C.A., & Albain, K.S. (1999). Underrepresentation of patients 65 years of age or older in cancer-treatment trials. *New England Journal of Medicine, 341*, 2061–2067.

International Conference on Harmonisation of Technical Requirements for Registration of Pharmaceuticals for Human Use. (1996, June 10). *ICH harmonised tripartite guideline: Guideline for good clinical practice, E6(R1)*. Retrieved from http://www.ich.org/fileadmin/Public_Web_Site/ICH_Products/Guidelines/Efficacy/E6/E6_R1_Guideline.pdf

Jenkins, J., & Hubbard, S. (1991). History of clinical trials. *Seminars in Oncology Nursing, 7*, 228–234.

Jenkins, J.F., & Lake, P.C. (1988). Celebration of an era of public service at the National Institutes of Health and the National Cancer Institute. *Cancer Nursing, 11*, 58–64.

Kaitlin, K.I., & DiMasi, J.A. (2011). Pharmaceutical innovation in the 21st century: New drug approvals in the first decade, 2000–2009. *Clinical Pharmacology and Therapeutics, 89*, 183–188.

Kelly, P.J., & Cordell, J.R. (1996). Recruitment of women into research studies: A nursing perspective. *Clinical Nurse Specialist, 10*, 25–28.

La Rosa, J.H. (1994). Office of Research on Women's Health: National Institutes of Health and the women's health agenda. *Annals of the New York Academy of Sciences, 736*, 196–204.

Lewis, J.H., Kilgore, M.L., Goldman, D.P., Trimble, E.L., Kaplan, R., Montello, M.J., ... Escarce, J.J. (2003). Participation of patients 65 years of age or older in cancer clinical trials. *Journal of Clinical Oncology, 21*, 1383–1389. doi:10.1200/JCO.2003.08.010

Lilienfeld, A.M. (1982). Ceteris paribus: The evolution of the clinical trial. *Bulletin of the History of Medicine, 56*, 1–18.

McCarthy, C.R. (1994). Historical background of clinical trials involving women and minorities. *Academic Medicine, 69*, 695–698.

Merkatz, R.B., & Junod, S.W. (1994). Historical background of changes in FDA policy on the study and evaluation of drugs in women. *Academic Medicine, 69*, 703–707.

Millon-Underwood, S., Sanders, E., & Davis, M. (1993). Determinants of participation in state-of-the-art cancer prevention, early detection/screening, and treatment trials among African-Americans. *Cancer Nursing, 16*, 25–33. Retrieved from http://journals.lww.com/cancernursingonline/Citation/1993/02000/Determinants_of_participation_in_state_of_the_art.2.aspx

Murthy, V.H., Krumholz, H.M., & Gross, C.P. (2004). Participation in cancer clinical trials: Race-, sex-, and age-based disparities. *JAMA, 291*, 2720–2726. doi:10.1001/jama.291.22.2720

National Cancer Institute. (n.d.). NCI's Clinical Trials Cooperative Group Program. Retrieved from http://www.cancer.gov/cancertopics/factsheet/NCI/clinical-trials-cooperative-group

National Cancer Institute. (2005). *Cancer clinical trials: The in-depth program* [NIH Publication No. 05-5051]. Bethesda, MD: Author.

National Cancer Institute. (2007, June 4). New approaches to cancer drug development and clinical trials: Questions and answers. Retrieved from http://www.cancer.gov/newscenter/pressreleases/PhaseZeroNExTQandA/print?page=&keyword

National Cancer Institute. (2011). A closer look: Cancer clinical trials system restructuring moves forward. *NCI Cancer Bulletin, 8*(24). Retrieved from http://cancer.gov/ncicancerbulletin/121311/page8/print

National Cancer Institute. (2012). *Cancer: Changing the conversation—The nation's investment in cancer research*. Retrieved from http://www.cancer.gov/aboutnci/budget_planningleg/plan-2012

National Cancer Institute. (2013). *Community Oncology Research Program guidelines*. Retrieved from http://prevention.cancer.gov/files/programs-resources/NCORPProgramGuidelines.pdf

National Cancer Institute. (2014a). Children's assent. Retrieved from http://www.cancer.gov/clinicaltrials/learningabout/patientsafety/childrensassent

National Cancer Institute. (2014b). NCI Community Cancer Centers program pilot: 2007–2010. Retrieved from http://ncccp.cancer.gov/Media/FactSheet.htm

National Commission for the Protection of Human Subjects of Biomedical and Behavioral Research. (1979, April 18). *The Belmont report: Ethical principles and guidelines for the protection of human subject of research.* Retrieved from http://www.hhs.gov/ohrp/humansubjects/guidance/belmont.html

National Institutes of Health. (1998, March 6). NIH policy and guidelines on the inclusion of children as participants in research involving human subjects. Retrieved from http://grants.nih.gov/grants/guide/notice-files/not98-024.html

National Research Act, Pub. L. No. 93-348 (1974). Retrieved from http://history.nih.gov/research/downloads/PL93-348.pdf

Nuremberg Code. (1949). In *Trials of war criminals before the Nuremberg military tribunals under Control Council Law No. 10* (Vol. 2, pp. 181–182). Retrieved from http://www.hhs.gov/ohrp/archive/nurcode.html

Phillips, C. (2010). Insurance coverage expanding for cancer clinical trials. *NCI Cancer Bulletin, 7*(10). Retrieved from http://www.cancer.gov/ncicancerbulletin/051810/page5

Pinn, V.W. (1994). The role of the NIH's Office of Research on Women's Health. *Academic Medicine, 69,* 698–702. Retrieved from http://journals.lww.com/academicmedicine/pages/articleviewer.aspx?year=1994&issue=09000&article=00003&type=abstract

Repucci, N. (2012). A step-by-step checklist for conducting a clinical trial Medicare coverage analysis. *Medical Research Law and Policy Report,* pp. 1–9. Retrieved from http://www.dentons.com/en/insights/articles/2012/october/4/a-stepbystep-checklist-for-conducting-a-clinical-trial-medicare-coverage-analysis

Sateren, W.B., Trimble, E.L., Abrams, J., Brawley, O., Breen, N., Ford, L., ... Christian, M.C. (2002). How sociodemographics, presence of oncology specialists, and hospital cancer programs affect accrual to cancer treatment trials. *Journal of Clinical Oncology, 20,* 2109–2117.

Skloot, R. (2010). *The immortal life of Henrietta Lacks.* New York, NY: Broadway Paperbacks.

Sparks, J. (2002). Timeline of laws related to the protection of human subjects. Retrieved from http://history.nih.gov/about/timelines_laws_human.html

Swann, J.P. (1998). The Food and Drug Administration. In G.T. Kurian (Ed.), *A historical guide to the U.S. government* (pp. 248–254). New York, NY: Oxford University Press.

Talarico, L., Chen, G., & Pazdur, R. (2004). Enrollment of elderly patients in clinical trials for cancer drug registration: A 7-year experience by the U.S. Food and Drug Administration. *Journal of Clinical Oncology, 22,* 4626–4631. doi:10.1200/JCO.2004.02.175

U.S. Department of Health and Human Services. (2004). *Clinical research and the HIPAA Privacy Rule* [NIH Publication No. 04-5495]. Bethesda, MD: Author.

U.S. Department of Health and Human Services. (2014a). Federal policy for the protection of human subjects. Retrieved from http://www.hhs.gov/ohrp/humansubjects/commonrule/index.html

U.S. Department of Health and Human Services. (2014b). Federalwide Assurances FWAs. Retrieved from http://www.hhs.gov/ohrp/assurances/assurances/index.html

U.S. Food and Drug Administration. (1996, April). *Guidance for industry E6 good clinical practice: Consolidated guidance.* Retrieved from http://www.fda.gov/downloads/Drugs/GuidanceComplianceRegulatoryInformation/Guidances/UCM073122.pdf

White-Hershey, D., & Nevidjon, B. (1990). Fundamentals for oncology nurse/data managers—Preparing for a new role. *Oncology Nursing Forum, 17,* 371–377.

World Medical Association. (n.d.). Declaration of Helsinki: Recommendations guiding physicians in biomedical research involving human subjects. Retrieved from http://www.wma.net/en/60about/70history/01declarationHelsinki

World Medical Association. (1996). Declaration of Helsinki. *BMJ, 313,* 1448–1449. doi:10.1136/bmj.313.7070.1448a

Chapter 2

Drug Development

David Gillogly, BS, MBA, Pamela Perry, MS,
and Joan G. Westendorp, RN, MSN, OCN®, CCRP, CIM

Introduction

Drug development has been a work in progress for centuries. Pasteur's work on the germ basis of infectious diseases in the 1800s (Gallin, 2012) is only one example of the great drug developments in the United States' early history. There is a tremendous medical need for new treatments in oncology to augment the existing therapies available to patients with cancer today. Although the role for biologic and device development in oncology is extremely important, this chapter will specifically focus on small molecule development.

Before describing the drug development process, defining what is considered a drug or biologic is important. The Federal Food, Drug, and Cosmetic Act, 21 U.S.C. § 321(g)(2) (2010) classifies *drugs* specifically as
  (A) articles recognized in the official United States Pharmacopoeia, official Homoeopathic Pharmacopoeia of the United States, or official National Formulary, or any supplement to any of them; and (B) articles intended for use in the diagnosis, cure, mitigation, treatment, or prevention of disease in man or other animals; and (C) articles (other than food) intended to affect the structure or any function of the body of man or other animals; and (D) articles intended for use as a component of any article specified in clause (A), (B), or (C).

According to the Public Health Service Act, 42 U.S.C. § 262(i) (1999), a *biologic product* is
  A virus, therapeutic serum, toxin, antitoxin, vaccine, blood, blood component or derivative, allergenic product, or analogous product, or arsphenamine or derivative of arsphenamine (or any other trivalent organic arsenic compound), applicable to the prevention, treatment, or cure of a disease or condition of human beings.

In the United States, oncology drug development has two key players: the sponsor and the U.S. Food and Drug Administration (FDA). The sponsor, most often a pharmaceutical or biopharmaceutical company, is responsible for ensuring the compound being developed is manufactured and investigated in such a way that reasonable data supporting the efficacy and safety can be provided to FDA for evaluation. FDA offers guidance for the industry in how to develop adequate clinical investigations, and it reviews all of the sponsor-provided data to decide whether or not to grant licensing approval. The context of drug development refers to the following specific areas:
* The process of bringing new drugs or therapies to the market, which includes basic science, drug discovery, and sources of drugs
* The process of expanding a current drug into new patient indications, dosages, and delivery systems.

For simplicity, drug development as discussed here will be viewed from a U.S. context.

Where Does It All Begin?

When a promising compound is identified, preclinical investigations take place in animals. These data are carefully evaluated by the sponsor investigators so they can identify signs of targeting a disease state. Often, at this point, the mechanism of action is not well understood.

Basic science is vital for the development of a drug. There needs to be an understanding of the disease to be treated, and investigators must unravel the underlying cause of the condition. When studying a disease, investigators must understand how genes are altered: how it affects the proteins, how those proteins interact with each other, how those affected cells change the specific tissue they are in, and how the disease affects the entire patient. Investigators consider known molecules that affect the disease and decide which to target. Typically, a single molecule is chosen that is involved in a particular disease. The target on the molecule needs to be one that can potentially interact with and be affected by a drug/biologic.

Basic research refers to the process of discovery within the laboratory, which is the next step after basic science. The two stages of basic research are lead compound generation and lead compound optimization. *Lead generation* is when a promising molecule could become a drug by acting on one or multiple targets to alter a disease. This lead generation could be from plant, animal, mineral, microbiology, or semisynthetic/synthetic or recombinant DNA sources.

Lead optimization begins once the laboratory scientists discover a molecule or compound with a specific therapeutic or disease target (lead generation). During lead optimization, preclinical and animal testing occurs in the laboratory to determine if the drug is safe enough for human testing. The testing at this stage is in vitro ("vitro" is "glass" in Latin), which is conducted in the laboratory in test tubes and beakers. The other type of testing that occurs is in vivo ("vivo" is "life" in Latin), which is conducted in living cell cultures and animal models. During this series of testing, researchers conduct an early assessment of safety, which includes absorption, distribution, metabolism, excretion, and toxicology.

During the rigorous testing in the preclinical phase, a drug is considered successful if it is (a) absorbed into the bloodstream, (b) distributed to the proper site of action in the body, (c) metabolized efficiently and effectively, (d) successfully excreted from the body, and (e) demonstrated to be nontoxic. If a compound survives this preclinical phase (many do not), it is then ready for introduction for use in humans. At this point, an application is made to the FDA to begin "first in man" or phase I (see Chapter 4) testing. The application to begin human testing is part of the process known as an investigational new drug application (IND).

The Investigational New Drug Application

It is an exciting time when a new molecular entity seems viable enough to be targeted for consideration for first-in-man early-phase trials. This is accomplished through an IND and must be completed before the drug is administered to any humans.

Per U.S. law, any drug shipped across a state line must be the subject of an approved marketing application (U.S. FDA, 2014). The IND is the legal authorized exemption by the FDA allowing the drug sponsor to ship the chemical entity to sites within the United States for research purposes. The regulation is found in 21 C.F.R. §§ 312.23 and 312.24. Final guidance can be found on the FDA website regarding oncology exemptions: *Guidance for Industry: IND Exemptions for Studies of Lawfully Marketed Drug or Biological Products for the Treatment of Cancer.*

The two IND categories are commercial and research (noncommercial). A *commercial IND* is representative of a compound sponsored by a corporation or received from the National Institutes of Health (NIH). The objective is to bring a new drug to market. In the noncommercial arena, four different types of INDs can be submitted to the FDA, as follows.

- **Investigator-held IND.** When a physician is interested in conducting an investigation of either a compound in development or a new indication for an approved drug, he or she applies for this IND. Typically, he or she will request the investigational drug from the manufacturer, but the physician retains responsibility for the trial development and conduct. Often called investigator-initiated trials, these studies are commonly conducted in the oncology therapeutic arena and can bring great value to the understanding of a compound and potential indications for further study.
- **Emergency use IND.** When there is not enough time to follow the regulated submission pathway for an IND, this mechanism allows for the use of an investigational drug in an emergency situation. Subjects may not meet the requirements for inclusion into the protocol being conducted, or the investigational drug may be indicated when an approved study protocol is not in place. The FDA website has tools that will support the physician while ensuring the subject meets the established criteria for an emergency use IND, as well as a checklist that can be used by a physician when compiling the FDA-required information. The IND is obtained via a phone call to the FDA, with phone numbers provided for regular business and after-business hours.
- **Treatment IND.** This IND can be submitted when an investigational compound is at the end of its promising late-stage testing and it is under review by the FDA for a serious or immediately life-threatening condition. This would allow for restricted use of the investigational compound per the scope of the IND.
- **Exploratory IND (screening or microdose).** As defined by the FDA, this IND is for clinical trials that are conducted early in phase I development, with extremely limited human exposure and no therapeutic or diagnostic intent, such as screening or microdose studies.

U.S. Food and Drug Administration Review of the Application

The Center for Drug Evaluation and Research has a specialized program that supports pre-IND communication between the new drug review divisions and the IND applicant. The intent is to ensure that the sponsor is clear on the scope of data the agency requires for the IND submission. This is formally called the Pre-Investigational New Drug Application Consultation Program (Center for Drug Evaluation and Research, 1998).

The scope of the IND must include information that supports the FDA's understanding of the potential safety of the compound in question for human use. The following information must be provided in the initial IND.

- Preclinical data from animal pharmacology and toxicology studies. If the applicant has any additional data related to use in humans, they must also be submitted. This can happen when a compound is being researched or is approved in a foreign country.
- Information from the manufacturer. This includes details about the chemical composition of the compound, manufacturer location, stability data for the drugs, and information regarding good manufacturing practices.
- Initial clinical protocols and investigator information to ensure that the initial development plan is scientifically rigorous and valid from a regulatory perspective to protect subject safety. Investigators are expected to be qualified, as confirmed through submission of their curriculum vitae, and committed to conducting sound research following U.S. regulation and good clinical practice. This is confirmed by the principal investigator–signed Form FDA 1572 (U.S. FDA Office of Good Clinical Practice, 2010).

FDA requires a 30-day period from the time of IND submission to clinical trial initiation. There is no formal "approval" of the IND by FDA, but it is understood that the agency uses the 30 days to review the submission details so that it can consider the safety and applicability of the protocol from a medical, chemical, pharmacologic, and statistical perspective. If the reviewers feel that not enough evidence demonstrated that the compound is safe to administer in humans, they will institute a "clinical hold," and the trial cannot move forward until the additional data are submitted.

Maintaining and Amending an Investigational New Drug Application

Once an IND is filed, and FDA does not institute a clinical hold, the clinical trial investigation can begin as indicated in the IND. These are expected to be managed per good clinical practices (see Chapter 9) and applicable regulations.

There are three key reasons to amend or update an active IND.

- Studies that require a change or are new studies with the same indication can be submitted by the IND holder as an IND amendment.
  - This applies if there is a change in a current protocol, a new study to be held under the active IND in question, or a new investigator.
  - FDA offers guidance on the structure and the time frame allotted for this reporting activity.
- A sponsor must report any safety data that are not expected or foreseen for all studies operating under an IND. These are called IND Safety Reports, and they are to be issued when unexpected adverse events occur during the conduct of a clinical trial. This report is documented on a form called *MedWatch*, and an associated cover letter to FDA must be completed. FDA expects the report no more than 15 days after the original serious adverse event is made known to the investigator, sponsor, or the sponsor representative. An adverse event is classified as a *suspected adverse reaction* if evidence supports a causal relationship between the drug and the adverse event. An adverse event is classified as *serious* under 21 C.F.R. § 312.32 if it results in (IND Safety Reporting, 2013)
  - Death
  - A life-threatening adverse event
  - Inpatient hospitalization or prolongation of hospitalization
  - Persistent or significant incapacity or substantial disruption of the ability to conduct normal life functions
  - A congenital or anomalous birth defect.
- The sponsor is required to submit an annual report each year, even if no active studies are being conducted under the IND. This is a progress report of all activity conducted under the IND, which is due within 60 calendar days of the anniversary date that the IND went into effect.

The investigational agent under the IND goes through the clinical trial process of phase I and phase II. If successful in phase II and an optimal dosage is determined, the compound may move into larger phase III trials in patients with the disease to gain more data regarding the drug's efficacy and safety. If the drug shows efficacy with acceptable safety in adequate and well-controlled studies, the data may be submitted to FDA as a new drug application (NDA). Figure 2-1 illustrates an overview of the drug development process that has been reviewed.

Upon approval of the NDA, a company may begin marketing the drug to consumers. Additional drug testing may continue after the NDA is approved to gain additional data regarding the subjects' quality of life, as well as cost-effectiveness of treatments and other epidemiologic parameters. Further clinical trial work may continue after NDA approval to support new dosages and new forms or routes of administration (e.g., patch, IV, oral tablets, oral suspension). Testing in pediatric patients may begin after the NDA approval because additional patent protection is allowed under parts of drug legislation for drugs that have conducted pediatric trials.

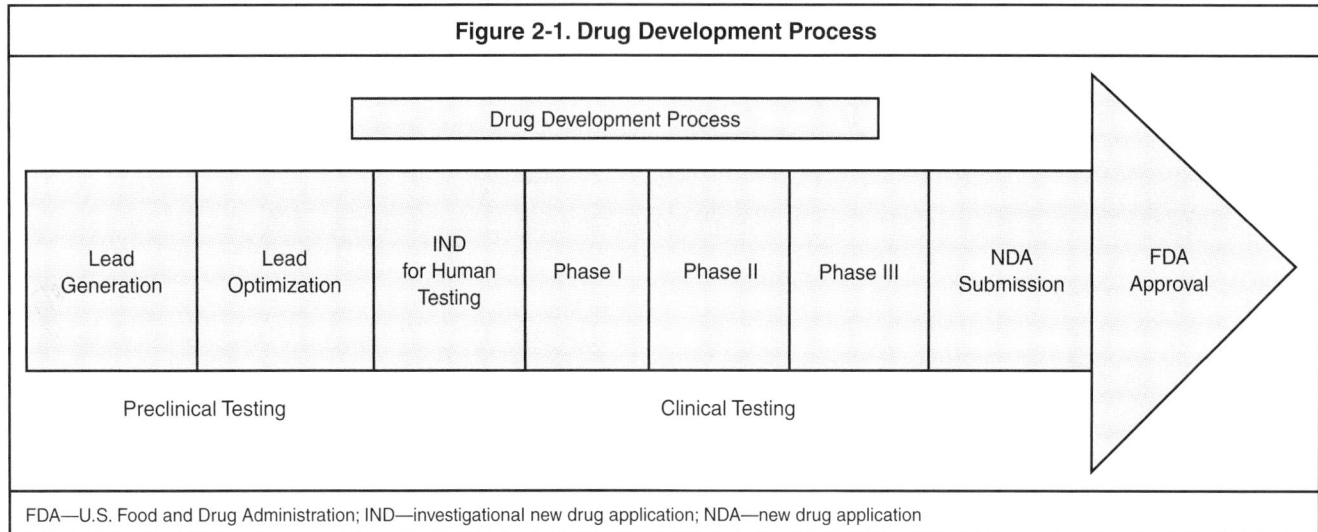

Figure 2-1. Drug Development Process

FDA—U.S. Food and Drug Administration; IND—investigational new drug application; NDA—new drug application

Naming of Drugs

As the investigational agent goes through the drug development process, it has likely been given a number of names, which is very confusing. The agent receives a chemical, generic, and brand name. The chemical name is the scientific name based on the compound's chemical structure and is almost never used to identify the drug in a clinical or marketing situation. The generic name is granted by the International Union of Pure and Applied Chemistry (www.iupac.org/home/about.html) and is commonly used to identify a drug during its clinical lifetime. This is the name that appears with the company's trade name on drug labels, advertisements, and other information. The brand name is created by the company that patents the drug. The brand name identifies the drug during the years that the company has exclusive rights to make and sell the drug.

Summary

Despite the considerable hurdles in developing drugs, the new oncology drugs that have been approved in recent years have been novel and commercially successful. The development process of an investigational agent is vital for the safety and potential therapeutic outcomes for patients with cancer.

Key Points

- FDA and the sponsor have essential roles in U.S. drug development.
- Drug development requires basic science and research.
- Preclinical testing for agents is necessary to determine a successful drug for human use.
- INDs and NDAs are necessary for the process of drug development.

References

Center for Drug Evaluation and Research. (1998, May 1). *Manual of policies and procedures: Review management—IND process and review procedures (including clinical holds)* [MAPP 6030.1]. Retrieved from http://www.fda.gov/downloads/AboutFDA/CentersOffices/CDER/ManualofPoliciesProcedures/ucm082022.pdf

Federal Food, Drug, and Cosmetic Act, 21 U.S.C. § 321 (2010). Retrieved from http://www.gpo.gov/fdsys/pkg/USCODE-2010-title21/html/USCODE-2010-title21-chap9-subchapII.htm

Gallin, J.I. (2012). A historical perspective on clinical research. In J.I. Gallin & F.P. Ognibene (Eds.), *Principles and practice of clinical research* (3rd ed., pp. 1–18). San Diego, CA: Elsevier Academic Press.

IND Safety Reporting, 21 C.F.R. § 312.32 (2013). Retrieved from http://www.accessdata.fda.gov/scripts/cdrh/cfdocs/cfcfr/cfrsearch.cfm?fr=312.32

Public Health Service Act, 42 U.S.C. § 262 (1999). Retrieved from http://www.fda.gov/RegulatoryInformation/Legislation/ucm149278.htm

U.S. Food and Drug Administration. (2014, February 13). How drugs are developed and approved. Retrieved from http://www.fda.gov/drugs/developmentapprovalprocess/howdrugsaredevelopedandapproved

U.S. Food and Drug Administration Office of Good Clinical Practice. (2010, May). Information sheet guidance for sponsors, clinical investigators, and IRBs: Frequently asked questions—Statement of investigator (Form FDA 1572). Retrieved from http://www.fda.gov/downloads/regulatoryinformation/guidances/ucm214282.pdf

Chapter 3

Types of Clinical Research: Background

Teresa Knoop, MSN, RN, AOCN®, Pamela Carney, MSN, RN, OCN®,
and Joan G. Westendorp, RN, MSN, OCN®, CCRP, CIM

Introduction

Clinical research is evolving. Although the time-honored designs of experimental and observational studies continue to provide the foundation for clinical research, the field recognizes that the rapid translation of scientific advances to the clinical setting is increasingly important. Medical, scientific, and research experts agree that the evolution of clinical research methods and designs must occur to keep pace with the need for efficient and expedient translation of scientific research findings to patient care in order to continually improve treatment of serious illnesses, especially cancer. Newer designs, such as comparative effectiveness research (CER), may provide an avenue for expanding the medical knowledge base in an expeditious manner.

Additionally, efforts are underway to develop and optimize an infrastructure that will transform the clinical research enterprise. Advisory groups such as the Institute of Medicine (IOM) have provided several reports in the past five years related to clinical research. The IOM reports provide a vision for the future of clinical research (IOM, n.d.; Mack & Nass, 2011; Nass, Moses, & Mendelsohn, 2010; Weisfeld, English, & Claiborne, 2012).

Experimental Versus Observational Clinical Research

Clinical research involves the study of voluntary human participants, with the ultimate goal of increasing medical knowledge that leads to efficacious disease prevention, diagnosis, and treatment and patient care management. Clinical research sets the stage for subsequent study and discovery. One type of traditional clinical research is experimental, which may also be referred to as a clinical trial or interventional research. The hallmark of an experimental study is the use of a research intervention, which may be a drug, a medical device, a procedure, or a change in behavior. Typically, experimental research proceeds in a stepwise fashion through a series of phases that test concepts related to safety, optimal dosing or scheduling, adverse event identification, efficacy, risks and benefits compared to standard treatment, and long-term safety (National Cancer Institute [NCI], n.d.; National Institutes of Health [NIH], 2012).

The gold standard of an experimental design is the randomized controlled trial (RCT), which provides the highest level of evidence-based medicine, particularly in the development of new drugs. However, conducting and completing experimental research, particularly RCTs, can be expensive, time consuming, and labor intensive (Weisfeld et al., 2012).

A second type of traditional clinical research is defined as observational, and although this type of research does include voluntary human participants, it does not involve a planned research alteration or intervention. Participants may be receiving interventions, such as standard medical care or routine procedures, but no experimental interventions or agents are assigned. Subjects in observational studies provide data related to health outcomes and allow the researcher to define the outcomes in specific groups of participants (NCI, n.d.; NIH, 2012).

Comparative Effectiveness Research

Healthcare providers depend on clinical research for information regarding the natural history of a disease, clinical presentation, diagnosis, and treatment options. Consumers, patients, and caregivers require reliable, current information to help them evaluate their disease and treatment options. Unfortunately, the information needed to guide these medical decisions is often incomplete or unavailable. According to IOM, more than 50% of the treatments delivered today lack clear evidence of effectiveness. This uncertainty contributes to variability in clinical practice as well as cost and outcomes, which differ across the United States (IOM, 2009).

CER has captured the attention of a wide array of stakeholders, including providers, investigators, patients, payers, and policy makers. This keen interest is partially because of the hope that CER will provide patient-centered information to guide clinical decisions and ultimately improve the quality of care while controlling cost (Golub & Fontanarosa, 2012). CER is defined as

> the generation and synthesis of evidence that compares the benefits and harms of alternative methods to prevent, diagnose, treat, and monitor a clinical condition or to improve the delivery of care. The purpose of CER is to assist consumers, clinicians, purchasers, and policy makers to make informed decisions that will improve health care at both the individual and population levels. (IOM, 2009, p. 29)

In the American Recovery and Reinvestment Act of 2009 (ARRA), U.S. Congress allocated $1.1 billion to CER to stimulate the national effort toward effectiveness research. The legislation created a national council on CER and directed IOM to identify high-priority topics for research. IOM sought input from a variety of stakeholders and received more than 2,000 nominations for topics over a three-week period. Following a three-step voting process, IOM identified 100 high-priority topics for consideration and support by ARRA funds. Cancer was the focus of several high-priority topics that encompassed screening technologies for breast and colon cancer, strategies for early breast and prostate cancer management, interventions aimed at reducing health disparities, and comparison of the effectiveness of genetic and biomarker testing (Sox & Greenfield, 2009).

Research Methodologies

CER encompasses both evidence generation and synthesis. Generation of comparative effectiveness evidence uses experimental and observational methods. RCTs compare outcomes across groups of participants who are randomly assigned to different interventions that often include a placebo or control arm. RCTs are considered the gold standard of experimental methodology, but the evidence is limited in its application to real-world decision making. RCTs will contribute significantly to CER as innovative study designs are emerging, which are aimed at improving translation to everyday practice (Hahn & Schilsky, 2012).

Observational trials compare outcomes between patient groups who receive different interventions through some process other than randomization (Armstrong, 2012). Observational studies represent an increasing proportion of CER because of their applicability to various settings and the opportunity to investigate differences in effectiveness across subgroups (Lyman, 2012). Synthesis of evidence is accomplished by systematic review and clinical decision models. Systematic review is a high-level overview of all high-quality evidence available on a particular research question. Systematic reviews can be tailored to CER by broadening the type of studies and evaluating the full range of benefits and harm of alternative strategies (Brouwers, Thabane, Moher, & Straus, 2012). Decision modeling is an approach to evidence synthesis that brings together data from a range of sources to estimate expected outcomes of different interventions. Many factors influence the selection of study design, including time, logistical constraints, data availability, and ethical dimensions of the study (Armstrong, 2012).

Patient Involvement

The goal of CER is to provide stakeholders, including patients and physicians, with evidence-based information to make informed healthcare decisions. In the past, researchers designed CER studies, and patients provided relatively little input. Patient engagement is rapidly gaining acceptance and is considered by many as being essential to the successful translation of CER (Mullins, Abdulhalim, & Lavallee, 2012).

The Patient Protection and Affordable Care Act of 2010 created the Patient-Centered Outcomes Research Institute (PCORI, n.d.-b) to fund and promote CER. PCORI's mission is to help "people make informed healthcare decisions and improve healthcare delivery and outcomes, by producing and promoting high-integrity, evidence-based information that comes from research guided by patients, caregivers, and the broader healthcare community" (PCORI, n.d.-a). PCORI approved 25 awards, totaling $40.7 million over three years, to fund patient-centered clinical CER projects under the first four areas of its National Priorities for Research and Research Agenda (Fischer, 2012). Engaging patients in CER requires additional effort compared to the traditional research process, but if the result is patient-centered evidence that is useful to clinical practice and decision making, then the outcome is well worth the extra effort (Mullins et al., 2012).

Importance to Oncology

Although cancer was only included in a limited fashion in the IOM's top CER priorities, nowhere are the need and potential for CER greater than in oncology. Scientific advances in molecular biology and genetics have led to the identification of countless potential targets for diagnostic, prognostic, and predictive assays, as well as targets for treatment and prevention of cancer. Driven by new technologies and therapies, healthcare spending has risen dramatically, and cancer diagnosis and treatment accounts for a substantial portion of the overall increase (Lyman, 2012). CER provides the means to bridge the gap between clinical research and real-world clinical practice.

Nursing Companion Studies

Companion studies offer nurses the opportunity to conduct independent research within a supportive framework through collaboration with other investigators that will advance the specialty of oncology nursing. Nursing companion studies may be performed with a variety of disciplines but most often are associated with medical research. Two general types of companion studies exist: collaborative and parallel.

Collaborative Companion Studies

Collaborative companion studies are conducted in association with an ongoing medical study. These can be associated with observational or experimental clinical research. The studies are initiated and implemented by a nurse researcher, although interdisciplinary effort by the nurse and physician investigator is imperative. In this situation, two or more studies are carried out jointly; subject accrual, day-to-day management, data collection, and analysis often overlap between the two. Collaborative studies are the most successful type of companion studies (Ferrell & Cohen, 1991).

Parallel Companion Studies

A parallel companion study is one in which a nurse investigator implements a study as a result of a nursing concern that may have arisen from observations of patients enrolled in a trial, usually in an experimental clinical trial. Parallel studies typically address general nursing issues, such as nausea, stomatitis, quality of life, fatigue, and pain (Ferrell & Cohen, 1991).

Barriers and Benefits of Companion Studies

Regardless of the type of study conducted, the success of companion studies depends on positive interdisciplinary collaboration. Lancaster (1985) first described the importance of teamwork in carrying out these types of studies by introducing the "six C's" of companion research. She defined these characteristics as (a) contribution, (b) compatibility, (c) communication, (d) consensus, (e) commitment, and (f) credit. For a companion study to be successful, all healthcare members involved in the research project must embrace these attributes, have the ability to work well together, possess mutual respect for each other's efforts, and be coauthors on any publication (see Chapter 44). A nurse researcher may initiate a companion study as an investigator or participate as a member of a multidisciplinary team designing a companion study.

Companion studies have many potential benefits, but barriers to conducting these studies exist, as well. Researchers must be aware of the potential challenges and benefits prior to embarking on this endeavor. Benefits of conducting companion studies include gaining access to a larger population of subjects than would be available to nurse researchers conducting an independent study. Through collaboration, access to subjects is enhanced, and opportunities for enrollment at multiple sites may be possible. Patient accrual, therefore, might be accomplished in a shorter period of time, or a larger and more diverse sample size may be made a reality. Frequently, companion studies can be conducted at a lower cost because expenses can be shared between studies. Shared expenses might pertain to patient screening, accrual, and follow-up; data collection and management; and blood sampling.

Another advantage to conducting companion research studies is the opportunity for interdisciplinary collaboration. These studies allow novice investigators to take an active role in the research process, affording them an opportunity they otherwise might not have had to evaluate patient outcomes. Companion studies also can provide a challenge to the experienced researcher because they may extend beyond the individual's scope of research.

Keeping in mind that companion studies have potential drawbacks is important. Although medical studies and companion studies may be implemented at the same time, they are, in reality, two separate trials based on complete and separate protocols that must stand alone in terms of scientific merit and patient safety. Each study requires extensive, comprehensive planning before implementation, just as if each had been implemented independently. Each must meet the institution's research and human rights committee requirements and receive approval. A principal investigator who will assume accountability for the study must be identified for each study. When planning these studies, investigators must be aware that although some costs may be shared, each study requires a separate budget. Also, each must have a time frame established before initiation and be monitored closely. Analysis of study results, ownership of the data, and plans for dissemination through publication or presentation must be negotiated in advance.

Institute of Medicine Reports: Efforts to Improve the Clinical Trials Enterprise

Background of the Institute of Medicine

The four branches of the National Academies are (a) the National Academy of Sciences, (b) the National Academy of Engineering, (c) IOM, and (d) the National Research Council. With the first academy (Sciences) chartered by Congress in 1863, these four branches serve to advise the U.S. government about issues related to science, engineering, and medicine. IOM, established as a separate branch in 1970 by the National Academy of Sciences, functions to advise the federal government on public health policy by identifying and examining issues related to medical care, research, and education (IOM, n.d.).

To accomplish its goals, IOM organizes workshops and invites experts in the field to tackle specific issues identified in areas of health care. One such priority identified in the past five years was the area of clinical trials. After each workshop, the team publishes a summary report (IOM, n.d.). Three of these reports are especially important for those working in the area of cancer clinical trials.

2010 Report: *A National Cancer Clinical Trials System for the 21st Century: Reinvigorating the NCI Cooperative Group Program*

Since 1956, the NCI Clinical Trials Cooperative Group Program (also known as the Cooperative Groups) has contributed greatly to positively affect the lives of patients with cancer; however, it became apparent to NCI that the system needed to undergo changes to improve efficiency, effectiveness, and productivity. Although three previous analyses were made of the Cooperative Group Program—the Armitage Report in 1996, the Clinical Trials Working Group Report in 2004, and the Operational Efficiency Working Group in 2010—additional efforts were needed (Mack & Nass, 2011; Nass et al., 2010). Recognizing that the Cooperative Group system was complex, redundant, and underfunded and that only 60% of NCI-sponsored trials are completed and published, the NCI director requested that IOM make recommendations for an overhaul of the Cooperative Group Program that would incorporate the strengths of the system with a redesign of the areas that did not work as well (Nass et al., 2010).

The IOM group of experts published their first report in 2010 by focusing on four overreaching goals (Nass et al., 2010):

- Improve speed and efficiency in the design, launch, and conduct of trials
- Incorporate innovative science and trial design
- Improve prioritization, selection, support, and completion of cancer clinical trials
- Increase and incentivize patient and physician participation.

The identified goals generated 12 recommendations and required the IOM-led group to take a broader view of cancer clinical trials that included a vision for the Cooperative Group Program to join forces with academic, government, industry, insurance, physician, and patient partners. To reach the goals, six needs were identified for cancer clinical trials in 2015:

- Rapid translation of scientific discoveries into public health benefits
- Strong publicly supported clinical trials system in the United States that complements industry trials to develop drugs and devices
- Robust, standardized, and accessible clinical trials infrastructure
- Harmonized and synchronized rules and guidelines across federal regulatory agencies
- Support for clinical investigators
- Broad patient involvement in clinical trials. (Nass et al., 2010, pp. 8–9)

2011 Report: *A National Cancer Clinical Trials System for the 21st Century: Reinvigorating the NCI Cooperative Group Program*

Building upon the 2010 IOM report, a second group of cancer experts, including members of IOM's National Cancer Policy Forum and the American Society of Clinical Oncology, met in March 2011 to develop a plan to address the goals and recommendations from the 2010 IOM report (Mack & Nass, 2011).

Based on the IOM reports, the dialogue among stakeholders in cancer research has begun to build the foundation for transformation. Evidence of systemic change is already apparent in the Cooperative Group Program with the consolidation of the front and back office operations along with consolidation of the various groups from 13 cooperative groups into four adult groups and one pediatric group. Additionally, funding issues are being addressed so that financial resources are appropriately allocated. With a truly concerted effort among cancer research stakeholders, the implementation of the IOM recommendations will guide the way to transformation (Mack & Nass, 2011).

2012 Report: *Envisioning a Transformed Clinical Trials Enterprise in the United States: Establishing an Agenda for 2020*

In 2011, a team of research and healthcare experts gathered to lay the groundwork for transformation of the clinical trials enterprise (CTE) in the United States by focusing on drug discovery and development and translation; the full report was published in 2012. At this meeting, the CTE was defined as the "full spectrum of clinical trials and their applications" (Weisfeld et al., 2012, p. 1), inclusive of processes, institutions, and individuals that use clinical trial outcomes as the basis for clinical patient care. The belief that RCTs are the underpinning of the CTE and serve as the basis for drug development and evaluations of existing therapies made RCTs the main topic of discussion. The team of experts also discussed other types of clinical research in a broader context encompassing nonrandomized trials, observational studies, non-interventional studies, and CER (Weisfeld et al., 2012). Current challenges to the CTE were identified, as were stakeholders such as

- Federal agencies
- Nongovernmental organizations that fund or conduct clinical trials (academic institutions, patient advocacy groups, philanthropic foundations)
- Industry (pharmaceutical, biotechnology, and medical devices companies)
- Clinical trial regulators.

The workshop was divided into four sessions. A fifth session provided an opportunity for summaries and subsequent discussions. To develop a vision for CTE transformation, it was proposed that the path forward should include the following perspectives: healthcare delivery systems, health sciences policy, research organization, NIH, and international perspectives. The workshop concluded with a discussion surrounding an agenda for implementation: long-term goals, priorities, short-term goals, workforce, infrastructure, and stakeholder engagement (Weisfeld et al., 2012).

Summary

Clinical research allows the discipline of medicine to provide excellence in patient care and drives the improvement of disease prevention, detection, and treatment. The oncology specialty is experiencing rapid scientific advances, particularly in the area of personalizing and predicting approaches to precision treatment. Currently, more than 800 cancer therapies are being developed, which provide hope for patients with cancer and implore those with an interest in cancer research to transform practices, which will allow scientific advances to reach the clinical setting as expeditiously as possible (Nass, Balogh, & Mendelsohn, 2011). By thoroughly examining and analyzing current clinical research designs and processes and working together with all stakeholders in cancer research, medical experts can aid in the transformation of clinical trials and their positive impact in cancer care.

Key Points

- Experimental and observational studies have historically provided the foundation for clinical research.
- Clinical research methods and designs are evolving to keep pace with the need for efficient and expedient translation of scientific research findings to patient care.
- Newer designs such as CER may provide an avenue for expanding the medical knowledge base in an expeditious manner.
- CER encompasses both evidence generation and evidence synthesis.
- The goal of CER is to provide the means to bridge the gap between clinical research and real-world clinical practice.
- Patient involvement is a central element in the generation of clinically useful CER evidence.
- Collaborative and parallel companion studies provide a means for nurses to conduct independent research to advance oncology nursing knowledge.
- Advisory groups such as IOM provided several reports in the past five years that present a vision to develop and optimize an infrastructure that will transform the clinical research enterprise.

References

Armstrong, K. (2012). Methods of comparative effectiveness research. *Journal of Clinical Oncology, 30,* 4208–4214. doi:10.1200/JCO.2012.42.2659

Brouwers, M.C., Thabane, L., Moher, D., & Straus, S. (2012). Comparative effectiveness research paradigm: Implications for systematic reviews and clinical practice guidelines. *Journal of Clinical Oncology, 30,* 4202–4207. doi:10.1200/JCO.2012.45.9792

Ferrell, B., & Cohen, M. (1991). Cancer clinical trials. Companion studies. *Seminars in Oncology Nursing, 7,* 252–259.

Fischer, E. (2012, December 18). PCORI announces funding for first comparative effectiveness research projects [Press release]. Retrieved from http://www.pcori.org/2012/funding-awards

Golub, R.M., & Fontanarosa, P.B. (2012). Comparative effectiveness research. *JAMA, 307,* 1643–1645. doi:10.1001/jama.2012.490

Hahn, O., & Schilsky, R. (2012). Randomized controlled trials and comparative effectiveness research. *Journal of Clinical Oncology, 30,* 4194–4201. doi:10.1200/JCO.2012.42.2352

Institute of Medicine. (n.d.). About the IOM. Retrieved from http://www.iom.edu/About-IOM.aspx

Institute of Medicine. (2009). *Initial national priorities for comparative effectiveness research.* Retrieved from http://www.iom.edu/reports/2009/comparativeeffectivenessresearchpriorities.aspx

Lancaster, J. (1985). The perils and joys of collaborative research. *Nursing Outlook, 33,* 231–232.

Lyman, G. (2012). Comparative effectiveness research in oncology: An overview. *Journal of Clinical Oncology, 30,* 4181–4184. doi:10.1200/JCO.2012.45.9792

Mack, A., & Nass, S. (2011). *Implementing a national cancer clinical trials system for the 21st century: Workshop summary.* Washington, DC: National Academies Press.

Mullins, C.D., Abdulhalim, A.M., & Lavallee, D.C. (2012). Continuous patient engagement in comparative effectiveness research. *JAMA, 307,* 1587–1588. doi:10.1001/jama.2012.442

Nass, S., Balogh, E., & Mendelsohn, J. (2011). A national clinical trials network: Recommendations from the Institute of Medicine. *American Journal of Therapeutics, 18,* 382–391. doi:10.1097/MJT.0b013e3181ff7e23

Nass, S., Moses, H., & Mendelsohn, J. (Eds.). (2010). *A national cancer clinical trials system for the 21st century: Reinvigorating the NCI Cooperative Group Program.* Washington, DC: National Academies Press.

National Cancer Institute. (n.d.). Clinical trials reporting program. Retrieved from http://www.cancer.gov/clinicaltrials/conducting/ncictrp/resources/glossary

National Institutes of Health. (2012). Learn about clinical studies. Retrieved from http://clinicaltrials.gov/ct2/about-studies/learn

Patient-Centered Outcomes Research Institute. (n.d.-a). Mission and vision. Retrieved from http://www.pcori.org/about/mission-and-vision

Patient-Centered Outcomes Research Institute. (n.d.-b). PCORI funding awards. Retrieved from http://pfaawards.pcori.org

Sox, H., & Greenfield, S. (2009). Comparative effectiveness research: A report from the Institute of Medicine. *Annals of Internal Medicine, 151,* 203–205. doi:10.7326/0003-4819-151-3-200908040-00125

Weisfeld, N., English, R.A., & Claiborne, A.B. (2012). *Envisioning a transformed clinical trials enterprise in the United States: Establishing an agenda for 2020: Workshop summary.* Retrieved from http://www.nap.edu/catalog.php?record_id=13345

Chapter 4

Types of Clinical Research: Experimental

Elizabeth Ness, RN, MS, and Georgia Cusack, MS, RN, AOCNS®

Introduction

Clinical research involves research conducted on humans. Clinical research studies can be divided into either observation/descriptive or experimental/interventional. This chapter will cover basic concepts associated with experimental clinical trials, including phase 0–IV clinical trials. Tips for the clinical trial nurse (CTN) will be highlighted. For more information on ethical issues and protocol development, including statistical analysis related to clinical trial designs, please refer to Chapters 12 and 15, respectively.

Key Concepts to Understanding Clinical Trial Designs

A basic understanding of clinical trials involves understanding key concepts and terminology related to trial design, including randomization, stratification, blinding/masking, control groups, trial designs, and stages (see Table 4-1).

Randomization

Randomization is the process of assigning research patients to a treatment group or a control group to assess differences in treatment outcomes that can be attributed to the intervention versus other characteristics. Each group is referred to as an *arm* of the study (National Institutes of Health, 2012). Randomized controlled trials (RCTs) remain the gold standard in clinical research and hold many advantages, including (Shaw, Johnson, & Borkowf, 2012)
- Allowing treatment allocation to be free from selection bias by the investigator, either intentionally or unintentionally
- Ensuring that the difference in baseline characteristics of the research patients were by chance only
- Increasing the likelihood of comparable study groups
- Balancing prognostic variables, both known and unknown
- Ensuring that statistically significant differences in the treatment groups are due to the actual treatment rather than other external reasons.

Several methods of randomization are described in Table 4-2. Simple and complex software programs can be used to complete the task. Implementing randomization can be done via sealed opaque envelopes with sequential numbers; a telephone answering service, coordinating center, or interactive voice response system; or a local computer network or a computer system through a coordinating center.

Once the implementation is determined and the randomization occurs, the randomization code (i.e., the treatment) is shared with the pharmacist, and for an unmasked study, with the research team (Shaw, Johnson, & Borkowf, 2012). It is important for the CTN to understand the randomization process for a clinical trial prior to enrolling a patient. This information is found in the protocol or in a separate manual of operations. Through patient education, the CTN should reinforce the process of randomization. With reinforcement of the rationale for randomization and why it is being used to answer specific scientific study questions, patients may be less likely to withdraw from participation.

Blinding/Masking

Blinding/masking studies helps to minimize biases that might result from differences in patient assessment and management or interpretation of a result by the patient, investigator, or others (International Conference on Harmonisation of Technical Requirements for

Registration of Pharmaceuticals for Human Use [ICH], 2000; Miller & Steward, 2011). The two terms are often used interchangeably (Stoney & Johnson, 2012a). The three types of blinded studies are single, double, and triple (see Table 4-1). Double-blinded studies are the most common. The protocol should clearly specify
- Who is to be blinded
- The purpose of the blinding
- Under what circumstances unblinding will occur
- The procedure to be used for unblinding, including to whom the unblinded information is to be provided.

Studies that are not blinded are referred to as an *unblinded, open study,* or *open label* (Miller & Steward, 2011; Stoney & Johnson, 2012b). The CTN should understand the rationale for the type of blinding used and under what clinical situations unblinding may be needed (e.g.,

Table 4-1. Selected Experimental Design Concepts and Terminology	
Term	Definition
ADME	Used in pharmacokinetic studies to describe how the drug or biologic is absorbed (A) by the body, distributed (D) throughout the body, metabolized (M), and excreted (E) by the body
Blinded/masked	Intended to ensure that subjective assessment is not affected by knowledge of treatment assignment, and minimizes the potential biases resulting from differences in management, treatment, or assessment of patients or interpretation of results. Types include • Single blind—subject does not know treatment • Double blind (recommended)—Neither subject nor healthcare providers know treatment • Triple blind—subject, healthcare providers, and statistician/monitors do not know treatment.
Control group	The set of patients randomized to receive either a standard treatment or a placebo
Direct endpoint	Clinically meaningful endpoints that directly measure how the research participant feels and functions or survives. These endpoints characterize the clinical outcome of interest as either an objective endpoint (e.g., survival, disease exacerbation, clinical event) or a subjective endpoint (e.g., symptom score, health-related quality of life). Customarily, the basis for approval of new drugs.
Dose-limiting toxicity (DLT)	Unacceptable toxicity for a specific dose level as predefined in the protocol (e.g., grade 3 or higher adverse event that is related to the intervention) for a specified amount of time (e.g., one cycle)
Investigational agent	A drug or biologic used in a clinical trial. The drug or biologic may be unapproved for commercial use in the United States (i.e., being conducted under an Investigational New Drug Application or commercially available).
Maximum tolerated dose (MTD)	Dose level at which 0–1 patients out of 6 develop a DLT
Microdose	A dose that is less than 1/100th of the animal dose calculated to yield a pharmacologic effect of a test agent
Mouse equivalent lethal dose (MELD) 10	Using a mouse model, it is the quantity of an agent that kills 10% of the mice
Pharmacodynamics (PD)	What the drug/biologic does to the body
Pharmacokinetics (PK)	What the body does to the drug/biologic
Randomization	The process of assigning research participants to a group (e.g., control group or intervention group) by chance
Recommended phase II dose (RP2D)	Dose determined in a phase I clinical trial to be the safe dose used in a phase II clinical trial
Surrogate endpoint	Endpoint used as an alternative to a direct endpoint so that it becomes the surrogate for clinical benefit (e.g., laboratory measure or a physical sign used as a substitute for a direct endpoint). Surrogate endpoints can be used for drug approval if well validated.
Stratification	Partitioning subjects by a factor other than the treatment (e.g., gender, age, disease severity, risk factors, prior treatments, or concomitant illness)
Therapeutic index	Based on animal studies, the level of drug to achieve a therapeutic effect is below the level at which the drug becomes toxic or caused death

Note. Based on information from National Institutes of Health, 2012; Shaw, Johnson, & Borkowf, 2012; Stoney & Johnson, 2012a.

Table 4-2. Types of Randomization	
Type	Description
Simple randomization	Equivalent to tossing a coin for each subject that enters a trial where heads will receive Treatment A and tails will receive Treatment B
Gives each treatment arm equal probability of being selected
Treatment assignment is completely unpredictable
May lead to an imbalance in the treatment assignment (e.g., there are more patients in Treatment A than Treatment B), which might reduce statistical power, especially with smaller trials
Even if treatment is balanced at the end of a trial, it may not be balanced at some time during the trial.
Block randomization	Divides patients into small blocks of equal sample sizes
Blocks are small and balanced with predetermined group assignments keeping the numbers of patients in each group similar at all times (e.g., 24 treatment assignments will be assigned in six blocks of four patients each: AABB, ABAB, BABA, ABBA, BBAA, BAAB)
Ensures equal treatment allocation within each block if the complete block is used
Stratified randomization or stratification	Partitioning of research patients by factors other than treatment
Creates a balance between baseline characteristics of a relatively homogenous group of research patients to produce more comparable groups providing more confidence that the outcomes are a result of the treatment effect
Examples of stratification factors include demographic factors (e.g., gender, age) or prognostic factors (e.g., estrogen receptor/progesterone receptor/nodal status in breast cancer)

Note. Based on information from Shaw, Johnson, & Borkowf, 2012.

patient hospitalization or unexpected death) and should provide ongoing patient education as needed as part of the informed consent process.

Control Groups

Randomized clinical trials need a control group. A *control group* is a group of research patients who do not receive the treatment being studied. The group receiving the treatment under investigation is referred to as the *experimental group*. The purpose of a control group is to distinguish the patient treatment outcomes (e.g., change in symptoms or disease status) from outcomes caused by other factors (e.g., natural progression of the disease or other treatment). The selection of a control group is critical and sometimes challenging. When considering a control group, one should consider what standard therapies are available for the study patient population, the goal of the clinical trial, the significance of the control group, and ethical considerations. Some control groups will receive no treatment while others may receive the standard of care (ICH, 2000; Stoney & Johnson, 2012a). See Table 4-3 for more information about types of control groups.

Clinical Trial Designs

Parallel Design

With parallel design, the patient is randomized to one of several treatment groups. The simplest parallel design uses two groups: one experimental group and one control (see Figure 4-1). However, more than one experimental group or control group can be used. Multiple concurrent groups can be used to study different doses or different treatments (Stoney & Johnson, 2012a).

Crossover Design

Crossover designs allow each patient to receive more than one treatment that is being investigated. A patient would be randomized to Treatment A and then, after meeting a specific outcome (e.g., disease progression, completion of a predetermined number of cycles), cross over to Treatment B, while another patient would be randomized to Treatment B and then cross over to Treatment A once the outcome was met (see Figure 4-2). As a result, patients are used as their own control, which reduces variability between subjects and requires a smaller sample size. A few disadvantages with a crossover design include the carryover effects (e.g., toxicity or response) may be difficult to assess and measure for the second treatment, and patients are required to be on the clinical trial for a longer period of time, which might affect retention (Stoney & Johnson, 2012a).

Factorial Design

Factorial design allows for multiple factors (e.g., different treatments) to be studied simultaneously, thus allowing multiple hypotheses to be tested. It is comparable to combining multiple parallel design studies into one study. The simplest is a 2 × 2 factorial design, which involves two fac-

Table 4-3. Common Types of Control Groups	
Control Group	Description
Placebo control	Inactive drug made to physically resemble the treatment being investigated (i.e., same color pill and same packaging). Both interventions are given in the same setting (e.g., one-hour IV infusion for both the experimental treatment and the placebo administered in the same setting, the same way, and with the same tubing) Inactive portion of the intervention typically used in device trials to mimic the experimental intervention (e.g., acupuncture study where the needles look and feel the same as the standard treatment, but they do not penetrate the skin); referred to as a *sham control* Almost always double-blinded Note that a placebo effect is still possible, depending upon the question being studied and the patient population (e.g., chronic pain study)
Nontreatment control	Patients randomly assigned to experimental intervention or no study treatment, not even a placebo Used when it would be difficult to use a double-blinded study design (e.g., easily recognizable side effects with experimental intervention or when the standard of care is observational)
Active concurrent control	Patients randomly assigned to experimental treatment or an active treatment Often used in oncology trials where the blinding of the experimental treatment is difficult due to differing side effects, routes of administration, or regimens Used to show that the experimental treatment is as effective as or superior to it (i.e., current standard) or to compare the safety and efficacy of two experimental treatments
Historical control	Use of external control group that was either treated at a different time or treated during the same time but in a different setting Nonrandomized Rapid, inexpensive, and good for initial testing of new intervention Vulnerable to biases because of differences in underlying populations, criteria for selecting patients in another study, standards of care, and diagnostic or evaluation criteria
Multiple controls	Use of more than one control in a study (e.g., active control and placebo) Can use several doses of the active control having multiple treatments

Note. Based on information from International Conference on Harmonisation of Technical Requirements for Registration of Pharmaceuticals for Human Use, 2000; Stoney & Johnson, 2012a.

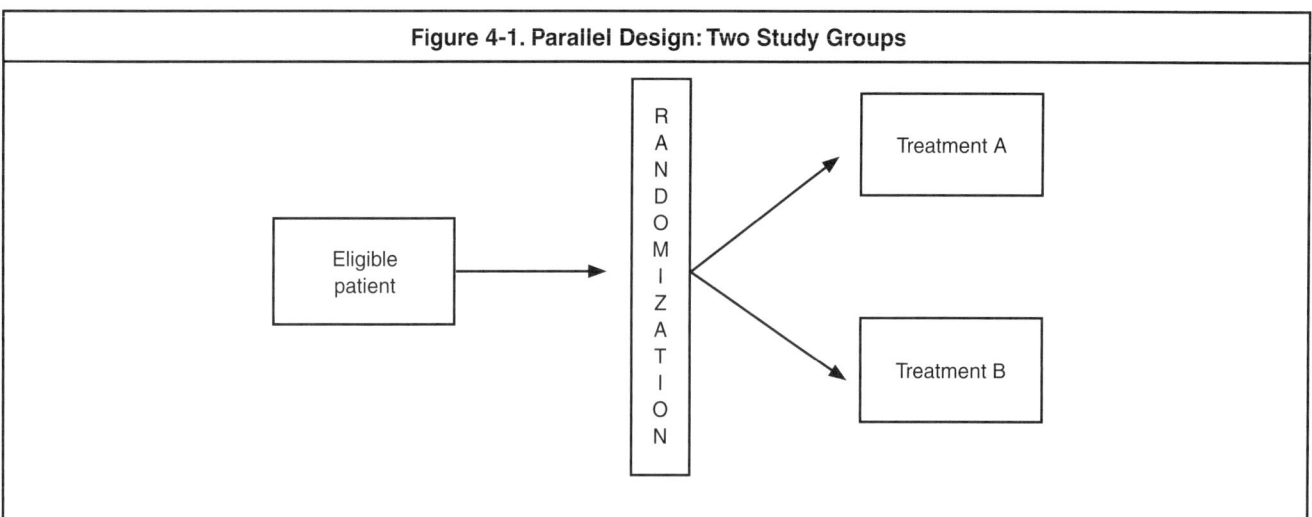

Figure 4-1. Parallel Design: Two Study Groups

Examples of Treatment A and Treatment B:
- Treatment A can be standard of care and Treatment B can be the experimental intervention (drug, biologic, surgery, radiation).
- Treatment A and Treatment B can use the same drug at different doses (e.g., high dose, low dose).
- Treatment A can be the experimental drug/biologic and Treatment B can be a placebo.
- Treatment A can be the experimental drug/biologic + standard of care and Treatment B can be the experimental drug/biologic alone.

Note. Based on information from Stoney & Johnson, 2012a.

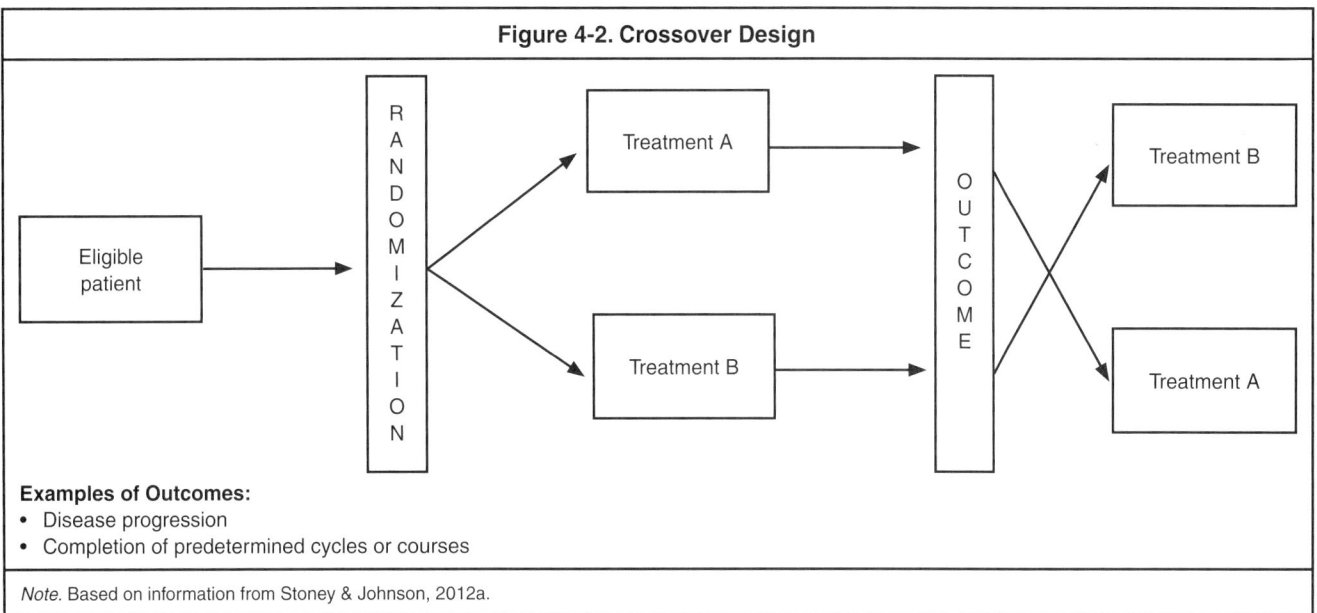

tors each with two levels (see Figure 4-3). Though patients have an increased opportunity to get an active treatment, they have to be willing and able to receive any of the treatments, and dose modification strategies may be more difficult to determine (Stoney & Johnson, 2012a).

Randomized Discontinuation Design

In a randomized discontinuation design, all patients start out receiving the experimental treatment for a predetermined period of time. After that time period has concluded, those patients with a significant response or stable disease without significant adverse events will then be blindly randomized to either continue or discontinue the experimental treatment (see Figure 4-4) (Stadler, 2009).

Adaptive Design

An adaptive design creates an opportunity to make changes to the design of the clinical trial after seeing the data without compromising the integrity and validity of the trial. These planned prospective changes include modifying
- Eligibility criteria for new patients or subset of already enrolled patients
- Randomization procedures
- Treatment dose levels or dosing schedules
- Sample size
- Primary or secondary objectives
- Analytic methods.

One type of adaptive design is continual reassessment, also referred to as Bayesian adaptive design. Initially, this design used a mathematical model to determine an individual patient's dose level based on toxicities experienced by patients treated with prior dose levels. Interest is increasing in using adaptive designs in drug development that may lead to more efficient trials that improve the understating of treatment effects (Ivy, Siu, Garrett-Mayer, & Rubinstein, 2010; Shaw, Johnson, & Proschan, 2012; U.S. Food and Drug Administration [FDA], 2010).

Basket Trials

The ability to classify tumors based on genetic and genomic alterations in addition to tumor histology has resulted in a new type of trial: the basket trial. A basket trial tests the effect of a targeted agent (i.e., drug or biologic) on the same genetic/genomic alteration across multiple types of cancer. This is different than the traditional study design where one or more agents are used to assess the effect on one tumor type. In a sense, basket trials are multiple parallel phase II trials conducted using one clinical trial protocol. Basket trial designs are evolving. As with other adaptive designs, the goal of basket trials is to more efficiently develop targeted agents (Menis, Hasan, & Besse, 2014; Redig & Jänne, 2015). According to Willyard (2013), basket trials "may be particularly useful when the cancer type or the mutation is rare" (p. 655), but he cautioned that grouping patients based on genomic profiling may be burdensome and not completely address disease management needs.

Phases of Clinical Trials

Clinical trials, specifically trials for drug or biologic development, occur in phases (see Table 4-4). Many of these trials are conducted under an investigational new drug application (IND) (see Chapter 2). For the purposes of the chapter, drugs and biologics will both be referred to as drugs. It is important for the CTN to have a basic understanding of these phases, including goals, design, subject selection, endpoints, and limitations.

Phase 0

Phase 0 clinical trials, also called first-in-human trials, are typically conducted under an exploratory IND before phase I studies. They are the result of the FDA 2004 white paper titled *Challenge and Opportunity on the Critical Path to New Medical Products,* which looked at bringing drugs to the market faster while continuing to ensure safety and efficacy. The three types of phase 0 studies are (Takimoto, 2009)

- Pharmacokinetic (PK) or imaging studies where microdoses of an investigational agent are given to evaluate biodistribution or to evaluate through imaging if the agent reached the targeted cells (e.g., cancer cell)
- PK-relevant dosing studies to look at bioavailability but not to determine the maximum tolerated dose (MTD)
- Pharmacodynamic (PD) endpoint studies to see if and how the body is altered by the agent.

Goals

Phase 0 studies have many goals, including but not limited to determining relevant dose ranges and

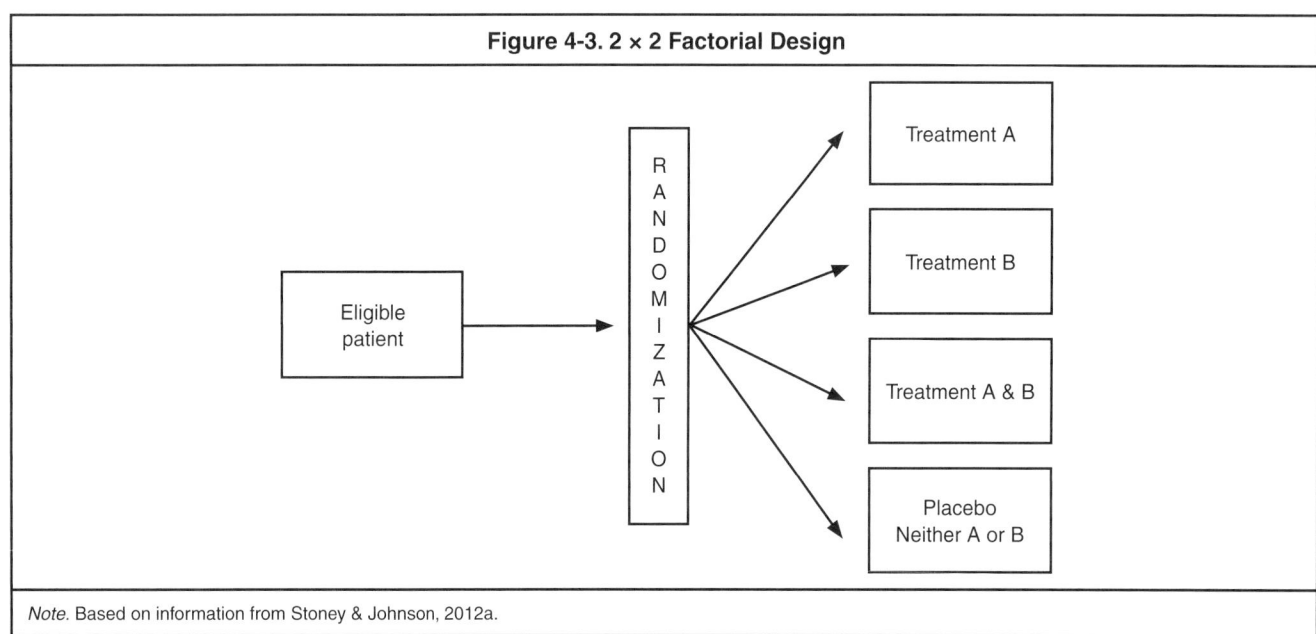

Figure 4-3. 2 × 2 Factorial Design

Note. Based on information from Stoney & Johnson, 2012a.

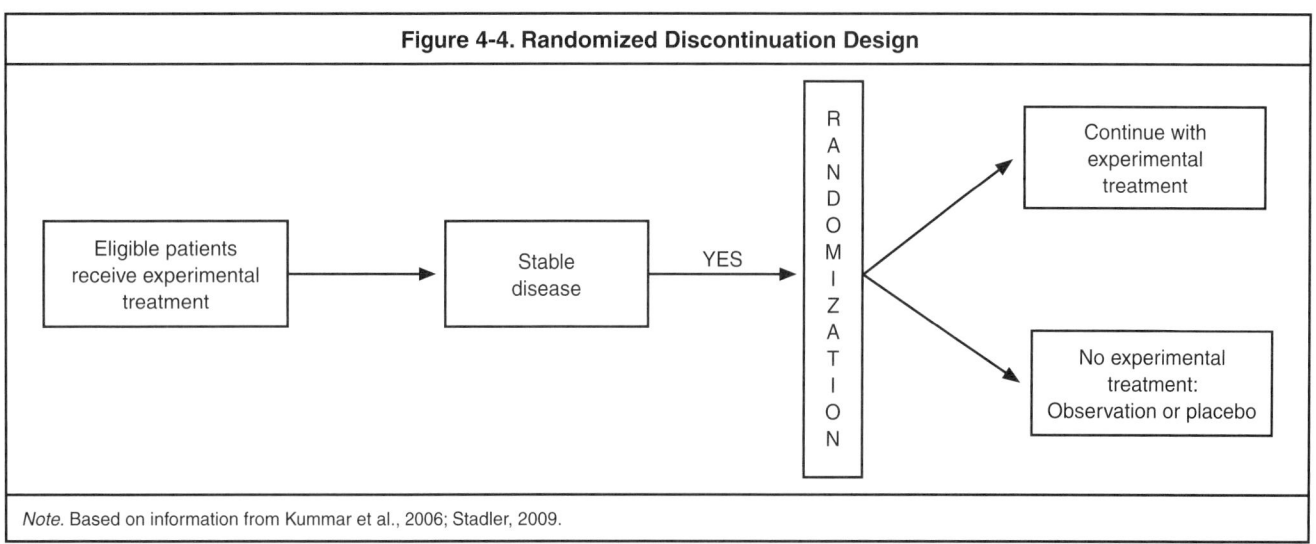

Figure 4-4. Randomized Discontinuation Design

Note. Based on information from Kummar et al., 2006; Stadler, 2009.

Table 4-4. Overview of Phase 0–IV Clinical Trials

Phase	Description	Goals	Subjects	Study Design
0	Exploratory study using small doses of investigational agent (i.e., microdosing for a drug or biologic) Very limited drug exposure with limited duration of dosing (approximately 7 days or less) No therapeutic (or diagnostic) intent	Provide human pharmacokinetic (PK)/ pharmacodynamic (PD) data prior to definitive phase I–II testing Determine whether mechanism of action defined in preclinical models can be observed in humans Refine biomarker assay using human tumor tissue and/or surrogate tissue Enhance efficiency and increase chance of success of subsequent development of the agent	Limited number of participants (about 10–15)	Dose escalation Open label Nonrandomized
I	Traditional first-in-human dose-finding study for a single agent Dose-finding study when using multiple agents or multiple interventions (e.g., drug + radiation)	Evaluate the safety and tolerability Determine the maximum tolerated dose (MTD): • Single agent • Combination of agents • Combination of interventions Determine dose-limiting toxicity (DLT) Define optimal biologically active dose Evaluate PK/PD Observe preliminary response (e.g., antitumor activity)	Limited number of subjects (20–100) Healthy volunteer Patient volunteer Usually many cancer types (e.g., solid tumors) Refractory to standard therapy or no remaining standard therapy Adequate organ function (e.g., bone marrow, liver, kidney) Pediatric studies conducted after safety and toxicity evaluation in adults	Dose escalation • Traditional 3 + 3 • Accelerated titration • Adaptive Open label Randomized (healthy volunteer) Nonrandomized (patient volunteer)
II	Phase IIA: Proof of concept study to provide initial information on activity of intervention to justify conducting a larger study Phase IIB: Optimal dosing study to target population	Phase IIA • Demonstrate activity of the intervention in the intended patient condition/ targeted population • Establish proof of concept Phase IIB • Establish optimal dosing for the intended patient condition/ targeted population to be used in phase III study Evaluate for safety	Moderate number of subjects (80–300) More homogenous population that is deemed likely to respond based on • Phase I data • Preclinical models and/or mechanisms of action Subject needs to have disease that can be accurately reproduced and measured May limit number of prior treatments	Open label or blinded Nonrandomized or randomized One-stage, two-stage, or crossover Nonstratified or stratified
III	Randomized controlled study	Compare efficacy of intervention being studied to a control group Evaluate for safety	Large number of subjects (hundreds to thousands) Homogenous population May be used for initial treatment	Open label or blinded Randomized Nonstratified or stratified Multi-institution/ multisite
IV	Postmarketing studies	Evaluate safety during postmarketing period May be initiated voluntarily or required by the U.S. Food and Drug Administration Compare the drug to another similar product that is already being marketed Monitor for long-term and additional safety, efficacy, and quality-of-life data Assess drug-food interactions Assess effect in specific populations (e.g., pregnant women, children), or determine cost-effectiveness	Large number of subjects with the labeled indication of the newly marketed drug/biologic	Open label Multi-institution/ multisite

Note. Based on information from Doroshow & Kummar, 2009; Kummar et al., 2006; Lertora & Vanevski, 2012.

sequence of administration of biomodulators, developing model imaging probes, and selecting the most promising candidate drugs for further development (Doroshow & Kummar, 2009; Kummar & Doroshow, 2011; Lertora & Vanevski, 2012) (see Table 4-4). Drugs must have a wide therapeutic index, the target must be known, and a valid assay must exist or be developed during the course of the study (Rowan, 2009). Patients have limited drug exposure (usually one dose) and duration of dosing (less than seven days), and doses should be nontoxic. With phase 0 studies, there is no *therapeutic intent*, which means no therapeutic benefit to the patient, which needs to be clearly stated in the informed consent document. Phase 0 studies may accelerate clinical testing of experimental drugs (Doroshow & Kummar, 2009; Takimoto, 2009).

Design

Rubenstein et al. (2010) recommend three trial designs for phase 0 studies based on 80%, 60%, or 40% PD response rate per dose level. For an 80% response rate, a one-stage design is used with three patients per dose level, needing two of the three to have a PD response to increase to the next dose level. A two-stage design is used for both 60% and 40% response rates. Five patients are enrolled to determine the 60% PD response rate, and eight patients are enrolled to determine the 40% response rate. All designs incorporate PK and/or PD sampling and use varying microdose levels depending upon the primary objective of the study.

Subjects

A limited number of participants are enrolled in phase 0 studies, approximately 10–15 total patients (Kummar et al., 2009).

Endpoints

Phase 0 endpoints include PK or PD data, or the drug's ability to reach its target (Rowan, 2010). This means that serial blood draws would occur around drug dosing and, for PD, patients would undergo tumor biopsies before and after drug dosing.

Benefits and Limitations

Benefits of phase 0 studies include enrollment of smaller numbers of patients, reduced initial pharmacologic and toxicology testing requirements, lower overall costs of drug development, quicker comparison of potential new drugs, and streamlined design for phase I trials (Eliopoulos et al., 2008). Limitations include the fact that microdosing does not always predict drug behavior or safety, and phase 0 studies are not expected to replace phase I studies (Eliopoulos et al., 2008; Takimoto, 2009). Another consideration is that if the target is incorrectly identified, an effective drug may not be recognized. An additional limitation is *therapeutic misconception*, where patients may think that they will benefit from the treatment, even when the goal of phase 0 studies does not include therapeutic benefit (Rowan, 2010).

Phase I

Phase I clinical trials are also referred to as first-in-human studies, especially when no phase 0 clinical trial preceded it (see Table 4-4). These trials can be conducted in patient volunteers (i.e., individuals with cancer) or healthy volunteers. A healthy volunteer is someone who consents to participate in a clinical trial and whose physiologic parameters and laboratory assessments are within the normal range. For most cancer drugs, patient volunteers are used, although the use of healthy volunteers in oncology targeted therapy drug development has gained support recently (Iwamoto, Iannone, & Wagner, 2012).

Goals

The goals for phase I studies are to determine the MTD for an investigational agent, assess safety, evaluate PK and PD, and explore drug metabolism and drug interactions (Gupta et al., 2012; LoRusso, Boerner, & Seymour, 2010; Yuan & Yin, 2011) (see Table 4-4). Phase I studies may be used to evaluate new treatment schedules, new drug combination strategies using IND agents or commercial drugs, and new multimodality regimens (e.g., IND agent and concurrent radiation therapy). They may provide early evidence of response, but this is not the primary aim. For molecular-targeted agents, clinical activity and target modulation are the endpoints; therefore, determining the biologically active dose is the goal, not the MTD (LoRusso et al., 2010). In healthy volunteer trials, the goals include assessing drug interactions, determining food effect, understanding safety parameters for specific populations such as the elderly, or evaluating the QT interval (Iwamoto et al., 2012).

Design

The two types of designs used for phase I studies are rule-based and model-based. *Rule-based designs* allow dose escalation and de-escalation based on toxicities. Patients are assigned to dose levels based on observations from clinical data.

Model-based designs assign patients to dose levels and define phase II doses based on target toxicity (Le Tourneau, Lee, & Siu, 2009). The standard design for a phase I study is an open label, nonrandomized dose escalation design. The 3 + 3 design is the most widely-based design in use (see Figure 4-5). Patients receive a low starting dose, typically based on one-tenth of the lethal dose, the dose at which 10% of the animals die, using the most sensitive species of animals tested or defaulting to the mouse model (if equivalent). Usually three to six patients are entered onto a dose level or cohort, and the dose is increased gradually until a predetermined (i.e., stated in the protocol) dose-limiting toxicity (DLT) occurs in any dose level. With a 3 + 3

Chapter 4. Types of Clinical Research: Experimental   31

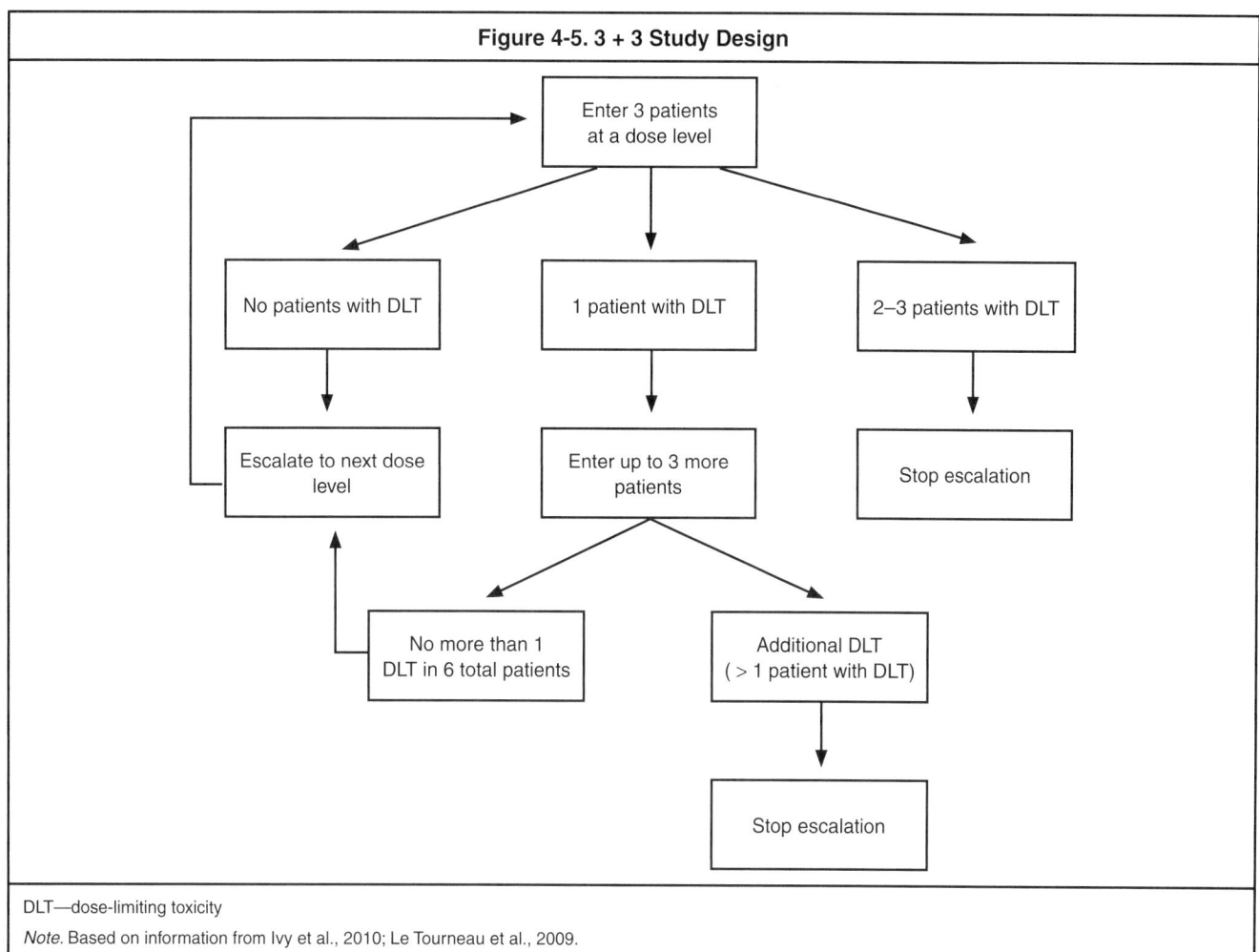

Figure 4-5. 3 + 3 Study Design

DLT—dose-limiting toxicity
Note. Based on information from Ivy et al., 2010; Le Tourneau et al., 2009.

design, three patients receive dose level 1. If none of the patients develop a DLT, three patients are then enrolled at dose level 2. If one patient in dose level 1 or subsequent dose level develops a DLT, then up to three additional patients receive that same dose. Dose escalation continues until the MTD is achieved, which is defined as the dose at which 0–1 patients experience a DLT. Dose escalation is based on a Classic Modified Fibonacci Dose Escalation Scheme (see Table 4-5) (Ivy et al., 2010). CTNs who coordinate phase I trials need to pay particular attention to the protocol to ensure they understand the definitions for DLT and MTD based on the protocol. Pediatric phase I clinical trials do not start until the adult studies are completed. Typically, the pediatric starting dose will be 80% of the adult MTD (Lee, Skolnik, & Adamson, 2005).

Several alternative designs may be used in phase I clinical trials, including accelerated titration design (ATD) and intrapatient dose escalation. In ATD, one patient is enrolled per dose level with dose levels increasing by 100% until a grade 2 Common Terminology Criteria for Adverse Events (CTCAE) toxicity occurs, and then the design returns to the 3 + 3 design.

The two types of *intrapatient escalation studies* are (a) patients can be escalated to a higher dose once the current dose level has been proven "safe" (i.e., without DLT) or (b) the patient can be used as the control and can be escalated to a higher dose level if the lower dose was tolerated without DLT (Ivy et al., 2010). Not all studies will use toxicity as an endpoint. Studies that are used to find the dose that is considered to be safe and have optimal biologic or immunologic effect (e.g., showing inhibi-

Table 4-5. Classic Modified Fibonacci Dose Escalation Scheme

Dose Level	Increase Above Preceding Dose
1	Starting dose
2	100% increase from level 1
3	67% increase from level 2
4	50% increase from level 3
5	40% increase from level 4
6+	30%–35% increase from level 5+

Note. Based on information from Le Tourneau et al., 2009.

tion of the target) are referred to as using the biologically active dose or optimal biologic dose. This dose is associated with an inhibition or prespecified amount of a biomarker that is needed to inhibit a target (Ivy et al., 2010; Le Tourneau et al., 2009).

Phase I healthy volunteer trials use a variety of randomized designs with or without blinding and a placebo group. Dosing can be either a single dose per volunteer with increasing dose levels (single ascending dose) or with the volunteer receiving multiple doses (multiple ascending dose) (Buoen, Bjerrum, & Thomsen, 2005).

Subjects

Phase I studies are conducted on small numbers of participants (20–100). Research participants may have advanced cancer with few, if any, options for treatment and a low prospect of personal benefit. This is an opportunity to receive intervention and may pose more than minimal risk. Eligibility usually requires good performance status, adequate organ function, and absence of concomitant medical illnesses that could confound interpretation of adverse events or place patients at unacceptable risk (Kummar, Gutierrez, Doroshow, & Murgo, 2006).

Healthy volunteers can provide data around safety, PK/PD, and drug interactions for molecular-targeted agents. Healthy volunteers must be illness-free, and the intervention should be considered no more than minimal risk (see Chapter 40 for more on risk assessment). There is no anticipated personal benefit, and the subject may receive monetary compensation.

Endpoints

Endpoints for phase I cytotoxic agents include DLT and MTD. DLT is determined using the CTCAE. Endpoints for biologics include plasma drug concentrations and target inhibition in tumor tissue (Le Tourneau et al., 2009). Additional endpoints include having specifics assays to measure PK and PD. The protocol should clearly describe how these endpoints will be measured and how biospecimens are to be handled.

Limitations

Limitations of phase I studies include potential risks without benefits; initial patients may be treated at low doses; slow accrual to complete trial; toxicities may be influenced by extensive prior therapy; minimal data about cumulative toxicity, imprecise definition of MTD; and interpatient variability.

Phase II

Goals

Phase II studies further define safety and toxicity, provide an initial assessment of efficacy or clinical activity, screen out ineffective drugs, and identify promising new drugs for additional evaluation. Phase II studies may be divided into two more phases: Phase IIA explores *proof of concept* and evaluates if the drug has any activity against the disease or condition under study, and phase IIB establishes optimal doses for phase III studies (Lertora & Vanevsky, 2012) (see Table 4-4).

Design

The most common design for a phase II study is the two-stage design with an early stopping rule for lack of activity or response to therapy. If the drug shows significant activity in the first stage of the study, the study will proceed to the second stage (Ratain & Sargent, 2009). The National Cancer Institute Clinical Trial Design Task Force recommends that the design of a study should be based on the endpoints of the study (Seymour et al., 2010). Single-arm designs with randomization may be used for single agents to assess tumor response. For combination therapy, randomization should be considered (e.g., blinded designs or placebo-controlled trials). For progression-free survival endpoints, randomization is required. Crossover designs may be used to increase patient access to investigational agents. Adaptive designs may be used to modify enrollment for predictive biomarkers (Seymour et al., 2010).

Subjects

Phase II studies require 80–300 subjects. Subjects may need to have measureable disease and a limited number of prior treatments. Subjects are a more homogenous population, selected based on phase I data, the preclinical model, animal model activity or response, or the mechanism of action for the drug or drugs being studied.

Endpoints

Phase II endpoints include response and additional safety data. Response-based endpoints are used if measuring tumor activity. Secondary endpoints include tumor markers, novel imaging, and molecular biomarkers and patient-reported outcomes. Imaging tools, such as positron-emission tomography, digital contrast-enhanced magnetic resonance imaging, and magnetic resonance spectroscopy, should be used to measure response rates for novel agents. Biomarker assays should be measured for drug activity if a strong correlation exists between assay results and clinical correlations (Adjei, Christian, & Ivy, 2009). Chapter 15 highlights the various endpoints (e.g., progression-free survival, objective response) and the measurement tools used in oncology clinical trials.

Limitations

Phase II studies are not without limitations. Because measurement of the disease is crucial, patients with unmeasurable disease (e.g., bone lesions, malignant ascites) may not be eligible. A lack of activity may not be valid and prematurely stop a drug or intervention from further development. Barriers to participation in phase II trials may include poorly designed trials, lack of insurance coverage, and regulatory policies (Adjei et al., 2009).

Phase III

Phase III clinical trials proceed once phase II studies have demonstrated activity in a specific disease or condition.

Goals

The goals of phase III studies include assessing the efficacy of the drug or new intervention compared to standard therapy and providing further evaluation of safety. Dosing ranges are assessed for safety in multiple patients as well as in special populations (e.g., children, patients with impaired renal or hepatic function) (Lertora & Vanevski, 2012).

Design

Phase III trial designs are randomized using a control group or groups. Investigators may employ blinding and further stratification in the protocol (Lertora & Vanevski, 2012).

Subjects

Phase III studies incorporate hundreds to thousands of subjects. The study is usually conducted on a single cancer type with well-defined eligibility criteria and may be used as frontline therapy. Because of the large number of subjects, phase III trials require multi-institutional participation to reach targeted accrual goals.

Endpoints

Endpoints for phase III trials include efficacy, overall survival, disease-free survival, symptom control, and quality of life (see Chapter 15).

Limitations

Limitations of phase III studies include the large number of patients required, the study complexity, the expense to conduct it, and the slow integration of results into frontline therapies.

Phase IV

Phase IV clinical trials, also referred to as postmarketing surveillance trials, are conducted after the drug has been approved for commercial marketing. These studies are conducted for a variety of reasons, including to compare the drug to another similar product that is already being marketed; monitor for long-term and additional safety, efficacy, and quality-of-life effects; assess drug-food interactions; assess effect in specific populations (e.g., pregnant women, children); and determine cost-effectiveness. Postmarketing studies may be voluntary (i.e., pharmaceutical company decides to conduct) or required (i.e., FDA-mandated as part of drug approval) and can be either observational or experimental ("FDA Drugs for Human Use Investigational New Drug Application," 2013).

Summary

There are many concepts related to experimental studies that the CTN will need to understand. Once proficient in these concepts and the basic goals, objectives, and study designs associated with phase 0–IV clinical trials, the CTN will find that core responsibilities will be easier, including understanding study requirements, study coordination, case report form development, the informed consent process, and staff and patient education.

Key Points

- A basic understanding of clinical trials involves an understanding of key concepts and terminology related to trial design.
- Randomization and blinding/masking are techniques to help minimize investigator bias.
- It is important for the CTN to understand the randomization and blinding process for a clinical trial before enrolling a patient, including what situations would trigger unblinding and the procedure for unblinding.
- With understanding of the rationale for randomization and blinding and its use to answer specific scientific study questions, the patient may be less likely to withdraw from participation.
- Many clinical trials are conducted in phases: 0, I, II, III, and IV. Once proficient in understanding the basic goals, objectives, and study designs associated with each phase, the CTN will find that core responsibilities will be easier.

References

Adjei, A., Christian, M., & Ivy, P. (2009). Novel designs and end points for phase II clinical trials. *Clinical Cancer Research, 15*, 1866–1872. doi:10.1158/1078-0432.CCR-08-2035

Buoen, C., Bjerrum, O.J., & Thomsen, M.S. (2005). How first-time-in-human studies are being performed: A survey of phase I dose-escalation trials in healthy volunteers published between 1995 and 2004. *Journal of Clinical Pharmacology, 45*, 1123–1136. doi:10.1177/0091270005279943

Doroshow, J.H., & Kummar, S. (2009). Role of phase 0 trials in drug development. *Future Medicinal Chemistry, 1*, 1375–1380. doi:10.4155/fmc.09.117

Eliopoulos, H., Giranda, V., Carr, R., Tiehen, R., Leahy, T., & Gordon, G. (2008). Phase 0 trials: An industry perspective. *Clinical Cancer Research, 14*, 3683–3688. doi:10.1158/1078-0432.CCR-07-4586

FDA Drugs for Human Use Investigational New Drug Application, 21 pt. C.F.R. 312 (2013). Retrieved from http://www.accessdata

.fda.gov/scripts/cdrh/cfdocs/cfcfr/CFRSearch.cfm?CFRPart=312&showFR=1

Gupta, S., Hunsberger, S., Boerner, S.A., Rubinstein, L., Royds, R., Ivy, P., & LoRusso, P. (2012). Meta-analysis of the relationship between dose and benefit in phase I targeted agent trials. *Journal of the National Cancer Institute, 104,* 1860–1866. doi:10.1093/jnci/djs439

International Conference on Harmonisation of Technical Requirements for Registration of Pharmaceuticals for Human Use. (2000, July 20). *ICH harmonised tripartite guideline: Choice of control group and related issues in clinical trials, E10.* Retrieved from http://www.ich.org/fileadmin/Public_Web_Site/ICH_Products/Guidelines/Efficacy/E10/Step4/E10_Guideline.pdf

Ivy, S.P., Siu, L.L., Garrett-Mayer, E., & Rubinstein, L. (2010). Approaches to phase I clinical trial design focused on safety, efficacy, and selected patient populations: A report from the Clinical Trial Design Task Force of the National Cancer Institute Investigational Drug Steering Committee. *Clinical Cancer Research, 16,* 1726–1736. doi:10.1158/1078-0432.CCR-09-1961

Iwamoto, M., Iannone, R., & Wagner, J.A. (2012). Use of healthy volunteers drives clinical oncology drug development decision making. *Clinical Pharmacology and Therapeutics, 92,* 571–574. doi:10.1038/clpt.2012.157

Kummar, S., & Doroshow, J. (2011). Phase 0 trials: Expediting the development of chemoprevention agents. *Cancer Prevention Research, 4,* 288–292. doi:10.1158/1940-6207.CAPR-11-0013

Kummar, S., Doroshow, J.H., Tomaszewski, J.E., Calvert, A.H., Lobbezoo, M., & Giaccone, G. (2009). Phase 0 clinical trials: Recommendations from the task force on methodology for the development of innovative cancer therapies. *European Journal of Cancer, 45,* 741–746. doi:10.1016/j.ejca.2008.10.024

Kummar, S., Gutierrez, M., Doroshow, J., & Murgo, A. (2006). Drug development in oncology: Classical cytotoxics and molecularly targeted agents. *British Journal of Clinical Pharmacology, 62,* 15–26. doi:10.1111/j.1365-2125.2006.02713.x

Lee, D.P., Skolnik, J.M., & Adamson, P.C. (2005). Pediatric phase I trials in oncology: An analysis of study conduct efficiency. *Journal of Clinical Oncology, 23,* 8431–8441. doi:10.1200/JCO.2005.02.1568

Lertora, J.J.L., & Vanevski, K.M. (2012). Clinical pharmacology and its role in pharmaceutical development. In J.I. Gallin & F.P. Ognibene (Eds.), *Principles and practice of clinical research* (3rd ed., pp. 627–639). doi:10.1016/B978-0-12-382167-6.00043-6

Le Tourneau, C., Lee, J.J., & Siu, L.L. (2009). Dose escalation methods in phase I cancer clinical trials. *Journal of the National Cancer Institute, 101,* 708–720. doi:10.1093/jnci/djp079

LoRusso, P., Boerner, S., & Seymour, L. (2010). An overview of the optimal planning, design, and conduct of phase I studies of new therapeutics. *Clinical Cancer Research, 16,* 1710–1718. doi:10.1158/1078-0432.CCR-09-1993

Menis, J., Hasan, B., & Besse, B. (2014). New clinical research strategies in thoracic oncology: Clinical trial design, adaptive, basket and umbrella trials, new end-points and new evaluations of response. *European Respiratory Review, 23,* 367–378. doi:10.1183/09059180.00004214

Miller, L.E., & Stewart, M.E. (2011). The blind leading the blind: Use and misuse of blinding in randomized controlled trials. *Contemporary Clinical Trials, 32,* 240–243. doi:10.1016/j.cct.2010.11.004

National Institutes of Health. (2012, August). Glossary of common site terms. Retrieved from http://clinicaltrials.gov/ct2/about-studies/glossary#wrapper

Ratain, M.J., & Sargent, D.J. (2009). Optimising the design of phase II oncology trials: The importance of randomisation. *European Journal of Cancer, 45,* 275–280. doi:10.1016/j.ejca.2008.10.029

Redig, A.J., & Jänne, P.A. (2015). Basket trials and the evolution of clinical trial design in an era of genomic medicine. *Journal of Clinical Oncology, 33,* 975–977. doi:10.1200/JCO.2014.59.8433

Rowan, K. (2009). Oncology's first phase I trial. *Journal of the National Cancer Institute, 101,* 978–979. doi:10.1093/jnci/djp213

Rubinstein, L.V., Steinberg, S.M., Kummar, S., Kinders, R., Parchment, R.E., Murgo, A.J., ... Doroshow, J.H. (2010). The statistics of phase 0 trials. *Statistics in Medicine, 29,* 1072–1076. doi:10.1002/sim.3840

Seymour, L., Ivy, S.P., Sargent, D., Spriggs, D., Baker, L., Rubinstein, L., ... Berry, D. (2010). The design of phase II clinical trials testing cancer therapeutics: Consensus recommendations from the Clinical Trial Design Task Force of the National Cancer Institute Investigational Drug Steering Committee. *Clinical Cancer Research, 16,* 1764–1769. doi:10.1158/1078-0432.CCR-09-3287

Shaw, P.A., Johnson, L.L., & Borkowf, C.B. (2012). Issues with randomization. In J.I. Gallin & F.P. Ognibene (Eds.), *Principles and practice of clinical research* (3rd ed., pp. 243–253). doi:10.1016/B978-0-12-382167-6.00020-5

Shaw, P.A., Johnson, L.L., & Proschan, M.A. (2012). Intermediate topics in biostatistics. In J.I. Gallin & F.P. Ognibene (Eds.), *Principles and practice of clinical research* (3rd ed., pp. 295–320). doi:10.1016/B978-0-12-382167-6.00024-2

Stadler, W. (2009). Other paradigms: Randomized discontinuation trial design. *Cancer Journal, 15,* 431–434. doi:10.1097/PPO.0b013e3181bd0431

Stoney, C.M., & Johnson, L.L. (2012a). Design of clinical studies and trials. In J.I. Gallin & F.P. Ognibene (Eds.), *Principles and practice of clinical research* (3rd ed., pp. 225–242). doi:10.1016/B978-0-12-382167-6.00019-9

Stoney, C.M., & Johnson, L.L. (2012b). Development and conduct of studies. In J.I. Gallin & F.P. Ognibene (Eds.), *Principles and practice of clinical research* (3rd ed., pp. 381–394). doi:10.1016/B978-0-12-382167-6.00029-1

Takimoto, C. (2009). Phase 0 clinical trials in oncology: A paradigm shift for early drug development? *Cancer Chemotherapy and Pharmacology, 63,* 703–709. doi:10.1007/s00280-008-0789-4

U.S. Food and Drug Administration. (2004, March). *Challenge and opportunity on the critical path to new medical products.* Retrieved from http://www.fda.gov/downloads/ScienceResearch/SpecialTopics/CriticalPathInitiative/CriticalPathOpportunitiesReports/ucm113411.pdf

U.S. Food and Drug Administration. (2010, February). *Guidance for industry adaptive design clinical trials for drugs and biologics draft guidance.* Retrieved from http://www.fda.gov/downloads/Drugs/.../Guidances/ucm201790.pdf

Willyard, C. (2013). 'Basket studies' will hold intricate data for cancer drug approvals. *Nature Medicine, 19,* 655. doi:10.1038/nm0613-655

Yuan, Y., & Yin, G. (2011). Bayesian phase I/II adaptively randomized oncology trials with combined drugs. *Annals of Applied Statistics, 5,* 924–942. doi:10.1214/10-dAOAS433

Chapter 5

Types of Clinical Research: Observational

Geri L. Schmotzer, RN, MSN, MPH, PhD

Introduction

Observational research includes several study designs in which populations are observed within clinical practices or community settings. These study types are significant in healthcare research because they offer additional methods to answering important research questions (Yang et al., 2010).

Observational studies are a start to the process of confirming that something believed to be true may have some objective data to indicate that it actually may be true. Observational studies provide data, which then aid the investigator with developing future theories and ideas for possible interventions that can be studied in forthcoming research (Hannan, 2008; Yang et al., 2010).

In an observational study, the investigator assesses health outcomes or conditions in participants according to a protocol or research plan. Participants may receive an intervention, which may include drugs, devices, or procedures as part of their routine medical care, but the participants are not assigned to a specific intervention by the investigator as in a clinical trial. For instance, researchers may observe a group of older adults to learn more about the influences of lifestyles on cardiac health (Yang et al., 2010).

The common types of study design that fall within the category of observational research include (Hulley, Cummings, Browner, Grady, & Newman, 2007; Ligthelm et al., 2007; Noordzij, Dekker, Zoccali, & Jager, 2009; Stewart, 2004)
- Case report and case series studies
- Cross-section descriptive and analytical studies
- Case-control studies
- Cohort studies, prospective and retrospective
- Outcome studies.

Table 5-1 indicates study characteristics, strengths, and weaknesses. The purpose of observational studies is to establish one of the following: incidence, prevalence, cause, association, or outcomes (Mann, 2003). Table 5-2 displays the objective and type of study.

Study Types

Case Report/Case Series Studies

A *case report* is a type of observational study where a single individual (case report) or small group (case series) is explored to determine the likelihood of an association between an observed effect and a specific event, such as an environmental exposure. Findings are based on a comprehensive clinical evaluation and history of the individual or individuals. This type of study is usually conducted when the disease is uncommon and caused entirely or almost entirely by a single kind of exposure. Case report or case series studies may be the first to provide a clue in detecting a new disease or adverse health effect from an exposure (Castillo, Scharfstein, & MacKenzie, 2012; Hess, 2004; Noordzij et al., 2009). An example of a case report is Rosenfeld and Bronson's (1980) discovery of a relationship between diethylstilbestrol (DES) and reproductive difficulties in females who were exposed to DES in utero.

Cross-Sectional Studies

A *cross-sectional* study is a descriptive study where the disease or condition of interest and exposure are measured at the same time in a given population. Simply, the goal of this type of study is to describe the association between a disease or another health-related condition and other characteristics as they exist in a specific group at a certain point in time, without regard for what may have preceded the health status found in the

Table 5-1. Purpose, Characteristics, Strengths, and Weaknesses of Observational Studies				
Study Design	Purpose	Characteristics	Strengths	Weaknesses
Case report/ case series	Determine an association between an event and an effect	One or a few subjects Detailed description of a case(s) without a control group	First form of publication Fast, inexpensive Hypothesis-generating	Very limited potential to establish causal effects Selection bias*
Cross-sectional	Measure prevalence	Exposure and outcome measured at same point in time Subjects with and without outcome are compared	Useful to describe the prevalence of disease Fast, inexpensive Hypothesis-generating	Very limited potential to establish causal effects Selection bias* Survival bias*
Case-control	Identify risk factors	Cases (those with the outcome of interest) are compared with controls (those without the outcome of interest) with respect to exposure	Efficient Suitable to study rare outcomes and multiple exposures Relatively inexpensive Hypothesis-generating	Some potential to establish causal effects Can only study one outcome Choice of control group can be difficult Selection bias* Recall bias*
Cohort	Assess associations between exposure and outcomes	A cohort of subjects free of the outcome is followed and compared based on the exposure	Suitable to study multiple exposures, rare exposures, and multiple outcomes Hypothesis-generating High generalizability	Some potential to establish causal effects Can take a long period of time Can be expensive Selection bias*
Outcomes	Improve quality of care	Study of healthcare delivery	Provides better information to inform patient decisions Guides healthcare providers and informs policy decisions	Very limited potential to establish causal effects Selection bias* Recall bias*

* Each study design may suffer from specific types of bias.
Note. From "Study Designs in Clinical Research," by M. Noordzij, F.W. Dekker, C. Zoccali, and K.J. Jager, 2009, Nephron Clinical Practice, 113, p. c219. doi:10.1159/000235610. Copyright 2009 by Karger. Adapted with permission.

group at the time of the study. For this reason, cross-sectional studies can be thought of as providing a "snapshot in time." Because exposure and disease status are measured at the same point in time, it is not possible to distinguish whether the exposure preceded or followed the disease, and thus a causal relationship cannot be determined (Levin, 2006; Noordzij et al., 2009). Therefore, the main outcome measure obtained from a cross-sectional study is prevalence (Levin, 2006). An example of a cross-sectional study is the National Health Interview Survey (Centers for Disease Control and Prevention, 2013).

The two types of cross-sectional studies are *descriptive* and *analytical*. A descriptive cross-sectional study describes what occurs in a specific group but does not try to quantify what occurs. It is used to assess the prevalence of a disease or health condition in a specific population (Donovan, McDowell, & Hunter, 2007). An example of a descriptive study is one that would look at the prevalence of certain health behaviors in cancer survivors (Bellizzi, Rowland, Jeffery, & McNeel, 2005). Analytical cross-sectional studies attempt to quantify the relationship between two factors, such as an exposure and a health outcome. They are normally used to test a hypothesis (Donovan et al., 2007).

One of the most common cross-sectional analytical studies is the *survey*, in which a random sample is drawn to give an accurate representation of the population. It is similar to a descriptive survey except that the purpose

Table 5-2. Observational Study Purpose and Design	
Objective	Common Design
Prevalence	Cross-sectional
Incidence	Cohort
Cause	Cohort, case-control, case report/case series
Association	Cross-sectional, cohort
Outcomes	Outcomes

Note. From "Observational Research Methods. Research Design II: Cohort, Cross Sectional, and Case-Control Studies," by C.J. Mann, 2003, Emergency Medicine Journal, 20, p. 54. doi:10.1136/emj.20.1.54. Copyright 2003 by BMJ Publishing Group. Adapted with permission.

of the analysis is to record associations between variables rather than merely to report frequencies of their occurrence. An example of an analytic cross-sectional study is shown in the study by Polonijo and Carpiano (2013), where the researchers analyzed results from the 2008, 2009, and 2010 U.S. National Immunization Survey–Teen to test whether the odds of receiving a human papillomavirus vaccine recommendation from a healthcare provider were associated with low socioeconomic status.

Case-Control Studies

A *case-control* study is a type of retrospective study in which an investigator compares a group of subjects with a disease or condition to a group of similar subjects who do not have the disease or condition. The investigator looks back to compare how frequently the exposure to a risk factor is present in each group. The purpose of this type of study is to determine if a relationship exists between the risk factor and the disease (Castillo et al., 2012; Hess, 2004; Noordzij et al., 2009). An example of a case-control study is Wynder and Graham's (1950) determination that cigarette smoking caused lung cancer.

Cohort Studies

A *cohort* study is one in which observations of a group of subjects are made over a period of time. A key point of cohort studies is that the study participants are identified at the starting point of the study, and then their exposure to risk is assessed either in the past or the future. Figure 5-1 denotes study types and the occurrence of time. The two types of cohort studies are *prospective* and *retrospective*. Prospective studies are when a group of subjects are selected in the present and followed into the future. Examples of prospective studies include the Framingham Heart Study and the Wom-

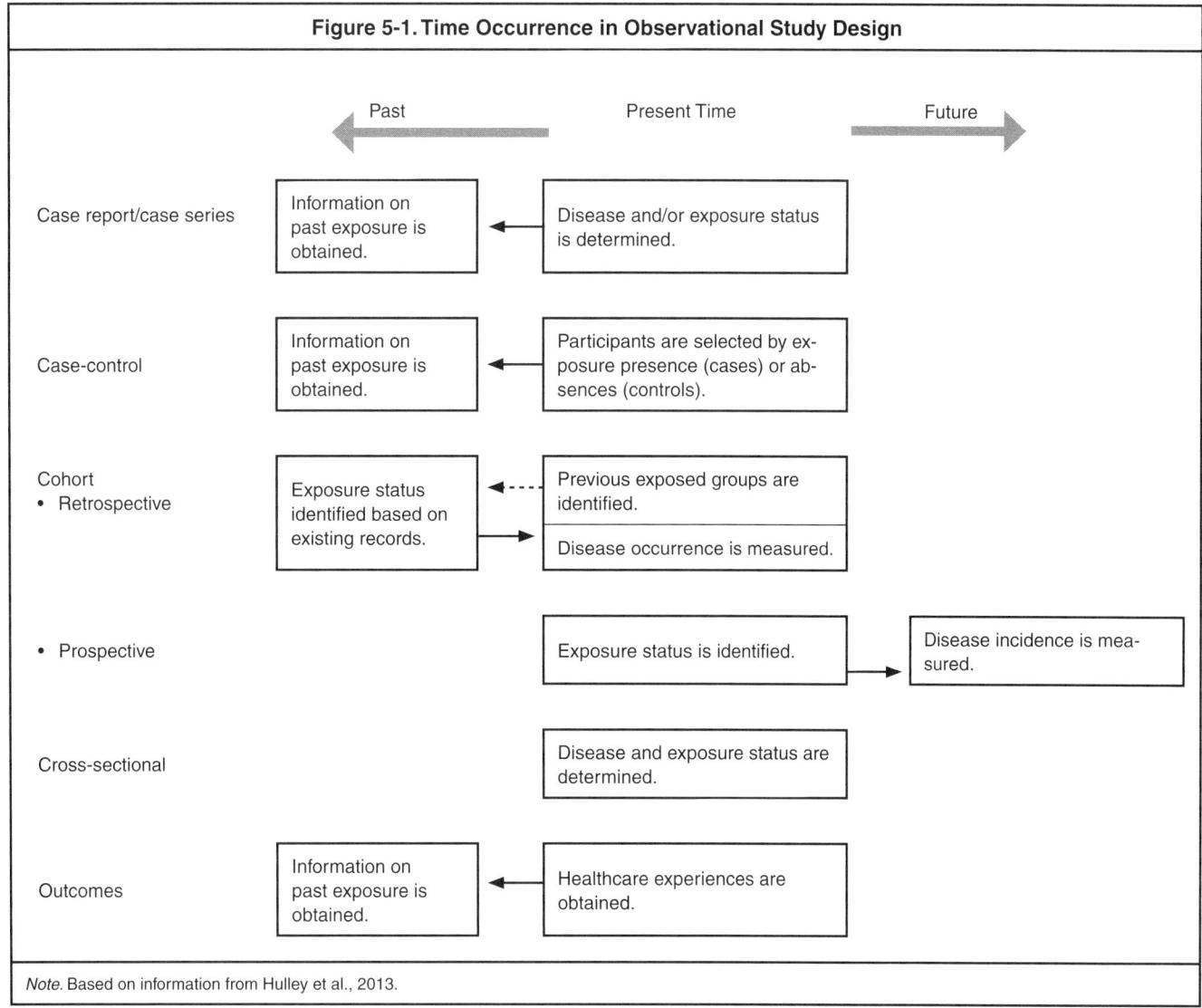

Figure 5-1. Time Occurrence in Observational Study Design

Note. Based on information from Hulley et al., 2013.

en's Health Initiative. A retrospective study examines information or specimens that were collected in the past (Hess, 2004). Cohort studies are done to assess associations between multiple exposures and multiple outcomes. These studies help to determine risk factors for diseases or conditions.

Outcomes Research

An *outcome study* explores the results of healthcare practices and interventions. Outcomes research consists of patient-based outcomes as well as the study of populations, databases, and the delivery of health care. Outcomes research differs from traditional clinical research where outcomes such as quality of life and cost-effectiveness are usually measured from the patient's perspective (Stewart, 2004). Results include issues that people experience and are concerned about, such as change in the ability to function or the cost-effectiveness of health care. By relating the care people receive to the results they experience, outcomes research has become a central method to developing better ways to monitor and improve the quality of care. Figure 5-2 lists the focus of outcomes research, whereas Figure 5-3 lists some suggested benefits of outcomes research.

Summary

Observational studies are conducted to observe groups to assess study participants' health status or con-

---

Figure 5-3. Suggested Benefits of Outcomes Research

Consumer
- Increased participation in decision making
- Increased choice regarding hospital/practitioner/treatment options
- Assurance regarding effectiveness of interventions
- Assessment and development of interventions to improve well-being, not just survival

Healthcare Provider
- Greater certainty regarding the benefit of an intervention
- Standards/guidelines to guide clinical practice
- Shared responsibility in decision making
- Protection from malpractice suits (if complying with above)

Healthcare Organization Management
- Greater use of effective interventions
- Discontinuation of ineffective interventions/practices
- An organizational culture emphasizing quality
- Cost savings as inappropriate use is eliminated (i.e., interventions, medications, hospitalizations)

Government
- Cost savings as inappropriate use is eliminated (i.e., interventions, medications, hospitalizations)
- Greater ability to plan health services
- Only effective pharmaceuticals and services are subsidized
- Target research in areas of greatest potential impact based on examination of databases, etc.

Note. From "Outcomes Research: What Is It and Why Does It Matter?" by M. Jefford, M.R. Stockler, and M.H.N. Tattersall, 2003, *Internal Medicine Journal, 33,* p. 113. doi:10.1046/j.1445-5994.2003.00302.x. Copyright 2003 by John Wiley & Sons. Reprinted with permission.

Figure 5-2. The Scope of Outcomes Research

Outcomes research may focus on:
- Quality-of-life measures
- Effectiveness
- Cost
- Quality of care
- Patient preferences
- Appropriateness
- Access
- Health status

In areas such as:
- Disease prevention
- Screening
- Drug treatment
- Medical procedures
- Medical practices
- Diagnostic tests
- Guidelines
- Healthcare policy

Note. From "Outcomes Research: What Is It and Why Does It Matter?" by M. Jefford, M.R. Stockler, and M.H.N. Tattersall, 2003, *Internal Medicine Journal, 33,* p. 112. doi:10.1046/j.1445-5994.2003.00302.x. Copyright 2003 by John Wiley & Sons. Reprinted with permission.

---

dition. The researcher selects what exposure to study, but does not influence them, and then notes who in the group develops the disease or condition of interest. Several study designs are considered observational research. Each design has its own purpose, characteristics, strengths, and weaknesses. No interventions are given to the study participants. Use of observation studies permits the investigation of incidence, prevalence, associations, causes, and outcomes.

Key Points
- Observational studies are a type of study in which individuals are observed and outcomes are measured. No attempt (e.g., treatment or intervention) is made to affect the outcome.
- Case series and case reports consist of collections of reports on the treatment of individual patients or a report on a single patient.
- Case-control studies are studies in which patients who already have a specific condition are compared with people who do not.
- Cohort studies take a large population and follow patients who have a specific condition or receive a particular treatment over time and compare them with another group that has not been affected by the condition or treatment being studied.

- Cross-sectional studies are when data are collected on the whole study population at a single point in time to examine the relationship between disease (or another health-related state) and other variables of interest.
- Outcomes research examines the end results of particular healthcare practices and interventions to monitor and improve the quality of health care.

References

Bellizzi, K.M., Rowland, J.H., Jeffery, D.D., & McNeel, T. (2005). Health behaviors of cancer survivors: Examining opportunities for cancer control intervention. *Journal of Clinical Oncology, 23*, 8884–8893. doi:10.1200/jco.2005.02.2343

Castillo, R.C., Scharfstein, D.O., & MacKenzie, E.J. (2012). Observational studies in the era of randomized trials: Finding the balance. *Journal of Bone and Joint Surgery, 94*(Suppl. 1), 112–117. doi:10.2106/jbjs.l.00242

Centers for Disease Control and Prevention. (2013). National Health Interview Survey. Retrieved from http://www.cdc.gov/nchs/nhis.htm

Donovan, D., McDowell, I., & Hunter, D. (Eds.). (2007). *AFMC primer on population health*. Retrieved from http://phprimer.afmc.ca/Part2-MethodsStudyingHealth/Chapter5AssessingEvidenceAndInformation/Observationalstudies

Hannan, E.L. (2008). Randomized clinical trials and observational studies: Guidelines for assessing respective strengths and limitations. *JACC: Cardiovascular Interventions, 1*, 211–217. doi:10.1016/j.jcin.2008.01.008

Hess, D.R. (2004). Retrospective studies and chart reviews. *Respiratory Care, 49*, 1171–1174. Retrieved from http://rc.rcjournal.com/content/49/10/1171.full.pdf+html

Hulley, S.B., Cummings, S.R., & Newman, T.B. (2007). Getting started: The anatomy and physiology of clinical research. In S.B. Hulley, S.R. Cummings, W.S. Browner, D.G. Grady, & T.B. Newman (Eds.), *Designing clinical research* (3rd ed., pp. 5–15). Philadelphia, PA: Lippincott Williams & Wilkins.

Levin, K.A. (2006). Study design III: Cross-sectional studies. *Evidence-Based Dentistry, 7*, 24–25. doi:10.1038/sj.ebd.6400375

Ligthelm, R.J., Borzì, V., Gumprecht, J., Kawamori, R., Wenying, Y., & Valensi, P. (2007). Importance of observational studies in clinical practice. *Clinical Therapeutics, 29*, 1284–1292. doi:10.1016/j.clinthera.2007.07.004

Mann, C.J. (2003). Observational research methods. Research design II: Cohort, cross sectional, and case-control studies. *Emergency Medicine Journal, 20*, 54–60. doi:10.1136/emj.20.1.54

Noordzij, M., Dekker, F.W., Zoccali, C., & Jager, K.J. (2009). Study designs in clinical research. *Nephron Clinical Practice, 113*, c218–c221. doi:10.1159/000235610

Polonijo, A.N., & Carpiano, R.M. (2013). Social inequalities in adolescent human papillomavirus (HPV) vaccination: A test of fundamental cause theory. *Social Science and Medicine, 82*, 115–125. doi:10.1016/j.socscimed.2012.12.020

Rosenfeld, D.L., & Bronson, R.A. (1980). Reproductive problems in the DES-exposed female. *Obstetrics and Gynecology, 55*, 453–456.

Stewart, M.G. (2004). Outcomes research: An overview. *ORL: Journal for Oto-Rhino-Laryngology and Its Related Specialties, 66*, 163–166. doi:10.1159/000079872

Wynder, E., & Graham, E. (1950). Tobacco smoking as a possible etiologic factor in bronchiogenic carcinoma: A study of six hundred and eighty-four proved cases. *JAMA, 143*, 329–336. doi:10.1001/jama.1950.02910390001001

Yang, W., Zilov, A., Soewondo, P., Bech, O.M., Sekkal, F., & Home, P.D. (2010). Observational studies: Going beyond the boundaries of randomized controlled trials. *Diabetes Research and Clinical Practice, 88*, S3–S9. doi:10.1016/S0168-8227(10)70002-4

Chapter 6

Expanded Access to Investigational Drugs

Deborah A. (Lindberg) Standafer, RN-C, BSN, MBA, CCRC

Introduction

Expanded access to and compassionate exemption for investigational drugs make it possible for a person or group of people with a serious disease such as cancer to receive a drug being studied in a controlled clinical trial before the research investigation is completed. Expanded access is reserved for patients who otherwise would not be eligible to enroll in the clinical trial investigating a drug that may help them. Today, the terms *expanded access* and *compassionate use* are used interchangeably; however, their meanings are slightly different and will be discussed in this chapter.

In August 2009, the U.S. Food and Drug Administration (FDA) revised its rules governing access to investigational drugs for patients and physicians outside the setting of enrollment in a clinical trial ("Expanded Access to Investigational Drugs for Treatment Use," 2009). These regulatory revisions, which were originally put in place in 1987, were designed to make drug access easier and guidelines for use clearer. The original regulations were established in response to the HIV/AIDS epidemic (Mack, 2009).

Clinical trial nurses (CTNs) routinely encounter the use of investigational drugs as part of a clinical study and need to be well educated about expanded access and compassionate use of the drugs for patients who are not able or not qualified to participate in a formal research study. This chapter will provide information about access programs to drugs that have not yet received full FDA approval (the final step in drug development) and thus are still considered investigational.

Expanded Access Programs

In the drug development process, clinical trials are used to establish the safety and efficacy of new medications, new combinations of medications, or new indications for existing medications. However, seriously ill patients may not qualify for or be able to enroll in a clinical trial. Many are too ill to wait for the investigational treatment to become available. Expanded access protocols (EAPs) provide a means for patients and their physicians to use an investigational drug outside of a designated clinical trial (National Cancer Institute [NCI], 2009). However, this avenue is restricted to patients with a serious condition or disease who no longer have satisfactory medical options available and who may benefit from the investigational therapy (see Figure 6-1). The purposes of EAPs are diagnosing, monitoring, and treating, rather than amassing data, as would be the purpose of a clinical trial ("FDA Investigational New Drug Application [IND]: Expanded Access to Investigational Drugs for Treatment Use," 2013; U.S. National Library of Medicine, 2009).

The FDA EAP regulation (2013) allows sponsors of a drug still in development to provide access to patients not enrolled in a designated clinical trial (see Figure 6-2). Sponsors are not required to allow their drugs to be available through an EAP; however, if they choose to provide this access, they must apply to FDA. FDA

Figure 6-1. Common Patient Criteria for Access to an Investigational Drug Through an Expanded Access Protocol

To be considered for treatment with an investigational drug outside a clinical trial, patients must meet the following criteria:
- Have undergone standard treatment that has not been successful
- Be ineligible for any ongoing clinical trials of this drug
- Have no acceptable treatment alternatives
- Have a cancer diagnosis for which the investigational drug has demonstrated activity
- Be likely to experience benefits that outweigh the risks involved.

Note. From "Access to Investigational Drugs" (Fact Sheet) by National Cancer Institute, 2009. Retrieved from http://www.cancer.gov/cancertopics/factsheet/Therapy/investigational-drug-access.

> **Figure 6-2. Criteria for an Investigational Drug Given Under an Expanded Access Protocol or Compassionate Use Exemption**
>
> - There must be substantial clinical evidence that the drug may benefit persons with particular types of cancer.
> - The drug must be able to be given safely outside a clinical trial.
> - The drug must be in sufficient supply for ongoing and planned clinical trials.
>
> *Note.* From "Access to Investigational Drugs" (Fact Sheet) by National Cancer Institute, 2009. Retrieved from http://www.cancer.gov/cancertopics/factsheet/Therapy/investigational-drug-access.

approves the application only if there are no other adequate and satisfactory treatments for the disease and if all other requirements in the regulation are met (see Figure 6-3).

Under the final rule of the 2009 changes that were made to the regulations, expanded access is available to individual patients, intermediate-sized patient populations of the same disease or condition, and larger populations under an IND ("Expanded Access to Investigational Drugs for Treatment Use," 2009; "FDA IND Expanded Access to Investigational Drugs for Treatment Use, General," 2013). Each have additional criteria to those listed in Figure 6-3 that must be met before FDA will grant approval for expanded access or compassionate use.

Individual Patients, Including Emergency Use

When an individual patient accesses investigational therapy, the process is referred to as *compassionate use* or *special exemption* (NCI, 2009). Despite these terms' connotations, a single patient receiving an investigational drug through an EAP is relatively common. Only after the patient's physician has determined that the risk from the investigational drug to the patient is not greater than the risk from the disease can the physician apply for special access on the patient's behalf ("FDA IND: Individual Patients, Including for Emergency Use," 2013). The patient's physician or the sponsor of the investigational drug submits the application with supporting medical information to FDA. If the required conditions are met, the physician's determination for risk to the patient is satisfactory, and FDA determines that the patient cannot obtain the drug under another IND or protocol, approval is granted ("FDA IND: Individual Patients, Including for Emergency Use," 2013). In emergency situations, approval from FDA may be obtained within 24 hours (American Cancer Society, 2013). In some situations, even with EAP convenience, the manufacturer may not have enough of the drug to fulfill every request for expanded access or compassionate use.

Intermediate-Sized Patient Populations

FDA may permit an investigational drug in the late stages of development to be used for treatment in a group of patients with similar health needs but not large enough to establish a treatment protocol or treatment IND. The EAP submission must satisfy FDA requirements (Figure 6-3), as well as the additional requirements identified in Figure 6-4.

FDA may ask a sponsor to consolidate expanded access when the agency (FDA) has received a significant number of requests for individual patient expanded use for an investigational drug for the same use ("FDA IND: Intermediate-Size Patient Populations," 2013) (see Figure 6-5).

> **Figure 6-3. Criteria for All Expanded Access Uses**
>
> Food and Drug Administration must determine that:
> - The patient or patients to be treated have a serious or immediately life-threatening disease or condition, and there is no comparable or satisfactory alternative therapy to diagnose, monitor, or treat the disease or condition.
> - The potential patient benefit justifies the potential risks of the treatment use and those potential risks are not unreasonable in the context of the disease or condition to be treated.
> - Providing the investigational drug for the requested use will not interfere with the initiation, conduct, or completion of clinical investigations that could support marketing approval of the expanded access use or otherwise compromise the potential development of the expanded access use.
>
> *Note.* From "FDA Investigational New Drug Application: Requirements for All Expanded Access Uses," 21 C.F.R. § 312.305(a), 2013. Retrieved from http://www.accessdata.fda.gov/scripts/cdrh/cfdocs/cfcfr/CFRSearch.cfm?CFRPart=312&showFR=1&subpartNode=21:5.0.1.1.3.9.

> **Figure 6-4. Additional Criteria for Expanded Access Use of an Investigational Drug for Intermediate-Sized Populations**
>
> - The expanded access submission must state whether the drug is being developed or is not being developed and describe the patient population to be treated.
> - If the drug is not being actively developed, the sponsor must explain why the drug cannot currently be developed for the expanded access use and under what circumstances the drug could be developed.
> - If the drug is being studied in a clinical trial, the sponsor must explain why the patients to be treated cannot be enrolled in the clinical trial and under what circumstances the sponsor would conduct a clinical trial in these patients.
>
> *Note.* From "FDA Investigational New Drug Application: Individual Patients, Including for Emergency Use," 21 C.F.R. § 312.315(c), 2013. Retrieved from http://www.accessdata.fda.gov/scripts/cdrh/cfdocs/cfcfr/CFRSearch.cfm?CFRPart=312&showFR=1&subpartNode=21:5.0.1.1.3.9.

Treatment Investigational New Drug Application or Treatment Protocol

The FDA final rule allows for a third category of use while the drug is still considered investigational: widespread treatment use ("FDA IND: Treatment IND or Treatment Protocol," 2013). The FDA will allow an investigational drug to be used under a Treatment IND if there is evidence of drug effectiveness and patients are not eligible for other ongoing clinical trials. Additional criteria address trial status, marketing status, and evidence (see Table 6-1).

An example of an EAP is one issued through the NCI Treatment Referral Center (TRC).

> NCI program staff establishes a TRC protocol when clinical evidence suggests that an investigational drug should be made more widely available to patients, even though the FDA approval process has not been completed.
>
> The TRC protocol is made available at NCI-designated cancer centers and other institutions selected to provide wide geographic availability of the drug to patients. (NCI, 2009, Question 3, para. 5)

Charging Rules

The revised FDA regulations of 2009 allowed drug manufacturers to bill patients for the investigational drugs made available through an EAP. The regulation described how to charge for an investigational drug based on the program type. FDA cited that charging the patient allows the manufacturer to be able to develop new drugs and offer those drugs through an access program (U.S. FDA, 2009). However, smaller drug companies may find the regulations concerning charging for investigational drugs onerous and burdensome (Mack, 2009).

Availability in Community Health Organizations

EAPs are usually based in academic medical centers. Although this allows some patients to enroll in a program at a large institution, social and financial barriers preclude access for many patients (Weiser, Welch, & Calman, 2010). Weiser and colleagues' (2010) study demonstrated that an expanded access program could effectively be established in a community setting, even with the additional administrative requirements needed to do so.

Figure 6-5. Situations Where Expanded Access Might Be Needed

- Drug is not being developed because the disease or condition is extremely rare, and the drug manufacturer is unable to recruit subjects for enrollment into a clinical trial.
- Drug is under investigation in a clinical trial, but sizable patient populations are unable to participate in the study, or the study is closed to enrollment.
- Drug was approved but is no longer available due to safety concerns.

Note. From "FDA Investigational New Drug Application: Intermediate-Size Patient Populations," 21 C.F.R. § 312.315(a), 2013. Retrieved from http://www.accessdata.fda.gov/scripts/cdrh/cfdocs/cfcfr/CFRSearch.cfm?CFRPart=312&showFR=1&subpartNode=21:5.0.1.1.3.9.

Table 6-1. Additional Criteria for Expanded Access Use of an Investigational Drug for Large Populations Under a Treatment IND or a Treatment Protocol

Topic	Criteria
Trial status	• Drug is being investigated in a controlled clinical trial under an IND designed to support a marketing application for the expanded access use. • All clinical trials of the drug have been completed.
Marketing status	• The sponsor is actively pursuing marketing approval of the drug for the expanded access use with due diligence.
Evidence	• There is sufficient clinical evidence of safety and effectiveness to support the expanded access use for a serious disease or condition. Evidence would consist of data from phase III trials or compelling evidence from completed phase II trials. • The available scientific evidence provides a reasonable basis to conclude that the investigational drug may be effective for expanded access use in an immediately life-threatening condition. – Patients would not be exposed to an unreasonable risk or injury. – Evidence would usually consist of data from phase III or phase II trials but could be based on more preliminary clinical evidence.

IND—investigational new drug application

Note. Based on information from "FDA Investigational New Drug Application: Treatment IND or Treatment Protocol," 21 C.F.R. § 312.320, 2013. Retrieved from http://www.accessdata.fda.gov/scripts/cdrh/cfdocs/cfcfr/CFRSearch.cfm?CFRPart=312&showFR=1&subpartNode=21:5.0.1.1.3.9.

Implications for Clinical Trial Nurses

CTNs need to be able to locate information about available clinical trials and established access programs. Information about these can be found at ClinicalTrials.gov; through FDA documents and www.fda.gov; NCI Cancer Information Service (800-4-CANCER); and directly from drug manufacturers. CTNs are responsible for ensuring ongoing formal and informal communication regarding clinical trials with team members. Therefore, when prepared with information on expanded access of investigational drugs, the nurse can astutely discuss with team members and patients the available options and assist with connecting patients to available resources.

Summary

Novel therapies for serious medical conditions and diseases progress through clinical trials, and, if proven to be safe and effective, receive FDA approval for use in specific indications. Prior to FDA approval, patients and providers can access these experimental treatments through a clinical trial or an EAP if one exists. CTNs can be key facilitators for information about these options.

Key Points

- Investigational drugs are those that are still being studied and have not received final FDA approval.
- Investigational drugs are typically accessed through enrollment in a controlled clinical trial.
- Expanded access programs allow drug manufacturers under specific circumstances and, with FDA approval, to make an investigational drug available to a patient or group of patients outside the setting of a clinical trial.
- More information about expanded access programs can be found through NCI (www.cancer.gov), drug manufacturers, or at
  - FDA website (www.fda.gov/ForConsumers/ByAudience/ForPatientAdvocates/AccesstoInvestigationalDrugs/default.htm)
  - FDA website (www.fda.gov/Drugs/default.htm): Emergency Use Investigational New Drug Program for Oncology Drugs
  - ClinicalTrials.gov (see "How do I find information on Expanded Access Studies in ClinicalTrials.gov?")
  - Pharmaceutical Research and Manufacturers of America (www.phrma.org).

References

American Cancer Society. (2013). Compassionate drug use. Retrieved from http://www.cancer.org/treatment/treatmentsandsideeffects/clinicaltrials/compassionate-drug-use

Expanded access to investigational drugs for treatment use. (2009, July 20). *Federal Register, 74*, 40900–40943. Retrieved from http://www.gpo.gov/fdsys/pkg/FR-2009-08-13/pdf/E9-19005.pdf

FDA Investigational New Drug Application: Expanded Access to Investigational Drugs for Treatment Use, General, 21 C.F.R. § 312.300 (2013). Retrieved from http://www.accessdata.fda.gov/scripts/cdrh/cfdocs/cfcfr/CFRSearch.cfm?CFRPart=312&showFR=1&subpartNode=21:5.0.1.1.3.9

FDA Investigational New Drug Application: Individual Patients, Including for Emergency Use, 21 C.F.R. § 312.310 (2013). Retrieved from http://www.accessdata.fda.gov/scripts/cdrh/cfdocs/cfcfr/CFRSearch.cfm?CFRPart=312&showFR=1&subpartNode=21:5.0.1.1.3.9

FDA Investigational New Drug Application: Intermediate-Size Patient Populations, 21 C.F.R. § 312.315 (2013). Retrieved from http://www.accessdata.fda.gov/scripts/cdrh/cfdocs/cfcfr/CFRSearch.cfm?CFRPart=312&showFR=1&subpartNode=21:5.0.1.1.3.9

FDA Investigational New Drug Application: Treatment IND or Treatment Protocol, 21 C.F.R. § 312.320 (2013). Retrieved from http://www.accessdata.fda.gov/scripts/cdrh/cfdocs/cfcfr/CFRSearch.cfm?CFRPart=312&showFR=1&subpartNode=21:5.0.1.1.3.9

Mack, G.S. (2009). Expanded access rules pose quandary for drug developers. *Nature Biotechnology, 27*, 871–872. doi:10.1038/nbt1009-871

National Cancer Institute. (2009, August 4). Access to investigational drugs. Retrieved from http://www.cancer.gov/cancertopics/factsheet/Therapy/investigational-drug-access

U.S. Food and Drug Administration. (2009, August 12). FDA expands access to investigational drugs. Retrieved from http://www.fda.gov/ForConsumers/ConsumerUpdates/ucm176845.htm

U.S. National Library of Medicine. (2009, October 24). FAQ: ClinicalTrials.gov—What is "expanded access?" Retrieved from http://www.nlm.nih.gov/services/ctexpaccess.html

Weiser, J., Welch, A., & Calman, N. (2010). From bench to clinic: Accessing promising investigational medications for patients with HIV infection in an urban family health center. *Journal of the American Board of Family Medicine, 23*, 566–570. doi:10.3122/jabfm.2010.05.090257

Chapter 7

Sponsoring Agencies

Joan G. Westendorp, RN, MSN, OCN®, CCRP, CIM

Introduction

Clinical trials are vital to advance medical science; however, sponsoring agencies are required so that the trials are available to investigators and patients. In U.S. Food and Drug Administration (FDA) investigational new drug application (IND) regulations ("Definitions and Interpretations," 2013, 21 C.F.R. § 312.3[b]), a *sponsor* is defined as "a person who takes responsibility for and initiates a clinical investigation." Some of the responsibilities of the sponsor also are indicated in the FDA IND regulations (General Responsibilities of Sponsors, 2013, 21 C.F.R. § 312.50):

> Sponsors are responsible for selecting qualified investigators, providing them with the information they need to conduct an investigation properly, ensuring proper monitoring of the investigation(s), ensuring that the investigation(s) is conducted in accordance with the general investigational plan and protocols contained in the IND, maintaining an effective IND with respect to the investigations, and ensuring that FDA and all participating investigators are promptly informed of significant new adverse effects or risks with respect to the drug.

This indicates that the sponsor is essentially responsible for all operational aspects of the clinical trials it sponsors.

The most common sponsors of clinical trials are government agencies, pharmaceutical companies, individual researchers, healthcare institutions, nonprofit organizations, and international programs. All sponsors have the same responsibilities; however, they may develop and conduct clinical trials in varying ways. The sponsor may transfer any or all of the responsibilities to a *contract research organization* (CRO). According to the International Conference on Harmonisation of Technical Requirements for Registration of Pharmaceuticals for Human Use (ICH), a CRO is "a person or an organization (commercial, academic, or other) contracted by the sponsor to perform one or more of a sponsor's trial-related duties and functions" (ICH, 1996, p. 4). If the sponsor uses a CRO, the ultimate responsibility for the quality and integrity of the trial data always resides with the sponsor. Any trial-related duties and functions that are transferred to and assumed by a CRO should be specified in writing. All references to a sponsor, with regard to responsibility, are applied to a CRO to the extent that a CRO has assumed the trial-related duties and functions of a sponsor (U.S. FDA, 1996).

Types of Sponsors

Government Agencies

Government agencies, such as the National Cancer Institute (NCI) and other parts of the National Institutes of Health (NIH), the Department of Defense, and the Department of Veterans Affairs, sponsor and conduct clinical trials. These agencies sponsor a large number of clinical trials each year and have developed a variety of programs to make cancer clinical trials widely available in the United States. See Figure 7-1 for a list of programs.

The NCI Office of Cancer Centers provides support to research-oriented institutions that have been recognized as NCI-designated cancer centers for their scientific excellence. An NCI-designated cancer center has vigorous interactions across its research areas, facilitating collaboration between basic laboratory, clinical, and prevention, control, and population-based science investigators, and a formal research program. The Office of Cancer Centers is the source of funding for the research within those cancer centers (NCI Office of Cancer Centers, n.d.).

The Clinical Trials Cooperative Group Program is a program that brings researchers from all types of institutions together into cooperative research groups. These groups work with NCI to identify important questions in cancer research and design. This program provides clin-

---

Figure 7-1. Government Programs

- Clinical Trials Cooperative Group Program
- National Cancer Institute Community Oncology Research Program
- National Cancer Institute Office of Cancer Centers
- Specialized Programs of Research Excellence
- National Institutes of Health Clinical Center
- National Cancer Institute International Collaboration

Note. Based on information from National Cancer Institute, 2013a, 2013b.

---

ical trials to a large number of investigators throughout the United States, therefore allowing a large number of individuals access to clinical trials. See Chapter 1 for more information.

The NCI Community Oncology Research Program (NCORP) was approved by the NCI Board of Scientific Advisors on June 24, 2013, to create a network for cancer care delivery research. NCORP's goal is to bring state-of-the art cancer prevention, control, treatment, and imaging clinical trials; cancer care delivery research; and disparities studies to individuals in their own communities. NCORP components include (a) research bases, (b) community sites, and (c) minority/underserved sites (NCI, 2013b). Research bases will be National Clinical Trials Network groups or cancer centers that design, develop, and conduct cancer prevention and control trials and cancer care delivery research. NCORP community sites will be single-community organizations or consortiums of community hospitals and private practices with the capacity to support cancer care delivery research that can enroll at least 80 people in NCI studies each year. Minority/underserved sites must have at least 30% of their patients with cancer and accrual from racial/ethnic minority or other underserved populations and must have the potential to contribute data on disparities outcomes and care (NCI, 2013b). NCORP is based at the Division of Cancer Prevention. The former Community Clinical Oncology Program, Minority-Based Community Clinical Oncology Program, and NCI Community Cancer Centers Program were replaced by the NCORP network in 2014 (NCI, 2013b).

Specialized Programs of Research Excellence (SPOREs) are the cornerstone of NCI's efforts to promote collaborative, interdisciplinary translational cancer research. The Translational Research Program is the home of the SPOREs within the NCI. SPOREs grants involve clinical/applied science and support projects that will result in new and diverse approaches to the prevention, early detection, and treatment of cancer.

The objective for all SPOREs is to reduce cancer incidence and mortality and to improve survival and quality of life for patients with cancer. SPOREs encourage the advice of patient advocates in SPORE activities.

Each SPORE is focused on a specific organ site, such as breast or lung cancer, or on a group of related cancers such as gastrointestinal cancers and sarcomas. SPOREs are designed to enable the rapid and efficient movement of basic scientific findings into clinical settings, as well as to determine the biologic basis for observations made in individuals with cancer or in populations at risk for cancer (NCI, 2013a).

Government agencies collaborate with pharmaceutical companies in a number of ways to be able to provide the best scientific clinical trials to individuals. One of their collaborations is with the Clinical Trials Cooperative Group Program and pharmaceutical companies. This is fostered by NCI as long as the proposed clinical trial is consistent with the goals of the cooperative group and is scientifically reasonable. The pharmaceutical or biotechnology company holds the initial IND for the investigational agent, but the sponsoring organization (in this case the cooperative group) must submit an IND to FDA for the particular clinical trial. Being the sponsor of the clinical trial, it is responsible for meeting FDA's IND regulations. The pharmaceutical or biotechnology company and the cooperative group collaborate in the planning and writing of the protocol document. The NCI Cancer Therapy Evaluation Program (CTEP) protocol review committee must review and approve the protocol document before activation.

Once the protocol is activated, the pharmaceutical or biotechnology company cannot directly contact the cooperative group to discuss any protocol matters (e.g., obtain protocol information, conduct data audits, discuss protocol amendments) without CTEP Regulatory Affairs Branch's prior approval (NCI, 2008). CTEP provides support, funding, and investigational drug per its standard procedures. The cooperative group may accept additional funding from the pharmaceutical or biotechnology company for the specific clinical trial only if the funds are to support additional costs, such as extra laboratory tests or data collection, as a result of work requested by the pharmaceutical or biotech company (NCI CTEP, 2014).

Government agencies also collaborate with investigational agent co-development via CTEP. The co-development of an investigational agent with CTEP may begin with the drug being developed at either CTEP or at a pharmaceutical or biotechnology company. If CTEP discovers a new agent, an industry sponsor is sought early because NCI does not market new agents. Pharmaceutical and biotechnology companies may seek CTEP co-development at any point in the process (e.g., antitumor screening, preclinical toxicology, clinical trials). If the investigational agent is proprietary to the pharmaceutical or biotechnology company, NCI negotiates and executes one of two types of contracts: either a cooperative research and development agreement (CRADA) or a clinical trials agreement (CTA). The Federal Technology Transfer Act of 1986 created CRADA agreements, which provide a means for the government to collaborate with industry. CTAs are an NCI initiative (NCI CTEP, 2008). After either agreement is initiated, CTEP will submit an IND, a legal mechanism under which investigational drug research is conducted in the United States, to FDA. CTEP then seeks investigators through a request for proposals (RFP), a competitive peer-review process in which the merits of the scientific question, which dictate support and funding, are decided (NCI CTEP, 2008).

The investigational agent can be used only within the scope of the protocol, though it may involve the study of a combination of other agents, including investigational or commercial anticancer agents. Expenses, protocol development, and data are shared in this partnership. Data are made available to the sponsoring pharmaceutical or biotechnology company, NCI, and FDA. The pharmaceutical or biotechnology company may use the clinical trial results for future trial development or in its FDA drug approval application. This is either a new drug application for cytotoxic or cytostatic agents or a biologics license application for biologic agents (NCI CTEP, 2008).

NCI recognized the need for expanded international collaboration in cancer clinical trials and developed the Center for Global Health. The National Cancer Act of 1971 authorized NCI to support collaborative international research and training. The goal of this program is to build expertise and leverage resources across nations to address the challenges of cancer and reduce cancer deaths worldwide. Enabling the open exchange of scientific knowledge is a critical goal in the fight against cancer (NCI, n.d.). The primary functions of the Center for Global Health are to (NCI, n.d.)

- Develop and implement plans to inform cancer control and provide technical assistance as countries work to implement cancer control programs
- Strengthen U.S. national, regional, multilateral, and bilateral collaboration in global health research, cancer research, and cancer control
- Train investigators and help develop research capacity in global health across the cancer continuum in the United States and in the developing world
- Develop and validate new agents and devices for cancer prevention, screening, diagnostics, treatment, and symptom management appropriate for use in the developing world
- Develop new scientific initiatives and implement plans relevant to global health and cancer control.

Pharmaceutical Industry Sponsorship

Pharmaceutical industry sponsorship is when a pharmaceutical or biotechnology company is responsible for the clinical trial. These sponsorships have become a major source of funding for research. A review of industry-sponsored clinical trials over 20 years noted that the percentage of industry-sponsored clinical trials increased to 62% between 1997 and 2000 (Buchkowsky & Jewesson, 2004). Pharmaceutical industry-sponsored clinical trials are frequently phase I and II, along with postmarket registry studies. From an institutional perspective, the most labor-intensive clinical trials are conducted in collaboration with a pharmaceutical or biotechnology company. This is the result of the numerous procedures, forms, data points, and quick timelines that are required. These are based on the pharmaceutical or biotechnology company's operating procedures and goals; for example, a study that may be used to obtain FDA approval will require more data (i.e., more work) than a study that will not be used to gain or extend an existing FDA approval.

The pharmaceutical or biotechnology company, with little (if any) input from the institutional principal investigators, frequently drafts the actual clinical trial design and protocol document. The pharmaceutical or biotechnology company will hold the IND for the trial and must comply with all FDA requirements. However, the standard steps for obtaining protocol approval from the institutions must be followed.

Unless a prior working relationship exists with a specific pharmaceutical or biotechnology company, the institution's principal investigator and the study coordinator will meet with a representative of the company for a prestudy site visit. During this visit, the parties discuss the protocol concept, thereby ascertaining the institution's (a) interest in the study, (b) ability to execute the study based on the number of patients, and (c) potential accrual estimates and patterns. The visit includes pharmaceutical or biotechnology company representatives touring the site where the research will be conducted, paying particular attention to the patient care areas, pharmacy, and laboratories.

Pharmaceutical industry-sponsored clinical trials include investigator-initiated clinical trials. Clinical investigators may wish to perform clinical trials with or without company drugs within or outside the approved product license or prior to marketing authorization. Industry may consider requests, which must be initiated by the clinical investigator as spontaneous, unsolicited, and not by industry, to support such clinical trials pre- and post-first marketing authorization. Support for these clinical trials may be in the form of drug product, comparator drug, financial resources, or all of these (Suvarna, 2012).

Nonprofit Organizations

Nonprofit organizations are frequent sponsors of clinical trials. These organizations usually sponsor clinical trials that match the goal or purpose of the organization (e.g., elimination of breast cancer). When looking at nonprofit organizations' goals, one will know what type of studies they will support. The nonprofit organizations usually develop foundations within the organization so that the clinical trials can be conducted via this avenue. Figure 7-2 features some of the nonprofit organizations that provide funding for research and their websites. This is not an all-inclusive list.

Figure 7-2. Nonprofit Organizations
American Cancer Society: www.cancer.org
Breast Cancer Research Foundation: www.bcrfcure.org
Colon Cancer Alliance: www.ccalliance.org
Leukemia and Lymphoma Society: www.lls.org
Lung Cancer Alliance: www.lungcanceralliance.org
Lymphoma Research Foundation: www.lymphoma.org
Multiple Myeloma Research Foundation: www.themmrf.org
Susan G. Komen: http://ww5.komen.org

Summary

Whether the clinical trial sponsor is NCI, a cooperative group, the pharmaceutical industry, or a nonprofit organization, the requirements of an individual investigator and research staff may vary. However, all sponsors are held to the same regulations. Clinical trial nurses must be aware of potential clinic trial sponsors because they may need to identify clinical trials on specific disease sites for their organization. Because clinical trial nurses are well versed in clinical trial procedures, they are able to take a leadership role in implementing the trial as written and in contributing to the timely completion of the study, no matter who the sponsor is. The clinical trial nurses' primary responsibilities involve patient education, patient recruitment, administration of protocol treatment, protocol compliance, data collection, coordination of required testing, and documentation of test results according to what the sponsor requires. (See Chapter 10 for more information about the CTN roles within a research team.) This is particularly labor intensive in today's healthcare environment. Strict attention to detail regarding the sponsoring agency's requirements will help ensure successful clinical trials that validate interventions that may translate into improvements in care for patients with cancer.

Key Points

- A sponsor is defined as "a person who takes responsibility for and initiates a clinical investigation" and is necessary to have clinical trials available to investigators and patients.
- Government agencies are sponsors of clinical trials and collaborate with industry organizations.
- Investigators, nonprofit organizations, and pharmaceutical and biotechnology companies are sponsors of clinical trials.
- The NCI Center for Global Health has been established to advance global cancer research, build expertise, and leverage resources to address the challenges of cancer and reduce cancer deaths worldwide.

References

Buchkowsky, S.S., & Jewesson, P.J. (2004). Industry sponsorship and authorship of clinical trials over 20 years. *Annals of Pharmacotherapy, 38,* 579–585. doi:10.1345/aph.1D267

Definitions and Interpretations, 21 C.F.R. § 312.3 (2013). Retrieved from http://www.accessdata.fda.gov/scripts/cdrh/cfdocs/cfcfr/CFRSearch.cfm?CFRPart=312&showFR=1

General Responsibilities of Sponsors, 21 C.F.R. § 312.50 (2013). Retrieved from http://www.accessdata.fda.gov/scripts/cdrh/cfdocs/cfcfr/CFRSearch.cfm?CFRPart=312&showFR=1

International Conference on Harmonisation of Technical Requirements for Registration of Pharmaceuticals for Human Use. (1996, June 10). *ICH harmonised tripartite guideline: Guideline for good clinical practice, E6(R1).* Retrieved from http://www.ich.org/fileadmin/Public_Web_Site/ICH_Products/Guidelines/Efficacy/E6/E6_R1_Guideline.pdf

National Cancer Institute. (n.d.). NCI Center for Global Health. Retrieved from http://www.cancer.gov/about-nci/organization/cgh

National Cancer Institute. (2013a, February 22). Cancer clinical trials. Retrieved from http://www.cancer.gov/cancertopics/factsheet/clinicaltrials/clinical-trials

National Cancer Institute. (2013b, June 24). NCI Community Oncology Research Program approved. Retrieved from http://ccop.cancer.gov/news-events/news/20130625

National Cancer Institute Cancer Therapy Evaluation Program. (2008, May 29). NCI—Cooperative Group—Industry relationship guidelines. Retrieved from http://ctep.cancer.gov/industryCollaborations2/guidelines.htm

National Cancer Institute Cancer Therapy Evaluation Program. (2014). *A handbook for clinical investigators conducting therapeutic clinical trials supported by CTEP, DCTD, NCI.* Retrieved from http://ctep.cancer.gov/investigatorResources/docs/InvestigatorHandbook.pdf

National Cancer Institute Office of Cancer Centers. (n.d.). Cancer centers. Retrieved from http://cancercenters.cancer.gov/cancer_centers/index.html

Suvarna, V. (2012). Investigator initiated trials (IITs). *Perspectives in Clinical Research, 3,* 119–121. doi:10.4103/2229-3485.103591

U.S. Food and Drug Administration. (1996, April). *Guidance for industry: E6 good clinical practice: Consolidated guidance.* Retrieved from http://www.fda.gov/downloads/Drugs/Guidanc%20eComplianceRegulatoryInformation/Guidance%20s/ucm073122.pdf

SECTION II.

Clinical Trials: Fundamental Information

Chapter 8

Legal, Regulatory, and Legislative Issues

Sally Brown, RN, BSN, MGA, OCN®, CBCN®, CCRP, Susan Markus, RN, BSN, MS, OCN®, and Carol Anne Bales, RN, MSN, CCRP

Introduction

Knowledge and understanding of research-related laws and regulations are expected of all individuals involved in the conduct of clinical research. Past wrongdoings in the treatment of research participants have led to the development of legal and regulatory systems that scrutinize every aspect of clinical research. Everyone associated with research on humans, regardless of their role, is expected to comply with the laws and regulations that govern the conduct of clinical research practices. It is important to note that regulations, guidance documents, and standards for conducting research are not stagnant; they are living documents that change and evolve.

The regulations and guidance documents that affect the conduct of clinical trials are designed to protect human participants in clinical research and ensure the accuracy of the data being collected. The history of the development of the regulations and guidance documents may be obtained from peer-reviewed articles or books written about clinical trials or from the regulatory groups that developed them. This chapter is intended to introduce and familiarize clinical trial nurses (CTNs) with the overarching legal and regulatory components of conducting clinical research, specific to research conducted in the United States (see Section XI for country-specific information). The aspects of clinical research to which these principles and standards apply are presented in depth in other chapters of this manual.

Selected Historical Events

Over the past 70 years, several instances of abuse of research participants have occurred. These incidents led to the development of laws, regulations, and guidelines that protect research participants and form the foundation for best clinical research practices in the United States and internationally.

Nuremberg Code

The beginning of the modern era for protecting human subjects can be traced to after World War II (WWII). During WWII, pseudoscientific experiments were performed on unwilling—and often unwitting—prisoners in German concentration camps. Nazi doctors performed extraordinarily cruel acts in the name of medical research. These acts were malicious in nature and unethical. The United States and its WWII allies developed the Nuremberg Code (1949), a set of 10 standards used by the Nuremberg Military Tribunal to evaluate experimentation on humans conducted by the Nazis.

Some limited rules and protocols for human medical experimentation existed before WWII. One of these, interestingly enough, was developed in Germany in 1931 in reaction to a failed vaccination experiment. However, none of these carried the force of law or was subjected to advanced legal scrutiny. This changed during the Nuremberg War Crimes Trials (Weindling, 2006).

The Allies held these trials in 1946–1947 to prosecute German war criminals. German doctors who had conducted the experiments on prisoners were among those on trial. In the ruling of the tribunal in the case of *United States of America v. Karl Brandt et al.*, the court laid out a list of 6 (later expanded to 10) characteristics of legitimate human research. The document went well beyond the existing American Medical Associa-

The authors would like to acknowledge Denise Dearing, RN, BSN, OCN®, for her contribution to this chapter that remains unchanged from the previous edition of this book.

tion directives and the German Guidelines for Human Experimentation of 1931 (Sass, 1983) and became the foundation for the Nuremberg Code (Weindling, 2006). Since it was first published in 1949, the Nuremberg Code has not been revised or updated. However, it has served as a template for subsequent laws, rules, codes, and guidance documents. The principles of the Nuremberg Code, and later the Declaration of Helsinki, have been incorporated into U.S. law in Title 45 of the *Code of Federal Regulations* (C.F.R.), specifically Part 46, Protection of Human Subjects (Weindling, 2006).

Declaration of Helsinki

The principles of the Nuremberg Code were reinforced when the World Medical Association (WMA) developed and adopted the *Declaration of Helsinki: Recommendations Guiding Medical Doctors in Biomedical Research Involving Human Subjects*. The Declaration of Helsinki, first issued in 1964, is a statement of ethical principles developed by WMA to be used as guidance in the conduct of medical research. The declaration builds upon the 10 principles of the Nuremberg Code and added that identifiable human material and identifiable data are considered medical research (WMA, 2013a). The document provides numerous ethical principles.

In 2013, the 10th version of the Declaration of Helsinki was proposed. For the first time, the public was asked to comment on the draft version (WMA, 2013a). The 10th version was adopted by the 64th WMA General Assembly in October 2013, just in time for the 50th anniversary of the original declaration a few months later (WMA, 2013b).

National Institutes of Health

In 1953, the National Institutes of Health (NIH) developed a policy to protect human subjects by requiring an independent prospective review of clinical research studies on healthy volunteers conducted at the NIH Clinical Center. The initial policy only applied to healthy volunteers; patients who were enrolled in clinical trials had no additional protection, which was in line with the general opinion of the medical community at that time. In the 1960s, as federal funding for research grew, interest in protecting the rights and well-being of research participants did as well. In 1966, NIH developed the first Public Health Service policy for the protection of human subjects, which applied to all clinical research conducted and funded by the Department of Health, Education and Welfare (DHEW), later renamed the U.S. Department of Health and Human Services (U.S. DHHS) (Wichman, 2012).

U.S. National Research Act

Regulations protecting human subjects did not exist in the United States until the National Research Act required DHEW to codify its human subject protection policy, which occurred on May 30, 1974 (Office for Human Research Protections [OHRP], 1993; Wichman, 2012). The Protection of Human Research Subjects (2009) regulations include information on the role and responsibilities of the institutional review board (IRB), as well as the informed consent process (see Chapter 14). The National Research Act established the National Commission for the Protection of Human Subjects of Biomedical and Behavioral Research (National Commission) (OHRP, 2008). The Belmont Report is a result of the National Commission's work.

The Belmont Report

Laws, regulations, and ethics are closely related but have some distinct differences. The Belmont Report, written by the National Commission in 1978 and published in the *Federal Registry* in 1979, is the standard for the ethical conduct of clinical trials. The full official name of the Belmont Report is *Ethical Principles and Guidelines for the Protection of Human Subjects of Research*. The report was named after the Belmont Conference Center in Elkridge, Maryland, where the 12-member commission met to develop the report. These guidelines and the DHHS human subject protection regulations constitute the basis for existing human subject protection standards in the United States (OHRP, 2008).

The Belmont Report outlines the distinction between research and practice and identifies basic ethical principles for the conduct of clinical research, including remarks about the application of each principle (National Commission, 1979).

Distinction Between Research and Practice

Boundaries between clinical practice and clinical research may become blurred when the objective of research is to test hypotheses concerning treatment modalities. The objective of clinical *practice* is generally to diagnose and provide preventive, curative, or palliative treatment to improve the health of individuals. The objective of clinical *research* is to test a hypothesis or hypotheses concerning the use of a clinical intervention and draw conclusions about the hypothesis based on the responses of study participants (captured in the form of data), and then report generalized conclusions from the research, thereby contributing to the knowledge base of healthcare science (see Table 8-1) (National Commission, 1979).

Basic Ethical Principles

The Belmont Report identifies the three unifying ethical principles for the conduct of clinical research as respect for persons, beneficence, and justice (see Table 8-2).

Respect for persons acknowledges the autonomy of study participants and incorporates a requirement to protect study participants with diminished autonomy, such as children and individuals with mental illness, senility, or dementia. *Autonomy* is a term meaning the ability of an individual to freely and voluntarily make his or her own decisions based on sound judgment. Respect for the autonomy of study participants includes ensuring that participants have sufficient knowledge of the study to enable them to make an informed decision about participating (i.e., the informed consent process). The Belmont Report includes descriptions of the required elements of the informed consent form, as well as consideration of ethical standards undergirding the process of informed consent (National Commission, 1979). For detailed information about the informed consent process, refer to Chapter 14.

The report defines *beneficence* by dividing the concept into two general principles: not harming study participants, and protecting them against possible harm while maximizing the possible benefits of their participation. Although beneficence is generally understood to apply to individuals, it also applies to society at large and to the institutions in which the research is conducted.

The Belmont Report addresses the nature of risks and benefits as they apply to clinical research and their disclosure in the informed consent document. *Risk* is defined as the probability of harm to participants and the potential severity of that harm. The report also lists harms other than physical and psychological harm (e.g., legal, social, financial, economic) that should be considered when comparing the risks and benefits of a study. *Benefit* in clinical research is defined as the positive value related to health or welfare. Benefits should be examined, as they affect not only the study subject but also society in general—in particular, people with the health condition under study (National Commission, 1979). The risk-benefit assessment is conducted as part of the ethical review of a study (i.e., conducted by an IRB or ethics review committee).

The report addresses the concept of *justice* against a historical background. It addresses the responsibility of researchers to ensure that the population from which study participants are recruited will be able to benefit from the research.

The Belmont Report further examines the fairness of participant selection in terms of the population that is most likely to benefit from the results of the research and, in particular, vulnerable populations such as those who are mentally impaired, institutionalized, or part of a minority population that is economically disadvantaged. The report calls for those involved in the conduct of clinical research to make a concerted effort to protect these vulnerable participants from exploitation because of the ease with which they might be recruited into a study (National Commission, 1979).

Table 8-1. Distinction Between Practice and Research

Concept	Description
Clinical practice	Diagnosis, provision of preventive, curative, or palliative treatment to improve the health of individuals
Clinical research	Testing hypothesis/hypotheses concerning the use of a clinical intervention, drawing conclusions based on responses of study subjects, and reporting conclusions, thereby contributing to the knowledge base of healthcare science (to hopefully improve the health of other individuals) and allowing for replication of the research
Clinical research of clinical practice interventions	Combines clinical practice and clinical research

Note. Based on information from National Commission for the Protection of Human Subjects of Biomedical and Behavioral Research, 1979.

Table 8-2. Application of the Belmont Report

Principle	Application

Respect for persons
• Individuals are autonomous agents.
• Individuals should be treated with respect.
• Persons with diminished autonomy need additional protection.
	Informed consent
	• Participants must be given the opportunity to choose what shall or shall not happen to them.
	• The consent process must include three elements:
	  – Information sharing
	  – Comprehension
	  – Voluntary participation.

Beneficence • Human participants should not be harmed. • Research should maximize possible benefits and minimize possible risks.	Assessment of risks and benefits by investigator and the institutional review board or ethics review committee
Justice • The benefits and burdens of research must be distributed fairly.	Selection of participants • Procedures and outcomes in the selection of research participants should be fair. • Eligibility criteria should include those who may benefit and exclude those who may be harmed.

Note. Based on information from National Commission for the Protection of Human Subjects of Biomedical and Behavioral Research, 1979.

U.S. Regulatory Authority

Several groups with regulatory authority are involved in the conduct of clinical trials both in the United States and in other countries. Even if the CTN does not live in the United States, he or she may be working on a study that is either funded by the U.S. government or, in the case of drug development, being used to support a drug marketing application in the United States. In the United States, the conduct of clinical trials is governed at the federal level by regulations that are enacted by DHHS and other agencies (e.g., Department of Defense, Department of Veterans Affairs). DHHS is the principal agency that protects the health of Americans. This agency consists of 11 operating divisions, including the Agency for Healthcare Research and Quality, the Centers for Medicare and Medicaid Services, the Centers for Disease Control and Prevention, the U.S. Food and Drug Administration (FDA), and NIH (see Figure 8-1) (U.S. DHHS, n.d.).

The two main regulatory groups within DHHS with whom the CTN could interact are OHRP and FDA. The interaction will be either direct or indirect depending upon the type of research, who funds the research, and how the CTN role is implemented at the research site. Table 8-3 presents various categories of clinical trials and the regulatory agency or center/office providing oversight. The content covered by these regulations is compared in Table 8-4. Although Title 45 Part 46 and Title 21 regulate different types of research, the human subject protection regulations are similar. A table of comparison is available online at http://www.fda.gov/ScienceResearch/SpecialTopics/RunningClinicalTrials/EducationalMaterials/ucm112910.htm.

Both OHRP and FDA have regulations and several guidance documents that the CTN will need to review.

By definition, *guidance documents* are intended to provide a framework for conduct and recommendations for managing an operation, such as conducting clinical trials, but are not legally binding. In many instances, they serve as the foundation for the development of standard operating procedures (see Chapter 11) and may be incorporated into legally binding requirements at a later date. Compliance with guidance documents represents adherence to the current standards of practice. The CTN needs to be aware of the guidance documents that apply to the type of research being conducted and the research setting. These may include international, national, and local documents.

Office for Human Research Protections

OHRP was established in 2000 by DHHS for protecting the rights, welfare, and well-being of research participants conducted or supported by DHHS. OHRP is part of the Office of the Assistant Secretary of Health in the Office of the Secretary. Before 2000, DHHS human subject protection was limited to NIH-funded studies with oversight from the NIH Office for Protection From Research Risks (Wichman, 2012).

OHRP focus is on the IRBs and the informed consent process. OHRP is the regulatory authority for 45 C.F.R. pt. 46, which includes
- Subpart A: Basic HHS Policy for Protection of Human Research Subjects (the Common Rule)

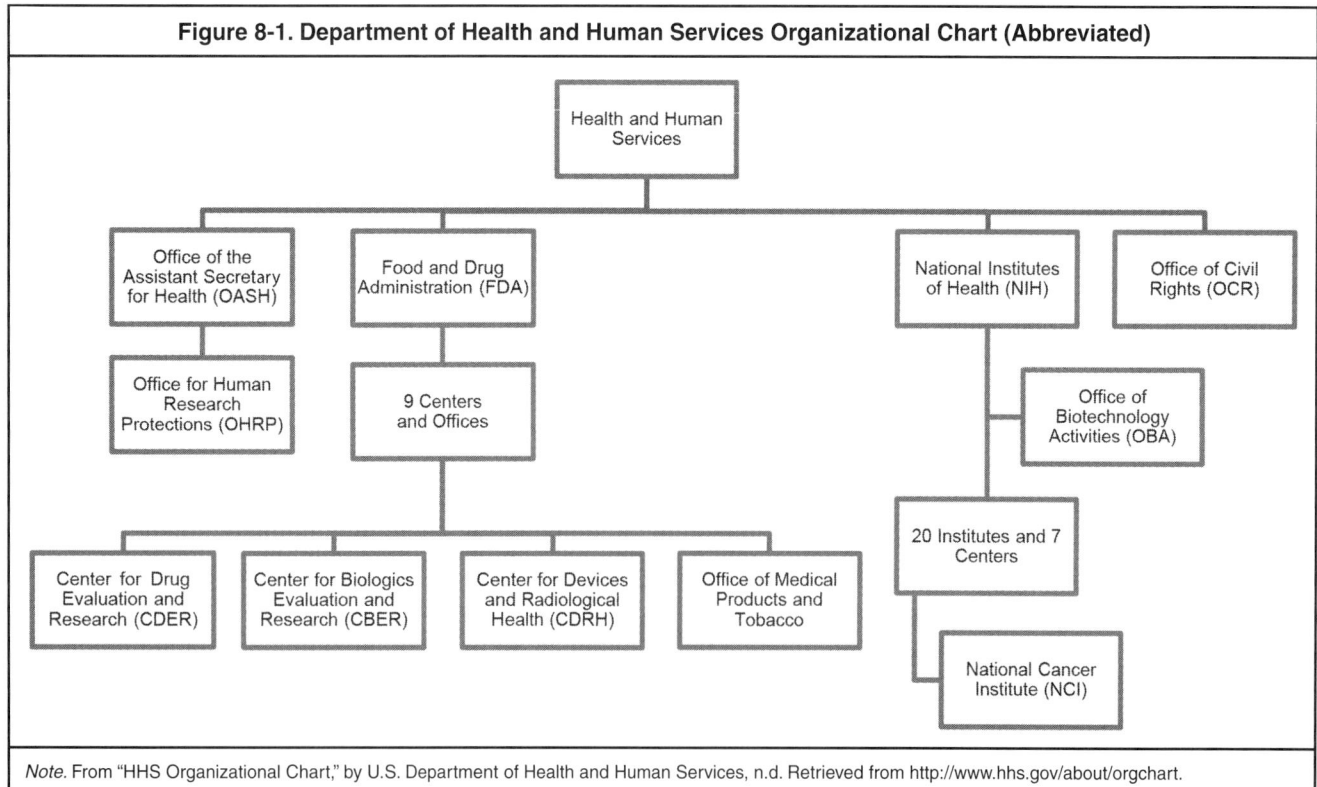

Figure 8-1. Department of Health and Human Services Organizational Chart (Abbreviated)

Note. From "HHS Organizational Chart," by U.S. Department of Health and Human Services, n.d. Retrieved from http://www.hhs.gov/about/orgchart.

Table 8-3. Regulatory Authority Based on Type of Study and Sponsor*						
	Federal Agencies With Clinical Trial Oversight					
	FDA Title 21 C.F.R.		OHRP Title 45 C.F.R. Part 46		DOD 32 C.F.R. Part 219	
Type of Study						
Biologic agents conducted under an IND: • Vaccines • Blood and blood products for transfusion and/or manufacturing into other products • Allergenic extracts, which are used for both diagnosis and treatment (for example, allergy shots) • Human cells and tissues used for transplantation (for example, tendons, ligaments, and bone) • Gene therapies • Cellular therapies • Tests to screen potential blood donors for infectious agents such as HIV	✓	CBER	✓	If DHHS funded For gene therapy, OBA oversight	✓	If DOD funded
Devices conducted under an IDE	✓	CDRH	✓	If DHHS funded	✓	If DOD funded
Drugs conducted under an IND: • Any article intended for use in the diagnosis, cure, mitigation, treatment, or prevention of disease • Any article, other than food, intended to affect the structure or any function of the body of man or other animals • New indication of an already marketed drug (known as a supplemental IND)	✓	CDER	✓	If DHHS funded	✓	If DOD funded
Type of Sponsors for Oncology Clinical Trials						
DOD	✓	CDER, CBER, CDRH if using an IND or IDE	–		✓	–
NIH- and NCI-sponsored, including cooperative group studies	✓	CDER, CBER, CDRH if using an IND or IDE	✓	–	–	
Private (e.g., biopharmaceutical industry, foundations)	✓	CDER, CBER, CDRH	–		–	

* Depending upon the study sponsor, two sets of regulations may have to be followed. For example, an NCI study using an IND agent needs to adhere to both OHRP and FDA regulations.

CBER—Center for Biologics Evaluation and Research; CDER—Center for Drug Evaluation and Research; CDRH—Center for Devices and Radiological Health; DOD—Department of Defense; FDA—U.S. Food and Drug Administration; IDE—investigational device exemption; IND—investigational new drug application; NCI—National Cancer Institute; NIH—National Institutes of Health; OBA—Office of Biotechnology Activities; OHRP—Office for Human Research Protections

Note. Based on information from Food and Drugs, 2013; Protection of Human Research Subjects, 2009; Protection of Human Subjects, 2013.

- Subpart B: Additional Protections for Pregnant Women, Human Fetuses, and Neonates Involved in Research
- Subpart C: Additional Protections Pertaining to Biomedical and Behavioral Research Involving Prisoners as Subjects
- Subpart D: Additional Protections for Children Involved as Subjects in Research
- Subpart E: Registration of Institutional Review Boards.

The first codified federal policy for the protection of human subjects was established in 1974. In 1991, this policy, informally known as the Common Rule, was issued by 15 other federal agencies and departments. The Common Rule is 45 C.F.R. pt. 46, subpt. A (OHRP, 2009).

As with any law or regulation, the Common Rule may need to be revised. In 2011, OHRP issued an Advance Notice of Proposed Rulemaking for changes and comments of the *Common Rule for Human Subject Research Protections: Enhancing Protections for Research Subjects and Reducing Burden, Delay, and Ambiguity for Investigators* (U.S. Food and Drug Administration Office of the Secretary, 2011). CTNs should be aware that 45 C.F.R. pt. 46 may change again and should check the OHRP website for the most current regulations.

Table 8-4. Content of Titles 21 and 45 of the U.S. Code of Federal Regulations Related to Clinical Trials

Title	Part	Topic Addressed
Title 21 (U.S. Food and Drug Administration): Food and Drugs	Part 11	Electronic records and signature
	Part 50	Protection of human subjects
	Part 54	Financial disclosure by clinical investigators
	Part 56	Institutional review boards
	Part 312	Investigational new drug application
	Part 314	Application for Food and Drug Administration approval to market a new drug
	Part 601	Licensing
	Part 812	Investigational device exemptions
	Part 814	Premarket approval of medical devices
Title 45 (Common Rule): Public Welfare and Human Services	Part 46	Protection of human subjects
	Part 46, subpart A	Basic Health and Human Services policy for protection of human research subjects (Common Rule)
	Part 46, subpart B	Additional protection pertaining to research development and research activities involving fetuses, pregnant women, and human in vitro fertilization
	Part 46, subpart C	Additional protection pertaining to research development and research activities involving prisoners as research subjects
	Part 46, subpart D	Additional protection pertaining to research development and research activities involving children as research subjects

OHRP is also responsible for compliance agreements and registration of IRBs. Institutions that conduct federally funded human subject research are required to obtain a Federalwide Assurance (FWA) for compliance with 45 C.F.R. pt. 46 prior to initiation of any clinical research. All IRBs listed on the FWA and IRBs in the United States who review FDA-regulated clinical trials must register with OHRP (n.d.-b). For more on FWAs and IRB registration, see Chapter 16.

U.S. Food and Drug Administration

Not all clinical research conducted in the United States is funded by DHHS. FDA has oversight for the laws for which they have authority (e.g., foods, drugs, biologics, devices, tobacco) regardless of who funds the research. FDA obtains its statutory authority through several acts of Congress (i.e., sets of laws). The acts of Congress include the Federal Food, Drug, and Cosmetic Act, the Prescription Drug User Fee Act, the Prescription Drug Marketing Act, and the FDA Modernization Act of 1997. FDA is composed of centers and offices (see Figure 8-2) that ensure all regulations are followed.

FDA also has regulations related to human subject protection: Title 21 Part 50, Protection of Human Subjects, and Title 21 Part 56, Institutional Review Boards, codified in 1980 and 1981, respectively. The rules and regulations are developed by departments and agencies of the government based on the laws passed by Congress. The regulations are published in the *Code of Federal Regulations* and given citations such as 21 C.F.R. pt. 50. Each agency then provides nonbinding guidance documents, published in the *Federal Register*, which represent the agency's current stance on a particular subject to provide further direction. The U.S. agencies involved in clinical research provide an overview of their involvement in clinical research, the regulations, and various guidance documents on their websites (see Figure 8-3). For more legal terms CTNs may encounter related to the development of regulations, see Figure 8-4.

The FDA regulations that apply to clinical research include electronic records and electronic signatures, informed consent, humans subject protection, financial disclosure by clinical investigators, investigational new drugs, approval of new drugs, investigational device exemptions, and premarket approval of medical devices (see Table 8-3).

In addition to the regulations, FDA has several guidance documents. FDA's description of guidance documents states,

> Guidance documents represent the agency's current thinking on a particular subject. They do not create or confer any rights for or on any person and do not operate to bind FDA or the public. An alternative approach may be used if such approach satisfies the requirements of the applicable statutes, regulations, or both. (U.S. FDA, 2012a)

FDA guidance documents may be found by searching the Division of Drug Information Database, available online at www.fda.gov/regulatoryinformation/guidances/default.htm.

Figure 8-2. Organizational Structure of the U.S. Food and Drug Administration

- Center for Biologics Evaluation and Research
- Center for Devices and Radiological Health
- Center for Drug Evaluation and Research
- Center for Food Safety and Applied Nutrition
- Center for Tobacco Products
- National Center for Toxicological Research
- Office of the Commissioner
- Office of Regulatory Affairs

Note. Based on information from U.S. Food and Drug Administration, 2014.

Figure 8-3. Websites for Overview of U.S. Regulations Involved in Clinical Research

- U.S. Food and Drug Administration (Title 21): www.fda.gov/AboutFDA/WhatWeDo/History/Overviews/ucm304485.htm
- Privacy Rule: www.hhs.gov/ocr/privacy/index.html and http://privacyruleandresearch.nih.gov/clin_research.asp
- Office for Human Research Protections 45 C.F.R. 46 FAQs: http://answers.hhs.gov/ohrp/categories/1562
- GINA (Genetic Information Nondiscrimination Act): www.genome.gov/24519851

International Conference on Harmonisation

The International Conference on Harmonisation of Technical Requirements for Registration of Pharmaceuticals for Human Use (ICH), established in 1990, developed and maintains major international standards for the conduct of research involving human subjects. ICH brings together the drug regulatory authorities of the European Union, Japan, and the United States (represented by FDA), along with the pharmaceutical trade associations from these three regions, to discuss scientific and technical aspects of product registration. ICH's mission is to achieve greater harmonization in the interpretation and application of technical guidelines and requirements for product registration, thereby reducing duplication of testing and reporting carried out during the research and development of new medicines. This harmonization is to ensure that safe, effective, and high-quality medicines are developed and registered in the most resource-efficient manner (ICH, 2010).

The scope of ICH guidelines covers a broad range of topics related to conducting clinical research. In 2005, ICH divided the guidelines into four categories: quality (Q), efficacy (E), safety (S), and multidisciplinary (M) with numbered revisions to each guideline (e.g., R1, R2). The ICH topics are contained within one of these categories. Examples of guidelines located within the "M" category include the Medical Dictionary for Regulatory Activities (known as MedDRA), the Common Technical Document, and Electronic Standards for the Transfer of Regulatory Information (known as ESTRI) (ICH, n.d.). Another example is in the "E" category, specifically *Guideline for Good Clinical Practice: E6* (ICH, 1996). This guideline is critical for CTNs to read and incorporate into practice. Refer to Chapter 9 for additional information.

International Standards, Laws, and Guidelines

Internationally conducted clinical trials are becoming increasingly more prevalent as the communication and technical capacities for these endeavors increase, and CTNs will have more opportunities to coordinate trials at an international level.

For example, a Spanish-speaking man from South America wants to be considered for a clinical trial at a U.S. site. From the initially available information, the investigators determine that his medical conditions satisfy the study's eligibility criteria. The patient agrees to come to the site for disease assessment visits every eight weeks. He plans to be followed by his local oncologist and have his required laboratory tests done at home. The study requires that tumor samples be collected and sent to the sponsor's laboratory in England. Before this patient is considered for the study, the international aspects of patient care, specimen processing, and data collection must be addressed.

Being aware of the legal and regulatory standards of other countries and jurisdictions is one of the obligations to be met by members of the research team. Although internationally conducted research offers the potential for tremendous benefit, it compounds the requirements for ensuring accountability and compliance. Annually, OHRP updates a compilation of international human research standards, which can be found at www.hhs.gov/ohrp/international/index.html. This serves as a comprehensive reference for international research.

Privacy and Confidentiality

Health Insurance Portability and Accountability Act

In response to the public's concern about potential abuse of confidentiality of health information, the U.S. Congress passed the Health Insurance Portability and Accountability Act of 1996 (HIPAA). As required by Congress, DHHS was to establish regulations that would determine how the health information was to be protected. These regulations, 45 C.F.R. Part 160 and Part 164, Subparts A and D, are titled Standards for Privacy of Individually Identifiable Health Information, commonly known as the Privacy Rule. Compliance was required as of April 14, 2003. The regulations resulted in new terminology, such as protected health information (PHI)

Figure 8-4. Glossary of U.S. Legal Terms

Act
Something done or performed (esp. voluntarily), a deed (Garner, 2011).

Act of Congress
A law that is formally enacted in accordance with the legislative power granted to Congress by the U.S. Constitution (Garner, 2011).

Administrative Agency
An agency that is authorized by the legislature to establish and enforce rules regulating its particular area of concern or regulatory agency (Wood, 2011).

Code
A complete system of positive law carefully arranged and officially promulgated; a systematic collection or revision of laws, rules, or regulations (the Uniform Commercial Code). Strictly, a code is a compilation not just of existing statutes but also of much of the unwritten law on a subject, which is newly enacted as a complete system of law (Garner, 2011).

Code of Federal Regulations **(C.F.R.)**
The annual collection of executive agency regulations published in the daily *Federal Register*, combined with previously issued regulations that are still in effect (Garner, 2011). The code is divided into titles, parts, and sections. Titles are general categories; parts are broad topics; and sections are specific areas within the topic. For example, 21 C.F.R. § 56.107 translates to Title 21 (Food and Drugs) of the *Code of Federal Regulations,* part 56 (Institutional Review Boards [IRBs]), section 107 (IRB membership).

Common Rule
45 C.F.R. pt. 46; governs the conduct of human subject research funded through any one of 17 federal agencies (OHRP, n.d.-a).

Federal Register
A daily publication containing presidential proclamations and executive orders, federal agency regulations of general applicability and legal effect, proposed agency rules, and documents required by law to be published (Garner, 2011).

Guidance Document
Current thinking by a U.S. agency, viewed as recommendations unless regulatory requirements are included (U.S. FDA, 2012a).

Guidelines
Documents that provide directives. Guidelines are not legally binding but contain expectations of conduct. Guidelines must be followed as strictly as regulations because they represent the standard of practice that should be maintained. Breaching them is not punishable by law; however, failure to comply can have disciplinary consequences or can lead to legal liability. Examples of legal liability include breach of protocol, noncompliance with standard operating procedures, and negligence to participants (Jones-Wright, 2006). Documents that describe an agency's interpretation of a policy on a regulatory issue. These are prepared for agency staff, applicants, sponsors, and the public (Zoon & Yetter, 2012).

Law
(1) The regime that orders human activities and relations through systematic application of the force of a politically organized society or through social pressures, backed by force in such a society; the legal system; (2) the aggregate legislation, judicial precedents, and accepted legal principle; the body of authoritative grounds of judicial and administration action, especially the body of rules, standards, and principles that the courts of a particular jurisdiction apply in deciding controversies brought before them; (3) the set of rules and principles dealing with a specific area of a legal system (e.g., copyright law); (4) the judicial and administrative process, legal actions, and proceedings; (5) a statute; (6) common law; (7) the legal profession (Garner, 2011).

Legal
(1) Of or pertaining to law, falling within the province of law; (2) established, required, or permitted by law; (3) of or relating to law as opposed to equity (Garner, 2011).

Negligence
Failure to exercise the standard of care that a reasonably prudent person would have exercised in a similar situation; any conduct that falls below the legal standard established to protect against unreasonable risk of harm except for conduct that is intentionally wanton or willfully disregardful of risk to others (Garner, 2011).

Regulation
A rule or order, having legal force, usually issued by an administrative agency (Garner, 2011).

Rule
All or part of a statement (as a regulation) by an administrative agency that has general or particular applicability and future effect and that is designed to implement, interpret, or prescribe law or policy or that describes the organization, procedure, or practice of the agency itself (Wood, 2011).

Statute
A law passed by a legislative body, specifically legislation enacted by any lawmaking body, including legislatures, administrative boards, and municipal courts. The term *act* is interchangeable as a synonym (Garner, 2011).

and covered entities. PHI relates not only to the individual but also include relatives, employers, and household members. The data considered PHI include (NIH, 2004; U.S. DHHS, 2013)
- Names
- Geographic information (e.g., street address, city, county, zip code)
- Dates related to the individual (e.g., date of birth, date of admission/discharge, date of death)
- Telephone numbers, including fax numbers
- Email addresses and other Internet identifiers
- Social Security number
- Medical record number
- Health plan beneficiary number
- Account number
- Certificate/license numbers
- Vehicle identifiers, including license plate number
- Device identifiers
- Biometric identifiers
- Full-face photographic images.

Covered entities are health plans, healthcare clearinghouses, and healthcare providers that transmit health information electronically in connection with transactions defined by HIPAA. An independent researcher is not considered a covered entity and does not have to comply with HIPAA privacy policies. However, very few researchers are totally independent. A researcher is part of a covered entity if he or she is the healthcare provider engaging in covered electronic submissions or is employed by a covered entity. The Privacy Rule *does* allow disclosure for research purposes. The rule established conditions for disclosure or use of PHI. These conditions include preparatory review for research, research on decedents' information, and de-identification of PHI. Research involving data and biospecimens are subject to this rule. The disclosure of PHI requires authorization either by waiver or participant authorization. The authorization for disclosure of PHI for research has required elements. In some instances, the core elements may be included in the informed consent document (NIH, 2004; U.S. DHHS, 2013). CTNs should refer to the Office of Civil Rights, NIH websites, and their institution's compliance and privacy division for specific information.

Genetic Information Nondiscrimination Act

On May 21, 2008, the Genetic Information Nondiscrimination Act (GINA) was signed into law in the United States, thereby affecting how clinical researchers handle genetic information. GINA prohibits discrimination based on genetic information for health coverage or employment. The Office of Civil Rights collaborated with the Department of Labor, Centers for Medicare and Medicaid Services, the Department of the Treasury, the Equal Employment Opportunity Commission, and NIH before issuing regulations for the enforcement of GINA. The regulations are found in 29 C.F.R. pt. 1635 (U.S. DHHS, 2009).

GINA has two specific areas of implication in research: (a) IRB criteria for approval and (b) requirements for informed consent. IRBs should consider the provisions of GINA when assessing whether genetic research satisfies the criteria required for IRB approval of research. In particular, IRBs should consider whether the risks are minimized and reasonable in relation to anticipated benefits and whether adequate provisions are in place to protect the privacy of subjects and maintain the confidentiality of the data. GINA is also relevant to informed consent. When investigators develop and IRBs review the consent processes and documents for genetic research, they should consider whether and how the protections provided by GINA should be reflected in the consent document's description of risks and provisions for ensuring the confidentiality of the data (OHRP, 2009).

Clinical Trials Registration and Patient Open Access

The need for a reliable way for the public to find the status of ongoing clinical trials and the results of completed clinical trials was addressed in the late 1990s. The FDA Modernization Act of 1997 mandated a registry of federal and private funded clinical trials of experimental treatments for serious or life-threatening diseases or conditions (Hathaway, Hass, & Scherer, 2009). In 2007, the FDA Amendments Act, specifically Section 801, expanded the scope of required trials (e.g., device trials) and required the reporting of clinical trial results (e.g., primary outcome, adverse events, demographics). For a detailed explanation, see Chapter 26.

Patient *open access* to clinical trials refers to patients knowing the outcome of ongoing and recently completed/analyzed studies. The importance of knowing negative as well as positive study outcomes has been identified as an unmet expectation. While study sponsors, whether private or public, are eager to share the positive outcomes, the publishing of negative results is often delayed or absent in the literature. The Cochrane Collaboration, which publishes widely respected data reviews and meta-analyses of available clinical trials, reports that selective reporting of investigational drug studies by companies needs to end, as it could be harming patients. Cochrane urges changes in policy and law to make it mandatory for researchers to publish all data after a 12-month period, and it calls for punitive measures to be taken against those who fail to comply (Adams, 2011).

In 2008, Congress passed the Consolidated Appropriations Act, which directed NIH to create a public access policy for NIH-funded research. The result, PubMed Central, is a free full-text archive with more than 2.4 million biomedicine and life science articles. It is a valuable and free resource for eletronic references (National Library of Medicine, 2008).

One concern of providing open access is the potential lack of understanding by the lay public of the difference between peer-reviewed publications and what one reads in social media. Historically, research papers that undergo peer review are scrutinized by experts in the field to ensure compliance with scientific method, use of established research processes, accurate statistical and mathematical evaluations, and that the papers are well written. This was, and still is, done to ensure the quality of the research being reported. The reports in social media are not required to provide the same level of compliance with scientific method or justifications for how the study was conducted. Potentially, social media and open access may impact the evaluation of research quality. Actions are being taken to ensure that the information is intelligible, meaning that it is understandable by readers who are not scientists, researchers, or clinicians without loss of the essence of the study particulars (Curry, 2013).

Another form of public access is access to information about types of cancer, clinical trials, and eligibility criteria for specific trials. Both NCI's website (www.cancer.gov) and the National Library of Medicine's public registry (www.clinicaltrials.gov) provide the public and healthcare professionals easy access to information on clinical trials for a wide range of diseases, conditions, and health problems. The commercial-based website CenterWatch (www.centerwatch.com) has a mission to provide reliable information concerning clinical trials to healthcare professionals and the public. It is important for CTNs to visit these sites to ensure that the information is accurate.

Federal Clinical Trial Legislation

Proposed legislation (bills) concerning clinical trials is submitted into both houses of the U.S. Congress. The submission of a bill does not guarantee that the bill will become law. In 2005, Senator Christopher Dodd (D-CT) submitted the Fair Access to Clinical Trials (FACT) Act (S. 470, 2005). The bill did not pass. It was resubmitted the following year and again was not passed (S. 467, 2007).

Although the FACT Act failed, others have passed. In 2000, a presidential memorandum introduced access to clinical trials to Medicare subscribers. The Improving Access to Clinical Trials Act of 2009 was signed into law in October 2010 (S. 1674, 2010). In this law, Congress recognized that in order to advance medical treatments, increased participation in clinical trials is required. The primary focus was improved access for individuals receiving Supplemental Security Income and Medicaid benefits. Before this law, individuals receiving these benefits might not have been allowed to receive any monetary compensation for participating in clinical trials. Although their compensation may be nominal, the additional income could have been enough to increase the individual's income above that required to receive Medicaid or Supplemental Security Income benefits. The Improving Access to Clinical Trials Act allows these individuals to receive payments without threat of loss of benefits (S. 1674, 2010).

The Patient Protection and Affordable Care Act (commonly referred to as the Affordable Care Act) was signed into law in March 2010. The intent of the act is to increase access to healthcare insurance, increase consumer protection, improve quality care and system performance, increase access to prevention and screening, provide assistance to increase or reorganize the healthcare workforce, and address rising healthcare costs. The clinical trials coverage in the Affordable Care Act incorporated many points from the Improving Access to Clinical Trials Act of 2009. This act expands requirements for health insurance plans (e.g., commercial plans, plans through the Federal Employee Health Benefit Program, self-insured employer-sponsored plans, and state self-insured plans) to cover some costs associated with participation in clinical trials. These plans are required to cover routine costs, including all items and services that are typically covered for a patient who is not enrolled in a clinical trial, that are associated with high-quality, phase I–IV trials for cancer and other life-threatening diseases (American Cancer Society Cancer Action Network, 2010). The coverage also must be available to the individual if the clinical trial is conducted out of the individual's state of residence (National Conference of State Legislatures [NCSL], 2011).

Finding the status of ongoing national legislation in any aspect of research involving human subjects is always possible by checking the Federal Register (www.federalregister.gov) for recent activity. Additional current information is available on websites related to the FDA, Centers for Medicare and Medicaid Services, clinical trials, law, and the Code of Federal Regulations.

State Clinical Trial Legislation

State laws and regulations have an impact on clinical trials. If state laws are stricter than federal regulations, then the state law must be followed (Kaltman & Isidor, 2006). Regulations that affect the conduct of clinical trials are very diverse on the state level. Most state regulations are related to insurance coverage and payment for "standard of care" costs while the insured is participating in a clinical trial; however, this can include the frequency of having the subject re-sign the informed consent document (i.e., reconsenting). As of September 2010, 27 states and the District of Columbia had laws addressing access to and payment for clinical trials (NCSL, 2010).

The NCSL website (www.ncsl.org/issues-research/health/clinical-trials-what-are-states-doing-2010.aspx) includes a page titled "Clinical Trials: What Are States Doing?" This page contains a list, by state, of the current status of laws in that state affecting clinical trials (NCSL, 2010).

Information provided by NCI concerning coverage for clinical trials in individual states can be found at www.cancer.gov/clinicaltrials/learningabout/payingfor/laws. In addition to a section on "States Requiring Coverage of Clinical Trial Costs," the website provides information about clinical trials in general.

Since 1989, the State Cancer Legislative Database, a program of NCI, has monitored and analyzed cancer-related state legislation. In 2005, NCI began offering online access to the searchable database. State Cancer Legislative Database data allow examination and comparison of cancer-related legislation across the United States (MayaTech Corporation, n.d.).

Laws and agreements are not consistent across the United States; coverage varies widely. However, in 2014, the Affordable Care Act started requiring health insurers to pay for routine costs of care in approved clinical trials for cancer and other life-threatening diseases. Covered clinical trial activities include treatment, prevention, and early detection trials (NCSL, 2011).

Retention of Records

All study-related records must be retained after the study is completed. "Completed" in this context means that all subjects have been recruited and have completed the study and all data have been collected and analyzed. The ICH GCP, OHRP, and FDA have varying requirements (see Figure 8-5). If local record retention policies are stricter than federal requirements, it is necessary to comply with the stricter local policy.

Shipment of Research Specimens

Some clinical studies require that specimens be shipped to laboratories specified by the sponsor for analysis. The specimens contain body fluids or human tissue that might be stored on dry ice or in formalin and are considered hazardous materials. The specific regulations for the packaging and shipment to prevent spillage during transport of these specimens are listed in Category B Infectious Substances (2013). The Occupational Safety and Health Administration, the U.S. Department of Transportation, and the International Air Transport Association (IATA), a multinational regulatory organization, regulate the shipment of these materials. The Federal Aviation Administration, the Federal Highway Administration, the Federal Railroad Administration, and the U.S. Coast Guard enforce the regulations within the United States.

Although research specimens are exempt from more stringent shipping requirements, the specific packaging and labeling requirements listed in Category B Infectious Substances (IATA, 2013) must be followed. IATA provides an exemption for patient specimens from IATA's dangerous goods regulations. IATA considers research specimens to be patient specimens. These specimens are designated for shipping as biologic substance Category B or commonly referred to as UN 3373 (IATA, 2011).

Although training is required by IATA for anyone who is packaging and shipping materials that meet the IATA description of dangerous goods, this requirement does not apply to those packing and shipping Category B specimens (IATA, 2013). The required training consists of knowing the specifics of the regulations for packaging and shipping the specimens. IATA does encourage obtaining an understanding of the dangerous goods regulations for packaging and shipping. Some sponsors will require training specific to a given study.

Compliance Issues

Because regulations and guidelines are constantly evolving, compliance with these regulations and guidelines requires awareness of ongoing changes. The moni-

---

Figure 8-5. Comparison of Duration of Record Retention Among ICH GCP and U.S. Governing Bodies

ICH GCP	45 C.F.R. § 46.115	21 C.F.R.

• At least two years after last approval of marketing application
• At least two years after formal discontinuation if no marketing application is submitted
	• Three years after completion of study (institutional review board records and informed consent documents)	• Part 56.115: IRB Record—At least three years after completion of research
		• Part 312.57: Sponsor and Investigators
		  – Two years after a marketing application is approved for the drug; or
		  – If an application is not approved for the drug, until two years after shipment and delivery of the drug for investigational use is discontinued and FDA has been notified

FDA—U.S. Food and Drug Administration; ICH GCP—International Conference on Harmonisation of Technical Requirements for Registration of Pharmaceuticals for Human Use Good Clinical Practice

Note. Based on information from Basic HHS Policy for Protection of Human Research Subjects, 2009; Institutional Review Boards, 2013; International Conference on Harmonisation of Technical Requirements for Registration of Pharmaceuticals for Human Use, 1996.

toring of clinical research activities for compliance with regulatory measures is an evolving field and has raised awareness of the importance of protection of research subjects. See Table 42-2 for OHRP and FDA electronic mailing list information. By subscribing to these email lists, CTNs can easily stay current with regulatory updates.

Noncompliance

Not adhering to regulations or the protocol may be regulatory noncompliance. Noncompliance may be discovered during a sponsor's monitoring visit, during a routine scheduled audit, or by someone involved in the research organization that may later become identified as a whistle-blower. The reporting of the event will initiate a more in-depth investigation. The investigation is conducted by the appropriate government agency, such as the FDA or Office of Research Integrity. Intent, awareness, and regard for what was being done carry great weight when determining whether misconduct has occurred.

Consequences of Noncompliance

The consequences of noncompliance with federal regulations depend on the severity of noncompliance. Both OHRP and FDA will take action against the sponsor of the study, the institution, or the investigator in order to ensure compliance. In recent years, OHRP has addressed issues of noncompliance related to the conduct of the IRB, including inappropriate expedited review, inappropriate composition of IRB, inadequate record keeping, and inadequacies in the informed consent document. When FDA finds regulatory noncompliance, it can obtain a court order requiring that the study be stopped at the site, institution, or sponsor level; charge the violator with a crime; seize the goods involved; bar the violator from future participation in a new drug application; impose a civil monetary penalty; or issue a written notice or warning (Rozovsky & Adams, 2003). Consequences can include

- Temporary suspension of investigator
- Lifetime suspension of investigator
- Names of disqualified or restricted investigators listed in the *Federal Register*
- Names of disqualified or restricted investigators listed on the FDA website indefinitely, even after the restriction has been lifted
- Penalties including fines or prison sentences.

Misconduct can be pursued using federal statutory, criminal, and civil law (Rozovsky & Adams, 2003). The institution also may be affected by noncompliance. The functions of the IRB may be suspended by OHRP for DHHS-funded research if the IRB procedures are found to be deficient (Wichman, 2012). This can result in loss of funding, damaged reputation, and expensive corrective actions (Rozovsky & Adams, 2003).

Research Misconduct

According to the Office of Research Integrity (2011), "research misconduct means fabrication, falsification, or plagiarism in proposing, performing, or reviewing research, or in reporting research results."

- *Fabrication* is making up data or results and recording or reporting them.
- *Falsification* is manipulating research materials, equipment, or processes or changing or omitting data or results such that the research is not accurately represented in the research record.
- *Plagiarism* is the appropriation of another person's ideas, processes, results, or words without giving appropriate credit.
- *Research misconduct* does not include honest error or differences of opinion (Office of Research Integrity, 2011).

Research misconduct may involve issues of disclosure about the researchers, being forthcoming with information about the conduct of the study or the study findings, or inclusion of appropriate study subjects.

In the 1980s, as a result of increased public concern about research integrity, a committee of the Institute of Medicine (1989) examined the issue and released *The Responsible Conduct of Research in the Health Sciences*. Institutions were given the responsibility of preventing and handling misconduct (Colbert, 2012) (see Table 8-5).

In 1996, the White House Office of Science and Technology Policy organized meetings with multiple agencies to discuss the definition of scientific misconduct. Each of these agencies participates in research, and each had a different definition of misconduct. In 1999, the National Sciences and Technology Council of the Office of Science and Technology Policy proposed a common statement regarding research misconduct. The document, *Research Misconduct Defined*, with common procedures

Table 8-5. Categories of Research Misconduct	
Category	Examples
Misconduct in science	Fabrication, falsification, plagiarism
Questionable research practices	Failure to retain data, inadequate records, honorary authorship, premature release of results
Other types of misconduct	Financial irregularities, sexual harassment, criminal activities

Note. Based on information from Colbert, 2012.

and policies, was supported by all federal agencies that support scientific research. After a positive review by the scientific community, the final federal policy for federally sponsored research was published in the *Federal Register* (Colbert, 2012).

FDA's website lists 8 warnings letters in 2012 and 13 in 2011 concerning the conduct of clinical trials. The warning letters, sent to investigators and institutions, addressed various issues, including falsification of data, the submission of the falsified data, failure of the IRB to comply with 21 C.F.R. § 56.111 (e.g., not requiring informed consent from prospective subjects), failure of the IRB to establish and maintain written operating policies, noncompliance with protocol-required testing, failure to ensure continuing approval by the IRB, and falsification of documentation of continuing IRB approval on the informed consent form (U.S. FDA, 2012b).

Financial Fraud and Abuse

Financial fraud and abuse occur when the management of clinical trial funds is not handled honestly and accurately. It occurs when Medicare or any insurance party is billed for services that are to be paid by the sponsor of a clinical trial. Billing more than one source for a service is known as *double dipping*; only one party is to be billed for a service. It is necessary to know which clinical trial activities or procedures are standard of care and which are research-related in order to determine the appropriate payer. Ensuring insurance coverage is mandated by some institutions before allowing patients to be screened. In addition, fraud and abuse occur when a report is filed that indicates additional funding is necessary to conduct the study when, in fact, it is not. The fiscal management of clinical trials must be done with *knowledge, accuracy, accountability,* and *integrity*.

The Office of Management Assessment investigates concerns of fraud and abuse in NIH-sponsored research. Reimbursement fraud can be prosecuted under the False Claims Act. This requires knowledge that false or fraudulent claims and false statements were made to the government. The False Claims Act primarily is enforced through the Department of Justice (Kalb & Koehler, 2002).

Financial fraud and abuse in clinical trials may occur related to the Stark Law. The Stark Law addresses the prohibition of physician health service referrals to an entity with which the physician has a financial relationship (Centers for Medicare and Medicaid Services, 2013; Stark Law, n.d.). This could include a compensation arrangement. According to Rusczek and Rusczek (2010), "a compensation arrangement is any arrangement involving remuneration, direct or indirect, between a physician (or a member of the physician's immediate family) and an entity." Funds forwarded by an institution to a principal investigator not employed by the hospital would fall under the umbrella of the Stark Law. For more information on financial fraud and abuse, see Chapter 21.

Negligence

Negligence can be described as *contributory negligence, criminal negligence,* or *culpable negligence*. Several elements must be proved to establish negligence. These elements are that the healthcare provider owed a duty to the patient, this duty was breached, damages occurred, and the damages were caused by the breach of duty.

Although CTNs adhere to a written, IRB-approved protocol, the potential exists for malpractice or negligence to occur. As individuals licensed by the state, CTNs must work within the scope of that state's nurse practice act. This means that CTNs may not assume roles that are not assigned to their level of license.

Implications for Clinical Trial Nurses

CTNs are required to comply with the nurse practice act for their state and institution and must comply with the most stringent regulations. CTNs acting as study coordinators, site managers, clinical research associates, study monitors, regulatory associates, or project managers have an obligation to know the current regulatory and compliance standards and when changes are being considered. One way to obtain information is to read the *Federal Register* (U.S. National Archives and Records Administration, n.d.).

Although the legal and legislative processes are not common areas of expertise for CTNs, they are areas that should not be ignored. These processes should be taken seriously. CTNs are able to provide a unique perspective and knowledge base to elected officials and their staff. The elected officials are not the experts in the field; the CTNs are. Involvement in these processes can range from sending comments to the officials to visiting the officials and their staffs and vocally advocating for a cause.

There are several ways to approach this challenging role and take steps in the legislative process:
- Make or obtain a list of your current federal representatives and senators, state senators and representatives, and local elected officials. The list should include contact information for each government official on the list (address, phone numbers, email addresses, and sites on social media networks). A listing of the U.S. senators and representatives may be found at www.house.gov/representatives/find. State representatives may be found on each state's website.
- Seize the opportunity to express your opinion directly to representatives by
  – Voting

– Writing a letter and sending it "return receipt requested"
– Sending an email
– Making use of the Internet, especially a blog page
– Attending meetings related to clinical trials attended by your representatives.
• Join or establish a government or legislative committee within a local chapter of a professional organization. For example, the Oncology Nursing Society offers a number of ways for members to get involved. Information is available in the "Advocacy and Policy" section on www.ons.org.

Reading beyond nursing literature and subscribing to professional journals will provide increased exposure to proposed changes in clinical trial regulatory and compliance issues. Journals from nursing or clinical trials–related organizations may contain articles of interest to CTNs.

Summary

This chapter discussed the origin, development, and application of laws, regulations and guidelines concerning clinical trials. This is a complex subject that has moral, ethical, and legal implications and is an ongoing issue in federal and state legislation. The U.S. government has a number of systems in place to ensure the safety and well-being of research participants. State governments and local healthcare institutions have developed measures to guide the conduct of clinical trials. It is the steadfast commitment of those involved in clinical research to provide for the protection of individual research participants while on the quest for knowledge that will reinforce the public's trust.

Key Points
• CTNs need to be knowledgeable and understand research-related laws and regulations.
• In the United States, regulations are developed from laws passed by Congress and are legally binding.
• Existing laws and regulations may change to address new issues or concerns for the well-being of human research subjects. Guidelines provide direction on how to follow the regulations. Guidelines are not legally binding in the United States but may be in other countries.
• All U.S. federally conducted or funded research must follow Title 45 C.F.R. Part 46. The regulatory authority for this regulation is the OHRP.
• Laws, regulations, and guidelines for the conduct of clinical research are based on the premise that human research subjects are to be protected. Every aspect of the development, conduct, and evaluation of clinical trials is subject to examination for compliance with established ethical and legal standards.
• Legal compliance with the most stringent law or regulation is required, whether it is the national or local jurisdiction's standard.

References

Adams, B. (2011, June 10). Call for open access to all clinical trial data. Retrieved from http://www.pharmafile.com/news/168665/call open-access-all-clinical-trial-data

American Cancer Society Cancer Action Network. (2010, April). Affordable Care Act: Clinical trials. Retrieved from http://www.acscan.org/pdf/healthcare/implementation/factsheets/hcr-clinical-trials.pdf

Basic HHS Policy for Protection of Human Research Subjects, 45 C.F.R. 46 (2009). Retrieved from http://www.hhs.gov/ohrp/humansubjects/guidance/45cfr46.html

Category B Infectious Substances, 49 C.F.R. § 173.199 (2013). Retrieved from http://www.ecfr.gov/cgi-bin/text-idx?SID=896a3753546d08d27b6dec6a226cd272&node=49:2.1.1.3.10.5.25.36&rgn=div8

Centers for Medicare and Medicaid Services. (2013, November 27). Physician self-referral. Retrieved from http://www.cms.gov/Medicare/Fraud-and-Abuse/PhysicianSelfReferral/index.html

Colbert, M.C. (2012). Integrity in research: Individual and institutional responsibility. In J.I. Gallin & F.P. Ognibene (Eds.), *Principles and practice of clinical research* (3rd ed., pp. 43–52). Boston, MA: Elsevier Academic Press. doi:10.1016/B978-0-12-382167-6.00004-7

Curry, S. (2013, March 22). Open access for the people. Retrieved from http://www.theguardian.com/science/occams-corner/2013/mar/22/1

Fair Access to Clinical Trials Act of 2005, S. 470, 109th Cong. (2005). Retrieved from https://www.govtrack.us/congress/bills/109/s470/text

Fair Access to Clinical Trials Act of 2007, S. 467, 110th Cong. (2007). Retrieved from https://www.govtrack.us/congress/bills/110/s467/text

Food and Drugs, 21 C.F.R. (2013). Retrieved from http://www.accessdata.fda.gov/scripts/cdrh/cfdocs/cfcfr/cfrsearch.cfm

Garner, B.A. (Ed.). (2011). *Black's law dictionary* (4th pocket ed.). St. Paul, MN: Thomson Reuters West.

Hathaway, C., Hass, J.B., & Scherer, C. (2009, May). FDA issues clarification of U.S. clinical trials registry requirements. *ABA Health eSource, 5*(9). Retrieved from https://www.americanbar.org/newsletter/publications/aba_health_esource_home/Hathaway.html

Improving Access to Clinical Trials Act of 2009, S. 1674, 111th Cong. (2010) (enacted). Retrieved from https://www.govtrack.us/congress/bills/111/s1674/text

Institute of Medicine. (1989). *The responsible conduct of research in the health sciences*. Retrieved from http://www.nap.edu/openbook.php?record_id=1388&page=R1

Institutional Review Boards, 21 C.F.R. 56 (2013). Retrieved from http://www.accessdata.fda.gov/scripts/cdrh/cfdocs/cfcfr/cfrsearch.cfm?cfrpart=56&showfr=1

International Air Transport Association. (2011). *Dangerous goods regulations* (52nd ed.). Retrieved from https://www.iata.org/whatwedo/cargo/dgr/Documents/DGR52_InfectiousSubstances(DGR362).pdf

International Air Transport Association. (2013, September 10). Dangerous goods training FAQ. Retrieved from http://www.iata.org/whatwedo/cargo/dgr/Documents/training-faq.pdf

International Conference on Harmonisation of Technical Requirements for Registration of Pharmaceuticals for Human Use. (n.d.). History. Retrieved from http://www.ich.org/about/history.html

International Conference on Harmonisation of Technical Requirements for Registration of Pharmaceuticals for Human Use. (1996, June 10). *ICH harmonised tripartite guideline: Guideline for good clinical practice, E6(R1)*. Retrieved from http://www.ich.org/fileadmin/Public_Web_Site/ICH_Products/Guidelines/Efficacy/E6_R1/Step4/E6_R1__Guideline.pdf

International Conference on Harmonisation of Technical Requirements for Registration of Pharmaceuticals for Human Use. (2010).

The value and benefits of ICH to drug regulatory authorities—Advancing harmonization for better health. Retrieved from http://www.ich.org/fileadmin/Public_Web_Site/News_room/C_Publications/ICH_20_anniversary_Value_Benefits_of_ICH_for_Regulators.pdf

Jones-Wright, P. (2006). Guiding principles and regulations. In C.A. Fedor, P.A. Cola, & C. Pierre (Eds.), *Responsible research: A guide for coordinators* (pp. 11–34). London, United Kingdom: Remedica.

Kalb, P.E., & Koehler, K.G. (2002). Legal issues in scientific research [Electronic version]. *JAMA, 287*, 85–91. doi:10.1001/jama.287.1.85

Kaltman, S.P., & Isidor, J.M. (2006). State law. In E.A. Bankert & R.J. Amdur (Eds.), *Institutional review board management and function* (pp. 304–307). Burlington, MA: Jones & Bartlett Learning.

MayaTech Corporation. (n.d.). About SCLD. What is SCLD? Retrieved from http://www.scld-nci.net/about/about-what-is-SCLD.cfm

National Commission for the Protection of Human Subjects of Biomedical and Behavioral Research. (1979, April 18). *The Belmont report: Ethical principles and guidelines for the protection of human subjects of biomedical and behavioral research*. Retrieved from http://www.hhs.gov/ohrp/humansubjects/guidance/belmont.html

National Conference of State Legislatures. (2010, September). Clinical trials: What are states doing? Retrieved from http://www.ncsl.org/issues-research/health/clinical-trials-what-are-states-doing-2010.aspx

National Conference of State Legislatures. (2011, March). The Affordable Care Act: A brief summary. Retrieved from http://www.ncsl.org/portals/1/documents/health/hraca.pdf

National Institutes of Health. (2004, June 22). Clinical research and the HIPAA Privacy Rule. Retrieved from http://privacyruleandresearch.nih.gov/clin_research.asp

National Library of Medicine. (2008, October 21). ClinicalTrials.gov to include basic results data. *NLM Technical Bulletin, 364*. Retrieved from http://www.nlm.nih.gov/pubs/techbull/so08/so08_clinicaltrials.html

Nuremberg Code. (1949). In *Trials of war criminals before the Nuremberg military tribunals under Control Council Law No. 10* (Vol. 2, pp. 181–182). Retrieved from http://www.hhs.gov/ohrp/archive/nurcode.html

Office for Human Research Protections. (n.d.-a). Federal Policy for the Protection of Human Subjects (Common Rule). Retrieved from http://www.hhs.gov/ohrp/humansubjects/commonrule/index.html

Office for Human Research Protections. (n.d.-b). IRBs and assurances. Retrieved from http://www.hhs.gov/ohrp/assurances/index.html

Office for Human Research Protections. (1993). *Institutional review board guidebook*. Retrieved from http://www.hhs.gov/ohrp/archive/irb/irb_introduction.htm

Office for Human Research Protections. (2008, November 13). The Belmont report. Retrieved from http://archive.hhs.gov/ohrp/belmontArchive.html#histReport

Office for Human Research Protections. (2009, March 24). *Guidance on the Genetic Information Nondiscrimination Act: Implications for investigators and institutional review boards*. Retrieved from http://www.hhs.gov/ohrp/policy/gina.pdf

Office of Research Integrity. (2011, April 25). Definition of research misconduct. Retrieved from http://ori.dhhs.gov/definition-misconduct

Protection of Human Research Subjects, 45 C.F.R. 46 (2009). Retrieved from http://www.hhs.gov/ohrp/humansubjects/guidance/45cfr46.html

Protection of Human Subjects, 32 C.F.R. 219 (2013). Retrieved from http://www.gpo.gov/fdsys/pkg/CFR-2013-title32-vol2/pdf/CFR-2013-title32-vol2-sec219-101.pdf

Rozovsky, F.A., & Adams, R.K. (2003). *Clinical trials and human research: A practical guide to regulatory compliance*. San Francisco, CA: Wiley.

Rusczek, J.M., & Rusczek, A.P. (2010). Fraud and abuse in clinical research: Three case studies. *ABA Health eSource, 6*(10). Retrieved from http://www.americanbar.org/newsletter/publications/aba_health_esource_home/Rusczek.html

Sass, H.-M. (1983). Reichsrundschreiben 1931: Pre-Nuremberg German regulations concerning new therapy and human experimentation. *Journal of Medical Philosophy, 8*, 99–112. doi:10.1093/jmp/8.2.99

Stark Law. (n.d.). Stark law. Retrieved from http://starklaw.org/stark_law.htm

U.S. Department of Health and Human Services. (n.d.). *Historical highlights*. Retrieved from http://www.hhs.gov/about/hhshist.html

U.S. Department of Health and Human Services. (2009, April 6). "GINA": The Genetic Information Nondiscrimination Act of 2008—Information for researchers and health care professionals. Retrieved from http://www.genome.gov/Pages/PolicyEthics/GeneticDiscrimination/GINAInfoDoc.pdf

U.S. Department of Health and Human Services. (2013, June 5). Understanding HIPAA privacy—Research. Retrieved from http://www.hhs.gov/ocr/privacy/hipaa/understanding/special/research/index.html

U.S. Food and Drug Administration. (2012a, November 19). Drugs: Research list of guidance documents. Retrieved from http://www.fda.gov/Drugs/GuidanceComplianceRegulatoryInformation/Guidances/ucm310704.htm

U.S. Food and Drug Administration. (2012b, January 25). Warning letters and notice of violation letters to pharmaceutical companies. Retrieved from http://www.fda.gov/Drugs/GuidanceComplianceRegulatoryInformation/EnforcementActivitiesbyFDA/WarningLettersandNoticeofViolationLetterstoPharmaceuticalCompanies/default.htm

U.S. Food and Drug Administration. (2014, April 11). FDA organization. Retrieved from http://www.fda.gov/AboutFDA/CentersOffices/default.htm

U.S. Food and Drug Administration Office of the Secretary. (2011, July 26). Human subjects research protections: Enhancing protections for research subjects and reducing burden, delay, and ambiguity for investigators. *Federal Register, 76*, 44512–44531. Retrieved from http://www.gpo.gov/fdsys/pkg/FR-2011-07-26/pdf/2011-18792.pdf

U.S. National Archives and Records Administration. (n.d.). Federal Register. Retrieved from http://www.archives.gov/federal-register

Weindling, P.J. (2006). *Nazi medicine and the Nuremberg trials: From medical war crimes to informed consent*. New York, NY: Palgrave Macmillan.

Wichman, A. (2012). Institutional review boards. In J.I. Gallin & F.P. Ognibene (Eds.), *Principles and practice of clinical research* (3rd ed., pp. 53–65). Boston, MA: Elsevier Academic Press. doi:10.1016/B978-0-12-382167-6.00005-9

Wood, L.P. (Ed.). (2011). *Merriam-Webster's dictionary of law*. Springfield, MA: Merriam-Webster.

World Medical Association. (2013a, April 6). Public to be consulted over changes to the WMA's Declaration of Helsinki. Retrieved from http://www.wma.net/en/40news/20archives/2013/2013_08

World Medical Association. (2013b, October). WMA Declaration of Helsinki—Ethical Principles for Medical Research Involving Human Subjects. Retrieved from http://www.wma.net/en/30publications/10policies/b3/index.html

Zoon, K.C., & Yetter, R.A. (2012). The regulation of drugs and biological products by the Food and Drug Administration. In J.I. Gallin & F.P. Ognibene (Eds.), *Principles and practice of clinical research* (3rd ed., pp. 79–90). Boston, MA: Elsevier Academic Press. doi:10.1016/B978-0-12-382167-6.00007-2

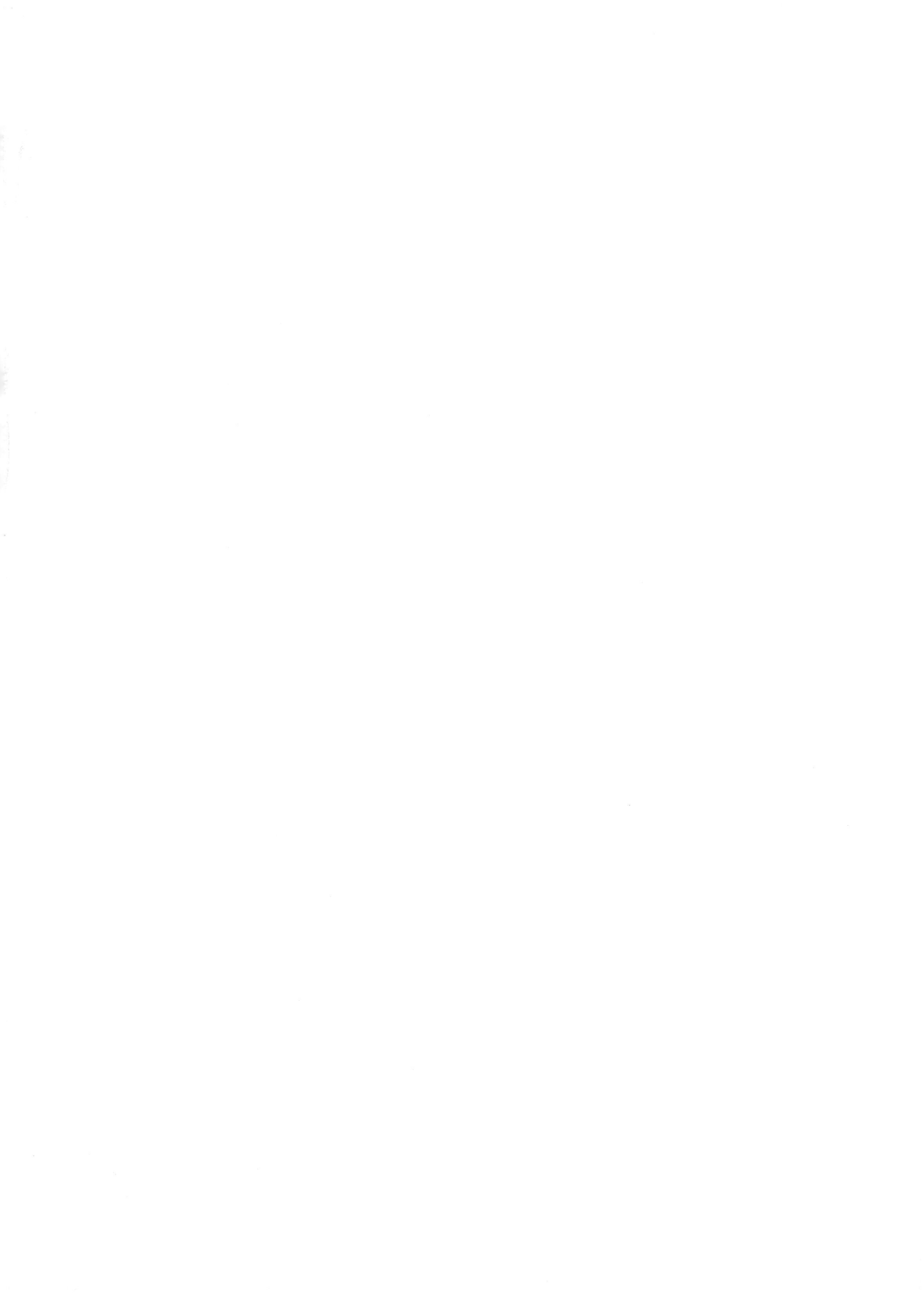

Chapter 9

Good Clinical Practice

Patricia C. Woltz, PhD, RN, and Anita Cizek Moore, MS, RN, CCRP

Introduction

How do clinicians know whether the new knowledge reported from a clinical study was based on valid data or whether the research was conducted in an ethical manner? *Good clinical practice* (GCP) in conducting research refers to a standard that ensures ethical and scientific quality in human subject research. GCP includes laws and regulations as well as internationally recognized standards that must be observed to ensure study quality. Thus, understanding GCP is critical for clinical trial nurses (CTNs) and others who are involved in clinical research operations.

This chapter reviews the origins of GCP to help readers understand how GCP is defined by institutional review boards (IRBs), the U.S. Food and Drug Administration (FDA), and the international research community. Key aspects of GCP are reviewed and resources are provided.

Background

The overarching objectives of GCP are to (a) protect study participants' rights, safety, and well-being and (b) ensure that trial data are credible. The evolution of providing these assurances of quality in human subject research has been guided by two forces that provide insight into the proscriptive nature of GCP: historical events of scientific misconduct and, more recently, economic globalization (see Figure 9-1).

In the aftermath of World War II, the Nuremberg Trials exposed horrific medical experiments carried out by doctors on concentration camp victims in Nazi Germany. The Nuremberg Code (1949) was the first internationally adopted document outlining a code of ethics and standards to which physicians were expected to conform when carrying out experiments on human subjects. Later, in 1964, the World Medical Association published the first version of the Declaration of Helsinki, which built upon the Nuremberg Code and emphasized the ethical principles of biomedical research with therapeutic intent involving human trial participants (World Medical Association, 2013).

Milestones in U.S. regulations governing protection of human subjects include passage of the Kefauver-Harris Amendments to the U.S. Food, Drug, and Cosmetic Act in 1962, following the discovery of a tragic link between fetal abnormalities and the use of thalidomide. The Kefauver-Harris Amendments required that written informed consent be obtained to participate in experimental treatments and that drug manufacturers demonstrate efficacy prior to obtaining market approval (U.S. FDA, 2014d), and, thus began the investigational new drug application (IND) process in the United States.

In 1979, the Belmont Report established boundaries between practice and research and served as an essential reference for IRBs reviewing federally funded human subject research proposals (National Commission for the Protection of Human Subjects of Biomedical and Behavioral Research [National Commission], 1979). The U.S. Department of Health and Human Services (DHHS) policy for the Protection of Human Research Subjects (2009) was revised in 1991 and codified in separate regulations by 15 federal departments and agencies; Subpart A is commonly referred to as the Common Rule (Protection of Human Research Subjects, 2009). In addition to DHHS regulations, FDA, a division of the DHHS, regulates clinical investigations of products under its jurisdiction (e.g., drugs, biologics, devices). FDA regulations are published in Title 21 Food and Drugs of the Code of Federal Regulations (C.F.R.) Part 50 (Protection of Human Subjects), Part 56 (Institutional Review Boards), Part 312 (Investigational New Drug Application), and Part 812 (Investigational Device Exemptions) (Office for Human Research Protections, n.d.).

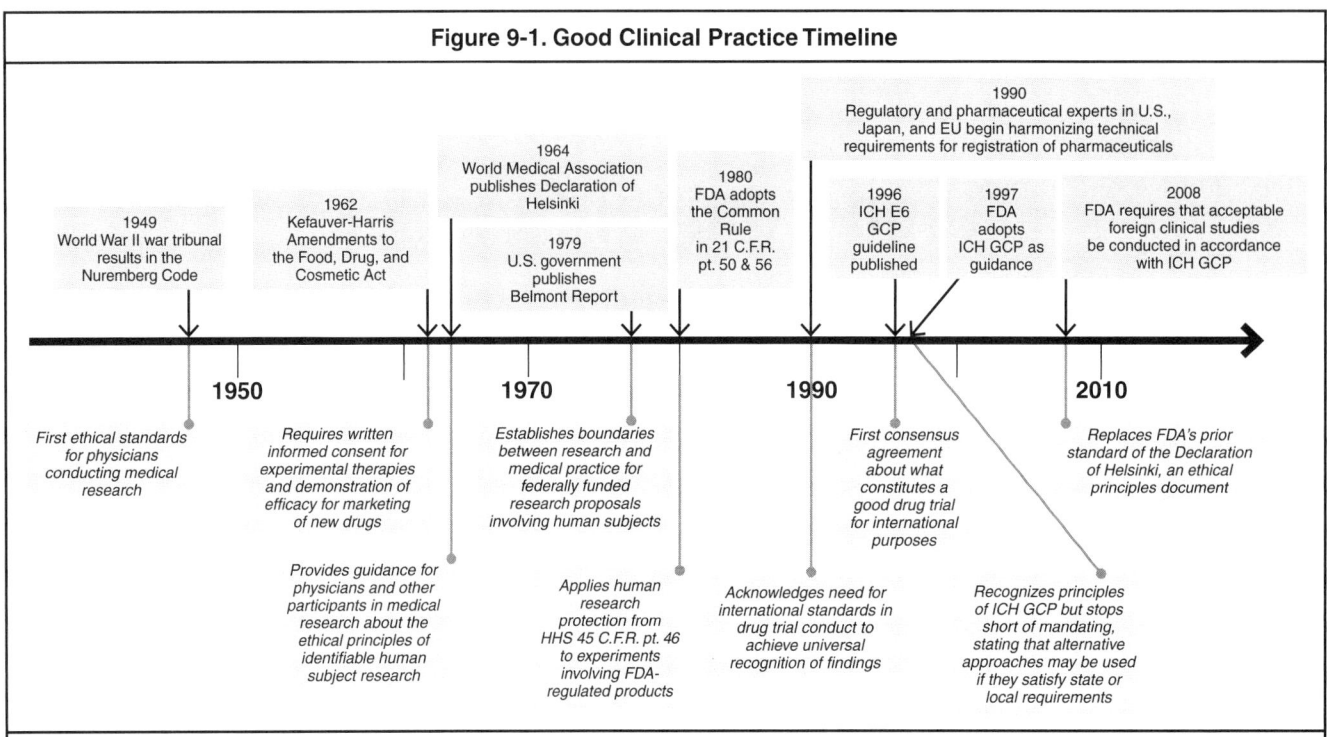

Figure 9-1. Good Clinical Practice Timeline

C.F.R.—*Code of Federal Regulations*; EU—European Union; FDA—U.S. Food and Drug Administration; GCP—good clinical practice; ICH—International Conference on Harmonisation of Technical Requirements for Registration of Pharmaceuticals for Human Use

Good Clinical Practice in a Global Economy

Economic globalization has affected the evolution of GCP. As costs associated with pharmaceutical research have risen, more industry-sponsored trials are being conducted overseas where trials are less expensive to conduct and participants may be more readily recruited (Glickman et al., 2009; U.S. FDA, 2004). Traditionally, strict FDA regulations rejected foreign study data as inferior; that led other countries interested in a share of the economic and intellectual drug development market to review their procedures for trial quality (Brynner & Stephens, 2001; Shah, 2003).

To streamline drug development and reduce or obviate duplicate testing, representative experts from regulatory bodies and the pharmaceutical industry in the European Union, Japan, and the United States embarked on a process in 1990 to develop a unified standard and harmonize the technical requirements for registration of pharmaceutical products in their collective countries. Using a process of expert working groups and consensus decision making, the collaboration gave rise to the International Conference on Harmonisation of Technical Requirements for Registration of Pharmaceuticals for Human Use (ICH, 2013b). ICH has created more than 50 harmonized guidelines organized in four topical categories: quality (Q), safety (S), efficacy (E), and multidisciplinary (M) (ICH, 2013a). These documents are maintained on the ICH website (www.ich.org).

The efficacy guideline, *ICH Harmonised Tripartite Guideline: Guideline for Good Clinical Practice* (ICH, 1996), is the experts' opinion about what constitutes best practices for clinical research conduct. The guideline was approved by the ICH Steering Committee in 1996. Within the year, the three ICH regions (the European Union, Japan, and the United States) had adopted similar, but not identical, versions of the ICH GCP. The European Union implemented the ICH GCP guideline as a legal directive in 1996 (ICH, 1996); Japan translated the document and legally enacted its version in 1997 (ICH, 2013a); and FDA adopted the E6 guideline as a guidance document (U.S. FDA, 1996). Following a controversial revision to the Declaration of Helsinki regarding the use of placebos in 2000, the FDA requirement for foreign studies that are used to support an IND or marketing application changed; the trials now need to be conducted in accordance with ICH GCP (U.S. FDA, 2008).

ICH defines *GCP* as "an international ethical and scientific quality standard for designing, conducting, recording and reporting trials that involve the participation of human subjects" (ICH, 1996, p. 1). Thus, the GCP guidelines provide a standard. A *standard* can be defined as that which represents accepted or mandated obligations, behaviors, and ethical expectations for one's profession (Duke Clinical Research Institute, 2010). The standard for clinical research conduct has evolved and is viewed as necessary to provide public assurance of trial participant protection and public and policymaker assurance that credible and reliable evidence exists for making informed decisions about medical practice and public health.

Despite differences among the versions of ICH GCP in the European Union, Japan, and the United States, the three regions agree that the underlying principles do not differ by region; most of the differences are without any real impact for the users (ICH, n.d.), and adherence to the standard is nevertheless crucial to maintaining the harmonization reached. Adherence to ICH GCP is required for all international submissions that are approved by regulatory agencies in the European Union, Japan, the United States, and Canada.

The ICH GCP standards are organized in eight sections: Glossary, Principles of ICH GCP, IRB, Investigator, Sponsor, Trial Protocol and Amendments, Investigator's Brochure, and Essential Documents. Key aspects of ICH GCP for investigative sites are outlined in Figure 9-2.

U.S. Food and Drug Administration Good Clinical Practice

FDA uses the term *GCP* somewhat differently than ICH. At FDA, *GCP* refers to a collection of regulations, guidance, and recommendations for clinical trials involving drugs, biologics, and medical devices that are under FDA authority (U.S. FDA, 2014c). The ICH GCP guideline is but one of many GCP guidance documents for FDA-regulated clinical trials (U.S. FDA, 2013). FDA chose to adopt the ICH GCP guideline without making it a regulation under the assumption that everything in the guideline is already contained in FDA regulations (U.S. FDA, 2014a). Unlike Title 21 of the C.F.R., which is legally binding and enforceable, implementation of ICH GCP is not mandatory for FDA-regulated research. For FDA, the ICH GCP document is to be used as a guide that represents its current thinking. FDA recognizes that an alternative approach to the guidance may be used if such an approach satisfies local and state requirements. FDA maintains a website (www.fda.gov/ScienceResearch/SpecialTopics/RunningClinicalTrials/GuidancesInformationSheetsandNotices/default.htm) that references its GCP requirements and recommendations. FDA also uses information sheets, which are guidance documents that give detail and instruction (U.S. FDA, 2014b).

Good Clinical Practice in Practice

Because FDA GCP is composed of regulations and guidances, FDA GCP and ICH GCP are not entirely equivalent. Generally, ICH GCP requirements are more rigorous and detailed than FDA regulations, but not always. See Table 9-1 for selected differences between ICH GCP and FDA requirements. These distinctions become important for CTNs who are involved in FDA-regulated research. However, it is increasingly true that even for research that is not FDA regulated, more IRBs are requiring that studies under their purview comply with ICH GCP. In particular, IRBs accredited by the Association for the Accreditation of Human Research Protection Programs require ICH GCP E6 guideline adherence (Kiskaddon, 2010). If CTNs are unsure of whether a study must comply with ICH GCP, they should check with the IRB and, if applicable, the study sponsor. The list of ICH GCP essential documents in the guideline individually and collectively are viewed as necessary for compliance with GCP to permit audit of study conduct; data quality is especially helpful in planning for operational procedures at study start-up (ICH, 1996). Other GCP resources that CTNs will find helpful are provided in Table 9-2.

Investigators, CTNs, and study team members must be fully aware of their obligations and responsibilities required by the sponsors, local oversight bodies, and applicable federal regulatory agencies prior to conducting research. Being fully educated and using checklists that provide a summary of responsibilities pertinent to data and document management in accordance with GCP guidance are highly recommended. GCP checklists provide a helpful starting point for preparing tools for adherence (see Figure 9-3).

Figure 9-2. Key Aspects of ICH Good Clinical Practice for Investigative Sites

- The objectives, design, conduct, analysis, and reporting of a clinical trial should be defined in a written protocol before the study starts. After it is approved, the protocol should be strictly followed.
- Protection of subjects is the shared responsibility of the investigator, the sponsor, and the institutional review board.
- Select, train, and keep a log of study team members with delegated responsibilities by investigator.
- Predict recruitment accurately and keep an up-to-date subject enrollment log.
- Pay particular attention to the ethical considerations of vulnerable populations and informed consent and scrupulously follow informed consent procedures.
- Report serious adverse events immediately to the sponsor.
- Precisely document product accountability.
- Diligently collect and record reliable study data.
- Keep all source documents and maintain organized files and archives.
- Keep everyone fully informed.
- The rights, safety, and well-being of the trial subjects should prevail over the interests of science and society.

Note. Based on information from International Conference on Harmonisation of Technical Requirements for Registration of Pharmaceuticals for Human Use, 1996.

Summary

Clinical trials are the scientific foundation for improving patient and public health outcomes. The ICH GCP guideline was established to provide international standardization for the conduct of clinical trials, to assure participants that they are properly protected and that trial data are credible, and to facilitate submission and approval of new medical products. It details the expectations of those who are responsible for the conduct of clinical research for FDA-regulated products. Although they do not address all trial situations (e.g., natural history, observational, non–investigational new drug trials), the guideline and the FDA resources and guidance documents provide ethical and scientific reference standards

Table 9-1. Selected Differences Between ICH GCP and FDA GCP Requirements		
Both ICH GCP and FDA GCP	**ICH GCP Guidelines**	**FDA GCP Requirements**
IRB reviews the informed consent, protocol, advertisements, and investigator's brochure.	IRB reviews recruitment procedures, written information provided to subjects, information about compensation, investigator's CV, and other documents evidencing qualifications (3.1.2).	Form FDA 1572 Statement of Investigator—requires investigator information, CV, lab, and IRB information and a signed statement of commitment (in accordance with 21 C.F.R. pt. 312, 21 C.F.R. pt. 50, and 21 C.F.R. pt. 56)
		Investigator agreement—Sponsors of device studies to obtain a signed investigator agreement (containing information similar to that requested on Form FDA 1572) from each participating investigator, per 21 C.F.R. § 812.43(c).
IRB is composed of at least five members, including one nonscientific member and one member not affiliated with the institution.	–	Diversity in race, gender, cultural backgrounds, and varying professional backgrounds (21 C.F.R. §§ 56.107(a)–(f))
–	Investigators maintain a list of appropriately qualified persons who have been delegated significant trial-related duties (4.1).	–
–	Investigators demonstrate potential for recruiting the required number of patients within the agreed recruitment period (4.2.1).	–
–	Investigators make every reasonable effort to ascertain the reason(s) for subject early withdrawal (4.3).	–
–	Investigators document and explain any deviation from the approved protocol (4.5.3).	–
Subjects sign, date, and receive a copy of the informed consent.	The copy that subjects receive must be signed and dated by the patient and the person obtaining consent (4.8.8).	The subject receives a copy of the consent. The subject (or LAR) signs and dates the informed consent form (21 C.F.R. § 50.25(a)(5)).
–	The informed consent should include the probability for random assignment (4.8.10(c)) and an explanation of the subject's responsibilities (4.8.10(e)).	–
–	The protocol identifies any data to be recorded directly on the CRF that will be considered source data (6.4.9).	–
–	Essential documents include Subject Screening Log, Subject Identification Code List, and Signature Sheet of persons authorized to make CRF entries (8.3).	Sponsors, IRBs, and investigators are required to permit FDA access to inspect and copy all records to an investigation (21 C.F.R. § 312.68; 21 C.F.R. § 812.145).

C.F.R.—Code of Federal Regulations; CRF—case report form; CV—curriculum vitae; FDA—U.S. Food and Drug Administration; GCP—good clinical practice; ICH—International Conference on Harmonisation of Technical Requirements for Registration of Pharmaceuticals for Human Use; IRB—institutional review board; LAR—legally authorized representative

Note. Based on information from Institutional Review Boards, 2013; International Conference on Harmonisation of Technical Requirements for Registration of Pharmaceuticals for Human Use, 1996; Investigational Device Exemptions, 2013; Investigational New Drug Application, 2013; Protection of Human Subjects, 2013.

Table 9-2. Recommended Good Clinical Practice (GCP) Resources		
Organization	GCP Information	Source
Association for the Accreditation of Human Research Protection Programs	Tip sheets and document library; training, IRB certification; free bimonthly newsletter; annual conference	www.aahrpp.org/apply/resources
Association of Clinical Research Professionals	Training and certification; membership services; free bimonthly and quarterly publications; annual global conference	www.acrpnet.org/FunctionalMenuCategory/AboutACRP_1.aspx
The Collaborative Institutional Training Initiative at the University of Miami	Training and certification	www.citiprogram.org/citidocuments/forms/Good
Office for Human Research Protections	Education; guidance; regulatory oversight; advice on regulatory and ethical issues	www.hhs.gov/ohrp
Oncology Nursing Society	Clinical trials nurse competencies that incorporate GCP concepts into behavioral activities	Lubejko, B., Good, M., Weiss, P., Schmieder, L., Leos, D., & Daugherty, P. (2011). Oncology clinical trials nursing: Developing competencies for the novice. *Clinical Journal of Oncology Nursing, 15*, 637–643. *Oncology Clinical Trials Nurse Competencies.* Retrieved from www.ons.org/sites/default/files/ctncompetencies.pdf
Public Responsibility in Medicine and Research	Training; certification; membership; public policy initiatives	www.primr.org/AboutUs.aspx?id=32
Society of Clinical Research Associates	Training, certification; membership services; quarterly publication; open access to selected past articles online; annual conference	www.socra.org
U.S. Food and Drug Administration	Guidance documents; information sheets; educational materials with references; conferences, meetings, and workshops	www.fda.gov/ScienceResearch/SpecialTopics/RunningClinicalTrials/default.htm www.fda.gov/ScienceResearch/SpecialTopics/RunningClinicalTrials/GuidancesInformationSheetsandNotices/default.htm www.fda.gov/ScienceResearch/SpecialTopics/RunningClinicalTrials/EducationalMaterials/ucm112925.htm
World Health Organization	GCP handbook	*Handbook for Good Clinical Research Practice: Guidance for Implementation.* Retrieved from www.who.int/medicines/areas/quality_safety/safety_efficacy/gcp1.pdf

from which best practices may be formulated. CTNs play an instrumental role in ensuring research participant safety and integrity in studies that lead to improved care. Knowledge of GCP is critical for all those involved in clinical research.

Key Points
- Use of GCP in clinical trial conduct is designed to protect participants' rights, safety, and well-being and ensure that the trial data are credible.
- ICH defines GCP as an international ethical and scientific quality standard for the design, conduct, performance, monitoring, auditing, recording, analyzing, and reporting of clinical trials.
- FDA GCP refers to a collection of regulations, guidances, and recommendations for clinical trials involving drugs, biologics, and medical devices that are under FDA authority.
- Investigators, CTNs, and other research team members conducting human subject research are required to know what constitutes proper study conduct as defined by local and federal oversight bodies and study sponsors.
- Recommended resources for GCP training and a sample GCP checklist have been provided.

References

Brynner, R., & Stephens, R. (2001). *Dark remedy: The impact of thalidomide and its revival as a vital medicine.* Cambridge, MA: Basic Books.

Duke Clinical Research Institute. (2010). Trial participation: Keys to building a successful research site. Retrieved from https://www

Figure 9-3. Sample Good Clinical Practice Review Checklist

Investigator:	Protocol:	Review Date:			Reviewer:
Institutional Review Board	Please check responses appropriately	Y	N	N/A	Comments
Dates	Initial submission to the IRB on file				
	Initial IRB approval letter				
	Protocol amendments? (keep all versions on file)				
	IRB approval letters?				
	IRB approval of advertising, questionnaires, other documentation				
	Full IRB approval of continuing review?				
	IRB annual approval letter?				
	Informed consent form approved? (keep all versions on file)				
	New approval dates on consent?				
	IRB has approved all study personnel?				
	Notification of restriction, suspension, or termination of study on file?				
Essential Documents	Please check responses appropriately	Y	N	N/A	Comments
Dates	FDA 1572 current, signed, dated, complete, correct? (keep all versions on file)				
	All subinvestigators listed?				
	CVs on file and updated every 2 years?				
	Site initiation training is documented?				
	Required training is current?				
	CITI, HIPAA, GCP?				
	Current medical licenses on file?				
	Financial disclosures on file?				
	Signatures and appropriate delegation of responsibility log of key personnel on file?				
	Protocol and accompanying SOPs available and current?				
	Signed agreement between investigator and sponsor on file?				
	Clinical laboratory certifications and normal ranges on file?				
	Current investigator brochure on file?				
	All communication with sponsor (electronic and written) kept with study records?				
	Progress reports to sponsor or other sites present in records?				

(Continued on next page)

	Figure 9-3. Sample Good Clinical Practice Review Checklist *(Continued)*				
	Screening and enrollment logs are present and reflect the conduct of the study?				
	Randomization procedures and participant logs are present and reflect the conduct of the study?				
Informed Consent Forms	**Please check responses appropriately**	**Y**	**N**	**N/A**	**Comments**
Dates:	Original signed and dated consent form found for each participant?				
	Consent form adequate (required elements present)?				
	Valid (IRB-approved) consent form used?				
	Patients re-consented when required?				
	HIPAA authorization signed and dated?				
	Appropriate use of LAR?				
	Evaluation of signed consent used?				
	Consent process documented in record?				
	Documentation that a copy of signed and dated consent form given to participant?				
	Consent obtained prior to study procedures?				
Eligibility	**Please check responses appropriately**	**Y**	**N**	**N/A**	**Comments**
Dates:	Eligibility checklist signed by investigator?				
	Did the participant meet all inclusion and exclusion criteria (and does source documentation authenticate this)?				
	Were all pre–enrollment/screening/baseline activities completed per protocol?				
	Is the actual number of enrolled subjects less than or equal to the total number of subjects IRB approved to enroll in study?				
	Did participant maintain eligibility?				
Protocol Adherence	**Please check responses appropriately**	**Y**	**N**	**N/A**	**Comments**
Date signed:	Copy of informed consent form on file?				
	Medical record alerted to notify patient's participation in a study to clinic staff?				
	Failure to meet inclusion/exclusion criteria?				
	Failure to perform study procedures or to obtain sponsor and IRB approval to deviate?				
	Unauthorized concomitant therapy used?				
	Other protocol nonadherence noted?				

(Continued on next page)

\multicolumn{7}{c}{Figure 9-3. Sample Good Clinical Practice Review Checklist *(Continued)*}

Treatment	Please check responses appropriately	Y	N	N/A	Comments
	Documentation of study arm patient randomized to?				
	Was the correct treatment regimen given?				
	Do all drug orders and administration records match (patients dosed properly per protocol)?				
	Correct treatment schedules followed? (correct days, doses, up and down times, dose modifications per protocol)				
	Diaries signed and dated by subject on file?				
Adverse Events	**Please check responses appropriately**	**Y**	**N**	**N/A**	**Comments**
	Master adverse event log available, current, and accurate (and matches source)?				
	Were type, grade, dates, duration, and investigator attribution of adverse events adequately recorded?				
	Were unanticipated events and serious adverse events reported correctly to the sponsor, IRB, FDA, and DSMB and within the required time frame per reporting requirement?				
	Out-of-range labs attributed as adverse events by the investigator?				
	Were adverse event–induced dose adjustments done per protocol and reasons documented for dose adjustments provided?				
	Were adverse events recorded on CRFs?				
Laboratory Tests	**Please check responses appropriately**	**Y**	**N**	**N/A**	**Comments**
	Were tests and procedures implemented approved by the IRB?				
	Were the labs and procedures documented in the study record (copy of test on file)?				
	If procedure was missed, was the reason properly documented on the master deviation log and reported to the sponsor, IRB, and DSMB?				
	Documentation of lab specimen collection and storage or shipping?				

(Continued on next page)

Figure 9-3. Sample Good Clinical Practice Review Checklist *(Continued)*					
Drug, Device, Test Article	**Please check responses appropriately**	**Y**	**N**	**N/A**	**Comments**
	Copy of drug order signed/dated by investigator listed on FDA 1572 in study record?				
	Medication administration record of study drug, pre- and post-drugs given per protocol (source documentation) in record?				
	Investigational drug or device used only on eligible subjects enrolled in the study after approved consent was signed?				
	Test article dispensed correctly (i.e., correct subject, drug, dose, route, time, frequency)?				
	All test article shipping and inventory records are present in the investigational drug services pharmacy or in study records?				
	Test article is stored in a secure location accessible only to study personnel or pharmacy?				
	Drug or device is stored according to conditions specified in protocol?				
	Adequate records of patient dispensing and returns?				
	Adequate documentation of transfers from pharmacy, study personnel, patients (chain of custody)?				
	Drug accountability properly documented with appropriate approvals from FDA or manufacturer?				
	Adequate records of disposition?				
General	**Please check responses appropriately**	**Y**	**N**	**N/A**	**Comments**
	Is follow-up of participants being done per protocol?				
	Are research charts and medical records organized?				
	Are data accurately recorded on the CRFs/database within 30 calendar days?				
	Reporting requirements per sponsor, IRB, FDA, and DSMB being followed?				
	Operating under SOPs written specifically for this protocol or for clinic operations?				
	Maintaining records of staff training on protocol, GCP, and area of research specialty?				
	Evidence of investigator involvement in conducting or supervising trial?				

(Continued on next page)

Figure 9-3. Sample Good Clinical Practice Review Checklist *(Continued)*

	Failure to document transfer of investigator responsibility for each research member (permitted tasks not listed)?				
	Continuing review with IRB did not expire?				
	Sponsor or monitoring reports on file?				
	Annual progress reports to sponsor, IRB, FDA, and DSMB on file?				
	Other (specify)?				

CITI—Collaborative Institutional Training Initiative; CRFs—case report forms; CVs—curricula vitae; DSMB—data and safety monitoring board; FDA—U.S. Food and Drug Administration; GCP—good clinical practice; HIPAA—Health Insurance Portability and Accountability Act of 1996; LAR—legally authorized representative; IRB—institutional review board; N—no; N/A—not applicable; SOPs—standard operating procedures; Y—yes

.dcri.org/trial-participation/KeysBuildingSuccessfulResearchSite.pdf/view

Glickman, S.W., McHutchison, J.G., Peterson, E.D., Cairns, C.B., Harrington, R.A., Califf, R.M., & Schulman, K.A. (2009). Ethical and scientific implications of the globalization of clinical research. *New England Journal of Medicine, 360,* 816–823. doi:10.1056/NEJMsb0803929

International Conference on Harmonisation of Technical Requirements for Registration of Pharmaceuticals for Human Use. (n.d.). E6 good clinical practice. Retrieved from http://www.ich.org/products/guidelines/efficacy/efficacy-single/article/good-clinical-practice.html

International Conference on Harmonisation of Technical Requirements for Registration of Pharmaceuticals for Human Use. (1996, June 10). *ICH harmonised tripartite guideline: Guideline for good clinical practice, E6(R1).* Retrieved from http://www.ich.org/fileadmin/Public_Web_Site/ICH_Products/Guidelines/Efficacy/E6/E6_R1_Guideline.pdf

International Conference on Harmonisation of Technical Requirements for Registration of Pharmaceuticals for Human Use. (2013a). Frequently asked questions: Work products. Retrieved from http://www.ich.org/about/faqs.html

International Conference on Harmonisation of Technical Requirements for Registration of Pharmaceuticals for Human Use. (2013b). History. Retrieved from http://www.ich.org/about/history.html

Institutional Review Boards, 21 C.F.R. pt. 56 (2013). Retrieved from http://www.accessdata.fda.gov/scripts/cdrh/cfdocs/cfcfr/CFRSearch.cfm?CFRPart=56&showFR=1

Investigational Device Exemptions, 21 C.F.R. pt. 812 (2013). Retrieved from http://www.accessdata.fda.gov/scripts/cdrh/cfdocs/cfcfr/CFRSearch.cfm?CFRPart=812&showFR=1

Investigational New Drug Application, 21 C.F.R. pt. 312 (2013). Retrieved from http://www.accessdata.fda.gov/scripts/cdrh/cfdocs/cfcfr/CFRSearch.cfm?CFRPart=312&showFR=1

Kiskaddon, S. (2010). From the president and CEO: Shift from Helsinki to ICH-GCP leads to single world standard. *AAHRPP Advance Newsletter.* Washington, DC: Association for the Accreditation of Human Research Protection Programs.

National Commission for the Protection of Human Subjects of Biomedical and Behavioral Research. (1979, April 18). *The Belmont report: Ethical principles and guidelines for the protection of human subject of research.* Retrieved from http://www.hhs.gov/ohrp/humansubjects/guidance/belmont.html

Nuremberg Code. (1949). In *Trials of war criminals before the Nuremberg military tribunals under Control Council Law No. 10* (Vol. 2, pp. 181–182). Retrieved from http://www.hhs.gov/ohrp/archive/nurcode.html

Office for Human Research Protections. (n.d.). Regulations. Retrieved from http://www.hhs.gov/ohrp/humansubjects

Protection of Human Research Subjects, 45 C.F.R. pt. 46 (2009). Retrieved from http://www.hhs.gov/ohrp/humansubjects/guidance/45cfr46.html

Protection of Human Subjects, 21 C.F.R. pt. 50 (2013). Retrieved from http://www.accessdata.fda.gov/scripts/cdrh/cfdocs/cfcfr/CFRSearch.cfm?CFRPart=50&showFR=1

Shah, S. (2003). Globalization of clinical research by the pharmaceutical industry. *International Journal of Health Services, 33*(1), 29–46.

U.S. Food and Drug Administration. (1996, April). *Guidance for industry E6 good clinical practice: Consolidated guidance.* Retrieved from http://www.fda.gov/downloads/Drugs/GuidanceComplianceRegulatoryInformation/Guidances/UCM073122.pdf

U.S. Food and Drug Administration. (2004, March). *Innovation or Stagnation: Challenge and opportunity on the critical path to new medical products.* Retrieved from http://www.fda.gov/downloads/ScienceResearch/SpecialTopics/CriticalPathInitiative/CriticalPathOpportunitiesReports/UCM113411.pdf

U.S. Food and Drug Administration. (2008, October 27). Human subject protection: Foreign clinical studies not conducted under an investigational new drug application—Notice of final rule. Retrieved from http://www.regulations.gov/#!documentDetail;D=FDA-2004-N-0061-0002;oldLink=false

U.S. Food and Drug Administration. (2013). ICH guidance documents. Retrieved from http://www.fda.gov/ScienceResearch/SpecialTopics/RunningClinicalTrials/GuidancesInformationSheetsandNotices/ucm219488.htm

U.S. Food and Drug Administration. (2014a, July 15). Clinical trials and human subject protection. Retrieved from http://www.fda.gov/ScienceResearch/SpecialTopics/RunningClinicalTrials/default.htm

U.S. Food and Drug Administration. (2014b). Information sheet guidance for institutional review boards (IRBs), clinical investigators, and sponsors. Retrieved from http://www.fda.gov/ScienceResearch/SpecialTopics/RunningClinicalTrials/GuidancesInformationSheetsandNotices/ucm113709.htm

U.S. Food and Drug Administration. (2014c, June 4). Selected FDA GCP/clinical trial guidance documents. Retrieved from http://www.fda.gov/ScienceResearch/SpecialTopics/RunningClinicalTrials/GuidancesInformationSheetsandNotices/ucm219433.htm

U.S. Food and Drug Administration. (2014d, March 25). Significant dates in U.S. food and drug law history. Retrieved from http://www.fda.gov/AboutFDA/WhatWeDo/History/Milestones/ucm128305.htm

World Medical Association. (2013). Declaration of Helsinki: Recommendations guiding physicians in biomedical research involving human subjects. Retrieved from http://www.wma.net/en/60about/70history/01declarationHelsinki

Chapter 10

The Research Team

Geri L. Schmotzer, RN, MSN, MPH, PhD, and Elizabeth Ness, RN, MS

Introduction

As the field of oncology has become increasingly complex, there has been a progressive movement toward the development of interdisciplinary teams to facilitate the development of research studies (Choi & Pak, 2007). The skills of many different experts are essential to effectively design and conduct a clinical trial. The key component of a successful clinical research program is a team of individuals who are committed to advancing patient care through the conduct of high-quality clinical trials. This team is responsible for the selection and implementation of good scientific protocols to meet the needs of specific patient populations. At the same time, the team must ensure the collection of quality data and the protection of the rights, interests, and safety of the patients, which remains the number-one priority in clinical research.

Central to the successful functioning of an interdisciplinary research team are seven key attributes: team purpose, goals, leadership, communication, cohesion, mutual respect, and reflection (Lakhani, Benzies, & Hayden, 2012). As Corbett et al. (2013) noted, successful interdisciplinary teams (a) have staff members who devote adequate time and energy, (b) conscientiously accept their significant responsibilities, (c) are suitably trained, committed members with appropriate time allocation, and (d) have the availability of adequate facilities to support clinical research activities. All members are essential across the board—whether the principal investigator (PI), subinvestigators, clinical trial nurses (CTNs), clinical trials office staff, clinical staff who perform patient assessment and treatment administration, pharmacy personnel, or laboratory personnel—as each plays a pivotal role and must possess the integrity, knowledge, and expertise necessary to conduct high-quality clinical trials. This chapter will highlight the roles and responsibilities of the key members of the clinical research team and the primary organizations involved in clinical trial conduct.

The clinical research team consists of professionals who are required to test the safety and efficacy of medicines, medical devices, and interventions so that the results of the investigational intervention can be made available for use with confidence on the public. Numbers and types of individuals may vary per clinical setting, but the primary functions needed to support good clinical practice (GCP) remain the same. All research teams are led by a PI and will have other key staff, including nurses, a study coordinator, and a clinical data manager, as well as research participants who are patients or healthy individuals who choose to participate in the clinical trial.

Additional members on the interdisciplinary team include all other individuals involved with clinical research activities: a statistician; personnel from the pharmacy, radiology department, and infusion center; and those who work in administrative roles such as contracting and billing (Baer, Zon, Devine, & Lyss, 2011).

Investigator

The only research team roles defined in the regulations and guidance documents are the investigator and subinvestigator. However, when multiple investigators are involved in a clinical trial, one is ultimately responsible for the overall conduct of the trial and the supervision of other research team members. This individual is referred to as the PI or investigator (with others referred to as subinvestigators) (see Table 10-1). For the purposes of this chapter, *PI* will be used.

The primary responsibility of the PI is to ensure the ethical conduct of the research study. This includes protecting research participants' rights, safety, and general welfare; complying with the protocol; providing valid quality data; and adhering to all institutional, state, and federal regulations. The PI is responsible for ensuring informed consent is appropriately obtained from each participant and for appropriately maintaining study records (Baer, Devine, Beardmore, & Catalano, 2011).

Table 10-1. Regulatory Definitions of Investigator

Position	Office for Human Research Protections	U.S. Food and Drug Administration	International Conference on Harmonisation
Investigator	Individual performing tasks related to the conduct of human subject research activities, such as obtaining informed consent from subjects, interacting with subjects, and communicating with the institutional review board. Any individual who is involved in conducting human subject research studies, including physicians, scientists, nurses, administrative staff, teachers, and students, among others.	An individual who actually conducts a clinical investigation under whose immediate direction the test article (i.e., drug, biologic, device) is administered, dispensed, or used on a subject. If the investigation is conducted by a team of individuals, the investigator is the responsible leader of the team.	A person responsible for the conduct of a clinical trial at a trial site.
Principal investigator	For research studies conducted by more than one investigator, one investigator is designated the "principal investigator" with overall responsibilities.	N/A	If a trial is conducted by a team of individuals at a trial site, the investigator is the responsible leader of the team and may be called the principal investigator.
Subinvestigator	N/A	Any individual member of the clinical trial team designated and supervised by the investigator at a trial site to perform critical trial-related procedures or to make important trial-related decisions (e.g., associates, residents, research fellows, clinical trial nurses).	Any individual member of the clinical trial team designated and supervised by the investigator at a trial site to perform critical trial-related procedures and/or to make important trial-related decisions (e.g., associates, residents, research fellows).

Note. Based on information from International Conference on Harmonisation of Technical Requirements for Registration of Pharmaceuticals for Human Use, 1996; Investigational Device Exemptions, 2013; Office for Human Research Protections, n.d.; Responsibilities of Sponsors and Investigators, 2013.

Office for Human Research Protections

According to the Office for Human Research Protections (OHRP), the role of all investigators is focused on protecting research participants. The PI is ultimately accountable for ensuring the conduct of the research study, including (OHRP, n.d.)
- Designing and implementing ethical research that is consistent with the three ethical principles delineated in the Belmont Report
- Complying with all applicable federal regulations related to the protection of human subjects
- Ensuring that all research involving human subjects is submitted to and approved by the appropriate institutional review board (IRB)
- Complying with all applicable IRB policies, procedures, decisions, conditions, and requirements
- Implementing research as approved and obtaining prior IRB approval for changes
- Obtaining and documenting informed consent and assent in accord with federal regulations and as approved by the IRB
- Reporting progress of approved research to the IRB as often and in the manner prescribed by the IRB
- Reporting to the IRB any injuries, adverse events, or other unanticipated problems involving risks to subjects or others
- Retaining signed consent documents and IRB research records for at least three years after completion of the research activity.

U.S. Food and Drug Administration

The U.S. Food and Drug Administration (FDA) regulations define the role of the investigator conducting clinical investigations of drugs or biologics in 21 C.F.R. pt. 312, subpt. D (Responsibilities of Sponsors and Investigators, 2013). However, many of those are included in section 9 of Form FDA 1572, *Statement of Investigator*, which lists the investigator's commitments (U.S. FDA, 2013). By signing this form, the PI agrees to
- Conduct the study with the current protocol and only make changes after notifying the sponsor
- Personally conduct or supervise the study
- Comply with informed consent requirements regarding the use of control participants and investigational drugs

- Report adverse events and understand the risks and potential side effects of the study drugs
- Ensure that all members of the investigation team understand their obligations regarding the aforementioned commitments
- Maintain and make available thorough and accurate records
- Communicate and seek IRB approval regarding changes in research activity and report unanticipated hazards to human subjects or others involved in the investigation.

FDA regulations define the role of the PI conducting clinical investigations of devices in 21 C.F.R. pt. 812, specifically §§ 812.43(c)(4) and 812.100, and include the requirement that there be a signed agreement between the PI and sponsor. Device regulations do not require the use of Form FDA 1572, although the agreements do contain similar information (Investigational Device Exemptions, 2013).

FDA has additional resources outlining the investigator's responsibilities, which are important for all research team members to review—specifically the investigators and CTNs. The first resource, *Guidance for Industry: Investigator Responsibilities—Protecting the Rights, Safety, and Welfare of Study Subjects* (U.S. FDA, 2009), provides an overview of the responsibilities of the PI who conducts a clinical investigation of a drug, biologic, or medical device. This guidance document provides information for the PI about supervisory activities associated with the conduct of a clinical trial, such as

- Appropriate delegation of study-related tasks (see section on delegation log), including
  - Adequate training for team members
  - Adequate supervision of the conduct of an ongoing clinical trial
  - Investigator's responsibilities for oversight of other parties involved in the conduct of a clinical trial
- Issues related to protecting the rights, safety, and welfare of study subjects, including
  - Reasonable medical care
  - Definition of reasonable access to medical care
  - Protocol violations that present unreasonable risk to research participants.

The second resource, *Information Sheet—Guidance for Sponsors, Clinical Investigators, and IRBs: Frequently Asked Questions—Statement of Investigator (Form FDA 1572)* (U.S. FDA, 2010), contains helpful tips to assist in the completion of the Form FDA 1572 and a device agreement. The CTN may be asked to assist in the completion of either type of agreement.

International Conference on Harmonisation Good Clinical Practice Guideline

The International Conference on Harmonisation of Technical Requirements for Registration of Pharmaceuticals for Human Use (ICH) *Guideline for Good Clinical Practice* (ICH, 1996) describes in detail the responsibilities of the PI. The CTN, as well as all research team members, should review the ICH CGP guidelines. The 13 general categories are as follows.

- Investigator qualifications and agreements
- Adequate resources
- Medical care of trial subjects
- Communication with the IRB
- Compliance with the protocol
- Investigational product
- Randomization procedures and unblinding
- Informed consent
- Records and reports
- Safety reporting
- Progress reports
- Premature termination or suspension of a trial
- Final report

National Cancer Institute

The National Cancer Institute (NCI) Division of Cancer Treatment and Diagnosis (DCTD) is responsible for funding and sponsoring (i.e., having regulatory accountability to the FDA) cancer research, specifically clinical trials to evaluate new anticancer agents. One of DCTD's major programs is the Cancer Therapy Evaluation Program (CTEP). Many oncology CTNs will be involved in CTEP-funded or sponsored clinical trials. The CTEP website (http://ctep.info.nih.gov) is an excellent resource. One item provided on the website is *A Handbook for Clinical Investigators Conducting Therapeutic Clinical Trials Supported by CTEP, DCTD, NCI* (NCI, 2014). This handbook provides very useful, practical information for anyone involved in CTEP clinical trials, including phases of clinical trials, protocol drafting and submissions (e.g., the letter of intent process), reporting requirements (e.g., adverse event reporting using the CTEP Adverse Event Reporting System), agent accountability, PI and research sites' responsibilities for single-site or multisite research, and audit procedures (NCI, 2014).

All investigators participating in NCI-sponsored clinical trials must register with NCI and renew their registration annually. Registration requires completion and submission of the following documents:

- Form FDA 1572 specific for CTEP studies (OMB No. 0925-0613)
- Supplemental investigator data form
- Financial disclosure form
- Current curriculum vitae.

Specific forms are found at http://ctep.cancer.gov/investigatorResources/investigator_registration.htm.

The Pharmaceutical Management Branch, a branch within CTEP, manages the registration for physician investigators. An NCI investigator number will be assigned to the investigator. The investigator number is necessary to obtain investigational agents that are supplied through NCI (2013).

Delegation Log

Although the PI is responsible for the oversight of clinical trials, certain tasks can be delegated to other appropriately trained staff. The challenge is to know what tasks can be delegated because it can vary based on the staff member's experience and licensure. To ensure that program resources are being appropriately used, personnel should be matched to tasks based on training and licensure so that they continue to enjoy and be challenged by the work and their responsibilities (Baer, Zon, et al., 2011). Each staff member's responsibilities should be documented in a task delegation log. The purpose of this log is to ensure that the individuals performing study-related tasks and procedures are appropriately trained and authorized by the PI. This log should be completed before the initiation of any study-related tasks and procedures for all individuals' delegated tasks. The PI is responsible for maintaining the delegation log of qualified study personnel to whom trial-related duties have been assigned. According to the FDA guidance document,

> This list should also describe the delegated tasks, identify the training that individuals have received that qualifies them to perform delegated tasks (e.g., can refer to an individual's CV on file), and identify the dates of involvement in the study. An investigator should maintain separate lists for each study conducted by the investigator. (U.S. FDA, 2009, pp. 2–3)

The PI often delegates this activity to the CTNs.

Subinvestigator

Some research studies may be conducted by more than one investigator; however, only the PI has primary responsibility for the study conduct. The subinvestigator, also referred to as a co-investigator, may perform all or some of the PI functions. A subinvestigator works under the supervision of the PI and is responsible for conducting all study-related procedures and making important study-related decisions in compliance with the ethical conduct of the study (ICH, 1996; Responsibilities of Sponsors and Investigators, 2013). Subinvestigators may include associate physicians, research fellows, residents, or even CTNs.

Research Participant

Every study will have research participants who are an essential part of the research team. A patient or a healthy volunteer may choose to participate in research for many reasons (Shannon-Dorcy & Drevdahl, 2011). Trust in the study physician, ability to receive medical care, and advancing medical science are noted by Truong, Weeks, Cook, and Joffe (2011) as reasons for participating in clinical trials. Because clinical research is a partnership between the participants and the research team, when individuals enroll in a research study, they agree to follow the study requirements. The following is a list of research participant responsibilities as proposed by Resnik and Ness (2012).

- Respect investigators, research staff, and other participants.
- Read the consent form and other documents. Ask questions if something about the study or the rights of the research participants are not understood or if more information is needed.
- Carefully weigh the risks and benefits when deciding whether to participate in the study.
- Refrain from signing the consent document until content is understood and the decision to participate feels comfortable.
- Follow directions for proper use, dosing, and storage of self-administered study medications; providing biologic samples; and preparing for tests, procedures, or examinations.
- Follow directions for abstaining from non-study-related medications or other contraindicated medications or procedures.
- Know when the study begins and ends. This is particularly important for an intervention trial that has a follow-up period after the intervention is completed.
- Attend scheduled appointments on time and inform the staff within a reasonable time if an appointment needs to be rescheduled.
- Provide truthful answers to questions asked during screening and enrollment and during the study.
- Inform staff if other medical care is needed while on the study.
- Inform staff if there are questions they would rather not answer.
- Report pain, discomfort, nausea, dizziness, and other problems and symptoms experienced during the study.
- Keep information about the study confidential if asked to do so.
- Keep staff informed when contact information (e.g., phone number, address) changes.
- Inform staff and follow the procedures if they decide to withdraw from the study.

Promoting participant responsibility is a task best accomplished by everyone on the research team. Participants should be provided with accurate study information and their questions should be answered honestly; the team should stress the importance of following the study protocol. Nurses have always excelled at patient education; for CTNs, this is in the context of clinical research.

The Nurse's Role

Nurses have held a strong role in clinical research that has been integral to research conduct at every level, from providing patient care, to coordinating studies, to designing and implementing their own programs of research (i.e., nurse scientists). Nurses are involved in research in both the public and private sectors, and the role varies considerably depending on the setting (Grady & Edgerly, 2009).

Historical Perspective

Despite a dramatic increase in the complexity and number of clinical trials over the past 25–30 years, the role of the nurse in research, outside of that of the nurse scientist, remains poorly defined and underrecognized (Bell, 2009). The first roles for oncology nurses in the United States were those associated with cancer research in the 1960s, during the very early clinical trials of chemotherapy. Nurses needed to develop new skills and knowledge and assume a new, collaborative role with physicians in the care of patients enrolled in clinical trials (Hubbard & DeVita, 1976; Moore, 1978; Suppers, Yarbro, & Mayer-Scogna, 1979).

In the 1980s, the integral role of the research nurse in the cancer research setting in relationship to other nursing roles was fully described (Gross, 1986; Henke, 1980; Hubbard, 1982; Hubbard & Donehower, 1980). The responsibilities of the research nurse were made explicit and described as they related to the development of a new cancer chemotherapeutic agent. Other nursing specialties began to describe this emerging role (Mullin, 1984).

The early 1990s saw further descriptions of the oncology research nurse role and activities (Cassidy & Macfarlane, 1991; Engelking, 1991, 1992; Hazelton, 1991; McEvoy, Cannon, & MacDermott, 1991; Melink & Whitacre, 1991). Wheeler (1991) described the process of preparing nursing staff for successful implementation of a protocol, whereas other authors focused on the oncology nurse's emerging role in data management (Cassidy, 1993; White-Hershey & Nevidjon, 1990). Subsequent articles identified and acknowledged research nurse involvement in the informed consent process (Berry, Dodd, Hinds, & Ferrell, 1996; Rosse & Krebs, 1999). Others began to investigate the research nurse's role, responsibilities, and contributions to clinical research (Freedman, 1998; Xanthos, Carp, & Geromanos, 1998). Although the amount of literature surrounding the role of the research nurse increased during the 1990s, it remained primarily anecdotal.

In early 2000, a shift was evident as more critical and substantive literature began to emerge surrounding the role of the research nurse. Ocker and Pawlik-Plank (2000) used a case study to explain how the research nurse role was systematically developed and integrated into a clinic-based oncology research setting. During the development phase, they identified several research nurse roles that incorporated the nursing process: educator, patient advocate, and protocol manager. Final implementation and integration of the research nurse in their setting led to increased job satisfaction for both research nurses and oncology nurse clinicians. In another study, Burnett et al. (2001) surveyed nurses' attitudes and beliefs toward cancer clinical trials at a comprehensive cancer center.

The CTN Special Interest Group of the Oncology Nursing Society (ONS) provided a major contribution to the literature by publishing the first edition of the *Manual for Clinical Trials Nursing* in 2000 (Klimaszewski et al., 2000). This was the first comprehensive nursing work that included CTNs from across the globe. The manual was designed to address the needs of novice CTNs while appealing to the sensibilities of experts.

Also in 2000, a CTN SIG working group began looking at developing a valid and reliable tool to assess the role of the research nurse within oncology. The outcome of this work was the development of the Clinical Trial Nurse Questionnaire (CTNQ) (Ehrenberger & Lillington, 2004). The CTNQ has since been used by others to further define the roles and responsibilities of nurses in clinical research (Catania et al., 2011; Catania, Poire, Dozin, Bernardi, & Boni, 2008; Nagel, Gender, & Bonner, 2010; Wilkes, Jackson, Miranda, & Watson, 2012).

In 2007, the National Institutes of Health (NIH) Clinical Center Nursing Department began a four-year initiative to define and delineate the practice within the specialty of clinical research nursing. One of the first activities they pursued was to develop a taxonomy for the specialty of clinical research nursing practice. Using a Delphi approach, the researchers developed and validated the overall domain of practice for clinical research nursing to include care provided to research participants, as well as coordination of care and services, and activities to support protocol implementation, data collection, human subject protection, and participation in team science (see Table 10-2). Within the 5 domains of practice, 52 activities were identified within the specialty of clinical research nursing. The clinical research nursing practice domain was further conceptualized to define and name two distinct roles and responsibilities performed by nurses practicing in clinical research settings. These represent the two main nursing roles in the clinical research setting: one largely involved with patient care (clinical research nurse) and the other role mainly engaged with study coordination (research nurse coordinator) (Bevans et al., 2011; Castro et al., 2011; Hastings, Fisher, & McCabe, 2012).

What's In a Name?

Confusion over the titles and responsibilities of nurses working in the research arena has persisted. Until recently, no standardized terminology delineated the roles of nurses within the clinical research infrastructure, with respect to nurses who provide direct patient care in a research setting or those who coordinate studies in a clinical setting (Hastings et al., 2012). Titles for licensed nurses working in clinical research vary greatly and have included research nurse, research nurse coordinator, clinical trial nurse, clinical research nurse, study coordinator, clinical research coordinator, and study nurse. Some of these titles (e.g., study coordinator, clinical research coordinator) can apply to either licensed nurses or unlicensed personnel who coordinate or support clinical research (Bevans et al., 2011; Hastings et al., 2012).

In order to achieve the best possible outcomes for study participants, all nurses involved in clinical research need well-developed critical-thinking skills, expert clinical skills, and an understanding of the complex regulatory, ethical, and scientific aspects of clinical research. To ensure the study objectives are met, the clinical research nurse or CTN manages activities listed in subsequent sections while maintaining the principles of participant rights, patient safety, and continuity of care (Hastings et al., 2012).

Clinical Trial Nurse

CTNs are nurses who safeguard the clinical trial's integrity while managing the activities of the study participants, often providing case management activities for patient participants. The role currently varies within each research site, as may the job title (e.g., research nurse coordinator, clinical research nurse, study coordinator, protocol coordinator). Figure 10-1 indicates CTNs' primary responsibilities and key team members with whom they interact to manage the clinical trials.

CTNs are usually responsible for study coordination and data management activities, including subject recruitment and enrollment, eligibility screening, informed consent education or counseling, and ensuring that informed consent was obtained. They maintain consistent activities in relation to the study's implementation, data integrity and management, and compliance with regulatory requirements and reporting. Some CTNs may also provide direct patient participant care.

Given the complex nature of cancer clinical trials, it is the position of ONS that the coordination of clinical trials (e.g., coordination of clinical sites, development of standardized treatment orders, symptom management, patient education and advocacy, facilitation of informed consent, assistance with participant accrual and retention) is accomplished best by nurses who have been educated and certified in oncology nursing (ONS, 2009).

As a result, members of the ONS CTN SIG formed a project team that developed core competencies for a comprehensive curriculum on clinical trials and the standardization of the CTN role, which were published in 2010. Here, *CTN* is defined as "the specialty nursing role requiring a unique framework of knowledge for working with patients involved in clinical research trials" (ONS, 2010, p. 5), with acknowledgment that the role has multiple names as previously identified.

Using the existing literature, the *Manual for Clinical Trials Nursing*, various job descriptions, training manuals from the cancer cooperative groups, and research management curricula, the project team proposed a draft set of CTN competencies. These competencies were distributed to ONS members who identified themselves as CTNs. After reviewing the surveys, the team defined 11 functional areas with more than 100 behaviors novice CTNs should acquire and possess during the first two years in their role as a CTN. After a field review, the competencies were further revised, resulting in 68 competencies. These competencies were sent for expert review, and the final core competencies, published in 2010, included 9 functional areas and 54 competencies (see Appendix 2) (Lubejko et al., 2011). CTNs should perform a self-assessment of the competencies to identify gaps. Throughout this manual, the role of the CTN will continue to be highlighted.

Clinical Research Nurse

The clinical research nurse, as defined by Hastings et al. (2012), is primarily concerned with the care of the research participant. This nurse supports the study activities within a patient care setting, such as the NIH Clinical Center, Clinical and Translational Science Award sites, General Clinical Research Centers, academic medical centers, or specialty care programs (e.g., oncology, cardiology) with a clinical research focus. Nurses who care for research participants may be the first to work with these patients on the actual delivery and management of a new experimental treatment. The clinical research nurse provides nursing care to research participants while taking into account the study requirements, as well as the collection of research data, the clinical indications, and patient care needs (Grady & Edgerly, 2009). In some settings, the clinical research nurse may be referred to as a staff nurse or a direct care nurse. Responsibilities include (Grady & Edgerly, 2009)
- Sharing clinical research information and general education with patients and other healthcare professionals outside the research team
- Collaborating with other facilities in the patient care of research participants

Table 10-2. The Domain of Clinical Research Nursing Practice

Dimension	Definition
Clinical practice	Provision of nursing care, education, and support, using the nursing process, to participants in clinical research and their families and significant others. Care requirements are determined by the scope of study participation, the clinical condition of the patient, and the requirements and clinical effects of research procedures and data collection.
Study management	Management of clinical and research support activities to ensure patient safety, address clinical needs, and ensure protocol integrity and accurate data collection.
Care coordination and continuity	Coordination of research and clinical activities to meet clinical needs, complete study requirements, and manage linkage with referring and primary care providers.
Human subjects protection	Facilitation of informed participation by diverse participants in clinical research.
Contributing to the science	Contributions as a research team member to the development of new ideas for study, explorations of innovations arising for clinical research, and application of clinical research findings to practice.

The overall domain of practice includes care provided to research participants, as well as coordination of care and services, and activities to support protocol implementation, data collection, human subject protection, and participation in team science.

Note. From "Clinical Research Nursing: A Critical Resource in the National Research Enterprise," by C.E. Hastings, C.A. Fisher, and M.A. McCabe, 2012, *Nursing Outlook, 60*, p. 152.e143. doi:10.1016/j.outlook.2011.10.003. Copyright 2012 by Elsevier. Reprinted with permission.

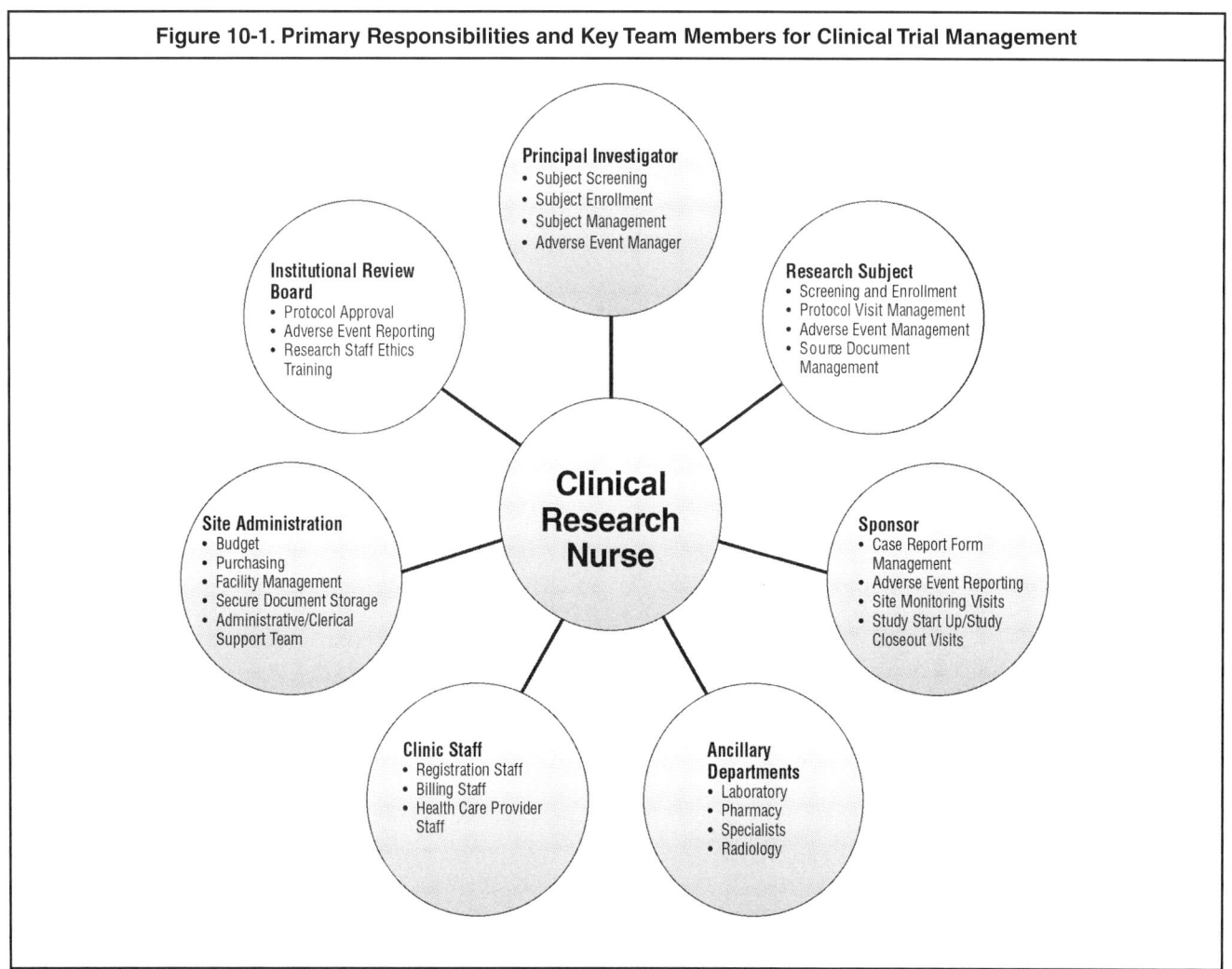

Figure 10-1. Primary Responsibilities and Key Team Members for Clinical Trial Management

Note. From "The Essential Role of the Clinical Research Nurse (CRN)," by R.D. Poston and C.R. Buescher, 2010, *Urologic Nursing, 30*, p. 56. Copyright 2010 by Society of Urologic Nurses and Associates, Inc. Reprinted with permission.

- Administering study medications, both investigational and those commercially available
- Performing detailed clinical assessments
- Collecting research samples
- Communicating with the research team study staff regarding observed results
- Reporting adverse events to the PI.

In 2007, the Research Society at the Royal College of Nursing in the United Kingdom began work formulating a framework to assist in the development of the skills, behavior, knowledge, and understanding required by nurses who support clinical research. The first edition of the *Competency Framework for Clinical Research Nurses* was published in 2008, followed by a second edition in 2011 and a revised second edition in 2013. In the context of this framework, *clinical research nurse* "refers to any nurse who is employed principally to undertake research within the clinical environment. This can include a variety of nursing roles, but they all share the common feature that research is a central part of their employment" (p. 9). The competency document defines current expectations of the clinical research nurse working at various levels, or bands, of seniority and is adaptable to meet the needs at all research settings and for various levels of seniority throughout the United Kingdom (Royal College of Nursing Research Society, 2013).

Clinical Research Coordinator

In some research settings, a non-nurse will provide study coordination activities. This role is often referred to as *clinical research coordinator*, though many aliases exist for this role as well (e.g., study coordinator). The clinical research coordinator has many roles similar to those of the CTN, primarily assisting with the management of multiple clinical trials and working directly with a PI or for a clinical trials office. Clinical research coordinators are responsible for the overall management and implementation of clinical research protocols while ensuring compliance, efficiency, and the safety and welfare of study participants (Speicher et al., 2012). Typical responsibilities are found in Figure 10-2. CTNs may see overlap with their activities. Both nurse and non-nurse study coordinators can benefit from learning more about project management, which provides knowledge, skills, and techniques to effectively and efficiently implement projects—the clinical research coordinator's project is study coordination.

Although the clinical research coordinator can assist in the management of a clinical trial, it is important for the CTN to know which research roles can be delegated. In some states, unlicensed personnel cannot administer or dispense medication or provide patient participant education; some organizations do not allow unlicensed personnel to document in the medical record. Therefore, prudent CTNs will become familiar with their state board of nursing's regulations regarding the use of unlicensed personnel (Weydt, 2010).

Clinical Data Manager

Some research teams will have a clinical data manager who is responsible for activities including data extraction, data entry, and data quality assurance. This role may have other aliases: clinical research associate, research assistant, or simply, data manager. The clinical data manager assists in the collection and management of subject data while complying with regulatory standards. The primary goal of the clinical data manager is to provide high-quality data by keeping the number of errors and delinquent data as low as possible and gathering maximum data for analysis (Kirishnankutty, Bellary, Kumar, & Moodahadu, 2012). See Chapter 38 for more details on the role of the clinical data manager and data management activities. The CTN may also take on the activities associated with this role.

The Interdisciplinary Team

The interdisciplinary team, as a whole, plays an integral role in the performance of specific requirements of designated clinical trials. These individuals are vital to the overall success of the clinical trial. Without their support, it would be extremely difficult, if not impossible, to ensure protocol compliance.

Pharmacy staff needs to be involved from the start of a clinical trial so that they know what is expected regarding drug preparation, storage, and accountability. The research pharmacist promotes patient safety, regulatory compliance, and safe conduct of human research with protocols involving investigational drugs and provides expert consultation to investigators. In addition, pharmacists prepare and dispense investigational medications, assist with the preparation of pharmacy budgets, serve as a resource for investigational drug-related questions, and maintain the drug inventory, accountability documentation, and study blinding (Formea, n.d.). Some organizations will have dedicated research pharmacies/pharmacists, or this may be delegated to others (e.g., another physician).

For any protocol in which an investigational agent is supplied, the PI is held accountable for ensuring its appropriate distribution and for meticulous record keeping with respect to storage, shipping, and distribution. This includes documentation of drug accountability demonstrating shipment (e.g., date and quantity received) and dispensing information (e.g., subject

Figure 10-2. Responsibilities of the Clinical Research Coordinator (CRC)	
Core CRC Responsibilities • Adherence to an IRB-approved protocol • Participation in the proper consenting of study subjects • Support of the safety of clinical research subjects • Coordination of clinical treatment, study visits, and follow-up care • Subject screening, recruitment, and enrollment • Maintenance of study source documents • Proper reporting of adverse events	**Additional CRC Responsibilities** • Submissions to regulatory authorities (e.g., IRB, FDA) • Regulatory documentation development and management • Completion of case report forms (paper and electronic data capture) • Coordination of prestudy, initiation, and monitoring visits • Collection, processing, and shipping of laboratory specimens • Maintenance of drug accountability documentation • Study budget preparation • Management of study finances, including resolving study subject billing issues • Acting as liaison for research subjects, investigator, IRB, sponsor, and healthcare professionals
FDA—U.S. Food and Drug Administration; IRB—institutional review board	
Note. From "The Critical Need for Academic Health Centers to Assess the Training, Support, and Career Development Requirements of Clinical Research Coordinators: Recommendations from the Clinical and Translational Science Award Research Coordinator Taskforce," by L.A. Speicher, G. Fromell, S. Avery, D. Brassil, L. Carlson, E. Steven, and M. Toms, 2012, *Clinical and Translational Science, 5,* p. 471. doi:10.1111/j.1752-8062.2012.00423.x. Copyright 2012 by John Wiley and Sons. Reprinted with permission.	

identifies, lot number, expiration date, date dispensed, quantity, who dispensed) (Responsibilities of Sponsors and Investigators, 2013). Although these responsibilities may be handled by anyone licensed to distribute medications, a designated research pharmacist has the capability, knowledge, and expertise to handle these responsibilities in the most efficient and thorough manner. A research pharmacist can also be instrumental in the initial review of the protocol and a tremendous resource with staff education and training.

Depending upon the nature of the protocol, other interdisciplinary team members may include physicians from other departments (e.g., other specialties such as radiation therapy, surgery, urology, and nuclear medicine), physicians within a specialized training program (e.g., residents, fellows), nurse practitioners, physician associates, and designated clinical support staff. These individuals provide treatments that are specific to their areas of expertise. Appropriate protocol information must be shared to ensure that all aspects of the protocol, with respect to the procedures and treatments, can be administered appropriately.

Diagnostic radiology frequently is part of the interdisciplinary team because of the ongoing disease assessments that are critical to the evaluation of the protocol treatment (e.g., tumor measurements). For many clinical trials, it is necessary to identify both a designated and a backup radiologist who will assume responsibility for all diagnostic evaluations at the site. These individuals need to be kept abreast of potential clinical trial candidates and the status and required evaluations for previously registered patients.

Central laboratory services personnel (e.g., pathologists, laboratory directors, technicians) provide protocol support for biopsies, tumor resections, and specimen collections. Before an institution decides whether to participate in a clinical trial requiring laboratory services, the protocol must be reviewed by a laboratory representative to ensure that the services involved can be provided. Because of the support they provide with respect to equipment and facilities, they often are called upon to collect and prepare specimens, centrifuge body fluids, provide specimen storage (e.g., –20°C or –70°C freezer space), handle or assist with specimen shipping, or provide necessary supplies (e.g., International Air Transport Association–approved containers, dry ice, packing materials, shipping labels). All protocol-specific instructions and supplies (e.g., containers, collection devices) must be given to the appropriate laboratory personnel either in bulk or on a per-patient basis—whichever is most suitable to meet their needs and ensure protocol compliance (National Institute of Allergy and Infectious Diseases, 2013).

Summary

Each team member has his or her own function, and developing a functional staff is essential to the success of a quality research program. Effective management is critical and requires a commitment to mutual respect, effective communication, and acknowledgment of each member's value to the team.

Key Points
- The ethical conduct of clinical research requires an interdisciplinary clinical research team.
- The overall success of a clinical trial depends upon the interdisciplinary team and can include professionals from radiology, pharmacy, laboratory services, and others (e.g., administrative personnel).
- The primary responsibility of the PI is to ensure the ethical conduct of the research study.

- Many different job titles describe the individual who provides study coordination activities and the individual who provides direct care to the research participant.
- Nurses have held a strong role in clinical research and have been integral to research conduct at every level from providing patient care to coordinating studies to designing and implementing their own programs of research.
- ONS *Oncology Clinical Trials Nurse Competencies* are available and should be reviewed and incorporated into practice.

The authors would like to thank Heidi E. Deininger, PhD, RN, AOCN®, for the beginning portion of the historical perspective section of this chapter, which was taken from Chapter 51 of the second edition of this book.

References

Baer, A.R., Devine, S., Beardmore, C.D., & Catalano, R. (2011). Clinical investigator responsibilities. *Journal of Oncology Practice, 7,* 124–128. doi:10.1200/jop.2010.000216

Baer, A.R., Zon, R., Devine, S., & Lyss, A.P. (2011). The clinical research team. *Journal of Oncology Practice, 7,* 188–192. doi:10.1200/jop.2011.000276

Bell, J. (2009). Towards clarification of the role of research nurses in New Zealand: A literature review. *Nursing Praxis in New Zealand, 25,* 4–16.

Berry, D., Dodd, M., Hinds, P., & Ferrell, B. (1996). Informed consent: Process and clinical issues. *Oncology Nursing Forum, 23,* 507–512.

Bevans, M., Hastings, C., Wehrlen, L., Cusack, G., Matlock, A.M., Miller-Davis, C., ... Wallen, G.R. (2011). Defining clinical research nursing practice: Results of a role delineation study. *Clinical and Translational Science, 4,* 421–427. doi:10.1111/j.1752-8062.2011.00365.x

Burnett, C., Koczwara, B., Pixley, L., Blumenson, L., Hwang, Y., & Meropol, N. (2001). Nurses' attitudes toward clinical trials at a comprehensive cancer center. *Oncology Nursing Forum, 28,* 1187–1192.

Cassidy, J. (1993). The role of the data manager in clinical cancer research: An opportunity for nurses. *Cancer Nursing, 16,* 131–138. doi:10.1097/00002820-199304000-00008

Cassidy, J., & Macfarlane, D.K. (1991). The role of the nurse in clinical cancer research. *Cancer Nursing, 14,* 124–131. doi:10.1097/00002820-199106000-00002

Castro, K., Bevans, M., Miller-Davis, C., Cusack, G., Loscalzo, F., Matlock, A., ... Hastings, C. (2011). Validating the clinical research nursing domain of practice [Online exclusive]. *Oncology Nursing Forum, 38,* E72–E80. doi:10.1188/11.ONF.E72-E80

Catania, G., Poire, I., Bernardi, M., Bono, L., Cardinale, F., & Dozin, B. (2011). The role of the clinical trial nurse in Italy. *European Journal of Oncology Nursing, 16,* 97–93. doi:10.1016/j.ejon.2011.04.001

Catania, G., Poire, I., Dozin, B., Bernardi, M., & Boni, L. (2008). Validating a measure to delineate the clinical trials nursing role in Italy. *Cancer Nursing, 31,* E11–E15. doi:10.1097/01.NCC.0000305761.11980.cc

Choi, B.C.K., & Pak, A.W.P. (2007). Multidisciplinary, interdisciplinary, and transdisciplinarity in health research, services, education and policy: 2. Promotors, barriers, and strategies of enhancement. *Clinical and Investigative Medicine, 30,* e224–e232. Retrieved from http://cimonline.ca/index.php/cim/article/viewFile/2950/1067

Corbett, C.F., Costa, L.L., Balas, M.C., Burke, W.J., Feroli, E.R., & Daratha, K.B. (2013). Facilitators and challenges to conducting interdisciplinary research. *Medical Care, 51,* S23–S31. doi:10.1097/MLR.1090b1013e31827dc31823c31829

Ehrenberger, H.E., & Lillington, L. (2004). The development of a measure to delineate the clinical trials nursing role [Online exclusive]. *Oncology Nursing Forum, 31,* E64–E68. doi:10.1188/04.ONF.E64-E68

Engelking, C. (1991). Facilitating clinical trials: The expanding role of the nurse. *Cancer, 67*(Suppl. 6), 1793–1797.

Engelking, C. (1992). Clinical trials: Impact evaluation and implementation considerations. *Seminars in Oncology Nursing, 8,* 148–155. doi:10.1016/0749-2081(92)90030-7

Formea, C. (n.d.). Research pharmacy. Retrieved from http://www.mayo.edu/ctsa/resources/clinical-research-unit/support-services/research-pharmacy

Freedman, T. (1998). The breast cancer prevention trial: Nurses' observations. *Cancer Nursing, 21,* 178–186. doi:10.1097/00002820-199806000-00004

Grady, C., & Edgerly, M. (2009). Science, technology, and innovation: Nursing responsibilities in clinical research. *Nursing Clinics of North America, 44,* 471–481. doi:10.1016/j.cnur.2009.07.011

Gross, J. (1986). Clinical research in cancer chemotherapy. *Oncology Nursing Forum, 13*(1), 59–65.

Hastings, C.E., Fisher, C.A., & McCabe, M.A. (2012). Clinical research nursing: A critical resource in the national research enterprise. *Nursing Outlook, 60,* 149.e143–156.e143. doi:10.1016/j.outlook.2011.10.003

Hazelton, J. (1991). The role of the nurse in phase I clinical trials. *Journal of Pediatric Oncology Nursing, 8,* 43–45. doi:10.1177/104345429100800108

Henke, C. (1980). Emerging roles of the nurse in oncology. *Seminars in Oncology, 7,* 4–8.

Hubbard, S.M. (1982). Cancer treatment research: The role of the nurse in clinical trials of cancer therapy. *Nursing Clinics of North America, 17,* 763–783.

Hubbard, S.M., & DeVita, V. (1976). Chemotherapy research nurse. *American Journal of Nursing, 76,* 560–566.

Hubbard, S.M., & Donehower, M. (1980). The nurse in the cancer research setting. *Seminars in Oncology, 7,* 9–17.

International Conference on Harmonisation of Technical Requirements for Registration of Pharmaceuticals for Human Use. (1996, June 10). *ICH harmonised tripartite guideline: Guideline for good clinical practice, E6(R1).* Retrieved from http://www.ich.org/fileadmin/Public_Web_Site/ICH_Products/Guidelines/Efficacy/E6/E6_R1_Guideline.pdf

Investigational Device Exemptions, 21 C.F.R. pt. 812 (2013). Retrieved from http://www.accessdata.fda.gov/scripts/cdrh/cfdocs/cfcfr/cfrsearch.cfm?cfrpart=812dsf

Kirishnankutty, B., Bellary, S., Kumar, N., & Moodahadu, L.S. (2012). Data management in clinical research: An overview. *Indian Journal of Pharmacology, 44,* 168–172. doi:10.43103/0253-7613.93842

Klimaszewski, A.D., Aikin, J.L., Bacon, M.A., DiStasio, S.A., Ehrenberger, H.E., & Ford, B.A. (Eds.). (2000). *Manual for clinical trials nursing.* Pittsburgh, PA: Oncology Nursing Society.

Lakhani, J., Benzies, K., & Hayden, K.A. (2012). Attributes of interdisciplinary research teams: A comprehensive review of the literature. *Clinical and Investigative Medicine, 35,* E260–E265.

Lubejko, B., Good, M., Weiss, P., Schmieder, L., Leos, D., & Daugherty, P. (2011). Oncology clinical trials nursing: Developing competencies for the novice. *Clinical Journal of Oncology Nursing, 15,* 637–643. doi:10.1188/11.CJON.637-643

McEvoy, M., Cannon, L., & MacDermott, M. (1991). The professional role for nurses in clinical trials. *Seminars in Oncology Nursing, 7,* 268–274. doi:10.1016/0749-2081(91)90065-W

Melink, T., & Whitacre, M. (1991). Planning and implementing clinical trials. *Seminars in Oncology Nursing, 7,* 243–251. doi:10.1016/0749-2081(91)90062-T

Moore, P. (1978). Beyond the protocol. *Oncology Nursing Forum, 5*(3), 12–14.

Mullin, S.M. (1984). An acute intervention trial: The research nurse coordinator's role. *Controlled Clinical Trials, 5,* 141–156. doi:10.1016/0197-2456(84)90120-X

Nagel, K., Gender, J., & Bonner, A. (2010). Delineating the role of a cohort of clinical research nurses in a pediatric cooperative clinical trials group [Online exclusive]. *Oncology Nursing Forum, 37,* E180–E185. doi:10.1188/10.ONF.E180-E185

National Cancer Institute. (2014). *A handbook for clinical investigators conducting therapeutic clinical trials supported by CTEP, DCTD, NCI.* Retrieved from http://ctep.cancer.gov/investigatorResources/docs/InvestigatorHandbook.pdf

National Institute of Allergy and Infectious Diseases. (2013). *DAIDS guidelines for good clinical laboratory practice standards.* Retrieved from http://www.niaid.nih.gov/LabsAndResources/resources/DAIDSClinRsrch/Pages/Laboratories.aspx

Ocker, B., & Pawlik-Plank, D. (2000). The research nurse role in a clinic-based oncology research center. *Cancer Nursing, 23,* 286–292. doi:10.1097/00002820-200008000-00005

Office for Human Research Protections. (n.d.). Investigator responsibilities—Frequently asked questions. Retrieved from http://www.hhs.gov/ohrp/policy/investigatorfaqsmar2010.pdf

Oncology Nursing Society. (2009, March). *Oncology Nursing Society position: Cancer research and clinical trials* (Retired). Pittsburgh, PA: Author.

Oncology Nursing Society. (2010). *Oncology clinical trials nurse competencies.* Retrieved from http://www.ons.org/sites/default/files/ctncompetencies.pdf

Resnik, D.B., & Ness, E. (2012). Participants' responsibilities in clinical research. *Journal of Medical Ethics, 38,* 746–750. doi:10.1136/medethics-2011-100319

Responsibilities of Sponsors and Investigators, 21 C.F.R. §§ 312.50–312.70 (2013). Retrieved from http://www.accessdata.fda.gov/scripts/cdrh/cfdocs/cfcfr/CFRSearch.cfm?CFRPart=312&showFR=1&subpartNode=21:5.0.1.1.3.4

Rosse, P., & Krebs, L. (1999). The nurse's role in the informed consent process. *Seminars in Oncology Nursing, 15,* 116–123. doi:10.1016/S0749-2081(99)80069-2

Royal College of Nursing Research Society. (2013, October). *Research nurse competency framework: A tool to promote patient safety and quality data.* Retrieved from http://www.rcn.org.uk/__data/assets/pdf_file/0019/201466/Research_Nurse_Competency_Framework_-_Version_2_-_Full_-_Oct_2011.pdf

Shannon-Dorcy, K.P., & Drevdahl, D.J. (2011). "I had already made up my mind": Patients and caregivers' perspectives on making the decision to participate in research at a U.S. cancer referral center. *Cancer Nursing, 34,* 428–433. doi:10.1097/NCC.0b013e318207cb03

Speicher, L.A., Fromell, G., Avery, S., Brassil, D., Carlson, L., Stevens, E., & Toms, M. (2012). The critical need for academic health centers to assess the training, support, and career development requirements of clinical research coordinators: Recommendations from the Clinical and Translational Science Award Research Coordinator Taskforce. *Clinical and Translational Science, 5,* 470–475. doi:10.1111/j.1752-8062.2012.00423.x

Suppers, V., Yarbro, C.H., & Mayer-Scogna, D. (1979). Nursing intervention in clinical research—A model program of nursing contributions to a cooperative study group. *Oncology Nursing Forum, 6* (4), 26–27.

Truong, T.H., Weeks, J.C., Cook, E.F., & Joffe, S. (2011). Altruism among participants in cancer clinical trials. *Clinical Trials, 8,* 616–623. doi:10.1177/1740774511414444

U.S. Food and Drug Administration. (2009, October). *Guidance for industry: Investigator responsibilities—Protecting the rights, safety, and welfare of study subjects.* Retrieved from http://www.fda.gov/downloads/Drugs/GuidanceComplianceRegulatoryInformation/Guidances/UCM187772.pdf

U.S. Food and Drug Administration. (2010, May). *Information sheet—Guidance for sponsors, clinical investigators, and IRBs: Frequently asked questions—Statement of investigator (Form FDA 1572).* Retrieved from http://www.fda.gov/downloads/regulatoryinformation/guidances/ucm214282.pdf

U.S. Food and Drug Administration. (2013, February). Statement of investigator. Retrieved from http://www.fda.gov/downloads/AboutFDA/ReportsManualsForms/Forms/UCM074728.pdf

Weydt, A., (2010). Developing delegation skills. *Online Journal of Issues in Nursing, 15*(2). doi:10.3912/OJIN.Vol15No02Man01

Wheeler, V.S. (1991). Preparing nurses for clinical trials: The cancer center approach. *Seminars in Oncology Nursing, 7,* 275–279. doi:10.1016/0749-2081(91)90066-X

White-Hershey, D., & Nevidjon, B. (1990). Fundamentals for oncology nurse/data managers: Preparing for a new role. *Oncology Nursing Forum, 17,* 371–377.

Wilkes, L., Jackson, D., Miranda, C., & Watson, R., (2012). The role of clinical trial nurses: An Australian perspective. *Collegian, 19,* 239–246. doi:10.1016/j.colegn.2012.02.005

Xanthos, G.J., Carp, D., & Geromanos, K.L. (1998). Recognizing nurses' contributions to the clinical research process. *Journal of the Association of Nurses in AIDS Care, 9*(1), 39–48. doi:10.1016/S1055-3290(98)80075-7

Chapter 11

Standard Operating Procedures

Cecilia Petrowsky, RN, MSN, CCRC, OCN®

Introduction

Standard operating procedures (SOPs) are written documents that describe, in detail, the procedures for a specific operation or process. "An important aspect of conducting clinical trials involves developing, maintaining, and adhering to standard operating procedures that are consistent with regulatory standards and guidelines" (Bains, 2009, p. 195). Consistent use of an approved SOP ensures compliance with organizational practices, reduces work effort, reduces errors, and improves data comparability, credibility, and defensibility (U.S. Environmental Protection Agency [EPA], 2007). The International Conference on Harmonisation of Technical Requirements for Registration of Pharmaceuticals for Human Use (ICH, 1996) defines SOPs as "detailed, written instructions to achieve uniformity of the performance of a specific function" (p. 8). The ICH good clinical practice guideline also states that the sponsor is responsible for implementing and maintaining quality assurance and quality control systems with written SOPs to ensure that trials are conducted and data are generated. This chapter will provide clinical trial nurses (CTNs) with an understanding of the value of research site SOPs, describe the relationship between SOPs and quality management, provide an overview of the development and maintenance of SOPs, and provide a recommended list of topics for SOP development for research sites.

Standard Operating Procedures and Quality Management

A *quality management plan* describes an organization's quality system. It identifies the organizational structure, policies and procedures, functional responsibilities of management and staff, lines of authority, and processes for planning, implementing, documenting, and assessing all activities conducted under the organization's quality system. *Quality assurance* includes routine self-audits, modification of existing SOPs or implementation of new SOPs for issues identified during the internal quality assurance process, recording of minor and major violations, and implementation of corrective action plans (Manghani, 2011).

The importance of properly established and managed quality control and quality assurance systems with their integral well-written SOPs provides a systematic and consistent approach to quality and performance improvement at the clinical trial site. SOPs provide an infrastructure that ensures quality controls and quality assurance systems are integrated within the research sites' overall operations.

Benefits of Quality Systems

SOPs generate group cohesion and support of coworkers, provide clear direction and guidance, foster staff confidence and autonomy in their roles, facilitate cross-training, measure quality and performance, and reduce risk and liabilities (Kleppinger & Ball, 2010). Other benefits of SOPs include (Amare, 2012)
• Standardizing activities of specific procedures
• Facilitating integration of new employees
• Improving transparency within the organization
• Serving as a valuable structure for internal communication
• Creating and supporting an infrastructure for the research site
• Sharing best practices within the organization
• Providing valuable background information for policy development and change and assisting with the transfer of knowledge and skills.

Clinical research sites that have quality management plans in place with effective SOPs demonstrate their understanding of research regulations and a commitment to quality research. For sponsors who view SOPs as necessary administrative support, efficient research site SOPs may be the favorable attribute that ensures site selection for a given clinical trial (Kee, 2011). Protocol-specific SOPs, often called a *manual of operations*, outline protocol procedures in great detail so that anyone at the site can follow the necessary steps for a specific study (Kleppinger & Ball, 2010).

Standard Operating Procedure Development

The development and use of SOPs minimizes variation and promotes quality through consistent implementation of a process or procedure within the organization, even with temporary or permanent personnel changes. "If not written correctly, SOPs are of limited value. In addition, the best written SOPs will fail if they are not followed" (U.S. EPA, 2007, p. 1). SOPs should be organized to ensure ease and efficiency in use and to be specific to the organization where they are developed. Internal formatting will vary with each organization as well as the type of SOP written. The level of detail provided in the SOP may differ based on whether the process is critical and the frequency and number of people involved for a specific procedure (U.S. EPA, 2007).

The organization should have a procedure in place for determining which procedures or processes need to be documented. Individuals knowledgeable with the activity and the organization's internal structure should write these SOPs. A team approach can be followed, especially for multitasked processes where the experiences of a number of individuals are critical; this method promotes adoption by potential end users (U.S. EPA, 2007).

It is helpful to organize a site's operations by key business components or core operational functions when determining categories and topics and resources for SOP development. Several resources have recommendations for specific SOP development for clinical research sites. The U.S. Food and Drug Administration and the Office for Human Research Protections have guidance documents that interpret regulations available on their websites (see Figure 11-1). The American Society of Clinical Oncology has a position statement on minimum standards and exemplary attributes of clinical trial sites, which recommends topics for SOP development (Zon, Meropol, Catalano, & Schilisky, 2008). Figure 11-2 outlines the key business components or core operational functions of an organization's clinical trial operations and a list of related

---

Figure 11-1. Resources for Developing Standard Operating Procedures

International Conference on Harmonisation Guidelines
- www.ich.org/products/guidelines.html

U.S. Department of Health and Human Services Office for Human Research Protections (OHRP)
- OHRP Policy and Guidance: www.hhs.gov/ohrp/policy/index.html
- International Compilation of Human Research Standards: www.hhs.gov/ohrp/international/index.html

U.S. Food and Drug Administration (FDA)
- Good Clinical Practice (GCP) Program Guidance documents: www.fda.gov/ScienceResearch/SpecialTopics/RunningClinicalTrials/GuidancesInformationSheetsandNotices/default.htm
- Selected FDA GCP Clinical Trial Guidance Documents: www.fda.gov/ScienceResearch/SpecialTopics/RunningClinicalTrials/GuidancesInformationSheetsandNotices/ucm219433.htm
- FDA Office of Good Clinical Practice query email account: gcp.questions@fda.hhs.gov
- Archived replies to GCP queries indexed by topic: www.fda.gov/ScienceResearch/SpecialTopics/RunningClinicalTrials/RepliestoInquiriestoFDAonGoodClinicalPractice/default.htm
- Compliance Program Guidance Manual for FDA Staff, Bioresearch Monitoring: Clinical Investigators and Sponsor-Investigators: www.fda.gov/ICECI/EnforcementActions/BioresearchMonitoring/ucm133562.htm
- FDA Code of Federal Regulations: www.accessdata.fda.gov/scripts/cdrh/cfdocs/cfcfr/cfrsearch.cfm

Other Regulations and Standards
- The Health Insurance Portability and Accountability Act of 1996 Privacy and Security Rules: www.hhs.gov/ocr/privacy
- American College of Surgeons Commission on Cancer Standard 1.9 Clinical Trial Accrual: www.facs.org/cancer
- Association for the Accreditation of Human Research Protection Programs Accreditation Standards: www.aahrpp.org
- Department of Transportation hazardous materials shipping guidelines: http://hazmat.dot.gov
- American Society of Clinical Oncology Statement on Minimum Standards and Exemplary Attributes of Clinical Trial Sites: http://jco.ascopubs.org/content/26/15/2562.full.pdf+html
- American Society of Clinical Oncology Research Program Quality Assessment Tool: www.asco.org/practice-research/asco-research-program-quality-assessment-tool

National Cancer Institute (NCI)
- NCI Division of Cancer Treatment Cancer Therapy Evaluation Program Guidelines and Policies: http://ctep.cancer.gov/investigatorResources/default.htm#guidelines_policies
- NCI Investigator's Handbook: http://ctep.cancer.gov/handbook/index.html

topics based on the aforementioned resources to assist with SOP development.

Developing a set of SOPs can be overwhelming; it is a time-intensive process requiring commitment from all levels of the organization. It is a multilayered process that is well worth the effort in the long run. The organization needs to identify the key areas where SOPs are necessary and determine the standards, regulations, guidelines, and evidence-based/best practices that are applicable to its quality management plan and SOP development. Figure 11-1 provides a partial list of resources for regulations, standards, policies, and best practices to refer to when developing SOPs for conducting clinical research. Consider the following steps when organizing an effort to create SOPs (U.S. EPA, 2007).

- Prioritize the list based on risk or need.
- Develop a standard approach to SOP development and writing.
- Follow a team-based approach for SOP development and problem solving whenever possible. Form a task force or focus group to map the current process, identify gaps in the process and opportunities for improve-

Figure 11-2. Example of a Standard Operating Procedures (SOPs) Table of Contents and Document Management								
Policy #	Categories	Title/Description	Effective Date	Revision Date	Last Literature Review	Associated Documents
	General and Administrative	• Development of SOPs • Site Research Mission, Organization, Scope, and Responsibilities • Research Staff Qualifications and Training • Research Site Communication Plan • Affiliate Institutional Network • Conflict of Interest in Research • Clinical Trial Patient Education and Outreach				Training materials; reference to related SOPs within the institution
	Protocol Management	• Protocol Activation and Implementation Plan • Study Recruitment Plan • Protocol Training • Institutional Review Board (IRB) Submissions • Regulatory Files • Protocol Termination • Archiving Study Files • Investigational Drug Management				Reference to related IRB SOPs
	Patient Management	• Study Recruitment • Informed Consent Process • Study Participant Study File • Study Participant Case Management on a Trial • Investigational Drug Administration and Treatment plan • Adverse Event Reporting • Specimen Collection and Handling				Related clinical procedures
	Data Management	• Source Documents • Storage and Archiving • Information System Compliance				
	Quality Assurance	• Audits and Inspections • Monitoring Visits • Data Safety and Monitoring Committee • Electronic Medical Record Access for External Audits • Quality management program				Audit tools
	Protocol Financial Management	• Research Participant Billing Compliance • Financial Review Process • Contractual Review Process • Medicare Coverage Analysis				

Note. Based on information from U.S. Food and Drug Administration, 2009; Zon et al., 2008.

ment, and brainstorm and problem solve to further define the process.
- Incorporate end-user review to gain consensus that procedures and expectations are appropriate and achievable. Pilot the SOP if possible.
- Establish an evaluation and review system to ensure SOPs are adhered to and that the steps are correct and appropriate.

Figure 11-3 provides an example of a decision-making and planning matrix for SOP development.

Writing Standard Operating Procedures

SOPs should be created by individuals who are experienced in the topic and reviewed by external parties for clarity, comprehension, and reliability within the context of the organization. Team writing for SOPs ensures that comprehensive knowledge acquired from different perspectives is applied to the SOP. Writing teams do not have to sit together to write. They can write portions of an SOP and edit parts of the SOP independently; then one person can combine the individual contributions. Once combined, the draft SOP should be circulated for review among the writers before editing the final draft. Ideally, the writing team should meet at least once to establish the objectives. SOPs should be written with sufficient detail so that employees with limited experience or knowledge of the procedure can successfully reproduce the procedure when unsupervised. For detailed and complex procedures, mapping the process is helpful. *Mapping* involves taking each step in the procedure and making it more efficient and easy to follow. Once the mapping is completed, the team will convert the process to an outline, diagram, flow chart, or any format that will make it easy to understand (U.S. EPA, 2007).

Whenever possible, an organization should pilot the SOP prior to broader use, as this will provide an opportunity to evaluate the effectiveness of the SOP. Subsequent revisions can then be made based on the feedback. Supplementing SOPs with checklists, work instructions, guidelines, and work flow charts will assist with SOP adoption and compliance. SOPs must be reviewed prior to their approval for release, adequacy, and completeness and compliance with all applicable legal, ethical, and regulatory requirements. The finalized SOPs should be approved by the organization's line of authority as outlined in the quality management plan (e.g., the director of the research office). See Table 11-1 for specific sections and items to include in the SOP documents.

Implementing Standard Operating Procedures

When possible, SOPs should be validated by one or more individuals with appropriate training and experience with the process. Develop a standard approach to the implementation or distribution of the SOP for broader use. Implementation should include a process for training current staff, as well as new staff, and should include documentation of training and metrics to evaluate effectiveness and compliance over time; this would be part of quality assurance. The training plan should include a regular annual review and staff competency review of SOPs to ensure compliance. It is helpful to use the individuals who were involved in SOP development as facilitators for implementation and ongoing quality assurance (U.S. EPA, 2007).

Maintaining Standard Operating Procedures

SOPs need to remain current to be useful; therefore, whenever procedures, standards, regulations, or guidelines are changed, SOPs should be updated and reapproved. SOPs should be reviewed on a regular basis (e.g., annual or biennial) to ensure that policies and procedures remain current and appropriate (U.S. EPA, 2007).

Revised SOPs should include a document identifier and a version date and status, and their distribution must always be documented and controlled. When obsolete SOPs are required to be retained for any purpose, they should be suitably identified to prevent unintended use. For historical and legal purposes, SOPs should be archived in the event they need to be referenced. Table 11-1 provides an example of a format to manage SOPs and related documents, which can easily be converted to an electronic data management system.

Summary

SOPs are integral to an organization's quality management plan, which ensures that the conduct and results of clinical trials meet regulatory and ethical standards. Effective SOPs provide the framework to ensure that quality controls and quality assurance systems are integrated within the research site's overall operations. An organizational commitment at all levels and participation from all individuals at the site are required for a quality system to succeed. CTNs need to know their organization's SOPs and quality management plan, and they should become involved in the development and implementation of SOPs. The national clinical research environment is changing rapidly, and a commitment to quality management by all is needed to ensure human subject protection, data integrity, and quality clinical research.

Figure 11-3. Example of a Decision-Making and Planning Matrix for Standard Operating Procedure (SOP) Development

Category	Subcategory/ Topics	Current Process	Current Documentation of Process	Process Not Defined and Needs to Be Developed	Regulatory/ Standards/ Guidelines/ Best Practice Resources for SOP Development	Content Expert Reviewer	SOP Developer(s) Key Personnel Involved in Process Development	SOP Required? Yes/No Cross-Reference (SOP available through another department)
Research specimen ordering, collection, processing, storing, and shipping	Staff training and competencies	Yes	Orientation checklist and annual competencies			Biohazard compliance officer	CRA and CTN	Yes
		Yes	Hazmat training		IATA	Compliance officer		No (see system policy for hazardous material shipment)
	Research study lab manual and supplies	Yes		Study specific				Yes
	General research lab supplies	Yes	Lab supply inventory and storage					Yes
		No	Ordering and disposal					
	Laboratory procedures	Yes	General lab manual	Study specific	Biohazard precautions	Lab manager		Yes
	Research lab patient orders and internal coordination	Yes	EMR instructions for ordering research samples		Research billing regulations	CTN		Yes
		Yes	Coordination instructions			Clinical manager		
		Yes	Central calendar—group wide					
		Yes	Calendar template					
	Research lab processing	No				Laboratory manager		Yes
	Research study lab shipping	Yes			Hazmat			Yes
	Laboratory specimen archiving/ freezer	No				Laboratory manager		Yes

CRA—clinical research associate; CTN—clinical trial nurse; EMR—electronic medical record; IATA—International Air Transport Association

Note. Based on information from U.S. Environmental Protection Agency, 2007.

Table 11-1. Items to Include in a Standard Operating Procedure (SOP) Document	
Item	Description
SOP document information	Policy identifier: SOP identification number and organization Category: If applicable Title: Clearly identifies the activity or procedure Date: Effective date and/or revision date
SOP author or reviewer and approver	Include name, title, and credentials of the person who created, reviewed, or revised the policy, as well as the person who approved the SOP. The determination of level of signature should be defined in the SOP for developing SOPs within the organization. The reviewers should be knowledgeable and experienced with the content of the SOP.
References or resources	Policy and procedure should be based on current evidence-based practice or a regulation, law, or accreditation that is mandating the policy. List related SOPs, supporting documentation, applicable regulations, and/or guidelines.
Table of contents	May be needed for quick reference for lengthy SOPs, for locating information, and to denote changes or revisions made only to certain sections of an SOP.
Purpose	The intent of the SOP. State the goal or purpose of the policy.
Scope	An overview of the process and the range of activities the SOP applies to, as well as any limitations or exceptions.
Responsibilities	The individuals and areas that are required to comply with the policy. For individuals, use titles or roles and avoid names.
Policy	A policy is a position statement that describes the organization's approach to a particular situation. It reflects the rules and is process based.
Definitions	Definitions or terminology that may need to be clarified. Include explanations of words or phrases unique to the document or topic that add to the readers' understanding of the basic policy.
Procedure	The definitive steps to carry out the policy. Procedures are action-oriented, outlining chronologically the specific steps needed to perform the action. Draft the SOP in a flow diagram or outline to assist in making the steps efficient or determining any gaps in the process or need for involving other people in developing the SOP. Content should be clear, concise, thorough, and comprehensive. Use tables, matrices, checklists, diagrams, and examples.
Effectiveness criteria/quality control measures	Describe all appropriate quality assurance and quality control measures or activities to ensure compliance with the procedure.
Policy dissemination	Develop a systematic approach to ensure SOP implementation and associated training and frequency of SOP review. Minimally, all SOPs should be reviewed during new staff orientation, annually, and at the time SOPs are revised.
Appendices	Additional documents that, given the situation, are the best method to accurately convey the necessary information and facilitate the consistent implementation of an SOP, such as examples, documentation tools, checklists, flow charts, diagrams, decision trees, and algorithms.

Note. Based on information from U.S. Environmental Protection Agency, 2007.

Key Points

- A quality management program will ensure compliance with good clinical practice guidelines to produce quality study results.
- SOPs are integral to an organization's quality management program.
- Establish a procedure for determining which SOPs should be developed.
- SOP development should include a team approach whenever possible and involve content experts and resources.
- Quality measures should be integrated within individual SOPs.
- SOPs should be reviewed regularly to ensure credibility and appropriate adherence to regulations, best practices, and standards.
- Investment in the development and maintenance of SOPs will save time and effort and ensure a quality operation.

References

Amare, G. (2012). Reviewing the values of a standard operating procedure. *Ethiopian Journal of Health Sciences, 22,* 205–208. Retrieved from http://www.ncbi.nlm.nih.gov/pmc/articles/PMC3511899

Bains, S., Bhandari, M., & Hanson, B. (2009). Standard operating procedures: The devil is in the details. *Journal of Long-Term Effects of Medical Implants, 19*, 195–199. doi:10.1615/JLongTermEffMedImplants.v19.i3.40

International Conference on Harmonisation of Technical Requirements for Registration of Pharmaceuticals for Human Use. (1996, June 10). *ICH harmonised tripartite guideline: Guideline for good clinical practice, E6(R1)*. Retrieved from http://www.ich.org/fileadmin/Public_Web_Site/ICH_Products/Guidelines/Efficacy/E6_R1_Guideline.pdf

Kee, A.N. (2011). Standard operating procedures for clinical research departments. *Journal of Medical Practice Management, 27*, 172–174.

Kleppinger, C.F., & Ball, L.K. (2010). Building quality in clinical trials with use of a quality systems approach. *Clinical Infectious Diseases, 51*(Suppl. 1), S111–S116. doi:10.1086/653058

Manghani, K. (2011). Quality assurance: Importance of system and standard operating procedures. *Perspectives in Clinical Research, 2*, 34–37. doi:10.4103/2229-3485.76288

U.S. Environmental Protection Agency. (2007, April). *Guidance for preparing standard operating procedures*. Retrieved from http://www.epa.gov/QUALITY/qs-docs/g6-final.pdf

U.S. Food and Drug Administration. (2009, October). *Guidance for industry: Investigator responsibilities—Protecting the rights, safety, and welfare of study subjects*. Retrieved from http://www.fda.gov/downloads/Drugs/.../Guidances/UCM187772.pdf

Zon, R., Meropol, N.J., Catalano, R.B., & Schilisky, R.L., (2008). American Society of Clinical Oncology statement on minimum standards and exemplary attributes of clinical trial sites. *Journal of Clinical Oncology, 28*, 2562–2567. doi:10.1200/JCO.2007.15.6398

Chapter 12

Ethics of Clinical Research

Connie M. Ulrich, PhD, RN, FAAN, and Gwenyth R. Wallen, PhD, RN

Introduction

All nurses who are involved with patients, but particularly clinical trial nurses (CTNs), must have a solid understanding of the ethics of clinical research. Clinical research is an important social and scientific goal; through research, the development of novel treatments can potentially reduce or mitigate life-altering illness. However, as Grady (2008) rightfully acknowledged, "Although clinical research has resulted in significant benefits for society, it continues to pose profound ethical questions" (p. 21). These ethical questions arise because clinical research relies on the voluntary consent of human participants. This includes concerns related to informed consent, respect for persons, scientific integrity, and patient-participants' expectations of research benefit. CTNs are an integral part of the research process because they are research team members responsible for the recruitment and retention of human participants, including informed consent, and coordinate the implementation of research procedures (Richmond & Ulrich, 2013).

Much of the history of research with human participants has been one of scandal (see Chapter 1). Other significant historical events, such as the Jewish Chronic Disease Hospital Study, the Willowbrook Hepatitis Study, and the U.S. Public Health Service Tuskegee Syphilis Study, all brought to light the unethical conduct of research with human participants and promulgated several significant ethical codes of conduct (Arras, 2008; Jones, 2008; Robinson & Unruh, 2008). Most notably, the Nuremberg Code, enacted after the Nazi war criminal trials, recognized the essential role of participants' voluntary consent in research (see Figure 12-1) (Annas & Grodin, 2008; Nuremberg Code, 1949; Weindling, 2008). Other important codes of conduct, such as the Belmont Report, denote guiding ethical principles in the conduct of research. These include beneficence, respect for persons, and justice (National Commission for the Protection of Human Subjects of Biomedical and Behavioral Research [National Commission], 1979). See Chapter 8 for more information about the Nuremberg Code and the Belmont Report. The purpose of this chapter is to highlight some of the ethical challenges that CTNs encounter in research and the strategies they can use to address these issues with patient-participants and other members of the research team.

Social and Scientific Value

For research to be ethical, it must address salient problems or important health-related questions (Emanuel, Wendler, & Grady, 2000). The Institute of Medicine (IOM, 2009), and others, suggest that limited-value studies (e.g., small, underpowered studies) make little impact to the overall goals of science (Saver, 2012). Furthermore, resources are limited; therefore, researchers need to carefully design studies that avoid unnecessarily exposing patient-participants to risk without the potential for individual or societal benefit. What, then, is a *high-value* study that contributes knowledge to the overall good of society?

Clinical research includes randomized controlled trials (RCTs)—treatment trials considered by many to be the gold standard because they randomly allocate patients to different treatments or experimental arms of the study (e.g., treatment versus control or placebo), thereby measuring the true effect of the intervention (Shaw, Johnson, & Borkowf, 2013). Participants and investigators are often blinded and do not know which participants in the trial receive the intervention (Joffe & Truog, 2008; Stolberg, Norman, & Trop, 2004). However, other types of clinical trials (e.g., prevention) and methodologic designs (e.g., epidemiologic, observational, historical) may also shed light on complex problems, thus being considered of scientific and societal value (Emanuel et al., 2000). Some examples of potential research questions that add social and scientific value are outlined in Figure 12-2.

> **Figure 12-1. Significant Ethical Codes of Conduct**
>
> **Nuremberg Code**
> Promulgated following the Nazi War Criminal trials in 1947 and stated that "The voluntary consent of the human subject is absolutely essential."
>
> **Declaration of Helsinki**
> Adopted by the World Medical Association General Assembly in Helsinki in 1964 with several revisions. Discusses informed consent, differentiates between therapeutic and nontherapeutic research, and addresses the role of surrogate decision making (World Medical Association, 1997).
>
> **Belmont Report**
> The National Commission for the Protection of Human Subjects of Biomedical and Biobehavioral Research identified three ethical principles in the conduct of research: beneficence, respect for persons, and justice.
>
> **Basic HHS Policy for Protection of Human Research Subjects (2009) 45 C.F.R. pt. 46, subpt. A, §§ 46.101–46.124 (also known as the "Common Rule")**
> Federal guidelines for the protection of human subjects. Subpart A also outlines requirements for informed consent and the function and composition of institutional review boards.
> Subparts B, C, and D address additional research protections for pregnant women, fetuses, neonates, children, and prisoners. (See www.hhs.gov/ohrp/humansubjects/commonrule/index.html and www.hhs.gov/ohrp/humansubjects/guidance/45cfr46.html)
>
> **Council for International Organizations of Medical Sciences (CIOMS)**
> Established in 1949 to provide ethical guidelines on the conduct of research developed for developing countries.
> See: Council for International Organizations of Medical Sciences. (1993). *International Ethical Guidelines for Biomedical Research Involving Human Subjects.* Geneva, Switzerland: CIOMS.

In order to be of social and scientific value, research must be methodologically rigorous. This means that instruments used to measure specific variables within the study are both reliable and valid. As such, the research is measuring what it intends to measure and this measurement is consistent (Waltz, Strickland, & Lenz, 2010). Providing an adequate power analysis is part of a rigorous scientific process because without this, the ability to detect significant differences in outcomes is compromised. Conducting a power analysis reduces the probability of a type II error (indicating that there is no statistical difference when, in fact, there is) and is necessary to determining the appropriate sample size for the study. Ethically, this is important because researchers do not want to expose patient-participants to unnecessary risk. In his sentinel article describing 22 instances of unethical or ethically questionable research at prominent academic institutions, Beecher (1966) concluded, "an experiment is ethical or not at its inception; it does not become ethical post hoc" (p. 372). This means that researchers need to be proactive and use critical-thinking skills throughout the research question formulation, design, methodology, analysis, and other important aspects of the protocol (e.g., multisite study, recruitment and retention of human participants, number of collaborators) prior to its implementation.

Other important research-related terms and processes that CTNs need to be aware of include *equipoise, randomization,* and *placebo-controlled.* These terms are important for several reasons. First, some evidence suggests that patients may not participate in research because they prefer a specific treatment or intervention and do not want to take a placebo (Ross et al., 1999). Second, patient-participants are often confused by study terms such as *randomization* and *placebo assignment* (Robinson et al., 2003; Welton, Vickers, Cooper, Meade, & Marteau, 1999); therefore, they may seek the advice of the CTN to help explain the specifics of these terms as part of the informed consent process.

Researchers designing an RCT, for example, and proposing to test the safety, efficacy, and effectiveness of an intervention must be in a state of equipoise. *Equipoise* is an important ethics-related term in RCTs because it represents a state of professional uncertainty regarding the superiority of the treatment arms. Ethically, physicians or nurse investigators cannot assign patient-participants to inferior care or treatment because of their professional codes of conduct and their therapeutic obligations to patient care (Miller & Joffe, 2011). With equipoise, there is a genuine consensus within the medical community (*clinical equipoise*) that it is not known whether treatment A is better than treatment B (Freedman, 1987). In RCTs, randomization is a method where study participants are assigned to a treatment group. This process of assigning groups by chance is explained to research participants as similar to flipping a coin. Researchers might propose a placebo-controlled trial in which the experimental drug is compared to placebo (inactive substance). Emanuel and Miller (2001) contended that placebo-controlled trials can be ethically

> **Figure 12-2. Examples of Research Questions That Add Social and Scientific Value**
>
> - What are the benefits and burdens of melanoma vaccine research?
> - What innovative strategies minimize health disparities in the recruitment and retention of human participants in clinical research?
> - What are the personal and societal costs of caregiving in light of an aging and chronically ill population?
> - What is the added value of community-based participatory research in meeting the healthcare goals of differing communities?
> - What is the role of interdisciplinary team science in translating research from the bench to the bedside?
> - What defines a "good death" from the point of view of individuals, families, and healthcare providers, and how is it different or similar among them?

justified for the following reasons: (a) there is a compelling methodologic argument to use a placebo, (b) a thorough and stringent ethical review has taken place, and (c) the risk of serious patient harm is null, and the risks of receiving a placebo are minimized to the greatest extent possible. Thus, these important ethics-related terms in RCTs must be outlined in the informed consent document as well as during the informed consent process and in a way that is understandable to patient-participants.

Informed Consent

Informed consent is a historical, regulatory, legal, and ethical concept. It respects the right of individuals to determine what is in their best interest. In fact, in *Schloendorff v. Society of New York Hospital*, 211 N.Y. 125, 105 N.E. 92 (1914), Justice Cardozo wrote the following opinion:

> Every human being of adult years and sound mind has a right to determine what shall be done with his own body; and a surgeon who performs an operation without his patient's consent commits an assault for which he is liable in damages. This is true except in cases of emergency where the patient is unconscious and where it is necessary to operate before consent can be obtained.

Thus, informed consent involves the voluntary consent and autonomous authorization of patients after they understand the purpose, risks, benefits, and other study-related aspects of the treatment or research that is being proposed. Informed consent consists of (a) disclosure of information, (b) decisional capacity (patient-participants' capacity to understand the information and make a decision), (c) voluntariness on behalf of patient-participants, and (d) comprehension of information (Emanuel et al., 2000; National Commission, 1979). Figure 12-3 describes what should be discussed with patients in research.

Unfortunately, a gap exists between what we ideally expect patient-participants to understand and what they actually comprehend. Many studies demonstrate that factors such as educational level, serious illness, age, and trust in the researcher influence informed consent (Flory & Emanuel, 2004; Joffe, Cook, Cleary, Clark, & Weeks, 2001). Moreover, the Office for Human Research Protections (OHRP) regulations, as defined in Figure 12-1, designate several groups of participants as vulnerable—those who have a diminished capacity to provide informed consent—and in need of additional safeguards (Protection of Human Research Subjects, 2009). This includes (a) adults with diminished capacity, (b) children, (c) pregnant women, neonates, and fetuses, and (d) prisoners (see Institutional Review Boards [IRBs] section). Although informed consent is an essential element

Figure 12-3. What Should Be Discussed With Potential Patient-Participants in Research?

- The nature and purpose of the study
- The risks and benefits
- The right to withdraw at any time without penalty
- The alternatives that might be available
- The name of the individual to contact in case of an emergency (generally the principal investigator or other study team members)
- The voluntariness of patients
- The remuneration of patients, if available
- The way that privacy and confidentiality of patient information will be handled (Certificate of Confidentiality), if needed for sensitive research

Note. Based on information from Appelbaum, Lidz, et al., 1987; Faden & Beauchamp, 1986.

for the ethical conduct of research with human participants, it is not sufficient (Emanuel et al., 2000; Faden & Beauchamp, 1986).

Peer review is vital in the protection of human participants and provides additional oversight that often includes an external panel of experts as well as lay individuals. Although it is often treated as a onetime event, informed consent is an ongoing process (Wendler & Rackoff, 2002). Indeed, Wendler and Rackoff (2002) suggested that investigators, as well as other team members, including CTNs and research coordinators, reaffirm patient-participants' willingness to continue in the research every few months through their verbal agreement. They further recommended that participants be reconsented when material and significant changes are made to the study protocol. See Chapter 14.

Therapeutic Misconception

Case Study 1

Jacob is a 75-year-old man diagnosed with stage III pancreatic cancer. He is enrolled in a phase II RCT that is evaluating the safety and efficacy of an experimental medication for his disease. His wife, Ruth, is the proxy decision maker for Jacob and indicates to the CTN, Anna, that she was very supportive of her husband enrolling in the trial because she knows that he will benefit from the medication; she completely trusts that Jacob's physician would not enroll him in the trial if it was not going to benefit him. Ruth tells the nurse that she really did not understand what was meant by *randomization* or *placebo* but that if her husband could remain stable with his disease by taking the new medication, she was all for it. Ruth also expressed her pleasure and gratitude for the constant monitoring that Jacob was receiving and valued the care and attention that was paid to him because it was sometimes difficult for her to address his care needs

at home. Anna now wonders whether Jacob and his wife understand what research is and have adequately assessed the benefits and risks or whether they are under a therapeutic misconception about the protocol.
- If you were Jacob's CTN, what would you do?

Therapeutic Misconception and Informed Consent

Research and clinical practice were defined and differentiated in the Belmont Report as both separate and distinct concepts, although they can and sometimes do overlap (see Figure 12-4). In fact, patient-participants may not perceive them differently, especially when research is conducted at the bedside where care is traditionally given and received. Much of the worry associated with research participation is that patients will not understand the difference between research and clinical care and will conflate the two, potentially undermining informed consent. Medical or clinical care is meant to benefit an individual; therefore, providers' primary commitment is to address the patient's immediate health and well-being. Conversely, research can potentially benefit individuals, but its goal is to improve care and treatment for future patients. Moreover, research represents a systematic process that is aimed at testing specific hypotheses meant to generalize knowledge.

Appelbaum, Roth, and Lidz (1982) first discussed the term *therapeutic misconception* in their seminal paper titled, "The Therapeutic Misconception: Informed Consent in Psychiatric Research" and argued that a therapeutic misconception exists when patient-participants believe that they will personally benefit or receive therapeutic gain from all aspects of research participation. In other work, Appelbaum, Roth, Lidz, Benson, and Winslade (1987) stated that "to maintain a therapeutic misconception is to deny the possibility that there may be major disadvantages to participating in clinical research that stem from the nature of the research process itself" (p. 20). Since the 1980s, however, therapeutic misconception has been defined and measured differently, only adding to the confusion surrounding this term in the research context and its implications for informed consent (Henderson et al., 2007; Horng & Grady, 2003; Kimmelman, 2007; Kim et al., 2009). Significant empirical research with differing groups of patient populations enrolled in clinical research (e.g., cancer, Parkinson disease, mental health) has highlighted several subject- and study-level factors that may place patient-participants at risk for therapeutic misconception (Appelbaum, Lidz, & Grisso, 2004; Kim et al., 2009). This includes those who are older, less educated, or in poorer health, as well as those with limited options and an increased sense of optimism (Appelbaum et al., 2004).

Horng and Grady (2003) delineated other aspects of patient-participants' misunderstanding beyond the therapeutic misconception that includes therapeutic misestimation and therapeutic optimism. An uneven risk-benefit assessment can lead to a therapeutic misestimation, either "underestimating the risks, overestimating the benefits, or both" (Horng & Grady, 2003, p. 13). In Case Study 1, it is not clear if Ruth and Jacob suffered from a therapeutic misconception, therapeutic misestimation, or both. It appears that Ruth, in particular, may not have understood the study design because she expressed a belief that her husband would directly benefit from the medication and explicitly reported her lack of understanding on important methodologic aspects of the study (i.e., randomization, placebo). It is possible that Ruth overestimated the benefits of the experimental drug in hopes that her husband's pancreatic cancer would respond in a positive fashion or at least remain stable.

Fostering optimism or hope in research participation is central to many patients' ability to cope with their illness and does not necessarily undermine their ability to make autonomous decisions (Horng & Grady, 2003; Jansen, 2006). However, therapeutic optimism can be unrealistic, and more data are needed to better understand the role of hope in the lives of patient-participants and at what point it biases their research-related decisions. Kim et al. (2009) called on researchers and others to refocus their attention on therapeutic misconception using a different lens. Indeed, CTNs should continue to foster hope, but at the same time, statements that reflect a misconception or misestimation should be carefully considered within the overall context of the patient-participant's decision-making process (Kim et al., 2009). CTNs can simply ask patient-participants to share with them their understanding of the purpose, aims, risks and benefits, and other procedural aspects of the study and how they arrived at a risk-benefit calculus for themselves. Open and consistent dialogue is the key to allay-

---

Figure 12-4. Definitions of Research and Clinical Practice Addressed in the Belmont Report

Research
Research designates an activity designed to test a hypothesis, permit conclusions to be drawn, and thereby to develop or contribute to generalizable knowledge (expressed, for example, in theories, principles, and statements of relationships). Research is usually described in a formal protocol that sets forth an objective and a set of procedures designed to reach that objective.

Practice
Practice refers to interventions that are designed solely to enhance the well-being of an individual patient or client and that a reasonable expectation of success. The purpose of medical or behavioral practice is to provide diagnosis, preventive treatment, or therapy to particular individuals.

Note. From *The Belmont Report: Ethical Principles and Guidelines for the Protection of Human Subjects of Research*, by National Commission for the Protection of Human Subjects of Biomedical and Behavioral Research, 1979. Retrieved from http://www.hhs.gov/ohrp/humansubjects/guidance/belmont.html.

ing misunderstandings and improving knowledge associated with the research process. Sometimes the CTN may worry that patient-participants are operating under a therapeutic misconception, therapeutic misestimation, or both. Figure 12-5 provides strategies the CTN can use when confronted with this situation.

Institutional Review Boards

The primary goal of the IRB review process is to protect the rights and welfare of human participants (Grady, 2010; Liu & Davis, 2001). See Chapter 16 for further information on the IRB's role. IRBs have the authority to approve, require modifications to, or disapprove research. IRB members are responsible for reviewing each study to assess whether the proposed research design is scientifically sound and will not unnecessarily expose subjects to risk. Risks to the participants must be deemed reasonable in relation to anticipated benefits, if any (Protection of Human Research Subjects, 2009). Members of the IRB must ensure that selection of subjects is equitable, informed consent is sought and documented, adequate data monitoring is provided, subject confidentiality is protected, and special provisions for ensuring the protection of vulnerable subjects are clearly delineated where applicable. The IRB provides investigators and institutions with written documentation of all decisions.

Minimum requirements exist that must be met in establishing an IRB. Each IRB must have at least five members (Hart & Belotto, 2010; Protection of Human Research Subjects, 2009). These members must have the appropriate professional and scientific background to review the anticipated research studies that will come up for review. Members often are physicians, pharmacologists, clergy, nurses, social workers, and bioethicists. An IRB must include one member who has a primary interest in a nonscientific area and one nonaffiliated member. Additionally, no IRB may have a member participate in the initial or continuing review of any project in which the member has a conflicting interest, except to provide information requested by the IRB.

Of note, nurses who sit on IRBs are generally considered scientific members. Nurses, particularly advanced practice nurses, who serve on IRBs often provide a broad lens by which to evaluate risks and benefits to the participants from both a clinical and human subject protection perspective. As knowledgeable care providers, they are often able to easily recognize or forecast procedural irregularities or potential for adverse events. For example, in reviewing a phase I clinical trial that involves serial blood testing and magnetic resonance imaging scans, an IRB member who is an oncology clinical nurse specialist may raise specific questions for the investigator related to clinical versus research-specific tests and undue burden on study participants. This member may also suggest consent language that specifies the process for each of these study procedures. Whether serving as an IRB member or as a nurse caring for research subjects, nurses in a variety of settings are responsible for promoting good science and for protecting the rights and welfare of their patients enrolled in clinical trials (Grady & Edgerly, 2009).

Scientific Integrity

Case Study 2

Emma is a CTN who is the coordinator for Dr. Plemma's randomized trial of integrative approaches for women diagnosed with advanced breast cancer. She is responsible for recruiting patient-participants and perceives tremendous pressure from Dr. Plemma to meet the study's goals because they only need a few more participants to complete trial enrollment. She interviews Claire, who was recently diagnosed with stage III bilateral breast cancer and subsequently underwent a bilateral mastectomy with follow-up chemotherapy and is potentially eligible for the study. Emma calls Dr. Plemma to inform her that Claire is emotionally distressed over her diagnosis and prognosis, and although she wants to participate in the study, she cannot commit at the present time. Dr. Plemma tells Emma to go ahead and enroll her so that she can take part in the possible benefits of the trial and that Dr. Plemma will backdate the informed consent document.
- What should Emma do in this situation?
- What would you do as Claire's CTN?

Foundation of Ethical Research

Beyond the role of the IRB in human subject protection, scientific integrity on the part of individual scien-

---

Figure 12-5. Strategies to Assist Clinical Trial Nurses in Addressing Concerns Related to a Therapeutic Misunderstanding in Clinical Research

- Revisit the study's purpose, aims, and research questions to address whether it still reflects patient-participants' goals and preferences.
- Clarify terms such as *randomization*, *placebo*, and *equipoise* or any other misunderstandings as needed.
- Inform patient-participants of any study changes as the protocol progresses.
- Discuss the risks and benefits of the study.
- Call a family and care team meeting to discuss ethical, procedural, or other concerns with the principal investigator and others integral to the protocol.
- Design informational brochures that can be shared with patient-participants to clarify aspects of the clinical trial. Remember, these brochures will need to be approved by the institutional review board of record.

Note. Based on information from Horng & Grady, 2003.

tists and institutions must remain a foundation for ethical research. Scientific integrity is at the core of ethical research and represents a measure of the public's trust in not only individual researchers but also the broader research enterprise. Integrity in science upholds ethical standards and promotes authenticity, transparency, and honesty in all aspects of the research process ranging from designing the actual study to disseminating the results. The IOM Committee on Assessing Integrity in Research Environments (2002) report on scientific integrity acknowledged the significance of intellectual honesty in the ethical conduct of research, including fairness in peer review, collegiality, and adherence to standards of practice as outlined between investigators and their research teams in the protection of human participants. Unfortunately, the public is often afraid to participate in research. In fact, less than 5% of adults with cancer, for example, actually participate in cancer clinical trials (Murthy, Krumholz, & Gross, 2004). Ulrich et al. (2012) interviewed 32 cancer clinical trial participants about what they believed helped or hindered research participation, and some expressed sentiments such as, "I often wonder if [the researcher] is not telling me everything" or "People are scared to death to participate." The ethical failings on the part of investigators and institutions seem more commonplace today, as instances of misconduct are highly publicized in media outlets with serious ramifications for all stakeholders.

Research Misconduct

The U.S. Office of Science and Technology Policy defines *research misconduct* as "fabrication, falsification, or plagiarism in proposing, performing, or reviewing research, or in reporting research results" (Steneck, 2007, p. 20) (see Figure 12-6). Research misconduct does not include differences of opinions. Actual reports of misconduct vary in the literature, with Pryor, Haberman, and Broome (2007) reporting 18% of research coordinators having knowledge of integrity violations.

Other areas that are not formally defined as research misconduct can create ethical concerns for the CTN. This may include protocol violations, inconsistencies in the process of informed consent, data collection and data management, pressures to recruit and retain patient-participants, failure to report adverse events in a timely fashion, modification of procedures without IRB approval, conflicts of interest, and authorship disputes. In fact, the CTN is a vital link between the patient-participant and the principal investigator. In their qualitative work on study coordinators' critical role in human subject protection (slightly more than two-thirds had nursing backgrounds), Davis, Hull, Grady, Wilfond, and Henderson (2002) reported that coordinators are often balancing patient, subject, and study advocacy, which can lead to

---

Figure 12-6. Definitions Related to Research Misconduct

Fabrication
Making up data or results and recording or reporting them

Falsification
Manipulating research materials, equipment, or processes, or changing or omitting data or results such that the research is not accurately represented in the research record

Plagiarism
The appropriation of another person's ideas, processes, results, or words without giving appropriate credit

Note. From *Federal Policy on Research Misconduct*, by U.S. Office of Science and Technology Policy, 2000. Retrieved from http://ori.dhhs.gov/education/products/RCRintro/c02/b1c2.html.

---

conflict. The IOM Committee on Assessing Integrity in Research Environments (2002) noted that individual scientists are the most unpredictable and influential variable within the research environment and, in some cases, have shifted blame to study coordinators for questionable practices (Davis et al., 2002). However, CTNs' proximal role to both the patient-participant and the protocol lends itself to immediately addressing any discrepancies before misconduct occurs. All CTNs should (Richmond & Ulrich, 2013)

- Conduct research with transparency, rigor, and truthfulness.
- Ask questions to clarify concerns related to the conduct of research and seek senior mentorship and support to address questionable research practices.
- Consult with an ethics committee as needed.
- Develop a memorandum of agreement that outlines the ethical standards of practice, authorship guidelines, and other intellectual interests associated with the research protocol.
- Have a basic understanding of the ethical codes of conduct and the ethical principles of research (i.e., beneficence, respect for persons, justice).
- Contact the IRB for any questions or uncertainty regarding reporting requirements, modifications, or amendments to the protocol.

Conflict of Interest

The ability to financially gain from one's research has been a source of intense discussion among the research community, the university academy, the pharmaceutical industry, and the public. In research, the secondary financial gain of investigators has the potential to undermine the primary protection of human participants and place them at undue risk. Moreover, Saver (2012) stated that "secondary interests can compromise the design, conduct, and reporting of research, while also threatening subject safety and undermining public trust" (p. 468). Thus, CTNs should be familiar with the Promoting Objectivity in Research (2011) regulations. These regulations specifically address financial conflicts of interest related to the conduct of research and address stock ownership and equity, consulting fees, paid authorship, and individual and institutional reporting requirements. "An individual has a conflict of interest when he or she has personal, financial, professional, or political interests that are likely to undermine his or her ability to meet or fulfill his or her primary professional, ethical, or legal obligations" (Shamoo & Resnik, 2009, p. 191). See Chapter 22 for more information.

Although individuals can disclose their financial conflicts of interest and develop sound management plans with institutional advisory oversight, there has been little focus on other types of conflicts, including nonfinancial conflicts of interests. These intellectual or intrinsic conflicts can undermine research because the pressures for success, including promotion and tenure or other accolades, may potentially bias one's judgment and contribute to hasty research-related decisions. Barrett (2010) speaks of a four-tiered system to promote the integrity of research, including personal and professional values, research mentorship, peer review, and IRB oversight. Maintaining research integrity requires a multifaceted approach, and the pragmatic abilities along with the scientific and healthcare expertise of CTNs provide a protective layer that is essential to the ethical conduct of research.

Ethics Consultation

Consultation with bioethicists and others who are not germane to the research study is sometimes warranted to provide expert and unbiased counsel on problematic issues that arise in the course of research. For example, a CTN might
- Question the capacity of an individual to provide informed consent
- Want help in communicating with difficult patient-participants, family members, or significant others
- Seek advice on end-of-life disagreements among study team members
- Want to better understand genetic risk implications for family members and determine when disclosure of risk to others is appropriate, if at all
- Need guidance in thinking through a study design that includes vulnerable population groups.

Regardless of position, all members of the study team, as well as students, patient-participants, family members, and significant others, can ask for an ethics consultation; sometimes this request might come from an IRB member. Some evidence suggests that nurses, in particular, fear retaliation for seeking ethics support, although Danis et al. (2008) did not find an association between fear of retaliation and decreased requests for ethics consultation.

Consultation provides not only a means of clarifying the ethical issues within the study but also an opportunity to hear all relevant stakeholder voices. As Danis et al. (2008) noted, assisting researchers and others "in the identification and analysis of ethical issues that arise in the course of conducting research—from the conception of a research question, throughout recruitment and enrollment of research participants, data collection, and even beyond a study's completion" (p. 7) is a primary goal of the consultation service. Since the 1980s, ethics consultation services have been widely available for practicing clinicians within hospital-based institutions (Danis et al., 2012), but more recently, bioethicists have lent their expertise to the research arena.

Not every institution will have a bioethicist or research ethics consultation service. The majority of academic institutions, however, have an office of research as well as IRB members who might be able to provide insight or guidance on ethics-related questions. CTNs who do not have access to an ethics consultation service can always call their IRB representative or check with their professional oncology society for guidelines that might assist them in addressing ethical questions. To some degree, patient-participants rely on CTNs to provide them with factual information about clinical trials and to help explain the treatment regimen because, as Dresser (2012) noted, "patients make trial decisions with a limited and sometimes inaccurate grasp of the facts" (p. 74). Patient-participants diagnosed with cancer are often scared; they face much uncertainty with their diagnosis and must make difficult treatment decisions.

Nurses have an ethical duty to protect patients from harm and advocate on their behalf; this extends to the research environment and sometimes requires an ethics consultation. Understanding the ethical principles of research, the relevant codes of conduct, the complicated terminology of clinical trials, the importance of informed consent with human participants, and the resources available to assist study team members and others with ethical questions in the protection of human participants reflects in the still-relevant words of Beecher (1966): "an ethical approach to experimentation with man [is] safeguarded by the presence of an intelligent, informed, conscientious, compassionate, responsible investigator" (p. 1360). This includes CTNs who are integral to research teams and foster critical dialogue among patient-participants, principal investigators, and other research team members.

Summary

Nurses caring for research participants are not called upon to act in place of the patient but rather as an advocate. Experience and knowledge of principles that guide the conduct of ethical research brings strength to the advocacy role of the CTN. Fear or uncertainty, including fear of the unknown, can become a barrier to advocacy (Thacker, 2008). As advocates, CTNs need to exercise ethical assertiveness during research team meetings and interdisciplinary rounds and advocate further for the role of the CTN as an active participant in ethical decisions (Norton & Joos, 2005). New knowledge and experience related to the ethical issues surrounding human subject research comes with the responsibility and accountability for CTNs, as caregivers and research advocates, to strive for full informed consent on the part of each research participant (Wallen & Baker, 2012).

Key Points

- CTNs are integral members of research teams responsible for the ethical conduct of research.
- CTNs face many ethical challenges in the implementation of clinical research.
- Ethical principles (beneficence, respect for persons, and justice) and ethical codes of conduct can guide CTNs in addressing ethical concerns that arise in clinical research.
- Ethics consultation services can provide support and objective counsel on difficult ethical issues that arise in clinical research.
- Knowledge of key ethical terms in clinical research (e.g., placebo, randomization, equipoise) can support CTNs' conversations with patient-participants on research participation.
- IRBs are part of the ethical oversight of clinical research and are responsible for protocol review.

References

Annas, G.J., & Grodin, M.A. (2008). The Nuremberg Code. In E.J. Emanuel, C. Grady, R.A. Crouch, R.K. Lie, F.G. Miller, & D. Wendler (Eds.), *Oxford textbook of clinical research ethics* (pp. 136–140). New York, NY: Oxford University Press.

Appelbaum, P.A., Lidz, C.W., & Meisel, A. (1987). *Informed consent*. New York, NY: Oxford University Press.

Appelbaum, P.S., Lidz, C., & Grisso, T. (2004). Therapeutic misconception in clinical research: Frequency and risk factors. *IRB: Ethics and Human Research, 26*(2), 1–8. doi:10.2307/3564231

Appelbaum, P.S., Roth, L.H., & Lidz, C. (1982). The therapeutic misconception: Informed consent in psychiatric research. *International Journal of Law and Psychiatry, 5*, 319–329. doi:10.1016/0160-2527(82)90026-7

Appelbaum, P.S., Roth, L.H., Lidz, C.W., Benson, P., & Winslade, W. (1987). False hopes and best data: Consent to research and the therapeutic misconception. *Hastings Center Report, 17*, 20–24.

Arras, J.D. (2008). The Jewish Chronic Disease Hospital case. In E.J. Emanuel, C. Grady, R.A. Crouch, R.K. Lie, F.G. Miller, & D. Wendler (Eds.), *Oxford textbook of clinical research ethics* (pp. 73–79). New York, NY: Oxford University Press.

Barrett, R. (2010). Strategies for promoting the scientific integrity of nursing research in clinical settings. *Journal for Nurses in Staff Development, 26*, 200–205. doi:10.1097/NND.0b013e31819b55dd

Beecher, H. (1966). Ethics and clinical research. *New England Journal of Medicine, 274*, 1350–1360. doi:10.1056/NEJM196606162742405

Danis, M., Farrar, A., Grady, C., Taylor, C., O'Donnell, P., Soeken, K., & Ulrich, C. (2008). Does fear of retaliation deter requests for ethics consultation? *Medicine, Health Care, and Philosophy, 11*, 27–34. doi:10.1007/s11019-007-9105-z

Danis, M., Largent, E., Grady, C., Wendler, D., Hull, S.C., Shah, S., ... Berkman, B. (2012). *Research ethics consultation: A casebook*. New York, NY: Oxford University Press.

Davis, A.M., Hull, S.C., Grady, C., Wilfond, B.S., & Henderson, G.E. (2002). The invisible hand in clinical research: The study coordinator's critical role in human subjects protection. *Journal of Law, Medicine, and Ethics, 30*, 411–419. doi:10.1111/j.1748-720X.2002.tb00410.x

Dresser, R. (2012). *Malignant: Medical ethicists confront cancer*. New York, NY: Oxford University Press.

Emanuel, E.J., & Miller, F.G. (2001). The ethics of placebo-controlled trials—A middle ground. *New England Journal of Medicine, 345*, 915–919. doi:10.1056/NEJM200109203451211

Emanuel, E.J., Wendler, D., & Grady, C. (2000). What makes clinical research ethical? *JAMA, 283*, 2701–2711. doi:10.1001/jama.283.20.2701

Faden, R., & Beauchamp, T. (1986). *A history and theory of informed consent*. New York, NY: Oxford University Press.

Flory, J., & Emanuel, E.J. (2004). Interventions to improve research participants' understanding in informed consent for research: A systematic review. *JAMA, 292*, 1593–1601. doi:10.1001/jama.292.13.1593

Freedman, B. (1987). Equipoise and the ethics of clinical research. *New England Journal of Medicine, 317*, 141–145. doi:10.1056/NEJM198707163170304

Grady, C. (2008). Clinical trials. In M. Crowley (Ed.), *From birth to death and bench to clinic: The Hastings Center bioethics briefing book for journalists, policymakers, and campaigns* (pp. 21–24). Garrison, NY: Hastings Center.

Grady, C. (2010). Do IRBs protect human research participants? *JAMA, 304*, 1122–1123. doi:10.1001/jama.2010.1304

Grady, C., & Edgerly, M. (2009). Science, technology, and innovation: Nursing responsibilities in clinical research. *Nursing Clinics of North America, 44*, 471–481. doi:10.1016/j.cnur.2009.07.011

Hart, R., & Belotto, M. (2010). The institutional review board. *Seminars in Nuclear Medicine, 4*, 385–392. doi:10.1053/j.semnuclmed.2010.03.007

Henderson, G.E., Churchill, L.R., Davis, A.M., Easter, M.M., Grady, C., Joffe, S., ... Zimmerman, C.R. (2007). Clinical trials and medical care: Defining the therapeutic misconception. *PLOS Medicine, 4*, e324. doi:10.1371/journal.pmed.0040324

Horng, S., & Grady, C. (2003). Misunderstanding in clinical research: Distinguishing therapeutic misconception, therapeutic misestimation, and therapeutic optimism. *IRB: Ethics and Human Research, 25*(1), 11–16. doi:10.2307/3564408

Institute of Medicine. (2009). *Conflict of interest in medical research, education, and practice*. Washington, DC: National Academies Press.

Institute of Medicine Committee on Assessing Integrity in Research Environments. (2002). *Integrity in scientific research: Creating an environment that promotes responsible conduct*. Washington, DC: National Academies Press.

Jansen, L.A. (2006). The problem with optimism in clinical trials. *IRB: Ethics and Human Research, 28*(4), 13–19. Retrieved from http://www.jstor.org/stable/30033204

Joffe, S., Cook, E.F., Cleary, P.D., Clark, J.W., & Weeks, J.C. (2001). Quality of informed consent in cancer clinical trials: A cross-sectional survey. *Lancet, 358*, 1772–1777. doi:10.1016/S0140-6736(01)06805-2

Joffe, S., & Truog, R.D. (2008). Equipoise and randomization. In E.J. Emanuel, C. Grady, R.A. Crouch, R.K. Lie, F.G. Miller, & D. Wendler (Eds.), *Oxford textbook of clinical research ethics* (pp. 245–260). New York, NY: Oxford University Press.

Jones, J.H. (2008). The Tuskegee syphilis experiment. In E.J. Emanuel, C. Grady, R.A. Crouch, R.K. Lie, F.G. Miller, & D. Wendler (Eds.), *Oxford textbook of clinical research ethics* (pp. 86–96). New York, NY: Oxford University Press.

Kim, S.Y.H., Schrock, L., Wilson, R.M., Frank, S.A., Holloway, R.G., Kieburtz, K., & de Vries, R.G. (2009). An approach to evaluating the therapeutic misconception. *IRB: Ethics and Human Research, 31*(5), 7–14. Retrieved from http://www.jstor.org/stable/25594887

Kimmelman, J. (2007). The therapeutic misconception at 25: Treatment, research, and confusion. *Hastings Center Report, 37*(6), 36–42. doi:10.1353/hcr.2007.0092

Liu, M.B., & Davis, K. (2001). *Lessons from a horse named Jim: A clinical trials manual from the Duke Clinical Research Institute*. Durham, NC: Duke Clinical Research Institute.

Miller, F., & Joffe, S. (2011). Equipoise and the dilemma of randomized clinical trials. *New England Journal of Medicine, 364*, 476–480. doi:10.1056/NEJMsb1011301

Murthy, V.H., Krumholz, H.M., & Gross, C.P. (2004). Participation in cancer clinical trials: Race-, sex-, and age-based disparities. *JAMA, 291*, 2720–2726. doi:10.1001/jama.291.22.2720

National Commission for the Protection of Human Subjects of Biomedical and Behavioral Research. (1979, April 18). *The Belmont report: Ethical principles and guidelines for the protection of human subjects of research*. Retrieved from http://www.hhs.gov/ohrp/humansubjects/guidance/belmont.html

Norton, C., & Joos, O. (2005). Caring for Catherine: A cry to support ethical activism. *Journal of Pediatric Oncology, 22*, 119–120. doi:10.1177/1043454204273771

Nuremberg Code. (1949). In *Trials of war criminals before the Nuremberg military tribunals under Control Council Law No. 10* (Vol. 2, pp. 181–182). Washington, DC: U.S. Government Printing Office. Retrieved from http://www.hhs.gov/ohrp/archive/nurcode.html

Promoting Objectivity in Research, 42 C.F.R. §§ 50.601–50.607 (2011). Retrieved from http://www.gpo.gov/fdsys/pkg/CFR-2011-title42-vol1/pdf/CFR-2011-title42-vol1-part50-subpartF.pdf

Protection of Human Research Subjects, 45 C.F.R. pt. 46 (2009). Retrieved from http://www.hhs.gov/ohrp/humansubjects/guidance/45cfr46.html

Pryor, E.R., Haberman, B., & Broome, M.E. (2007). Scientific misconduct from the perspective of research coordinators: A national survey. *Journal of Medical Ethics, 33*, 365–369. doi:10.1136/jme.2006.016394

Richmond, T., & Ulrich, C. (2013). *Ethical foundations for critical care nursing research*. Retrieved from http://www.aacn.org/wd/practice/docs/research/ethical-foundations-critical-care-nursing-research.pdf

Robinson, E.J., Kerr, C., Stevens, A., Lilford, R., Braunholtz, D., & Edwards, S. (2003). Lay conceptions of the ethical and scientific justification for random allocation in clinical trials. *Social Science and Medicine, 8*, 811–824. doi:10.1016/S0277-9536(03)00255-7

Robinson, W.M., & Unruh, B.T. (2008). The Hepatitis experiments at Willowbrook State School. In E.J. Emanuel, C. Grady, R.A. Crouch, R.K. Lie, F.G. Miller, & D. Wendler (Eds.), *Oxford textbook of clinical research ethics* (pp. 80–85). New York, NY: Oxford University Press.

Ross, S., Grant, A., Counsell, C., Gillespie, W., Russell, I., & Prescott, R. (1999). Barriers to participation in randomized controlled trials: A systematic review. *Journal of Clinical Epidemiology, 52*, 1143–1156. doi:10.1016/S0895-4356(99)00141-9

Saver, R.S. (2012). Is it really all about the money? Reconsidering nonfinancial interests in medical research. *Journal of Law, Medicine, and Ethics, 40*, 467–481. doi:10.1111/j.1748-720X.2012.00679.x

Schloendorff v. Society of New York Hospital, 211 N.Y. 125, 105 N.E. 92 (1914).

Shamoo, A.E., & Resnik, D.B. (2009). *Responsible conduct of research* (2nd ed.). New York, NY: Oxford University Press.

Shaw, P.A., Johnson, L.L., & Borkowf, C.B. (2012). Issues with randomization. In J.I. Gallin & F.P. Ognibene (Eds.), *Principles and practice of clinical research* (3rd ed., pp. 243–253). Boston, MA: Elsevier Academic Press. doi:10.1016/B978-0-12-382167-6.00020-5

Steneck, N.H. (2007). *ORI introduction to the responsible conduct of research*. Retrieved from https://ori.hhs.gov/sites/default/files/rcrintro.pdf

Stolberg, H.O., Norman, G., & Trop, I. (2004). Randomized controlled trials. *American Journal of Roentgenology, 18*, 1539–1544. doi:10.2214/ajr.183.6.01831539

Thacker, K. (2008). Nurses' advocacy behaviors in end-of-life nursing care. *Nursing Ethics, 15*, 174–185. doi:10.1177/0969733007086015

Ulrich, C.M., Knafl, K.A., Ratcliffe, S., Richmond, T., Grady, C., Miller-Davis, C., & Wallen, G. (2012). Developing a model of the benefits and burdens of research participation in cancer clinical trials. *American Journal of Bioethics: Primary Research, 3*(2), 10–23. doi:10.1080/21507716.2011.653472

Wallen, G.R., & Baker, K. (2012). Ethical challenges in transitioning to end-of-life care: Exploring the meaning of a "good death." In C.M. Ulrich (Ed.), *Nursing ethics in everyday practice* (pp. 151–161). Indianapolis, IN: Sigma Theta Tau International.

Waltz, C., Strickland, O., & Lenz, E. (2010). *Measurement in nursing and health research* (4th ed.). New York, NY: Springer.

Weindling, P.J. (2008). The Nazi medical experiments. In E.J. Emanuel, C. Grady, R.A. Crouch, R.K. Lie, F.G. Miller, & D. Wendler (Eds.), *Oxford textbook of clinical research ethics* (pp. 18–30). New York, NY: Oxford University Press.

Welton, A.J., Vickers, M.R., Cooper, J.A., Meade, T.W., & Marteau, T.M. (1999). Is recruitment more difficult with a placebo arm in randomised controlled trials? A quasirandomised, interview based study. *BMJ, 318*, 1114–1117. doi:10.1136/bmj.318.7191.1114

Wendler, D., & Rackoff, J. (2002). Consent for continuing research participation: What is it and when should it be obtained? *IRB: Ethics and Human Research, 24*(3), 1–6. doi:10.2307/3563787

World Medical Association. (1997). Declaration of Helsinki—Recommendations guiding physicians in biomedical research involving human subjects. *JAMA, 277*, 925–926. doi:10.1001/jama.1997.03540350075038

SECTION III.

Protocol Development, Review, and Approval Process

Chapter 13

Elements of a Protocol

Wendi Mitchell, RN, OCN®, and Zelda Smith, RN, CBCN®, OCN®

Introduction

A *protocol* is a detailed written plan of a clinical research study (National Cancer Institute Cancer Therapy Evaluation Program [NCI CTEP], 2014; National Institutes of Health [NIH], n.d., 2012). It is viewed as the "written agreement between the investigator, the subject, and the scientific community" (Friedman, Furberg, & DeMets, 1998, p. 10). To ensure consistency and enable communication among those working on the clinical trial, the same protocol is used at every participating site (NCI CTEP, 2014). Execution of the same protocol allows for the combination and comparison of data from multiple sites (NCI CTEP, 2014).

Every protocol has common or essential elements (see Figure 13-1). Protocol templates contain these essential elements and are used within a particular class of studies. The templates and applications enable investigators to easily insert research specifics into study documents. Template instructions are detailed and provide telephone, email, and fax contact information to reach the CTEP help desk. NCI encourages the use of a protocol template to facilitate rapid review when the protocol is submitted (NCI CTEP, 2014). NCI CTEP provides a sample of a general protocol template at http://ctep.cancer.gov/forms.

Several types of clinical trials exist; each is designed to answer different research questions (see Chapter 3). Examples of clinical trials include those that study treatment, prevention, screening, supportive care, biospecimens, palliative care, and translational research. Despite the differences in study focus, all clinical trials will have all of the basic elements of a protocol; however, industry-sponsored and other studies will have slight variations (NCI CTEP, 2014).

Figure 13-1. Essential Elements of a Protocol

- Title page
- Schema
- Objectives
- Background and rationale
- Patient eligibility criteria
- Pharmaceutical information
- Treatment plan
- Procedures for patient entry on study
- Adverse events list and reporting requirements
- Dose modifications for adverse events
- Criteria for response assessment
- Monitoring of patients
- Off-study criteria
- Statistical considerations
- Records to be kept
- Participation
- Multicenter trials

Note. From *A Handbook for Clinical Investigators Conducting Therapeutic Clinical Trials Supported by CTEP, DCTD, NCI* [v.1.2], by National Cancer Institute Cancer Therapy Evaluation Program, 2014. Retrieved from http://ctep.cancer.gov/investigatorResources/docs/InvestigatorHandbook.pdf.

Protocol Elements

The *title page* section of the clinical trial protocol is the primary source of identifying information for the CTEP Protocol and Information Office, the agent distribution system, the investigational new drug (IND) application file, and the U.S. Food and Drug Administration, as well as for listing of the protocol in the Clinical Trials Reporting Program (NCI CTEP, 2014). Therefore, the following sections are essential.
- Version date of the document
- Local protocol number (i.e., institution or group number) if applicable
- Title of study
- A single protocol/group chair who will be responsible for interactions with CTEP for the study, including his

---

The authors would like to acknowledge Angela D. Klimaszewski, RN, MSN, for her contribution to this chapter that remains unchanged from the previous edition.

or her name, institution/cooperative group, address, phone and fax numbers, and email addresses
- Full name of the institution/group submitting the study
- List of each participating institution/group/Community Clinical Oncology Program
- For agents supplied through the CTEP Pharmaceutical Management Branch, NCI Division of Cancer Treatment and Diagnosis, a list of each agent by name and National Service Center (NSC) number
- For non-CTEP IND agents, a list of each agent by name with NSC number (if applicable), IND number, and IND sponsor

Cooperative groups may summarize by specifying "all group members" or "restricted to . . ." and list institutions. All multicenter trials include the CTEP Multicenter Guidelines, which can be found on the CTEP website (http://ctep.cancer.gov/branches/ctmb/clinicalTrials/monitoring_multicenter.htm).

The *schema* section provides a brief description of the overall treatment plan, including the interventions to be administered, the length of time for each intervention (e.g., days, cycles), and an estimate of the number of patients exposed to the intervention (IND Content and Format, 2013; NCI CTEP, 2014). It often is provided in a diagram format. This section is a quick reference for treating physicians when reviewing patients for clinical trials. Because the overall treatment plan is simplified in this section, it is a useful tool when explaining the protocol to patients. This area may also outline required steps in a trial (see Chapter 4 for samples of the different types of study designs).

The *objectives* are the questions (hypotheses) to be answered by the clinical trial and may indicate what can be gained by performing the trial. Objectives guide what information will be collected and facilitates the development of the methodology (Masatu, 2012). Clinical trials will have primary objectives and may have secondary objective(s). *Primary objectives* are usually related to the target population and outcome being studied. For example, the primary objective for ECOG-ACRIN Cancer Research Group trial E1305 is "to compare the overall survival of patients with recurrent or metastatic head and neck cancer treated with standard platinum-based chemotherapy with or without bevacizumab" (ECOG-ACRIN Cancer Research Group, 2014).

Secondary objectives are usually related to other data that the researchers would like to gain from the specific population being studied. These could be in relationship to quality-of-life questions, ancillary laboratory tests, a specific subset of the population, tumor markers, or clinical correlation to a specific test. One secondary objective in E1305 is "to assess toxicities with the addition of bevacizumab to each platinum doublet and to compare the objective response rates and the progression-free survival achieved with each platinum doublet therapies" (ECOG-ACRIN Cancer Research Group, 2014).

The *background and rationale* section presents the earlier related studies that led to this study's hypothesis, and data from these studies are quoted in detail with references. This section gives a review of the rationale for the study and for evaluating correlations between tumor and patient outcome (e.g., response to intervention, overall survival). Information about ancillary studies (e.g., supportive care, quality of life) that may be included in the study and the implications for potential future studies are also presented (NCI CTEP, 2014).

Patient *eligibility criteria* are the unbiased requirements that the patient must meet in order to be enrolled into the trial. These requirements help ensure that patients in a trial are similar to each other in terms of specific factors such as age, type and stage of cancer, general health, and previous treatment. When all participants meet the same eligibility criteria, it gives researchers greater confidence that results of the study are caused by the intervention being tested and not by other factors (NCI, n.d.). Usually this part is divided into two sections: eligibility criteria and ineligibility (exclusion) criteria. Patients must meet all requirements in both areas. General questions requiring clarification of the criteria can be directed to the sponsor, cooperative group, or study chair.

Pharmaceutical information is required to provide details on the agents used in the clinical trial whether it is an investigational agent or a commercial agent. The following details should be provided for investigational agents: agent name, NSC number (if applicable), how the agent is supplied, stability, preparation instructions for the agent, storage requirements, route of administration, mechanism of action, formulation, adverse events, and unblinding procedures, if appropriate (NCI CTEP, 2014). Unblinding procedures are only included if the study is double blinded. Adverse events for the drug that is blinded are provided and should be included in the informed consent form and process.

The *treatment plan* section describes what treatment participants will receive. "Instructions for dose regimens should be complete, clear, and simple to follow. Treatment regimens should be expressed accurately, completely, and consistently throughout a protocol document" (NCI CTEP, 2008). This section includes all aspects of the treatment patients will receive, such as the dose, route, and schedule of all drugs or therapy, which includes whether any specific supportive therapies can or cannot be given while on the study.

Procedures for patient entry on study will provide detailed requirements needed to enroll patients on the trial. The number of steps and what is needed at each step will be specified, including stratification criteria and randomization. This section identifies the necessary regulatory documents and specifies if any credentialing needs to be completed prior to patient entry on study.

The *adverse events list and reporting requirements* section identifies what side effects have been previously reported in preclinical and clinical studies associated with the agents that will be used in the study. This information can be obtained from the investigator's brochure for investigational agents and the package insert for commercial agents. An *adverse event* is any unfavorable or unintended sign that occurs with the use of a medical intervention that may or may not be related to that intervention; it is a term used for medical documentation and scientific analyses (NCI CTEP, 2010). This section provides the guidelines (including the method and the time frame) for reporting adverse events or serious adverse events to the appropriate groups. Dose modifications for adverse events guide how to manage the agents in the clinical trial. Specific guidelines are given for each of the side effects that may occur and what should be done for each of the agents or treatment given. The Common Terminology Criteria for Adverse Events (CTCAE) is used to grade side effects to ensure that the same severity rating is used by all providers (NCI CTEP, 2010). See Chapter 28.

Criteria for response assessment is the section that provides objective study endpoints, including definitions of complete and partial response, stable disease, and progressive disease. These categories define the effect of the treatment that is being achieved. This section also provides details of when testing should be performed in order to determine the response.

Monitoring of patients is the section that guides investigators/clinical trial nurses on when a specific test (e.g., complete blood count, chemistry panels, liver enzymes, computed tomography scans, bone scans) is to be performed. It also gives detailed information on the time of these tests in relation to the treatment on the study. It includes the time period pre-entry, during treatment, and when the patient is in follow-up. This is usually provided in a table format with footnotes to provide further explanation and sometimes is referred to as *study parameters*.

Off-study criteria explain the circumstances in which patients should be removed from the clinical trial. The circumstances for removal from study could be because of progressive disease, adverse events, or delay in study treatment.

Statistical considerations are the statistical information, such as the uniform data method collection, the random variation, generalizability of the study population, the sample size, and design of the study rationale (Heavlin, 2006). It gives in-depth information on how the total enrollment was determined, along with the power calculations for the primary and secondary objectives. The projected distribution of gender and minorities are included in this section. The analysis plan for the clinical trial is discussed and whether there are any planned interim analyses.

Records to be kept are documents that are essential to validate the data that are being reported. This includes the specific forms that are to be used and time points for submission to the sponsor. Sponsors/groups mandate how long records need to be maintained after study completion.

Multicenter trials guidelines are for those sites that wish to collaborate with other institutions.

Summary

Clinical trials are one of the most valuable sources of evidence on the efficacy of treatments in humans. Evidence-based medicine seeks to apply findings from clinical trials to better evaluate and treat clinical populations across all domains of medicine (Ross, Tu, Carini, & Sim, 2010). Creating clearly organized protocol documents can be a monumental task. Investigators, clinical trial nurses, pharmacists, clinical research associates, and staff nurses, as well as others from many disciplines, use these documents daily. Clinical trial nurses working today with complex and comprehensive clinical trials ensure superior patient treatment and high-quality clinical trials through their knowledge of the protocol document.

Key Points
- Key elements are included in all clinical trial documents.
- Protocol documents protect participants on study.
- Protocol documents are a guideline for the clinical staff.
- Protocol documents provide consistency across all sites participating in the clinical trial.

References

ECOG-ACRIN Cancer Research Group. (2014, April 25). *A phase III randomized trial of chemotherapy with or without bevacizumab in patients with recurrent or metastatic head and neck cancer.* Retrieved from http://www.ecog.org/general/E1305_physician_study_summary.pdf

Friedman, L.M., Furberg, C.D., & DeMets, D.L. (1998). *Fundamentals of clinical trials* (3rd ed.). New York, NY: Springer-Verlag.

Heavlin, W.D. (2006). *The low-carb lecture on clinical trials.* Retrieved from http://home.comcast.net/~bill.heavlin/LowCarbLecture4CRA_nc.pdf

IND Content and Format, 21 C.F.R. § 312.23 (2013). Retrieved from http://www.accessdata.fda.gov/scripts/cdrh/cfdocs/cfCFR/CFRSearch.cfm?fr=312.23

Masatu, M.C. (2012, June 7). Research objectives [Slide presentation]. Retrieved from http://www.slideshare.net/MMASSY/research-objectives-13231506

National Cancer Institute. (n.d.). NCI dictionary of cancer terms: Eligibility criteria. Retrieved from http://www.cancer.gov/dictionary?cdrid=346518

National Cancer Institute Cancer Therapy Evaluation Program. (2008, May 29). *Protocol development: Guidelines for treatment regimens.* Retrieved from http://ctep.cancer.gov/protocolDevelopment/policies_nomenclature.htm

National Cancer Institute Cancer Therapy Evaluation Program. (2010, June 14). *Common terminology criteria for adverse events* [v.4.03]. Retrieved from http://evs.nci.nih.gov/ftp1/CTCAE/CTCAE_4.03_2010-06-14_QuickReference_5x7.pdf

National Cancer Institute Cancer Therapy Evaluation Program. (2014). *A handbook for clinical investigators conducting therapeutic clini-

cal trials supported by CTEP, DCTD, NCI. Retrieved from http://ctep.cancer.gov/protocolDevelopment/electronic_applications/docs/aeguidelines.pdf

National Institutes of Health. (n.d.). Glossary of common site terms. Retrieved from http://www.clinicaltrials.gov/ct2/about-studies/glossary#P

National Institutes of Health. (2012, August). Learn about clinical studies. Retrieved from http://www.clinicaltrials.gov/ct2/about-studies/learn

Ross, J., Tu, S., Carini, S., & Sim, I. (2010). Analysis of eligibility criteria complexity in clinical trials. *AMIA Summits on Translational Science Proceedings, 2010,* 46–50. Retrieved from http://www.ncbi.nlm.nih.gov/pmc/articles/PMC3041539

Chapter 14

Informed Consent

Angela D. Klimaszewski, RN, MSN

Introduction

The informed consent (IC) process is a continuing dialogue among the responsible investigator, the study participant, and the research team to ensure that the participant's consent is voluntary, is based on information and understanding, and does not in any way involve the participant relinquishing his or her legal rights (National Institutes of Health, n.d.). The consent form (CF), also referred to as the *informed consent form*, is an integral part of the IC process, documenting the exchange and understanding of (a) the protocol, (b) the risks and benefits to the potential participant, (c) the rights of the participant including the right to withdraw at any time, and (d) other treatment options available to the patient (Protection of Human Subjects, 2009; U.S. Food and Drug Administration [FDA], 2009). In the past two decades, clinical trials have moved from using a CF that fell short of protecting human subjects to an ongoing process of IC that truly captures the spirit and intent of the Declaration of Helsinki and the Belmont Report, the focus of each being the protection of human subjects. This chapter reviews the IC process and associated documents in clinical trials research involving human subjects in the United States.

Guiding Principles

The Belmont Report

The Belmont Report established three principles for the ethical conduct of clinical trials involving human subjects in the United States: (a) respect for persons, (b) beneficence, and (c) justice (National Commission for the Protection of Human Subjects of Biomedical and Behavioral Research [National Commission], 1979). *Respect for persons* means recognizing a participant's personal dignity and autonomy and the right of participants to act in their best interest, as well as recognizing that participants with diminished autonomy (e.g., children, older adults, prisoners) require additional protection. *Beneficence* protects research participants from harm and ensures their well-being. *Justice* means that benefits and burdens are fairly distributed among all participants (National Commission, 1979).

The Belmont Report (National Commission, 1979) identified IC as a process derived from the principle of respect for persons. It further delineated three elements of the IC process: (a) information, (b) comprehension, and (c) voluntariness. Because the participant's ability to understand is a function of intelligence, rationality, maturity, and language, it is necessary to adapt the presentation of the information to the participant's capacities and use an interpreter when necessary.

The investigators are responsible for determining whether participants have fully comprehended the information being presented. Key to that responsibility is determining that information about risk to participants is "complete and adequately comprehended, [and] when the risks are more serious, that obligation increases" (National Commission, 1979, part C.1., para. 7). Also key is ensuring that the patient understands all the viable options for appropriate alternative procedures or treatments (Protection of Human Subjects, 2009). An investigator may elect to give an oral or written test of comprehension to validate the participant's understanding (National Commission, 1979).

An individual's agreement to participate in research is considered a valid consent only if the individual gives that consent voluntarily. This means the individual agrees to participate in the research in conditions free of coercion and undue influence (National Commission, 1979).

Coercion occurs when an overt threat of harm is intentionally presented by one person to another in order to obtain compliance. *Undue influence*, by contrast, occurs through an offer of an excessive, unwarranted, inappropriate or improper reward or other overture in order to obtain compliance. (National Commission, 1979, part C.1., para. 10)

U.S. Department of Health and Human Services

The U.S. Department of Health and Human Services (DHHS) and its agencies, the Office for Human Research Protections (OHRP) and FDA, revised their regulations on clinical trials involving human subjects in response to the Belmont Report (Protection of Human Subjects, 2009). It is important for clinical trial nurses (CTNs) to know which agency regulations apply to a given clinical trial (OHRP or FDA), as specific agency regulations may have slight differences.

OHRP regulates *DHHS-funded* clinical research with regulations in Title 45 Part 46 of the *Code of Federal Regulations* (45 C.F.R. pt. 46), titled Protection of Human Subjects (2009). Trials that involve an investigational drug, biologic product, or medical device are generally, but not exclusively, *privately sponsored* and fall under FDA jurisdiction and Title 21 of the C.F.R. Of particular relevance to this chapter are the regulations outlined in Informed Consent of Human Subjects (2013), which are found in 21 C.F.R. §§ 50.20–50.27. Other FDA regulations that affect IC include portions of Investigational New Drug Application, found in 21 C.F.R. pt. 312, as well as portions of Investigational Device Exemptions, found in 21 C.F.R. pt. 812.

Federal regulations on clinical trials will share common characteristics with state and local regulations. When this occurs, the investigator and research staff must comply with the regulations that are most stringent (Kaltman & Isidor, 2006). Every member of the research team and the institutional review board (IRB) must be aware of state regulations. Therefore, the IRB is an excellent resource for CTNs regarding regulatory issues.

Investigators' Responsibilities

The FDA document *Guidance for Industry: Investigator Responsibilities—Protecting the Rights, Safety, and Welfare of Study Subjects* (2009) provides an overview of the general responsibilities of a person who conducts a clinical trial of an investigational drug, medical device, or biologic product; only the portions that pertain to IC will be addressed here. The investigator or a person designated by the investigator must obtain IC from the participant or the participant's legally authorized representative (LAR) prior to involving the participant in any aspect of research (International Conference on Harmonisation of Technical Requirements for Registration of Pharmaceuticals for Human Use, 1996; National Commission, 1979). Of note, CTNs should provide education about the clinical trial to patients and family members, reinforcing what the physician investigator has discussed; however, the physician investigator actually should obtain the consent. Mackintosh and Molloy (2003) noted that significant physician involvement is required for IC in studies where the science is technologically complicated. The physician will need more time to adequately explain the study requirements and answer questions. CTNs play a pivotal role in ascertaining the participant's understanding of the IC document, clarifying misconceptions, and being the liaison between the patient and the physician regarding IC issues.

Under 21 C.F.R. pt. 312 and 21 C.F.R. pt. 812, investigators have a responsibility to personally "supervise the conduct of the clinical investigation and to protect the rights, safety, and welfare of participants in drug and medical device clinical trials" (U.S. FDA, 2009, p. 2). As an extension of this, when an investigator delegates tasks, he or she is responsible for adequately supervising those to whom the tasks were delegated. Consequently, the investigator is accountable for any regulatory violations that occur during study activities as a result of inadequate supervision. See Chapter 8.

An investigator's plan for adequate supervision of designees as it pertains to IC might include procedures to ensure that the consent process is in accordance with Informed Consent of Human Subjects (2013) and that ethical and medical issues that occur during the study are promptly addressed (U.S. FDA, 2009). An example of an investigator's inappropriate delegation would be if the individuals who obtained IC lacked sufficient medical training, knowledge, and IC process training; knowledge of the clinical protocol; or familiarity of the investigational product or device necessary to be able to discuss the purpose, risks and benefits, adverse effects, and alternatives of a clinical trial with prospective participants.

FDA (2009) noted that the investigator is responsible for ensuring that all staff involved in the conduct of the study

- Have a general familiarity with the study and protocol
- Have a specific understanding of the details of the protocol and the investigational product, relevant to the tasks they will be performing
- Are aware of regulatory requirements and acceptable standards for the conduct of clinical trials, with respect to the conduct of the clinical trial and human subject protection
- Are competent to perform the tasks that they are delegated
- Are informed of any pertinent changes during the conduct of the trial and are educated or given additional training as appropriate.

General Requirements for Informed Consent (2009) stipulate that potential participants receive complete information about the study in the CF and have opportunities for the researcher and participant to exchange information and ask questions without coercion or undue influence. The information must be presented in language understandable to the participant or the LAR. Of note is the requirement that "no informed consent, whether oral or written, may include any exculpatory language through which the participant or representative is made to waive or appear to waive any of the subject's legal rights" (see Figure 14-1). The IC form also cannot include language that releases or appears to release the investigator, the sponsor, the institution, or its agents from liability for negligence.

The investigator must ensure that IC and a signed and dated CF are obtained from each participant in accordance with regulations (Elements of Informed Consent, 2013) and that the study is not started until it receives IRB approval.

The Process of Informed Consent

The IC process relies on the basic principles of the Belmont Report. Potential participants may begin the IC process when they read an advertisement, receive a phone call about a specific clinical trial, or are approached by an investigator after their case was presented at a tumor board. Once a patient is identified as a potential candidate for a study, physicians introduce the clinical trial, including the investigative procedures (e.g., blood and urine collection, biopsies, radiographic procedures) to the patient (Green & Rickles, 2007). Patients are encouraged to ask questions and take enough time to critically review their other treatment options.

Patients need to fully discuss the treatment plan, adverse reactions, and expected risks and benefits with professionals (i.e., principal investigator, CTN, referring physician) and significant others before consenting. It is important to have a relaxed conversation with the potential participant so that he or she has adequate time to review the CF. The researchers give the CF to the participants to take home, read, and consider away from the clinical setting. Providing patients with a CF to review before signing will foster patients' and significant others' critical review, allow the patients to circle and highlight sections to remind themselves to seek clarification, and provide a general guide for the discussion with the physician and CTN at the next visit. This entire process must be documented in the participant's medical record. Table 14-1 outlines the steps in the IC process.

Required Elements of the Consent Form

General Elements

The required CF elements for OHRP (General Requirements for Informed Consent, 2009) and FDA (Elements of Informed Consent, 2013) are nearly identical. Both include the following language (General Requirements for Informed Consent, 2009, § 46.116a, 1–8):
- A statement that the study involves research, an explanation of the purposes of the research and the expected duration of the subject's participation, a description of the procedures to be followed, and identification of any procedures which are experimental
- A description of any reasonably foreseeable risks or discomforts to the subject
- A description of any benefits to the subject, or to others, which may reasonably be expected from the research
- A disclosure of appropriate alternative procedures or courses of treatment, if any, that might be advantageous to the subject
- A statement describing the extent, if any, to which confidentiality of records identifying the subject will be maintained

---

Figure 14-1. Exculpatory Language in Informed Consent

No informed consent, whether oral or written, may include any exculpatory language through which the subject is made to waive or appear to waive any of the subject's legal rights, or releases or appears to release the investigator, the sponsor, the institution, or its agents from liability for negligence.—45 C.F.R. § 46.116

Examples of Exculpatory Language
- By agreeing to this use, you should understand that you will give up all claims to personal benefit from commercial or other use of these substances.
- I voluntarily and freely donate any and all blood, urine, and tissue samples to the U.S. Government and hereby relinquish all right, title, and interest to said items.
- By consent to participate in this research, I give up any property rights I may have in bodily fluids or tissue samples obtained in the course of the research.
- I waive any possibility of compensation for injuries that I may receive as a result of participation in this research.

Examples of Acceptable Language
- Tissue obtained from you in this research may be used to establish a cell line that could be patented and licensed. There are no plans to provide financial compensation to you should this occur.
- By consenting to participate, you authorize the use of your bodily fluids and tissue samples for the research described above.
- This hospital is not able to offer financial compensation nor to absorb the costs of medical treatment should you be injured as a result of participating in this research.
- This hospital makes no commitment to provide free medical care or payment for any unfavorable outcomes resulting from participation in this research. Medical services will be offered at the usual charge.

Note. From "Office for Protection From Research Risks Cooperative Oncology Group Chairpersons Meeting, November 15, 1996—Exculpatory Language in Informed Consent," by Office for Human Research Protections, 1996. Retrieved from http://www.hhs.gov/ohrp/policy/exculp.html.

Table 14-1. Elements of the Informed Consent Process	
Element	Details
Initial meeting	Provide the participant and family/significant others with the consent form (CF). Discuss the CF logically with the participant and one or more members of the research team. Encourage the participant and family to take notes. Provide adequate time for the participant and family members to consider participation and have all questions answered. Provide the participant with a video, audio recording, or interactive computer program to help them to understand the information in the CF. Ensure that parents or a legally authorized representative (LAR) will represent any participant younger than 18 years. If the participant is between ages 7 and 18 years, ask for assent to participate, and provide an assent form for signature.
Time to read and consider participation	Provide the participant adequate time to review the CF at his or her leisure. Encourage the participant to discuss the CF with family, friends, social workers, clergy, an LAR, or other trusted advisers. Ask the participant to record questions and concerns for discussion at the next meeting.
Assessment of understanding	Discuss the participant's questions and concerns that were recorded at home. Assess the participant's understanding with interactive questioning, through a written questionnaire, or by having the patient explain specific parts of the CF in his or her own words. Document the assessment of the participant's comprehension. Answer the participant's questions until the participant states that he or she has enough information to make a decision. Document the participant's statement regarding his or her decision.
Questions	Encourage the participant to ask questions until the participant is satisfied with his or her understanding of the CF. Encourage the participant to record questions while away from the clinic and either bring them to the next meeting or schedule a visit to have the questions discussed.
Verification before treatment	Ask the patient to verify that he or she still consents to the treatment he or she is about to receive immediately before administering the treatment.
New information	Assure the participant that any new information available will be shared. Follow up on assurance. Provide the participant with an updated CF for signature (as required). Document the participant's comprehension of new information in the presence of family. Document the participant's signing of the new CF, review of CF, and that all the participant's questions were answered. Provide a signed copy of the CF to the participant.
Communication techniques	Use more than one strategy to ensure understanding, including videos, audio recordings, interactive computer programs, and discussions with qualified professional and lay individuals.
Supplemental materials	Use multimedia formats to reinforce information in face-to-face conversations, including videos, audio recordings, written materials, and interactive computer programs.
Note. Based on information from National Cancer Institute, 2013a.	

- For research involving more than minimal risk, an explanation as to whether any compensation and an explanation as to whether any medical treatments are available if injury occurs and, if so, what they consist of, or where further information may be obtained
- Contact information for answers to pertinent questions about the research and research subjects' rights, and whom to contact in the event of a research-related injury to the subject
- A statement that participation is voluntary, refusal to participate will involve no penalty or loss of benefits to which the subject is otherwise entitled, and that the subject may discontinue participation at any time without penalty or loss of benefits to which the subject is otherwise entitled.

In regard to confidentiality, FDA requires disclosure that it may inspect participant records, whereas OHRP does not include this required notation. Additional elements that specifically address issues such as unforeseeable risks to the individual, consequences of withdrawal from the study, and sharing of significant new findings with the individual are delineated in Figure 14-2.

Registry Databank

An amendment to the IC regulations was required by the FDA Amendments Act of 2007 with the pur-

Figure 14-2. Additional Elements of Informed Consent*

When appropriate, one or more of the following elements of information shall also be provided to each subject:
- A statement that the particular treatment or procedure may involve risks to the subject (or to the embryo or fetus, if the subject is or may become pregnant) which are currently unforeseeable
- Anticipated circumstances under which the subject's participation may be terminated by the investigator without regard to the subject's consent
- Any additional costs to the subject that may result from participation in the research
- The consequences of a subject's decision to withdraw from the research and procedures for orderly termination of participation by the subject
- A statement that significant new findings developed during the course of the research which may relate to the subject's willingness to continue participation will be provided to the subject
- The approximate number of subjects involved in the study.

* U.S. Food and Drug Administration and the Office for Human Research Protections requirements are the same.

Note. From General Requirements for Informed Consent, 45 C.F.R. § 46.116 (2009). Retrieved from http://www.hhs.gov/ohrp/humansubjects/guidance/45cfr46.html#46.116.

pose of advocating transparency in clinical research to study participants. FDA initiated a requirement for additional language as part of the CF to inform participants that clinical trial information will be entered into the ClinicalTrials.gov databank. The rule became effective in 2011 with a compliance date of March 7, 2012 (Informed Consent Elements Rule, 2011). The language to be included in all applicable trials is as follows (Elements of Informed Consent, 2013, § 50.25(c)).

> A description of this clinical trial will be available on http://www.ClinicalTrials.gov, as required by U.S. Law. This website will not include information that can identify you. At most, the website will include a summary of the results. You can search this website at any time.

Consent Form Template

The National Cancer Institute (NCI) developed a CF template in 1998 and made it available to investigators. The updated version is reproduced in Appendix 3. CTNs should note that every sponsor and every institution's IRB generally has its own CF template for investigators to use as well.

The 2013 CF template has an additional section that describes four optional clinical research studies, any of which may be added by a principal investigator to a CF:
- Optional imaging study—extra scan
- Optional imaging study—research scan or procedure
- Optional quality-of-life study
- Optional sample collections for laboratory studies and/or biobanking for possible future studies (see the Genetic Testing and Human Genomic Research section).

The IRB must approve the final CF prior to use as stated in General Requirements for Informed Consent (2009).

The CF should be written using terminology that the participant understands. To that end, the NCI Cancer Therapy Evaluation Program (CTEP) has a website that provides a list of agents/drugs and associated side effects in table format (http://ctep.cancer.gov/protocolDevelopment/#informed_consent). Further, the National Comprehensive Cancer Network® (NCCN®) hosts an IC language database for researchers to use for writing or amending CFs. The database has lay descriptions of more than 1,500 risks and events that may be encountered in clinical research. A plan to expand the database includes adding lay terminology for drugs and medical procedures. The NCCN IC language database is available at www.nccn.org/clinical_trials/informed_consent.aspx. Registration is free but is required to access the database. Figure 14-3 presents a checklist of characteristics of easy-to-read IC document text and graphics prepared by NCI.

Assessing Comprehension and Improving Readability

Assessment of participants' understanding of the clinical trial and the CF is vital to the IC process (National Commission, 1979). Cumming, Sahni, and McClelland (2006) stressed that the IC process needs to ensure a two-way flow of information to address participants' understanding of the information. Documentation or preferably a recording of the conversation between the participant and the research team is crucial. Documentation in the medical record must include how the participant's understanding was assessed (e.g., oral question-and-answer session, written post-test) (Jaynes, 2005). Newton (2007) noted that having a patient repeat the information to the educator can validate the effectiveness of the education. Asking questions that require more than an affirmative or negative response will provide CTNs with a greater appreciation of what the participant truly understands. Hochhauser (2004) maintained that unless comprehension criteria have been established before the clinical trial is opened, no benchmark can exist for determining low, average, or above-average comprehension.

Although NCI (2013b) recommends writing consent documents at an eighth-grade level or lower, Rust, Rogers, and Joyce (2007) noted that 20% of U.S. adults read below a sixth-grade level. Therefore, any medical language, abbreviations, or jargon should be converted to

Figure 14-3. Checklist for Easy-to-Read Informed Consent Documents

Text
- Words are familiar to the reader. Any scientific, medical, or legal words are defined clearly.
- Words and terminology are consistent throughout the document.
- Sentences are short, simple, and direct.
- Line length is limited to 30–50 characters and spaces.
- Paragraphs are short. Convey one idea per paragraph.
- Verbs are in active voice (i.e., the subject is the doer of the act).
- Personal pronouns are used to increase personal identification.
- Each idea is clear and logically sequenced (according to audience logic).
- Important points are highlighted.
- Study purpose is presented early in the text.
- Titles, subtitles, and other headers help to clarify organization of text.
- Headers are simple and close to text.
- Underline, bold, or boxes (rather than all caps or italics) give emphasis.
- Layout balances white space with words and graphics.
- Left margins are justified. Right margins are ragged.
- Upper and lower case letters are used.
- Style of print is easy to read.
- Type size is at least 12 point.
- Readability analysis is done to determine reading level (should be eighth grade or lower).
- Avoid:
  - Abbreviations and acronyms.
  - Large blocks of print.
  - Words containing more than three syllables (where possible).

Graphics
- Graphics are:
  - Helpful in explaining the text.
  - Easy to understand.
  - Meaningful to the audience.
  - Appropriately located. Text and graphics go together.
  - Simple and uncluttered.
- Images reflect cultural context.
- Visuals have captions.
- Each visual is directly related to one message.
- Cues, such as circles or arrows, point out key information.
- Colors, when used, are appealing to the audience.
- Avoid graphics that won't reproduce well.

Note. Based on information from Doak et al., 1996; Meade & Howser, 1992; National Cancer Institute, 2003, 2008.

From "Simplification of Informed Consent Documents—Appendix 3: Checklist for Easy-to-Read Informed Consent Documents," by National Cancer Institute, 2013. Retrieved from http://www.cancer.gov/clinicaltrials/conducting/simplification-of-informed-consent-docs/page5.

Documenting Informed Consent

Researchers have two acceptable options for obtaining written IC from a clinical trial participant. The first is an IRB-approved written CF. This CF must contain all of the required elements and be IRB approved before the participant or LAR signs it. The CF may be read to the participant or the participant's LAR. The investigator is responsible for ensuring that the participant or LAR has adequate time to read it, has time to ask questions before signing it, and receives a written copy (Documentation of Informed Consent, 2009).

The second way to document IC involves an oral presentation of the CF to the participant or the participant's LAR in the presence of a witness. Before the form can be used, the IRB must approve a short, written form that clearly states that the required elements of the IC have been presented verbally to the participant or the participant's LAR. Only then may the participant or the LAR sign the CF. The participant or LAR signs only the short form, and the witness must sign both the short form and the summary. Additionally, the person giving the oral presentation must sign the summary. The participant receives copies of both the short form and the summary (Documentation of Informed Consent, 2009). It is

Figure 14-4. Communication Methods

Time to Read and Discuss the Form
Researchers should encourage the potential research participant to thoroughly read and re-read the consent form and supplemental materials, if provided, and to discuss the proposed research with others before signing the consent form. This may require a delay between the describing of the study and the signing of the consent document.

Assessment of Understanding
It may be helpful for the researcher to ask the potential research participant short questions, after the research has been described and the consent form read, in order to assess that the potential research participant has at least a basic understanding of what the research involves. Example questions include:
- Tell me in your own words what this study is all about.
- Tell me what you think will happen to you in this study.
- What do you expect to gain by taking part in this research?
- What risks might you experience by participating in the research?
- What are your alternatives (other choices or options to participating in this research)?

Communication Techniques
Video, audio, interactive computer programs, and discussions with qualified lay individuals may assist in educating the potential research participant about the clinical trial.

Note. Based on information from Titus & Keane, 1996.

From "Simplification of Informed Consent Documents—Appendix 4: Communication Methods," by National Cancer Institute, 2013. Retrieved from http://www.cancer.gov/clinicaltrials/conducting/simplification-of-informed-consent-docs/page5#appendix4.

layperson's language written at no higher than a sixth-grade reading level. Evaluating the participant's level of understanding may result in adapting the presentation of information to the participant's capacities (National Commission, 1979). See the Special Populations section of this chapter for additional information. Communication methods pertaining to IC are detailed in Figure 14-4.

important to note that each IRB will have its own policies regarding the use of the short-form consent process.

Risks of treatment must be weighed against the benefits before the participant decides to proceed with any treatment for any disease. In a clinical trial, some of the risks and benefits may not be known or may be observed during the course of the study. The principal investigator is responsible for providing participants with an adequate explanation of expected effects of the treatment on an ongoing basis throughout the study. If unexpected toxicities are observed during the course of the study, the investigator will amend the CF, and the IRB will review and approve (or not approve—an amended form does not guarantee IRB approval) the new form. From that point forward, only the amended CF may be used. Participants still engaged in therapy or otherwise affected by the new findings must sign an amended consent (Documentation of Informed Consent, 2009; General Requirements for Informed Consent, 2009).

Reconsent

New information that becomes available about an investigational drug (including biologics for this chapter) or device during the course of a clinical trial may necessitate reconsent, a part of the IC process that requires the signing of a new CF. The IRB must approve an amendment to the protocol and the new CF. If the new information might be relevant to the participant's decision to stay in the trial (continued consent) or may have affected his or her original decision to enroll in the trial, the participant should be notified and a new signed CF obtained and documented (Dal-Ré, Avendaño, Gil-Aguado, Gracia, & Caplan, 2008; NCI, 2013c). If the new information indicates a small risk of developing low-severity toxicity, the information could be shared verbally by phone and in writing at the next scheduled visit (NCI, 2013c). If the protocol stipulates that new information not requiring consent be mailed to all study participants, then an IRB-approved letter should be sent to every participant enrolled. If the procedure for reconsent is not stipulated in the protocol document, the principal investigator should assess the relevance of the new information and determine if patients should be called for an unscheduled visit or if the principal investigator can discuss the new information at the patient's next scheduled visit.

Types of information that would compel reconsent include, but are not limited to,
- If the information involves new toxicity data demonstrating that the toxicity is likely to develop and has a high risk of being severe
- If the IRB or sponsor requires reconsent based on new information.

Also, if a child or adolescent gave assent when they were enrolled in a trial and he or she reaches the state's legal age for healthcare decisions, the participant should be consented and a new CF signed.

A new or updated CF must have IRB approval and a notation that a review was completed and approval granted. From that point forward, only the most recent IRB-approved version may be used; the previous CF cannot (Documentation of Informed Consent, 2009; General Requirements for Informed Consent, 2009). Figure 14-5 lists the steps involved with reconsent of participants in a clinical trial.

The participant has the right to withdraw from a clinical trial at any time. However, if withdrawal endangers the participant's health, such as withdrawal from a high-dose chemotherapy regimen for bone marrow transplantation before rescue or stem cell reinfusion, the CF clearly must state the possibility of serious complications or death (General Requirements for Informed Consent, 2009).

Procedures for Consent of a Non–English-Speaking Participant

NCI emphasized the need to include diverse populations in cancer research:

This important and complex issue requires cultural sensitivity in developing the IC document and communicating with the potential research participant and family members. The standards for valid consent should not

---

Figure 14-5. Steps Involved in Reconsenting Study Participants

1. Explain the new information to all participants in the presence of significant others.
2. Provide participants with an updated consent form that reflects the new information in a manner consistent with what a reasonable person would need to know to make a decision about staying in the trial.
3. Discuss participants' initial questions and concerns.
4. Schedule a return visit for additional discussion if a participant needs more time and give a copy of the new consent form to the participant for review with significant others.
5. Discuss questions and concerns using the consent form to guide the discussion.
6. Assess participants' understanding when they state that they have enough information to make a decision.
7. Document in the progress note the participant's statement about his or her understanding and decision in the presence of the significant others.
8. Document in the progress note the participant's signing of the new consent form, review of the consent form, and that all of his or her questions were answered.
9. Provide participants with a copy of the new signed and dated consent form and place the originals in their research file.

Note. Based on information from Dal-Ré et al., 2008; National Cancer Institute, 2013b; Richmond, 2013.

be compromised in the face of language, cultural, or physical challenges. (NCI, 2013c, p. 2)

A non–English-speaking participant must be presented with a CF written in the participant's native language. Alternatively, an oral presentation of IC information by a translator in conjunction with a short-form written consent document (stating that the elements of consent have been presented verbally) and a written summary of what was presented verbally can be used. The short-form written CF should be in a language understandable to the participant. In this case, the IRB-approved English-language CF may serve as the summary, and the witness should be fluent in both English and the participant's language (General Requirements for Informed Consent, 2009).

At the time of consent, the participant or the participant's LAR should sign the short-form document. The investigator should sign the summary (i.e., the English-language IC document). The witness should sign the short-form document and the summary (General Requirements for Informed Consent, 2009). When a translator assists the person obtaining consent, the translator may serve as the witness.

Caution should be exercised when selecting an interpreter for IC. Each institution will have its own policy on the type and availability of interpreter services. Becze (2007) reported that several states have developed guidelines and standards regarding the training and certification of medical interpreters. The goal is to ensure that interpreters are proficient in both languages being used and medical terminology.

The IRB must receive all foreign-language versions of the short-form document as a condition of approval (General Requirements for Informed Consent, 2009). Expedited review of these versions is acceptable if the protocol, the full English-language CF, and the English version of the short-form document have already been approved by the convened IRB. In any case, each IRB will have its own set of policies on the use of the short-form process.

Source Documentation for the Informed Consent Process

The original signed CF must be kept in the patient's medical record for all (English- and non–English-speaking) participants. The participant receives a copy, and an additional copy may be kept in the participant's medical record (General Requirements for Informed Consent, 2009). Although not a regulatory requirement, the participant's medical record should include a notation of the time that the CF was signed. This is especially important for verifying that consent was obtained before initiation of the study when the date of consent and the date of initiation of study procedures or administration of study drug are the same.

Special Populations

The Belmont Report (National Commission, 1979) noted that involving vulnerable populations in research must be justifiable. Special provisions may need to be made if an individual's comprehension is limited by immaturity or mental disability. Respect for persons requires giving the individual the opportunity to choose whether to participate in research. The report stated that any objections to participation that are made by these individuals should be honored.

Federal regulations require that IRBs give special consideration to protecting the welfare of particularly vulnerable participants, such as children, institutionalized or incarcerated people, pregnant women, people with mental disabilities, or people who are economically or educationally disadvantaged (Protection of Human Subjects, 2009). A comparison of OHRP and FDA regulations for vulnerable populations may be found in Table 16-2.

CTNs need to be fully informed and aware of all aspects of a protocol. If issues arise related to the inclusion of vulnerable populations in a study design, CTNs should seek guidance from the institution's ethics committee (see Chapter 12) or IRB, if an ethics committee does not exist at an institution.

Procedures for Consent of a Child

Consent (or permission) for a minor participant is twofold: The participant must provide assent, and the participant's parent(s) must give consent. Parental permission is confirmed with their signature on the CF. The IRB must determine whether the permission of both parents is necessary and the conditions under which one parent may be considered "not reasonably available" (Requirements for Permission by Parents or Guardians for Assent by Children, 2009). Children do not need parental consent once they are 18 years old (or their state's legal age for healthcare decisions), and emancipated minors are consented as adults. In some lower-risk studies, adolescents will not need parental consent, but this must be at the discretion of the institution's IRB (Requirements for Permission by Parents or Guardians for Assent by Children, 2009).

Assent is obtained from all children who are old enough to consider the risks and benefits of their participation. The IRB is essential in determining whether a child is capable of providing assent. The IRB must consider the child's age, level of maturity, and current psychological state (Requirements for Permission by Parents or Guardians for Assent by Children, 2009). Barrett (2002) noted that a child's ability to assent should not be based exclusively on age because "many children with chronic disease and much experience of hospitals are more mature than their years" (Issues of Consent section, para. 5).

A child's failure to object does not indicate assent. Children should be provided with an explanation of what the study will involve and any alternatives available to them. Their right to refuse is evaluated based on factors such as their age and the severity of their illness. Although assent is confirmed with the child's signature on the CF, in cases of younger children who may not understand the implications of signing a legal document, having a third party sign for the child may be necessary to verify that assent was offered voluntarily (Additional Protections for Children Involved as Subjects in Research, 2009).

Special conditions, such as a child who is pregnant or one who is a ward of the state, may occur. If a child is pregnant, the child's assent and parental permission are obtained (Research Involving Pregnant Women or Fetuses, 2009). If a child is a ward of the state, the IRB must require the court to appoint an advocate for the child, in addition to anyone else who may be acting on the child's behalf.

Protection of Pregnant Women, Fetuses, and Neonates

The federal government provides additional protection to pregnant women, fetuses, and neonates involved in clinical research. Specific conditions must be met before these individuals may participate in research at all. Some of those conditions include but are not limited to (a) the risk to the fetus is a result of only the intervention and is anticipated to directly benefit the fetus or mother; (b) the risk to the fetus is minimal for interventions that will not directly benefit the fetus; and (c) the mother will not, in any way, be persuaded through the use of money, gifts, or other inducements to have an abortion (Research Involving Pregnant Women or Fetuses, 2009). IC for research involving pregnant women, fetuses, or neonates generally involves the pregnant woman or her LAR. However, in some circumstances, the father's consent may be required (Research Involving Pregnant Women or Fetuses, 2009).

Older Adult Participants

Competent older adult participants generally do not require special protections with regard to research. Obstacles to IC, such as hearing impairment and poor vision, can and should be overcome by using large-print forms and recorded consents (Klimaszewski, 2006). Some older adults, however, may be deemed ineligible for entry into specific clinical trials because of concurrent health problems.

Javid and colleagues (2012) studied the influence of older age (65 years and older) on physician and patient decision-making when considering enrollment in breast cancer clinical trials (SWOG trial S0316). Patients who met the criteria to participate in a survey (N = 1,079) were given one of two questionnaires: patients who participated in the clinical trial (n = 152) or patients who refused (n = 159). Participation rates among eligible patients were not significantly different based on age (34% for age 65 years and older vs. 40% for age younger than 65 years) (Javid et al., 2012). The researchers concluded that older patients were less likely to meet the eligibility requirements (65% vs. 78%, p = 0.004). However, those who were eligible participated at a rate similar to younger patients (34% vs. 40%, p = 0.32) (Javid et al., 2012).

A patient's decision-making capacities include being able to (a) communicate a choice, (b) understand relevant information, (c) appreciate the current medical situation and its consequences, and (d) reason through information rationally (Mayo & Wallhagen, 2009). Hoover-Regan, Becker, Williams, and Shenker (2013) interviewed a random sample of 570 clinical trial participants (24%) of 2,364 people admitted to a clinical research unit at a university hospital between 2005 and 2009. One focus of the interviews was determining the participants' understanding of clinical trials. Participants with cancer were older (mean age 60.1 [± 12.5] years vs. 46.4 [± 21.9] years, p < 0.001) than participants without cancer. Participants with cancer, overall, showed less understanding of research than participants without cancer (p = 0.001), and participants older than age 68 had less understanding than younger participants. The researchers concluded that older participants and those on oncology trials need to be better informed about research protocols (Hoover-Regan et al., 2013).

NCCN (2015) recommends assessing decision-making capacity of a patient based on those four criteria if the healthcare team or the patient and the patient's family have concerns about decision-making capacity or suspect cognitive impairment, or if cognitive impairment would affect the planning or delivery of care to the patient.

Two exceptions exist where older adults may need special protection: (a) if they have a cognitive impairment and (b) if they are institutionalized. Under those conditions, the same considerations are applicable as with any other participant in the same circumstances, regardless of the participant's age.

Participants With Mental Disabilities or Dementia

A few approaches may be employed when an older patient's decision-making capacity is diminished. NCCN (2015) recommends seeking information about the patient's goals and values for cancer care from the patient's LAR, advance directive, living will, healthcare power of attorney, or the healthcare provider documentation. Other approaches include consulting the institution's ethics committee, a social worker, or the palliative care team (NCCN, 2015).

The LAR's consent is required for a participant who is mentally ill, impaired, or has dementia. These participants may be institutionalized (voluntarily or involuntarily) in facilities such as psychiatric hospitals, halfway houses, nursing homes, or psychiatric inpatient units in general hospitals. As with minors, the CF must include a justification for offering the study to the specified participant population or a rationale for not using a less vulnerable group. Specific benefits to the selected group must be cited. The CF must clearly state what consequences may result from withdrawal, such as transfer to another institution or discontinuation of previous therapies. However, the rights of the potential participant to decline to participate without negative consequences must be honored (Stiles, Epstein, Poythress, & Edens, 2012).

Dresser (2001) suggested use of a research advance directive. Such a directive would delineate a person's preference in the event that a particular study would become available after the person develops cognitive impairment. Unlike research involving children, prisoners, and fetuses, however, no additional DHHS regulations specifically govern research that involves participants who are cognitively impaired. Thus, the IRB must make the final determination of who will provide consent.

As a general rule, all adults, regardless of their diagnosis or condition, should be presumed competent to consent unless documented evidence exists of serious mental disability that would impair reasoning or judgment. Even those who do have a diagnosed mental disorder may be perfectly able to understand the matter of being a research volunteer and may be capable of consenting or assenting to or refusing participation (National Commission, 1979).

CTNs explaining a proposed clinical trial to a patient who has not been deemed incompetent should present information in a way that affords the patient an opportunity to demonstrate his or her highest level of functioning, then accept the patient's decision to accept or decline participation (Mayo & Wallhagen, 2009; Plawecki & Amrhein, 2009). CTNs should inform the principal investigator and seek the advice of an ethics committee if the capacity of an individual to provide IC is questionable (NCCN, 2015) (see Chapter 12).

Mental disability alone should not disqualify a person from consenting to participate in research; rather, investigators should have specific evidence of an individual's incapacity to understand and to make a choice before he or she is deemed unable to consent. People formally deemed incompetent have a court-appointed guardian who must be consulted and will consent on their behalf. Officials of the institution in which incompetent patients reside (even if they are the patient's legal guardians) generally are not considered appropriate. Family members or others who are financially responsible for the patient may be subject to conflicting interests because of financial pressures, emotional distancing, or other ambivalent feelings that are common in such circumstances. IRBs should bear this in mind when determining appropriate consent procedures for cognitively impaired participants.

Prisoners

Protocols that are written for populations in prison must state so in the text of the written protocol. This, then, is reviewed by the institution's IRB. Prisoner advocates can be consulted to review the protocol and CF in order to prevent exploitation of a population that may not have full access to resources to guarantee their rights. These safeguards are in place to prevent involuntary or coerced participation of a prisoner (Stiles et al., 2012). Additionally, if a prisoner enrolled in a clinical trial completes the study and is required to have follow-up examinations, provisions must be made for that to occur. Before signing the consent document, the prisoner must be informed of and agree to the follow-up examinations. If a prisoner is being considered for a protocol written for the general population, the IRB must be informed, and an amendment to the CF may be required (Additional Protections Pertaining to Biomedical and Behavioral Research Involving Prisoners as Subjects, 2009).

Should a situation arise where prisoners fear negative consequences, such as sanctions from prison staff if they decline to participate in a research study, steps should be taken to protect the prisoners from the perceived consequences (Stiles et al., 2012). Ways to protect prisoners who decline might include adjusting recruitment procedures to allow for an information session with a prisoner and a researcher, to be followed by the prisoner contacting the researcher with his or her choice via telephone away from prison staff. Another way might be for the researcher to declare the prisoner ineligible to participate, thus freeing the prisoner from the responsibility of making a decision. Stiles et al. (2012) also suggested having a prisoner meet and spend time with research staff as if he or she were on study, but not collecting information from him or her, or having the patient sign a CF "with the understanding that the investigator will document in the research record that the individual was not permitted to enroll in the study due to concerns about voluntariness" (p. 17). In all instances, prisoners must be afforded the same right to voluntary consent as nonprisoners.

Genetic Testing and Genomic Research

Genetic testing involves analysis of DNA, RNA, or protein to detect variant genes linked to a disease. It can confirm a suspected diagnosis, predict the possibility of future illness, detect the presence of a carrier state in unaffected individuals (whose children may be at risk), and predict response to therapy (National Human Genome Research Institute, 2015b).

IC in the genetic testing process provides a means for the provider or investigator and the individual to confirm that the essential elements of testing, including the benefits and limitations associated with possible results of the specific test, were explained and accepted (American Society of Clinical Oncology, 2012). A second consent may be obtained before issuing test results to ensure that the individual still consents to receive the results.

Federal requirements for IC (General Requirements for Informed Consent, 2009) apply to consents for genetic testing and human genomic research. Chapter 32 discusses IC for genetic testing in detail. Figure 32-6 lists the elements of IC for genetic testing, and Figure 32-7 notes the IC elements tailored to genetic research. One of the optional clinical research studies that may be added to a CF by a principal investigator and included in the 2013 CF template is optional sample collections for laboratory studies or biobanking for possible future studies. See Chapter 35 for detailed information on consents for biobanking and data sharing.

The National Human Genome Research Institute (2015a) has links to model CFs from National Institutes of Health–sponsored research studies that show how to incorporate issues pertinent to genomics research in a CF.

Exemptions and Waivers

In special circumstances, the legal requirement for IC does not apply. A participant's right to self-determination is not absolute in those cases. The requirement to obtain IC may be waived by an IRB in special circumstances. OHRP (2004) provides graphic aids in the form of decision trees to assist investigators, IRBs, and others with questions regarding whether the IC, its elements, or IC documentation may be waived. These decision charts may be accessed at www.hhs.gov/ohrp/policy/checklists/decisioncharts.html.

Role of Clinical Trial Nurses

Perhaps the most important role for CTNs is educating patients about clinical trials and providing any significant new information about them during or after the trial (Oncology Nursing Society, 2010). CTNs must be patient advocates, supporting treatment decisions that reflect patients' personal values and preferences (Tariman, Berry, Cochrane, Doorenbos, & Schepp, 2012).

CTNs must confirm with the investigator that participants have had an adequate amount of time to review the CF and that all of the participants' questions have been answered. CTNs must verify that the IC forms have been signed, with the original in the research record and a copy in the medical record and also one given to the participant, before performing any study tests or administering any study treatments. They also ensure that the ongoing exchange of information in the consent process is performed and documented and that patient confidentiality is maintained.

Wujcik (2007) compared patient education with the IC process, stating, "Patients and family members need an ongoing assessment of their understanding and willingness to continue with the plan of care" (p. 5). Every time participants return for treatment, CTNs should verify or reaffirm that they truly wish to continue. Asking "Are you ready for your treatment today?" may evoke a humorous response from participants, a serious response, or one that will immediately alert CTNs to the possibility that a participant is considering withdrawing consent. Patients may indicate that their spouse wants them to continue with the clinical trial, although they admit to feeling tired and ready to stop. CTNs must notify the investigator if a participant has additional questions or decides to withdraw consent. By taking the additional time to verify consent, CTNs will protect and maintain the rights of participants and the integrity of the IC and the clinical trial.

Summary

The IC process may begin with an advertisement or a phone call, progress to a frank discussion about the contents of the IC document, and then develop into an ongoing relationship between the participant and the research team. Education must be tailored to the participant's level of understanding, ability, and learning styles and preferences. Reinforcement, updating, and reassessment promote fully informed decisions. Special vulnerable participant populations may require additional advocacy and aids to ensure that fully informed consent is obtained. In every case, the patient must decide whether to participate in a clinical trial, decline participation, or affirm or withdraw consent. It is the patient's disease and the patient's decision.

The past decade brought significant improvements worldwide in the protection of human rights in human subject research. CTNs can help protect human participants by being advocates and educators in the process of IC. By protecting patients' rights, remaining objective, and respecting whatever decisions patients make, CTNs will foster ethical and autonomous consent where the patients provide full IC to participate in a clinical trial.

Key Points
- Information, comprehension, and voluntariness are the major elements of the IC process.

- The IC process is a continuing dialogue between the responsible investigator, the study participant, and the research team.
- Federal regulations guide the IC process.
- Vulnerable populations may require additional safeguards for comprehension and truly voluntary consent.
- CTNs are advocates for patients and can foster IC by ensuring patients understand the clinical trial and any new information that arises from the clinical trial during or after its completion.

References

Additional Protections for Children Involved as Subjects in Research, 45 C.F.R. §§ 46.401–46.409 (2009). Retrieved from http://www.hhs.gov/ohrp/humansubjects/guidance/45cfr46.html#subpartd

Additional Protections Pertaining to Biomedical and Behavioral Research Involving Prisoners as Subjects, 45 C.F.R. §§ 46.301–46.306 (2009). Retrieved from http://www.hhs.gov/ohrp/humansubjects/guidance/45cfr46.html#subpartc

American Society of Clinical Oncology. (2012, March). Genetic testing. Retrieved from http://www.cancer.net/all-about-cancer/genetics/genetic-testing

Barrett, J. (2002, July 1). Why aren't more pediatric trials performed? *Applied Clinical Trials*. Retrieved from http://www.actmagazine.com/appliedclinicaltrials/content/printContentPopup.jsp?id=83729

Becze, E. (2007, March). Certified medical interpreters provide better services. *ONS Connect, 22*(3), 30.

Cumming, J.F., Sahni, A.R., & McClelland, G.R. (2006, March 1). The importance of the subject in informed consent. *Applied Clinical Trials*. Retrieved from http://www.actmagazine.com/appliedclinicaltrials/content/printContentPopup.jsp?id=310810

Dal-Ré, R., Avendaño, C., Gil-Aguado, Gracia, D., & Caplan, A.L. (2008). When should re-consent of subjects participating in a clinical trial be requested? A case-oriented algorithm to assist in the decision-making process. *Clinical Pharmacology and Therapeutics, 83*, 788–793. doi:10.1038/sj.clpt.6100357

Doak, C.C., Doak, L.G., & Root, J.H. (1996). *Teaching patients with low literacy skills* (2nd ed.). Philadelphia, PA: Lippincott Williams & Wilkins.

Documentation of Informed Consent, 45 C.F.R. § 46.117 (2009). Retrieved from http://www.hhs.gov/ohrp/humansubjects/guidance/45cfr46.html#46.117

Dresser, R. (2001). Advance directives in dementia research: Promoting autonomy and protecting subjects. *IRB: Ethics and Human Research, 23*(1), 1–6. doi:10.2307/3563979

Elements of Informed Consent, 21 C.F.R. § 50.25 (2013). Retrieved from http://www.accessdata.fda.gov/scripts/cdrh/cfdocs/cfcfr/CFRSearch.cfm?fr=50.25

General Requirements for Informed Consent, 45 C.F.R. § 46.116 (2009). Retrieved from http://www.hhs.gov/ohrp/humansubjects/guidance/45cfr46.html#46.116

Green, D., & Rickles, F.R. (2007). Enhancing participation in clinical research: Keys to obtaining informed consent. *Journal of Supportive Oncology, 5*, 48–50. Retrieved from http://www.oncologypractice.com/jso/journal/articles/0501048.pdf

Hochhauser, M. (2004, April 1). Informed consent: Reading and understanding are not the same. *Applied Clinical Trials*. Retrieved from http://www.actmagazine.com/appliedclinicaltrials/content/printContentPopup.jsp?id=90594

Hoover-Regan, M., Becker, T., Williams, M.J., & Shenker, Y. (2013). Informed consent and research subject understanding of clinical trials. *Wisconsin Medical Journal, 112*, 18–23. Retrieved from https://www.wisconsinmedicalsociety.org/_WMS/publications/wmj/pdf/112/1/18.pdf

Informed Consent Elements Rule, 76 Fed. Reg. 256–270 (proposed Jan. 4, 2011) (to be codified at 21 C.F.R. § 50.25c). Retrieved from http://www.gpo.gov/fdsys/pkg/FR-2011-01-04/html/2010-33193.htm

International Conference on Harmonisation of Technical Requirements for Registration of Pharmaceuticals for Human Use. (1996). *Guidance for industry—E6 good clinical practice: Consolidated guidance*. Retrieved from http://www.fda.gov/downloads/Drugs/Guidance/ucm073122.pdf

Javid, S.H., Unger, J.M., Gralow, J.R., Moinpour, C.M., Wozniak, A.J., Goodwin, J.W., ... Albain, K.S. (2012). A prospective analysis of the influence of older age on physician and patient decision-making when considering enrollment in breast cancer clinical trials (SWOG S0316). *Oncologist, 17*, 1180–1190. doi:10.1634/theoncologist.2011-0384

Jaynes, T. (2005, June 1). Informed consent: Imparting knowledge or signing a form? *Applied Clinical Trials*. Retrieved from http://www.actmagazine.com/appliedclinicaltrials/content/printContentPopup.jsp?id=165486

Kaltman, S.P., & Isidor, J.M. (2006). State law. In E.A. Bankert & R.J. Amdur (Eds.), *Institutional review board management and function* (pp. 304–307). Burlington, MA: Jones & Bartlett Learning.

Klimaszewski, A.D. (2006). Psychosocial aspects of experimental therapy: Clinical trials. In R.M. Carroll-Johnson, L.M. Gorman, & N.J. Bush (Eds.), *Psychosocial nursing care along the cancer continuum* (2nd ed., pp. 489–497). Pittsburgh, PA: Oncology Nursing Society.

Mackintosh, D.R., & Molloy, V.J. (2003, May 1). Opportunities to improve informed consent. *Applied Clinical Trials*. Retrieved from http://www.actmagazine.com/appliedclinicaltrials/content/printContentPopup.jsp?id=88095

Mayo, A.M., & Wallhagen, M.I. (2009). Considerations of informed consent and decision-making competence in older adults with cognitive impairment. *Research in Gerontological Nursing, 2*, 103–111. doi:10.3928/19404921-20090401-08

Meade, C.D., & Howser, D.M. (1992). Consent forms: How to determine and improve their readability. *Oncology Nursing Forum, 19*, 1523–1528.

National Cancer Institute. (2003, February 27). Clear and simple: Developing effective print materials for low-literate readers. Retrieved from http://www.cancer.gov/cancertopics/cancerlibrary/clear-and-simple/page1

National Cancer Institute. (2008). *Making health communications programs work* (Rev. ed.) Retrieved from http://www.cancer.gov/cancertopics/cancerlibrary/pinkbook/Pink_Book.pdf

National Cancer Institute. (2013a, June 3). Simplification of informed consent documents: Appendix 4: Communication methods. Retrieved from http://www.cancer.gov/clinicaltrials/conducting/simplification-of-informed-consent-docs/page5#appendix4

National Cancer Institute. (2013b, June 3). Simplification of informed consent documents: Checklist for easy-to-read informed consent documents. Retrieved from http://www.cancer.gov/clinicaltrials/conducting/simplification-of-informed-consent-docs/page5

National Cancer Institute. (2013c, June 3). Simplification of informed consent documents: Recommendations. Retrieved from http://www.cancer.gov/clinicaltrials/conducting/simplification-of-informed-consent-docs/page2

National Commission for the Protection of Human Subjects of Biomedical and Behavioral Research. (1979, April 18). *The Belmont report: Ethical principles and guidelines for the protection of human subjects of research*. Retrieved from http://archive.hhs.gov/ohrp/humansubjects/guidance/belmont.htm

National Comprehensive Cancer Network. (2015). *NCCN Clinical Practice Guidelines in Oncology (NCCN Guidelines®): Senior adult oncology* [v.1.2015]. Retrieved from http://www.nccn.org/professionals/physician_gls/pdf/senior.pdf

National Human Genome Research Institute. (2015a). Consent form examples and model consent language. Retrieved from http://www.genome.gov/27526660

National Human Genome Research Institute. (2015b). Regulation of genetic tests. Retrieved from http://www.genome.gov/10002335

National Institutes of Health. (n.d.). Glossary and acronym list: Informed consent. Retrieved from http://grants.nih.gov/grants/glossary.htm#I

Newton, S. (2007, May). Patients should be able to repeat key points. *ONS Connect, 22*(5), 14.

Office for Human Research Protections. (2004, September 24). Human subject regulations decision charts. Retrieved from http://www.hhs.gov/ohrp/humansubjects/guidance/decisioncharts.html

Oncology Nursing Society. (2010). *Oncology clinical trials nurse competencies.* Retrieved from http://www.ons.org/sites/default/files/ctncompetencies.pdf

Plawecki, L.H., & Amrhein, D.W. (2009). When "no" means no: Elderly patients' right to refuse treatment. *Journal of Gerontological Nursing, 35,* 16–18. doi:10.3928/00989134-20090706-03

Protection of Human Subjects, 45 C.F.R. pt. 46 (2009). Retrieved from http://www.hhs.gov/ohrp/humansubjects/guidance/45cfr46.html

Requirements for Permission by Parents or Guardians for Assent by Children, 45 C.F.R. § 46.408 (2009). Retrieved from http://www.hhs.gov/ohrp/humansubjects/guidance/45cfr46.html#46.408

Research Involving Pregnant Women or Fetuses, 45 C.F.R. § 46.204 (2009). Retrieved from http://www.hhs.gov/ohrp/humansubjects/guidance/45cfr46.html#46.204

Richmond, E. (2013, May 7). The Wednesday AccrualNet post (5-7-13): Top 12 informed consent dings. Retrieved from https://accrualnet.cancer.gov/communities/conversation/the_wednesday_accrualnet_post_5_7_13_top_12_informed_consent_dings#.U81iwJRdV8E

Rust, D., Rogers, B., & Joyce, M. (2007, May). Materials should be simplified and contain visuals. *ONS Connect, 22*(5), 14.

Stiles, P.G., Epstein, M., Poythress, N., & Edens, J.F. (2012). Protecting people who decline to participate in research: An example from a prison setting. *IRB: Ethics and Human Research, 34*(2), 15–18.

Tariman, J.D., Berry, D.L., Cochrane, B., Doorenbos, A., & Schepp, K. (2012). Physician, patient, and contextual factors affecting treatment decisions in older adults with cancer: A literature review [Online exclusive]. *Oncology Nursing Forum, 39,* E70–E83. doi:10.1188/12.ONF.E70-E83

Titus, S.L., & Keane, M.A. (1996). Do you understand?: An ethical assessment of researchers' description of the consenting process. *Journal of Clinical Ethics, 7,* 60–68.

U.S. Food and Drug Administration. (2009). *Guidance for industry: Investigator responsibilities—Protecting the rights, safety, and welfare of study subjects.* Retrieved from http://www.fda.gov/downloads/Drugs/GuidanceComplianceRegulatoryInformation/Guidances/UCM187772.pdf

Wujcik, D. (2007, May). Human interaction is the key to effective patient education. *ONS Connect, 22*(5), 5.

Chapter 15

Protocol Development and Response Assessment

Lydia T. Madsen, RN, PhD, OCN®, AOCNS®, and Elizabeth Ness, RN, MS

Introduction

The development of a clinical research protocol involves multiple interactions among the clinicians, statistician, and sponsor, if applicable. If the protocol involves the use of an investigational new drug, the U.S. Food and Drug Administration (FDA) may serve as the regulatory agency. Additional collaborators, such as clinical trial nurses (CTNs), may add valuable clinically applicable knowledge to the design and implementation of a protocol and should be included in the development process. Once the objectives and study design are determined, the statistician remains a key team member with the goal of developing the appropriate statistical considerations for the study. A greater understanding of the statistician's role and the statistical tools used in both clinical protocol development and response assessment will facilitate increased and more effective interaction between the statistician and the CTNs involved in the conduct of the study. The purpose of this chapter is to provide CTNs with the steps associated with writing and developing a research protocol, including statistical considerations and response assessment. See Chapter 13 for additional protocol components that are not addressed herein.

Determining Primary and Secondary Objectives

The principal investigator and others as appropriate (e.g., sponsor, study chair) define the study objectives as an initial step to the development of a clinical protocol. The primary objective is a short statement of the purpose of the study that should answer the following questions (Stoney & Johnson, 2012b).

- Is this to be a comparative or descriptive study?
- What are the endpoints of primary interest?
- What is the subject population?
- What are the treatments?

Most studies have more than one objective. Secondary objectives are, by definition, of secondary importance and exploratory and hypothesis-generating in nature. These objectives may sometimes involve additional aspects of study interest such as collection of biospecimens to answer correlative questions, quality-of-life (QOL) measurements, or compliance related to treatment (International Conference on Harmonisation of Technical Requirements for Registration of Pharmaceuticals for Human Use, 1997).

Regardless of how many objectives there might be, each one should have some method for measuring the outcome, such as

- Adverse event assessment using the Common Terminology Criteria for Adverse Events (CTCAE) (National Cancer Institute [NCI] Cancer Therapy Evaluation Program [CTEP], 2010)
- Participant well-being assessment using an established health-related QOL survey (NCI Coordinating Center for Clinical Trials, 2013)
- Compliance with self-administered study agents using a drug administration diary
- Laboratory assay for measuring pharmacokinetics or pharmacodynamics
- Computed tomography (CT) scan for measuring disease response.

CTNs can play a critical role during the protocol development to ensure that the objectives are measurable and have a tool or method for evaluating the outcome. They can review the procedures in the protocol document to ensure that all are related in some way to the objectives and the institution has the capability of executing the procedures outlined in the study.

CTNs may consider if aspects of the study, for example, medication adherence, are relevant to nursing practice as something to study during the trial. They should consider bringing forward concerns or questions during the protocol development stage to determine if additional objectives can be considered for incorporation into the protocol as a secondary survey or instrument (e.g., QOL) for data collection.

Selecting a Study Design

The statistical section should summarize the study design that was developed to answer the primary objective. The primary objective drives the study design used. The section should address
- Number of treatment arms
- How subjects are assigned treatment by randomization (i.e., by random choice usually directed by a computer-generated coin toss, by direct assignment, or by other means, such as physician or subject choice)
- How randomization is stratified so that each subgroup of participants, defined by entry characteristics, is balanced between treatment arms
- Phase of the study
- Mathematical calculations needed to determine the sample (U.S. FDA, 1998).

Efficient procedures are now available for both phase II and III studies that allow the team to stop accrual or follow-up because of clear, early evidence of the results (U.S. FDA, 2010). A simple example is that if the investigators decided that in a sample size of 30, 5 episodes of toxicity are unacceptable, then the study should stop if 5 episodes occur in the first 10 participants who enter the study. Similarly, if a study is designed to detect a 20% difference in survival between arms, and an early analysis indicates a 60% difference, perhaps the study should be terminated and the results published. Numerous procedures exist to allow the development of such adaptive designs. Consideration of adaptive designs is valuable because when trials are stopped early, clinical information of significance may be lost, and questions related to secondary outcomes may go unanswered. An adaptive design allows for modification of one or more aspects of the study design and hypotheses (e.g., study eligibility criteria, randomization procedure, treatment dose, treatment schedule, sample size, selection of secondary endpoints) based on analysis of interim data at predetermined time points (U.S. FDA, 2010). In-depth reading materials regarding adaptive trial designs are included in the list of additional resources at the end of this chapter for readers interested in more detailed sources and the large body of literature available on multistage and sequential designs.

Phase I studies are handled differently than phase II and III studies in that the purpose is to identify the maximum tolerated dose for use in other studies. Small cohorts of subjects are entered at a dose of drug, and depending on the toxicity observed and the escalation/de-escalation scheme, either the study is terminated at that dose, more subjects are entered at that dose or a lower dose, or accrual is commenced at a higher dose.

To develop the design, the team decides upon definitions of dose-limiting toxicity (DLT) and the true rate of DLT that would be unacceptable. The statistician uses exact binomial probabilities to develop an algorithm of subject numbers and dose levels. This algorithm has a high probability of allowing dose escalation if the true rate of DLT at that dose is low, yet also has a low chance of approving for further use a dose with an unacceptably high level of DLT. Some phase I studies randomize rather than sequentially assign subjects to doses, but the intent is always to ensure subject comparability, not to contrast the outcomes statistically. For more information on study designs, see Chapters 4 and 5.

Eligibility

When writing a protocol, much thought is given to the participant population. Ideally, participants enrolled will be those who will best answer the hypothesis of the study (Karp & Nussenblatt, 2012; Stoney & Johnson, 2012b). The protocol must specify through the eligibility requirements a clearly defined patient group, thereby minimizing any unnecessary or confounding variables in reaching the goals of the study. For example, if the study is measuring the efficacy of a standard adjuvant treatment regimen in breast cancer and comparing it to a higher dose or different schedule of chemotherapy, all patients must be free of metastatic disease. However, the histologic category, estrogen status, or other variables may need to be limited to answer a specific or additional research question.

Phase I trials are less concerned with histology or the extent of disease because the main goal is to establish a safe dose level. Organ function, however, plays an important part in testing drug tolerability and the extent of toxicities in these studies. Therefore, parameters of hepatic and renal function may be outlined in the eligibility requirements. Histology and the extent of disease become much more crucial in defining eligibility in phase II studies, where the response to the drug is being tested in a specific disease site. A staging workup completed within a specified time frame (e.g., two weeks) may be required prior to registration or randomization to ensure that the desired extent of disease has not changed.

Eligibility is written in a format that defines inclusion and exclusion criteria. *Inclusion criteria* are the elements that must be satisfied before a patient can enter into a trial, whereas *exclusion criteria* identify elements that, if met, will keep the patient from participating in the trial (Karp & Nussenblatt, 2012; Stoney & Johnson, 2012b). Once determined, eligibility criteria must be strictly followed. For example, if a platelet count of more than 100,000/mm³ is required, then a patient with a platelet count of 101,000/mm³ can be enrolled, and a patient with a platelet count of 99,000/mm³ cannot be enrolled. Similarly, if a hemoglobin level below 10 g/100 ml is identified in the exclusion criteria, then a patient with a hemoglobin level of 9.8 g/100 ml will not be eligible to participate in the trial. Although it is possible to have an exception granted for minimal variances, it is important to remember that the eligibility criteria were established after thoughtful deliberation, so exception requests should be uncommon.

Before enrolling a patient in a study, the CTN is responsible for confirming that all of the criteria have been met (Lubejko et al., 2011). This is accomplished by interviewing the patient, reviewing the medical record, and obtaining documentation of all required data prior to enrollment.

Pathology

Pathology reports are crucial in determining patient eligibility, particularly in phase II and III studies. Some institutions require a special review if the original pathology was performed at another facility. Clinical trial networks and sponsors sometimes require a centralized review of pathology specimens to ensure consistency. These requirements should be delineated clearly within the protocol.

Stage of Disease

Protocol eligibility criteria identify patients with a specific stage of disease for enrollment. The purpose of staging systems is to classify or describe the extent of disease to provide physicians with enough information to determine treatment options and prognostic indicators. The most common system for staging or categorizing the extent of disease for solid tumors is the TNM system, in which T is the primary tumor size, N indicates the regional lymph node involvement, and M represents distant metastasis. The TNM system is based on a clinical assessment and workup. It has been accepted by the Union for International Cancer Control and the American Joint Committee on Cancer (NCI, 2015c). TNM staging is essential to phase II and III studies, in which the primary goal of the study is to determine response in a specific stage of a specific disease. Other staging systems need to be considered based on the disease, such as

- Rai system (used predominantly in the United States) or the Binet system (used widely in Europe) for chronic lymphocytic leukemia (NCI, 2015e)
- Ann Arbor staging system for adult Hodgkin and non-Hodgkin lymphoma (NCI, 2015a, 2015b)
- St. Jude staging system for non-Hodgkin lymphoma in children (NCI, 2015d)
- International Staging System for multiple myeloma (NCI, 2015g)
- International Neuroblastoma Staging System for neuroblastoma (NCI, 2015f)
- International Retinoblastoma Staging System for retinoblastoma (NCI, 2015h).

When developing disease-specific inclusion criteria, it may be useful to include the actual staging criteria as an appendix in the protocol with the appendix referenced in the inclusion criteria.

The physician is responsible for assessing the clinical and pathologic stage of the patient's disease. Staging is discussed frequently at tumor board meetings or in consultation with physicians from related disciplines, such as pathology and radiology, and documentation is a requirement of the American College of Surgeons for accreditation. CTNs typically confirm that staging has been completed and documented in the medical record before enrolling the patient into the study.

Performance Status

In oncology trials, standard scales and criteria quantify patients' general well-being and assess patients' abilities to perform ordinary tasks (e.g., activities of daily living). These ratings of *performance status* have been shown to correlate fairly well with overall survival (Evers, Logan, Sills, & Chin, 2013; Lee et al., 2013; Sørensen, Klee, Palshof, & Hansen, 1993). Performance status is commonly used in the clinical oncology setting, so the CTN may already be familiar with this concept. When developing a protocol, selecting a performance status scale is typically a component of the inclusion criteria. The two most common performance status scales used for adults are Karnofsky (Karnofsky, Abelmann, Craver, & Burchenal, 1948) and Eastern Cooperative Oncology Group (Oken et al., 1982). The Lansky scale (Lansky, List, Lansky, Ritter-Sterr, & Miller, 1987) is used when a pediatric population is included in a clinical trial. In addition to inclusion criteria, performance status may also be used for stratification in either randomization or data analysis.

Study Intervention and Required Procedures

The protocol should be written to include clear and detailed descriptions of the study interventions (e.g., study drug administration, radiation therapy) and all procedures (e.g., physical exams, biospecimen collections, radiologic procedures) that will be required for both safety and efficacy assessments. Developing a schedule of events table is useful (see Figure 15-1). When determining the frequency of procedures, it is helpful to prioritize what is essential for meeting protocol objectives and assessing participant safety versus what would be valuable, but not essential, data because the participant will already be in for a visit. An example would be the value, but not necessity, of a monthly bone marrow biopsy when disease staging would routinely be needed every two months. It is important to remember that nonessential data, although valuable, may have an invasive or time-intensive component, which may affect accrual or retention.

All procedures should have specified time points that delineate when they are to be completed (Karp & Nussenblatt, 2012; Stoney & Johnson, 2012b). It is helpful to build in an allowable variance for these time points to accommodate an unforeseen circumstance that might result in deviation from the protocol. For example, if safety laboratory tests are needed weekly, the protocol should state that these must be done on day 8 plus or minus two days. This variance is based on the assumption that the variance will not compromise participant safety.

Biospecimen Collection

Many protocols require research-specific biospecimens to be collected throughout the study. Some of these samples may even be used for eligibility critera (e.g., vascular endothelial growth factor status), for treatment assignment, or as a stratification variable. It is important that the protocol clearly includes the following information (NCI Office of Biorepositories and Biospecimen Research, 2011).
- What types of test tubes or other specimen collection system is to be used
- Time points samples will be collected
- Storage of samples until processing (e.g., on ice for no more than 15 minutes, room air)

Figure 15-1. Sample Template for Schedule of Events Table

Procedure	Screening/ Baseline	Cycle 1						Subsequent Cycles		Post Therapy Follow-Up
		Day X	Day X	Day X	Day X	Day X	Day X	Day X	Day X	
History and physical exam										
Vital signs										
Performance score										
Labs (list specific labs)										
Biopsies										
Correlative research studies										
Pharmacokinetics/ pharmacodynamics										
Radiologic assessments (list specific studies)										
Other specific assessments (such as electrocardiogram/echocardiogram, audiology, pulmonary function tests)										
Response evaluation										
Adverse events		X								
Concomitant medications		X								

- Contact person for sample processing
- How samples will be processed (i.e., temperature, speed and duration of time for centrifuge, number of aliquots required)
- Sample storage, including location and freezer temperature
- How and when to ship samples, if applicable
- Identified or de-identified samples
- Description of when, if, and how results will be discussed with the participant

Off-Treatment Follow-Up

The frequency of study procedures once a participant is no longer receiving active study treatment is another consideration when writing a protocol. Including this information in the study calendar or even as a separate study calendar is helpful to ensure that the data are collected to meet study objectives.

For protocols that will have long-term follow-up (e.g., until participant death to measure overall survival), protocols need to identify
- What procedures will be conducted and when
- What data elements will be collected
- Who will be responsible for the continued follow-up
- What measures will secure follow-up for those participants who do not comply with the protocol-specified time (e.g., phone call, return-receipt letter)
- What determines whether a participant is to be deemed "lost to follow-up."

Additionally, the informed consent document should clearly outline the long-term follow-up period and what will be done during this time (Ness, 2013).

Oncology Trial Endpoints

The *endpoints* of a study are the clinical and biologic parameters that will be measured to evaluate the study's primary and secondary objectives (Gravetter & Wallnau, 2013). The endpoints of the study should be clearly defined so that they are reproducible and, where relevant, consistent with other studies in the same disease and population. *Reproducible* is when given the same data, different evaluators will code the endpoint the same way both within a site and across all the sites that might participate in a study. The purpose of publishing reproducible, detailed statistical results is to provide researchers with a set of standardized tests that are recognized and understood within the scientific community (Gravetter & Wallnau, 2013). This helps prevent, for example, having the response rate for one site or clinician be much higher than others because of a difference in evaluation rather than a true difference in the clinical result. Common endpoints of oncology trials include safety, disease response, and QOL indicators.

Safety Endpoints

All protocols will need to address safety. In oncology clinical trials, the standard tool used to measure adverse events is the CTCAE (NCI CTEP, 2010). Because of the size of the CTCAE, the protocol is often written with the Web address for accessing the latest version of the CTCAE. For example, a protocol template could state

> The descriptions and grading scales found in the revised Common Terminology Criteria for Adverse Events (CTCAE) version 4.0.3 will be utilized for adverse event reporting. All appropriate treatment areas should have access to a copy of the CTCAE version 4.03. A copy of the CTCAE version 4.03 can be downloaded from the CTEP website (http://ctep.cancer.gov/protocolDevelopment/electronic_applications/ctc.htm).

For more information about the CTCAE, see Chapter 28.

Disease Response

In the 1970s, FDA used overall response rate as the endpoint for approval of drugs used in oncology. The overall response rate endpoint relied solely on physical and radiologic exams to assess tumor status. However, in the 1980s, FDA began including other responses as endpoints that were considered during the drug approval process: disease-free survival, overall survival, improvement in QOL, and relief of tumor-related symptoms (U.S. FDA, 2007). See Table 15-1 for FDA's endpoints used for approval of cancer drugs and biologics.

Every protocol must include how disease response will be assessed (i.e., measured). In oncology clinical trials, standards for response criteria have been developed, usually by expert consensus, for both solid tumors and hematologic malignancies. This section should not only include a reference to the standard but also should describe in detail the definitions associated with response based on the procedures being used to assess disease response. Outside of the research setting, these standards have been used as a guide to assist the clinician and patient to make a decision about continuing with therapy.

When using radiologic assessments to assess disease response, it is important to maintain consistency to control for variation between practitioner interpretation and equipment. It is helpful to designate a radiologist to measure tumors at each site while using consistent methodology (e.g., CT, magnetic resonance imaging, plain films). Ideally, the same scanning equipment should be used, but this may not always be feasible.

Table 15-1. Clinical Trial Endpoints

Endpoint	Definition
Overall survival	• Time from randomization until death • Intent-to-treat population
Disease-free survival	• Randomization until recurrence of tumor or death from any cause • Adjuvant setting after definitive surgery or radiotherapy • Large percentage of patients achieve complete response after chemotherapy
Objective response rate	• Proportion of patients with reduction of tumor size of a predefined amount and for a minimum time period • Measure from time of initial response until progression • Sum of partial response patients and complete response patients • Uses standardized criteria when possible
Progression-free survival	• Randomization until objective tumor progression or death • Preferred regulatory endpoint • Assumes deaths are related to progression
Time to progression	• Randomization until objective tumor progression, excluding deaths
Time to treatment failure	• Randomization to discontinuation of treatment for any reason (e.g., progressive disease, toxicity, death) • Not recommended for regulatory drug approval

Note. Based on information from U.S. Food and Drug Administration, 2007.

Solid Tumor Response Assessment

Best practices for evaluating solid tumors include (Einsenhauer et al., 2009)
- Characterizing the overall tumor burden through quantitative evaluation of lesions
- Identifying lesions before initiating therapy
- Using the same method of investigation (e.g., using the same radiographic procedure and equipment) for each assessment time point
- Confirming complete and partial responses.

Initial attempts to standardize solid tumor assessment began in the 1960s. In 1979, the World Health Organization (WHO) developed standardized criteria for response assessment, which included measuring the sum of the area (i.e., length × width) of lesions. However, there were problems with the WHO criteria, specifically, interpretation of WHO guidelines varied among research groups, minimum lesion size and number of lesions to be recorded varied, and definition of progressive disease varied, which resulted in modifications to the WHO criteria (Einsenhauer et al., 2009; Therasse et al., 2000).

In 1994, an international task force was established to address these problems. The task force was composed of members from the European Organisation for Research and Treatment of Cancer, NCI, and the National Cancer Institute of Canada Clinical Trials Group. After a retrospective tumor response review of 4,000 patients, the task force made recommendations to simplify response evaluation for solid tumors by using longest diameter, identifying target and nontarget lesions, and standardizing the assessment of these lesions and new lesions to assess overall response. The new criteria, Response Evaluation Criteria in Solid Tumors (RECIST), were publicly presented and accepted at the American Society of Clinical Oncology meeting in 1999 and published in 2000. RECIST version 1.0 was intended for solid tumor response assessment in phase II clinical trials but actually was used for response assessment in all phases (Therasse et al., 2000).

The task force committed to continual review to improve RECIST as needed. After using RECIST, questions began to arise (Eisenhauer et al., 2009):
- Were 10 lesions needed?
- Was confirmation needed?
- How would progressive disease in subjects with nonmeasurable disease be assessed?
- Were lymph nodes being adequately assessed?
- Should functional imaging be used instead of anatomical imaging?

The task force once again met and, using an evidence-based approach, proposed changes to RECIST version 1.0 and published RECIST version 1.1 in January 2009. It is important when writing a protocol that the version of RECIST is identified and, ideally, should be the most current version (Eisenhauer et al., 2009).

Understanding how to use RECIST means understanding the measurability of lesions (i.e., measurable disease or nonmeasurable disease) and which lesions will be used to determine tumor response (i.e., target or nontarget). *Measurable disease* is a tumor lesion that is 10 mm or larger with CT scans (5 mm slice) or twice the thickness of slice measurement if CT scan measures more than 5 mm slices. This means that when reviewing a CT scan report, it is important to know the slices of the scanner. When measurements are taken by clinical exam (e.g., using calibers) or by chest x-ray, a measurable lesion is 10 mm or larger and 20 mm or larger, respectively. *Nonmeasurable disease* is all other lesions, including bone lesions, leptomeningeal disease, ascites, pleural/pericardial effusion, inflammatory breast disease, or cystic lesions (Eisenhauer et al., 2009).

Evaluating tumor response is determining the overall tumor burden. This evaluation includes lymph nodes. Target and nontarget lesions must be identified at baseline with the same lesions followed over time. A *target lesion* is a measurable lesion. There can be a total of five measurable lesions, and all organs with measurable lesions need to be represented with no more than two lesions per organ identified. Selection of target lesions is based on their size and suitability for accurate repeated measurements so that the sum of the diameters becomes the final measurement for target lesions. *Nontarget lesions* are any other lesions or sites of disease not classified as a target lesion that are measured as being present at baseline and either present or absent at follow-up. It is acceptable to record multiple nontarget lesions in the same organ or as a single item on a case report form. Lymph nodes are measured using the short axis. To be a target lesion, a lymph node must be 15 mm or larger; a nontarget lesion is a lymph node smaller than 15 mm. If the lymph node is smaller than 10 mm, it is considered normal (Eisenhauer et al., 2009).

Determining the overall response using RECIST combines the individual assessment for both target and nontarget lesions and assessment of the appearance of new lesions. The four response types for target lesions are as follows (Eisenhauer et al., 2009).

- Complete response is the disappearance of all target lesions, and any pathologic lymph nodes (whether target or nontarget) must have reduction in short axis to less than 10 mm.
- Partial response is at least a 30% decrease in the sum of the diameters of target lesions, taking as reference the baseline sum diameters.
- Progressive disease is at least a 20% increase in the sum of the diameters of target lesions, taking as reference the smallest sum on study (this includes the baseline sum if that is the smallest on study), and the relative increase of 20% must have the sum be an absolute increase of at least 5 mm. Progressive disease is also defined as the appearance of one or more new lesions.
- Stable disease is neither partial response nor progressive disease, taking as reference the smallest sum diameters while on study.

Because nontarget lesions have no associated measurements, their response is defined by their presence or absence or appearance of new lesions. Responses are defined as follows (Eisenhauer et al., 2009).

- Complete response is the disappearance of all nontarget lesions and normalization of tumor marker level. All lymph nodes must be nonpathologic in size (less than 10 mm at the short axis). If tumor markers are initially above the upper normal limit, they must normalize for a patient to be considered in complete clinical response.
- Non–complete response/non–progressive disease is the persistence of one or more nontarget lesions and/or maintenance of tumor marker level above the normal limits.
- Progressive disease is the appearance of one or more new lesions and/or *unequivocal progression* of existing nontarget lesions. Unequivocal progression should not normally trump target lesion status. It must be representative of overall disease status change, not a single lesion increase.

Overall response is best summarized by Table 15-2 for patient participants with measurable disease with or without nonmeasurable disease and in Table 15-3 for patient participants with only nonmeasurable disease. These

Table 15-2. Best Response Criteria for Patients With Measurable Disease				
Target Lesions	Nontarget Lesions	New Lesions	Overall Response	Best Overall Response When Confirmation Is Required*
CR	CR	No	CR	≥ 4 weeks confirmation**
CR	Non-CR/non-PD	No	PR	≥ 4 weeks confirmation**
CR	Not evaluated	No	PR	≥ 4 weeks confirmation**
PR	Non-CR/non-PD/not evaluated	No	PR	≥ 4 weeks confirmation**
SD	Non-CR/Non-PD/not evaluated	No	SD	Documented at least once ≥ 4 weeks from baseline**
PD	Any	Yes or no	PD	No prior SD, PR or CR
Any	PD***	Yes or no	PD	No prior SD, PR or CR
Any	Any	Yes	PD	No prior SD, PR or CR

* See RECIST 1.1 manuscript for further details on what is evidence of a new lesion.
** Only for non-randomized trials with response as primary endpoint.
*** In exceptional circumstances, unequivocal progression in nontarget lesions may be accepted as disease progression.
CR—complete response; PD—progressive disease; PR—partial response; SD—stable disease

Note. Patients with a global deterioration of health status requiring discontinuation of treatment without objective evidence of disease progression at that time should be reported as *symptomatic deterioration*. Every effort should be made to document the objective progression even after discontinuation of treatment.

From "CTEP Protocol Template," by National Cancer Institute Cancer Therapy Evaluation Program, 2015, p. 48. Retrieved from http://ctep.cancer.gov/protocol Development/templates_applications.htm.

Table 15-3. Best Response Criteria for Patients Who Only Have Nonmeasurable Disease

Nontarget Lesions	New Lesions	Overall Response
CR	No	CR
Non-CR/non-PD	No	Non-CR/non-PD*
Not all evaluated	No	Not evaluated
Unequivocal PD	Yes or No	PD
Any	Yes	PD

* Non-CR/non-PD is preferred over stable disease for nontarget disease since SD is increasingly used as an endpoint for assessment of efficacy in some trials, so to assign this category when no lesions can be measured is not advised.

CR—complete response; PD—progressive disease

Note. From "CTEP Protocol Template," by National Cancer Institute Cancer Therapy Evaluation Program, 2015, p. 49. Retrieved from http://ctep.cancer.gov/protocolDevelopment/templates_applications.htm.

tables, as well as other RECIST information, should be included the protocol. NCI CTEP (2015) has RECIST language that can be used when writing a protocol. It is helpful for CTNs to review this language to better understand RECIST because this manual cannot completely cover various nuances associated with the use of the criteria.

Hematologic Malignancy Response Assessment

Internationally agreed-upon response standards exist for certain hematologic malignancies. Bone marrow assessment is a key component in response assessment (see Table 15-4). This chapter will not review the specific details for each disease response because of the complexity of these standards and the diversity of hematologic malignancies. However, CTNs should refer to protocol specifics to determine the method for response criteria and review the references listed in Table 15-4.

Health-Related Quality of Life

QOL assessment is an additional oncology trial endpoint that is of continued, increasing interest. Although the measures of QOL are subjective (i.e., patient reported), the value of this endpoint cannot be overemphasized. With the increasing number of potential treatments available to subjects that could prolong life, QOL data as a trial endpoint will provide information that subjects may use for various treatment considerations. FDA has a guidance document to assist in using patient-reported outcome (PRO) measures to support a medical product label (U.S. FDA, 2009). This may serve as a useful resource when writing a protocol that has PRO-related objectives.

To determine how to measure a QOL- or PRO-related outcome, the principal investigator needs to select an appropriate QOL or PRO tool. Assessment tools are frequently under copyright, so permission is often required for both use and analysis of the data. When consideration is given to a tool, the developer's website will commonly have both the psychometrics and the population the tool has been previously used to evaluate. Tool development for a specific population QOL issue requires validation, which is beyond the scope of this manual. However, frequently the tool author or developer can be contacted and may be able to assist with adapting for the application and validation of the tool in the proposed study population.

Once the tools have been identified, consideration of when the assessment will be given is important (e.g., with clinical appointments or protocol procedure time points) along with the method of delivery (e.g., in person, by mail, electronically). The protocol should include

- Whether the tool can be completed by someone else on behalf of the participant, whether the participant can give verbal responses versus written, or if the response must be written
- Description of when the responses will be reviewed, especially if any items might have immediate clinical implications (e.g., suicidal ideation, harm to others)
- How responses will be returned (e.g., by secure electronic link, via a provided self-addressed, prepaid return envelope)
- Where or how the tools will be stored.

CTNs can assist in protocol development by ensuring that the protocol incorporates the information above.

Statistical Considerations

Statistical analysis of data helps to ensure that the information gathered in a study is organized, interpreted, and scientifically presented in an accurate and informative way (Gravetter & Wallnau, 2013). Essential purposes of the statistical section of each protocol are to state and justify the sample size and describe the planned statistical evaluation of the outcome data. Based upon the study's primary objectives, endpoints, and design, the statistician decides upon the basic type of statistical test that will be used to analyze the data.

The study team bases the research hypothesis on long-term clinical use of standard regimens and on extensive phase II or phase III use of experimental modalities and combinations. Generally, the null hypothesis states that the treatments are comparable; the alternative hypothesis states that the new treatment is better than the standard (a one-sided alternative) by a stated amount or that one is different from the other by a stated amount. The magnitude of the alternative hypothesis should be a ther-

Table 15-4. Summary of Selected Hematologic Response Assessments		
Disease	**History**	**Methods of Measuring Disease**
Malignant lymphomas	1987: Need for uniform reporting of clinical trial endpoints identified 1998: International Working Group consensus on standard guidelines for response assessment in adult patients with indolent and aggressive lymphomas 2007: International Harmonisation Project revised 1998 International Working Group guidelines to incorporate positron-emission tomography (PET), immunohistochemistry, and flow cytometry for definitions of response in non-Hodgkin and Hodgkin lymphoma	Disease response is based on • Nodal masses using fludeoxyglucose (FDG)-PET or PET/computed tomography (CT) • Recommendations for use of FDG and timing of imaging studies based on type of lymphoma • Spleen and/or liver assessed by physical exam or CT • Bone marrow biopsy for morphology or immunohistochemistry
Acute myeloid leukemia	1988: Consensus met to determine standards for response assessment in clinical trials. The standards were published in 1990. 2001: International group met to revise previous standards because of major advances in the biology and molecular genetics of acute leukemia. The revised standards were published in 2003.	Disease response is based on • Neutrophils • Platelets • Bone marrow biopsy for blasts • Cytogenetics • Extramedullary disease
Multiple myeloma	2006: International Myeloma Working Group published uniform response criteria to be used in clinical trials.	Disease response is based on • Serum and urine M protein • Serum free light chain • Bone marrow • Lytic lesion assessment • Calcium level

Note. Based on information from Cheson et al., 2003, 2007; Durie et al., 2006.

apeutic effect that is both clinically relevant and yet realistic. The difference between the null and alternative hypotheses has a direct effect on the sample size—the larger the difference, the smaller the sample size (see Figure 15-2).

Although hypothesizing a large difference to guarantee a small sample size may be tempting, if that difference is larger than that which is clinically of value (or even clinically possible), the resulting small sample size may fail to detect a less profound but still important treatment advance. The statistical section, therefore, must clearly state the alpha level, the power, and the null and alternative hypotheses. The statistician uses formulas, published tables, and computer programs to calculate the sample size needed in each arm of the study to detect the specified difference between the null and alternative hypotheses, given the stated values for alpha and power.

Power and Sample Size

The development and conduct of a trial may be expensive to the sponsoring agency, as well as labor intensive and time consuming at the clinical sites (e.g., data management activities, statistical analysis). For these reasons, determining the appropriate number of subjects needed for a study is important. By calculating the number of subjects needed to answer the proposed protocol research question, the goals of protecting subject safety, conserving resources, and completing the study in a timely manner can each be met. The results of a clinical protocol can then be statistically reported with confidence, and those results, whether positive or negative, can be disseminated to the scientific community.

A clinical trial must be large enough so that the results are statistically valid and can be generalized to the target population as a whole. If the study is too small, an important lifesaving advance in therapy could be missed (a statistical type II error), or a toxic or lethal regimen could be accepted for use in a large population (a statistical type I error) (Polit & Beck, 2012). A study that is too small may provide incomplete or incorrect information, potentially resulting in a waste of not only time and effort but also of limited subject and financial resources. This is particularly true for phase II and III clinical trials (see Figure 15-2).

The statistician works with the clinical investigators, review committees, and agencies to design a study that is large enough, or powered, to test the study questions. *Power* refers to the ability to detect meaningful or significant relationships between the variables of interest. The sample size is based on the stated objectives and must be large enough, with suitable adjustments, to account for the number of intended statistical tests. Power is an aspect of trial development that is of critical importance. Statistical power of a trial under development takes into consideration the size of the study sample population and requires a well-defined independent variable and a method for precise measurement of the study outcome

> **Figure 15-2. Definitions of Statistical Terms**
>
> The **null hypothesis**, or *H0*, is the outcome that the trial designers are trying to disprove or to "reject." The *H0* in most randomized studies is that a new therapy is not better than the standard treatment arm or that two experimental treatments have the same efficacy. *H0* in most single-arm studies is that the therapy under consideration has an unacceptable rate of the endpoint of interest (e.g., a specified unacceptably low rate of response, a stated unacceptably high rate of toxicity).
>
> The **alternative hypothesis**, or *HA*, is the outcome that the trial designers hope will occur: that the new therapy is better than the standard in a comparative study or that an investigative therapy has a better response rate (or lower toxicity) than the stated null unacceptable rate. Results of most statistical tests follow a known statistical distribution, such as the normal distribution or "bell-shaped curve" centered at zero. Other common distributions are the *t*, the χ^2 (chi-square), and the *F*. Values of the tests near zero are uninteresting because they are very likely, whereas large (positive or negative) values in the "tail" of the distribution are unlikely. The χ^2-value is the probability that the value of a statistical test of data could be that far from zero by chance. A χ^2-value of 0.003 means that there is a 0.3% chance that the results of a test were a random event rather than the result of interesting things happening in the data.
>
> The **type I error** or α-level (alpha-level) of a study is the probability that the overall results of the study will indicate that the null hypothesis is false or rejected when in fact it is true. The common α-level is 0.05, but other levels are employed when more- or less-stringent criteria are acceptable.
>
> The **type II error** or β-level (beta-level) of a study is the probability that the overall results of the study will fail to reject the null hypothesis when the alternative is in fact true. The power of the study, or chance of detecting a true effect, is $1 - \beta$. Commonly, studies are designed to have 80%–90% power (β of 0.10 or 0.20).
>
> The **significance level** is the maximum p-value of a test that will be taken to indicate statistical significance. When many tests are run on the same data, the significance level for any one test may need to be smaller than 0.05 to keep the overall α-level of the study at 0.05.
>
> *Note.* Based on information from Gravetter & Wallnau, 2013.

or objective. Power is important because insufficient power places the study at risk for a type II error, in which an existence of a relationship between variables remains undetected (Polit & Beck, 2012).

The procedure for calculating the sample size for a single-arm study or for each arm of a randomized, noncomparative phase II study follows the outline for a randomized study in that the statistician elicits the null and alternative hypotheses and the desired alpha-level and power for the study from the team. In single-arm evaluations, the null hypothesis comes from historical data about prior treatment and outcomes or from a clinical decision about what would constitute an unacceptable outcome. The null hypothesis generally is the therapy under investigation that is either ineffective or too toxic (i.e., the "bad" outcome). The alternative hypothesis is set by a medical decision about what would be a clinically meaningful result. It should be a therapeutic effect that is both clinically relevant and yet realistic.

To calculate the sample size for a randomized phase III study, the statistician identifies the test that will be used to compare the primary outcomes between the treatment arms on the study. The statistician then determines with the study team the values for the alpha-level for the study, the desired power, and the null and alternative hypotheses of interest.

A detailed discussion on the development for powering a study is provided later this chapter. For those who have an additional interest in how a proposed study sample size is calculated or want more detailed information on this aspect of clinical research, suggested reading materials are provided at the conclusion of the chapter.

Statistical Tests

Often, several different statistical tests will be used. For randomized studies, examples include the chi-square test, Fisher's exact test, and logistic regression for comparisons of categorical data; a log-rank test or Cox regression for comparisons of censored survival data; and a t-test or analysis of variance for comparisons of normally distributed data. Confidence intervals or one-sample tests generally are used for comparing the observed data with a hypothesized or historical control value in single-arm evaluations (U.S. FDA, 1998). Nonparametric analogs exist for most of these tests, as well (see Figure 15-2).

Descriptive Statistics

Descriptive statistics is another category of statistics that provides essential information to an interdisciplinary group conducting research. *Inferential statistics* are used by the scientific community to study samples and subsequently make generalizations about the population that is represented by the test or study population, whereas *descriptive statistics* describe the data and are necessary to first organize, summarize, and present the study information in a consistent manner (Gravetter & Wallnau, 2013). When the study results are reviewed and presented for publication, the descriptive statistics are always presented in the introductory information to help to frame the results of the study and define the study population. Thus, the descriptive statistics section provides information that allows members of the scientific community to determine whether the published results are applicable to their subject population.

Descriptive statistics are relevant at each interim analysis and may be hypothesis-generating for future studies. They are an important component of the research role that CTNs should be familiar enough with to discuss at study reviews. These commonly reported statistics include frequency, mean, median, mode, range, minimum, maximum, sum, and variance and are reported for each variable for which data points are collected during the course of the study (see Figure 15-3).

Analysis Plan

The analysis plan details the intended analyses of the primary and secondary endpoints and often is not included in a protocol document. However, it may be quite lengthy in an industry-sponsored study that will be part of an FDA filing. The analysis plan covers the particular statistical tests that will be used, with specific attention to issues such as handling stratification and missing data. The plan documents the rules that will be applied for the inclusion and exclusion of cases, in addition to special coding and transformations of the data.

The number and type of comparisons to be made need to be specified for a study that has more than one primary endpoint or for a phase III study with more than two treatment arms. Often, the type I error is divided by the number of comparisons. For example, a three-arm study with two comparisons (arm A versus arm B, and arm A versus arm C) might use 0.025 type I error for each comparison. Many statistical issues that arise during data analysis, such as post-randomization dropout or noncompliance to protocol therapy, cannot be foreseen at the time of the design. However, every attempt should be made to anticipate data problems that could compromise the analysis.

Monitoring

Safety is a vital endpoint in clinical trials (Polit & Beck, 2012). How safety is monitored and interpreted differs by the phase and objectives of each trial. Although disease outcome is not ignored in phase I studies, it is more important in phase II and III studies. Data from clinical trials are evaluated by internal and external reviewers on an ongoing basis to detect unexpected or unacceptable toxicity and to consider whether it is clear early in accrual that a treatment is ineffective and that subjects should not continue on that arm (U.S. FDA, 1998). It should be noted that at interim analysis, treatment might be stopped if the significance of the treatment benefit cannot be detected in the projected sample population,

---

Figure 15-3. Commonly Used Statistical Terms

Mean
The measure of central tendency that is most commonly used when defining a characteristic of the study population. Adding all the scores for the variable and dividing that total by the number of scores will provide the mean.

Median
The number value that is calculated by locating where exactly half of the data set scores have a value less than or equal to. The median is the 50th percentile. This number is used instead of the mean when the average does not provide a good representation of the study population.

Mode
The data score that occurs with the greatest frequency in a distribution of scores.

Range
The measure or value representing the variability within the data sample. The number is calculated by subtracting the lowest value (the minimum) from the highest value (the maximum) in the data score distribution.

Minimum
The lowest value represented in a data score distribution.

Maximum
The highest value represented in a data score distribution.

Sum
The total number reached when adding all the values (data) within a score distribution.

Variance
The "spread" or variability that is represented between data values in a data set. Variance is a mathematical calculation that is represented by the standard deviation when it is squared.

Note. Based on information from Gravetter & Wallnau, 2013; Polit & Beck, 2012.

---

or alternately, significant safety issues or superiority is detected in either study arm.

In 2011, FDA published draft guidelines related to risk-based approaches to clinical trial monitoring. In August 2013, they published the final guidance document titled *Guidance for Industry: Oversight of Clinical Investigations—A Risk-Based Approach to Monitoring* (U.S. FDA, 2013). Reviewing this guidance can help sponsors and investigators develop a thoughtful data and safety monitoring plan.

It is important to consider whether the study demonstrates early convincing evidence that one or more treatments are a significant advance in therapy. If so, the study should be stopped and the results made public. The monitoring section of the statistical considerations not only outlines the monitoring plan but, where not stated in the sample size section, provides the stopping rules that guide the reviewers. Note that for some protocols, the monitoring plan may be in a separate section.

In phase I studies, usually small numbers of subjects (three to six) are treated at each dose level. Monitoring the safety of subjects, occasionally on a subject-by-subject basis, is essential because the escalation/de-escalation scheme to determine the maximum tolerated dose depends on the toxicities observed in subjects at a particular dose level (Stoney & Johnson, 2012a).

In phase II studies, monitoring for both response rate and toxicity often occurs. Phase II studies can have two-stage designs in which a small number of subjects are entered and accrual is continued to the planned total only if a minimum number of responses are seen. The statistical section must state the number of responses needed for the accrual to continue to the second stage. Even if no rules are stated, a study can be paused or closed at any time because of unacceptable or unexpected toxicity (Stoney & Johnson, 2012a).

Outcomes of phase III studies often are monitored through group sequential methods. As an alternative to analyzing the data after the study has accrued all of the necessary subjects and had full follow-up, interim analyses may take place at prespecified fractions of the total planned study time, the total planned study accrual, or the number of events needed to obtain the power specified in the sample size section. The group sequential methods specify boundary values for statistical tests (which correspond to χ^2-values) in a way that preserves the overall alpha-level of the study.

The type I error (often 0.05) is spread throughout the number of interim analyses (commonly called *looks*), with the last look evaluated at a significance level less than 0.05. If at any analysis the statistical test for the primary endpoint exceeds the boundary established in the statistical design, then statistical significance can be declared, and the trial may be terminated. Procedures exist that allow termination because of a clear lack of a difference. Although these methods allow a study to close early if it shows convincing evidence that the study objectives have been met, the sample size has to be a bit larger (about 5%) to allow reuse of the data (Gravetter & Wallnau, 2013; U.S. FDA, 2010).

A data and safety monitoring board (DSMB) reviews the interim analysis and other administrative reports. DSMBs play an important role in reviewing interim data from a trial that may have implications for subject safety, the early termination of accrual, or greater treatment efficacy. The committee is composed of a variety of experts from different fields and may include clinicians, ethicists, subject advocates, and biostatisticians. The group meets periodically to consider a study's treatment-specific toxicity and outcomes in a strictly confidential, closed meeting. It is common to hold a planned yearly review of a study, even if the accrual has not yet reached a predetermined interim analysis review point. If no monitoring of phase III outcome data by a DSMB is planned, or if a prolonged delay in data review occurs, a justification must be given to the institutional review board. For more information about data and safety monitoring plans, see Chapter 40.

Summary

Interaction among the entire research team is important in establishing the design, hypotheses, and endpoints that will drive the sample size and power considerations for a clinical trial. The entire research team must have clearly defined plans for interim monitoring and the eventual analysis of the study, as all parts affect each other. The role of CTNs is critical, serving as gatekeeper to ensure that the study protocol follows a logical assessment plan, accurate response assessments are consistently recorded, and study enrollment and follow-up are not too burdensome on the patient. Each of these considerations must be implemented in an environment that fosters integrity of the study data obtained.

Issues evolving in clinical trials that bear watching in the next decade include flexible protocol design, proposed regulations to require electronic submission of study data, streamlining of clinical trial data collection, radiology-based endpoints, and merging of clinical trial phases. Evaluation and consideration of current statistical methods will be necessary as protocol design and data collection continue to evolve and CTNs remain essential members of the research team.

Key Points
- CTNs may add valuable, clinically applicable knowledge to the design and implementation of a protocol and should be included in the development process.
- CTNs plays a critical role during the protocol development to ensure that the objectives are both clinically measurable and that a tool or method for evaluating the outcome is included in both baseline and follow-up assessments.
- A critical function of the CTN role is adherence to study inclusion and exclusion criteria—those elements that define patient eligibility. Inclusion criteria are the elements that must be satisfied before a patient can enter into a trial, whereas exclusion criteria identify elements that, if met, will keep the patient from participating in the trial.
- When determining the frequency of procedures, it is helpful to delineate between what is essential for meeting protocol objectives and assessing participant safety versus what would be valuable, but not essential, data when the patient returns for a study visit.
- RECIST is intended for solid tumor response assessment; determining overall response using RECIST combines the individual assessment for both target and nontarget lesions while assessing for the appearance of new lesions.

- Statistically calculating the appropriate number of subjects needed for a study is a critical step to answering the proposed protocol research question while conserving resources and completing the study in a timely manner. Study results can then be statistically reported with confidence, and those results, whether positive or negative, can be disseminated to the scientific community.
- Descriptive statistics provide information that allows members of the scientific community to determine whether the published results may be applicable to their subject population.

References

Cheson, B., Bennett, J.M., Kopecky, K.J., Büchner, R., Willman, C.L., Estey, E.H., ... Bloomfield, C.D. (2003). Revised recommendations of the International Working Group for Diagnosis, Standardization of Response Criteria, Treatment Outcomes, and Reporting Standards for Therapeutic Trials in Acute Myeloid Leukemia. *Journal of Clinical Oncology, 21,* 4642–4649. doi:10.1200/JCO.2003.04.036

Cheson, B.D., Pfistner, B., Juweid, M.E., Gascoyne, R.D., Specht, L., Horning, S.J., ... Diehl, V. (2007). Revised response criteria for malignant lymphoma. *Journal of Clinical Oncology, 25,* 579–586. doi:10.1200/JCO.2006.09.2403

Durie, B.G.M., Harousseau, J.-L., Miguel, J.S., Bladé, J., Barlogie, B., Anderson, K., ... Rajkumar, S.V. (2006). International uniform response criteria for multiple myeloma. *Leukemia, 20,* 1467–1473. doi:10.1038/sj.leu.2404284

Eisenhauer, E.A., Therasse, P., Bogaert, J., Schwartz, L.H., Sargent, D., Ford, R., ... Verweik, J. (2009). New response evaluation criteria in solid tumours: Revised RECIST guideline (version 1.1). *European Journal of Cancer, 45,* 228–247. doi:10.1016/j.ejca.2008.10.026

Evers, P.D., Logan, J.E., Sills, V., & Chin, A.I. (2013). Karnofsky Performance Status predicts overall survival, cancer-specific survival, and progression-free survival following radical cystectomy for urothelial carcinoma. *World Journal of Urology,* 385–391. doi:10.1007/s00345-013-1110-7

Gravetter, F.J., & Wallnau, L.B. (2013). *Statistics for the behavioral sciences* (9th ed.). Belmont, CA: Wadsworth Cengage Learning.

International Conference on Harmonisation of Technical Requirements for Registration of Pharmaceuticals for Human Use. (1997, July 17). *General considerations for clinical trials, E8.* Retrieved from http://www.ich.org/fileadmin/Public_Web_Site/ICH_Products/Guidelines/Efficacy/E8/Step4/E8_Guideline.pdf

Karnofsky, D.A., Abelmann, W.H., Craver, L.F., & Burchenal, J.H. (1948). The use of nitrogen mustard in the palliative treatment of carcinoma. *Cancer, 1,* 634–656. doi:10.1002/1097-0142(194811)1:4<634::AID-CNCR2820010410>3.0.CO;2-L

Karp, B.L., & Nussenblatt, R.B. (2012). Writing a protocol. In J.I. Gallin & F.P. Ognibene (Eds.), *Principles and practice of clinical research* (3rd ed., pp. 483–489). Waltham, MA: Elsevier Academic Press. doi:10.1016/B978-0-12-382167-6.00032-1

Lansky, S.B., List, M.A., Lansky, L.L., Ritter-Sterr, C., & Miller, D.R. (1987). The measurement of performance in childhood cancer patients. *Cancer, 60,* 1651–1656. doi:10.1002/10970142(19871001)60:7<1651::AID-CNCR2820600738>3.0.CO;2-J

Lee, C.K., Simes, R.J., Brown, C., Gebski, V., Pfisterer, J., Swart, A.M., ... Friedlander, M. (2013). A prognostic nomogram to predict overall survival in patients with platinum-sensitive recurrent ovarian cancer. *Annals of Oncology, 24,* 937–943. doi:10.1093/annonc/mds538

Lubejko, B., Good, M., Weiss, P., Schmieder, L., Leos, D., & Daugherty, P. (2011). Oncology clinical trials nursing: Developing competencies for the novice. *Clinical Journal of Oncology Nursing, 15,* 637–643. doi:10.1188/11.CJON.637-643

National Cancer Institute. (2015a, April 22). Adult Hodgkin lymphoma treatment (PDQ®): Stage information for adult Hodgkin lymphoma [Health professional version]. Retrieved from http://www.cancer.gov/types/lymphoma/hp/adult-hodgkin-treatment-pdq#link/stoc_h2_2

National Cancer Institute. (2015b, April 24). Adult non-Hodgkin lymphoma treatment (PDQ®): Stage information for adult NHL [Health professional version]. Retrieved from http://www.cancer.gov/types/lymphoma/hp/adult-nhl-treatment-pdq#link/stoc_h2_5

National Cancer Institute. (2015c, January 6). Cancer staging. Retrieved from http://www.cancer.gov/cancertopics/factsheet/detection/staging

National Cancer Institute. (2015d, May 26). Childhood non-Hodgkin lymphoma treatment (PDQ®): Staging information for childhood NHL [Health professional version]. Retrieved from http://www.cancer.gov/types/lymphoma/hp/child-nhl-treatment-pdq#link/stoc_h2_2

National Cancer Institute. (2015e, April 2). Chronic lymphocytic leukemia treatment (PDQ®): Staging information for chronic lymphocytic leukemia [Health professional version]. Retrieved from http://www.cancer.gov/types/leukemia/hp/cll-treatment-pdq#link/stoc_h2_1

National Cancer Institute. (2015f, May 11). Neuroblastoma treatment (PDQ®): Stage information for neuroblastoma [Health professional version]. Retrieved from http://www.cancer.gov/types/neuroblastoma/hp/neuroblastoma-treatment-pdq#section/_14

National Cancer Institute. (2015g, May 22). Plasma cell neoplasms (including multiple myeloma) treatment (PDQ®): Stage information about plasma cell neoplasms [Health professional version]. Retrieved from http://www.cancer.gov/cancertopics/pdq/treatment/myeloma/healthprofessional#section/_45

National Cancer Institute. (2015h, May 11). Retinoblastoma treatment (PDQ®): Stage information. Retrieved from http://www.cancer.gov/types/retinoblastoma/hp/retinoblastoma-treatment-pdq#link/_613_toc

National Cancer Institute Cancer Therapy Evaluation Program. (2010, June 14). *Common terminology criteria for adverse events* [v.4.03]. Retrieved from http://evs.nci.nih.gov/ftp1/CTCAE/CTCAE_4.03_2010-06-14_QuickReference_5x7.pdf

National Cancer Institute Cancer Therapy Evaluation Program. (2015, May 15). CTEP protocol template. Retrieved from http://ctep.cancer.gov/protocolDevelopment/templates_applications.htm

National Cancer Institute Coordinating Center for Clinical Trials. (2013, November). BIQSFP '14 (Biomarker, Imaging, and Quality of Life Studies Funding Program) quality of life study evaluation guidelines. Retrieved from http://www.cancer.gov/aboutnci/organization/ccct/funding/BIQSFP/2014_BIQSFP_QOLStudyEvaluationGuidelines

National Cancer Institute Office of Biorepositories and Biospecimen Research. (2011). NCI best practices for biospecimen resources. Retrieved from http://biospecimens.cancer.gov/bestpractices/2011-NCIBestPractices.pdf

Ness, L. (2013, November). Documentation and document management in clinical research [PowerPoint presentation]. Retrieved from https://ccrod.cancer.gov/confluence/download/attachments/83530280/Documentation%20and%20Document%20Management.pdf?version=1&modificationDate=1385473200133&api=v2

Oken, M.M., Creech, R.H., Tormey, D.C., Horton, J., Davis, T.E., McFadden, E.T., & Carbone, P.P. (1982). Toxicity and response criteria of the Eastern Cooperative Oncology Group. *American Journal of Clinical Oncology, 5,* 649–655. doi:10.1097/00000421-198212000-00014

Polit, D.F., & Beck, C.T. (2012). *Nursing research: Generating and assessing evidence for nursing practice* (9th ed.). Philadelphia, PA: Lippincott Williams & Wilkins.

Sørensen, J.B., Klee, M., Palshof, T., & Hansen, H.H. (1993). Performance status assessment in cancer patients. An inter-observer variability study. *British Journal of Cancer, 67*, 773–775. doi:10.1038/bjc.1993.140

Stoney, C.M., & Johnson, L.L. (2012a). Design of clinical studies and trials. In J.I. Gallin & F.P. Ognibene (Eds.), *Principles and practice of clinical research* (3rd ed., pp. 225–242). Waltham, MA: Elsevier Academic Press. doi:10.1016/B978-0-12-382167-6.00019-9

Stoney, C.M., & Johnson, L.L. (2012b). Development and conduct of studies. In J.I. Gallin & F.P. Ognibene (Eds.), *Principles and practice of clinical research* (3rd ed., pp. 381–394). Waltham, MA: Elsevier Academic Press. doi:10.1016/B978-0-12-382167-6.00029-1

Therasse, P., Arbuck, S.G., Eisenhauer, E.A., Wanders, J., Kaplan, R.S., Rubinstein, L., ... Gwyther, S. (2000). New guidelines to evaluate the response to treatment in solid tumors. *Journal of the National Cancer Institute, 92*, 205–216. doi:10.1093/jnci/92.3.205

U.S. Food and Drug Administration. (1998, September). *Guidance for industry: E9 statistical principles for clinical trials*. Retrieved from http://www.fda.gov/downloads/Drugs/GuidanceComplianceRegulatoryInformation/Guidances/ucm073137.pdf

U.S. Food and Drug Administration. (2007, May). *Guidance for industry: Clinical trial end points for the approval of cancer drugs and biologics*. Retrieved from http://www.fda.gov/downloads/Drugs/GuidanceComplianceRegulatoryInformation/Guidances/ucm071590.pdf

U.S. Food and Drug Administration. (2009, December). *Guidance for industry: Patient-reported outcome measures: Use in medical product development to support labeling claims*. Retrieved from http://www.fda.gov/downloads/Drugs/Guidances/UCM193282.pdf

U.S. Food and Drug Administration. (2010). *Guidance for industry: Adaptive design clinical trials for drugs and biologics* [Draft guidance]. Retrieved from http://www.fda.gov/downloads/Drugs/.../Guidances/ucm201790.pdf

U.S. Food and Drug Administration. (2013, August). *Guidance for industry: Oversight of clinical investigations—A risk-based approach to monitoring*. Retrieved from http://www.fda.gov/downloads/Drugs/.../Guidances/UCM269919.pdf

Additional Resources

Englert, S., & Kieser, M. (2012). Adaptive designs for single-arm phase II trials in oncology. *Pharmaceutical Statistics, 11*, 241–249. doi:10.1002/pst.541

Seymour, L., Ivy, S.P., Sargent, D., Spriggs, D., Baker, L., Rubinstein, L., ... Berry, D. (2010). The design of phase II clinical trials testing cancer therapeutics: Consensus recommendations from the Clinical Trial Design Task Force of the National Cancer Institute Investigational Drug Steering Committee. *Clinical Cancer Research, 16*, 1764–1769. doi:10.1158/1078-0432.CCR-09-3287

Yuan, Y., & Uin, G. (2011). Bayesian phase I/II adaptively randomized oncology trials with combined drugs. *Annals of Applied Statistics, 5*, 924–942. doi:10.1214/10-AOAS433

Chapter 16

Protocol Review and Approval Process

Kelly Filchner, MSN, RN, OCN®, CCRC

Introduction

Although the institutional review board (IRB) has a vital role in the protection of research participants, other types of reviews may occur before the investigative team presents the study to the IRB. It is important to understand the significance of the pre-IRB reviews, such as scientific, institutional biosafety, and radiation safety reviews. Clinical trial nurses (CTNs) need to understand these protocol review processes, along with the IRB's role and responsibilities, so that the investigators can conduct a study in a manner that maintains the ethical rights and safety of the participants. This chapter will include information about the various types of reviews and approvals that a protocol has to undergo, as well as implications for CTNs.

Pre–Institutional Review Board Reviews and Approvals

Upon receipt of a new study, a CTN may be involved in preparing the study document for regulatory review. In addition to the required IRB approval, other reviews may be needed before the IRB review. These are categorized into three groups: scientific, safety, and sponsor reviews. CTNs must be familiar with each of these categories in addition to the site's standard operating procedures (SOPs) (see Chapter 11) regarding the submission and review process. Examples of additional site review requirements may include pharmacy, laboratory, or financial feasibility. CTNs must be aware of what local reviews and processes include.

Scientific Reviews

The primary focus of a scientific review and the scientific review committee is to evaluate the scientific value of the study. Questions that may be addressed during the scientific review include the following (National Cancer Institute [NCI], 2012a, 2012b).
- Are the primary and secondary aims clearly defined?
- Are the literature review and background material sufficient to support the study?
- Is the statistical method valid and sample size adequate to meet objectives?
- Is the research staff qualified to conduct the study?

Scientific review is a requirement for the NCI-designated cancer centers (NCI, 2012a, 2012b). This review is not required by the U.S. Food and Drug Administration (FDA) or the U.S. Department of Health and Human Services (DHHS) Office for Human Research Protections (OHRP). It is individualized to the institution or research site. For example, smaller community settings may not use scientific review; however, large academic centers most likely would have a scientific review process in place.

The scientific committee may serve as a resource for the IRB and may include protocol monitoring or assessing organizational resources as part of its responsibilities. Each committee sets the frequency of meetings and deadlines for submissions, as well as membership composition. The scientific review process should be used as a tool for the investigators for submission of complete information to the IRB, ultimately helping to avoid delays in the approval process.

Safety Reviews

Safety reviews may be specific to an institution or required, depending on the type of research (e.g., gene therapy). The reviews may need to be completed before submission to the IRB. A CTN may be directly involved with specific aspects of these reviews (e.g., document preparation) or be responsible for ensuring that the reviews occur and appropriate approval is secured and submitted to the IRB per the IRB SOPs.

Radiation Safety

If a study requires use of ionizing radiation beyond what is considered standard of care, some institutions will require approval by the institution's radiation safety committee. The institution's policies and procedures will guide the need for this review and the necessary steps to gain approval. CTNs should be aware of their institutional requirements, including using correct application forms.

Depending on the type of research conducted at the site, a radioactive drug research committee may also be in place. This committee is specific for oversight of radioactive drugs used for research and has specific requirements for membership and functions (Radioactive Drugs for Certain Research Uses, 2013). As the existence of this type of committee is generally specific to large academic institutions, CTNs should refer to the site's SOPs for guidance on how to submit protocols for approval.

Recombinant DNA Safety Review

Two reviewing bodies cover research involving recombinant DNA or synthetic nucleic acid molecules: an institutional biosafety committee (IBC) and the National Institutes of Health (NIH) Office of Biotechnology Activities (OBA). Institutions who receive funding from NIH for research involving recombinant DNA or synthetic nucleic acid molecules will need to follow the *NIH Guidelines for Research Involving Recombinant or Synthetic Nucleic Acid Molecules* (NIH OBA, 2013d), which include establishing an IBC for protocol review and submitting the protocol for OBA review. The NIH guidelines are detailed safety practices and containment procedures for basic and clinical research involving recombinant or synthetic nucleic acid molecules. Even if this only applies to one NIH-funded research project at the institution, all similar projects or protocols conducted at or sponsored by that institution must comply with the NIH guidelines. Adherence to these guidelines may be a condition of support from other federal agencies or private funders of research (NIH OBA, 2013a). Because these products are not yet approved for use, an investigational new drug application (IND) will need to be submitted to FDA (see Chapter 2 for more details).

IBCs are the foundation of institutional oversight of recombinant DNA research. They approve and oversee projects in accordance with appendix M of the NIH guidelines. An IBC may be institution-based, or the institution may need to use an external or commercial IBC. The IBC must register with OBA (2013b). CTNs may need to assist with some of the following activities surrounding use of an IBC.

- Application process, including
  - Obtaining necessary information from the sponsor, such as supporting research conducted on the study agent
  - Securing proper institutional signatures
  - Providing documentation of training for individuals that will be directly involved with the research (e.g., documentation of infection control training)
- Securing local representatives if an external IBC will be used
- Helping to identify a biologic safety officer for the institution (This is an individual appointed by an institution to oversee management of biosafety risks.)
- Submission of ongoing reviews, amendments, and serious adverse events to the IBC for review and approval
- Tracking adverse events and current patient status (on-study treatment, off-study treatment, completed) for submission at time of annual review

The OBA is responsible for developing, implementing, and monitoring NIH policies and procedures for the safe conduct of recombinant DNA activities, including human gene transfer research (NIH OBA, 2013a). The NIH Recombinant DNA Advisory Committee (RAC) was formed in 1974 with the primary responsibility of instituting guidelines that would govern the safe conduct of recombinant DNA research by outlining appropriate biosafety practices and containment measures. These guidelines were first published in 1976 and are known as *The NIH Guidelines for Research Involving Recombinant or Synthetic Nucleic Acid Molecules* (NIH OBA, 2013d). The RAC provides recommendation to the IBC for their consideration in approving the protocol (NIH OBA, 2013c).

It is important for CTNs to understand that the IBC and IRB will *not* review research involving gene therapy until after the RAC review is complete and the associated correspondence from the committee is submitted with the IBC application. Figure 16-1 provides IBC and OBA resources for CTNs.

Sponsor Approval

An investigator-initiated research project is one in which the study has been funded as a result of an investigator developing and writing his or her own protocol (NIH, n.d.). The funding may come in the form of securing the investigational agent by submitting a letter of

---

Figure 16-1. Office of Biotechnology Activities (OBA) Resources

- OBA website: http://oba.od.nih.gov/oba/index.html
- National Institutes of Health guidelines: http://osp.od.nih.gov/sites/default/files/NIH_Guidelines.html
- Institutional biosafety committees (IBCs): http://osp.od.nih.gov/office-biotechnology-activities/biosafety/institutional-biosafety-committees
- Training and educational materials for IBCs: http://oba.od.nih.gov/rdna_ibc/ibc_training.html
- Externally administered IBCs: http://osp.od.nih.gov/sites/default/files/resources/External_IBC_FAQs.pdf

intent to the sponsor or manufacturer of the agent (e.g., a pharmaceutical company or the NCI Cancer Therapy Evaluation Program [CTEP]). This means that the sponsor will need to review and approve the protocol. This approval may be documented by an informal communication, such as an email, or, as is the case with CTEP, a formal approval letter. For more information about CTEP letters of intent and protocol review and approvals, see sections 7.0 and 8.0 of *A Handbook for Clinical Investigators Conducting Therapeutic Clinical Trials Supported by CTEP, DCTD, NCI* (NCI, 2014). The protocol cannot proceed without the sponsor's approval and the IRB's approval of the same version of the protocol. Regardless of the sponsor, CTNs must be aware of the necessary documents that must accompany the protocol through the approval processes.

Institutional Review Board Ethical Review

The primary purpose of an IRB is to ensure that appropriate steps are taken to protect the rights and welfare of human subjects who participate in biomedical and behavioral research. The IRB involves a group process to review research protocols and related materials, such as informed consent documents, advertisements, and investigator brochures. The term *institutional review board* is primarily used in the United States because it is DHHS and FDA nomenclature. Internationally, other names that may be used for IRBs include *research ethics committee* and *ethical review board* (Amdur & Bankert, 2011).

Assurances and Institutional Review Board Registration

Obtaining or verifying the presence of an assurance and registering the IRB most likely will occur before submitting the study through the ethical review process.

Assurances

Any institution engaged in federally conducted or funded human subject research must have an assurance of compliance in place. An *assurance* is the written commitment by the institution to protect participants and follow the regulations in *Code of Federal Regulations* Title 45 Part 46 (45 C.F.R. pt. 46) (Protection of Human Subjects, 2009). This assurance must be in place (i.e., filed with and accepted by OHRP) before any DHHS funding is awarded or research has commenced (OHRP, 2011a).

A Federalwide Assurance (FWA) is the only type of assurance accepted for review and approval by OHRP as of January 1, 2006. Each legally distinct entity that is engaged in federally supported human subject research must file its own separate assurance. Once an FWA is obtained, all employees and agents of the institution are covered whenever they are involved in the conduct of research defined by the FWA. CTNs must be aware of the existence of the site's FWA because it is closely linked to the IRB process. This is especially true for international studies (i.e., when CTNs are coordinating multisite research with sites outside of the United States). All participating sites for DHHS-funded research, even those outside of the United States, need to comply with OHRP regulations, including securing an FWA and registering the IRB (Trocky & Ness, 2013).

Obtaining an FWA is a two-step process. The FWA process includes registering the IRB and completing the FWA application online (see Figure 16-2). Instructions and forms can be found on the OHRP website (www.hhs.gov/ohrp/assurances). Each FWA must be linked to an IRB (internal or external) (OHRP, n.d.-a, 2011a).

CTNs may be involved or at least should be aware of the following additional activities surrounding the FWA.
- Assurances are effective for five years and must be renewed at the end of that period to remain effective, even if no changes have occurred.
- Any changes to the FWA should be completed within 90 days of the change. An example is adding a facility owned or operated by the main institution where research activities may take place.
- Obtaining/collecting investigator-related documents:
  – An institution holding an OHRP-approved FWA may extend the applicability of its FWA to cover two types of collaborating individual investigators: collaborating independent investigators and collaborating institutional investigators.
  – The extension of an assured institution's FWA to cover a collaborating individual investigator should be documented using an individual investigator agreement (OHRP, 2011a, 2013).

Institutional Review Board Registration

The registration of an IRB applies to those IRBs that are designated on an FWA (45 C.F.R. pt. 46, subpt. E) and those IRBs in the United States reviewing clinical investigations for which FDA has regulatory oversight (21 C.F.R. pt. 56, subpt. B) (Institutional Review Boards, 2013; Registration of Institutional Review Boards, 2009). Each IRB must register electronically with OHRP using the electronic submission system. The registration process will require information such as primary contacts, IRB chairperson, IRB roster information, staff dedicated to IRB functions, and approximate number of active research protocols, including types of FDA-regulated products (OHRP, 2011b).

Each registered IRB will receive an IRB organization number. Similar to the FWA update process, any changes must be updated within 90 days of the

144   Section III. Protocol Development, Review, and Approval Process

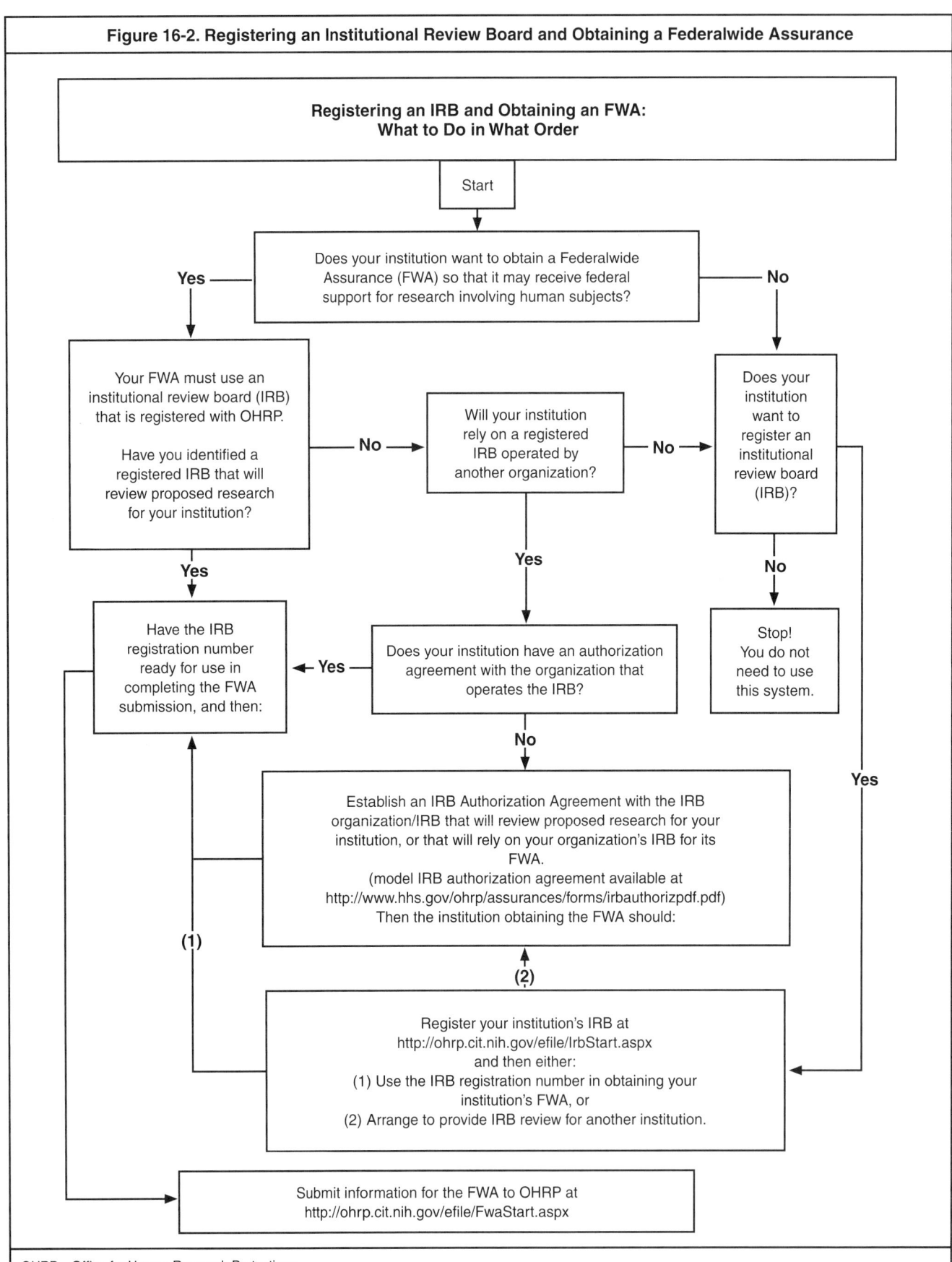

Figure 16-2. Registering an Institutional Review Board and Obtaining a Federalwide Assurance

OHRP—Office for Human Research Protections

Note. From "Registering an IRB and Obtaining an FWA: What to Do in What Order," by U.S. Department of Health and Human Services Office for Human Research Protections, n.d. Retrieved from http://www.hhs.gov/ohrp/assurances/irbfwasequence.pdf.pdf.

change. The registration must be renewed every three years (even if no changes have occurred) to maintain active status. Any update or renewal electronically submitted and approved by OHRP begins a new three-year effective period. Disbanding a registered IRB must be reported to OHRP in writing within 30 days after permanent cessation of the IRB's review of DHHS-conducted or supported research (OHRP, 2013). Visit OHRP's website for initial instructions (www.hhs.gov/ohrp/assurances/irb/register/index.html) and for registration updates or renewals (www.hhs.gov/ohrp/assurances/irb/update/index.html).

If the institution already has a registered IRB and FWA, CTNs may need to provide documentation to sponsors. If CTNs are coordinating a multi-institutional study, they will need to ensure that those sites' IRBs have an FWA. The status of active IRBs and FWAs can be checked online (OHRP, n.d.-b, n.d.-c). Instructions are located on the OHRP website (www.hhs.gov/ohrp/assurances/status/index.html), and the direct link to the registration status website is http://ohrp.cit.nih.gov/search.

Educational webinars (e.g., When the Assurance Comes a "Knockin": Everything You Need to Know About OHRP's FWA and IRB Registration Processes) are available on the OHRP website to review these procedures (www.hhs.gov/ohrp/education/training/ded_webinar.html).

Figure 16-3. Types of Institutional Review Boards (IRBs)

Internal IRB
Local IRB
- Affiliated with the institution or organization conducting the research
- Example: a university or hospital

External IRB
Commercial IRB
- Paid by institution or sponsor to conduct review of research
- Not affiliated with a specific institution
- Often used by industry to expedite activation of studies at sites
- May see use in physician practice setting
- May allow for rapid opening of a study for a specific patient as the study has already been centrally approved

Central IRB
- Used with research that involves large, multisite clinical trials
- Conducts review on behalf of all study sites that agree to participate in the centralized review process
- May be commercial (overlap with commercial IRB info)
- May be established by public research organizations such as the National Cancer Institute Central Institutional Review Board Initiative (www.ncicirb.org)

Note. Based on information from Moon & Khin-Maung-Gyi, 2009.

Types of Institutional Review Boards

Generally, the two main types of IRBs are internal or external (see Figure 16-3). These two categories can be known by other terms. Internal IRBs are often called *local* IRBs, and external IRBs can be known as *commercial, independent,* or *central* IRBs. Traditionally, IRBs were located where the investigator conducted research, such as an academic medical center. However, because of access of clinical trials in the community setting, external IRBs, which have no site affiliation, have evolved over time. All types of IRBs must follow the same regulations (Moon & Khin-Maung-Gyi, 2009). When using an external IRB, CTNs may need to facilitate local informed consent document creation and submission of a local IRB application. The site should have SOPs in place for the use of external IRBs. CTNs should be aware that depending upon the type of research, more than one IRB may be used (e.g., NCI Central Institutional Review Board used for phase III trials conducted through the National Clinical Trials Network and the local IRB used for investigator-initiated studies).

General Functions and Operations

For the IRB to fulfill its charge to protect human subjects, certain functions and operations must be upheld. These can be found in OHRP regulations 45 C.F.R. pt. 46, specifically §§ 46.101–46.124 (Protection of Human Subjects, 2009) and FDA regulations 21 C.F.R. pt. 56 (Institutional Review Boards, 2013). The general functions include following written procedures for (Institutional Review Boards, 2013; Protection of Human Subjects, 2009)

- Conducting initial and continuing review of research
- Reporting findings to the investigator and the institution
- Determining which projects need more frequent review and which projects need verification from sources other than the investigator
- Ensuring prompt reporting of changes and requiring that changes to the research may not occur until IRB review has taken place unless there are immediate hazards to the subjects
- Ensuring prompt reporting of unanticipated problems to appropriate regulatory authorities (e.g., IRB, FDA)
- Reporting noncompliance with regulations or IRB determinations
- Reporting suspension and termination of the research.

Institutional Review Board Membership

Regulations require IRBs to be composed of at least five members with varying backgrounds to promote complete and adequate review of research activities commonly conducted by the institution. The IRB must be sufficiently qualified through the expertise of its members to review the research proposals. This includes review of proposed research in terms of institutional commitment, applicable laws, and standards of professional conduct. The IRB membership criteria are (Institutional Review Boards, 2013; Protection of Human Subjects, 2009)

- Diversity of its members (e.g., male, female, various races, cultural backgrounds) so that there is sufficient sensitivity to the community in which the research is being conducted
- At least one member whose primary concern is in the scientific areas
- At least one member whose primary concern is nonscientific
- At least one member with no direct affiliation with the institution or part of the immediate family of any member
- If working with vulnerable populations (e.g., children, prisoners, mentally challenged), one member must have knowledge of or experience working with these populations
- IRBs may call in special members to review a specific study if no current member has experience with the population or study intervention. These special members may not vote with the IRB.

CTNs should be aware of the member composition of the IRBs in which they interact. If a special member is needed for review, it would be helpful for the IRB to have this information before receipt of the protocol. CTNs should also be familiar with the IRB's policies regarding conflicts of interest for IRB members. Any IRB member with a conflict (e.g., an investigator participating in a protocol being reviewed, an investigator holding stock in the pharmaceutical company sponsoring the trial) should not participate in the approval process for that research study.

Institutional Review Board Administrative Support

Although not part of the IRB, each IRB will most likely have some type of administrative support to assist in preparation of IRB documents and ensure meeting minutes are taken and approval documents are returned to the investigators. Most IRBs have an application process that is either on paper or electronic and often requires human subject protection training for key research staff prior to submission. Common elements of the application include

- Protocol documents with all appropriate appendices, including any patient surveys, questionnaires, or educational materials
- Abstract components of the protocol, including primary and secondary objectives, background and rationale, research participant characteristics, study procedures, summary of the statistical analysis plan, and how confidentiality and privacy will be maintained
- Informed consent documents
- Recruitment plan and materials, including advertisements
- Other approvals (e.g., radiation safety committee, OBA, NCI CTEP).

CTNs should be educated about the application process for each IRB based upon the type of study being submitted for approval (i.e., internal versus external).

Institutional Review Board Meetings

The IRB will set the frequency of meetings, which may be determined based on factors such as the IRB type or workload. Some local institutions may have more than one IRB to accommodate the workload. Every meeting will have an agenda and a due date for document submission (e.g., initial protocol, amendments, continuing review). This process allows IRB members to have sufficient time to adequately review the documents before the actual meeting. CTNs should know IRB meeting dates and submission deadlines.

Except where expedited review applies, the IRB members must review the research at a convened meeting that includes at least one member with a nonscientific background. A majority of members (or *quorum*) must be present at the meeting. For example, if the IRB has 20 members, at least 11 members must be present in order to conduct the business of the meeting. The quorum must be held throughout the entire meeting (Amdur & Bankert, 2011; Institutional Review Boards, 2013; Protection of Human Subjects, 2009).

Types of Institutional Review Board Reviews

Not all research requires IRB review. OHRP provides decision charts as a guide for IRBs, investigators, and others who need to determine if an activity is research involving human subjects that must be reviewed by an IRB under 45 C.F.R pt. 46 (Protection of Human Subjects, 2009).These charts can be found at www.hhs.gov/ohrp/policy/checklists/decisioncharts.html.

The three types of IRB reviews are full board, expedited, and exempt. A *full board* review is when the entire IRB, at least a quorum, convenes to conduct business. This is required for many of the activities for which the IRB is responsible (Amdur & Bankert, 2011). Certain types of research review may qualify for *expedited review*. This is defined as the ability to approve the research without a convened meeting of the IRB. Review of the research may be performed by the IRB chairperson or by one or more experienced members of the IRB desig-

nated by the chairperson. The reviewer has all authorities of the IRB except disapproval. An IRB may use the expedited review procedure for either of the following (Amdur & Bankert, 2011; Institutional Review Boards, 2013; Protection of Human Subjects, 2009).
- Some or all of the research involves no more than minimal risk to subjects.
- Minor changes are proposed in previously approved research during the period covered by the original approval.

Regulations are in place that provide for *exemption from IRB review*. The qualified research can include research conducted in an educational setting; tests, surveys, interviews, and public behavior observations; research on existing data, documents, records, and specimens; research for the public benefit or service programs; and research on food taste and acceptance studies. The following conditions need to be met in order to qualify for OHRP exemption (Institutional Review Boards, 2013; Protection of Human Subjects, 2009).
- Information will be recorded by investigators in a manner that subjects cannot be identified directly or through identifiers.
- Disclosure of subjects' responses cannot reasonably place the subject at risk of criminal or civil liability and cannot be damaging to the subjects' financial standing, employability, or reputation.

Different criteria apply when determining FDA exemption for emergency use of a test article. See 21 C.F.R. § 56.104 for specific information.

Each IRB can determine policies regarding exempt research (Institutional Review Boards, 2013; Protection of Human Subjects, 2009). Some IRBs may require all research in the institution to be reviewed in some manner by the IRB even though the study qualifies per the regulations as exempt. Others may require that exempt research be reviewed by the institution's human subject protection program. CTNs should follow their IRB policies regarding exempt research.

Risk-Benefit Analysis

In order for the IRB to review the research, there must be an understanding of risk and benefit. *Risk* is defined as a calculation of the probability of the magnitude of harm. OHRP defines *minimal risk* as the "probability and magnitude of harm or discomfort in the research is not greater in and of themselves than those ordinarily encountered in daily life or during the performance of routine physical or psychological examinations or test" (Definitions, 45 C.F.R. § 46.102(i), 2009). The regulations only define minimal risk; however, risk can be defined as the probability of harm or injury occurring as a result of participation in the research. This risk can be physical, psychological, social, or economic. For adults, one of the following risk categories will be determined by the IRB and included in the minutes (see Figure 16-4):
- Research involves no more than minimal risk to subjects
- Research involves greater than minimal risk (Wichman, 2012).

A research *benefit* is considered to be something of health-related, psychosocial, or other value to an individual research subject, or something that will contribute to the acquisition of generalizable knowledge. One of the following categories will be determined by the IRB and included in the minutes (see Table 16-1):
- Research involves the prospect of direct benefit to individual subjects
- No prospect of direct benefit to individual subjects, but benefit to others (e.g., further society's understanding of disorder or condition) (Wichman, 2012).

The risk level for children is slightly different and somewhat combines risk and benefit assessment (Amdur & Bankert, 2011; Protection of Human Subjects, 2009):
- Research not involving greater than minimal risk to subjects
- Research involving greater than minimal risk but presenting the prospect of direct benefit to the individual subjects

---

Figure 16-4. Institutional Review Board Risk-Benefit Assessment

RISK
Regulatory definition of minimal risk: Minimal risk means that the probability and magnitude of harm or discomfort anticipated in the research are not greater in and of themselves than those ordinarily encountered in daily life or during the performance of routine physical or psychological examinations or tests (45 C.F.R. § 46.102(h)(l)).
Check appropriate risk category:
1. _____ The research involves no more than minimal risk to subjects.
2. _____ The research involves more than minimal risk to subjects.
   a. _____ The risk(s) represents a minor increase over minimal risk, or
   b. _____ The risk(s) represents more than a minor increase over minimal risk.

BENEFIT
Definition: A research benefit is considered to be something of health-related, psychosocial, or other value to an individual research subject, or something that will contribute to the acquisition of generalizable knowledge. Money or other compensation for participation in research is not considered to be a benefit, but rather compensation for research-related inconveniences.
Check appropriate benefit category:
1. _____ The research involves no prospect of direct benefit to individual subjects, but is likely to yield generalizable knowledge about the subjects' disorder or condition.
2. _____ The research involves the prospect of direct benefit to individual subjects.

Note. Figure courtesy of Fox Chase Cancer Center. Used with permission.

Table 16-1. Components of Institutional Review Board (IRB) Meeting Minutes

Component	Comments
Meeting attendance	Presence of quorum
Summary of discussion	–
Controversial issues	Discussion and resolution
Conflicts of interest	Recusal of members as applicable
Accounting of the votes of each actionable item	Members voting for, voting against, or abstaining
Risk assessment	Minimal, greater than minimal
Benefit assessment	Prospect of direct benefit, no prospect of direct benefit
Stipulations	Determinations of IRB conditions for approval

Note. Based on information from Institutional Review Boards, 2013; Protection of Human Subjects, 2009.

- Research involving greater than minimal risk and no prospect of direct benefit to individual subjects but likely to yield generalizable knowledge about the subjects' disorder or condition
- Research not otherwise approvable which presents an opportunity to understand, prevent, or alleviate a serious problem affecting the health or welfare of children.

As part of the IRB application process, the investigator identifies a risk-benefit category.

The IRB's review standards should include
- Risk analysis and assessment
  - Identification of the risks associated with the research as separate from the risks of therapies that the subject would have if not in the research
  - Determination of minimization of risk to greatest extent possible (subject safety is maximized)
  - Determination that the risks are reasonable in relation to the benefits and the importance of the knowledge gained from the research
- Benefit assessment: Identification of probable benefits from the research
- Adequate scientific design to answer the study objectives
- Assurance that the subjects will be provided an accurate description of the risks and benefits (informed consent document and methods are acceptable)
- Adequacy of privacy and confidentiality
- Adequate rationale for research procedures and statistical analysis
- Equitable subject selection
- Assessment of compensation and cost for research participants
- Assessment of recruitment strategies and approvals as needed (e.g., for advertisements)
- Confirmation that FDA-regulated research meets FDA guidelines
- Determination of appropriate safeguards for vulnerable populations when appropriate
- Determination of the intervals of review by the IRB and, when appropriate, whether there is adequate monitoring of the data (Amdur & Bankert, 2011; Institutional Review Boards, 2013; Protection of Human Subjects, 2009; Wichman, 2012).

Risk for Vulnerable Populations

Regulations for risk involving vulnerable populations limit research that bears more than minimal risk (see Table 16-2). The Belmont Report recommends special limitations for people who are mentally disabled and institutionalized. For these populations, risk would be determined in relation to risks normally encountered in daily life. In other words, is the population more sensitive or vulnerable because of their general condition or disability? This rule could apply to other populations (National Commission for the Protection of Human Subjects of Biomedical and Behavioral Research, 1979). For example, having people with asthma perform outdoor exercise when the air has a heavy pollen count may constitute a greater degree of risk even though this would usually be considered an activity of daily life.

Certificates of Confidentiality

For some types of research, the IRB may direct an investigator to obtain a certificate of confidentiality (CoC). These certificates are issued by NIH, as directed by the Secretary of DHHS under the Public Health Service Act, to institutions or universities where sensitive biomedical, behavioral, clinical, or other research (e.g., collecting genetic information, collecting information on psychological well-being of subjects, collecting information on subjects' sexual attitudes, preferences, or practices) occurs to protect the privacy of individuals who are participating in that research. The CoC helps protect the privacy of the research participant by protecting investigators and institutions from being compelled to release information that could be used to identify the research participants (NIH, 2011). More information about the CoC can be found on the NIH website (http://grants.nih.gov/grants/policy/coc/background.htm).

Special Considerations for Device Research

Although medical device research is less common in cancer, it does occur. The IRB should be aware of the

Table 16-2. Regulations for Vulnerable Populations		
	Regulations	
Population	**Office for Human Research Protections**	**U.S. Food and Drug Administration**
Pregnant women, human fetuses, and neonates	45 C.F.R. pt. 46, subpt. B	No specific regulations
Prisoners	45 C.F.R. pt. 46, subpt. C	No specific regulations
Children (general)	45 C.F.R. pt. 46, subpt. D	21 C.F.R. pt. 50, subpt. D
Children (specific)		
• No greater than minimal risk	45 C.F.R. § 46.404	21 C.F.R. § 50.51
• Greater than minimal risk but presenting the prospect of direct benefit to individual research participant	45 C.F.R. § 46.405	21 C.F.R. § 50.52
• Greater than minimal risk and no prospect of direct benefit to individual research participant but likely to yield generalizable knowledge about the participant's disorder or condition	45 C.F.R. § 46.406	21 C.F.R. § 50.53
• Clinical investigations not otherwise approvable that present an opportunity to understand, prevent, or alleviate a serious problem affecting the health or welfare of children	45 C.F.R. § 46.407	21 C.F.R. § 50.54

Note. Based on information from Protection of Human Subjects, 2009, 2013.

additional requirements for reviewing studies using medical devices. Before reviewing device research, the IRB must identify and evaluate the regulatory status of the device: Is the device exempt from investigational device exemption (IDE) regulations, or does the study qualify as a non–significant risk (NSR) device study or a significant risk (SR) device? An *SR device* is any one of the following (Investigational Device Exemptions, 2013; U.S. FDA, 2006).
- Device is intended as an implant and presents a potential for serious risk to the health, safety, or welfare of a subject.
- Device is purported or represented to be for a use in supporting or sustaining human life and presents a potential for serious risk to the health, safety, or welfare of a subject.
- Device is for a use of substantial importance in diagnosing, curing, mitigating, or treating disease, or otherwise preventing impairment of human health and presents a potential for serious risk to the health, safety, or welfare of a subject.
- Device otherwise presents a potential for serious risk to the health, safety, or welfare of a subject.

If the device is NSR and the IRB agrees, then the IRB may go on to review the research. However, if the IRB disagrees, and finds the study to be SR and there is no IDE assigned, it will provide the investigator and, if appropriate, the sponsor, with its finding. The sponsor is responsible for notifying the FDA of the IRB's SR determination. The IRB will not review the research until the sponsor provides written proof that either the FDA has granted an IDE or that the FDA disagrees with the IRB's determination (Investigational Device Exemptions, 2013; U.S. FDA, 2006).

Payment

Paying subjects to participate in research poses an ethical dilemma. IRBs need to determine if the payment is a reimbursement or an inducement. *Reimbursement* is designed to help offset some of the costs that the subject incurs during participation, whereas *inducement* motivates a person to participate in the research for financial gains (Amdur & Bankert, 2011). Although payment to patients participating in oncology studies is not always utilized, there are instances where the participants are either paid directly for completion of certain procedures (i.e., possible inducement) or may be given certain privileges at the site for their participation, such as receiving a small monetary stipend to cover expenses related to travel to the site, free lunches, or parking passes (i.e., reimbursement). The IRB should review both the amount of the payment and the proposed method of disbursement to ensure that coercion or undue influence does not exist. Coercion and undue influence fall under inducements. Unusually large payments should be reviewed by the IRB. Payments should reflect degree of risk or discomfort and subject inconvenience (Protection of Human Subjects, 2013; U.S. FDA, 2010). IRBs will have established standards that apply to their own community. Some IRBs may have a limit on the amount of subject payments. CTNs should be aware of the IRB's policies regarding payments prior to submission and should also be aware that the informed consent document must clearly define payments for subjects.

Informed Consent

No investigator may involve a human being as a subject in research unless the investigator has obtained informed consent from the subject or the subject's legally authorized representative in accordance with regulations. The IRB must examine the informed consent document to ensure that all required elements of consent are included. The text must be in a language understandable to the subject, including appropriate reading levels. There may not be any exculpatory language through which the subject or legally authorized representative is made to waive or appear to waive the subject's legal rights or releases or appears to release the investigator, the sponsor, the institution, or its agents from liability from negligence (Protection of Human Subjects, 2009, 2013). CTNs must be aware of the requirements for the informed consent process and the IRB procedures for review. Each IRB may have specific language that must be included in the consent document. Informed consent is covered in depth in Chapter 14.

Institutional Review Board Review Outcomes

The IRB has the authority to approve, require modifications in, or disapprove all research activities covered by the regulations (Institutional Review Boards, 2013; Protection of Human Subjects, 2009). As part of the review process, the IRB will require the following.
- Information is given to subjects as part of the informed consent process in accordance with the regulations.
- Additional information is given to the subject if it is in the IRB's judgment that it would aid in the protection of the rights of the subject.
- Documentation of the informed consent process is done in accordance with the regulations with allowable exceptions, for example, emergency research.
  The IRB must provide
- Written notification to the investigators and the institution of the decision to approve or disapprove the research or of any modifications required to gain IRB approval. If disapproval is the outcome of review, the IRB must supply reasons in writing to the investigators and allow opportunity for investigator response.
- Continuing review of the research at intervals appropriate to the degree of risk but not less than one year from date of original approval
- Documentation in writing to a sponsor of research involving an exception of informed consent that the information was publicly disclosed (e.g., emergency research). This disclosure must be prompt and the sponsor must then provide this documentation to the FDA.
- Documentation that the IRB has determined that the research involving children is in compliance with the regulations.

CTNs should be aware of the actions resulting from the IRB review. The IRB will take one of the following actions when reviewing a study (OHRP, 2010a).
- Approve the research study as submitted without any changes or with conditions, often referred to as *stipulations*.
- Require modifications to secure approval and defer or table the research study for further review after the modifications have been completed (sometimes referred to as *stipulations*).
- Disapprove the research study or proposed changes.

If stipulations exist, the IRB may either preclude the research from any activity or may allow the research to commence as soon as certain conditions are met. This is known as *conditional approval* or *approval with contingencies*. As soon as the conditions are met, the IRB may designate the IRB chairperson or other individual with appropriate expertise to review the revised materials and release IRB approval documents without reviewing again at a full board IRB meeting.

If the study is tabled or deferred, it needs to return to a convened IRB meeting for review. Reasons a study may be deferred include pending contract approval, FDA review, or the investigator being unable to provide sufficient answers to questions posed by the IRB members, in turn requiring additional queries to the sponsor.

CTNs may be directly involved in obtaining additional requested information to meet the conditions. This may be in the form of correcting an informed consent document or obtaining specific clarifications from a sponsor. CTNs should be familiar with the IRB SOPs regarding this process.

Review of Changes to the Original Protocol Document

During the course of the study, changes may be made to the protocol document for various reasons. These can be relatively minor, such as clarifying grammatical errors, or can be more significant, such as changes to doses of study agents. These changes may be called *amendments, revisions, updates,* or *modifications*. OHRP (45 C.F.R. § 46.103) and FDA (21 C.F.R. § 56.108) regulations require that institutions have written IRB procedures for ensuring prompt reporting of proposed changes in a research activity and for ensuring that such changes in approved research, during the period for which IRB approval has already been given, may not be initiated without IRB review and approval except when necessary to eliminate apparent immediate hazards to the subject (Institutional Review Boards, 2013; Protection of Human Subjects, 2009). Revisions are written by the principal investigator or designee and may result from findings at the study sites or as result of a monitoring visit. Depending on the significance of the change, the revision may undergo expedited review or receive full board review and approval. Each IRB has the authority to determine the type of review based on the institution's SOPs.

Any modifications need to be reviewed prior to IRB approval for possible changes to the informed consent form. CTNs and the principal investigator would be involved in this procedure. CTNs may be involved in modifying the informed consent form, gaining sponsor approval of the revised document, and then submitting it to the IRB for final review. CTNs may also be involved in notifying appropriate research staff members and patients of changes. Patients may be required to sign a new consent form if changes are significant per the IRB SOPs.

Continuing Review

Continuing review of research is conducted to allow the IRB to reassess the study, including if the risk-benefit assessment has not changed, or if it has, that appropriate measures have been taken. It is used to ensure that changes in the approved research were promptly reported to and approved by the IRB. Continuing review allows for suspension or termination of approval of research that is not being conducted in accordance with the IRB's requirements (OHRP, 2010b; U.S. FDA, 2012).

The continuing review reports should specifically include (OHRP, 2010b; U.S. FDA, 2012)
- Number of subjects enrolled, including gender, race, and ethnicity
- Brief summary of any amendments or changes that occurred during the review period
- New information (published or unpublished) that may alter the risk-benefit assessment
- Summary of unanticipated risks or problems and updated information regarding adverse events
- New information that may alter the willingness of the subject to participate
- Copy of current consent document to ensure all new or updated information has been added and the information is still accurate and complete
- Summary of any withdrawal of research subjects and reasons for withdrawal
- Any updated investigator brochure or other significant information related to subject risk
- Summary of review by the data and safety monitoring board if available or appropriate.

Continuing review may not be conducted using an expedited review procedure unless

- The study was eligible for and reviewed initially using an expedited review procedure
- The study has changed such that the only activities remaining are eligible for expedited review
- The study is closed to accrual and patients are followed only for toxicity and survival data.

Continuation of research after expiration of IRB approval is a violation of the regulations; there are no grace periods. If approval has expired, no new subjects may be enrolled in the study; however, an IRB may allow current participants to continue the trial while continuing renewal is sought. If the investigator is pursuing renewal and the IRB believes there are overriding safety concerns, the IRB can stop the research activities.

The investigator is ultimately responsible to make sure the study remains in compliance; however, the IRB may have systems in place to prompt annual renewal data (e.g., a form may be generated from an IRB database and sent to the investigator two to three months before the expiration date, which helps to avoid any lapse in approval). CTNs will need to be aware of the IRB SOPs regarding continuing review as he or she may be directly involved in collecting the necessary information to submit with the continuing review report, including providing tables of adverse events that have occurred since study origination.

CTNs must be aware of the IRB procedures regarding length of approval. Many institutions use an 11-month review process to ensure compliance with the regulation of review not less frequently than one year from the last approval. For example, a study approved in March would have its annual review performed in February of the following year. Special contingencies may exist for length of review based on the degree of risk of the research (e.g., phase I first-in-human or gene therapy studies may be reviewed at shorter intervals per IRB SOPs). FDA continuing review regulations do not provide specific instructions to IRBs on how to set up review processes within the framework of the regulations.

Another important concept for CTNs is the awareness of the IRB's policies on the end date of approval for items related to the study, including any items that may be deferred or tabled. For example, if there was an amendment midway during the approval period, CTNs would need to know if the overall end date of the research changes to the date of approval of the amendment or if the original approval end date still applies.

Other Reportable Events

Other events that need to be reported to the IRB (see Table 16-3) include deviations, unanticipated problems that are adverse events and non–adverse events (see Chapter 28), suspension or termination of the study, and any serious or continuing noncompliance with 45 C.F.R. pt. 46 or the requirements or determinations of the IRB

Table 16-3. Other Reportable Events to the Institutional Review Board

Event	Description
Deviation	A departure from the protocol-specific procedures • Major—protocol variance that makes the resulting data questionable; factors having significant impact on eligibility, treatment, or toxicity reporting • Minor—does not affect the outcome or interpretation of the study Report per IRB SOPs
Unanticipated problems	Any unanticipated problems involving risks to subjects or others Reviewed for continued risk assessment Report per IRB SOPs Discussed in detail in Chapter 28
Serious adverse events	Reviewed for continued risk assessment Report per IRB SOPs Discussed in detail in Chapter 28
Termination	May occur for a variety of reasons. • Study completion • Lack of compliance with continuing review Research activities should be stopped. Patients should be notified as applicable. Procedures for withdrawal of enrolled subjects should take into account the rights and welfare of the subjects. If follow-up of subjects for safety reasons is permitted or required by the IRB, the subjects should be informed and any adverse events reported to the IRB and the sponsor. Study documents must be archived per federal regulations and IRB SOPs.

IRB—institutional review board; SOP—standard operating procedure

Note. Based on information from Institutional Review Boards, 2013; Protection of Human Subjects, 2009.

(OHRP, 2010b). CTNs must be aware of the IRB SOPs on reportable events as the IRB may have additional requirements.

Institutional Review Board Records

As a requirement of 45 C.F.R. § 46.103(b)(4) and (5) and 21 C.F.R. pt. 56, subpt. D, the IRB must maintain adequate documentation of IRB activities. This includes
- Copies of all research proposals reviewed and any accompanying scientific reviews, informed consent documents, progress reports, and reports of injuries, serious adverse events, or unanticipated problems
- Minutes of IRB meetings with sufficient details to show attendance, voting results, summary of discussions, and outcome (see Table 16-1)
- Documentation of continuing review activities
- Copies of correspondence between the IRB and investigators
- List of IRB members identified by name with associated qualifications
- Written SOPs
- Statements of significant new findings reported to subjects.

Records must be kept for at least three years after the completion of the research. The records must be accessible to authorized representatives of OHRP and FDA (Institutional Review Boards, 2013; Protection of Human Subjects, 2009).

CTNs may be directly involved in record keeping (e.g., maintaining informed consent documents) and should be aware of all regulations.

Additional Institutional Review Board Oversight Requirements

Principal Investigator Qualifications

In order to fulfill responsibilities of 21 C.F.R. § 56.107(a), the IRB needs information about the qualifications of the investigators who will be conducting and supervising the research. FDA regulations place responsibility on the sponsor to select appropriate investigators, though the IRB does a have a role in reviewing the investigator's qualifications. Identifying a qualified investigator may be simple or may involve a detailed assessment (for example, if the IRB is currently familiar with the investigator versus an investigator who has never conducted research at the facility). The IRB may need to assess protocol-specific training and experience, especially if the research involves high-risk populations or novel therapies. The IRB may elect to observe the consent process and research if any concerns about investigator qualifications or experience are present. IRBs may check publicly available information about an investigator's inspectional history in addition to other assessments (U.S. FDA, 2013). CTNs should be aware of the necessary documentation the IRB requires regarding investigator qualifications. This information would be submitted with the initial application for review.

Site Qualifications

Before an IRB can approve a research project, the IRB must be able to verify the institutional commitments and regulations, applicable law, and standards of professional practice and conduct. The IRB, most likely, will be familiar with the institution's capabilities, so this assessment can be simple, or more formal, depending on requirements of the study (U.S. FDA, 2013). CTNs may be involved in gaining approvals from key departments affected by the research study. For example, if a study involves complicated lab procedures, a formal acceptance by the lab department may be needed to be submitted along with the IRB application. The IRB could request a description of the facility where the research will take place. For example, the institution may have multiple infusion rooms where therapy could be delivered. All sites would need to be listed. CTNs may assist in determining the operational issues involved with the study and helping to provide additional supporting documentation to the IRB.

Verification of Investigational New Drug Application or Investigational Device Exemption

FDA regulations require sponsors and investigators to determine the need for an IND. The IRB should ask the investigator about the need for an IND and ask to have supporting documentation. If there are any questions regarding the need for the IND, the IRB should follow SOPs for resolution (U.S. FDA, 2013).

An IDE allows an investigational device to be used in a clinical study in order to collect safety and effectiveness data. As with drugs and biologics and IND, sponsors are responsible for submission of an IDE application to FDA. Sponsors are responsible for making risk determination of the device and presenting it to IRB. If the IRB disagrees with risk determination, the IRB must inform the investigator and the sponsor, as appropriate (Protection of Human Subjects, 2013). CTNs should be familiar with these processes, as they may be involved in obtaining the appropriate documentation from the sponsor and investigators to include with IRB applications.

Accreditation of Human Subject Protection Programs

Support is increasing for independent evaluation for accreditation of organizations that conduct clinical research. As the IRB is one component of each site's human subject protection program, a research site may choose to become accredited by the Association for the Accreditation of Human Research Protection Programs or the Alion Human Research Protection Program Accreditation. Accreditation can apply to programs in the United States or international sites. The primary purpose of this accreditation is to strengthen protections for research participants. It fosters and advances the ethical and professional conduct of professionals and organizations that engage in research with human participants (Wichman, 2012). Applying for accreditation is the responsibility of the human subject protection office or administrator at the site; however, CTNs may be involved in gathering some of the information for the application or even be interviewed during the accreditation site visit.

Summary

Many steps are necessary for protocol review and approval as outlined in this chapter. A plethora of information is available to help understand and apply the regulations regarding protocol review. CTNs should be familiar with the pre-IRB reviews that may need to occur as well as the role and responsibilities of the IRB. It is important for CTNs to remember that the goals of the review processes and associated regulations are for the protection of research participants. CTNs are the connection between the process and the participants.

Key Points

- Understand the sequence of reviews necessary for protocol approval, including pre-IRB and IRB reviews.
- Be aware of the general functions and responsibilities of IRBs.
- Be familiar with the necessary forms (paper or electronic) needed for submission through the regulatory process, which are unique to the study site.
- Know the site key personnel, such as the IRB coordinator or administrator, IRB chairperson, signatory officials, and administrative department leaders as they are an integral component to the approval process.
- Be familiar with the IRB SOPs.
- Understand the CTN's role within the approval process as determined by the site procedures.
- The best resources are the regulations.
  – OHRP: www.hhs.gov/ohrp/humansubjects/index.html

- FDA: www.accessdata.fda.gov/scripts/cdrh/cfdocs/cfcfr/cfrsearch.cfm
- The endpoint of these review processes is to have an IRB-approved protocol and related documents (such as the informed consent form or advertisements).

References

Amdur, R., & Bankert, E.A. (2011). *Institutional review board member handbook* (3rd ed.). Burlington, MA: Jones & Bartlett Learning.

Definitions, 45 C.F.R. § 46.102(i) (2009). Retrieved from http://www.hhs.gov/ohrp/humansubjects/guidance/45cfr46.html#46.102

Institutional Review Boards, 21 C.F.R. pt. 56 (2013). Retrieved from http://www.accessdata.fda.gov/scripts/cdrh/cfdocs/cfcfr/CFRSearch.cfm?CFRPart=56&showFR=1&subpartNode=21:1.0.1.1.22.2

Investigational Device Exemptions, 21 C.F.R. pt. 812 (2013). Retrieved from http://www.accessdata.fda.gov/scripts/cdrh/cfdocs/cfcfr/CFRSearch.cfm?fr=812.3

Moon, M.R., & Khin-Maung-Gyi, F. (2009, April). The history and role of institutional review boards. *Virtual Mentor, 11,* 311–321. Retrieved from http://virtualmentor.ama-assn.org/2009/04/pfor1-0904.html

National Cancer Institute. (2012a, September 25). Policies and guidelines relating to the P30 Cancer Center Support Grant. Retrieved from http://cancercenters.cancer.gov/documents/CCSG_Guidelines.pdf

National Cancer Institute. (2012b, November). Scientific review. Retrieved from http://www.cancer.gov/clinicaltrials/learningabout/patientsafety/scientificreview

National Cancer Institute. (2014). *A handbook for clinical investigators conducting therapeutic clinical trials supported by CTEP, DCTD, NCI* [v.1.2]. Retrieved from http://ctep.cancer.gov/investigatorResources/docs/InvestigatorHandbook.pdf

National Commission for the Protection of Human Subjects of Biomedical and Behavioral Research. (1979, April 18). *The Belmont report: Ethical principles and guidelines for the protection of human subjects of research.* Retrieved from http://www.hhs.gov/ohrp/humansubjects/guidance/belmont.html

National Institutes of Health. (n.d.). Glossary and acronym list. Retrieved from http://grants.nih.gov/grants/glossary.htm

National Institutes of Health. (2011, January 20). Certificates of confidentiality: Background information. Retrieved from http://grants.nih.gov/grants/policy/coc/background.htm

National Institutes of Health Office of Biotechnology Activities. (2013a, April). Frequently asked questions (FAQs) of interest to IBCs. Retrieved from http://osp.od.nih.gov/sites/default/files/IBC_FAQs.pdf

National Institutes of Health Office of Biotechnology Activities. (2013b, April). Frequently asked questions: NIH guidelines for research involving recombinant or synthetic nucleic acid molecules. Retrieved from http://oba.od.nih.gov/oba/faqs/Synthetic_FAQs_April_2013.pdf

National Institutes of Health Office of Biotechnology Activities. (2013c, April). Frequently asked questions about the NIH Review process for human gene transfer trials. Retrieved from http://oba.od.nih.gov/oba/ibc/FAQs/NIH_Review_Process_HGT.pdf

National Institutes of Health Office of Biotechnology Activities. (2013d, November). NIH guidelines for research involving recombinant or synthetic nucleic acid molecules. Retrieved from http://osp.od.nih.gov/sites/default/files/NIH_Guidelines_0.pdf

Office for Human Research Protections. (n.d.-a). Institutional review boards (IRBs). Retrieved from http://www.hhs.gov/ohrp/assurances/irb/index.html

Office for Human Research Protections. (n.d.-b). Office for Human Research Protections (OHRP) database for registered IORGs and IRBs, approved FWAs, and documents received in last 60 days. Retrieved from http://ohrp.cit.nih.gov/search

Office for Human Research Protections. (n.d.-c). Status of IRBs and FWAs. Retrieved from http//www.hhs.gov/ohrp/assurances/status/index.html

Office for Human Research Protections. (2010a, September 1). Guidance on IRB approval of research with conditions. Retrieved from http://www.hhs.gov/ohrp/policy/conditionalapproval2010.html

Office for Human Research Protections. (2010b, November 10). Guidance on IRB continuing review of research. Retrieved from http://www.hhs.gov/ohrp/policy/continuingreview2010.html

Office for Human Research Protections. (2011a, March). Assurance process: Frequently asked questions. Retrieved from http://www.hhs.gov/ohrp/policy/assurancefaqsmar2011.pdf

Office for Human Research Protections. (2011b, March). IRB registration process: Frequently asked questions. Retrieved from http://www.hhs.gov/ohrp/policy/registrationfaqsjun2011.pdf

Office for Human Research Protections. (2013, March 28). When the assurance comes a "knocking": Everything you need to know about OHRP's FWA and IRB registration processes. Retrieved from http://www.hhs.gov/ohrp/education/training/ded_webinar.html

Protection of Human Subjects, 21 C.F.R. pt. 50 (2013). Retrieved from http://www.accessdata.fda.gov/scripts/cdrh/cfdocs/cfcfr/CFRSearch.cfm?CFRPart=50&showFR=1

Protection of Human Subjects, 45 C.F.R. pt. 46 (2009). Retrieved from http://www.hhs.gov/ohrp/humansubjects/guidance/45cfr46.html

Radioactive Drugs for Certain Research Uses, 21 C.F.R. § 361.1 (2013). Retrieved from http://www.accessdata.fda.gov/scripts/cdrh/cfdocs/cfcfr/CFRSearch.cfm?fr=361.1

Registration of Institutional Review Boards, 45 C.F.R. §§ 46.501–46.505 (2009). Retrieved from http://www.hhs.gov/ohrp/humansubjects/guidance/45cfr46.html

Trocky, N., & Ness, E. (2013). Institution and IRB registration. *Monitor, 27*(5), 49–52.

U.S. Food and Drug Administration. (2006, January). Information sheet guidance for IRBs, clinical investigators, and sponsors: Significant risk and nonsignificant risk medical device studies. Retrieved from http://www.fda.gov/downloads/RegulatoryInformation/Guidances/UCM126418.pdf

U.S. Food and Drug Administration. (2010, October). Payment to research subjects—Information sheet: Guidance for institutional review boards and clinical investigators. Retrieved from http://www.fda.gov/regulatoryinformation/guidances/ucm126429.htm

U.S. Food and Drug Administration. (2012, February). Guidance for IRBs, Clinical investigators, and sponsors IRB continuing review after clinical investigation approval. Retrieved from http://www.fda.gov/downloads/RegulatoryInformation/Guidances/UCM294558.pdf

U.S. Food and Drug Administration. (2013, August). Guidance for IRBs, clinical investigators, and sponsors—IRB responsibilities for reviewing the qualifications of investigators, adequacy of research sites, and the determination of whether an IND/IDE is needed. Retrieved from http://www.fda.gov/downloads/RegulatoryInformation/Guidances/UCM328855.pdf

Wichman, A. (2012). Institutional review boards. In J.I. Gallin & F.P. Ognibene (Eds.), *Principles and practice of clinical research* (3rd ed., pp. 225–242). Boston, MA: Elsevier Academic Press. doi:10.1016/B978-0-12-382167-6.00005-9

SECTION IV.

Financial Factors

Chapter 17

Workload Determination and Resource Allocation

Wendy Cooper, RN, BSN, OCN®, CCRP, and Clement K. Gwede, PhD, MPH, RN

Introduction

The clinical research management profession continues to grow. Over the past several years there has been an increase in published data with respect to prospective workload determination and resource allocation; however, little in the literature validates this work in a way that would make it translatable. For purposes of this discussion, a *clinical research coordinator* (CRC) or *clinical trial coordinator* is defined as a research professional who may or may not have a nursing background. As a result, research administrators and clinical trial coordinators have wrestled for a long time with key issues, such as
- Assignment of studies to CRCs
- Appropriate coordinator-to-study ratios
- Appropriate patient-to-coordinator ratios
- Determining the cost of doing clinical trial "work" (budgeting)
- Determining cost recovery (billing and collection)
- Determining the most efficient staff mix to maximize clinical trial productivity and cost-effectiveness.

Fundamental questions remain unanswered despite long-standing interest and progress in the topic in recent years. Many in the field continue to ponder very basic workload questions:
- How many clinical trial protocols can each coordinator handle (based on acuity)?
- How many patients can each coordinator handle?
- How many coordinators does it take?
- How busy is coordinator A versus coordinators B or C?
- At what point should a coordinator be provided with ancillary resources?
- Can some of the clinical trial work be shared or integrated into the standard of care clinic flow?

The universal answer to these questions is, "It depends." Recognizing that both clinical trial workload measurement and resource allocation are monumental and that volatile issues have plagued the profession for decades, this chapter takes an evolutionary look at the past decades toward development of solutions for these questions. The chapter highlights and summarizes selected aspects of these topics and chronicles the progress toward development of solutions for managing workload and resources in an ever-changing landscape. Both historical studies about the need for tools, as well as the most recent published literature regarding validated tools for workload determination and resource allocation, are reviewed. This synthesis will illustrate how the field is changing to close the gaps between the recognized work of the research team and the successful measures to document it.

Factors Affecting Workload Determination and Resource Allocation

Factors that affect workload determination and resource allocation include but are not limited to
- The diversity of research personnel (roles, qualifications, and training) and heterogeneity in the organization of clinical research services within and across research centers (Gwede, Johnson, & Daniels, 2001; Gwede, Johnson, & Trotti, 2000a, 2000b)
- The type (e.g., sponsor type, therapeutic versus nontherapeutic, clinical phase) and acuity or complexity of protocols involved (Briggs, 2008; Fowler & Thomas, 2003; Good, Lubejko, Humphries, & Medders, 2013; Gwede et al., 2000a, 2000b; James et al., 2011a, 2011b; Roche et al., 2002; Smuck et al., 2011)
- The actual time it takes to do the work (Fowell & Wilson, 2002; Fowler & Thomas, 2003; Good et al., 2013;

James et al., 2011a, 2011b; Roche et al., 2002; Smuck et al., 2011). The time and intensity of work increases as the protocol implementation phase moves from setup/planning to screening and enrollment, with the highest workload values expected during the treatment phase. Then the workload begins to slowly decline in follow-up and at off-study.
- Associated costs and rate of cost recovery (Chirikos, 2003; Emanuel, Schnipper, Kamin, Levinson, & Lichter, 2003; Johnson, 2003).

Thus, determining the workload and resources needed for clinical trial management can be a challenging task. The CRC provides cohesiveness that holds together the clinical trial process. As the total number of cancer cases is expected to double by 2050 if current incidence rates remain stable (Edwards et al., 2002), and given projections that by 2030 one in five Americans will be 65 years or older (Yancik, 1997; Yancik & Ries, 2004), increased representation of older adults in clinical trials is an important consideration for CRCs. More importantly, having adequate resources to coordinate their care in clinical trials is paramount.

Over the past decade, many models for managing clinical trials have been developed, including a variety of administrative and organizational structures (Good et al., 2013; Gwede et al., 2001; James et al., 2011a, 2011b; Smuck et al., 2011), as well as an evolving and increasingly delineated role for CRCs (Ehrenberger & Lillington, 2004). Specifically, numerous distinct clinical trial tasks have been identified, and the expansive scope of the work of CRCs is now better understood (Devine, Nagel, Benson, & Krailo, 2005; Good et al., 2013; Fowler & Thomas, 2003; Gwede et al., 2000a, 2000b; James et al., 2011a, 2011b; Roche et al., 2002; Smuck et al., 2011).

The work of CRCs involves wide-ranging responsibilities, including regulatory processing, contracts management, patient accrual and monitoring, collection and processing of research specimens, dispensing of study drugs, data collection and management, auditing, and billing. As a result, new CRC roles/positions, such as regulatory specialist, clinical trial nurse, data manager, specimen processing specialist, and clinical trial pharmacist, have emerged and are evolving in research centers.

A critical mix of multidisciplinary personnel now exists to cover the different facets and many responsibilities of CRCs. Yet, despite these developments, many CRCs remain burdened by the vast scope of work required of them, as they sometimes feel as though they have to "do it all." A natural question is whether some of the roles fall under the usual care pathway and could be completed by other members of the care team. Depending on the culture of the organization, this may be a daunting challenge. Nevertheless, mutually beneficial role delineation can be achieved collaboratively across various departments when the affected parties agree on the value of such an effort.

Promise of a Prospective Comprehensive Workload Tool

Is a comprehensive workload measurement tool already realized, or is it just a promise? Earlier studies sought a direct answer to this question (Fowler & Thomas, 2003; Gwede et al., 2000a, 2000b, 2001; Gwede, Johnson, Roberts, & Cantor, 2005; Roche et al., 2002) and proposed a number of approaches. The conclusion from these earlier studies was that a quantitative system for measuring workload was feasible, but the data were not ready for general use without careful adaptation. That is, the validity and general applicability of data in the various research settings had not been established. After a notable gap, recent studies have moved the field forward and produced workload measurement tools building on the components proposed by earlier authors (Good et al., 2013; James et al., 2011a, 2011b; Smuck et al., 2011). These studies have produced three plausible tools: OPAL (Ontario Protocol Assessment Level) (Smuck et al., 2011), RETA (Research Effort Tracking Assessment) (James et al., 2011a, 2011b), and WPAT (Wichita Protocol Assessment Tool) (Good et al., 2013). These three tools approach workload in similar but disparate ways (see Tables 17-1 and 17-2).

The University of Michigan Comprehensive Cancer Center Clinical Trials Office developed the RETA, a web-based tool to assess and allocate effort (James et al., 2011a, 2011b) based on the number of hours expended and accruals on therapeutic trials over a four-year period. The Wichita Community Clinical Oncology Program developed the WPAT, a protocol-specific, acuity-based tool that assigns acuity scores based on six trial-related tasks. The final score is derived by multiplying the protocol acuity score by the number of active patients per research nurse (Good et al., 2013).

The Ontario Institute for Cancer Research developed the OPAL system based on trial complexity attributable to trial tasks and the time needed to complete the tasks (Smuck et al., 2011). The OPAL and RETA tools are fundamentally driven by both protocol task complexity or time expended (acuity) and number of active patients. The WPAT, on the other hand, is largely driven by consideration of trial type (treatment or cancer control) and patient category (active treatment, off treatment, or off study) to derive workload scores for an individual coordinator. Although these new measures extend the field and provide objective measurement tools, there remains variability. An important methodologic contribution of the early studies (Fowler & Thomas, 2003; Gwede et al., 2000a, 2000b, 2001, 2005; Roche et al., 2002) is the shift of measures from only considering number of patients to identification of protocol complexity based on actual work tasks and estimation of time it takes to do specific protocol tasks. This critical and paradigm-shifting effort proved seminal and laid the seeds for very promising

Table 17-1. Selected Workload Studies in Clinical Trial Management

Author/Year	Purpose/Key Findings	Author Conclusions/Utility in Workload Management
Gwede et al., 2000a, 2000b	To report the number of patients enrolled by a typical clinical research coordinator (CRC) in a cooperative group and to identify factors associated with this measure of workload. Self-reported workload (number of patients) varied widely by CRC and type of study. Focusing on the work tasks is perhaps a better measure of workload than number of patients. No definitive workload formula was provided or recommended.	In the absence of reliable, valid, and universally accepted clinical trial workload measures, administrators must take a broader approach and focus on the time required to do tasks rather than the number of patients.
Gwede et al., 2001	To document the structure and organization of clinical research services and to evaluate the impact on the workload of CRCs. Organization of clinical research services may account for efficiencies and productivity. Three primary data management models (centralized, decentralized, and mixed) were identified, and workload (number of patients) varied by data management model.	Within each of the three primary data management models, the challenges and determinants of workload vary. The data management model provides an all-important context and environmental milieu in which workload and resource utilization dynamics occur.
Roche et al., 2002	To measure time required to complete specific protocol tasks and identify factors associated with task times. Early-phase trials had longer task times than phase III trials, and industry-sponsored trials had longer task times than local or cooperative group studies. Task times were identified, but no definitive workload formula was provided or recommended.	The study showed the importance of consideration of sponsor type and study phase in estimating costs, workload, and resource allocation. A close examination of the time required for individual tasks may influence daily decisions about workload distribution among CRCs. Further research is needed to improve accuracy of time estimates.
Fowler & Thomas, 2003	To quantify protocol acuity and task times (workload threshold) based on actual coordinator time and activities in order to guide prospective staffing and budgetary decisions. Task times and acuity score were identified.	Each research center has to determine the acuity load for each coordinator or protocol. The preliminary tool presented here may be refined or adapted for other centers to generate a numbers-driven workload measurement system.
Devine et al., 2005	To determine what percentage of time CRCs spend on different work tasks. Results indicated that focusing on trial tasks rather than on enrollment numbers is the best approach. No definitive workload formula was provided or recommended.	For daily management, CRCs may be assigned based on appreciation of the tasks and percent effort required. This study informs role delineation to reduce scope of work.
Smuck et al., 2011	To develop a clinical trial complexity rating scale and workload measurement tool. The OPAL (Ontario Protocol Assessment Level) scoring system quantifies workload based on study protocol complexity and number of active cases. The OPAL system is recommended as an objective staffing tool among Ontario cancer centers.	The OPAL provides clinical trial departments with an objective method to quantify workload on the basis of protocol complexity and number accrued or active cases. The OPAL represents a *trial workload* score. The trial workload is in turn multiplied by the number of cases on the trial to yield a *case workload* score. *Total workload* for a coordinator is the sum of trial workload plus the case workload. The OPAL scoring system is being implemented and evaluated in Ontario among cancer research sites.
James et al., 2011a, 2011b	To develop and implement an effort tracking web-based application to quantify data management and regulatory workload. The RETA (Research Effort Tracking Application) was developed based on four key factors that influenced workload—accrual rate, accrual volume, sponsor type, and enrollment status. Task times are tracked per protocol. The RETA was successfully implemented in the Clinical Trials Office at University of Michigan Comprehensive Cancer Center.	The RETA provides an objective tool for data management and regulatory workload measurement to inform staffing decisions. It is used to inform budget negotiations and study-related expenses. Further refinement is underway at University of Michigan Comprehensive Cancer Center.

(Continued on next page)

Table 17-1. Selected Workload Studies in Clinical Trial Management *(Continued)*		
Author/Year	Purpose/Key Findings	Author Conclusions/Utility in Workload Management
Good et al., 2013	To develop an acuity-based workload measurement tool to guide staffing decisions in a community clinical oncology program. The Wichita Clinical Oncology Program successfully developed and tested an acuity-based system guided by points assigned by trial type (treatment or cancer control) and by patient category (active treatment, off treatment, or off study). The WPAT (Wichita Protocol Acuity Tool) has been implemented at a single institution.	The WPAT measures workload at the patient level. This acuity score is intended to estimate the workload of an individual coordinator. Its best utility is to measure trial workload and inform decisions about when a single coordinator needs workload adjustments. Its prospective application to estimate workload before a trial is opened has not been evaluated. The WPAT has not been fully evaluated for other stages of protocol management (e.g., regulatory, screening, enrollment) and has only been tested in one institution. Further evaluation is needed.

measures now realized: OPAL, RETA, WPAT, and others. Figure 17-1 summarizes the core work tasks identified in this literature.

Within these general or core work categories exist numerous time-intensive subtasks to be completed, which constitute an important part of the *actual* workload of CRCs. Although crude measures such as number of patients or number of protocols managed by a CRC are important and commonly recognized outcomes, they are not entirely accurate or direct measures of workload. The actual work should be measured. Nevertheless, these tools are, in essence, good *measures of productivity*, and should be considered in the context of the time and resources needed to produce those outcomes. Widely validated and reliable estimates of the time and resources required to perform the broad protocol-directed tasks, and the many distinct subtasks, are still needed.

Hence, a single universal specific "magic" number, metric, or formula is not provided in this chapter. Instead, readers can make their own assessment of the published data and adopt or adapt a selected metric for use in their own clinical setting (Fowler & Thomas, 2003; Good et al., 2013; Gwede et al., 2000a, 2000b, 2001, 2005; James et al., 2011a, 2011b; Roche et al., 2002; Smuck et al., 2011). Table 17-2 summarizes key elements of published time-, task-, and accrual-based metrics and identifies three quantitative workload components: protocol acuity score, task times, and number of patients managed (Fowler & Thomas, 2003; Good et al., 2013; James et al., 2011a, 2011b; Roche et al., 2002; Smuck et al., 2011).

The implications of reliable protocol task time estimates are clear. As a new protocol is developed locally or received from an external sponsor, it is possible to outline the tasks involved in the specific protocol, estimate the time and costs, and budget for the appropriate level of resources (see Chapter 18). In principle, prospective cost estimating and resource planning is ideal, but practical challenges in funding, hiring, training, and retention of experienced research personnel still remain. When trained CRCs are not available for hiring, the workload will continue to increase. Limited personnel still are expected to manage the work and to meet compliance and quality standards. Moreover, patient accrual and budget projections may not be accurate, and an overestimation or underestimation of either or both elements will result in undesirable workload and resource imbalances. Thus, qualitative approaches for day-to-day management of workload burden will remain a meaningful alternative until a robust quantitative workload measure is available. As the clinical research management arena continues to experience greater role delineation with increased separation of budgetary, regulatory, and trial and data management roles, the workload measurement methodologies predicated on complexity of task and time expended on tasks are plausible universal approaches for workload assessment. The global nature of this issue is now evident in Europe, particularly with the efforts of the European Organisation for Research and Treatment of Cancer. The results are promising (Berridge & Coffey, 2008; Coffey, Lyddiardc, Briggs, & Berridge, 2010).

Key Lessons Learned About Workload Measurement

Many lessons about clinical trial workload determination have been documented elsewhere (Fowler & Thomas, 2003; Good et al., 2013; Gwede et al., 2000a, 2000b; James et al., 2011a, 2011b; Neuer, 2002; Smuck et al., 2011). Three lessons that are most relevant as background for resource planning and allocation are summarized here.

- The workload of CRCs continues to increase despite greater role delineation in the field.
- Measuring protocol complexity and the actual work tasks (task times), rather than only the number of patients or protocols managed by a CRC, seems to be the better approach. The intensity and scope of work is a product of protocol-related acuity (complexity of tasks) *and* the number of patients managed.

- One size does not fit all. A customized approach that takes the local realities into consideration is needed at different centers or clinical research sites.

First, the workload of CRCs, as determined by crude measures such as the number of clinical trials or the number of patients actively managed by a single CRC, is increasing annually (Fowler & Thomas, 2003; Good et al., 2013; Gwede et al., 2000a, 2000b; James et al., 2011a, 2011b; Neuer, 2002; Smuck et al., 2011). Reasons for this include increasing costs of conducting clinical research, a growing trend in health care to do more work with fewer resources, and the growing recognition that more

Measure/Tool	Possible Final Outcome Product	Possible Utility in Workload Management
Protocol acuity score Task time estimates (Fowler & Thomas, 2003)	Protocol acuity score Hours per task/patient/protocol/coordinator	Prospective uses: • Budgeting • Comparison of individual studies or coordinators • Staff assignments Conclusions: • Is a preliminary measure • May be adapted for individual research centers
Protocol task time estimates (Roche et al., 2002)	Hours per task/patient/protocol/coordinator	Prospective uses: • Budgeting • Comparison of individual studies or coordinators • Staff assignments • Staff role delineation Conclusions: • Is a preliminary measure • Underestimates task times • Needs further development to better and more accurately capture the true scope of work • Not yet ready for dissemination or wide application
OPAL (Ontario Protocol Assessment Level) score Complexity of protocol-specific tasks Number of active cases (Smuck et al., 2011)	Protocol complexity score × Number of active cases	Proposed uses: • Estimating number of protocols and cases per staff • Estimating total workload per staff • Estimating workload distribution among staff • Determining reallocation of staff or resources Conclusions: • A useful objective and consistent tool • Further evaluation underway to evaluate broader applicability
RETA (Research Effort Tracking Assessment) tool Protocol complexity rating Task times (James et al., 2011a, 2011b)	RETA produces a score based on • Rating in four categories (accrual rate, size of accrual, sponsor type, study enrollment status) • Time it takes for data management or regulatory tasks.	Proposed uses: • Data management • Regulatory workload estimation • Protocol budgeting • Budget negotiations Conclusions: • Positive impact in workload measurement, budget processes, and related decision making • Further refinement anticipated but has potential generalizability and implications for clinical research operations at other centers
WPAT (Wichita Protocol Assessment Tool) Protocol acuity score Number of patients (Good et al., 2013)	WPAT is based on two components. Individual coordinator workload is calculated by multiplying protocol acuity score by number of patients per specific trial.	Proposed uses: • Monitoring of individual research coordinator workload • Staffing level projections and adjustment Conclusions: • Research nurse group average acuity score of 35.0–40.0 generally validated the need to consider an increase in staff. • Supported by 15 years (since 1999) of workload assessment data • Used by only one research program

Table 17-2. Empirically Developed Task-Based Workload Measures

Figure 17-1. Core Work Tasks of Clinical Research Coordinators

- Initial and continuing institutional review board regulatory processing
- Contracting, budgeting, and billing
- Patient eligibility screening, workup, and enrollment
- Patient monitoring during active treatment and follow-up
- Study drug dispensing and accountability
- Research lab specimen processing
- Data collection/management and case report completion
- Administrative and other coordination activities
- Audit preparation and clarification of data

Note. Based on information from Fowler & Thomas, 2003; Good et al., 2013; Gwede et al., 2000a, 2000b, 2001, 2005; James et al., 2011a, 2011b; Roche et al., 2002; Smuck et al., 2011.

patient participation in clinical trials improves quality of care. Many healthcare organizations seek to increase the number of patients participating in clinical trials (Good et al., 2013; James et al., 2011a, 2011b; Smuck et al., 2011; West, Wright, Tuffnell, Jankowicz, & West, 2005).

Given the increasing responsibilities of CRCs and the decreasing time allotted to complete them, mounting professional and social pressure creates a burden on CRCs. One study demonstrated that some CRCs experience employment-related distress and burnout (Gwede et al., 2005). Such distress may lead to coordinator turnover and loss of experienced personnel (Fowler & Thomas, 2003; Gwede et al., 2000a, 2000b; Neuer, 2002). Studies have found that the majority of CRCs have been in their current positions for less than three to five years (Gwede et al., 2000a, 2000b; Neuer, 2002). One analysis of CRCs (N = 500) found that 56% had been in their current positions for less than three years in 2002, compared to 40% in 1999 (Neuer, 2002). Although this change may reflect increased growth in the profession as well as staff turnover (Fowler & Thomas, 2003; Gwede et al., 2000a, 2000b; Neuer, 2002), it also demonstrates that the overall experience level of CRCs is declining. Consequently, the retention and training of clinical research staff is a paramount effort at investigative sites, and accurate determinations of workload with subsequent assignment of resources remain important priorities for the clinical research administrator.

Regarding how much workload one CRC can handle, the measurement of CRC workload does not entail measuring merely the number of patients or protocols managed (Devine et al., 2005; Fowler & Thomas, 2003; Gwede et al., 2000a, 2000b; Roche et al., 2002). Rather, it is best to identify specific work tasks and determine how much time it takes to complete them. Once the tasks and times have been delineated, the relevant costs and resources can be estimated and assigned (Devine et al., 2005; Fowler & Thomas, 2003; Good et al., 2013; Gwede et al., 2000a, 2000b; James et al., 2011a, 2011b; Roche et al., 2002; Smuck et al., 2011). Five studies have addressed this issue directly (Fowler & Thomas, 2003; Good et al., 2013; James et al., 2011a, 2011b; Roche et al., 2002; Smuck et al., 2011), but the findings are preliminary (see Tables 17-1 and 17-2) and have not been widely and rigorously evaluated in clinical research organization settings.

With regard to quantitative, objective workload measurement and determination, Tables 17-1 and 17-2 summarize selected chronologic studies aimed at addressing the clinical trial workload measurement gap with promising results (Good et al., 2013; James et al., 2011a, 2011b; Smuck et al., 2011). Workload determination and resource allocation are cornerstone issues in defining a profession. They are directly related to productivity, quality, and satisfaction—all important values for patients, CRCs, employers and managers, and study sponsors who have a financial stake in successful clinical trial management.

The third lesson is that one size does not fit all. It is not clear to what extent a system developed in one research center may be applicable (or adaptable) for use in other settings where research operations (i.e., organization, structure, culture) and resources differ significantly. For example, can a protocol acuity system developed for a cardiology practice also work in an oncology setting? Or, is a measurement system developed in a cancer center readily translatable to community clinical oncology program settings? What adaptations are required to refine and validate the system across disciplines (e.g., adult oncology, pediatric oncology)? Until the profession matures and a consensus is reached regarding uniform standards in role delineation, organization of clinical research operations, employment practices, and professional training, a need for customized approaches remains. Other qualitative solutions to match the structure and culture of each organization are needed. Administrators are faced with the challenge of how to create a sensible local solution that takes into account the many variables and realities of each center.

For example, staff mix and role delineation, type and phase of clinical trial protocols (i.e., industry-sponsored, cooperative group, or locally authored trials), organization of the clinical research operations, and the institutional culture and mindset about clinical research participation on the part of investigators and treating physicians vary widely among centers across the United States. These factors are important influences on both productivity and workload-related distress for CRCs (Fowler & Thomas, 2003; Good et al., 2013; Gwede et al., 2000a, 2000b, 2001, 2005; James et al., 2011a, 2011b; Roche et al., 2002; Smuck et al., 2011).

When a coordinator senses that his or her workload is increasing, few validated and widely accepted objective tools are available to help to quantify the workload and provide justification for additional resources. Much like other professions, such as nursing, where workload and acuity measures and resource allocation systems continue to evolve and attract scrutiny, workload systems for clinical research will see much contention and refinement (Jones, Cusack, & Chisholm, 2004; Rozich & Resar, 2002; Van Slyck, 1995; Walts & Kapadia, 1996). Even if a purely quantitative universal measure is not imminent, a practical, functional workload measurement approach that facilitates daily staffing decisions is now conceivable based on the growing body of work.

These are indeed exciting times in the field of clinical trial workload measurement. Recent progress has occurred in the development and successful testing of at least three elegant workload tools (Good et al., 2013; James et al., 2011a, 2011b; Smuck et al., 2011). The most promising aspect of these tools is their comprehensiveness because they move beyond the single dimension of tallying just the number of patients accrued or managed. The recent tools have answered an earlier call for task complexity and time-focused measures (Gwede et al., 2000a, 2000b, 2001; Roche et al., 2002). Several challenges remain even as we begin to see light at the end of the tunnel. Specific challenges include

- The need for further testing to evaluate generalizability of such tools beyond a single center or homogenous setting
- Head-to-head comparisons of these metrics with the goal of either determining comparative effectiveness or to develop consensus on a uniform and universal measure.

Because the field is still in its infancy, these laudable ideas may remain lofty goals, and incremental progress is expected over the next decade. Nevertheless, the discourse on clinical research workload measurement has shifted from conceptualization and debate to tangible and highly promising workload measurement products. Thus, the authors of this chapter ask the next natural question: Will clinical research operations programs begin testing the available tools in their own local environments and disseminate (publish) their experiences in an effort to contribute to and increase the evidence base?

Protocol-Directed Resource Planning

Several key variables must be considered when determining resource allocation. Variables such as the phase of the trial, type of protocol (therapeutic versus nontherapeutic), complexity of the trial, study sponsor (industry, government, or other), the type and stage of disease being studied, protocol implementation stage (planning, enrollment, treatment, follow-up), and anticipated personnel needs (qualifications, training, and expertise) all must be evaluated before beginning the process of determining and allocating resources. Other less obvious factors beyond these, such as patient quality-of-life issues, life expectancy, ethical values, and online data entry versus paper data collection via case report forms, also must be considered.

Depending on the institution that is planning to conduct the trial, resource allocation is presented to evoke ideas, lend suggestions, and provide a possible template for determining resource allocation in various clinical research settings. The key to this effort is recognizing the positive impact that protocol task–directed resource planning and allocation has in an institution's capacity when an appropriate workload and resource analysis is completed before protocol implementation.

The process begins by formulating questions addressing the "who, what, when, and why" of performing the resource analysis and allocation. A thorough analysis of specific protocol tasks and appropriate knowledge of the institutional resources to be used are required before accurate protocol task–based costs are determined. Outlining the steps and procedures a patient would go through to complete the protocol is a natural way to break down the protocol into smaller tasks (see Figure 17-2). In addition, a thorough analysis allows for evaluation of the specific tasks to see if they meet institutional standards or whether exceptions from the normal process and flow will have to be incorporated to accomplish protocol-specific tasks. Exceptions from the normal pro-

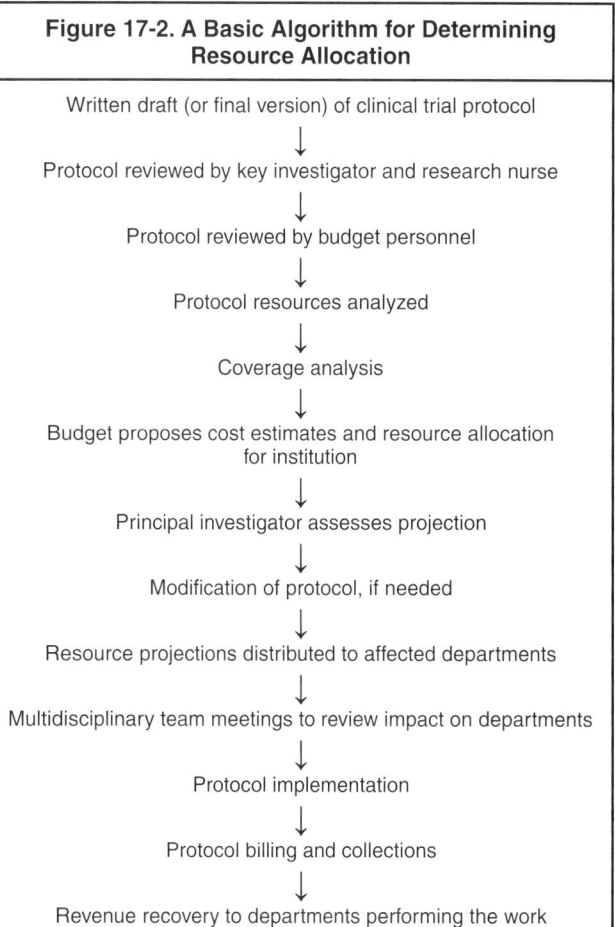

Figure 17-2. A Basic Algorithm for Determining Resource Allocation

Written draft (or final version) of clinical trial protocol
↓
Protocol reviewed by key investigator and research nurse
↓
Protocol reviewed by budget personnel
↓
Protocol resources analyzed
↓
Coverage analysis
↓
Budget proposes cost estimates and resource allocation for institution
↓
Principal investigator assesses projection
↓
Modification of protocol, if needed
↓
Resource projections distributed to affected departments
↓
Multidisciplinary team meetings to review impact on departments
↓
Protocol implementation
↓
Protocol billing and collections
↓
Revenue recovery to departments performing the work

cess and flow usually translate into increased research staff effort. This illustrates the need to integrate the flow of the research patient into the normal clinic flow so that the research work is not a distinct and separate workflow. Caution should be taken to not sequester information related to clinical trials into a database to which only selected personnel have access, as this limits resources and can create a duplication of effort in documenting the research process.

Identifying distinct subtasks creates a timeline of the life of the protocol. A picture of the scope of work is created when individual quantifiable events and their frequency and duration of occurrence are listed. This timeline can be divided into manageable segments of time, such as days, cycles, or admissions. Within a defined time frame, resources can be broken down by the department (or person) who will provide a specific service. This process culminates in a protocol budget and resource plan that will guide implementation of the project (Johnson, 2003). A protocol-based timeline or plan of work can be used to enhance the multidisciplinary approach to implementing a new clinical trial. Figure 17-3 lists questions to ask when designing a timeline. One should also consider the design of the trial and the anticipated rate of accrual when considering resource allocation. Many newer adaptive trial designs move through patient accrual at an accelerated rate but are totally dependent on real-time data entry, which can strain resources if not proactively planned.

Many clinical research centers have collected data, over varying time periods, related to research tasks and task/protocol complexity in an attempt to measure workload and, in so doing, allocate resources (Briggs, 2008; Good et al., 2013; James et al., 2011a, 2011b; Smuck et al., 2011). Validation of these tools is limited, and therefore, additional work is needed to add to the foundation of information now being created.

Graphics Used for Resource Planning and Allocation

Computer-generated graphics, formulas, or algorithms may be used to plot resource information. A flow chart or grid is an example of a graphic (see Figure 17-4). To facilitate implementation, financial billing, and collection, the activities are divided into sections of who provided the service, thus allowing the service provider to see at a glance what services are expected from each department and to guide a plan for cost recovery when collections are received. An example of this is the planned visit report that can be generated from the clinical trial tracking database called OnCore (the Online Collaborative Research Environment). In this database, calendars are created for each protocol. Each patient is then assigned to a study-specific calendar that preplans study visits for the individual patient. Each planned visit can later be marked as "occurred" or "missed," which in turns allows the finance department to bill for the activity.

Another example of a visual resource allocation graphic is the protocol planning map (see Figure 17-5). The planning map is an excellent tool to help departments visualize when their services are required. The protocol map can be several pages in length and depicts all of the costs that will be incurred, as well as costs related to unplanned events. The map's timeline starts at the beginning of the protocol and proceeds through long-term follow-up and the patient's discharge from the protocol (as applicable). The principal investigator and the research administrator or CRC are responsible for confirming that the map is an accurate reflection of the proposed protocol and associated work.

After the timeline is established for one patient to receive the full treatment of the protocol and estimates have been made for the number of patients who will go through each phase of the protocol, the next step is to develop a *master timeline*. A master timeline plots each participant's usage of critical, limiting threshold resources, such as specialized care areas, over time. How patients are accrued onto a protocol often will determine if certain resources will be overtaxed (see Figure 17-6).

Threshold resources guide the determination of what resources must be added to successfully implement the protocol as planned. It is important not to undercut this process by imposing unrealistic estimates. For example,

---

Figure 17-3. Questions to Ask When Designing a Timeline

- Does the protocol contain a table of assessments listing activities to be performed?
- Is there information to help understand how a patient goes through the entire protocol?
- Will the information be used as part of a recruitment tool that can be shown to referring physicians or prospective patients so that they can readily understand what the protocol will entail?
- Can this information be used to prospectively plan for resources to be put in place for a patient to successfully complete the protocol?
- Will a cost estimate be generated? If so, how will it be used?
  - Will it be used to create a budget for the protocol?
  - Will it be used as part of the analysis in determining whether the protocol is approved to be implemented?
- Will this information provide a sense of protocol intensity or extent of time required to implement?
- What additional information is needed (e.g., case report forms, lab manual, pharmacy manual) to make an assessment of workload and to complete cost estimates?
- Is the additional information forthcoming? Can the protocol be approved for implementation without this additional information?
- Is the method used to derive costs appropriate, adequate, and balanced for all involved?

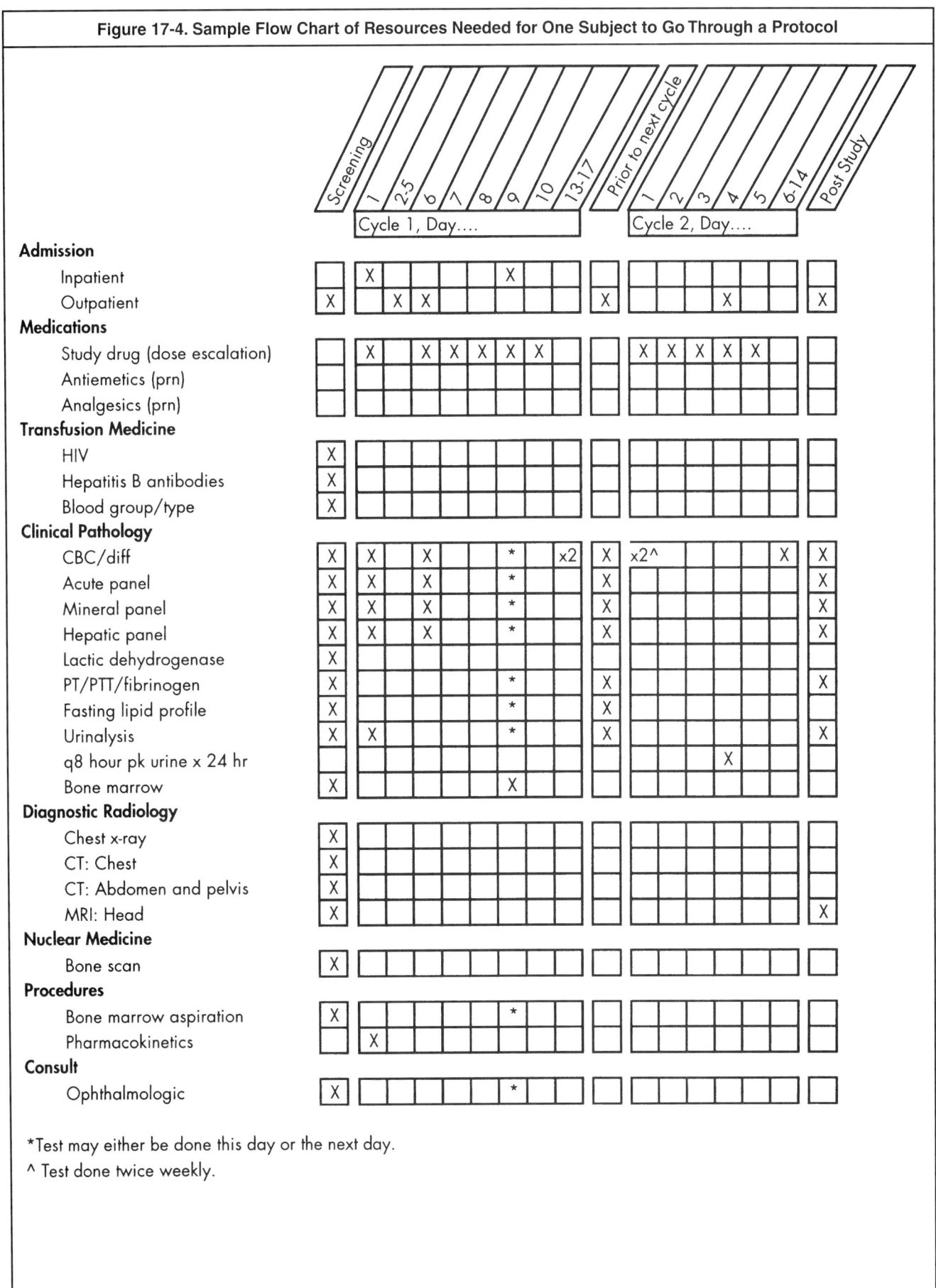

Figure 17-4. Sample Flow Chart of Resources Needed for One Subject to Go Through a Protocol

*Test may either be done this day or the next day.
^ Test done twice weekly.

__	__	__	__
<td colspan="4" align="center">**Figure 17-5. Sample Protocol Planning Map**</td>
<td colspan="4">Protocol Planning Map (Date) (For example, questions one would ask to complete map) Name of Protocol: Treatment of cancer Principal Investigator (PI): Dr. Smith   Branch: Medical Oncology Max N: 50 patients (entire study)   N (projected): 40   N (for first year): 15 Sign-off by PI: Electronic sign-off Clinical Research Coordinator: Ma Jones, RN, Phone #/Beeper #: 104-104-7</td>
Date	**Screening**	**Cycle 1**	**Post–Cycle 1 Follow-Up Visit**
Site	**Oncology Clinic**	**Inpatient Unit**	**Oncology Clinic**
Assessment and interventions	Eligibility requirements Life expectancy Karnofsky Performance Status Past medical history and treatment	Care requirements for staff Frequent vital signs or monitoring Special bed or equipment needs	Care requirements for staff Frequent vital signs or monitoring
Medications	List patient's medications. Will patient use his own supply or hospital's? Who is supplying treatment for protocol? Hospital pharmacy, drug company, grant-sponsored?	Chemotherapy Immunotherapy treatment of side effects (e.g., nausea and vomiting, diarrhea, headache, fatigue, neutropenia) Radiation therapy Wound care Mouth care	Chemotherapy Immunotherapy treatment of side effects (e.g., nausea and vomiting, diarrhea, headache, fatigue, neutropenia) Radiation therapy
Labs	Eligibility labs Tumor markers HIV Hepatitis profile 24-hour urine Pregnancy tests Type and cross Protocol research labs required	Pharmacokinetics: peripheral or venous access device Daily labs: phlebotomy or RN draw Urine specimen collection Transportation of specimens	Pharmacokinetics: peripheral or venous access device Daily labs: phlebotomy or RN draw Urine specimen collection Transportation of specimens
Diagnostic tests	Chest x-ray Electrocardiogram Multigated acquisition scan Computed tomography scans Magnetic resonance imaging Ultrasound Radiation simulation for treatment	Treatment of side effects Chest x-ray after line placement Restaging scans Follow-up scans	Treatment of side effects Restaging scans Follow-up scans
Consults	Surgery for line placement Biopsies needed for study or diagnosis Dental work before bone marrow transplant Vision or hearing tests Pain team consult Anesthesiology Radiation therapy Pathology labs Apheresis/department of transfusion medicine Neurology Anticipated intensive care unit admission	Blood product transfusions Pharmacy Nurse practitioner On-call physician Outpatient cancer center for follow-up	Long-term follow-up issues Pain control Surgery for future biopsies
Teaching	Informed consent and education about the protocol Treatment schema Admission procedure	Management of side effects Colony-stimulating factor injections Blood product transfusions Inpatient and outpatient procedures	Follow-up issues Management of long-term side effects
Miscellaneous	Bed space issues Sedation of patients Transportation issues Family support Social work issues Third-party reimbursement issues	Dietary issues Staffing issues 1:1 patient care Frequent pharmacokinetics Emotional support Advance directives	Fear of recurrence, emotional support issues Transportation Insurance coverage issues

														Figure 17-6. Sample Master Timeline for a Protocol													

Effect of Limited Resources on Rate of Patient Accrual Onto a Protocol
Example: One research magnetic resonance imaging (MRI) test space per week

													Week													
Patient	1	2	3	4	5	6	7	8	9	10	11	12	13	14	15	16	17	18	19	20	21	22	23	24	25	26
A	x									x																
B		x									x															
C			x									x														
D				x									x													
E					x									x												
F						x									x											
G							x									x										
H								x									x									
I																		x							x	
J																			x							x

Notes/Assumptions: Each patient needs baseline research MRI immediately prior to initiation of protocol therapy and a post-treatment MRI nine weeks later. In this example, the research team has only one opening for a research MRI per week. Patients I and J must wait until weeks 17 and 18 to begin the protocol.

some investigators may want to implement the protocol for academic gain and will waive investigator fees in order to meet a sponsor's arbitrary or predetermined funding level. Although such a practice may achieve important goodwill with sponsors, it may lead to poor project performance when resources are inadequate. The potential negative implications are far-reaching.

Of course, unexpected events do occur. Patients may develop complications related to their disease or to the interventions. It may be helpful to create and compare several timelines regarding a critical resource, with one indicating the worst-case scenario and the other demonstrating a timeline that goes according to the planned protocol. It can prove very valuable to do an early analysis of anticipated effort versus actual expenditure of effort after the first three to five patients are accrued. This allows the opportunity to reorganize the work, or renegotiate the budget, if there is a great discrepancy.

Once a listing of resources has been determined, the next step is to establish who will provide each service and whether the service provider has the resources to accommodate the request. Looking at these resources very early in the implementation process is important in order to optimally engage all stakeholders. For planning purposes, rewriting the list of resources and grouping them by service provider can be helpful. The service provider then can be notified of the requested resources, and provisions can be made to have the necessary resources available when the patient arrives. This communication process is a key factor in smooth and accurate implementation of the protocol, especially with issues of limited availability of resources. For example, what if it takes three weeks to get a computed tomography scan appointment and the protocol timeline requires an appointment in a week?

After a resource allocation proposal is designed, a cost estimate can be generated per task, per protocol interval, per patient, and for the entire protocol. Both direct and indirect costs must be included in the protocol budget. Direct costs will be identified as activity and resource allocation lists are generated and prepared. Indirect costs may include fees for the initiation of the trial, administrative costs, data management, institutional review board submissions, publicity and advertisements, pharmacy charges, and long-term follow-up (see Chapter 18). Many institutions have a preset percentage of total costs for indirect costs, and the percentages may vary based on the funding source (pharmaceutical company funding versus grant funding). These fees may be charged to the study sponsor above the cost of the direct patient services.

The complexity of this process requires the use of a clinical trial management software system to set up, track, and manage the process. Consequently, a host of homegrown and commercially developed software programs have emerged to address the need. Table 17-3 provides a limited list of software programs and data-

Table 17-3. Examples of Software Programs/Databases for Tracking Clinical Trial Activity and Metrics

Program/Database	Launch Date/ Current Version	Key Features	Developer Description
OnCore (Online Collaborative Research Environment) Electronic Patient Record Management System http://forteresearch.com/enterprise-research-oncore	Launched: 2002 Current version: 12.0	Electronic data capture Status and timeline tracking of protocol Individual subject tracking Financial console Business service management console	OnCore is an on-premise, eClinical solution for the clinical research enterprise that fully integrates clinical trial management system (CTMS), electronic data capture, data management, billing compliance, biospecimen management, and patient registry management functionality. The system has been developed to specifically address the needs of mid-sized to large research hospitals, cancer centers, academic medical centers, and staff working under the Clinical and Translational Science Award grant.
Allegro CTMS http://forteresearch.com/ctms-allegro	Launched: 2011	Management of study start-up and study conduct Subject tracking Financial tracking Multisite functionality	Allegro is a cloud-based CTMS that helps manage study start-up, study conduct, subject visits, budgets, and financials. Allegro CTMS@Site is designed for investigator sites and research groups. Allegro CTMS@Network is designed for multisite networks, contract research organizations, and site management organizations.
Velos http://velos.com	Launched: 1996 Current version: 9.1	Integrated modules that track administrative, financial, and clinical research activities Business service management tracking Compliance review	Flagship product, Velos eResearch, is the core of the clinical research management suite. This pure Internet platform connects essential financial, administrative, and clinical research activities and includes integrated modules to track and manage biospecimens and compliance review, as well as system administrator tools and integration tools for linking other applications.
eClinForce SmartStudy http://eclinforce.com	Launched: 2006	Patient databases Management of recruitment Subject tracking Financial management Clinical trial management functions	SmartStudy is a fully web-based clinical trial management software that provides clinical trial management functionalities for patient databases, recruitment, enrollment, visit planning and scheduling, and financial management, as well as complete oversight and reporting.
Intralinks Studyspace www.intralinks.com	Launched: 2010	Centralizes study documents Centralizes communication Standardizes processes Real-time activity dashboards for clinical operation Compliance and auditing functionality Data management Study management	Intralinks Studyspace specifically helps to • Centralize all study-related documents, communication, and activity history in an organized, consistent, and searchable fashion • Standardize and automate processes such as contract and budget negotiation, regulatory document distribution, and collection and ongoing document exchange • Eliminate repetitive and redundant site data entry and document submission • Provide sites with a personalized view of tasks, requests, and due dates, with reminder alerts and a secure communication channel to ensure timely site activation • Monitor process progress with real-time activity dashboards and meet regulatory compliance with detailed access reports and audit trails.

(Continued on next page)

Table 17-3. Examples of Software Programs/Databases for Tracking Clinical Trial Activity and Metrics *(Continued)*			
Program/Database	Launch Date/ Current Version	Key Features	Developer Description
IntelliTRIAL www.intellitrial.com	Launched: 2005	Budgeting Compliance Collections Regulatory reporting Workload scheduling Financial reporting	IntelliTRIAL is a CTMS designed to make research easier for coordinators, schedulers, finance directors, and the billing/compliance team.
Clinical Conductor CTMS http://bio-optronics.com/clinical-conductor	Launched: 2010	Streamlines workflows Financial management Patient recruitment	Designed specifically for clinical research sites, Clinical Conductor CTMS is today's most comprehensive CTMS. Clinical Conductor CTMS streamlines and enhances study setup, patient recruitment, financial management, staff and patient scheduling, marketing campaign tracking, patient payments, reporting, metrics, and other aspects of clinical trial management.

bases that track clinical trial activity and metrics. Most of the programs are similar in scope and functionality in that they track similar information via similar task-specific consoles. When exploring software options, issues to consider are the ease of adaptation and use, the cost required to license the software (initial and future updates), the amount of support provided by the vendor, the number of years the vendor has been in business, and the specificity of the product (i.e., do they only provide this service for oncology or do they accommodate other disease entities?).

The work of creating and validating tools has recently caught the attention of various special interest groups. The Association of American Cancer Institutes has a Clinical Research Initiative group that has regular teleconferences. The primary objective of the group is to review what each participating center is currently doing to track metrics and allocate resources. The anticipated outcome is to take the best practices and collaboratively develop a tool that can be validated and that is generalizable to the research community as a whole.

Summary

The future of clinical trial workload, funding, and staffing cannot be predicted; thus, workload measurement and resource allocation continue to be key concerns. It is increasingly clear that utilization of protocol task– and activity time–based resource planning can be a positive, proactive way to estimate and obtain appropriate levels of funding for clinical trials and can be an appropriate tool to manage resources. As the clinical research industry continues to experience rapid computerization and increasing use of electronic trial management and support systems, the integration of computer resources and technology is vital to managing clinical trials in the future.

Key Points

- The future of clinical trial workload determination and resource allocation looks bright. Several workload tools have been developed and successfully tested in limited settings. Nevertheless, further testing remains to be done to evaluate generalizability of such tools.
- The comparability of these measures has yet to be evaluated, with the goal of either developing a uniform/universal measure or uncovering how these tools measure up or perform head-to-head.
- The role of technology and clinical trial management software is a central consideration in any successful effort to delineate and manage workload and resources in small or large clinical trials enterprises.
- No one optimal software exists, and the multitude of options cause challenges for some centers in matching their needs with the appropriate software to deploy. These limitations are important for all scales of clinical research operations: local, regional, national, and global.
- A critical mass of studies is needed from a large number of sites working simultaneously (separately or together) to generate a sufficient evidence base to answer the persistent core questions outlined earlier.
- The increasing knowledge and recognized value of workload and resource determination provide momentum for greater successes in the next decade. This is an inspiring time, and the outlook is quite promising despite the prevailing global economic crunch.

References

Berridge, J., & Coffey, M. (2008). Workload measurement: How one workload study measured tasks, time, and resources necessary to run a cancer clinical trial today. *Applied Clinical Trials.* Retrieved from http://www.appliedclinicaltrialsonline.com/appliedclinicaltrials/article/articleDetail.jsp?id=522055&pageID=1&sk=&date=

Briggs, J. (2008). Real-world workload needs: Developing a process and management tool for scoring complexity in cancer clinical trials. *Applied Clinical Trials.* Retrieved from http://www.appliedclinicaltrialsonline.com/appliedclinicaltrials/article/articleDetail.jsp?id=513744

Chirikos, T.N. (2003). Three questions about costs and cancer clinical trials. *Cancer Control, 10,* 71–78. Retrieved from http://moffitt.org/research–clinical-trials/cancer-control-journal/high-dose-therapy

Coffey, M., Lyddiardc, J., Briggs, J., & Berridge, J. (2010). A workload measurement. *Applied Clinical Trials.* Retrieved from http://www.appliedclinicaltrialsonline.com/appliedclinicaltrials/article/articleDetail.jsp?id=681230

Devine, S., Nagel, K., Benson, L., & Krailo, M. (2005, April). CRA discipline time and effort study: Children's Oncology Group. *Applied Clinical Trials.* Retrieved from http://www.appliedclinicaltrialsonline.com/appliedclinicaltrials/article/articleDetail.jsp?id=154234

Edwards, B.K., Howe, H.L., Ries, L.A.G., Thun, M.J., Rosenberg, H.M., Yancik, R., ... Feigal, E.G. (2002). Annual report to the nation on the status of cancer, 1973–1999, featuring implications of age and aging on U.S. cancer burden. *Cancer, 94,* 2766–2792. doi:10.1002/cncr.10593

Ehrenberger, H.E., & Lillington, L. (2004). Development of a measure to delineate the clinical trials nursing role [Online exclusive]. *Oncology Nursing Forum, 31,* E64–E68. doi:10.1188/04.ONF.E64-E68

Emanuel, E.J., Schnipper, L.E., Kamin, D.Y., Levinson, J., & Lichter, A.S. (2003). The costs of conducting clinical research. *Journal of Clinical Oncology, 21,* 4145–4150. doi:10.1200/JCO.2003.08.156

Fowell, J.P., & Wilson, J.T. (2002, Summer). The six phases of a research site budget. *Monitor,* pp. 31–34.

Fowler, D.R., & Thomas, C.J. (2003). Protocol acuity scoring as a rational approach to clinical research management. *Research Practitioner, 4,* 64–71.

Good, M.J., Lubejko, B., Humphries, K., & Medders, A. (2013). Measuring clinical trial-associated workload in a community clinical oncology program. *Journal of Oncology Practice, 9,* 211–215. doi:10.1200/jop.2012.000797

Gwede, C.K., Johnson, D., & Daniels, S. (2001). Organization of clinical research services at investigative sites: Implications for workload measurement. *Drug Information Journal, 35,* 695–705.

Gwede, C.K., Johnson, D.J., Roberts, C., & Cantor, A.B. (2005). Burnout in clinical research coordinators in the United States. *Oncology Nursing Forum, 32,* 1123–1130. doi:10.1188/05.ONF.1123-1130

Gwede, C.K., Johnson, D., & Trotti, A. (2000a). Measuring the workload of clinical research coordinators, part I: Tools to study workload issues. *Applied Clinical Trials, 9*(1), 40–44.

Gwede, C.K., Johnson, D., & Trotti, A. (2000b). Measuring the workload of clinical research coordinators, part II: Workload implications for sites. *Applied Clinical Trials, 9*(2), 42–47.

James, P., Bebee, P., Beckman, L., Browning, D., Innes, M., Kain, J., ... Waldinger, M. (2011a). Effort tracking metrics provide data for optimal budgeting and workload management in therapeutic clinical trials. *Journal of the National Comprehensive Cancer Network, 9,* 1343–1352. Retrieved from http://www.jnccn.org/content/9/12/1343.long

James, P., Bebee, P., Beckman, L., Browning, D., Innes, M., Kain, J., ... Waldinger, M. (2011b). Effort tracking tool to improve therapeutic cancer clinical trials workload management and budgeting. *Journal of the National Comprehensive Cancer Network, 9,* 1228–1233. Retrieved from http://www.jnccn.org/content/9/11/1228.full?sid=dc124b64-f3f5-46ee-a0f1-1dff87e8200b

Johnson, G.P. (2003, May). Budget tool helps investigative sites calculate the cost of a coordinator's time for a typical outpatient study visit: Part II. *SoCRA SOURCE,* pp. 33–37. Retrieved from https://www.socra.org/assets/SoCRA-Source/InvestigativeSiteBudgetToolbyGuyJohnson.pdf

Jones, A., Cusack, G., & Chisholm, L. (2004). Patient intensity in an ambulatory oncology research center: A step forward for the field of ambulatory care—Part II. *Nursing Economics, 22,* 120–123, 107.

Neuer, A. (2002). The rising tide of CRC workload and turnover. *CenterWatch, 9,* 1–7.

Roche, K., Paul, N., Smuck, B., Whitehead, M., Zee, B., Pater, J., ... Walker, H. (2002). Factors affecting workload of cancer clinical trials: Results of a multicenter study of the National Cancer Institute of Canada Clinical Trials Group. *Journal of Clinical Oncology, 20,* 545–556. doi:10.1200/JCO.20.2.545

Rozich, J.D., & Resar, R.K. (2002). Using a unit assessment tool to optimize patient flow and staffing in a community hospital. *Joint Commission Journal on Quality Improvement, 28,* 31–41.

Smuck, B., Bettello, P., Berghout, K., Hanna, T., Kowaleski, B., Phippard, L., ... Friel, K. (2011). Ontario protocol assessment level: Clinical trial complexity rating tool for workload planning in oncology clinical trials. *Journal of Oncology Practice, 7*(2), 80–84. doi:10.1200/JOP.2010.000051

Van Slyck, A. (1995). Not all acuity systems are the same. *Nursing Management, 26*(7), 11.

Walts, L.M., & Kapadia, A.S. (1996). Patient classification system: An optimization approach. *Health Care Management Review, 21*(4), 75–82. doi:10.1097/00004010-199623000-00009

West, J., Wright, J., Tuffnell, D., Jankowicz, D., & West, R. (2005). Do clinical trials improve quality of care? A comparison of clinical processes and outcomes in patients in a clinical trial and similar patients outside a trial where both groups are managed according to a strict protocol. *Quality and Safety in Health Care, 14,* 175–178. doi:10.1136/qshc.2004.011478

Yancik, R. (1997). Epidemiology of cancer in the elderly. Current status and projections for the future. *Rays, 22*(Suppl. 1), 3–9.

Yancik, R., & Ries, L.A.G. (2004). Cancer in older persons: An international issue in an aging world. *Seminars in Oncology, 31,* 128–136. doi:10.1053/j.seminoncol.2003.12.024

Chapter 18

Billing, Budgets, and Funding

Kelly Willenberg, MBA, BSN, CCRP, CHRC, Lora Black, RN, MPH, OCN®, CCRP, and Brandy Troisi, BA, RN

Introduction

The key to a carefully prescribed clinical trial management plan starts with the development of a proper budget. This is a daunting task for even the most experienced research administrator. A clinical trial may be considered a success or failure in the minds of the research team depending on whether it makes or loses money. What are the guidelines to prepare a budget correctly? What are the key ingredients of a successful budget? According to Wright et al. (2005), "The study budget represents the total amount of money required to conduct a trial and is usually negotiated on a per patient basis" (p. 422). The financial impact of conducting a clinical trial in oncology can be mitigated by astute negotiation for proper reimbursement. This chapter will provide the proper tools needed to budget a clinical trial successfully. As Good (2002) noted, "Sweat the small stuff. Attorneys do it; so do CPAs. Don't just record major expenditures—air travel and outlays to advertising agencies—but track every phone call and the time your staff spends on it" (p. 163). The research team's success depends on the completeness of the plan at the beginning of the budget process—not after the study is open to accrual, when it is too late.

Administrative Components

First and foremost, the clear starting point for proper budgeting is reading and understanding the protocol. Second, the administrator must be familiar with the clinical trial budget process and institutional templates for budget creation. For the purposes of this chapter, the following definition will be used to describe the scope of a budget: "a detailed budget is an itemized list accounting for every expense required to complete the project" (Higdon & Topp, 2004, p. 924). The administrator must review what the sponsor provides, knowing his or her facility's costs and being secure in that knowledge. If something is unclear or confusing in the protocol regarding what has to be done, the administrator obtains clarification from the sponsor. In investigator-initiated studies, confusing items should be clarified with the principal investigator (PI) before opening the study for patient accrual. Knowing what is required before opening the trial shows that the administrator's review was thorough.

A careful review of both the study calendar that graphically depicts the timing of study events and the clearly defined parameters of what the sponsor considers to be covered under the reimbursement agreement and budget is vital to development of a successful budget. The administrator must provide sufficient justification for all components of the study, including materials and labor costs (Koren, 2005).

Delineating conventional care from what is considered to be part of the research for the protocol is extremely important. A *Medicare coverage analysis billing grid* should be used to build the patient care budget (see Figure 18-1). All research nurses and study coordinators or people responsible for billing need to be trained on how to interpret the billing grid, understanding that it displays how they will post charges for the study. The billing grid also is a guide for ordering supplies for each patient visit. The key to successful budget building is verifying at the beginning what constitutes conventional care versus care that is provided for research purposes only. This can include a *rating system* to estimate a budget per patient (see Figure 18-2) (Spear, 2005).

The administrator must schedule a meeting with the research team and calculate the complexity of the study to determine the amount of time that will be necessary to complete every aspect of the study. "Financial managers should collaborate with researchers and physicians in

Figure 18-1. Sample Billing Grid

Version: 2.0	Date of Visit						Contracted Subjects: 0		
Protocol Dtd: 12/27/07	Visit #s	1	2	3	4	5	6		
	ARMS	Screen	Procedure Stent Placement	Discharge	1-month follow-up	6-month follow-up	12-month follow-up		
	Windows	<1 Mo							
Clinical Activity	CPT Code	Baseline						Gross charges	% Disc	Net
ABI's-rest CPT 93922	93922	$537			$537	$537	$537	$2,148		$2,148
Abdominal aortic aneurism repair—endovascular	34800–34834	$0						$0		$0
Radiology for endovascular repair	75952							$0		$0
Angio-extremity—unilateral	75710							$0		$0
Catheter abdom/fem first order	36245							$0		$0
Angio select addl vessel S&I	75774							$0		$0
Guide wires/catheters	36245-36248							$0		$0
Transcatheter placement wireless sensor	34806							$0		$0
Contrast iodine 300–3991 ml Q9967	Dept 3606 92753473							$0		$0
Abdominal CT	74170	$1,000			$1,000	$1,000	$1,000	$4,000		$4,000
Subtotal (Clinical Activity)		$1,537	$0	$0	$1,537	$1,537	$1,537	$6,148		$6,148

(Continued on next page)

Figure 18-1. Sample Billing Grid (Continued)

Version: 2.0	Date of Visit									Contracted Subjects: 0	
Protocol Dtd: 12/27/07	Visit #s	1	2	3	4	5	6				
	ARMS	Screen	Procedure Stent Placement	Discharge	1-month follow-up	6-month follow-up	12-month follow-up				
	Windows	< 1 Mo									
		Baseline						Gross charges	% Disc	Net	
Lab Activity											
Venipunctures	36415	$12					$12	$24		$24	
Basic met panel	80048	$15					$15	$30		$30	
CBC w/diff & platelets	85025	$15					$15	$30		$30	
PT/INR	85610	$15					$15	$30		$30	
PTT	85730	$20					$20	$40		$40	
Subtotal (Lab Activity)		$77	$0	$0	$0	$0	$77	$154		$154	
Investigator Activity											
Physical exam	99215–99323	$0	$0	$0	$0	$0	$0	$0		$0	
Subtotal (Investigator-Driven Fees)		$0	$0	$0	$0	$0	$0	$0		$0	
Staff Activity											
Informed consent	CRC = 2 hr	**$100**						**$100**		**$100**	
Incl/exclu criteria check	CRC = 30 min	$25						$25		$25	
Medical history	CRC = 30 min	$25				$25		$50		$50	
Con meds review	CRC = 30 min	$25	$25	$25	$25	$25	$25	$150		$150	
Attendance at procedure	CRC = 2 hr		$100					$100		$100	
Walking questionnaire	CRC = 15 min	$13			$13	$13	$13	$52		$52	

(Continued on next page)

Figure 18-1. Sample Billing Grid (Continued)

		Date of Visit							Contracted Subjects: 0		
		Visit #s	1	2	3	4	5	6			
	Version: 2.0	ARMS	Screen	Procedure Stent Placement	Discharge	1-month follow-up	6-month follow-up	12-month follow-up			
	Protocol Dtd: 12/27/07	Windows	<1 Mo						Gross charges	% Disc	Net
			Baseline								
	Phone call	CRC = 30 min		$25	$25	$25	$25	$25	$0		$0
	Adverse event log	CRC = 30 min	$50	$50	$50	$50	$50	$50	$125		$125
	CRF time	CRC = 1 hr		$200	$100				$300		$300
	Subtotal (Staff-Driven Activity)		$238	$282	$141	$113	$138	$113	$902		$902
A	Direct expenses		$1,852	$52	$26	$429	$436	$450	$7,204		$7,204
B	Overhead	26%	$482						$1,875		$1,875
C	Subject stipend	N/A	$0	$0	$0	$0	$0	$0	$0		$0
D = A + B + C	Subtotal w/ overhead		$2,334	$252	$126	$2,079	$2,111	$2,177	$9,079		$9,079
E = A*%	PI protocol supervision	15%	$278	$30	$15	$248	$252	$260	$1,083		$1,083
F = D + E	Total budget per subject		$2,612	$282	$141	$2,327	$2,363	$2,437	$10,162		$10,162
X	Revenue		Subtotal w/ overhead (D) × estimated subjects						$0		$0
Y	PI revenue		PI protocol supervision (E) × estimated subjects						$0		$0
Z = X + Y	Total project revenue		Total revenue						$0		$0

Figure 18-2. Rating System to Estimate Budget Per Patient					
Acuity Level	Study Phase	Activity	Hours Per Week	Full-Time Employee % Per Week	Cost Per Subject
					$ complete based on annual salary
All levels	All phases	Prescreening	1	2.50%	
4	1	Screening	12	30.00%	
3	2	Screening	12	30.00%	
2	3	Screening	10	25.00%	
1	4	Screening	10	25.00%	
4	1	On treatment	8	20.00%	
3	2	On treatment	6	15.00%	
2	3	On treatment	4	10.00%	
1	4	On treatment	2	5.00%	
4	1	Withdraw/termination	5	12.50%	
3	2	Withdraw/termination	3	7.50%	
2	3	Withdraw/termination	2	5.00%	
1	4	Withdraw/termination	1	2.50%	
All levels	All phases	Auditing/reporting	5	12.50%	

4 = Highest intensity/complex
3 = Moderate intensity/complex
2 = Less intensity/complex
1 = Least intense/not complex

implementing and interpreting a standard costing format for clinical trials" (West, Balas, & West, 2000, p. 11).

One always must consider future cost and, therefore, price increases for services for the duration of the study. The administrative fees should include an analysis of protocol data to build a budget and negotiate a contract that will define the institutional overhead. The administrative components include all *nonrefundable fees* (see Figure 18-3). Travel expenses, investigator fees, and computer-related expenditures should be documented. In addition, the administrator should keep track of time spent on study-related tasks—including time spent on the telephone, which can be substantial (Good, 2002). It is vital to track everything because the data may be useful at a later time; electing not to open a study because the budget does not meet the site's budget feasibility is perfectly acceptable. Rowell (2005) noted that Louisiana State University handles about 100 studies a year but may turn away that many protocols because they do not meet the institution's budget feasibility. He stated, "One of the advantages of being a big site is [that] we turn some down before we get to the budget phase" (Rowell, 2005, p. 91).

Rowell (2005) further noted that it is not unusual for the budget he has generated to be twice the amount the sponsor originally said it would pay. "But I won't come down below our costs. We won't lose money doing research—we can't afford to" (p. 91). A breakeven point and the bottom line should be analyzed. The administrator needs to feel empowered to make a recommendation that a particular study will lose money and should not be opened. Many academic centers have review committees that have the authority to decide whether the institution will take a financial "hit" to do the study. The key to achieving success is being aware up front of what the study entails financially and planning how to accomplish it without a loss.

Online tools are available to assist in creating a budget. The National Cancer Institute Cancer Therapy Evaluation Program offers spreadsheet templates for a cooperative group common budget outline (see http://ctep.cancer.gov/protocolDevelopment/docs/coop_grp_budget.xls).

Estimating Accrual

Estimating accrual is complicated and must be done for the entire study. According to Iber, Riley, and Murray (1987), "Physicians new to drug and device investigations usually overestimate the ease of obtaining subjects, underestimate the time of complying with regulatory affairs, under-budget for the unexpected, and overestimate their own efficiency" (p. 53).

Administrators should be realistic when estimating accrual. To improve accuracy, they can check cancer registry data to note how many patients are diagnosed by the institution over a given time frame and ensure data from the registry are current and apply to the specific disease stage under study. In addition, referencing a site's past accrual to studies with similar diagnoses may be helpful. Administrators should not overestimate the total number of patients to be accrued and should know the average number of cycles or days that each patient will be on study and have a clear understanding of the timeline for finishing the study (see Chapter 17). Those preparing the budget should include assumptions within study-specific budget documents for future reference.

The number-one thing administrators should remember is to *never* agree to the sponsor's initial offer, regardless of how incredible the dollar amount sounds. All sponsors or clinical research organizations have a business plan, and making money is their goal. They may underestimate what it will cost the facility to complete the study. The offer may sound good, but unless the budget is prepared carefully, the administrator will have no idea how accurate it truly is. Overestimating accrual consistently can lead to a loss of revenue overall. An institution is paid on an accrual basis, and funding comes months afterward; therefore, the budget should be planned accordingly. In the end, it is best not to open a study if doubts exist about the feasibility of accruing the number of subjects needed to reach financial milestones set by the site.

Nonrefundable Fees

Nonrefundable fees are the only way to collect start-up costs. Examples of these costs include the pharmacy fees, institutional review board (IRB) fees, IRB preparation and consent form composition, RN coordinator time, budget preparation, contract negotiations, prestudy visits with the sponsor (which can be combined with the initiation visit to save time in some situations), and meetings to set up the protocol or review the budget (see Figure 18-3).

Figure 18-3. Nonrefundable/Onetime Fees

One-Time-Per-Study Nonrefundable Fees (insert as applicable)

Description	5-Digit Account #	Totals
IRB Preparation	61400	$5,000
Consent Form Development	61400	$50
IRB Submission and Review	61400	$400
IRB Amendments Processing	61400	$100
SAE Processing	61400	$250
IRB Annual Review	61400	$500
Total for Account 61400		**$6,300**
Pharmacy Protocol Management Fee	61910	$100
Archival Fee	61910	$0
Advertising Fee	61910	$250
Clinical Trial Operational Fee	61910	$400
Storage Fee	61910	$1,000
Shipping and Postage Fees	61910	$200
Auditing Fee	61910	$200
Coverage Analysis Fee	61910	$3,000
Total for Account 61910		**$5,150**
Duplication	60000	$785
Publication Costs	60010	$125
Printing	60020	$150
Postage	60030	$175
Office Supplies	60040	$700
Lab Supplies	60150	$1,500
Federal Express	60225	$45
Drug Floor Stock	60530	$1,000
Telephone	61300	$225
Misc. Expense	61900	$500
Meeting Expense	62100	$50
Subject Participation	63400	$400

Pharmacy fees should be included as nonrefundable. Doing so prevents the pharmacy fee from being connected to the price per patient, which can result in a loss of the protocol management fees if patient accrual is low. Regardless of the number of patients accrued, the pharmacy incurs fees, such as preparing an itemized budget, developing order entry sets, maintaining drug inventory records and binders established for the study, and carefully reviewing the protocol. The pharmacy expends time and effort before any patient is registered to the study and should be compensated regardless of whether there is accrual to the study. An alternative approach is to include a nonrefundable start-up fee for pharmacy in addition to a per-patient reimbursement (included as a line item in the per-patient cost). Separating the costs is reasonable in the event the sponsor is not willing to accept the initial request for increased pharmacy fees.

IRB fees are considered nonrefundable, may be predetermined by the research arm, and are nonnegotiable. These fees vary and can be associated with the number of adverse events or amendments submitted. Listing these as "pass-through," or *invoiceable*, costs can help in preparing an invoice for the sponsor.

Medicare coverage analysis (MCA) creation is considered a nonrefundable fee, as establishment is necessary before opening a study regardless of overall accrual. The administrator may augment negotiation for appropriate reimbursement regarding MCA development by including the site's standard procedure for MCA development with the start-up request. Ensure that the memo (on letterhead) outlines the institutional requirement to complete this step for compliant billing. A provision for invoicing an MCA "update fee" should be included for instances when protocol revisions require changes to the initial MCA.

Billing Compliance for Medicare and Third-Party Payers

An essential component to developing a comprehensive clinical trial budget is the completion of an MCA. The administrator may wish to finalize the MCA prior to beginning the budget. In doing so, clarity is given to what needs to be included in the budget for sponsor reimbursement.

Medicare established a National Coverage Decision (NCD) in 2000 addressing clinical trials under the Clinton administration. NCD 310.1 requires clinical trials to meet predefined criteria before being designated as *qualifying* (Centers for Medicare and Medicaid Services [CMS], 2000). *Qualifying status* is the most important step in determining whether items or services provided as part of the protocol may be considered billable to third-party payers. The process of coverage analysis not only encompasses determination of qualifying status but also documents the billable nature of tests and procedures included on the study calendar.

To determine qualifying status, a clinical trial must meet all of the following per NCD 310.1 (CMS, 2000): (a) services must fall within a benefit category, (b) the trial must be designed with therapeutic intent, and (c) patients must have a diagnosed disease. Qualifying trials also must meet the seven desirable characteristics outlined in the NCD. A careful understanding and review of what the regional Medicare contractor requires will help the site administrator to determine the billing status of a clinical trial.

Trials determined to be qualifying are eligible for expanded coverage under Medicare, defined in the NCD as *routine costs*. Routine costs within a qualifying clinical trial include

- Items or services that are typically provided absent a clinical trial (e.g., conventional care);
- Items or services required solely for the provision of the investigational item or service (e.g., administration of a noncovered chemotherapeutic agent), the clinically appropriate monitoring of the effects of the item or service, or the prevention of complications; and
- Items or services needed for reasonable and necessary care arising from the provision of an investigational item or service—in particular, for the diagnosis or treatment of complications. (CMS, 2000, p. 1)

Routine costs do not include services completed only for research purposes (i.e., not required for the clinical management of the patient). For example, a venipuncture completed only for collection of blood for pharmacokinetic analysis would not be covered.

Third-party private payers often follow Medicare's lead for coverage of a qualifying clinical trial. To ensure appropriate billing, it is essential to understand the institutional contract with third-party payers, as well as state law regarding clinical trial coverage. Not all states have legislation addressing this issue, and state-to-state variation is common. For more information about clinical trials and payment legislation at the state level, please see the National Conference of State Legislatures (www.ncsl.org/research/health/clinical-trials-what-are-states-doing-2010.aspx).

A provision within the Patient Protection and Affordable Care Act of 2010 was implemented in January 2014, mandating clinical trial coverage by private insurers in every state. Information regarding this act and clinical trial coverage is available at www.cms.gov/CCIIO/Resources/Fact-Sheets-and-FAQs/aca_implementation_faqs15.html.

Services billable to Medicare must be determined by reviewing NCD 310.1 requirements. Each item on the study calendar (attached to a charge) should be included on the MCA grid with clear documentation of the responsible payer, either the third party or the research account. It is absolutely crucial that *only* the responsible party be billed for services. Instances of "double dipping" occur when the third-party payer is billed in addition to the sponsor reimbursing the site. CMS classifies this offense as fraudulent billing, putting institutions at risk for financial and civil penalties under the False Claims Act.

In addition, Medicare Advantage Plans do not cover the routine costs in drug trials covered under the Clinical Trial Policy. This makes the reimbursement Medicare's responsibility, and it is time consuming.

Another requirement that began in January 2014 is that the clinical trial number assigned by the National Library of Medicine (available at http://clinicaltrials.gov) is required on government claims. As of 2015, dummy numbers can no longer be used.

Device Trials

Device trials need to be assessed up front so that the administrator has the U.S. Food and Drug Administration (FDA) exemption letter stating the category assigned and the investigational device exemption (IDE) number. This information must be submitted to the IRB and Medicare for approval for billing by the sponsor. The administrator must know the device category to determine whether it is billable under Medicare guidelines. Many different categories of devices exist. It is very important to understand the category of the device being used in the specific clinical trial, as the various categories are supplied and potentially billed differently.

Category A (Experimental) Devices— Innovative Medical Devices

Devices in category A do not have a functional equivalent that has already been proved to be safe and effective and, therefore, are considered experimental (CMS, 2000). The initial questions of safety and effectiveness have not been resolved, and FDA is unsure whether the device can be safe and effective. Billing may include *only* the conventional care costs in clinical trials involving IDE category A devices; this excludes billing for the device itself. It is important that the "Q1" *procedure code modifier* be applied to conventional care items billed to CMS. The Q1 modifier indicates that the "item or service is provided as routine care in a qualified clinical trial" (CMS, 2000).

Category B Devices— Investigational Devices

A category B classification means that incremental risk is being investigated and that the fundamental issues of safety and effectiveness have already been resolved (CMS, 2000). These devices are so similar to other devices on the market that regulators believe they are at least as safe and effective as the ones on the market. Payment for these devices is payable by Medicare. The device must be reasonable and necessary for the treatment or diagnosis of a medical condition or disease (CMS, 2000). Devices that are statutorily excluded from coverage are not covered simply because they are part of a clinical trial. *The payment for a category B investigational device is limited to the amount equal to or less than what Medicare would have paid for a comparable approved device.* Payment under Medicare for a category B device will be based on information provided in the IDE submission. The billing for this device must include a Q0 modifier and the IDE number. Sites get into trouble with category B devices when the study-required device is much more expensive than the comparable device. Reimbursement is not appropriate, and sites lose money on each patient accrued. Devices provided must be accounted for on claims.

Patient Care Costs

To determine the budget necessary to cover the cost of the study, the administrator must price each test and procedure that is not considered conventional care (see Figure 18-4). Knowing the procedures and where they will be performed is important. Are they cardiology, radiology, laboratory, or respiratory procedures? Are special readings to be taken, specific contrast used, or the x-rays copied? All of these items are budgeted in a detailed way. Laboratory shipment fees can be significant if labs must be shipped overseas or across the country. Tissue and pathology costs and professional/physician fees are part of the overall budget and should not be forgotten. The administrator should not only consider pathology but also radiology for examples of fees to be charged. A separate fee is assessed for the test and the interpretation.

Common items missed in budget preparation are pharmacy costs, a lengthy consent form process for the coordinator, follow-up visits not included in the original schedule of events, supplies to give IV medications, drawing labs that are sent to a central lab and shipping, screen failure payments, interval training (PI and coordinator), and sponsor communication. Other fees include advertising costs, storage of study documents, and RN coordinator time.

Laboratory Fees

Laboratory fees must be accounted for when determining a clinical trial budget. Iber et al. (1987) stated that in all studies, 5%–15% of tests that are performed can be expected to be abnormal, unsatisfactory, or simply confusing to interpret and must be repeated. They

Figure 18-4. Calculating Nonstandard Procedure Costs

Review items necessary but not standard of care. Find current procedural terminology code that correlates and institutional cost for each item. Budget appropriate number according to study requirements and do not bill to third-party payer or Medicare. See the following table for an example of how to formulate budget costs.

Procedure	Current Procedural Terminology Code	Cost Including Professional Fee	Research Frequency	Total Cost to Budget Per Subject
Chest x-ray, two views	71020	$185.00	4	$185 × 4 = $740

recommended budgeting $50 per subject to cover repeat test fees. Laboratory fees also may change during the course of a study. Market adjustments can put the budget into disarray. The administrator must know the high- and low-end amounts required to cover these costs.

If the protocol requires two tests but to obtain results the institution requires an additional test to be done, the additional test must be billed to the sponsor. These may be institutional facility fees or requirements and should be considered in budget preparation.

The itemized budget list includes not only the research-related patient care procedures but also the ancillary services that will be used in the facility. Will the patients be admitted to the general clinical research center? Will they be in the clinic or treatment room? Will they be admitted as inpatients? These questions must be considered during budget preparation.

Pharmacy Costs

Pharmacy costs can be included in the nonrefundable fees and are published and confirmed in writing to ensure that the pharmacy receives payment regardless of accrual to the study. The fees that usually comprise a per-patient amount are fees for dispensing based on number of visits or cycles. Do not forget supplies in this fee, such as fluid or a pump to administer the provided drug or a special type of tubing. Investigational drug pharmacies charge protocol management fees, which should be considered nonrefundable, and dispensing fees, which are patient-specific.

Pharmacokinetic Sampling

Pharmacokinetic sampling (PKS) is a necessary item in early-phase studies. The administrator must plan and know the number of hours at which samples will be drawn. If special supplies are needed to perform PKS, such as a special centrifuge, a freezer that the facility might not have, IV supplies, special syringes, dry ice, tubes, or even a microwave, do not fail to include them in the budget. The person preparing the budget should always consider the staffing necessary for PKS that must be drawn in the off hours when the clinic is not open. On-call coverage, as well as possible shift differential for physicians or research staff, also should be budget items.

Investigators should consider using the general clinical research center or an infusion center for PKS blood draws if the facility has these departments. This is a cost to the budget, and the pharmaceutical sponsor should cover the costs of the staff to draw samples. Thus, it is important to know who will draw off-time labs and who will be responsible for spinning down, separating, and storing them.

If PKS must be conducted, the time needed to package and ship the samples should be included in the budget. If special items are needed, for example, storage boxes, tubes, Styrofoam containers, popcorn pellets for shipping, or the actual payment for shipping, these items should be secured up front from the sponsor. If items such as these are not accounted for in the initial budget, the facility will incur the costs later. These can be rather expensive, especially if the study requires only a small number of samples.

Staff Effort and Budgeting

Principal Investigator

A minimum number of hours should always be budgeted for the PI's effort based on his or her time needed to complete the study requirements. Overseeing the daily operations of a clinical trial can be significant, especially if the institution is acting as the coordinating center for a large study. For example, the PI may sometimes be responsible for reviewing eligibility for patients from all sites studywide. The administrator should consider whether the PI helped to develop the study with the sponsor. Some institutions have a minimum percent effort that must be included in each study budget. The PI's true effort in the study completion is what should be budgeted. Documenting the justification for reimbursement within the internal study budget template is an important and evolving aspect of regulatory compliance.

The other area where the PI may be required to put in large amounts of time, especially for phase I studies, is conference calls. These sometimes may require an hour or two per week in between cohorts for safety analysis or discussions with the sponsor. As noted by Wujcik and Willenberg (1999), "the same process and template are used for each review in order to identify procedures that exceed standard care and the percent effort by the PI" (p. 5).

A PI's time can be budgeted by different methods. One way is to calculate a percentage of the PI's overall annual salary by taking the number of hours necessary to do the study multiplied by the annual salary, and then divide by 2080 (the number of hours in a year of full-time work). The second way to calculate PI time is based on a timeline per visit. This provides a budget amount. Some pharmaceutical sponsors will send a template to the administrator to calculate salary. Either way is acceptable as long as the administrator feels that the PI's actual time is accurately reflected.

On government grants, justification and certification of time and effort are equally important. "In general, all budgets should include estimates for (a) personnel, including consultations if needed, (b) the purchase of rental equipment, (c) local and long distance travel, (d) supplies, and (e) other miscellaneous expenditures" (Ingersoll & Eberhard, 1999, p. 132).

Investigator meetings are a high-dollar time necessity, and not all sponsors cover the travel costs and time to complete these. Consider all of this when building a budget if the sponsor is not covering the time needed to attend.

Study Coordinator

The effort of the study coordinator or research nursing staff should be budgeted by *hours* (see Figure 18-5) or *time points* necessary for the staff to be with the patient (see Figure 18-6). Review prestudy activities for protocol feasibility and budget preparation. Baseline eligibility for each patient should be carefully considered. Phase I studies might require up to two days for review of the patient's eligibility criteria. How long does it take to obtain informed consent from a potential participant? Allow ample time to do a thorough job with each patient. Consider what it takes to create a calendar, patient information packet, or checklist(s) for each patient. Remember to include the time it takes to discuss with each study participant activities, such as quality-of-life surveys and questions or phone calls they might require, and budget for the coordinator's time to see the patient as well.

Screen failures (i.e., patients who are screened for eligibility but are deemed ineligible) take time as well. Administrators learn to rely on the past experience of the team and patient population to sufficiently budget for these, considering how many patients will need to be screened to enroll one. Enrollment log completion should always be included among the budgeted items. Some studies will require that numerous logs be completed (prescreening, screening, and enrollment). The administrator should ask if they must be completed within a certain time frame and faxed to the sponsor because the study site should be compensated for the coordinator's time to complete. This will help to cover the institution's expenses. When budgeting for screen failures, a minimum number of hours should be budgeted. General assumptions allow for at least three to four hours for screening a patient and at least one to two hours per cycle or time point in the study for the study coordinator. This total can be shown as a percentage of their total annual hours in a budget.

Screening for accrual can be a time-consuming process. If the study coordinator says that 10 patients will need to be screened in order to accrue one patient, budget for that time. Screen failures should always be a part of the budget, and any sponsor that will not cover screening costs should be considered as not really understanding the clinical trial process. The budget should include wording to invoice the maximum amount up to the total dollar amount of a screening visit based on what is completed in each instance of a screen failure. Some sponsors will allow for a limited number of screenings; however, a 20% screen failure rate is considered to be fair, and most sponsors abide by this figure in their contracts and legal agreements. The manager should not agree to be paid for five screen failures if the plan is to accrue 100 patients, and the amount of time required for chart screenings and logs should be fully accounted for as well. These can take a significant amount of time, and the institution should be paid to complete this work. Assessment of work can be crucial, and a manager should evaluate at time points (see Figure 18-5).

The staff will require time to complete treatment activities. The coordinator's time at the physician visit should be included, as well as the coordinator visit alone. The RN coordinator's time in relation to the PI should be included in the budget as well. The RN's time spent with monitors when the study has begun to accrue patients must be considered. This may require a large block of time weekly or monthly with high-accruing studies.

The administrator preparing the budget should remember to include the lab-only visits if the coordinator will perform the lab tests and should keep in mind that reporting adverse events and serious adverse events will take time, which is based on the type of drug involved. The time involved in scheduling lab tests, biopsies, and cardiology or radiology procedures should be considered. The time it takes to assemble scans or films and to order supplies or equipment for the study should be

---

Figure 18-5. Calculating Staff Effort

Nurse/Coordinator
Annual salary budget entry = $XX/per hour × 2,080 hours/year

Data Manager/Clinical Research Associate
Annual salary budget entry = $XX/per hour × 2,080 hours/year

Figure 18-6. Workload Summary for Study Coordinators

Time Assessment	Number	Comments
Therapeutic study accrual this month		
Correlative accrual this month		
Open protocols this team manages		
Patients on study		
Patients in follow-up		
Queries received		
Queries pending		
Queries completed		
Outside safety reports processed		
Patients with data > 1 month		

recorded. The coordinator's time must be covered in order to do all of these tasks. The administrator should work with the coordinator to ensure that his or her effort to complete the study is covered in the budget. Encourage coordinators to notify the administrator with new developments in the study workflow that may affect the budget (e.g., time, supplies). Revisions to the contract can and should be requested when the initial assumptions are no longer accurate.

Data Management/ Clinical Research Associate

Every study requires someone to enter data either into a case report form (CRF) or into a web-based data collection system. Administrators will find that their staff will require a minimum number of hours for complex studies, which is based on the activities of doing eligibility reviews, screening, performing routine visits, and conducting patient teaching, as well as other activities associated with the clinical trial. Thus, tracking all activities in monthly reports, which document the amount of work done within a certain time frame, can create benchmarks for standards. The time needed for coordinators to prepare for monitor and patient visits, the time spent with a patient for each visit, the number of hours it takes to complete adverse event reports for each patient, and the review and preparation of outside safety reports that come in from sponsors prior to submitting to the IRB should always be considered when preparing the budget. (Workload assessment is covered in Chapter 17.)

Whether the data manager or research associate must travel for training or go to investigator meetings should be determined because this can be a substantial amount of time if they have to be away from the workplace for a lengthy period. Many sponsors cover some expenses of personnel to travel, but not all. If the institution must contract the work out of a department, or if personnel must travel on a weekend, additional money should be included in the budget to cover these institutional expenses.

The data management piece may comprise the largest amount of time put into any study that is performed at an institution. Knowing up front whether a study will be done in paper or electronic format is crucial to successful budgeting for the study. The administrator preparing the budget should ask to see the CRFs before putting the budget together. In doing so, the administrator may include estimated time to create site-specific source documents. If a data log is to be maintained, the time necessary to do so should be included. If a database has to be maintained, including a file server, storage, and archiving, the administrator must not hesitate to project the true time that is needed to maintain these items. The follow-up schedule will need to be determined, and if the sponsor asks for more follow-ups than are in the CRFs, the administrator should verify it and include this time in the budget. The data manager's or clinical research associate's needs might be under-reimbursed if the administrator does not review all of the items necessary to complete the CRFs.

Hidden Costs

Every budget includes expenses that cannot be predicted. These can result in a budget shortfall and possibly poor budget management by the study administrator. Incorporating an adjusted cost or administrative rate into the budget will help to account for unexpected market adjustments in salaries or increases in hospital ancillary expenses, such as lab or x-ray costs.

Increasing attention is being concentrated on *regulatory compliance*. Therefore, it is crucial to include billing statement reviews and staff time essential to append appropriate modifiers to claims. Interval audits of billing practices are indispensable; hence, the administrator should consider adding time for one standard audit per study. For device studies, submission to the regional Medicare contractor for approval is mandatory. Staff time for this activity can be incorporated into fixed start-up costs. Equally as important is regulatory work that must be done to receive initial and ongoing IRB approval. Staff time, both regulatory and coordinator staff, for completing documents and engaging in follow-up communication should be included as budget items.

Other items that are not tangible costs but that will add to the bottom line are staff training, source document design, obtaining a second or revised consent, phone calls, query resolution, enrollment log completion, advertising and Internet fees, and screening of patient charts. Moreover, it is wise to include the ability to invoice for potential situations. For example, an hourly, invoiceable fee should be included if the sponsor requests materials for remote monitoring. Figure 18-1 displays all of the budget items together, showing where to include personnel costs and patient care costs in one budget for a sponsor. Costs can be calculated by reviewing itemized bills and planning for contingencies, such as price increases. Contracts are negotiable; the administrator should not hesitate to approach the sponsor for a revision when confronted with unanticipated circumstances after opening the study.

The following checklist may be used to prepare a clinical trial budget.
- Compensation and personnel costs (e.g., salaries, fringe benefits, professional fees)
- Supplies and document storage (e.g., office supplies, tubes for blood draws, shipping materials such as special boxes or cartons)
- Travel (e.g., investigator meetings not covered by the sponsor)
- Budgeting services, including invoicing of sponsors
- Equipment (e.g., dry ice, document storage, beepers)
- Other (e.g., phone, fax, shipping, subject payments, records retention)
- Research pharmacy
- Administrative costs (e.g., IRB fee, clinical trials office fee)
- University fringe and administrative costs (industry sponsors must pay anywhere from 20%–35%)
- Start-up fees (including all screening costs)
- Nonreimbursable start-up fees
- Interim monitoring visit fees (for time the research coordinator spends during the visit)
- Query resolution fees
- Close-out costs (e.g., long-term storage fees, queries)
- Decision of what is conventional care and what is being done for research purposes only
- Advertising fees
- Investigator oversight fees

Summary

Clinical trial budgeting is an art. A person who does it daily becomes very savvy at it. The one item to keep in mind is that once actual expenses are tracked, bad budget decisions will be apparent. The administrator should look at the institution's history with certain types of trials and consider this information when preparing a budget. By accurately tracking expenditures, an administrator can minimize the chances of problems developing.

Key Points
- Administrative costs for clinical trials, both routine and study-specific, should be identified and continually added as regulations and best practices change.
- Identifying hidden costs will ensure proper budgets. Including the research team in budget review is beneficial in exposing unanticipated costs.
- Administrators must know drug and device billing rules for compliance.
- Study costs for patient care and staff effort for each visit should be itemized in detail.
- A Medicare coverage analysis should be used for budget development.

References

Centers for Medicare and Medicaid Services. (2000, September). *September 2000 final national coverage decision*. Retrieved from http://www.cms.hhs.gov/ClinicalTrialPolicies/Downloads/finalnationalcoverage.pdf

Good, P.I. (2002). *A manager's guide to the design and conduct of clinical trials*. New York, NY: Wiley-Liss.

Higdon, J., & Topp, R. (2004). How to develop a budget for a research proposal. *Western Journal of Nursing Research, 26*, 922–929. doi:10.1177/0193945904269291

Iber, F.L., Riley, W.A., & Murray, P.J. (1987). *Conducting clinical trials*. New York, NY: Plenum Medical Book Company. doi:10.1007/978-1-4419-1586-3

Ingersoll, G.L., & Eberhard, D. (1999). Grants management skills keep funded projects on target. *Nursing Economics, 17*, 131–141.

Koren, G. (2005). How to increase your funding chances: Common pitfalls in medical grant applications. *Canadian Journal of Clinical Pharmacology, 12*, e182–e185.

Rowell, J.P. (2005). Fair budgets lead to better research. *Clinical Trials Administrator, 3*, 91–93.

Spear, L. (2005). *Effort calculator*. Durham, NC: Duke Comprehensive Cancer Center.

West, D.A., Balas, E.A., & West, T.D. (2000). Financial managers' costing expertise is needed in clinical trials. *Journal of Health Care Finance, 27*(1), 11–20.

Wright, J.R., Roche, K., Smuck, B., Cormier, J., Cecchetto, S., Akow, M., … Pritchard, K.I. (2005). Estimating per patient funding for cancer clinical trials: An Ontario based survey. *Contemporary Clinical Trials, 26,* 421–429. doi:10.1016/j.cct.2005.03.003

Wujcik, D., & Willenberg, K. (1999). Vanderbilt workload assessment tool validated by nursing committee. *Quarterly Newsletter for the Eastern Cooperative Oncology Group, 4,* 5.

Additional Resource

Kulakowski, E.C., & Chronister, L.U. (Eds.). (2006). *Research administration and management.* Burlington, MA: Jones & Bartlett Learning.

Chapter 19

Agreements and Contracts

Kelly Willenberg, MBA, BSN, CCRP, CHRC, and Mariel D. Norton, JD

Introduction

Clinical trial agreements are a very important part of the clinical trial process. For many people negotiating a clinical trial agreement, it is neither easy nor well understood. The contract between the sponsoring agency and a site (e.g., hospital, physician practice, research facility) must be established to protect both entities. The negotiation process is vital for a smooth and productive relationship from the beginning. All clinical trial studies should have a contract, if one is necessary with the sponsoring agency, in order to protect the clinical trials office, hospital administration, principal investigator, and clinical trial nurse.

The Agreement

The eight key areas that must be addressed with sponsors for a good clinical trial agreement are as follows (Model Agreements and Guidelines International, 2014).
- Confidentiality
- Indemnification
- Scope of work
- Intellectual property
- Dispute resolution
- Termination
- Medicare secondary payer clause regarding subject injury
- Health Insurance Portability and Accountability Act of 1996 (HIPAA)

Other areas that may be included are principal investigator responsibilities and compliance with various local, state, and federal laws. It is best practice to have agreements reviewed by a legal representative, or hospital representative, before signing them to ensure that the terms are understood. If an administrative or clinical person reviews the contract, he or she must be trained to understand the implications when negotiating contract language.

Confidentiality

The privacy of patient information, research development, and resulting data must be a critical aspect of the negotiation. Confidentiality considerations for a clinical trial contract need to focus on what information will be exchanged between the parties and how such information may be used, the roles of any and all individuals participating in the clinical trial, and the participants' concerns that may arise with use of confidential information. Protections for the security of confidential information need to be in place both during the clinical trial and after when the underlying contract has come to an end (National Institute of Environmental Health Sciences, n.d.; U.S. Department of Health and Human Services [DHHS] Office for Civil Rights, n.d.-a).

Indemnification

Indemnification and the potential ramifications for such a provision can become a source of dispute in any contract negotiation process. Under an indemnification provision or section, the parties set out the process by which one or both parties may *indemnify* or compensate the other party under particular circumstances. Specifically, the act of *indemnifying* is defined as the process "of providing reimbursement (to another) for a loss suffered because of a third party's or one's own act or default" (Garner, 2009, p. 337).

An indemnification clause or provision normally takes the form of a promise or agreement for one or both par-

Note. The authors are not providing legal advice, nor does this chapter create an attorney-client relationship. This may not be specific to your situation.

ties to compensate the other under particularly provided circumstances, such as damages caused by a party's breach of the contract or injuries and/or death occurring as a result of the acts of a party. The sponsoring agency and site must discuss which party will indemnify the other, what circumstances and damages must arise for the indemnification provisions to be triggered, and what injuries or damages may be reimbursed.

Scope of Work

Under any contractual arrangement, the parties should clearly set forth the nature and intent behind the contract. Specifically, the sponsoring agency and site should provide a *scope of work* provision or similar clauses, which specifically detail (a) the intent of the clinical trial contract, (b) the goals of the trial, (c) any and all deliverables to be created during the course of the contract, and (d) the tasks to be undertaken by each party for purposes of the clinical trial's completion. Although one section regarding the scope of work in a clinical trial contract may be all that is necessary, the nature of the underlying agreement may necessitate additional and numerous definitions of the scope of work. For example, if the contract is a partial agreement rather than a complete contract for purposes of the entire clinical trial, additional smaller definitions of the scope of work may be considered and negotiated separately as the clinical trial develops over time. During the negotiation process, it is important to consider the nature of the potential development in the scope of work as to both the sponsoring agency and site, and the parties may wish to consider smaller separate clinical trial agreements in combination with a master agreement, providing for smaller, separately defined scope of work provisions over the course of the clinical trial. Whether the scope of work is found in one individual section of the clinical trial contract or in the form of smaller gradually defined sections in separate phases of the contract over the course of the trial, parties should focus on negotiating and defining within the terms of their agreement a clear scope of work for both parties.

Intellectual Property

Clinical trial contract negotiation should address the issue of intellectual property rights. *Intellectual property* is defined in the U.S. Patent and Trademark Office (2013) glossary as "creations of the mind—creative works or ideas embodied in a form that can be shared or can enable others to recreate, emulate, or manufacture them; protected by trademark, trade secret or copyright." Because of the extensive nature of intellectual property law, the advice of specialized legal counsel should be considered.

Dispute Resolution

Similar to other contractual agreements, parties to a clinical trial contract must consider any potential disputes, disagreements, or misunderstandings that may arise after the negotiation and contract process is completed. During the life of a clinical trial and the underlying contract, disagreements and disputes may develop between the sponsoring agency and the site. Although some contractual disputes result in eventual legal action within the court system, additional methods for the resolution of disagreements currently exist to allow for any number of contractual terms regarding dispute resolution. Additionally, the parties may want to consider provisions regarding the choice of law or courts for resolution of disputes. Parties may also negotiate for costs associated with any resulting dispute resolution so that the prevailing party may receive a reimbursement of all legal fees, or parties may agree to split arbitrator or mediator costs under certain circumstances. Of course, the validity and applicability of such terms may change depending on state versus federal law implications or recognition of the provisions as valid under state law. In any event, parties to a clinical trial contract should consider the expansive contractual options for purposes of dispute resolution techniques to allow for a simplified and efficient method for resolving conflict in combination with, and potentially before, the need for legal action (ClinicalTrials.gov, n.d.; National Institute of Environmental Health Sciences, n.d.).

Payments

Payment sections can be problematic with regard to the revenue cycle and billing for both payers and sponsors. Some agreements will have flat-rate or fixed payments and should not be tied to the outcome of the trial. These tend to be more complicated in deciding what the sponsor is actually paying for in the patient care cost. A fee-for-service or line-item budget tends to be more transparent for compliance. This enables the site to be able to defend what the sponsor covered for each subject and what it paid for the staff time, including the principal investigator. In order to prepare a proper budget, a site should perform a coverage analysis. Reimbursable costs are usually part of the agreement or contract as well when items are not known or required for all subjects. Sites tend to find this demanding, as someone then must be responsible to actually produce invoices for payments. This arduous task can take hours to complete if the site has no method for tracking each subject or patient electronically. However, the process *must* be tracked in order to validate payments from sponsors at the site level. Investigators must be compensated based on the trial work (Pharmaceutical Research and Manufacturers of America, 2011).

Termination

Clinical trial agreements should address the circumstances and effects of termination. Although the completion of the clinical trial under the terms set forth in the original contract may provide one event triggering a termination of a contract, consideration for other circumstances should be negotiated and set out in a clinical trial contract. Termination should be allowed by both sides and should not be one-sided. Although the hope of any contract is for the terms and conditions to be performed in the entirety until final completion of the contract, the reality of contracting, as well as the logistics of research and funding, may necessitate a contract to be terminated by one or both parties before the agreed-upon end date. As a result, additional grounds for termination should be negotiated within the clinical trial contract to accommodate the potential need and resulting consequences of early termination of the contractual terms. Several things should be considered when preparing for additional termination conditions, for example, (a) the reasons for a termination of the contract, (b) the terms of payment in each circumstance, and (c) what must be considered if the reasons for termination were to arise for purposes of the underlying research and the participants. The valid ground for termination could be either ineffective treatment (to protect subjects from receiving the experimental drug) or clearly effective treatment (to give benefit of effective treatment to the control group). The other reasons for termination could be safety concerns if the side effects of the treatment are found to be unacceptable. Negotiations for the terms of termination in a clinical trial contract should address the process a termination will follow, considering the steps to be taken with pending research data, exchanged information and/or confidential documents, and the finalization of any clinical trial work. Whether termination clauses will be mutually applicable to both parties or not may also need to be explored during the negotiation process.

Medicare Secondary Payer Issues

Medicare secondary payer (MSP) issues continue to be a difficult issue for sponsors to understand. Often (sponsors are actually getting better not worse), the language in agreements contradicts MSP statutes, and the study site must insert proper language. Typical subject injury language in a clinical trial agreement may include the following: *Sponsor shall pay for all medically necessary services to diagnose and treat injury arising from participation in the trial if the subject's insurance rejects or denies coverage of the service.* The MSP statute states that Medicare is never a primary payer (e.g., payer of first resort) when another entity can be billed. If the above language is included, the sponsor must be billed. If the site bills Medicare instead, Medicare will consider that an overpayment, and the site will be required to reimburse Medicare or be subject to triple damages under the False Claims Act. Medicare views the sponsor as the liability plan or payer. Sponsors are insurers when they agree to pay for injuries arising from the trial (e.g., subject injury) in their clinical trial agreement (Centers for Medicare and Medicaid Services, 2014). Although such contract language obligates the sponsor to pay for related injuries, the sponsor may be able to limit their obligations by including language that excludes those manifestations of known and disclosed side effects. The sponsor is obligated only if there is an injury clause and the informed consent form states that medical care will be provided. The issue for most sites is properly billing an injury when it occurs. Another issue that sites encounter is ensuring that the agreement language does not match the informed consent language. Conscientious coordinators should watch for language in the body of the clinical trial agreement that limits payment. The clinical trial agreement should be very clear about the sponsor's responsibilities for covering subject injury.

Health Insurance Portability and Accountability Act

As in any contract associated with health information and documents, clinical trial contracts must include a set of provisions or entire sections regarding HIPAA (1996). Specific reporting requirements and instructions should be included in all contracts that may require the creation, access, transmission, or storage of information considered to be protected health information (PHI).

If a sponsoring entity of a clinical trial is deemed to be a covered entity or a business associate, the entities are responsible for meeting all requirements of the HIPAA Security Rule, the requirements of the Breach Notification Rule, and many of the provisions of the HIPAA Privacy Rule (HIPAA, 1996). Contracts related to clinical trials must address these requirements.

A *business associate* is an individual or company that performs any function or activity involving the creation, controlled access, use, disclosure, storage, or destruction of PHI. Business associates must also manage their subcontractors by having business associate agreements in place. Subcontractors must meet HIPAA requirements included in the Omnibus Rule. Business associates are subject to audit under the Office for Civil Rights ongoing auditing program that was defined in the Health Information Technology for Economic and Clinical Health (HITECH) law (U.S. DHHS Office for Civil Rights, n.d.-b).

Determining covered entity or business associate status is different in the research arena, where the Common Rule also applies. A researcher may be a business associate if the researcher performs a function, activity, or service for a covered entity that falls under the definition of business associate (e.g., healthcare operations such as creating a de-identified or limited data set for a covered entity). When an individual functions in both the researcher and business associate roles, that individual must return or destroy patient identifiers when the business associate role ends and the researcher role begins.

Before any contract award, the clinical trial sponsor should determine if and how any third parties will provide services deemed to involve PHI. When a vendor is identified, the sponsor must determine if the vendor has sufficient experience, knowledge, and infrastructure to provide the services and to satisfy the security, privacy, and breach notification requirements that must be included in the contract. Acting as a business associate, the vendor must meet requirements of 45 C.F.R. § 164.504(e) (Standard: Business Associate Contracts, 2009).

- The contract should include references to appropriate and timely data life cycle management procedures (i.e., procedures to be followed by both parties upon initial acquisition and use of data through the analysis and reporting of results, data storage and archival, and data destruction).
- The contract should require that the vendor supporting the project perform periodic audits and provide results to the contracting entity.
- The contract should provide that upon request, the contracting entity may obtain the business associate's privacy and security policies and documentation that the vendor's staff members have received appropriate HIPAA training before they access or use PHI on behalf of the contracting entity. The contracting entity may want to request a copy of an annual Statement on Standards for Attestation Engagements No. 16 audit or summary, if the vendor is responsible for administering and maintaining internal financial controls in protecting information assets.
- The contract should specify that upon termination or expiration of the contract, the business associate will destroy any PHI that is within its possession or control at that time. The contract also should specify the minimum standards that the vendor must follow to destroy any PHI and specify the allocation of costs for destruction of PHI upon termination or expiration of the contract.

Before execution, the contract for clinical trials should be reviewed for standard legal obligations, such as indemnification, right to audit, confidentiality, executed business associate agreement if PHI is involved, and appropriate support of duty performance (e.g., billing, certificate of accomplishment, progress reports, invoices) as required by the contracting entity to meet its various regulatory requirements.

It is critical that covered entities and business associates develop and manage effective working relationships and meet their contractual obligations to each other. As in any relationship, understanding the goals and regulatory requirements of the other party is important. Information regarding HIPAA compliance requirements for covered entities and business associates is available on the Phyllis A. Patrick & Associates LLC website (www.phyllispatrick.com).

Implications for Clinical Trial Nurses

In consideration of the competencies necessary to be a clinical trial nurse, bear in mind that many nurses do not receive adequate training in the area of agreements. The National Institutes of Health (NIH) Clinical Research Nursing Model of Care states, "The primary clinical research nurse is a clinical research nurse with expertise in clinical research implementation who practices in a specific clinical care area" (NIH Clinical Center Nursing and Patient Care Services, 2011, p. 3). The basic tenets of practice for primary clinical research nurses are expertise, accountability, continuum of care, and advocacy (NIH Clinical Center Nursing and Patient Care Services, 2011).

Protocol compliance includes the contract because it affects participants' consent process and how reimbursement will be handled by sites. A good clinical trial nurse will become familiar with and identify the protocol issues that are essential to the conduct of the study. This includes oncology clinical trial nurse competencies surrounding the requirements of the research protocol and good clinical research practice while remaining cognizant of the needs of diverse patient populations (Oncology Nursing Society, 2010). Understanding the regulations and guidance that mandate research agreements will assist clinical trial nurses in many ways while protecting and caring for patients.

Summary

The best advice is to *never* sign an agreement without knowing the meaning of the clauses and provisions written in it. Grasping the importance of regulations and guidance in the areas that impact an agreement will help not only the site but also the principal investigator. Encourage the principal investigator to understand the legalities of clinical trial agreements and seek counsel when necessary. Signing anything that is sent without a review by a specialized legal representative or adequate training is not recommended, and learning the meaning of what is signed will have a lasting impact.

Key Points
- Clinical trial nurses should be familiar with the legal obligations for the parties involved in the clinical trial.
- Clinical trial agreements contain specific language to address regulatory issues, such as HIPAA and PHI.
- Investigators should be aware of considerations when contracting with sponsors.

- The clinical trial agreement should include indemnification and protection for the site and the sponsor.
- Clinical trial nurses should be familiar with Medicare secondary payer clauses and how to bill in the case of participant injury.
- The scope of work for the site should be clearly defined within the clinical trial agreement.

References

Centers for Medicare and Medicaid Services. (2014, July 10). Mandatory insurer reporting (NGHP). Retrieved from http://www.cms.gov/Medicare/Coordination-of-Benefits-and-Recovery/Mandatory-Insurer-Reporting-For-Non-Group-Health-Plans/Overview.html

ClinicalTrials.gov. (n.d.). For study record managers. Retrieved from http://clinicaltrials.gov/ct2/help/for-manager

Garner, B.A. (Ed.). (2009). *Black's law dictionary* (9th ed.). St. Paul, MN: West Thomson Reuters.

Health Insurance Portability and Accountability Act of 1996, Pub. L. No. 104-191 (1996). Retrieved from http://www.cms.gov/Regulations-and-Guidance/HIPAA-Administrative-Simplification/HIPAAGenInfo/downloads/hipaalaw.pdf

Model Agreements and Guidelines International. (2014, August 13). MAGI's model clinical trial agreement [M1012 v.1.36]. Retrieved from https://magiworld.org/standards

National Institute of Environmental Health Sciences. (n.d.). Office of Human Research Compliance: Clinical research. Retrieved from https://www.niehs.nih.gov/research/clinical/join/ohrc/index.cfm

National Institutes of Health Clinical Center Nursing and Patient Care Services. (2011, July 6). Building the foundation for clinical research nursing: A clinical research nursing model of care. Retrieved from http://clinicalcenter.nih.gov/nursing/crn/CRN_Model_of_Care.pdf

Oncology Nursing Society. (2010). *Oncology clinical trials nurse competencies*. Retrieved from https://www.ons.org/sites/default/files/ctncompetencies.pdf

Pharmaceutical Research and Manufacturers of America. (2011, July). *Principles on conduct of clinical trials and communication of clinical trial results*. Retrieved from http://www.phrma.org/sites/default/files/pdf/042009_clinical_trial_principles_final_0.pdf

Standard: Business Associate Contracts, 45 C.F.R. § 164.504(e) (2009). Retrieved from http://www.gpo.gov/fdsys/pkg/CFR-2011-title45-vol1/pdf/CFR-2011-title45-vol1-sec164-504.pdf

U.S. Department of Health and Human Services Office for Civil Rights. (n.d.-a). Health information privacy. Retrieved from http://www.hhs.gov/ocr/privacy

U.S. Department of Health and Human Services Office for Civil Rights. (n.d.-b). Health information privacy: HITECH Act enforcement interim final rule. Retrieved from http://www.hhs.gov/ocr/privacy/hipaa/administrative/enforcementrule/hitechenforcementifr.html

U.S. Patent and Trademark Office. (2013). Intellectual property. Retrieved from http://www.uspto.gov/main/glossary/index.html#i

Chapter 20

Financial Risk Assessment and Monitoring

Connie M. Szczepanek, RN, BSN, and Lyndon Vestal Evans, RN, BS

Introduction

Healthcare providers and institutions are increasingly challenged with improving the response rate and quality of life of patients with cancer while reducing the costs of care. The cost of treating and caring for patients with cancer consumes 5% of the overall healthcare costs in the United States but involves only 0.5% of the population (Emanuel, 2013). As the population grows older and the healthcare workforce decreases, a crisis in delivering quality cancer care ensues. Clinical trial outcomes that affect and improve the practice of oncology care while containing costs are paramount in the battle against cancer. Oncology clinical trials need to be completed in a timely fashion and designed to answer pertinent questions to improve response rates, survival, and quality of life (Kurzrock et al., 2009).

Participation in clinical trials requires infrastructure that incurs financial investment and risk for the research site. The science and benefits of improving patient care and outcomes are often perceived to outweigh, but not eliminate, these risks. The margin between costs and revenue is typically very tight. Industry- or pharmaceutical-sponsored trials reimburse at a higher rate than cooperative or federally supported protocols, but even with a carefully analyzed budget in place, the funding may fail to cover the actual costs. Many clinical trial sites rely on supplemental financial support provided by their institutions to sustain operations, as the funding generated by the research itself may not be enough to fully fund operations (Seow et al., 2012).

Financial risks are present partially because of the variables outside the control of the investigative site. At the time of trial activation, unknowns include the number of study amendments, reconsents, adverse events, and serious adverse events that will occur during the life of the trial. These lead to increased salary costs because of time for trial oversight, regulatory burden, and clinical trial staff.

Financial risks are also associated with predictable factors, such as extra procedures, specimens, and rigorous scheduling of study-required events. The benefit of assessing the risk of predictable factors may substantially reduce the financial burden of the investigative site. No literature was found to measure the downstream financial effect of clinical trial activities at the investigative site, but research supports implementation of processes to evaluate and reduce the known financial risks of conducting oncology clinical trials (Snyder, 2008).

Answering research questions is dependent on timely enrollment of patients to well-designed trials, as well as efficient data collection and analysis; both are keys to addressing response rates and quality of life (Nass, Moses, & Mendelsohn, 2010). Cancer care must be affordable (Institute of Medicine [IOM], 2013). To keep investigative sites engaged in trial activities and enrolling subjects, the financial risks for the clinical trials department or team must be balanced with the benefits of participation. The ability of the site to periodically measure the financial risks and benefits helps the site build a sustainable research program.

Areas of Potential Financial Risks and Risk Reduction Strategies

One common theme noted in recent literature is the negative effect of opening clinical trials that do not meet either the overall or site-specific accrual goals (IOM, 2012b; Kanarek, Kanarek, Olatoye, & Carducci, 2012). Clinical trials that are unable to meet accrual goals cost the industry millions of dollars. Even more critical is the time lost in improving cancer care.

Although the literature did not specify the cost, experience of the authors would estimate the research site's cost to start up a clinical trial, even before enrolling the first subject, as between $2,000 and $8,000. Federally funded National Cancer Institute trials do not typically reimburse start-up or regulatory costs. Thorough evaluation of industry budgets and contracting for start-up fees can offset up-front costs for pharmaceutical trials.

Costs are also incurred to maintain regulatory and institutional review board (IRB) approvals. Every year of regulatory submissions without corresponding new patient enrollments results in an additional financial burden. Failure to enroll patients to trials opened or to meet accrual goals guarantees that the clinical research department will operate at a financial deficit and will be at risk of not being sustainable as an operation. One of the most common reasons for slow or no accrual is finding that clinical trials of interest are not actually feasible at the site level. If that discovery is made after a significant investment of resources, the degree of financial risk increases.

Strategies to Reduce Risk

A thorough feasibility review of each potential protocol prior to opening the study should help to identify if a site has the patient population, tools, and commitment to enroll, conduct, and complete the study. Effective risk reduction strategies include setting the program's direction (e.g., goals, timelines, priorities), partnering with research bases/sponsors that best fit, choosing protocols strategically, putting processes and tools in place, being aware of hidden costs, identifying invisible institutional barriers, and monitoring research finances.

Setting Program Direction: Goals, Timelines, and Priorities

The initial step in reducing financial risk is defining the mission, goals, and priorities for the research program that are agreed upon by the stakeholders. The stakeholders include the institution, the site researchers and team, medical providers, the community, and the patient base. Financial outcome measures and funding sources should also be agreed upon. These decisions will help guide setting the strategic plan and building the program structure needed to effectively conduct the selected clinical trials.

If the research program is primarily focused on participation in practice-changing phase III trials, a research protocol menu composed primarily of National Cancer Institute Cooperative Group trials may be a good fit. Infrastructure would most likely be built on a nonprofit funding model, which counts on additional in-kind support from the institution. These trials are generally funded with federal monies and have to be managed according to strict grants management rules.

If the expectation is to generate revenue, then a higher volume of industry-sponsored clinical trials may be a better fit. These trials tend to require significantly higher regulatory time and effort, which adds to costs.

If the mission is geared toward academics and a priority goal is publication, the clinical trials chosen may be very different from the institution whose mission and goals are to offer compassionate-use drugs to an indigent population. Budgeting for dedicated time—both for investigators and research staff—is essential. Funding for this type of research work may come out of general operational funds and is difficult to extract directly from accrual-driven payments.

Along with determining the type of research, balanced goals should be set regarding the number of clinical trials that the research team can manage at one time. The investigator and research team should meet regularly to review the status of studies being considered and then rank order priority in setting time frames. It is important to weigh the need for the trial and the science behind it with the cost of opening and sustaining the trial. It is critical to consider study acuity and complexity when laying out the timeline for opening new studies so that the research team can realistically meet deadlines.

It is also important to regularly reevaluate continuation of clinical trials. If there is no accrual after a specified time, the investigators should stop and ask questions: Is the study still relevant to the investigators, institution, and patients? Are additional education and recruitment strategies needed? Are there barriers that need to be addressed? At a minimum, it is wise to evaluate study activity at the time of each annual/continuing review.

Partnering With Research Bases and Sponsors That Best Fit the Institution's Mission

Develop partnerships and memberships with research bases and sponsors that will provide clinical trials that match the program goals. The community, patient base, clinical sites, community interests, and priorities are important factors to help guide the selection of research partners and protocols. Setting up a file with this information will enhance efficiency.

When identifying the best potential research base affiliations, determine if a single research base and sponsor will serve the needs of the program or if membership in several groups will be required. A particular sponsor or pharmaceutical company may focus on a specific disease site or type of trial (e.g., symptom management) or investigator-initiated research. Research sponsor offerings should match the needs of the population and program goals and be in step with the site's strategic plan.

One common perception is that the bigger the research membership or protocol list, the stronger a program will be. Although this outcome may follow long-term program growth, it should not be a starting point for a program. Investigators must be selective and judicious, choose trials that the institution can successfully implement to build a strong base, and work closely with selected sponsors to mutually understand expectations, set up membership structure, put agreements in place, and build a successful track record. This will reduce unexpected study implementation delays and prevent failure to meet study goals, which add to costs and increase financial risk. A strategic approach can open doors for future trials, further enhancing the funding stream.

Choosing Protocols Strategically

The first step in selecting protocols is to know what is needed by reviewing the types of cancers of the patients in the service area. Once potential trials to explore are decided upon, the investigators should start with a high-level assessment. Examples of questions to be considered include

- Is the patient base adequate to open and implement the clinical trials being considered?
- What will it take to reach these patients and to provide them with access (Penberthy, Dahman, Petkov, & DeShazo, 2012)?
- Are physician investigators interested in the study? Without physician champions, accrual to a study can be difficult.
- Are other clinical trials open that would compete?

This first-glance, in-depth review should be done for every study being considered, even before exploring the specifics of feasibility. Ideally, the decision to proceed to full feasibility review should be made through discussion with the site's principal investigator and program leadership.

It is important to periodically analyze the protocol menu to identify potential overlap as well as gaps; screening and accrual data should be regularly evaluated to ensure whether active protocols are being used and to determine why they are not before opening additional protocols.

Once high-level interest in a study concept is confirmed, a comprehensive feasibility review should be conducted. Although this process can be time-intensive, the up-front investment results in improved efficiency and better use of valuable resources. Some questions to consider are listed in Figure 20-1. Additional strategies to enhance protocol selection include

- Monitoring research base protocol lists and setting time to periodically review available clinical trials, as well as pending concepts, so as to maximize opportunities to participate in studies that fit the program goal. This will also allow proactive anticipation of studies that can prevent gaps in the protocol menu.
- Reevaluating studies that were ruled out in the past. Perhaps an original decision was made to decline or defer opening a clinical trial based on other trials currently open or concerns regarding logistics, such as staffing or workload balance. By tracking every study considered, as well as noting the rationale for decisions made, time will be saved in the long run and the base of available trials will broaden.
- Looking for innovative opportunities. Examples of strategies for long-term program viability include professional networking with other regional and national research organizations, active participation in protocol design and development with research base committees and thought leaders, working with young investigators, and partnering with research groups interested in the types of studies the institution is hoping to implement.

Putting Processes and Tools in Place

Standardizing processes and developing workflows will strengthen quality and consistency as well as reduce redundancy. The time saved is time that can be reallocated to program priorities. The use of a site-specific template or worksheet to document the elements of feasibility review will help standardize processes and prevent oversights that could later cause delays and result in patient and site burden and additional costs. This documentation can also serve as a guide for research team

Figure 20-1. Sample Comprehensive Feasibility Review Questions

- Does the study fill a need or gap, and does it match program vision and goals?
- Does the patient base at your site correlate with the projected accrual?
- Is there physician buy-in and support?
- Is it feasible from the research staff perspective?
- Are the recruitment plan and tools in place?
- What is the projected accrual? Are the accrual goals feasible? Your site may decide to open a trial for a rare cancer type with limited accrual expectations; by knowingly planning for that, you can balance the effort expended with trials that are more likely to accrue.
- What start-up activities will need to be completed (e.g., kits ordered, training, site initiation visit scheduled, drug on hand, agreements in place)?
- Is any nonroutine care involved?
- What other clinical care or other departments need to be involved (pathology, surgery, radiology)?
- Are correlative studies required?
- Does your site have the required technology?
- Is credentialing (procedural, site, staff, investigator) a prerequisite?
- What is the availability and expertise required of research staff?
- Has a study budget been completed, and is the funding sufficient to cover costs?
- Has a financial coverage analysis been completed?
- Are there special billing or coding concerns?
- Are the monitoring or auditing expectations realistic?

members once the study is opened (see Figure 20-2 for an example).

Efficiency can be enhanced by batching activities that need to be done multiple times, such as making educational packets, prepping mailings, shipping specimens, prepopulating form headers, and making labels. Developing standard operating procedures is a must. Creation of worksheets and documentation tools for repeated or tracked processes helps streamline the team's efforts and improves consistency.

It is important to verify the expectations of the research sponsors so as to design effective tracking and report tools. Commercial clinical trial software products are becoming more available but are not created equal. Principal investigators should select a product that best helps the site track and run reports in a manner consistent with research sponsor expectations and designate a site leader to serve as a resource and to monitor deadlines.

The site administrator should set up financial worksheets and reports to aid in tracking revenues due as well as actual costs. Setting up invoice templates and tracking spreadsheets is helpful when opening a clinical trial while the feasibility assessment is still fresh in everyone's minds. Not only will this enhance revenue capture, but the information also can be used to develop future study budgets.

Periodic mission evaluation, strategic planning, goal setting, and performance review will help keep a program dynamic. Investigators should anticipate holes in the protocol menu to prevent gaps and track previously declined trials for potential fit in the future. Evaluating the success of partnerships is a two-way process: ensuring that each sponsor meets the program goals and that the institution meets the expectations of the sponsor. Physician investigators, administrators, and research team members should be involved in clinical trial planning to build engagement. Innovative strategies should be considered for recruitment and to streamline processes. Process improvement tools and methods may be helpful to reduce the number of steps that do not add value (Pope, 2012).

Being Aware of Hidden Costs

Constructing and evaluating a study budget is a critical piece in a maintainable research program, as described in Chapter 18. The industry sponsor often provides a budget, but the institution must evaluate the proposal to ensure local institutional costs are covered. The costs of specific study procedures can be estimated, but staff time is more difficult to anticipate and predict. The assessment of staffing costs commonly includes time for consenting, enrolling, conducting required tests, administering agents, and collecting data, but additional hidden costs should be considered (see Table 20-1). Investigative sites will benefit by monitoring the hidden costs of staff and investigators' time over the course of the study (Emanuel, Schnipper, Kamin, Levinson, & Lichter, 2003). Time and effort logs are valuable tools to help identify these costs. Berridge and Coffey (2008) conducted a workload study to measure tasks and the associated time for an oncology study. As a result of their work, an instrument was developed and validated in 2011. The exercise of recording time for tasks through an instrument such as Berridge and Coffey's is of great assistance in identifying hidden costs.

Identifying Invisible Institutional Barriers

Invisible barriers may exist when steps and tasks are duplicated or perceived as wasteful. Tasks should be evaluated to ensure they add value to study activities and organizational mission. A process map may give a snapshot of these tasks and help identify and minimize activities that do not add value (Dilts & Sandler, 2006). Lean Six Sigma principles or other methods of process improvement may offer a manner to reduce wasteful steps and improve efficiency in the process of taking a trial from initial consideration to closure (Schweikhart & Dembe, 2009). Lean Six Sigma focuses on root cause so that effective change can be implemented. Pope (2012) detailed the success of employing this methodology with an IRB and a sponsor.

Key decision makers should consider the point at which the clinical trial is introduced to the institution and ensure that the person taking the call has the knowledge and authority to reject a trial when the objectives fail to meet the goals set by the stakeholders. The ability to turn down a trial during the first phone call of introduction saves valuable time. Sponsors frequently request completion of lengthy feasibility forms, confidentiality disclosure agreements requiring multiple signatures, and possible conference calls only to lead to the site turning down the trial because of competing studies. A knowledgeable person at the first point of contact, therefore, should be identified.

Contract and budget review may involve more than one party. All parties involved should identify absolute deal-breakers and triage these key items before the in-depth review. For example, the financial team may have minimum start-up fees in the budget, and legal may only accept the local state of law in the contract review. These deal-breaker items could be assigned to one party as the initial step. Simultaneous reviews can reduce the time from receiving a study to the first enrollee, but a careful evaluation of what points need to be agreed upon prior to initiating simultaneous reviews is critical. For example, if budget and contract review and IRB submission occur simultaneously, at what point will the investigators compare the consent to the budget? A change in the budget

Figure 20-2. Protocol Feasibility Review Worksheet	
PROTOCOL NUMBER/TITLE:	
Study start-up issues	
Recruitment and tools needed	
Projected accrual	
Pre-study requirements	
Registration requirements	
Treatment issues	Surgery
	Chemotherapy
	Radiation therapy
	Other
Nonroutine care issues	Radiology
	Tumor measurements
	Lab
	Other
Drug ordering/management	
Data management/case report forms	
Ancillary or correlative studies	Pathology
	Specimen collection
	Quality of life
	Other
Credentialing or training needed	
Feasibility issues	Clinical
	Finance
	Billing/coding
	Regulatory
	Monitoring/auditing
	Other
Funding issues	
COMMENTS:	
Reviewed by: Team Member Name_____ Date_____	

Note. The authors would like to express their gratitude to the Research Team at the Grand Rapids Clinical Oncology Program, who continue to learn and grow together as a team to develop best practices and tools similar to these particular tools in order to enhance clinical trials research.

Table 20-1. Hidden Costs in the Start-Up Process

Element	Description
Obtaining the protocol	This involves taking calls from sponsors; completing the confidentiality disclosure agreement; obtaining signatures; legal review (if required); submitting the confidentiality disclosure agreement to the sponsor; reading, responding, and redirecting multiple emails; and answering phone calls related to obtaining the protocol.
Completing the sponsor's feasibility review and associated forms	The feasibility review may require running reports from the cancer registry or medical records, calls, or meetings with the investigator and sponsor.
Obtaining team consensus	The team or stakeholders meeting may be necessary to assess feasibility and gain consensus to move forward with opening the trial.
Scheduling and preparation for the qualification visit and site initiation visit	Multiple phone calls and emails may be required to confirm attendees and block facilities and schedules. Assessing study materials that are available for the site initiation visit should occur. Rescheduling the visit because of unforeseen changes in travel plans may have to occur as well.
Obtaining contract and legal review	This requires obtaining multiple signatures, performing local document management, and returning executed documents to the sponsor.
Preparing institutional review board and regulatory submissions	Regulatory preparation includes the time to present and follow up with the institutional review board of record.
Obtaining pharmacy review	The pharmacy department will review for feasibility, development of order sets, and storage setup.
Preparing for enrolling patients	This involves obtaining interactive voice response system passwords, credentialing, and Web data training follow-up to ensure all parties have the tools needed for the study.
Conducting Medicare coverage analysis and billing setup	The number of departments and staff involved in this process increases the cost.
Opening the study	This involves staff announcement, addition to the website, adding to pocket cards or booklets, alerting referring physicians, and training and documentation of training.
Screening activities	If study subjects will be identified through the current patient pool, less screening costs may be incurred than in a population requiring a detailed recruitment plan. In a study requiring a specific pathologic marker, estimating the number of screen fails to identify an eligible patient may assist in identifying a hidden cost.
Informed consent process	Time involved with the informed consent process varies based on protocol complexity. A registration study may take additional minutes of the investigator's time and one hour of the research staff time as compared to a three-arm randomized trial, which may take an hour of the investigator's time and many hours of research staff time.
Scheduling extra procedures	The time involved in scheduling and notifying patients of tests and follow-up of test results should be noted. Accounting for the time involved with locating space and preparing for ancillary tests such as neurocognitive testing or quality-of-life questionnaires is necessary for the conduct of the trial.
Communicating eligibility questions	Telephone calls and emails to the project manager and internal quality assurance activities are completed to confirm eligibility.
Pharmacy staff activities	The staff order, receive, log, store, and reconcile investigational items. The pharmacy may be responsible for training associated staff at multiple locations on the investigational product.
An unreliable patient population	Patients who miss appointments or have transportation issues and require rescheduling increase the risk of filing deviation reports.
Reporting adverse events	Studies requiring reporting of all adverse events cost more in staff time than those requiring reporting of only grade 3 or 4 events. A phase I or II study may have more adverse events than a phase III study.
Capturing the details of all prior cancer treatments	The case report form may ask for a summary versus list of each drug and dose, which affects data management time.
Reporting all subsequent cancer treatments	Studies requiring survival information during the follow-up period will involve less work than those asking for subsequent treatment details.

(Continued on next page)

Table 20-1. Hidden Costs in the Start-Up Process *(Continued)*	
Element	Description
Monitor the visits (change in monitors and multiple monitors)	The sponsor-required monitoring plan can affect staff time. Consider the number of times the monitor needs to meet with the investigator and pharmacy and the percent of chart monitored.
Close-out	Hidden costs associated with close-out include time for preparation, scheduling attendees, and participating in the close-out visit; pharmacy staff reconciling, returning investigational drugs, and meeting with monitor; packing and sending study materials to storage as well as notifying the sponsor of this activity; IRB and subject notification of study closure; fielding calls from subjects and study team due to study closure; and updating website, pocket cards or protocol booklets, medical records, and study team of change in protocol status.

can cause a change in the consent, leading to an additional IRB submission. Does the pharmacy or other ancillary departments review the study at the time of feasibility review or at the time of IRB submission? Each task to open a study should build upon the previous step.

IRB review and tasks related to protection of human subjects may occur at multiple institutions and on federal and state levels as required by the local institution. Multiple reviews may be perceived as duplicative or as an unavoidable obligation to human subjects. The literature supports the view that a multiple review process is costly, and appropriately reducing regulatory costs is necessary for the clinical trial system (IOM, 2012a).

Monitoring Research Finances

Financial reporting and monitoring are rarely topics in the training of oncology nurses. Clinical research departments may set expected metrics or key indicators, such as new accrual per full-time employee, number of weighted subjects per full-time employee, or number enrolled as compared to number of new patients with cancer. Although hospital administration may question research revenue, workload measurement—not financial performance—is the more commonly generated report (Snyder, 2008). Research teams may find it beneficial to set defined benchmarks to measure their work, so as to have data to share with administration to support their efforts. Oncology clinical research departments rarely, if ever, include financial profit as a primary mission. Net profit can be useful to trend and can be measured for the overall clinical research department and for each study.

Snyder (2010) recommended that research institutions consider the use of a clinical trial management system as a tool for managing productivity and finances. These products are available from multiple sources and can often be tailored to the needs of the local department. Clinical trial management systems are designed to automate many of the financial tasks for the research nurses and clinical investigators (see Chapter 38). Billing errors and subsequent loss of revenue or fines is addressed in Chapter 18. A research department should have processes to monitor, report, and correct billing errors.

Profit and loss analysis may give a snapshot, but it fails to truly capture the full financial effect of research in an institution. Methods to comprehensively monitor research finances are complicated, and the literature does not identify proven methodology for cancer clinical trial programs. The downstream effect of a research program may be the primary benefit to the institution, which is difficult, if not impossible, to measure. A few downstream effects include fees for protocol procedures, patients choosing an institution over a competitor because of research offerings, patients' perception that a research institution offers the best care on- or off-study, and increased team experience with investigational agents, which results in efficient care to patients after the drug is on the market.

Summary

Each institution has unique processes for obtaining, reviewing, opening, and conducting clinical trials. The involved parties at the institution may have different points of view and different goals during the process. The foundation of a successful program lies in developing a well-defined mission and goals and a strategic plan all agreed upon by the stakeholders.

Ensuring that accrual goals can be met through an in-depth feasibility process is critical. Building awareness of potential hidden costs and proactively reducing those expenses can ease the department's financial risk. Comprehensive monitoring of research finances is a challenge and is worth further study and investigation to ensure oncology research is positioned for success.

Key Points
- All stakeholders should be involved in setting goals and completing periodic evaluations.
- Research partners should be identified to provide appropriate studies for the institution.

- Feasibility review tools should be implemented to conserve resources.
- Hidden costs and institutional barriers can be identified and addressed through process mapping.
- Methods to monitor research finances should be investigated.

References

Berridge, J., & Coffey, M. (2008, June). Workload measurement: How one workload study measured tasks, time, and resources necessary to run a cancer clinical trial today. *Applied Clinical Trials.* Retrieved from http://www.appliedclinicaltrialsonline.com/appliedclinicaltrials/article/articleDetail.jsp?id=522055

Dilts, D.M., & Sandler, A.B. (2006). Invisible barriers to clinical trials: The impact of structural, infrastructural, and procedural barriers to opening oncology clinical trials. *Journal of Clinical Oncology, 24,* 4545–4551. doi:10.1200/JCO.2005.05.0104

Emanuel, E. (2013, March 23). A plan to fix cancer care [Opinion]. *New York Times Online.* Retrieved from http://opinionator.blogs.nytimes.com/2013/03/23/a-plan-to-fix-cancer-care

Emanuel, E.J., Schnipper, L.E., Kamin, D.Y., Levinson, J., & Lichter, A.S. (2003). The costs of conducting clinical research. *Journal of Clinical Oncology, 21,* 4145–4150. doi:10.1200/JCO.2003.08.156

Institute of Medicine. (2012a). *Envisioning a transformed clinical trials enterprise in the United States: Establishing an agenda for 2020* [Workshop summary]. Retrieved from http://www.nap.edu/catalog.php?record_id=13345

Institute of Medicine. (2012b). *Public engagement and clinical trials: New models and disruptive technologies* [Workshop summary]. Retrieved from http://www.nap.edu/catalog.php?record_id=13237

Institute of Medicine. (2013). *Delivering affordable cancer care in the 21st century* [Workshop summary]. Retrieved from http://books.nap.edu/catalog.php?record_id=18273

Kanarek, N.F., Kanarek, M.S., Olatoye, D., & Carducci, M.A. (2012). Removing barriers to participation in clinical trials: A conceptual framework and retrospective chart review study. *Trials, 13,* 237. doi:10.1186/1745-6215-13-237

Kurzrock, R., Pilat, S., Bartolazzi, M., Sanders, D., Hood, J.V., Tucker, S.D., ... Bast, R.C., Jr. (2009). Project Zero Delay: A process for accelerating the activation of cancer clinical trials. *Journal of Clinical Oncology, 27,* 4433–4440. doi:10.1200/JCO.2008.21.6093

Nass, S.J., Moses, H.L., & Mendelsohn, J. (Eds.). (2010). *A national cancer clinical trials system for the 21st century: Reinvigorating the NCI Cooperative Group Program.* Retrieved from http://www.nap.edu/catalog.php?record_id=12879

Penberthy, L.T., Dahman, B.A., Petkov, V.I., & DeShazo, J.P. (2012). Effort required in eligibility screening for clinical trials. *Journal of Oncology Practice, 8,* 365–370. doi:10.1200/JOP.2012.000646

Pope, D. (2012, October 9). Lean Six Sigma in the clinical trial industry: Two perspectives. *Applied Clinical Trials.* Retrieved from http://www.appliedclinicaltrialsonline.com/appliedclinicaltrials/article/articleDetail.jsp?id=791938

Schweikhart, S.A., & Dembe, A.E. (2009). The applicability of Lean and Six Sigma techniques to clinical and translational research. *Journal of Investigational Medicine, 57,* 748–755.

Seow, H.-Y., Whelan, P., Levine, M.N., Cowan, K., Lysakowski, B., Kowaleski, B., ... Arnold, A. (2012). Funding oncology clinical trials: Are cooperative group trials sustainable? *Journal of Clinical Oncology, 30,* 1456–1461. doi:10.1200/JCO.2011.37.2698

Snyder, A. (2008, July 1). A Dow Jones for sites: Real-time financial performance indicator for clinical research sites that answers the question, "How are we doing?" *Applied Clinical Trials.* Retrieved from http://www.appliedclinicaltrialsonline.com/appliedclinicaltrials/Articles/A-Dow-Jones-for-Sites/ArticleStandard/Article/detail/527740

Snyder, A. (2010, July 1). CTMS can provide business intelligence for sites. *Applied Clinical Trials.* Retrieved from http://www.appliedclinicaltrialsonline.com/appliedclinicaltrials/Articles/CTMS-Can-Provide-Business-Intelligence-for-Sites/ArticleStandard/Article/detail/678140

Chapter 21

Internal Financial Audit and Quality Assurance

D. Marie Jackson, PhD, MBA, and Douglas C. Stahl, PhD, MBA

Introduction

The clinical trial life cycle can be described as a complex series of process steps, many of which involve various forms of financial management. Each financial process step can generate one or more defects or *failure modes* that vary in terms of severity, likelihood of detection, and frequency of occurrence. As the complexity of clinical research increases over time, organizations are increasingly dependent upon the design, implementation, and continuous improvement of internal financial control systems. This chapter summarizes a broad range of issues and recommendations for clinical trial financial management and quality assurance. It also presents a technique called *failure mode and effects analysis* (FMEA) that can be used to characterize, prioritize, and minimize the most significant risks in your organization.

Definitions of Terms

Clinical trial nurses should understand the definitions of the following terms to fully grasp the purpose of a clinical trial internal financial audit.
- *Audit* is a systematic and independent examination of trial-related activities and documents to determine whether the evaluated trial-related activities were conducted and the data were recorded, analyzed, and accurately reported according to the protocol, the sponsor's standard operating procedures, good clinical practice, and the applicable regulatory requirements (International Conference on Harmonisation of Technical Requirements for Registration of Pharmaceuticals for Human Use [ICH], 1996).
- *Failure mode and effects analysis* (FMEA) is a systematic method of identifying and preventing product and process problems before they occur (McDermott, Mikulak, & Beauregard, 2009).
- *Quality assurance* is a system of planned and systematic actions established to ensure that a clinical trial is performed and data are generated, documented (recorded), and reported in compliance with good clinical practice and all applicable regulatory requirements (ICH, 1996).
- *Quality system* is the sum of all aspects of a system that implements quality policy and ensures that quality objectives are met (ICH Steering Committee, 2005).

Background

Financial audit and quality assurance are key components of an overall quality system that can be used to assess and improve performance in
- Compliance with applicable policies, procedures, regulations, and contractual obligations
- Efficiency and cost of operations
- Effectiveness of internal controls.

At the U.S. federal level, the Centers for Medicare and Medicaid Services (CMS) issued a National Coverage Determination (NCD) for Routine Costs in Clinical Trials in the *Medicare National Coverage Determinations Manual* (Boyd & Meade, 2007; CMS, 2014). The NCD sets policy and provides the basic framework for establishing a compliant research billing program, including separate billing for research versus conventional care, and the categories of items and services covered by Medicare for patients on clinical trials. For items and services furnished on or after July 9, 2007 (CMS, 2007a), Medicare covers the routine costs of qualifying clinical trials, along with items and services deemed necessary for the diagnosis and treatment of complications arising from study participation. Medicare coverage generally excludes the investigational item or service itself, other items and services used solely for research purposes, and anything provided free of charge by clinical trial sponsors for research subjects.

In addition to federal regulations, some states have laws that provide coverage for conventional care tests, procedures, and services provided during a patient's participation as a research subject. For example, the state of California requires all California insurers, including the state's Medicaid program, to provide this level of coverage (California Senate, 2001). The National Cancer Institute (2012) maintains a summary of state-level legislation and agreements requiring health plans to pay the cost of routine medical care received by patients participating in a clinical trial.

The financial management of clinical trial tests, procedures, and services often involves many people and functional areas (see Figure 21-1). It is important to integrate and coordinate roles, responsibilities, policies, procedures, and information among the functional areas. General guidelines and best practices can be found in Figure 21-2.

The Financial Audit Process

A clinical research financial audit begins with the collection and review of important documents (see Figure 21-3). The symptoms of many financial process defects present as discrepancies within and among documents. The budget grid should include all billable tests, procedures, and services defined within the protocol. The consent form should clarify the patient's financial responsibilities and the sources of funds for all other research items, including subject injuries and adverse events. Any items listed as *free* in the consent documentation cannot be billed to the patient. The clinical trial agreement and the notice of grant award must align with the budget grid and consent documentation.

The list of patients enrolled on a protocol and their on- and off-study dates can be used with the budget grid to establish a chronologic time frame for reviewing patient bills. Some organizations have automated charge filtering and bill scrubbing systems, whereas others perform these processes manually. In either scenario, each item on each patient bill must be reviewed to confirm that it was charged to the correct payer. While comparing each bill with the budget grid, the medical record should be reviewed to confirm accurate documentation and coding.

Additional checks should include who has access to the financial systems and whether their access is appro-

---

Figure 21-2. General Guidelines for Financial Management of Clinical Trials

- Identify all sources of financial support (e.g., insurance, industry, grant, internal).
- Perform a coverage analysis to determine if/how charges will be reimbursed.
- Create a budget grid from the protocol study calendar (see Chapter 18). Ensure that all components of a covered procedure are included—for example, if breast biopsies are being done under ultrasound guidance, be certain that the ultrasound is included as well as the breast biopsy, or if a bone marrow aspiration and biopsy are being done, all testing done on that bone marrow needs to be included in the charge because the tests will not be paid for if no procedure is associated with them.
- Ensure adherence to policies and procedures for registration and scheduling of study-related tests, procedures, and services.
- Notify all applicable staff, hospitals, ancillary departments, and other entities that the patient is on a clinical trial.
- Track all research subjects in real time to document when they go on and off a clinical trial.
- Identify all tests, procedures and services as "research" or "standard of care" at the time they are ordered (Centers for Medicare and Medicaid Services, 2007b).
- Reconcile all bills and invoices with the budget grid before submitting for third-party reimbursement.
- Create a robust internal audit program to ensure processes are efficient, effective, and compliant.

Figure 21-1. Examples of Staff and Departments Involved in the Financial Management of Clinical Trials

- Physicians/investigators
- Clinical trials office (clinical research associates, study coordinators, nurses)
- Institutional review board
- Contracting/technology transfer
- Research finance and billing
- Medical center billing/physician professional billing and coding
- Department administrators and study fund managers
- Information technology
- Registration
- Scheduling
- Medical records and coding
- Pharmacy, lab, and other ancillary services
- Compliance
- General counsel
- Internal audit

Figure 21-3. Documents Used in a Clinical Trial Financial Audit

- Clinical trial research protocol
- Informed consent: Identify anything listed as *free of charge*
- Coverage analysis
- Budget grid, including the delineation of research and standard-of-care items
- Clinical trial agreement and/or notice of grant award
  - Who pays for subject injury and adverse events?
  - If grant funded, time and effort reports
- List of patients on and off study and their bills
- Source documentation in medical record
- Access to the systems that transmit and store financial data
- Complaints and feedback from stakeholders (e.g., patients, sponsors, third-party payers)

priate. Review the storage and backup plan for the financial data. Stakeholder feedback and patient complaints may provide additional insights about process defects and opportunities for improvement.

The audit process should be documented using a standardized format, and the final report should be reviewed with all stakeholders. All findings, recommendations, responsible individuals, and action item due dates should be clearly communicated, acknowledged, and tracked. Figure 21-4 lists components of a standard audit report.

Failure Mode and Effects Analysis as a Quality System Framework

In addition to an internal audit program, organizations can benefit from a more systematic approach for identifying, prioritizing, and eliminating process defects. Through the application of FMEA, defects are documented, scored, and prioritized according to the severity of consequences, frequency of occurrence, and ease of detection (McDermott et al., 2009). The FMEA for an organization's clinical research financial management processes would proceed through the following general steps (Tague, 2005).

- Identify all key process steps of interest.
- List the potential failure modes for each step.
- For each failure mode, list all potential effects, causes, and current process controls, if any.
- Rate the severity (S) of each effect on a scale from 1–10, where 1 is insignificant and 10 is catastrophic.
- Rate each failure mode's frequency of occurrence (O) on a scale from 1–10, where 1 is extremely unlikely and 10 is inevitable.
- Rate the likelihood of detection (D) for each process control on a 1–10 scale, where 1 means the control is certain to detect the problem and 10 means the control will not detect the problem or no control exists.
- Calculate the *risk priority number* (RPN) by multiplying S × O × D. RPN values provide guidance for ranking potential failures in the order they should be addressed.

- Identify countermeasures to lower severity, improve detection, and reduce frequency of occurrence. Note who is responsible for the countermeasures and target completion dates.
- As actions are completed, recalculate RPN values and reprioritize risks as necessary.

See Figure 21-5 for an example of a FMEA that a bank might use for an automated teller machine.

Although the individual category scores, recommended actions, responsible parties, and target completion dates will vary by institution, FMEA can be applied to a broad range of processes and products. To further illustrate this approach for clinical research financial management, a FMEA grid is presented in Table 21-1. Note that the scores for each failure mode are not included because these will be institution dependent. The countermeasures are possible solutions to consider for each failure mode but will be institution specific based on the potential causes.

Summary

According to Ratti (2009),

> A strong proactive approach, rather than a reactive approach, may alleviate the problem of billing errors and provide much-needed clarity to the labyrinthine billing process. Not only does the risk of becoming liable for civil and criminal penalties warrant scrupulously accurate billing activities, but also the associated potential for a tarnished reputation of the research enterprise from negative federal audits, whistleblower suits, and expensive fines. (p. 47)

Through careful integration of audit and quality assurance processes, organizations can decrease wasteful spending, increase cost recovery, and improve billing compliance.

Key Points
- As the complexity of clinical research increases over time, organizations are increasingly dependent upon the design, implementation, and continuous improvement of internal financial control systems.
- Financial audit and quality assurance are key components of an overall quality system that can be used to assess and improve performance.
- The financial management of clinical trial tests, procedures, and services often involves many people and functional areas. It is, therefore, important to integrate and coordinate roles, responsibilities, policies, procedures, and information.
- The symptoms of many financial process defects present as discrepancies within and among documents.
- FMEA can be used to characterize, prioritize, and minimize risks and process defects.

Figure 21-4. Components of a Standard Audit Report

- Purpose
- Background
- Audit approach/methodology
- Executive summary of findings
- Recommendations
- Conclusions
- Planned action log
- Detailed findings and supporting data
- List of auditors, contributors, process participants, and report recipients

Figure 21-5. An Example of Failure Mode and Effects Analysis (FMEA) for the Cash Dispensing Function of an Automated Teller Machine (ATM)

Process	Potential Failure Mode	Potential Effect(s) of Failure	S	Potential Cause(s) of Failure	O	Current Process Controls	D	RPN	Recommended Action(s)	Responsibility and Target Completion Date
Dispense amount of cash requested by customer	ATM does not dispense cash	Very dissatisfied customer	8	Out of cash	5	Internal low cash sensor	5	200		
		Cash balance discrepancy		Machine jams	3	Internal jam alert	7	168		
				Power failure during transaction	2	None	10	160		
	ATM dispenses too much cash	Bank loses money	6	Bills stick together	2	Shuffle bills before loading	7	84		
		Cash balance discrepancy		Bills in wrong trays	3	Two-person visual inspection	4	72		
	ATM takes too long to dispense cash	Customer somewhat annoyed	3	Heavy computer network traffic	7	None	10	210		
				Power interruption during transaction	2	None	10	60		

D—detection rating; O—occurrence rating; RPN—risk priority number; S—severity

Potential failure modes, causes, effects, and process controls are documented and scored on a scale from 1–10 to calculate each failure mode's RPN. As recommended actions are completed, RPN values are recalculated to reprioritize risks and risk mitigation projects.

Note. From *The Quality Toolbox* (2nd ed., p. 238), by N.R. Tague, 2005, Milwaukee, WI: ASQ Quality Press. Copyright 2005 by ASQ Quality Press, http://asq.org. Adapted with permission. No further distribution allowed without permission.

Table 21-1. Failure Mode and Effects Analysis Grid for Clinical Trials

Process	Potential Failure Mode	Effects of Failure	Potential Causes	Possible Countermeasures
Budget construction	Failure to properly identify standard of care versus research Failure to build budget grid for all study sponsors	Incorrect billing: leaving money on the table; double billing Increased financial burden to patients with co-pays and deductibles Possible violation of laws and regulations Insufficient budget to cover costs	Budget grid not constructed properly Lack of understanding by investigator, research staff, or support staff Lack of clarity on budget legend	Conduct a coverage analysis, which allows for accurate and consistent decisions. Standardize budget grid definitions and construction process. Conduct mandatory training for staff. Create a budget grid for every study that generates patient charges.
	Failure to identify that a study is deemed qualifying	Incorrect billing	Lack of knowledge regarding when a study is deemed qualifying or not in the eyes of CMS	Create a standard template interpreting the CMS guidelines that outlines what studies are deemed qualifying.

(Continued on next page)

Table 21-1. Failure Mode and Effects Analysis Grid for Clinical Trials *(Continued)*				
Process	Potential Failure Mode	Effects of Failure	Potential Causes	Possible Countermeasures
Research administration/finances (RAF)	Failure to invoice sponsor for pass-through costs (invoiceables) or research-only tests or procedures	RAF unaware that invoiceable item occurred	Loss of revenue Clinical staff unaware of budget grid Lack of communication between clinical staff and RAF RAF backlogged in sending invoices Ancillary services unaware that patient is on clinical trial	Utilize preprinted research order sets. Implement software solutions such as alerts or flags.
	Failure to allocate surpluses or cover deficits appropriately after study closure	Spend money on unallowable expenses, such as luncheons, travel, or gifts Can be viewed as a kickback	Lack of internal controls for spending Possible incentives for questionable billing practices to cause nondisclosure of conflicts	Develop, provide training on, and implement an institutional residual policy.
	Failure to locate payments	Decrease in revenue	Check misplaced or misdirected Lack of process for billing and debiting against the study budget	Establish a central location for checks to be placed, such as a lockbox.
Billing staff	Failure to apply codes and modifiers	Incorrect billing: leaving money on the table; double billing Denials from Medicare	Billing staff unaware that patient is on clinical trial Billing staff unaware that test or service is associated with a clinical trial	Register patient twice: once as a patient and then as a subject. Utilize separate research order sets. Develop a good relationship with local Medicare medical director.
	Failure to follow Medicare rules	Office of Inspector General audit Pay fines/jail time Reputation damage Loss of Medicare funding	Lack of knowledge regarding rules Lack of knowledge on how to interpret or apply rules	Establish a coverage analysis. Train staff on coverage analysis.
Contracting	Failure of principal investigator/staff to follow terms of contract	Incorrect billing Potential insurance fraud or false claims	Staff unaware Lack of knowledge or training	Develop a template for distilling and communicating terms that affect study execution.
Clinical staff documentation	Failure to document tests and procedures	Incorrect billing Unable to bill what is not properly documented	Overburdened clinical staff with competing priorities Lack of knowledge that patient is on a clinical trial	Create standard dictation templates for research.
Hospital billing or physician billing	Failure to segregate bill properly	Incorrect billing	Staff unaware Lack of knowledge or training	Create a research charge master. Train staff.
Legal	Failure to manage physician referrals when a financial conflict of interest is present	Physicians receive money from referrals, directly or indirectly	Staff unaware of Stark Law Misinterpret law Willfully breaking law	Educate physicians and staff on Stark Law.

References

Boyd, C.E., & Meade, R.D. (2007). Clinical trial billing compliance at academic medical centers. *Academic Medicine, 82,* 646–653. doi:10.1097/ACM.0b013e318065bb4d

California Senate. (2001). California Senate Bill SB37. Retrieved from http://info.sen.ca.gov/pub/01-02/bill/sen/sb_0001-0050/sb_37_bill_20010810_chaptered.html

Centers for Medicare and Medicaid Services. (2007a, July 9). Decision memo for clinical trial policy (CAG-00071R). Retrieved from http://www.cms.gov/medicare-coverage-database/details/nca-decision-memo.aspx?NCAId=186&ver=26&NcaName=Clinical+Trial+Policy+(1st+Recon)&bc=BEAAAAAEAAA&&fromdb=true

Centers for Medicare and Medicaid Services. (2007b, September 21). *Unlabeled use for anti-cancer drugs: Medical literature used to determine medically accepted indications for drugs and biologicals used in anti-cancer treatment* [Pub. 100-02 Medicare Benefit Policy]. Retrieved from http://www.cms.gov/Regulations-and-Guidance/Guidance/Transmittals/downloads/R78BP.pdf

Centers for Medicare and Medicaid Services. (2014, May 28). *Medicare national coverage determinations manual: Coverage determinations.* Retrieved from http://www.cms.gov/Regulations-and-Guidance/Guidance/Manuals/Downloads/ncd103c1_Part4.pdf

ICH Steering Committee. (2005). ICH Q9: Quality risk management. Retrieved from http://ec.europa.eu/health/files/eudralex/vol-10/3cc1aen_en.pdf

International Conference on Harmonisation of Technical Requirements for Registration of Pharmaceuticals for Human Use. (1996, June 10). *ICH harmonised tripartite guideline: Guideline for good clinical practice, E6(R1).* Retrieved from http://www.fda.gov/downloads/Drugs/Guidances/ucm073122.pdf

McDermott, R.E., Mikulak, R.J., & Beauregard, M.R. (2009). *The basics of FMEA* (2nd ed.). New York, NY: Productivity Press.

National Cancer Institute. (2012). States requiring coverage of clinical trial costs. Retrieved from http://www.cancer.gov/ncicancerbulletin/051810/page5

Ratti, P. (2009, October). Billing errors in clinical research. *Monitor,* pp. 42–47. Retrieved from http://www.lsuhospitals.org/Documents/news/11823-09-Ratti_42.pdf

Tague, N.R. (2005). *The quality toolbox* (2nd ed.). Milwaukee, WI: ASQ Quality Press.

Chapter 22

Financial Conflict of Interest

Tammie L. Bain, BS, JD

Introduction

Healthcare providers and institutions of higher education have a strong duty to protect the general public, especially patients. The public must be able to trust that the health care provided by, and the information disseminated from, these entities is accurate and unbiased. Therefore, federal agencies, particularly those that provide funding for research activities, are generating and tightening regulations related to conflict of interest (COI). On its grants and funding website, the National Institutes of Health (NIH) quotes its director, Dr. Francis Collins: "The public trust in what we do is just essential, and we cannot afford to take any chances with the integrity of the research process" (NIH, 2014). It is because of this trust that for-profit entities are so keen to partner with independent healthcare providers and academics within the United States. The public is far more willing to participate in research activities or believe a claim if provided by an independent healthcare provider or institution of higher education than if provided directly by a pharmaceutical company.

Background

Since passage of the Bayh-Dole Act in 1980, which allowed individuals and institutions to retain rights to intellectual property developed using federal funds, research collaborations between industry and institutions of higher education have been increasing. Along with these collaborations come increasingly complex financial relationships. According to Henderson and Smith (2002) in their law review article on COI in medical research,

Industry funding of medical research increased from $1.5 billion in 1980 to $22.4 billion in 2000. The number of patents awarded from research conducted at universities increased from approximately 250 annually in 1980 to 4,800 in 1998. Furthermore, [as of 2002] over 2,200 new companies have been formed around the licensing of these inventions by universities. (p. 46)

The Federation of American Societies for Experimental Biology (n.d.) discusses the benefits of academic institutions working with industry in its definition of academic-industry relationships, which includes the statement that these relationships "are a fundamental and beneficial part of modern biomedical science" (Benefits of Academic-Industry Relationships section, para. 1).

With stronger financial incentives to shepherd innovation from the bench to the benefit of the general public via commercialization, the potential for COI has increased. In 1995, the U.S. Public Health Service (PHS) enacted regulations to ensure that policies and procedures were in place to minimize or eliminate COIs that could adversely affect the conduct of research and results therefrom. In addition to PHS, many federal agencies have rules—via federal regulations or agency policies and guidelines—that address COI, including the U.S. Department of Health and Human Services (DHHS), the U.S. Food and Drug Administration (FDA), and the Centers for Medicare and Medicaid Services (CMS).

The concept of *conflict* is not consistently defined in regulations and federal guidelines. In their law review article, Henderson and Smith (2002) discussed COI in medical research as existing when "external relationships influence, or appear to influence, an individual's or institution's attitude or behavior toward particular research" (p. 445). *Black's Law Dictionary* (Garner, 2009) defines

---

The author would like to acknowledge Mary E. Brimer, RN, MSN, OCN®, for her contribution to this chapter that remains unchanged from the previous edition of this book.

conflict as "a real or seeming incompatibility between one's private interests and one's public or fiduciary duties." Although not totally consistent, most federal definitions of conflict speak to instances when other relationships could *bias* or *influence* internal activities such as research, teaching, or the provision of health care. This chapter will identify and briefly discuss the various types of COI but will focus primarily on financial COI.

Identifying Conflicts of Interest

A multitude of potential COIs exist. While this list is by no means comprehensive, a few examples of COIs are
- Conflict of commitment
- Patient advocacy conflict
- Academic and institutional conflict
- Personal conflict
- Professional conflict.

Conflict of Commitment

At institutions of higher education with federal funding for their research projects, this is a hot topic. Conflicts of commitment are governed under the dreaded "effort reporting" concept. As frustrating as this process can be, it is imperative that there is a reliable system to report and manage researchers' commitment to the entities that engage them. The institutional responsibilities of researchers may include clinical (including training residents engaged in providing health care), research, teaching, administrative, management, student recruiting, and mentoring duties—all in addition to writing proposals and publishing research results. As one might expect, it is difficult to realistically identify the level of effort researchers spend on each of their duties, and it is easy for researchers to promise far more than they are able to provide. Therefore, it is crucial that researchers honestly report all of their commitment and effort. Not only will this allow their institutions to appropriately report effort to federal sponsors (and other sponsors who might request the same), but it also helps the researchers and administration to identify overcommitment and possible well-intended but unrealistic objectives.

In addition to duties owed to their employers, researchers often have supplementary duties outside the institution, which may include private practice, sitting on a board of directors, other professional associations or committees, consulting, and speaking engagements. Many researchers are prolific writers for both journals and textbooks. As one might imagine, this is not something easily managed through institutional COI offices. Therefore, it is imperative that researchers take an honest look at all commitments and evaluate whether their outside activities may affect their ability to meet their internal obligations or their duty to their patients.

Patient Advocacy Conflict

For some individuals, participating in research-related activity provides their best source of health care. Under these circumstances, it can be difficult for healthcare providers to exclude a patient from participation in a research project that could benefit that patient. One can easily imagine a scenario in which a well-intended individual ignores an exclusion criterion, repeats a test until the result is adequate, or unintentionally coaches a patient toward an answer that would allow inclusion in the clinical trial. Although the healthcare provider or study coordinator may consider such an action benign, it can very easily introduce bias into research results.

Academic and Institutional Conflict

One type of academic and institutional COI is when a significant financial interest exists between the parties. Although it may be disputed, any time an entity receives significant funding from any single source, there is the perception of a financial incentive to provide research results that are favorable to the source of those funds. Most reasonable people would doubt true objectivity if they learned that a healthcare provider or institution receives millions of dollars from a particular sponsor (e.g., a cancer center working on multiple clinical trials funded by only one or two pharmaceutical companies). Most individuals working in this field understand the concept of "arm's length negotiations" (a bona fide transaction in which all parties are not only independent but also have equal bargaining power) and that payments are determined by the fair market value for the work performed; in fact, many funding agreements specifically state that the consideration provided is not to influence the outcome of the study. However, the public may wonder how objective healthcare providers can be in providing research results to an entity that pays them millions of dollars per year. Even if the public believes that the healthcare provider holds their individual health care paramount, it is easy to imagine a scenario in which healthcare providers would bias results in a manner favorable to the source of funds (i.e., giving the benefit of doubt to the drug or device provided by that sponsor). Double-blind studies are designed to reduce this potential bias, but no system is failproof.

Another COI issue is when conflicting studies are being conducted within a single institution, for example, when one study is attempting to prove a theory that another research project is attempting to disprove, or when studies are competing for the same patients and their participation in another study is part of the exclusion criteria.

This topic would be particularly vexing for institutions of higher education with large medical research portfolios. Except when it may violate law or the fundamental mission of the institution, or not adequately protect the rights of the study subjects, faculty typically are not censored related to the subject matter of their research projects. Faculty projects usually are not approved or rejected based on subject matter; if projects are declined by an academic institution, the rejection is characteristically based on financial feasibility, cost share, or other resource limitations. Rarely, if ever, is there an individual within an academic institution who is aware of every active study and has the training to fully understand the subject matter of these studies to identify potential scientific overlap or other conflict. However, smaller healthcare institutions, physician practices, or companies engaging in research activities with greater control over research subject matter should be sensitive to this type of COI and develop policies and procedures that would enable them to identify and eliminate such conflict.

Personal Conflict

Perhaps the most difficult potential influence to identify and manage is personal beliefs. How many of us can be truly objective when it comes to our personal belief system? Could we proceed in an objective manner if our research is leading to a discovery that contradicts a strongly held personal ideology? Might a researcher with strong convictions related to sexuality question results that support the conclusion that homosexuality is genetically determined? The mere action of questioning results based on nonscientific criteria can introduce bias in the outcome and dissemination of results. Fortunately, the vast majority of scientists throughout the world make valiant efforts to eliminate personal bias, and science would not have had such significant advances over the years if this was not true. However, all researchers and healthcare providers must still maintain conscious vigilance against their own conflicts personally.

Professional Conflict

Professional conflict can include conflicts—real or perceived—created when a program director/principal investigator (hereafter referred to as either *PD/PI* or *PI*) is working with a spouse, life partner, or relative. In such circumstance, can the PI be truly objective and free from influence when working on a research project? Would the PI value the input of a relative over that of an unrelated individual? Or, conversely, might the PI improperly minimize the input from a relative with the intent to avoid influence, thereby introducing bias? A reasonable person could certainly question objectivity when such apparent potential for influence exists, even if the influence is unintentional. Many of these conflicts can be managed by removing the relative from the project or devising a management plan whereby the relative does not report directly to the PI.

This type of conflict is even more complex when the relative is working on independent projects with related subject matter. Could a PI doubt his or her results if they are inconsistent with the results generated by a relative on a separate project? Might a PI hesitate to publish results that would obviate or contradict the work of a relative? Even if the hesitation is unintentional, it certainly introduces some bias. Not only is this more difficult to identify, but it also is far more difficult to manage. Therefore, we must rely on the *scientific integrity* of the related individuals, as well as their administration. Furthermore, this highlights the need for a safe environment in which PIs, or any other person working on the project, may openly discuss these issues with their COI officers or committees.

Although it is not often discussed, potential COI exists in collaborations between colleagues. If a co- or subinvestigator is in a position of higher professional authority than the PI, might the PI, intentionally or unintentionally, report results in such a manner that the colleague approves, or that would benefit the research efforts of the other party? Might a PI hesitate to publish results that would obviate or contradict the work of his or her superior?

Yet another example of professional conflict is when multiple open clinical trials at an institution are covering the same subject matter. It would be tempting, consciously or not, for healthcare providers to suggest their own study, although the other might be more appropriate. Again, consciously or not, it is plausible that healthcare providers might favor the trial under their direction or which is sponsored by an entity with a stronger tie to the institution or employee (i.e., a company that funds more research, or one which the institution or employee would like to fund more studies).

Although these types of COIs are relevant to research and warrant policies and procedures to educate the faculty and staff who are involved in research, as well as guidance on how to manage, reduce, or eliminate these types of conflicts, the balance of this chapter will be devoted to financial COIs.

Definition of Financial Conflict of Interest

Before we can define *financial conflict of interest* (FCOI), we must first consider the parties affected by the rules relating to it. Most rules and regulations apply to "investigators." Most institutions, and many other agencies, use the NIH definition. Part I of the NIH Grants Policy Statement defines the PD/PI as the person whom the institution (the official applicant) has deemed to have "the appropriate level of authority and responsibility to direct the project or program to be supported by the award" (NIH, 2013). The policy statement further states that an institution may designate more than one person as a PD/PI if the other individual(s) "share the authority and responsibility for leading and directing the project, intellectually and logistically" (NIH, 2013). In the case of multiple PD/PIs, each is responsible for the project and for meeting all compliance obligations. If the institution decides that certain study staff (i.e., nurses or coordinators) have the authority and responsibility for leading and directing the project, those individuals may be considered investigators for the purposes of complying with certain regulations. Therefore, it is important for all study staff to check with their institution's policy to determine their individual level of responsibilities and obligations regarding compliance. For the purposes of this chapter, the NIH definition of PD/PI will be used, and text will refer to these individuals as either *PD/PI* or simply *PI*.

FCOI is by far the most "interesting" type of COI for the federal government. DHHS, FDA, PHS, and CMS have enacted regulations related to the disclosure, elimination, and management of FCOI.

One should understand that *consideration* (the value received for participating in the research) is not always provided in dollars, or immediately. Consideration could be something as simple as allowing a researcher to participate in the publication of groundbreaking research or giving access to a drug or device that would benefit the researcher's patients. Some device companies, for a limited period of time, allow only sites that had participated in clinical trials to purchase the new devices. This provides limited monopolies to the participating sites, which is a secondary, but possibly substantial, benefit to the healthcare providers. Therefore, although not required by all federal regulations governing this topic, it is important that each institution address all types of consideration in its policies and procedures for eliminating or managing personal COIs.

Henderson and Smith (2002) captured the true spirit of FCOI, describing it as financial interests that have "the potential to undermine the integrity of medical research results, threaten the safety of research subjects, and diminish public trust" (p. 445). However, the various federal agencies do not share a single definition of FCOI. FDA has codified its requirements in the *Code of Federal Regulations*, specifically 21 C.F.R. pt. 54. Although neither COI nor FCOI are clearly defined, the Purpose statement in 21 C.F.R. pt. 54 captures the intent of FDA, and one can infer that the FDA definition of COI is interests that could bias the design, conduct, reporting, and analysis of research. Furthermore, because FDA is under the purview of PHS, one can rely on the PHS definition when evaluating FCOI associated with projects funded by FDA (U.S. FDA, 2014). Fortunately, many of the federal funding agencies fall under PHS, which defines FCOI as "a significant financial interest that could directly and significantly affect the design, conduct, or reporting of PHS-funded research" (42 C.F.R. § 50.603).

The National Science Foundation (NSF) has now clearly defined COI. In its *Award and Administration Guide*, NSF states that "a conflict of interest exists when the reviewer(s) reasonably determines that a significant financial interest could directly and significantly affect the design, conduct, or reporting of NSF-funded research or educational activities" (NSF, 2014, section A, para. 4).

Office of Management and Budget Requirements for Researchers

The Office of Management and Budget (OMB) sets the standards for all federal grants. Circulars issued by OMB are actually regulations. These regulations are clarified in the newly issued Uniform Guidelines. OMB Circular A-110, which is applicable to colleges, universities, nonprofits, and hospitals, is codified at 2 C.F.R. pt. 215 (formerly under 45 C.F.R. pt. 74). The regulations at 2 C.F.R. § 215.0 require federal agencies to apply the rules set forth in the circular to recipients, and those recipients must apply the same to their subrecipients. As to federal contracts, recipients must maintain written standards of conduct for individuals administering a contract providing federal funds. Furthermore, no one involved in the administration of a contract providing federal funds should have a "real or apparent" COI. This regulation does not expressly prohibit the recipient from having COIs directly related to the contract provided to it by the federal government; however, it does prohibit conflicts between the primary recipient and any subrecipient by stating that a conflict would arise if

> the employee, officer, or agent, any member of his or her immediate family, his or her partner, or an organization which employs or is about to employ any of the parties indicated herein, has a financial or other interest in the firm selected for [a subcontract]. (OMB, 2005, Codes of Conduct)

To avoid conflicts, recipients are expected to
> set standards for situations in which the financial interest is not substantial or the gift is an unsolicited item of nominal value. The standards of conduct shall provide for disciplinary actions to be applied for violations of such standards by officers, employees, or agents of the recipient. (OMB, 2005, Codes of Conduct)

Although this type of activity is not expressly defined as FCOI, it should be addressed in an organization's policy (see Figure 22-1).

Figure 22-1. National Science Foundation Strategies to Manage, Reduce, or Eliminate Conflicts

- Public disclosure of significant financial interests
- Monitoring of research by independent reviewers
- Modification of the research plan
- Disqualification from participation in the portion of the National Science Foundation–funded research that would be affected by significant financial interests
- Divestiture of significant financial interests
- Severance of relationships that create conflicts

Note. From "Chapter IV—Grantee Standards" in *Award and Administration Guide* (NSF 15-1), by National Science Foundation, December 26, 2014. Retrieved from http://www.nsf.gov/pubs/policydocs/pappguide/nsf15001/aag_4.jsp#IVA.

U.S. Food and Drug Administration Requirements for Researchers

FDA requirements have been codified in 21 C.F.R. pt. 54. The Purpose clause of this regulation discusses the importance of research being free from bias. Unlike some agencies, which leave training, monitoring, and oversight to the institutions, FDA actually uses the information provided in certifications (disclosures) when evaluating marketing applications for human drugs, biologic products, or devices. It will use the FCOI disclosure form, along with other information related to the design and purpose of the study, in evaluating the reliability of the data (U.S. FDA, 2014). This regulation is applicable to the entity submitting the marketing application, the sponsor. Therefore, for PI-initiated clinical trials, the institution is the sponsor and must comply with this regulation. Even when a for-profit entity is the sponsor, the regulation clearly states that the sponsor is responsible for obtaining appropriate certifications from other sites by requiring full disclosure of any clinical investigator not employed by that sponsor (U.S. FDA, 2014). Therefore, investigators must provide this information to any external sponsor in a timely and accurate manner. An interesting note is that, when evaluating marketing applications, FDA does not evaluate apparent or potential COI, but *actual* conflicts.

FDA does not rely on applicants or institutions to manage conflicts; rather, it reviews the certifications and disclosure provided to it when evaluating a marketing application to ascertain the size and nature of the conflict, and the steps taken to minimize potential bias, to determine the impact of the COI (U.S. FDA, 2014).

This may appear to be a redundant process, and to some extent it is, but one must remember that FDA reviews and approves marketing applications. In this capacity, it is not providing funding for research and it is more appropriate for 21 C.F.R. pt. 54 to apply. In instances where FDA is providing funding for research, it will fall under the PHS requirements codified under 42 C.F.R. pt. 50 and 45 C.F.R. pt. 94, both of which are discussed in the following sections.

U.S. Public Health Service Requirements for Researchers

PHS falls under DHHS. Quite a few agencies under PHS provide funding for research, including Centers for Disease Control and Prevention, FDA, Health Resources and Services Administration, Substance Abuse and Mental Health Services Administration, and, most importantly, NIH. PHS has the most comprehensive FCOI definition and management plan of any of the federal agencies, codified at 42 C.F.R. pt. 50, subpt. F, and 45 C.F.R. pt. 94, both of which are applicable to entities receiving research funding from PHS. The regulations at 42 C.F.R. pt. 50, subpt. F, were last revised in 2000. The regulations at 45 C.F.R. pt. 94 have much more recently been modified (August 25, 2011) and implemented (August 25, 2012).

While these regulations are relevant primarily to the actual investigator(s), if an institution defines *investigator* broadly enough, other study staff, such as study coordinators or study nurses, may be required to comply with these regulations.

One should be very much aware of the fact that many nongovernmental funding entities, predominantly nonprofit organizations, such as the American Heart Association and the Lupus Foundation, may require recipients of their research funding to follow PHS requirements for FCOI training, disclosure, and management. Although these regulations are not directly applicable by force of law, by accepting the terms and conditions of the award, the institution is agreeing to comply. The requirements are typically on the funding entity's website or in the funding opportunity announcement. Therefore, because obligations attach at the point of application submission, it is essential to check the funding opportunity announcements, as well as the guidelines of nonprofit organizations, well in advance of submission.

Grants and Cooperative Agreements Issued by Public Health Service Agencies

The regulation found at 42 C.F.R. pt. 50, subpt. F, was codified to promote "objectivity in research by establishing standards to ensure there is no reasonable expectation that the design, conduct, or reporting of research funded under PHS grants or cooperative agreements will be biased by any conflicting financial interest of an Investigator" (42 C.F.R. § 50.601). This regulation applies to funding provided under *grants or cooperative agreements*, as opposed to federal contracts, and is applicable to institutions that receive and *apply for* research funding from PHS through grants or cooperative agreements, and to investigators by implementation of this regulation by their institutions. It is important to note the distinction between applying for and receiving funds. Even if an institution has never received funding from a PHS agency, the mere act of applying for funding establishes the requirement to comply with this regulation, even as a subrecipient.

> For the purpose of this regulation, an *investigator* is the principal investigator and any other person who is responsible for the design, conduct, or reporting of research funded by the PHS, or proposed for such funding. For purposes of the requirements of this subpart relating to financial interests, "Investigator" includes the Investigator's spouse and dependent children. (42 C.F.R. § 50.603)

An "investigator" need not have that title to be subject to this regulation. For instance, graduate students, postdoctoral researchers, or study nurses, even if not named as Key Personnel on the proposal, may be deemed investigators if they help to design, conduct, or report (even coauthoring publications) the research funded by PHS.

Most of the duties under this regulation fall to the institution, and most institutions will follow the PHS definition of investigator and not expand it to include study staff. However, many study staff will assist in maintaining compliance by assisting their PIs and/or obtaining required certifications from other sites. Therefore, it is wise to have a general understanding of these regulations.

42 C.F.R. pt. 50 clearly identifies *significant financial interest* as

> anything of monetary value, including but not limited to, salary or other payments for services (e.g., consulting fees or honoraria); equity interests (e.g., stocks, stock options or other ownership interests); and intellectual property rights (e.g., patents, copyrights and royalties from such rights). (42 C.F.R. § 50.603)

Not only is it important to understand what is construed as a significant financial interest, but it also is essential to understand what a significant financial interest is *not* by consulting the regulations for the comprehensive listing found in this section of the regulation.

42 C.F.R. pt. 50 sets the standards for policies and enforcement relating to COI within institutions that seek funding from PHS. One should consult the regulations for a complete list, but the highlights of the requirements for each institution are (42 C.F.R. § 50.604)

- Generate, maintain, and enforce a policy on COI that complies with the regulation
- Inform the investigators of the regulations, policies, and reporting responsibilities
- Take reasonable steps to ensure that all subrecipients and collaborators, including the investigators, comply with 42 C.F.R. pt. 50
- Ensure that, *at the point of application submission*, each investigator has submitted to the designated official a list of the investigator's known significant financial interests and entities whose financial interests would appear to be affected by the research.

At the application stage, each institution must provide certain certifications, including that it has a written and enforced policy, will report any COI found, and will reduce, manage, or eliminate any COI *prior to spending any funds* awarded by PHS (42 C.F.R. § 50.604).

Institutions must manage identified COI by having the official review all disclosures to determine whether a conflict exists and what action is required by the institution to reduce, manage, or eliminate the conflict. Some examples are as follows (42 C.F.R. § 50.605):

- Publicly disclosing the COI
- Engaging independent reviewers to monitor the research
- Modifying the proposal, scope of work, or research plan
- Disqualifying the conflicted investigator from participating in the research, in whole or in part
- Causing the conflicted investigator to divest (get rid of) the conflicting financial interest
- Severing the relationship that created the conflict.

It should be noted that other DHHS regulations may apply to PHS-funded research governed by 42 C.F.R. pt. 50, including

- 42 C.F.R. pt. 50, subpt. D: Public Health Service Grant Appeals Procedure
- 45 C.F.R. pt. 16: Procedures of the Departmental Grant Appeals Board
- 45 C.F.R. pt. 74: Uniform Administrative Requirements for Awards and Subawards to Institutions of Higher Education, Hospitals, Other Nonprofit Organizations, and Commercial Organizations; and Certain Grants and Agreements with States, Local Governments and Indian Tribal Governments
- 45 C.F.R. pt. 76: Governmentwide Debarment and Suspension (Nonprocurement)
- 45 C.F.R. pt. 79: Program Fraud Civil Remedies
- 45 C.F.R. pt. 92: Uniform Administrative Requirements for Grants and Cooperative Agreements to State, Local, and Tribal Governments.

Contracts Issued by Public Health Service Agencies

Similar to 42 C.F.R. pt. 50, 45 C.F.R. pt. 94 "promotes objectivity in research by establishing standards that provide a reasonable expectation that the design, conduct, and reporting of research performed under PHS contracts will be free from bias resulting from Investigator financial conflicts of interest" (45 C.F.R. § 94.1). However, 45 C.F.R. pt. 94 governs funding provided under a *contract* issued by a PHS agency as opposed to *grants or cooperative agreements*. As with 42 C.F.R. pt. 50, this regulation is applicable to institutions that *apply for* (not just those that receive) research funding from PHS and to investigators through implementation of this regulation by their institutions. Remember, even if an institution has never received funding by means of a contract from a PHS agency, the mere act of applying for funding, even as a subrecipient, establishes the requirement to comply with this regulation.

Additional similarities between the two regulations include definition of FCOI; definition of investigator; requirement to ensure compliance by any subrecipient or collaborator; establishing, maintaining, and enforcing institutional policy; and informing investigators of their responsibilities and obligations (45 C.F.R. § 94.3).

45 C.F.R. pt. 94 has a comprehensive definition of *significant financial interest*, with a relatively low dollar threshold. The definition states that a significant financial interest exists when the investigator (or his or her spouse or dependent children) has a financial interest that reasonably *appears to be related* to the investigator's institutional responsibilities (45 C.F.R. § 94.3). For exact guidelines and differences between publicly traded and non–publicly traded entities, as well as information concerning income from intellectual property, one should consult the full regulation.

Unlike 42 C.F.R. pt. 50, the definition of significant financial interest found in 45 C.F.R. pt. 94 includes disclosure requirements for travel costs reimbursed or sponsored (i.e., not paid directly to the investigator, but on his or her behalf, so the total value cannot be easily determined) by another party. Investigators must disclose the occurrence of any such travel related to their institutional responsibilities. However, the regulation includes some exceptions. Furthermore, the institution's FCOI policy must specify the details of this disclosure and must include, at minimum, the purpose of the trip, the destination, the duration, and the identity of the sponsor/organizer. The institution's FCOI policy should empower institutional officials to (a) determine if additional information is needed, including monetary value, and (b) obtain that information to determine if the travel constitutes an FCOI. Therefore, if study staff are included in the institution's definition of *investigator*, they may be asked to provide detailed information on travel funded by entities other than their institution.

Similar to 42 C.F.R. pt. 50, 45 C.F.R. pt. 94 establishes institutional responsibilities (see Figure 22-2). Institutions must certify in each proposal that it (a) has a process to identify and manage FCOI, (b) will enforce compliance by investigators, (c) will manage FCOI and provide required reports, (d) agrees to make available to DHHS information relating to any FCOI disclosure and

Figure 22-2. Examples of Institutional Responsibilities Established by 45 C.F.R. Pt. 94

- Maintain a current written and enforced policy on financial conflict of interest (FCOI).
- Make policy available on a website accessible to the general public (with provisions in the absence of a website).
- If institutional policy is more restrictive than the regulation, the institution must follow its policy and provide FCOI reports in accordance with this more stringent policy.
- Inform each investigator of the regulations, institutional policy, and his or her responsibilities and duties.
- Provide and require investigators to complete FCOI training.
- Take reasonable measures to ensure that all subrecipient investigators comply with the regulation with contractual obligations for subrecipients to (a) mandate that its investigators follow the FCOI policy of either the prime institution or the subrecipient institution, with certification that it is compliant with this regulation; (b) establish time periods for reporting all identified FCOI; and (c) provide FCOI reports.
- Designate an institutional official with the authority to require and evaluate FCOI disclosures and provide that official with guidelines.
- Require investigators to disclose FCOI annually at minimum, or within 30 days of discovering or acquiring a new FCOI.
- Manage any FCOI, including those of any subrecipient investigator, by developing a management plan and, if required, a retrospective review and mitigation report.
- Provide all required FCOI reports to the U.S. Public Health Service agency that is providing funding.
- Maintain records for a minimum of 3 years, or as specified in 48 C.F.R. pt. 4, subpt. 4.7.
- Provide for sanctions or other actions to ensure compliance by investigators.

Note. Based on information from 45 C.F.R. pt. 94.

its review and response to such disclosure, and (e) will fully comply with this regulation (45 C.F.R. § 94.4).

45 C.F.R. pt. 94 sets out a comprehensive plan for managing COI by establishing certain requirements that institutions must meet prior to spending any PHS funds for research projects (see Figure 22-3). Section 94.5(a)(1) provides examples of how to manage FCOI (see Figure 22-4).

45 C.F.R. pt. 94 provides specific remedies (consequences) for instances of noncompliance. If an investigator fails to comply with the institution's policy or management plan, and the noncompliance appears to have biased the research design, conduct, or reporting, the institution must create a corrective action plan and submit it to the funding agency. The agency may take action or refer the matter back to the institution to take further action (45 C.F.R. § 94.6). This section states that the agency may "include directions to the Institution on how to maintain appropriate objectivity in the PHS-funded research project." Furthermore, the agency or DHHS may, at any time, inquire into any disclosure and any records related to the disclosure, even if the institution did not deem the conflict to be an FCOI. After review of disclosures and/or associated records, the agency may

determine that an FCOI will bias a PHS-funded research project and action is required, or that the institution has not adequately managed an FCOI. If this occurs, the agency may issue a stop-work order or other enforcement action until the issue is resolved. Depending on the nature of the research, a stop-work order or significant delay could render useless the work already completed—a very serious consequence for a PD/PI who is planning to publish the results. Furthermore, if DHHS determines that PHS-funded research related to a clinical trial was biased, the investigator may be obligated to report the FCOI in any public presentation and request an addendum to any previously published presentations to disclose the FCOI.

Centers for Medicare and Medicaid Services Requirements

CMS released the final rule on February 1, 2012, which became effective April 9, 2013, to implement the Transparency Reports and Reporting of Physician Ownership or Investment Interests section of the Patient Protection and Affordable Care Act (ACA). This section, now commonly known as the Physician Payments Sunshine Act and codified at 78 Fed. Reg. 9457, implements part of the ACA in an effort to make health care more affordable and to ensure that health care is accessible for every U.S. citizen. Another goal of the ACA is to make certain that the public is aware of potential COIs generated by financial benefits provided to certain healthcare providers by certain manufacturers of covered drugs, devices, biologic products, and medical supplies (Medicare, Medicaid, Children's Health Insurance Programs; Transparency Reports and Reporting of Physician Ownership or Investment Interests, 2013).

Although these obligations relate primarily to physicians, it is wise for clinical trial staff to understand institutional policy as it relates to their role and to have a general idea of how this affects PIs and their participation in clinical research.

Applicable manufacturers and group purchasing organizations (collectively referred to as *manufacturers*) must now report certain information about physicians and teaching hospitals (collectively referred to as *covered recipients*). Manufacturers began capturing data (effective August 1, 2013) concerning certain payments or other transfers of value to covered recipients and began providing annual reports on March 31, 2014. The information reported reflects data for the prior calendar year. Section I.A.2.b states that manufacturers also must report "information about certain ownership or investment interests held by physicians and the immediate family members of physicians in such entities, as well as payments and other transfers of value to such physicians" (Medicare, Medicaid, Children's Health Insurance Programs; Transparency Reports and Reporting of Physician Ownership or Investment Interests, 2013). CMS began providing this information on a publicly

---

Figure 22-3. Examples of Requirements That Institutions Must Meet Prior to Spending PHS Funds for Research Projects Per 45 C.F.R. Pt. 94

- Institutional official will review disclosures and determine if an FCOI exists and, if so, develop and implement a plan that identifies specific actions to manage the FCOI.
- For any investigator new to the project who discloses an FCOI, or newly identified FCOI of an existing investigator, the institutional official must, within 60 days, review disclosure, determine if it is related to the PHS-funded research, and determine if it is actually an FCOI. If so, a management plan with specific actions to be taken to manage conflict should be implemented.
- If an investigator did not submit a disclosure or the institution did not review a disclosure (including those of subrecipients), the official will, within 60 days, follow the steps above.
- If an FCOI is not disclosed, reviewed, identified, or managed in a timely manner, or there is noncompliance with a management plan, the institution must, within 120 days of discovery of noncompliance, complete a retrospective review of investigator's activities and research to determine if there was bias in the design, conduct, or reporting of the research.
- In the event of noncompliance, the institution must submit an updated FCOI report and, if bias was found, notify the agency through a mitigation report.
- The institutional official must monitor management plans until completion of the project.
- Institutions must make FCOI information publicly accessible, and in great detail, through a website (with instructions for institutions without a publicly available website).
- Institutions may generate and enforce a more rigorous policy.
- Institutions must report to the awarding agency any instances of FCOI relating to PHS-funded research prior to expending funds, and in great detail.

FCOI—financial conflict of interest; PHS—U.S. Public Health Service
Note. Based on information from 45 C.F.R. pt. 94.

Figure 22-4. Examples of How to Manage Financial Conflict of Interest

- Public disclosure of financial conflicts of interest (e.g., when presenting or publishing the research)
- For research projects involving human subjects research, disclosure of financial conflicts of interest directly to participants
- Appointment of an independent monitor capable of taking measures to protect the design, conduct, and reporting of the research against bias, resulting from the financial conflict of interest
- Modification of the research plan
- Change of personnel or personnel responsibilities, or disqualification of personnel from participation in all or a portion of the research
- Reduction or elimination of the financial interest (e.g., sale of an equity interest)
- Severance of relationships that create financial conflicts.

Note. From "Management and Reporting of Financial Conflicts of Interest," 45 C.F.R. § 94.5(a)(1)(i)–(vii). Retrieved from http://www.ecfr.gov/cgi-bin/text-idx?tpl=/ecfrbrowse/Title45/45cfr94_main_02.tpl.

available website in September 2013, and the information is available by June 30 each year.

Reportable payments include payments for research-related activities. One should consult the regulation for a comprehensive list of what must be reported. Reportable payments or other transfers of value that may not be intuitive include charitable contributions (e.g., providing textbooks without receiving anything of value in exchange); travel and lodging; entertainment; education; royalties (other than royalties paid to a physician from the physician's employer); and food and beverage (other than buffet meals provided in large-scale settings such as conferences) (Medicare, Medicaid, Children's Health Insurance Programs; Transparency Reports and Reporting of Physician Ownership or Investment Interests, 2013). Some payments or transfers of value excluded from reports include educational materials intended for patients and that would directly benefit patients, discounts and rebates for covered items, items provided for charity care, samples provided for patient use, and payments or transfers of value that are $10 or less per payment or less than $100 in aggregate. Study staff should consult the regulation for a comprehensive list of exclusions.

It is interesting to note that manufacturers are not required to report payments or transfers of value to interns, nurses, physician assistants, nurse practitioners, physical therapists, or others who are not within the definition of covered recipient but have significant influence on healthcare decisions. However, it is important to understand that if consideration is provided to a person or entity that is not a covered recipient for the benefit of a covered recipient (e.g., textbooks given to a nurse to pass along to students at the teaching hospital), that transaction will be construed as *indirect payment* to the covered recipient (the teaching hospital in this example) and reportable under the final rule. It also should be noted that if a covered recipient directs a payment or transfer of value to another party that would not be the subject matter of a manufacturer's report, that payment or transfer of value must be reported as if made directly to the covered recipient; this is considered a *directed payment*.

The reports provided by manufacturers must include the name and business address of covered recipients (e.g., physicians or teaching hospitals). If the covered recipient is a physician, the manufacturer must include the physician's National Provider Identifier (referred to as NPI) and specialty. This will allow CMS to match multiple sources of income to a single physician and will facilitate public searches, as well as monitoring of the website by physicians and/or teaching hospitals. Furthermore, rather than reporting specific categories of consideration, the manufacturer must report the form and nature of payments for each payment or transfer of value (a list from which to choose is provided). Lastly, CMS allows manufacturers to provide some information as to the context of the payment or transfer of value (e.g., honorarium for speaking engagement) (Medicare, Medicaid, Children's Health Insurance Programs; Transparency Reports and Reporting of Physician Ownership or Investment Interests, 2013).

Unfortunately, the rule set forth at 78 Fed. Reg. 9457 does not mandate prior approval from the individual or teaching hospital before any disclosure by a manufacturer. It merely recommends that manufacturers voluntarily provide covered recipients an opportunity to review the information prior to disclosure, but it does require manufacturers to provide an attestation certifying that the data submitted are accurate, complete, and timely. Section I.A.1 provides a process for physicians and institutions to "review, dispute, and propose corrections to reported payments or other transfers of value, or ownership or investment interests, attributed to them" (Medicare, Medicaid, Children's Health Insurance Programs; Transparency Reports and Reporting of Physician Ownership or Investment Interests, 2013).

If covered recipients are registered with CMS, they will receive a notification alerting them to the fact that a manufacturer has provided information about them. It should be noted that although registration is not mandatory, without registration, CMS will not provide covered recipients the ability to review data attributed to them.

Once a covered recipient initiates a dispute, manufacturers will have an additional 15 days to correct data and submit corrected data (with additional attestation) to CMS. It is critical that covered recipients review the data immediately; if a dispute is not initiated early enough for the manufacturer to resolve and update the data, it may not be corrected prior to public disclosure. If there is insufficient time to correct the data or the manufacturer does not agree with the covered recipient, the manufacturer's information will be published along with the modified information provided by the covered recipient. In the event of an indirect payment to a nonphysician recipient, it will be reported under the name of the physician and/or teaching hospital. Therefore, all study staff must keep track of anything of value received from any manufacturer.

Unfortunately, CMS will not intervene or attempt to resolve disputes. However, CMS will monitor the rate of disputes and take note of any manufacturer with an abnormal amount or rate of unresolved disputes.

As this regulation went into effect, some issues have been discovered. Many institutions of higher education, as well as other healthcare providers, are working with CMS to resolve these issues.

Consequences of Noncompliance

Managing, reducing, or eliminating COI is paramount to good research. Figure 22-5 contains suggestions for the development of policies and procedures, including performing random audits and establishing enforcement procedures and remedies for noncompliance. Bias and influence can be insidious—the researchers may be completely unaware that their work is affected by certain relationships. Little by little, the objectivity of those involved in research activities may be reduced. By the time the researcher or institution becomes aware of the bias, the research results could be useless. If a researcher purposefully fails to disclose real or apparent COI, and the results of the research

---

Figure 22-5. Suggestions for Policies and Procedures

- The best way to ensure compliance with applicable regulations and policies of funding entities is to evaluate each and make certain the most restrictive requirement is adopted.
- It is advisable that institutions and physicians read the Physician Payments Sunshine Act (Medicare, Medicaid, Children's Health Insurance Programs; Transparency Reports and Reporting of Physician Ownership or Investment Interests, 2013) and evaluate the effect on the institution and/or its physicians. They should decide if they will register with Centers for Medicare and Medicaid Services (CMS) to receive updates, who will monitor the disclosures of manufacturers, and how they plan to address any discrepancies. Because this could be a daunting task for larger institutions with a significant physician workforce, it is likely that they will expect physicians to monitor the reports relating to them individually.
- It would be prudent for institutions to, at minimum, engage in random audits to ensure that the information reported on the CMS website does not conflict with the information disclosed to it by the physicians. In their rush to complete yet another set of paperwork, physicians could overlook a seemingly insignificant source of funds. However, if auditors (evaluating conflict of interest [COI] compliance) identify the discrepancy, they may issue a finding. If there truly is an unreported value provided to a physician, the auditing agency could determine that the institution was on notice of the discrepancy because the information was on a publicly available website, and the institution should have required the physician to provide an updated/corrected disclosure. Failure to do so could be seen as willful ignorance, something the federal agencies do not tolerate.
- Once the institution determines the procedures for monitoring disclosures by manufacturers, they should be captured in its policy on COI.

Helpful websites for identifying, managing, and eliminating COI, as well as for policy development, are
- National Institutes of Health: http://grants.nih.gov/grants/policy/coi
  - Presentation with Case Studies—under "Resources" on this page
  - Checklist for Policy Development—also under "Resources"
  - Frequently Asked Questions: http://grants.nih.gov/grants/policy/coi/coi_faqs.htm
- National Council of University Research Administrators: www.ncura.edu/content (membership may be required to access all information)
- Society of Research Administrators International: www.srainternational.org (membership may be required to access all information)
- Council on Governmental Relations: www.cogr.edu (membership may be required to access all information)
- Federation of American Societies for Experimental Biology: www.faseb.org/coi

Institutions may want to consider the following items when establishing written policies and procedures related to any type of conflict, including financial COI:
- Determine which agencies one wishes to fund research projects—both current and potential sponsors.
- Determine which funding mechanisms (i.e., contract versus grant) one is willing to accept.
- Determine whether the institution conducts, or plans to conduct, any clinical trial that is
  - Initiated by an external entity (other party is the sponsor), or
  - Initiated by a faculty member (institution is the sponsor).
- Read, evaluate, and compare all applicable policies, guidelines, and regulations, including those established by nonfederal funding sources.
- Establish a policy, or conform existing policy, to ensure that it complies with the most restrictive requirement of each, making certain that each and every requirement is addressed (i.e., U.S. Food and Drug Administration requirements for principal investigator–initiated research as well as U.S. Public Health Service requirements for contracts).
- Consult both the *Proposal and Award Policies and Procedures Guide*, January 2013 NSF 13-1, OMB Control Number: 3145-0058, and 45 C.F.R. § 94.5(a)(1) to help you determine how the institution will
  - Convene and manage COI committee(s) and determine level/flow of authority
  - Designate an institutional official and determine level of authority
  - Establish a process to train employees and manage records relating to same
  - Establish a process to obtain disclosures and manage records relating to same
  - Establish a process to evaluate disclosures and manage records of determinations/decisions made
  - Establish a process to manage, reduce, or eliminate conflicts
  - Establish a process for subrecipients
  - Establish a website to make information publicly available (or other special requirements if a publicly accessible website is not possible)
  - Establish process to provide reports to applicable parties (funding entity, primary recipient, etc.)
  - Establish process to provide any required notifications
  - Establish enforcement procedures and remedies for any noncompliance.
- Last, and far from least, evaluate the institution's policy on all COI. Many institutions have more restrictive policies than what is established by regulation or sponsor policies/guidelines. For instance, some institutions require all employees to report any and all income generated outside the scope of their employment, with no exclusions. Some institutions allow no gifts whatsoever from for-profit entities. In these cases, federal agencies encourage institutions to follow their own policy when setting thresholds.

are compromised, reporting those results could be considered *scientific misconduct*. Reports of failure to meet responsible conduct of research standards could seriously damage an open and trusting relationship between researchers and the public. Institutional COI officers will assist researchers working through these problems.

Probably the worst-case scenario would be the inadvertent harm to a patient created by a biased medical decision made by a conflicted healthcare provider. The general public does, and should be able to, rely on unbiased care. Even if no patient is harmed, if the public becomes aware of a COI that is not appropriately managed, the public trust would be greatly diminished. The resulting lack of confidence would affect not only the institution, but all of the individual healthcare providers within that institution. Patients may choose another physician, practice group, or hospital if they learn that decisions related to their personal care have been influenced by drug companies.

Neither the Common Rule nor FDA policies establish specific sanctions or remedies levied against institutions in the event of noncompliance. However, this does not mean there would be no consequences—one can always expect some penalty when violating federal regulations, guidelines, or policies. Perhaps the most significant would be the loss of confidence in the institution by the funding entity. If sponsors question a PI's ethics, freedom from bias or influence by external parties, or ability to manage COI, their likelihood of providing future funding to the PI, and even the institution as a whole, will be greatly diminished.

The regulations established at 42 C.F.R. pt. 50, subpt. F, provide for remedies in the event an institution fails to comply and the design, conduct, or reporting of the PHS-funded research has been biased. Per section 50.606, the agency will either take appropriate action or allow the institution to take action, including guidance on how to maintain objectivity in the research. Furthermore, the agency has the right to make inquiries to the institution and to review any records related to the research funded by that agency. In situations where the COI has not been adequately reduced, managed, or eliminated, the agency may suspend funding until the matter is resolved. Section 50.606 goes on to state that if the research involves evaluation of

> the safety or effectiveness of a drug, medical device, or treatment [and the research] has been designed, conducted, or reported by an Investigator with a conflicting interest that was not disclosed or managed as required by this subpart, the Institution must require the Investigator(s) involved to disclose the conflicting interest in each public presentation of the results of the research.

Such a disclosure could reduce the author's standing in the research community. And, if any study staff are named authors, their reputation also could be greatly diminished.

CMS has published guidance documents for all parties affected by this new legislation. For additional information related to open payments, the CMS website provides links to fact sheets for manufacturers, physicians, and teaching hospitals, among other resources; see www.cms.gov/Regulations-and-Guidance/Legislation/National-Physician-Payment-Transparency-Program/index.html.

Summary

Like any other compliance issue associated with sponsored research, FCOI regulations are expanding. Everyone can expect all governmental sponsors to eventually follow suit. Therefore, everyone must constantly evaluate guidelines, policies, and regulations and compare them with institutional policies and procedures. One should never forget professional contacts, professional organizations, email distribution list contacts, and other resources for ideas, advice, guidance, and compassion. Collectively, a wealth of information is available.

Key Points

- Many types of COIs exist, including conflict of commitment, patient advocacy conflict, academic and institutional conflict, personal conflict, and professional conflict.
- *FCOI* is defined as a significant financial interest that could directly and significantly affect the design, conduct, or reporting of research.
- Institutions and investigators have responsibilities to disclose and manage COI and FCOI.
- 42 C.F.R. pt. 50 governs research funded by grants and cooperative agreements issued by PHS agencies, whereas 45 C.F.R. pt. 94 governs research performed under PHS contracts.
- Key requirements for compliance vary depending on specific regulations and policies, but include conducting training on COI, disclosing and identifying COI in a timely manner, and having a plan to manage COI.
- Evaluating the applicable regulations and policies of funding entities and being familiar with the Physician Payments Sunshine Act may help in establishing written policies and procedures.
- Many online sources provide materials to aid in identifying and managing COI, including resources from NIH (http://grants.nih.gov/grants/policy/coi).

References

Federation of American Societies for Experimental Biology. (n.d.). COI toolkit. Retrieved from http://www.faseb.org/coi/Introduction.aspx

42 C.F.R. §§ 50.601–50.605. Retrieved from http://www.ecfr.gov/cgi-bin/text-idx?c=eC.F.R.&SID=f9f92d186b8c240b11381766f6

4b2cc8&rgn=div5&view=text&node=42:1.0.1.4.23&idno=42#42:1.0.1.4.23.6.19.3

45 C.F.R. pt. 94. Retrieved from http://www.ecfr.gov/cgi-bin/text-idx?tpl=/ecfrbrowse/Title45/45cfr94_main_02.tpl

Garner, B.A. (Ed.). (2009). *Black's law dictionary* (9th ed.). St. Paul, MN: Thomson Reuters.

Henderson, J., & Smith, J. (2002). Financial conflict of interest in medical research: Overview and analysis of federal and state controls. *Food and Drug Law Journal, 57*, 445–456. Retrieved from http://www.fdli.org/resources/resources-order-box-detail-view/financial-conflict-of-interest-in-medical-research-overview-and-analysis-of-federal-and-state-controls

Medicare, Medicaid, Children's Health Insurance Programs; Transparency reports and reporting of physician ownership or investment interests [Final rule], 78 Fed. Reg. § 9457 (2013). Retrieved from https://www.federalregister.govarticles/2013/02/08/2013-02572/medicare-medicaid-childrens-health-insurance-programs-transparency-reports-and-reporting-of

National Institutes of Health. (2013, October 23). Grants and funding: NIH Grants Policy Statement, part I: NIH Grants—General information, section 1.2: Definitions of terms. Retrieved from http://grants.nih.gov/grants/policy/nihgps_2013/nihgps_ch1.htm#definitions_of_terms

National Institutes of Health. (2014, September 29). Grants and funding: Financial conflict of interest. Retrieved from http://grants.nih.gov/grants/policy/coi

National Science Foundation. (2014, December 26). Chapter IV—Grantee standards. In *Award and administration guide*. Retrieved from http://www.nsf.gov/pubs/policydocs/pappguide/nsf15001/aag_4.jsp#IVA

Office of Management and Budget. (2005). Uniform administrative requirements for grants and agreements with institutions of higher education, hospitals, and other nonprofit organizations (OMB Circular A-110) (2 C.F.R. § 215). Retrieved from http://www.gpo.gov/fdsys/pkg/C.F.R.-2005-title2-vol1/html/C.F.R.-2005-title2-vol1.htm

U.S. Department of Health and Human Services. (2009). Protection of human subjects (45 C.F.R. pt. 46). Retrieved from http://www.ecfr.gov/cgi-bin/text-idx?SID=0defa0a582923f8a97ea4e0682a7f1a8&node=pt45.1.46&rgn=div5

U.S. Food and Drug Administration. (2014). Financial disclosure by clinical investigators (21 C.F.R. pt. 54). Retrieved from http://www.accessdata.fda.gov/scripts/cdrh/cfdocs/cfcfr/CFRSearch.cfm?CFRPart=54

SECTION V.

Recruitment and Retention

Chapter 23

Public and Patient Education

David Leos, MBA, RN, OCN®,
and Norma Sheridan-Leos, RN, MSN, AOCN®, CPHQ, CPPS

Introduction

For patients with cancer, participating in clinical trials provides access to research with the hope of extending survival time, greater access to healthcare professionals, and altruistic satisfaction (Biedrzycki, 2010). Effective communication of information is an essential prerequisite for enabling patients to make informed decisions about their care (Cox, Jenkins, Catt, Langridge, & Fallowfield, 2006). A common trajectory of care for patients with cancer will often include an option for participation in a clinical trial.

Healthcare providers have a professional and moral responsibility to provide patients with cancer with complete and comprehensive information regarding their disease and encourage them to be as involved as they wish in decisions regarding their treatment and care (Cox et al., 2006). However, providing a level of information sufficient for patients to make informed decisions remains a challenge for healthcare providers. Therefore, the ability of clinical trial nurses (CTNs) to identify effective public and patient health education methodologies can prove instrumental to ensuring the delivery of adequate healthcare services while facilitating clinical trial participation in their communities. This is of great utility to the overall success of clinical trials. Considering the interest of society as a whole, enhanced rates of participation in cancer clinical trials should not only hasten the testing and development of effective treatments but also save costs and energy by eliminating ineffective treatments more efficiently (Biedrzycki, 2010).

CTNs, among other healthcare providers, face challenges in providing clinical trial education for patients, staff, and the public, particularly in how and what information is disseminated. Some of the challenges include providing consistent information, involving the collective efforts of many, and securing resources to meet the needs of patients, staff, and the public (Stepan, Gonzalez, Pyle, Villejo, & Cantor, 2010). This chapter will review the literature on methods and resources that CTNs can use in the quest to create awareness about clinical trials among various populations.

Clinical Trial Nurses' Role in Education

Providing education is a cornerstone in the foundation of the nurse's role in patient care. The subspecialty of oncology clinical trials nursing allows practitioners to apply this core competency in an expanded fashion. A synthesis of all that makes a competent clinical oncology nurse added with the ability to master and coordinate clinical trial–related communication for any audience is what makes CTNs a preferred provider for clinical trial education. The ongoing evolution of the CTN role has resulted in a shift away from being a simple data collector to being an integrated member of the clinical trial team and, in most cases, the coordinator of the clinical trial process (Green, 2011). Providing clinical trial education is a communication-related component of the Oncology Nursing Society (ONS) *Clinical Trials Nurse Competencies* (ONS, 2010). These competencies were developed as the framework for the confluent demonstration by CTNs of critical-thinking skills and implementation of the nursing process to provide leadership in the successful conduct of clinical trials. As such, CTNs must understand and incorporate into their daily practice a philosophy of continually adding to their knowledge base to further develop their clinical and educational skills. The next step in this process is to seek ways to improve lay, and in some cases professional, education about clinical trials. In their pivotal role of overseeing every aspect of the protocol, CTNs are the key member of the research team most appropriately situated to undertake and achieve this task. Although oncology nurses in the CTN role work in unison with other oncology care professionals to provide treatment-related care and information, their singular focus is on treatment via clinical trials. With this teaching opportunity, oncology nurses should ascertain patients' perceived and actual knowledge gaps to improve the adequacy of research information (Biedrzycki, 2011).

Effect of Education on Accrual

Patient education is only the first step toward increasing clinical trial enrollment rates (Du, Mood, Gadgeel, & Simon, 2008). Meeting the accrual target is the vital capability that allows clinical trial to successfully play their part in the development of more effective cancer treatments (Jacobsen et al., 2012). CTNs are often the de facto members of the clinical trial team for education delivery over the long term. The challenge of this delivery is made increasingly complex by having to analyze a vast array of clinical, technical, and, at times, legal information related to cancer research protocols and distill it into a message that is appropriate and comprehensible to the intended audience. The effectiveness with which this is done is a critical yet often underrecognized contributing factor in the overall outcome of clinical trials. The effort can run the gamut from providing an individual patient with detailed information on a specific study to an introductory-level presentation to a public audience. The intent of the latter approach may be to create awareness of a clinical trial program within the community or to advertise a study better suited to the community at-large, such as a prevention study. In either situation, oncology CTNs must convey certain basic information to aid audiences' understanding of the implications of clinical trial participation.

The literature varies on whether educational efforts have a significant positive impact on accrual outcomes. In some cases, the educational effort reverses an informational deficit. In doing so, this effort may eliminate distrust or, perhaps, fear that is based on actual or unfounded accounts of research-related misdeeds or the burdens and risks imposed by participation in clinical trials. Quinn et al. (2007) found that their educational interventions led to increased clinical trial accruals of 8%–33%. Conversely, Vanderpool, Kornfeld, Mills, and Byrne (2011) recognized that a discussion of a clinical trial does not necessarily lead to participation and that many barriers to clinical trial participation exist besides lack of awareness. Stiles et al. (2011) found that their educational interventions, while serving to increase the level of satisfaction attained from the information received, could not demonstrate an increase in subsequent enrollment in clinical trials. Therefore, a recommendation would be to ascertain patients' perceived and actual knowledge and close the gaps to improve the adequacy of research information (Biedrzycki, 2011).

Individual, Group, and Public Education

Oncology CTNs have opportunities to provide clinical trial education in three settings: individual, group, and public, each having its own communication needs. Such communication can be fraught with challenges. Dellson, Nilbert, Bendahl, Malmström, and Carlsson (2010) found that no specific method for communicating information has yet proven superior to another. In light of this finding, a recommendation would be to focus on some basic tenets of effective communication as outlined by Rodin et al. (2009). These include (a) the use of lay terms, (b) tailoring the discussion to recipients' need for informational content and detail, (c) offering a variety of media formats (when available) for the information provided (e.g., written, audio, video), and (d) asking if the recipients have questions or concerns about the information presented. Follow-up to the initial discussion should reinforce information and allow for addressing subsequent questions or concerns.

Individual Education

A review of the literature finds that there have been numerous efforts to improve clinical trial education through enhancement of patient-provider communication. The communication interventions were aimed at fostering better dialogue that, hopefully, would lead to better patient understanding. Several of these published efforts included the use of video or related multimedia approaches (Du, Mood, Gadgeel, & Simon, 2009; Hoffner et al., 2012; Strevel, Newman, Pond, MacLean, & Siu, 2007; Wells et al., 2012). Consistent with prior work, the results of these studies were generally mixed in terms of increasing knowledge and less favorable in terms of positively affecting patient accruals. On a more fundamental level of information delivery, Rodin et al. (2009) observed that patients varied in their preferences for information and decision making, thus indicating the need to tailor the communication based on needs of the individual.

Armed with these data, oncology CTNs should consider the population and circumstances under which any adult educational activities are carried out, as well as the variables associated with each. Individually oriented education is perhaps the most common example and typically is based at the bedside for inpatient settings or in the clinic for ambulatory settings. CTNs must be adept at and comfortable in carrying out this effort in either setting while acknowledging that the information recipient may not be well situated to learn this way. They can confidently address possible barriers to education by having supplemental resources (e.g., pamphlets, videos) at hand when delivering clinical trial information.

Timing of Education

Providing clinical trial education to a patient is a process, not a singular event. Although the value of providing such education is not a disputed issue, much like other essential tasks for oncology CTNs, it requires advance planning in order to achieve its intended purpose. Commonly, the process is initiated early on in the clinician-patient relationship. Conventional wisdom would hold that early intervention would be optimal and even preferred. However, Biedrzycki (2011) found that although patients have indicated that receiving desired information in advance reduces stress, the author suggested that the time when a patient is being evaluated for anticancer therapy may not be the ideal teachable moment.

Steps that can be taken to educate a patient about a specific clinical trial include an initial assessment of the patient's level of comprehension and emotional-receptive status, especially because the discussion often coincides with the initial disclosure of a cancer diagnosis or treatment failure. The opportunity for the prospective study patient to meet with another patient who is currently on or who has completed a particular study offers valuable insight as to what the patient might expect in terms of side effects, all relayed from a point of experience.

Group and Public Education

Although literature on group or public education for cancer clinical trials remains scarce, such efforts can generally be presumed to take place in healthcare facilities or nonhealthcare settings within the community. Healthcare settings outside of CTNs' own practice area, such as community clinics and offices, offer a venue to reach study subjects closer to where they reside. The group setting can offer the advantage of a greater audience, which can make individuals within that group feel more comfortable among similarly interested participants. Nonhealthcare settings, such as places of employment or worship and other community-based centers, can provide information recipients with the advantage of familiarity, proximity, and convenience. In this situation, a potential sense of trust can occur with what can be interpreted as an implied endorsement from the hosting facility. Conversely, mistrust of the healthcare system is an important barrier to research participation regardless of prior experience or socioeconomic status (Scharff et al., 2010). This concept must be acknowledged as a legitimate concern for certain populations in order to enact a diversity-sensitive approach to education efforts in the community. Such a nursing-led effort is augmented by a community-derived sense of trust toward nurses, as evidenced by Gallup (2014) poll findings that have consistently found the profession rated at the top in honesty and ethics. In nonhealthcare group settings, recipients have the opportunity to be exposed to diverse perceptions and questions beyond their own experiences about the provided information. CTNs should consider this as an opportunity to both support an open dialogue and to provide information that will dispel any misconceptions related to clinical trial participation. This should lead toward a better understanding of the educational message and to the likelihood of more informed decision making among recipients.

The choice of setting for an educational session is a factor in the public's receptiveness to the message. Despite some compelling instances, the volume of recent literature on this issue is, unfortunately, scant. For example, Linnan et al. (2005) found that beauty shops represent an innovative setting where health promotion interventions may be planned, delivered, and evaluated. Similarly, anecdotal information suggested that traditional community gathering places for men, such as barbershops, can provide an environment conducive for health education.

CTNs can readily identify patients within their healthcare setting for whom clinical trial education would be appropriate. Identifying appropriate patient groups that typically are outside of one's practice setting is more of a challenge but can be achieved by collecting community demographic information (such as census data). This can lead to the identification of residential areas and social gathering locations of groups that may be receptive to clinical trial education among a population consistent with that being targeted by the protocol. From there, the particular requirements and eligibility criteria of the protocol will be the determining factors in whether a patient is eligible for, and ultimately provides consent to, registration on the study.

Opportunities and Preparation for Speaking to the Public

Opportunities to take clinical trial education to the public audience will vary. One approach involves presenting the information to the audience in a non–protocol-specific manner as a public service. This effort could involve making an educational presentation to a school or vocational audience, club, or civic organization or to the public at large at health fairs or through the use of radio, television, and increasingly, social media. Regardless of the venue, a basic approach is to focus on providing the history of clinical trials and an explanation of key concepts of the clinical trial process, as well as the implications of study participation, all with an emphasis on the audience achieving, at least, a basic understanding. The presenter should allow time for and invite questions from the audience.

In preparation for the event, the presenter should create learning objectives for the presentation and conduct pre- and post-testing to gauge the didactic effect, remembering not to assume that merely providing educational material for patients in an accessible form is sufficient to address information needs. An excellent downloadable resource is the National Cancer Institute workbook, available at www.cancer.gov/publications/health-communication/pink-book.pdf. This book is a revision of the original *Making Health Communication Programs Work*, first printed in 1989. The key is reading all the steps and adapting those relevant to a specific program. The tips and sidebars throughout the book suggest ways to tailor the educational event to meet the learning needs of the audience.

A public presentation on clinical trials can be used to bring attention to a specific protocol. Such opportunities come up when the protocol involves a patient population not found within the typical practice setting. Examples of this would be a cancer prevention study or a study related to the emerging field of proteomics research, wherein prospective study participants are healthy volunteers without a cancer diagnosis. Outside of cancer care settings, the healthy population most likely would be limited to family members and visitors of patients at most other clinical practice areas. Therefore, one would have to seek speaking venues outside of his or her practice setting to reach the necessary audience in meaningful quantities.

Funding typically is an issue for most health-related educational outreach activities. If funding for such activities is insufficient, options include (a) working with volunteers from the community or from the healthcare organization sponsoring the event, (b) starting with a small venue first that would attract a smaller audience as a pilot test prior to reaching a larger audience, and (c) working with other interested organizations, such as church or civic groups (National Cancer Institute, 2008).

Michaels et al. (2012) described a community partnership to change knowledge, attitudes, and role behaviors among community leaders, primary care providers, and clinical researchers about cancer clinical trials. More than 70 trainers were recruited; trainers were expected to deliver workshops to community leaders and primary care providers. They found that programmatic efforts were effective in increasing knowledge and training community leaders and primary care providers to disseminate education about clinical trials and ultimately increasing patient inquires about local clinical trials. They found increased cultural competency skills of the staff involved in the study and the generation of effective partnerships. The community partnership showed a potential to reduce key barriers to cancer clinical trials (Michaels et al., 2012).

Mackenzie et al. (2010) described a media campaign to raise public awareness of clinical research called "Get Randomized." This campaign was the first of its kind and was set in the United Kingdom. Television, radio, and newspaper advertising showed leading clinical researchers, general practitioners, and patients informing the public about the importance of randomized clinical trials. After the intervention, public awareness of clinical trials improved, wherein 56.7% recalled seeing or hearing advertising following the campaign. However, when asked if they would personally take part in a clinical trial, little difference was noted between pre- and postintervention responses. The authors concluded that it is possible to raise awareness of clinical trials, but additional efforts may be needed to influence a person's decision to take part in them.

Credibility

Potential obstacles that can be encountered when making a public-wide attempt at either protocol-specific or non–protocol-specific education include having a credible message and being a credible messenger. Message credibility can be achieved with many audiences through a straightforward, user-friendly presentation of factual and relevant information. It is when the messenger's credibility is either not already established within the audience (i.e., through messenger or institution name recognition) or when the presentation fails to establish a credible message that the overall educational objective is not achieved. A preventive action plan for this situation could include (a) identifying a receptive and appropriate audience for the educational presentation and (b) having the information presented by or mediated through a known credible messenger, such as a trusted community figure.

Explain the Importance of Eligibility Criteria

As part of public education efforts, a good approach should include pointing out how and why most clinical trials have specific eligibility criteria that define a limited patient population. With the advent and expanded use of new targeted, personalized therapies, this often means that in order to meet increasingly rigid eligibility criteria, a patient's disease must, in certain cases, express specific surface biomarkers or have certain mutational profiles related to that therapy. Patients who do not meet the specific requirements of a study, especially if the trial has received publicity that is encouraging, may feel that they have been denied opportunity and, consequently, hope. In settings where patients with similar diagnoses can exchange health histories, such as in treatment waiting areas, the necessity for an individualized treatment approach can be misconstrued. It may contribute to an overall misunderstanding or perhaps even negative attitudes on the part of patients or the public toward the process by which clinical trials are conducted. They may not understand how randomized clinical trials are the "gold standard" for testing new treatment concepts and instead see them as arbitrary and favoring scientific principle over patient care because of the necessity for such rigidity to satisfactorily evaluate the protocol's endpoints. The situation can be exacerbated for patients or for the public by disagreement within or between the medical and political communities or those with a vested interest when the response rate of a new treatment is not deemed acceptable for regulatory approval. This could, and has, stemmed from a test agent's marginal disease response that appears to benefit some but not enough study patients to be more widely applicable later on to everyday practice or when the treatment's benefits have not outweighed the risks taken. Beyond these controversies, the principle remains that one must ensure compliance with eligibility criteria as evidence of competent protocol management as outlined in the ONS (2010) *Clinical Trials Nurse Competencies*.

Informational Materials

As limitations in human resources and program infrastructure can often affect the capacity to conduct clinical trial education, it is beneficial to be aware and take advantage of more simplistic, yet readily available, resources that will meet education objectives. Printed materials, such as brochures supplied by the study sponsor, in particular from the National Cancer Institute and some of the cancer cooperative groups, remain a common approach for the delivery of protocol-specific information. These materials represent a peer-reviewed and often no-cost communication tool. However, the use of informational brochures, as pointed out earlier, has its limitations. A recent study by the University of Leicester (Mayor, 2012) looked at the use of patient information leaflets for 13 cancer clinical trials. Out of the 26 patients surveyed, 18 found that scientific terms made the trial leaflets too detailed and difficult to understand. Most of the patients made decisions on the basis of their relationships with members of the clinical team. The research group suggested the patient information sheets are influenced more by the needs of the institution rather than the education needs of the patients.

The use of consumer technology is a common means worldwide to provide and acquire health information. According to statistics from Pew, 81% of U.S. adults use the Internet, and 59% said they had looked online for health information in the previous year (Fox & Duggan, 2013). The rapid assimilation of smart handheld devices has enabled a point-of-service informational capability. Many patients are using Internet-derived health information gathered personally or by family or friends. In a sense, the Internet and its enabling devices can help to level the healthcare playing field and mitigate the barrier to entry by providing information at the click of a key or swipe of a screen. Vigilance must be exercised in order to recognize the strengths and weaknesses that this medium poses as a source of information for clinical trial education. How best to leverage the Internet's potential as a conduit for valid and forthright information about clinical trials, as well as how to deal with the potential barrage of questions from technology-equipped and savvy patients or members of the public, should motivate CTNs to sharpen their information technology skill set. Challenges aside, this informational medium is in common use and has been embraced as an essential tool in navigating today's clinical research landscape. CTNs must balance Internet opportunities with the negative aspects that come with the plethora of health-related information, some of which is either misleading or outright false, done in the guise of offering hope.

Most cancer institutions provide their own Internet-based information related to cancer care for the public. A mainstay of these websites is information related to clinical trials in general and about those offered through that institution. Although the sites provide viewers with information on clinical trials, the availability typically is limited to that vicinity, unless patients are willing to travel to the sponsoring institution for care. To reach a wider geographic audience, several publicly or privately sponsored websites are available that provide accurate and current information on all aspects of clinical trial participation, along with registries for listings of actively accruing clinical trials being conducted across the country. See Figure 23-1 for a listing of Internet resources that may be applicable to the learning objectives for one-to-one education or a particular group educational program.

Simon, Schramm, and Hillis (2010) conducted an explorative survey to assess how cancer care providers view and respond to patient Internet use related specifically to cancer clinical trials. The study was done on the premise that clinician perceptions may be important to future efforts to improve patient knowledge about clinical trials. They found that clinicians thought the Internet had a mostly positive effect on patient decision making but that the clinicians' communication efforts did not always follow this positive perception. Patient-provider discussions about Internet use may be an opportunity for clinicians to contribute to improved patient knowledge regarding clinical trial enrollment.

Figure 23-1. Clinical Trial Educational Resources

- **AccrualNet:** Sponsored by the National Cancer Institute. Focus of the site is for professionals caring for clinical trial participants. Offers resources, strategies, and tools. Contains descriptions and links to professional and patient education resources about clinical trials.
  https://accrualnet.cancer.gov
- **American Cancer Society Asian Pacific Islander Cancer Education Materials Tool:** Allows users to search clinical trial and other oncology-related material in Asian or Pacific Islander languages.
  www.cancer.org/apicem/default
- **American Cancer Society Clinical Trials: What You Need to Know:** A downloadable educational booklet that explains clinical trials to patients who are considering a clinical trial.
  www.cancer.org/treatment/treatmentsandsideeffects/clinicaltrials/whatyouneedtoknowaboutclinicaltrials/clinical-trials-what-you-need-to-know-toc
- **American Cancer Society Clinical Trial Patient Worksheet:** A downloadable worksheet with questions for patients to ask regarding clinical trials and a place to document the information for review later.
  www.cancer.org/acs/groups/content/@nho/documents/webcontent/clinicaltrialpatientworksheetp.pdf
- **Center for Information and Study on Clinical Research Participation Educational Brochures:** Information for patients considering a clinical trial and for professional use. Educational booklets that provide potential research participants an introduction to clinical trials.
  www.ciscrp.org/professional/store/brochures_main.html
- **CenterWatch:** Offers information regarding clinical trials for a variety of diseases and conditions.
  www.centerwatch.com/health-resources
- **National Heart, Lung, and Blood Institute:** Offers information for the public and healthcare professionals regarding enrolling a child in a clinical trial.
  www.nhlbi.nih.gov/childrenandclinicalstudies/index.php
- **National Institutes of Health (NIH) National Institute on Aging:** Site addresses older adults' concerns regarding entering a clinical trial. Free educational pamphlet downloads.
  www.nia.nih.gov/health/publication/clinical-trials-and-older-people
- **NIH Clinical Research Trials and You:** Provides basic information, patient stories, and educational materials. Spanish language materials available.
  www.nih.gov/health/clinicaltrials/index.htm

Underrepresented Populations

Oncology clinical trials represent an opportunity for improvements in cancer treatment and prevention. Studies have shown that only a small portion of the general oncology patient population participate in clinical trials (Banda, St. Germain, McCaskill-Stevens, Ford, & Swain, 2012). Population groups of racial minorities, the poor, and the elderly participate in clinical trials at even lower rates (Banda, St. Germain, et al., 2012; Evans, Lewis, & Hudson, 2012; Sprague, Russo, LaVallie, & Buchwald, 2012). Treatment and prevention data from studies based on a homogenous population do not allow for understanding the therapeutic response and safety profile for novel therapies and exacerbate racial/ethnic and age differences in cancer treatment and survival (Banda, St. Germain, et al., 2012).

Patients' ability to make an educated decision to participate in a clinical trial is based on a combination of skills: (a) patients having an understanding of research and science, (b) patients being able to seek out and evaluate health information, and (c) healthcare providers giving health education interventions that are appropriate for the populations served (Evans et al., 2012). Education interventions have been shown to be more effective when they are culturally appropriate for the population being served (Banda, Libin, Wang, & Swain, 2012). Interventions that have a reported success in reaching underrepresented groups are discussed as follows.

Older Adults

The risk of being diagnosed with cancer increases with age; most cases occur in adults who are middle-aged or older. About 78% of all cancers are diagnosed in people 55 years of age and older (American Cancer Society [ACS], 2015). Hence, the need to include older adults in clinical trials to enable the results to be applicable to them is clear. However, the expeditious recruitment of an appropriate number of patients that reflects the reality of the population of patients with cancer is a constant challenge. As cancer generally is accepted to be a disease most frequently found in the older adult population, CTNs most likely will find that their educational efforts will be directed toward this group. Despite that fact, older patients are disproportionately underrepresented in clinical trials (Bellera et al., 2013). Care of older patients is often complicated by comorbidities and other physiologic factors. This makes it difficult to apply information from cancer clinical trials based on a younger population to older patients. To completely understand how to correctly administer cancer treatment and to increase the use of cancer services by older adults, clinical trials with adequate representation of older patients need to be performed (Briggs, Robinson, & O'Neill, 2012).

Patients With Low Incomes

Unger and colleagues (2012) found that patients with cancer and annual household incomes less than $50,000 were less likely to participle in clinical trials than patients with annual incomes of $50,000 or higher. The study was done to better understand the impact of socioeconomic status and decision making about clinical trials. The results showed those with an annual income less than $50,000 participated at 7.6%, whereas those with an income greater than $50,000 participated at 10%. The researchers found that patients with low incomes were more likely to be concerned about how to pay for the care they would receive as a clinical trial participant than those with a higher income.

Specific educational strategies for these patients, such as how to deal with indirect and hidden costs (e.g., unpaid leave from work, more co-pays for visits, hotel costs), could be learning objectives to help patients with low incomes participate in clinical trials. Lack of insurance coverage for routine patient care costs is a barrier to enrollment of patients who might otherwise take part in a clinical trial. Lack of coverage makes it harder for researchers to successfully conduct clinical trials that could improve prevention and treatment options (Phillips, 2010). However, the Patient Protection and Affordable Care Act requires health insurers to pay for routine costs of care in approved clinical trials for cancer and other life-threatening diseases. Covered clinical trials may include treatment, prevention, and early detection trials.

Hispanics/Latinos

Data that describe clinical trial participation among Latinos, a population that has poor cancer outcomes, are lacking. Latinos are one of the fastest growing and largest minority groups in the United States. A study by Wallington et al. (2012) described the correlates of awareness and willingness to participate in clinical trials among a population of Central, North, and South American immigrant Latinos using safety net clinics (those that provide services on a sliding-scale fee system). The study population (N = 944) had a low acculturation level. Although only 48% of the study population knew what a clinical trial was when educated about clinical trials in a culturally sensitive manner, 65% indicated a willingness to participate. Study participants stated that healthcare providers were the most common source of information, but this was not associated with knowledge or intent to participate in clinical trials, suggesting a missed opportunity for educating this vulnerable population.

African Americans

According to ACS (2013), the overall cancer death rate has steadily decreased for African American men and women. In fact, the most recent data show that death rates dropped faster for African American men than for men in any other racial or ethnic group (ACS, 2013). That has caused the disparity in cancer death rates between African American and White men to shrink considerably. Cancer death rates among African American women are declining at a similar rate as those of White women. Despite these declines, however, death rates for all cancers combined remain 33% higher in Black men and 16% higher in Black women compared to White men and women (ACS, 2013).

African Americans continue to have lower overall five-year survival than White patients with cancer (60% versus 69%) and for each stage of diagnosis for most cancer sites (ACS, 2013). Much of the difference in survival is believed to be because of barriers that limit access to timely, high-quality medical care. Furthermore, African Americans are more likely to be diagnosed at a later stage of disease when treatment choices are more limited and less effective (ACS, 2013). This makes accrual to clinical trials very important for this population. However, Black patients with cancer participate in clinical trials at lower rates than the general population (Banda, Libin, et al., 2012). The most frequently cited barrier to Black participation in clinical trials that can be addressed through education is lack of information. A study by Banda, Libin, et al. (2012) was designed to address specific attitudes of Black patients to clinical trials and to increase participation through the development of a 15-minute culturally sensitive narrative video. Patients' likelihood of enrolling in a clinical trial after watching the educational video showed 34% of the patients had a positive change in the intent to enroll.

American Indians and Alaska Natives

American Indians and Alaska Natives have some of the highest cancer-related mortality rates of all U.S. ethnic groups; however, they are underrepresented in cancer clinical trials (Sprague et al., 2012). Lung and colorectal cancer incidence rates for men and women in this group are significantly higher than for Whites. Sprague and colleagues (2012) described a project to identify factors that influenced willingness to participate in cancer clinical trials in a population of tribal college students (N = 489). Using a questionnaire, they examined 10 factors that influence participation and found that 80% of the students were willing to participate in a clinical trial if (a) the clinical trial would lead to new treatments or help others with cancer in their community, (b) the clinical trial doctor was experienced in treating American Indians and Alaska Natives, and (c) they received payment for enrolling in a study. Older nonstudent adults were more likely to participate based on the doctor's expertise than were younger students. The authors concluded that patients in this population are willing to participate in clinical trials. The findings from this study could be used as an educational platform for CTNs in working with American Indians and Alaska Natives.

Summary

Educating patients and the public about their potential role in clinical trials is essential to achieving progress in the overall treatment of cancer. The challenges in meeting this objective are significant and present oncology CTNs with opportunities for professional skills development and improved patient care and public relations. This skill was recognized during the formulation of the ONS (2010) *Clinical Trials Nurse Competencies* and was therefore included as a key function in competent practice of a CTN. As highly trusted members of the community, oncology nurses honor that trust in their role by assessing for and reducing health-related knowledge deficits in diverse patient populations through teaching. By recognizing the need to use an evidence-based approach in disseminating information to their patient population as well as to the general public, CTNs can foster better informed and conceivably better engaged healthcare consumers. Patient and public outreach education helps to build and strengthen a research-supportive relationship with the CTN's healthcare colleagues through enlightenment and continuous updates on clinical trials. Oncology CTNs should expand that role to include devising, implementing, and assessing population-appropriate techniques to effectively present accurate and up-to-date information about cancer clinical trials upon which patients can base their treatment decision or that the public can use to formulate an informed opinion.

Key Points

- Effective communication skills on the part of CTNs are an essential prerequisite for enabling patients to make informed decisions about their care.
- Education is a process, not a singular event.
- Message credibility can be achieved through a straightforward, user-friendly presentation of factual and relevant information.
- Healthcare providers have a professional and moral responsibility to provide patients with cancer complete and comprehensive information regarding their disease and clinical trial options.
- CTNs are the key member of the clinical trial team most appropriately situated to undertake education regarding clinical trials.
- CTNs should ascertain patients' perceived and actual knowledge and close the gaps to improve the adequacy of research information.
- Educational efforts that increase awareness of clinical trials do not necessarily lead to increased clinical trial enrollment.

References

American Cancer Society. (2013). *Cancer facts and figures for African Americans 2013–2014*. Retrieved from http://www.cancer.org/acs/groups/content/@epidemiologysurveilance/documents/document/acspc-036921.pdf

American Cancer Society. (2015). *Cancer facts and figures 2015*. Retrieved from http://www.cancer.org/research/cancerfactsstatistics/cancerfactsfigures2015/index

Banda, D.R., Libin, A.V., Wang, H., & Swain, S.M. (2012). A pilot study of a culturally targeted video intervention to increase participation of African American patients in cancer clinical trials. *Oncologist, 17*, 708–714. doi:10.1634/theoncologist.2011-0454

Banda, D.R., St. Germain, D., McCaskill-Stevens, W., Ford, J.G., & Swain, S.M. (2012). A critical review of the enrolment of Black patients in cancer clinical trials. *American Society of Clinical Oncology Educational Book, 2012*, 153–157. doi:10.14694/EdBook_AM.2012.32.153

Bellera, C., Praud, D., Petit-Monéger, A., McKelvie-Sebileau, P., Soubeyran, P., & Mathoulin-Pélissier, S. (2013). Barriers to inclusion of older adults in randomized controlled clinical trials on non-Hodgkin's lymphoma: A systematic review. *Cancer Treatment Reviews, 39*, 812–817. doi:10.1016/j.ctrv.2013.01.007

Biedrzycki, B.A. (2010). Decision making for cancer clinical trial participation: A systematic review [Online exclusive]. *Oncology Nursing Forum, 37*, E387–E399. doi:10.1188/10.ONF.E387-E399

Biedrzycki, B.A. (2011). Research information knowledge, perceived adequacy, and understanding in cancer clinical trial participant [Online exclusive]. *Oncology Nursing Forum, 38*, E291–E296. doi:10.1188/11.ONF.E291-E296

Briggs, R., Robinson, S., & O'Neill, D. (2012). Ageism and clinical research. *Irish Medical Journal, 105*, 311–312. Retrieved from http://www.imj.ie/ViewArticleDetails.aspx?ArticleID=9214

Cox, A., Jenkins, V., Catt, S., Langridge, C., & Fallowfield, L. (2006). Information needs and experiences: An audit of UK cancer patients. *European Journal of Oncology Nursing, 10*, 263–272. doi:10.1016/j.ejon.2005.10.007

Dellson, P., Nilbert, M., Bendahl, P.-O., Malmström, P., & Carlsson, C. (2010). Towards optimised information about clinical trials; identification and validation of key issues in collaboration with cancer patient advocates. *European Journal of Cancer Care, 20*, 445–454. doi:10.1111/j.1365-2354.2010.01207.x

Du, W., Mood, D., Gadgeel, S., & Simon, M. (2008). An educational video to increase clinical trials enrollment among lung cancer patients. *Journal of Thoracic Oncology, 3*, 23–29. doi:10.1097/JTO.0b013e31815e8bb2

Du, W., Mood, D., Gadgeel, S., & Simon, M. (2009). An educational video to increase clinical trials enrollment among breast cancer patients. *Breast Cancer Research and Treatment, 117*, 339–347. doi:10.1007/s10549-009-0311-7

Evans, K.R., Lewis, M.J., & Hudson, S.V. (2012). The role of health literacy on African American and Hispanic/Latino perspectives on cancer clinical trials. *Journal of Cancer Education, 27*, 299–305. doi:10.1007/s13187-011-0300-5

Fox, S., & Duggan, M. (2013, January 15). Health online 2013. Retrieved from http://www.pewinternet.org/Reports/2013/Health-online.aspx

Gallup. (2014). Honesty/ethics in professions. Retrieved from http://www.gallup.com/poll/1654/honesty-ethics-professions.aspx

Green, L. (2011). Explaining the role of the nurse in clinical trials. *Nursing Standard, 25*(22), 35–39. doi:10.7748/ns2011.02.25.22.35.c8316

Hoffner, B., Bauer-Wu, S., Hitchcock-Bryan, S., Powell, M., Wolanski, A., & Joffe, S. (2012). Entering a clinical trial: Is it right for you? *Cancer, 118*, 1877–1883. doi:10.1002/cncr.26438

Jacobsen, P.B., Wells, K.J., Meade, C.D., Quinn, G.P., Lee, J., Fulp, W.J., ... Sullivan, D. (2012). Effects of a brief multimedia psychoeducational intervention on the attitudes and interest of patients with cancer regarding clinical trial participation: A multicenter randomized controlled trial. *Journal of Clinical Oncology, 30*, 2516–2521. doi:10.1200/JCO.2011.39.5186

Linnan, L.A., Ferguson, Y.O., Wasilewski, Y., Lee, A.M., Yang, J., Solomon, F., & Katz, M. (2005). Using community-based participatory research methods to reach women with health messages: Results from the North Carolina BEAUTY and Health Pilot Project. *Health Promotion Practice, 6*, 164–173. doi:10.1177/1524839903259497

Mackenzie, I.S., Wei, L., Rutherford, D., Findlay, E.A., Saywood, W., Campbell, M.K., & MacDonald, T.M. (2010). Promoting public awareness of randomized clinical trials using the media: The "Get

Randomized" campaign. *British Journal of Clinical Pharmacology, 69,* 128–135. doi:10.1111/j.1365-2125.2009.03561.x

Mayor, S. (2012). Patient information leaflets about cancer trials are too complicated, finds study. *BMJ, 344,* e2356. doi:10.1136/bmj.e2356

Michaels, M., Weiss, E.S., Guidry, J.A., Blakeney, N., Swords, L., Gibbs, B., … Patel, S. (2012). The promise of community-based advocacy and education efforts for increasing cancer clinical trials accrual. *Journal of Cancer Education, 27,* 67–74. doi:10.1007/s13187-011-0271-6

National Cancer Institute. (2008). Making health communications work. Retrieved from http://www.cancer.gov/cancertopics/cancerlibrary/pinkbook

Oncology Nursing Society. (2010). *Oncology clinical trials nurse competencies.* Retrieved from https://www.ons.org/sites/default/files/ctncompetencies.pdf

Phillips, C. (2010). Insurance coverage expanding for cancer clinical trials. *NCI Cancer Bulletin, 7*(10). Retrieved from http://www.cancer.gov/ncicancerbulletin/051810/page5

Quinn, G.P., Bell, B.A., Bell, M.Y., Caraway, V.D., Conforte, D., Graci, L.B., … Bepler, G. (2007). The guinea pig syndrome: Improving clinical trial participation among thoracic patients. *Journal of Thoracic Oncology, 2,* 191–196. doi:10.1097/JTO.0b013e318031cdb6

Rodin, G., Zimmerman, C., Mayer, C., Howell, D., Katz, M., Sussman, J., … Brouwers, M. (2009). Clinician-patient communication: Evidence-based recommendations to guide practice in cancer. *Current Oncology, 16,* 42–49. doi:10.3747/co.v16i6.432

Scharff, D.P., Mathews, K.J., Jackson, P., Hoffsuemmer, J., Martin, E., & Edwards, D. (2010). More than Tuskegee: Understanding mistrust about research participation. *Journal of Health Care for the Poor and Underserved, 21,* 879–897. doi:10.1353/hpu.0.0323

Simon, C., Schramm, S., & Hillis, S.T. (2010). Patient Internet use surrounding cancer clinical trials: Clinician perceptions and responses. *Contemporary Clinical Trials, 31,* 229–234. doi:10.1016/j.cct.2010.03.003

Sprague, D., Russo, J., LaVallie, D.L., & Buchwald, D. (2012). Barriers to cancer clinical trial participation among American Indian and Alaska Native Tribal College students. *Journal of Rural Health, 29,* 55–60. doi:10.1111/j.1748-0361.2012.00432.x

Stepan, K.A., Gonzalez, A.P., Pyle, N.D., Villejo, L.A., & Cantor, S.B. (2010). Initiative to standardize a clinical trial program. *Oncology Nursing Forum, 37,* 535–539. doi:10.1188/10.ONF.535-539

Stiles, C.R., Johnson, L., Whyte, D., Nergaard, T.H., Gardner, J., & Wu, J. (2011). Does increased patient awareness improve accrual into cancer-related clinical trials? [Online only]. *Cancer Nursing, 34*(5), E13–E19. doi:10.1097/NCC.0b013e31820254db

Strevel, E.L., Newman, C., Pond, G.R., MacLean, M., & Sui, L.L. (2007). The impact of an educational DVD on cancer patients considering participation in a phase 1 clinical trial. *Supportive Care in Cancer, 15,* 829–840. doi:10.1007/s00520-006-0199-2

Unger, J.M., Hershman, D.L., Burg, K., Moinpour, C., Albain, K.S., Petersen, J.A., & Crowley, J. (2012). *Patterns of decision making about cancer clinical trials participation among online cancer treatment community: A collaboration between SWOG and NexCura®.* Paper presented at the American Society of Clinical Oncology Annual Meeting, Chicago, IL. Abstract retrieved from http://meetinglibrary.asco.org/content/97158-114

Vanderpool, R.C., Kornfeld, J., Mills, L., & Byrne, M.M. (2011). Rural-urban differences in discussions of cancer treatment clinical trials. *Patient Education and Counseling, 85,* 69–74. doi:10.1016/j.pec.2011.01.036

Wallington, S.F., Luta, G., Noone, A.-M., Caicedo, L., Lopez-Class, M., Sheppard, V., … Mandelblatt, J. (2012). Assessing the awareness of and willingness to participate in cancer clinical trials among immigrant Latinos. *Journal of Community Health, 37,* 335–343. doi:10.1007/s10900-011-9450-y

Wells, K.J., Quinn, G.P., Meade, C.D., Fletcher, M., Tyson, D.M., Jim, H., & Jacobsen, P.B. (2012). Development of a cancer clinical trials multi-media intervention: "Clinical Trials: Are They Right for You?" *Patient Education and Counseling, 88,* 232–240. doi:10.1016/j.pec.2012.03.011

Chapter 24

Accrual Base, Recruitment, and Promotion Strategies

Marjorie J. Good, RN, BSN, MPH, OCN®

Introduction

Clinical trials have proven to be essential to the advancement of cancer care. However, patient recruitment to cancer clinical trials has continued to be challenging. Only a small proportion of adult patients with cancer participate, as evidenced by frequently quoted participation rates of approximately 2%–5% (Comis, Miller, Aldigé, Krebs, & Stoval, 2003; Ford et al., 2008; Murphy, Krumholz, & Gross, 2004), and ethnic minorities and underserved populations are even less likely to be participants (Ford et al., 2008). An estimated 20%–40% of cancer clinical trials are reported to close early because of inadequate accrual (Cheng, Dietrich, & Dilts, 2010; Korn, Freidlin, Mooney, & Abrams, 2010; Nass, Moses, & Mendelsohn, 2010).

Lengthy, ineffective, and inefficient recruitment to a clinical trial threatens to compromise its scientific, financial, and ethical integrity (Gul & Ali, 2010). Failing to enroll the required number of participants to a trial affects the statistical power, which has the potential for inaccurate reporting of clinically important effects as less than statistically significant. This results in a delay or failure to implement a clinically effective intervention and further delays the identification of ineffective interventions (Kaur, Smyth, & Williamson, 2012). Lengthy recruitment periods increase time and expense as well as put clinical trials in jeopardy of being terminated prematurely. Clinical trials that are terminated prematurely also pose ethical questions as enrolled participants have been exposed to an intervention unnecessarily without producing definitive results (Treweek et al., 2010).

Recruitment of appropriate and adequate numbers of research participants is an essential component of successful trial completion and the subsequent generation of results. However, the task of recruiting research participants is often challenging and multifaceted. This chapter will address the challenges and will provide strategies that can be used to increase the number of participants enrolled to cancer trials.

Recruitment Considerations

Barriers

Having a basic understanding and awareness of the challenges and barriers that affect accrual is essential before attempting to develop and implement recruitment strategies. The awareness of the potential predictors of high or low accrual is important so that appropriate strategies can be established to overcome or address the barriers, thereby facilitating successful trial accrual (Kaur et al., 2012).

Barriers to clinical trial participation are many and often involve multiple levels, including barriers attributable to such categories as patient, provider, system, and community perspectives (Baquet, Henderson, Commiskey, & Morrow, 2008; Paskett et al., 2008). For example, patient-related barriers may include lack of awareness, fear of side effects, additional costs, a desire to select the treatment, and added time required. Provider barriers often include lack of availability of appropriate trials, associated time and costs, and disinterest in study design. Table 24-1 lists examples of commonly reported barriers categorized by area of impact.

Other factors may negatively affect accrual but are not commonly addressed in recruitment literature. Dilts and Sandler (2006) reported on what they considered *invisible* barriers, or *administrative* barriers, that take place outside of the patient-provider interaction. The authors divided administrative barriers into three types: procedural, structural, and infrastructural. *Procedural* barriers are associated with the processes or series of steps

Table 24-1. Commonly Reported Barriers to Participation in Clinical Trials by Category

Category	Barrier

Patient	• Lack of awareness
	• Lack of education/understanding
	• Fear of experimentation
	   – Mistrust of research
	   – Being a "guinea pig"
	   – Being given a placebo
	• Fear of side effects
	• Lack of insurance coverage or inadequate insurance coverage
	• Additional costs
	   – Travel/transportation
	   – Time away from work
	• Poor access to healthcare facility
	   – Inaccessible locations
	   – Limited hours of operation
	   – Inadequate organization and delivery of healthcare services
	• Low socioeconomic status
	• Older age
	• Comorbidities
	• Desire to select treatment
	• Sociocultural aspects
	   – Language, literacy
	   – Lack of family/social support
	   – Spiritual/religious beliefs

Physician	• Lack of awareness • Concern regarding study validity and design • Lack of compensation, reward, and recognition • Increased time required • Lack of experienced and/or dedicated research support staff • Anxiety regarding influencing patient-physician relationship • Loss of professional autonomy

Trial related	• No available trial
	• Lack of equipoise in clinical trial design
	• Eligibility and exclusion criteria
	   – Overly restrictive
	   – Prohibits comorbidities
	• Complex study design
	   – Multiple randomizations and study arms
	   – Biospecimen collection and submission requirements
	   – Need to screen many patients to enroll small number (e.g., targeted therapy trials)
	• Consent document length and language

Research staff	• Lack of administrative support
	• No or limited prior research-related education
	• No formal mechanism established to conduct eligibility screening
	• Research is only part of job role
	   – Staff has multiple other competing responsibilities
	   – No formal time devoted to research
	• Lack of buy-in for clinical trial system ("not-my-job" mentality)
	• No one in research staff representative of ethnic populations
	• No or limited physical space provided to conduct research activities
	• Perceived as "outsider" within oncology practices

Administrative	• Procedural: Complex process/steps required to open trial (multiple departmental or board approvals required)
	• Structural: Organizational design that leads to delays in approval (poor communication between departments, e.g., radiology and grants/contracts office)
	• Infrastructural
	   – Lack of sufficient institutional review board (IRB) support staff
	   – Infrequently held IRB meetings

Note. Based on information from Dilts & Sandler, 2006; Ford et al., 2008; Gul & Ali, 2010; Joseph & Dohan, 2009; Kaur et al., 2012; Paskett et al., 2008; Rooney et al., 2011; Spaar et al., 2009; Ulrich et al., 2010; Unger et al., 2013; Wujcik & Wolff, 2010.

required to open a clinical trial within an institution or research program. Dilts and Sandler (2006) provided the example of the commonly occurring approval process within academic centers, which often requires a large number of consecutive departmental and other levels of approval before a clinical trial can be opened. The levels of approvals may begin with the department or unit where the trial will be conducted, and then it must be submitted to an institutional review board, a scientific review committee, a contracts and grants office, and others before the trial is approved for activation. *Structural* barriers are created by the design of the organization when different groups or departments within the organization have different steps to follow, which often leads to confusion and misunderstandings. One department, such as the grants and contracts office, requires a condition to be met, but the sponsor cannot agree to the condition unless the radiology department agrees to another condition. *Infrastructural* barriers are associated with how the core institutional system is designed and how it interconnects. An example may be an organization that has insufficient resources to have regularly scheduled, timely institutional review board meetings, which causes a delay in evaluation of potential clinical trials. These invisible barriers are very real for many research programs.

Minority and Underserved Populations

Despite improvements in cancer treatments and survival rates, disparities in cancer outcomes continue to exist, particularly for African Americans (Patel et al., 2012). African Americans have the highest death rate and shortest survival of any racial and ethnic group in the United States for most cancers (American Cancer Society [ACS], 2013). The causes of these inequalities are complex and are thought to reflect social and economic disparities more than biologic differences associated with race (ACS, 2013). Between 1975 and 2009, the death rate for all cancers combined continued to be higher among African Americans than Whites, with the gap much larger for men than for women (ACS, 2013). These statistics reflect a critical need to recruit African Americans and other minority populations to research studies, particularly studies assessing cancer-specific characteristics and genetic alterations (Patel et al., 2012). Minority and underserved populations, however, often have increased levels of mistrust or misunderstanding of clinical research in addition to healthcare access issues such as lack of insurance, transportation issues, and language barriers. Added to these barriers are institutional barriers where care is delivered and recruitment occurs, which, in the case of minority and underserved populations, are often resource-constrained safety net hospitals and clinics (those that provide care to low-income, uninsured, and vulnerable populations at little or no cost) (Joseph & Dohan, 2009). Moreover, minority and underserved patients with cancer are often ineligible for clinical trials because of advanced disease at presentation and the presence of comorbidities (Ford et al., 2008).

Before trial initiation, every effort should be made to identify potential recruitment barriers and to choose potential strategies to reduce them. Some measures to reduce potential recruitment barriers may be resource intense, requiring significant amounts of time as well as financial resources, and as a result, it may be impossible to address all of them. Therefore, it is important to focus on the most important barriers and to choose effective measures to minimize them as much as possible (Spaar, Frey, Turk, Karrer, & Puhan, 2009).

Trial Focus

Recruiting participants to treatment-focused clinical trials may entail different recruitment and planning strategies than cancer control, symptom management, quality-of-life, prevention, screening, or early detection trials. Potential participants for treatment trials are primarily patients with cancer who have a compelling motive to treat their disease and are generally accessible in oncology clinics and physician practices. Patients with cancer often experience an array of disease- or cancer treatment-associated symptoms; therefore, they are motivated to participate in a clinical trial that may alleviate that symptom. Research staff should be aware that presenting both a symptom management trial and a treatment trial to a patient may be an overwhelming amount of information for a patient to consider (Berger, Neumark, & Chamberlain, 2007).

Unlike treatment and cancer control trials, potential participants for prevention, screening, or early detection trials usually include healthy subjects from the general population or from a defined high-risk group. Accessing these healthy individuals, who may not be as motivated as patients with a disease to take part in a clinical research study, requires additional recruitment planning, strategizing, and effort.

Eligibility screening for clinical trials is often time intensive with associated costs that sponsors typically do not cover. Many of today's trials include ancillary components requiring the submission of specimens for the examination of biomarkers. Biomarkers are needed as a means of predicting clinical outcomes, including the ability to stratify patients by risk, predict responses to treatment, and give a more accurate prognosis (Dunn, Jegalian, & Greenwald, 2011); however, screening for biomarker-focused trials increases time-associated efficacy challenges because many patients may need to be screened before actual enrollment of an eligible patient, particularly if the biomarker used for patient selection is of low prevalence in the tumor type of focus.

Estimation of the costs associated with identifying and screening patients is important to evaluate. Considering time requirements without considering the implications of associated costs does not provide an accurate assessment of the actual costs incurred (Ota et al., 2006). In a prospective evaluation of time spent on screening by research staff using a real-time tracking system, Penberthy, Dahman, Petkov, and DeShazo (2012) found substantial variation in attributed costs by study type and phase with the average time spent per patient ranging from 3.4 to 8.8 hours and costs ranging from $129 to $336. This translated to an estimated uncompensated annual screening cost of more than $90,000 for the institution, demonstrating how substantial the cost of screening can be. Institutions conducting more phase I trials than other phase trials were considered to have substantially higher screening-associated costs (Penberthy et al., 2012).

Research Team Perspectives

Team-based care, such as multidisciplinary disease-oriented care programs, is currently considered to be essential to meeting the supply and demand imbalance of today's workforce and is considered to be a critical element of improving healthcare delivery (Coniglio, 2013). The team-based care concept can also be applied to cancer clinical trial programs. The core research team may include a variety of personnel, such as a research manager and coordinator, clinical trial nurses (CTNs), clinical research associates, regulatory specialists, and quality assurance personnel, who conduct the day-to-day research activities and are employees of the research program. In addition to the physician investigators, the core team is essential to accrual. However, when considering recruitment efforts for cancer clinical trials, the research team should extend beyond these individuals to include institutional administrators, other oncology nurses, private practice personnel, pharmacists, laboratory and finance personnel, and patient navigators and advocates. Figure 24-1 illustrates the potential components of the broader cancer research team. Engaging the broader community from the onset can strengthen the research program's recruitment and accrual efforts (National Cancer Institute [NCI], 2010).

It is important for the entire research team to commit to making research a foundation of its culture—a culture that brings people together to share responsibility with a sense of ownership for clinical trials. A clinical trial culture needs to be supported from the top down, including institution and practice administration, the research program principal investigator, management, and support staff. But most importantly, it must be a thought process for the research team. If the research team does not portray the culture of accrual, no one will. A classic example of understanding the vision of a team culture occurred when President John F. Kennedy was touring NASA and asked a janitor what his job was. "Sending a man to the moon" was the janitor's reply. Everyone from the top to the bottom knew the goal of NASA (NCI, 2009). It is vital that a clear message of the team's expectations and its predefined, measureable goals be communicated to everyone on the team. The leader of a research team must make every effort to acknowledge the value of each of its members while promoting a culture of teamwork and commitment to delivering high-quality care to patients (Baer, Zon, Devine, & Lyss, 2011).

An important aspect of recruitment success is having a research staff that is devoted and responsible to the research process, including recruitment planning, implementation, and maintaining follow-up. Research programs are most effective when research staff is assigned solely to the research program. When one position is split between both research and clinical practice, the research tasks often are neglected (Baer et al., 2011). Special consideration should be allowed for sufficient time and staffing for recruiting patients from minority and low socioeconomic populations (Gul & Ali, 2010). Having devoted research staff increases the likelihood of improved accrual rates. Bradley and colleagues (2006) found having a full-time research assistant resulted in a more systematic and persistent assessment of eligibility of patients for entry into clinical trials, ensuring nonbiased sampling and selection of patients and that all patients had the opportunity to participate.

Clinical trial recruitment literature historically has reported the relationship between patients and their doctors as crucial to the success of recruitment into clinical research; therefore, recruitment should occur as part of the therapeutic alliance between doctors and patients (Symonds, Lord, Mitchell, & Raghavan, 2012). The patient and physician have been described as the "healthcare team" (Coniglio, 2013). There is no doubt that the relationship between the physician and patient is important to participation in cancer research. In fact, Comis, Miller, Colaizzi, and Kimmel (2009) found that patient participation in a clinical trial was directly related to the level of physician involvement reported by the patient. Rooney et al. (2011) reported that the most effective method of recruitment was a personal invitation from a trusted general practitioner, hospital consultant, or community/faith leader. Schilsky (2011) supported this concept, indicating that the one factor that most greatly influences a patient's decision to participate in a clinical trial is his or her oncologist's recommendation to do so. However, physician participation in cancer clinical trials is hampered by increased time and effort required to find a clinical trial, determine eligibility, explain the trial to potential participants, obtain informed consent, and then ensure the additional testing and study-related procedures are completed (Spaar et al., 2009). It is unrealistic to expect the physician alone to undertake all of the activities associated with clinical trial participation.

The Oncology Nursing Society (2010) *Oncology Clinical Trials Nurse Competencies* state that CTNs are able to provide leadership in the conduct of clinical trials,

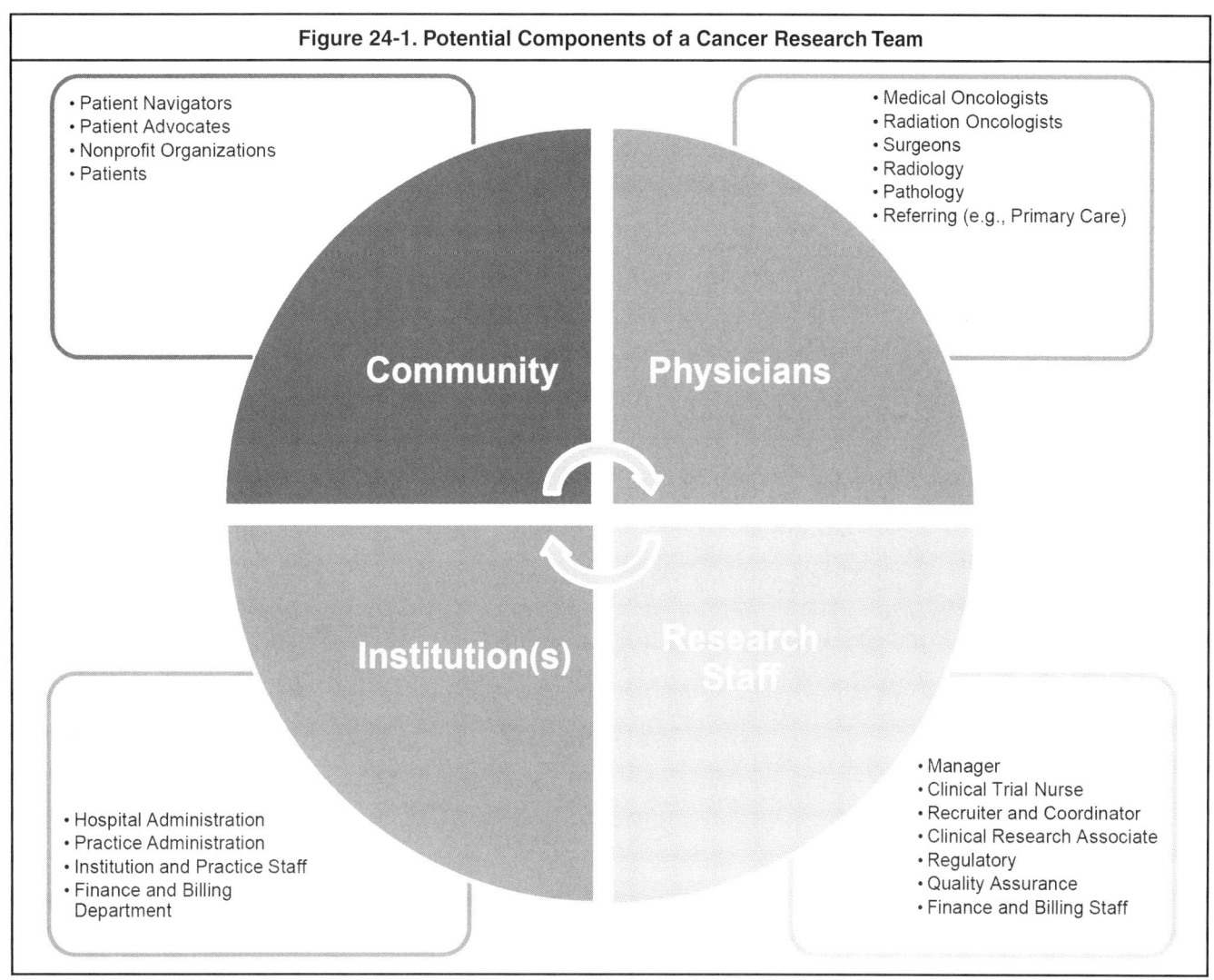

Figure 24-1. Potential Components of a Cancer Research Team

thereby improving outcomes for patients and enhancing study integrity. As a leader and a vital component of the research team, CTNs can play a key role in reducing the time and effort required of physicians, a significant barrier to recruitment efforts.

CTNs, working as a team members in tandem with the physicians, can reduce physicians' burden by pre-screening patient charts and, when a potential participant is identified, have the consent document and study-required information available for discussion with the physicians before their encounter with the patient. After the physicians introduce the clinical trial to patients, physicians could rely on CTNs to provide the additional trial- and disease-related information to the patients and their significant others. Physicians could then be free to visit with other scheduled patients while CTNs provide patient education and consent information. After the patients have had time to consider their decision, usually at a follow-up visit, CTNs can ensure trial eligibility criteria are met and, after obtaining signed consent, order any outstanding research-related tests. The physi-

cians would follow up with patients to answer any further questions and concerns. Physicians, CTNs, and patients become a team throughout the process of enrollment, treatment, and follow-up.

Wujcik and Wolff (2010) described a similar example of applied team-based care that they reported improved accrual to cancer clinical trials at their institution. Their research staff actively participates in the patient screening and assessing process, advising physicians of potential clinical trial options, eligibility requirements, and potential hurdles to overcome early in the patient evaluation process, thereby limiting the physician burden.

CTNs can also consider a variety of strategies to enhance recruitment, such as playing a leadership role in the implementation of recruitment plans, identifying and developing processes to overcome patient-related barriers, and identifying institutional or community-based resources or groups that can assist in achieving identified recruitment goals (Oncology Nursing Society, 2010).

Constant monitoring of recruitment activities and accrual by a dedicated management team that is willing to proactively investigate problems and barriers encountered and invest resources toward potential solutions is key to successful recruitment efforts (McCaskill-Stevens et al., 2013; Menon et al., 2008). Accrual graphs that are updated on a monthly basis indicating accrual goals in relation to actual accrual can be maintained and shared with research staff, investigators, and support personnel (see Figure 24-2). Reports indicating accrual by investigators may be considered as a means of promoting a competitive spirit. Regularly held research staff meetings provide an opportunity for the team to collectively assess accrual trends, discuss any barriers or problems encountered, and develop possible options for reducing them as well as providing an opportunity for team building and collaboration.

Effective communication and motivation are keys to soliciting crucial nonresearch staff (McSweeney, Pettey, Fischer, & Spellman, 2009). When nonresearch staff members have a clear understanding of clinical trials research, what will be required of them, and how the research could benefit them and their community, recruitment will be less burdensome. The research team may consider multiple methods to increase awareness and support for clinical research at their research sites, such as flyers, posters, in-service trainings, and attendance at staff meetings (Chlan, Guttormson, Tracy, & Bremer, 2009). Research staff should be aware of the clinic or site environment when they are there for research-related purposes and be sympathetic to the clinic staff's day-to-day workload and activities. Every effort should be made not to place unnecessary additional demands on site staff as a result of research endeavors. A consistent visibility of the research team helps the clinic staff to become familiar with research and has the potential to promote and nurture a partnership between the clinic staff and research team. It will be invaluable for the research team to identify a research site contact person or site champion who can serve as a point of contact for potential comments about staff concerns or barriers and possible solutions (Berger et al., 2007; Chlan et al., 2009).

Recognizing a clinic staff individual's or the entire staff's efforts can prove to be a successful engagement strategy (McCaskill-Stevens et al., 2013; Segre, Buckwalter, & Friedemann, 2011). Possible recognition methods could include handwritten thank-you notes placed in personnel files and certificates of appreciation presented at staff meetings or gatherings, gift certificates to a coffee shop, and recognition in newsletters or interoffice communications. Physician investigators, particularly those with high accrual, can be recognized through mechanisms such as newsletters, tumor board conferences, and other cancer program meetings and events. Furthermore, every effort should be made to share the results of clinical trials with the research and nonresearch staff when available, as an additional opportunity to provide education and also to reinforce the importance of clinical

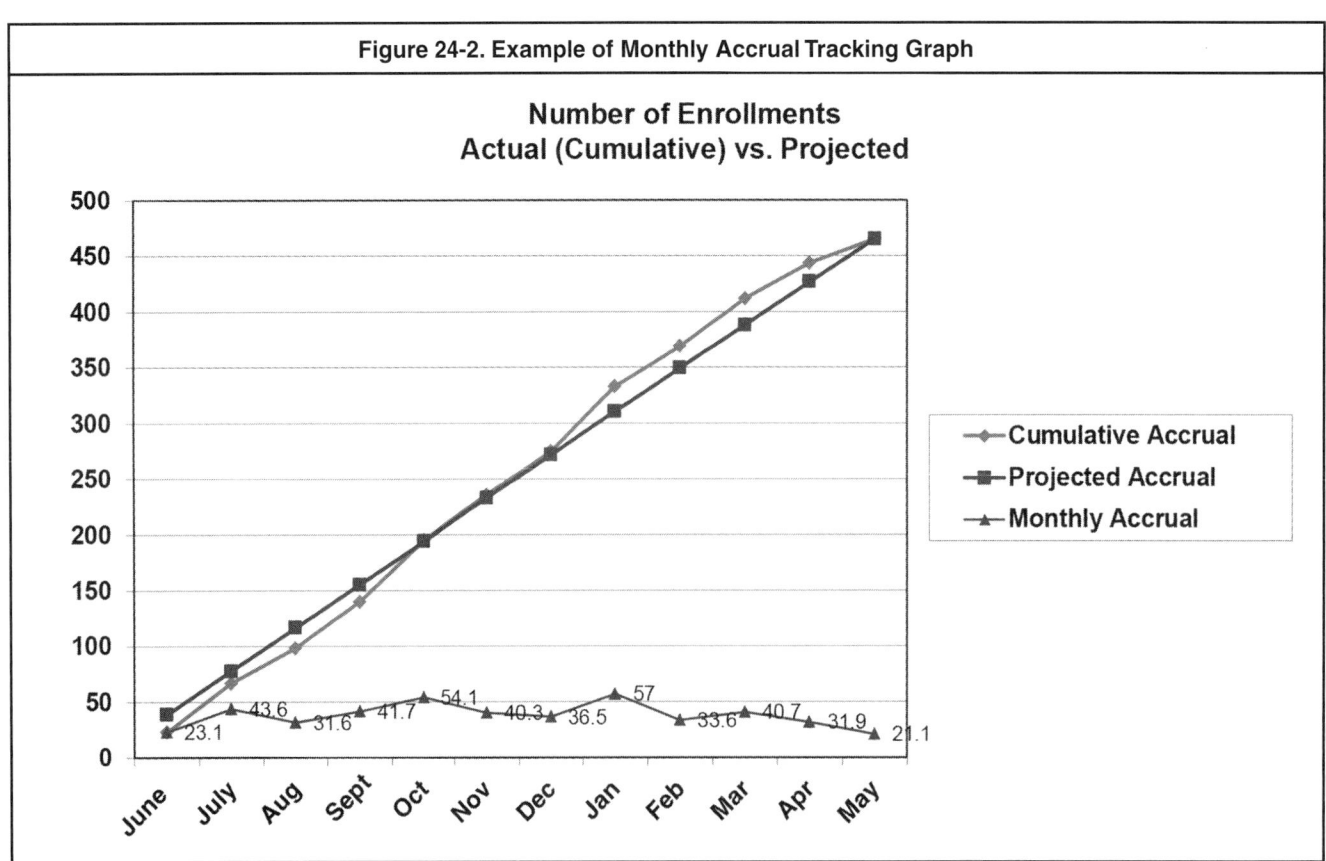

Figure 24-2. Example of Monthly Accrual Tracking Graph

research and the important role they played in contributing to the research efforts.

The research staff should be adequately and properly educated regarding clinical trials research. As the complexity of clinical trials continues to increase, it will become even more important for the research staff to understand and explain study details and consent documents (Gerber et al., 2012). Berger and colleagues (2007) emphasized the importance of research staff valuing the research being conducted. In order to value the research, they must not only understand the rationale behind clinical research in general but also should understand the trial objectives before discussing the trial with patients or potential participants. The importance of the first contact with potential participants cannot be ignored (Gul & Ali, 2010). The individual making the first contact must not only be educated about the study and able to answer all concerns and questions but also must portray an attitude that is culturally aware. Gerber and colleagues (2012) studied 922 participants, of which 872 patients were consented by 187 consenters. Patients were more likely to agree to participate in a clinical trial when the consenter was more experienced (had obtained consent multiple prior times). They attributed this finding to the consenter being more familiar with the trial rather than simply their communication skills.

Research staff education can be enhanced by attending national and local research meetings and participating in professional development (Baer et al., 2011). National research meetings not only provide education but also provide an opportunity for networking and sharing of experiences with staff from other research programs. If attending national meetings is too challenging because of budgetary constraints, another option for furthering the opportunity for education and networking is online resources, such as NCI's website devoted to clinical trial accrual called AccrualNet (https://accrualnet.cancer.gov). It is a web-based resource and collaboration tool that supports professionals involved in the process of recruiting and retaining participants to clinical trials. AccrualNet provides a continually updated collection of resources, training materials, and tools, as well as an environment for collaborative work, professional development, and dissemination of accrual best practices. By joining AccrualNet, research staff can be connected to others in the recruitment community facing the same issues.

The Recruitment Process

Successful recruitment of participants to cancer clinical trials requires a well-designed process that defines the tasks, approaches, and team member responsibilities (NCI, 2010). The NCI (2010) training module "Including Clinical Trials in Your Practice" describes a five-step process to be followed for each trial's recruitment efforts:
- Step 1: Identify the number of participants needed for the trial.
- Step 2: Determine the site's strategies for recruiting participants.
- Step 3: Screen potential participants.
- Step 4: Enroll eligible participants.
- Step 5: Continually evaluate recruitment efforts for all trials at the site.

All of these steps of the recruitment process are important; however, ensuring enough patients or potential participants are available for specific clinical trials and the strategies to consider for recruitment and enrollment are vital.

Before undertaking the process of activating a clinical trial, the research program should verify that sufficient numbers of potential patients or participants will be available to justify the activation of the trial and that predefined accrual goals are likely to be attained. Cancer registries, programs supported by the Centers for Disease Control and Prevention and the NCI Surveillance, Epidemiology, and End Results Program, collect information about cancer cases diagnosed and deaths from cancer. Registries are a source for identifying cancer incidence rates by disease site for a specific institution or region as a means of assessing cancer burden, informing and evaluating prevention efforts, and addressing disparities (Centers for Disease Control and Prevention, 2011). Registries can prove to be a valuable resource for research programs as they assess the availability of specific cancer populations for specific clinical trials.

Recruitment Strategies

Multiple recruitment methods and tools are required in recruiting patients to clinical trials (Gul & Ali, 2010; Gren et al., 2009; Longbottom et al., 2012). Patients and research sites are heterogeneous, indicating that individual methods and tools may vary in effectiveness; a strategy that works for one research program may not be effective for another. According to Longbottom and colleagues (2012), the more tools in place, the better, but they suggested that the implementation of multiple methods requires full-time personnel.

Population-specific barriers need to be considered, and attempts should be made to reduce or eliminate as many barriers as possible. To successfully recruit minority populations into cancer clinical trials, the research team needs to be culturally competent. Having research staff of the same ethnicity as potential trial participants has been recommended and has been credited with improving accrual of minority populations to clinical trials (Carpenter & Ziner, 2008; Marcus, Lenz, Sammons, Black, & Garg, 2012; Wujcik & Wolff, 2010).

Recruitment strategies that have worked for prevention trials may or may not help in treatment trial accrual. Figure 24-3 lists potential recruitment strategies for consideration.

Tumor Boards

Tumor-specific or multidisciplinary tumor boards provide an option for improving clinical trial recruitment rates. In a study conducted by McNair and colleagues (2008), clinical trial recommendation by a multidisciplinary tumor board significantly increased the likelihood that patients were screened for trial entry, and as a result, clinical trial recruitment rates improved. Flagging potential participants in tumor board meetings allowed CTNs an easy and quick means to identify potentially eligible patients; it also served as a reminder to tumor board members to discuss the trial with the patient (McNair et al., 2008).

Electronic Screening

Automated systems for eligibility screening using health information technology tools are becoming more commonplace in today's clinical trial arena. They have the potential to reduce the burden of manual chart reviews and may ensure that more patients have the opportunity to be evaluated for participation in clinical trials (Penberthy, Brown, Puma, & Dahman, 2010). Properly configured electronic screening systems can be used to conduct prescreening for the research staff, leaving the staff to conduct a more detailed eligibility determination on a less burdensome number of manual chart reviews (Thadani, Weng, Bigger, Ennever, & Wajngurt, 2009). Electronic screening systems not only have the potential to assist in evaluating potential participants but also may have the capability to capture information on all screened patients into an electronic screening log, including important information such as reasons for ineligibility. The knowledge obtained can inform the research program staff of barriers being encountered, for which possible solutions can be developed (Virginia Commonwealth University Massey Cancer Center, n.d.).

Clinical Trials as a Business

Regarding clinical trials from a business perspective is another idea that has been considered by some authors assessing methods to improve accrual to clinical trials (Longbottom et al., 2012; McDonald et al., 2011). Initially, the idea of applying business models to medicine may seem inappropriate; however, they share common goals: businesses strive to find customers and encourage them to buy what is being offered, and clinical trials strive to find physicians and patients and encourage them to participate (McDonald et al., 2011). McDonald

---

Figure 24-3. Selected Recruitment Strategies

- Marketing research program and/or specific clinical trials
  - Unique and recognizable logo
  - Public website with members-only component
  - Brochures and recruitment materials (in applicable languages for population served)
  - Have public and professional level slide presentations prepared in advance explaining research program and specific trials (as needed)
  - Participation in community-based health fairs, events, and conferences
  - Direct mailings using commercial mailing lists, community outreach, and mass media for applicable trials (e.g., prevention and early detection trials)
- Repeated communication to research sites
  - Congratulatory emails, certificates of appreciation, and/or written thank-you notes for clinical trial referrals
  - Newsletters provided on consistent basis recognizing accrual achievements, success stories, and protocol updates
  - Accrual summaries in graph format or other methods indicating projected accrual goal and current accrual
  - Monthly updated listing of available open trials (e.g., pocket card, electronic app)
- Weekly research team strategy meetings
  - Accrual rates
  - Barriers encountered and possible solutions
  - New trial activations and development of recruitment plans
- Regularly scheduled meetings with physician investigators and ancillary staff
- Solicitation of funding to address participant barriers such as transportation, parking, etc.
- Patient specific
  - Include family members and significant others in patient visits (particularly the consent discussion).
  - If patients are experiencing fatigue and/or other symptoms, allow time to respond to requests, provide rest breaks, and be willing to space collection of data over time.
  - Show interest in other aspects of their lives.

Note. Based on information from Chlan et al., 2009; Goode et al., 2008; Gren et al., 2009; Longbottom et al., 2012; McCaskill-Stevens et al., 2013; McDonald et al., 2011; Segre et al., 2011.

and colleagues (2011) applied a business model that was developed using insights from a marketing theory to improve accrual to a national trial assessing treatment options for trauma patients. They applied multiple business model components, including concepts such as developing a brand value, devising strategies to overcome resistance, adopting a marketing plan, engaging champions, developing multi-audience messages, achieving buy-in, providing frequent positive reinforcements, and ensuring that trial procedures are simple and can be incorporated into a participating site's established routine. The model provided a consistent framework for planning and managing recruitment and provided the researchers valuable information that positively influenced accrual to the trial. Longbottom and colleagues (2012) also used marketing strategies within a recruitment plan for a cardiology-focused trial. Using multiple strategies such as the development of a unique study logo, trial-specific recruitment materials (posters, brochures, pocket cards, template press releases), funds for patient transportation, and flexible appointment schedules proved to be of benefit in successfully completing the trial.

Social Media

Recruitment to cancer clinical trials may be enhanced through the use of new and continuously evolving social media technology. Social media, or social networking sites, are web-based sites where conversations can take place between two or more people with the opportunity to exchange information (Andrews, 2012). People within these virtual communities often have common interests and are connecting to one another from all over the world to have conversations and exchange knowledge. The impact of social media is extensive and has fundamentally changed how professional and personal business is conducted. Within the medical world, nurses can now access educational meetings via Facebook, Twitter, or other social networking sites and are able to get immediate responses from colleagues around the world, not just in the local conference room (Andrews, 2012). The use of social media within the context of recruitment has many advantages. It is cost-effective, fast, interactive, easily accessible, and convenient. Specific patient populations may be targeted through such social networking sites as Facebook, through which a sponsor can establish an account focusing on a specific drug or disease, as well as can be customized to provide clinical trial–specific information, including how a potential participant can learn more (Andrews, 2012). Social media can be used to provide support and direct compliance efforts for participants during the trial and after the trial is completed during the follow-up period. It can also serve as a means of communication between participants and research program staff to keep participants motivated and to provide feedback or to ask questions. Confidentiality issues related to the use of social networking sites need to be considered, however. Even with the use of antivirus software, there is a risk of the website being invaded by "hackers," potentially putting participants' confidential information into inappropriate hands. Additionally, the content to be used within a social media network will need institutional review board approval before it goes live online (Andrews, 2012).

Patient Navigators

According to the Center to Reduce Cancer Health Disparities (2009), patient navigators are trained, culturally sensitive healthcare workers who provide support and guidance throughout the cancer care continuum. They essentially help people navigate through their cancer care, which may involve interactions with multiple doctors' offices, clinics, hospitals, outpatient centers, insurance and payment systems, patient-support organizations, and other components of the healthcare system. Originally used to increase poor diagnostic follow-up rates among minorities, patient navigation is currently being widely implemented by many healthcare facilities as a means of enhancing their cancer programs. How the institution's navigation program is structured depends on the needs of the target populations and the resources of the providers (Esparza & Calhoun, 2011). Frequently involved with cancer screening processes, patient navigators may be one of the first institutional contacts a newly diagnosed patient with cancer encounters.

An essential part of the patient navigation process should include the introduction of participation in a clinical trial as a viable treatment option; however, patient navigators generally are not provided trial-related training. In an effort to educate lay patient navigators, Bryant, Williamson, Cartmell, and Jefferson (2011) developed an evidence-based clinical trial training curriculum for patient navigators, which resulted in the navigators having an increased sense of confidence. Holmes, Major, Lyonga, Alleyne, and Clayton (2012) were successful in improving African American women's accrual to breast cancer clinical trials by merging the traditional oncology research nurse and patient navigator into a single role as an oncology nurse navigator. The nurse navigator interacted and collaborated with community-based physicians while engaging the African American patients with breast cancer. Not only did the nurse navigator guide the patients around the barriers of the healthcare system, but the navigator also played a key role in all phases of the clinical trial process (e.g., eligibility screening, consent process, research forms). As a result, 51 of 59 eligible patients enrolled in one or more clinical trials (Holmes et al., 2012).

Patient Advocates

Similar to patient navigators, patient advocates can play a role in a research program's recruitment efforts. The Institute of Medicine supported the use of patient advocates by recommending greater participation by patient advocates in the design of clinical trials and in patient recruitment for trials (Nass et al., 2010). Advocates for patients with cancer have been working with NCI cooperative groups since the early 1990s, including contributing to activities such as providing patient and family perspectives to the development of patient education and recruitment materials (Collyar, 2008).

Clinical trial research programs should invite patients to serve as advisers to the research team and as potential resources to other patients and families. Community advisory boards may also be considered as an option for local patients with cancer to provide insights about what measures of outcomes may be meaningful to potential participants as well as to contribute to the clinical trial education and recruitment process (Gul & Ali, 2010).

Summary

Recruitment to cancer clinical trials can be challenging. Many factors need to be considered before recruitment and during the study phase and follow-up. This chapter shared some of these factors, as well as steps and strategies to assist CTNs in their efforts to improve accrual to these important studies. As history has shown, nurses are often the ones who make the difference when it comes to patient and family care. CTNs have that opportunity again when promoting and supporting cancer clinical trials.

Key Points

- Recruitment of appropriate and adequate numbers of research participants to cancer clinical trials is an essential component of successful trial completion and the subsequent generation of results.
- Barriers to clinical trial participation are many and often involve several levels and factors. Before trial initiation, every effort should be made to identify potential trial-specific recruitment barriers and choose and implement options to reduce them.
- It is important for the entire research team to commit to making research a foundation of its culture—a culture that brings people together to share responsibilities with a sense of ownership for clinical trials.
- CTNs, vital members of research teams, play a key role in reducing barriers to clinical trial recruitment.
- Multiple recruitment strategies are often needed for successful clinical trial accrual.

References

American Cancer Society. (2013). *Cancer facts and figures for African Americans 2013–2014*. Retrieved from http://www.cancer.org/acs/groups/content/@epidemiologysurveilance/documents/document/acspc-036921.pdf

Andrews, C. (2012, November). Social media recruitment. *Applied Clinical Trials*. Retrieved from http://www.appliedclinicaltrialsonline.com/appliedclinicaltrials/Articles/Social-Media-Recruitment/ArticleStandard/Article/detail/796687

Baer, A.R., Zon, R., Devine, S., & Lyss, A.P. (2011). The clinical research team. *Journal of Oncology Practice, 7*, 188–192. doi:10.1200/JOP.2011.000276

Baquet, C.R., Henderson, K., Commiskey, P., & Morrow, J.N. (2008). Clinical trials: The art of enrollment. *Seminars in Oncology Nursing, 24*, 262–269. doi:10.1016/j.soncn.2008.08.006

Berger, A.M., Neumark, D.E., & Chamberlain, J. (2007). Enhancing recruitment and retention in randomized clinical trials of cancer symptom management [Online exclusive]. *Oncology Nursing Forum, 34*, E17–E22. doi:10.1188/07.ONF.E17-E22

Bradley, N.M.E., Chow, E., Tsao, M.N., Danjoux, C., Barnes, E.A., Hayter, C., ... Sinclair, E. (2006). Reasons for poor accrual in palliative radiation therapy research. *Supportive Cancer Therapy, 3*, 110–119. doi:10.3816/SCT.2006.n.007

Bryant, D.C., Williamson, D., Cartmell, K., & Jefferson, M. (2011). A lay patient navigation training curriculum targeting disparities in cancer clinical trials. *Journal of the National Black Nurses Association, 22*(2), 68–75.

Carpenter, J.S., & Ziner, K. (2008). A process to manage recruitment to multiple competing studies. *Western Journal of Nursing Research, 30*, 515–526. doi:10.1177/0193945907310644

Center to Reduce Cancer Health Disparities. (2009, July 23). What are patient navigators? Retrieved from http://crchd.cancer.gov/pnp/what-are.html

Centers for Disease Control and Prevention. (2011). National Program of Cancer Registries. Retrieved from http://www.cdc.gov/Features/CancerRegistries

Cheng, S.K., Dietrich, M.S., & Dilts, D.M. (2010). A sense of urgency: Evaluating the link between clinical trial development time and the accrual performance of Cancer Therapy Evaluation Program (NCI-CTEP) sponsored studies. *Clinical Cancer Research, 16*, 5557–5563. doi:10.1158/1078-0432.CCR-10-0133

Chlan, L., Guttormson, J., Tracy, M.F., & Bremer, K.L. (2009). Strategies for overcoming site and recruitment challenges in research studies based in intensive care units. *American Journal of Critical Care, 18*, 410–417. doi:10.4037/ajcc2009400

Collyar, D. (2008). An essential partnership: Patient advocates and cooperative groups. *Seminars in Oncology, 35*, 553–555. doi:10.1053/j.seminoncol.2008.07.009

Comis, R.L., Miller, J.D., Aldigé, C.R., Krebs, L., & Stoval, E. (2003). Public attitudes toward participation in cancer clinical trials. *Journal of Clinical Oncology, 21*, 830–835. doi:10.1200/JCO.2003.02.105

Comis, R.L., Miller, J.D., Colaizzi, D.D., & Kimmel, L.G. (2009). Physician-related factors involved in patient decisions to enroll onto cancer clinical trials. *Journal of Oncology Practice, 5*, 50–56. doi:10.1200/JOP.0922001

Coniglio, D. (2013). Collaborative practice models and team-based care in oncology. *Journal of Oncology Practice, 9*, 99–100. doi:10.1200/JOP.2012.000859

Dilts, D.M., & Sandler, A.B. (2006). Invisible barriers to clinical trials: The impact of structural, infrastructural, and procedural barriers to opening oncology clinical trials. *Journal of Clinical Oncology, 24*, 4545–4552. doi:10.1200/JCO.2005.05.0104

Dunn, B.K., Jegalian, K., & Greenwald, P. (2011). Biomarkers for early detection and as surrogate endpoints in cancer prevention trials: Issues and opportunities. *Recent Results in Cancer Research, 188*, 21–47. doi:10.1007/978-3-642-10858-7_3

Esparza, A., & Calhoun, E. (2011). Measuring the impact and potential of patient navigation: Proposed common metrics and beyond. *Cancer, 117*(Suppl. 15), 3535–3536. doi:10.1002/cncr.26265

Ford, J.G., Howerton, M.W., Lai, G.Y., Gary, T.L., Bolen, S., Gibbons, M.C., ... Bass, E.B. (2008). Barriers to recruiting underrepresented populations to cancer clinical trials: A systematic review. *Cancer, 112*, 228–242. doi:10.1002/cncr.23157

Gerber, D.E., Rasco, D.W., Skinner, C.S., Dowell, J.E., Yan, J., Sayne, J.R., & Xie, Y. (2012). Consent timing and experience: Modifiable factors that may influence interest in cancer research. *Journal of Oncology Practice, 8*, 91–96. doi:10.1200/JOP.2011.000335

Goode, P.S., FitzGerald, M.P., Richter, H.E., Whitehead, W.E., Nygaard, I., Wren, P.A., ... Weber, A.M. (2008). Enhancing participation of older women in surgical trials. *Journal of the American College of Surgeons, 207*, 303–311. doi:10.1016/j.jamcollsurg.2008.03.012

Gren, L., Broski, K., Childs, J., Cordes, J., Engelhard, D., Gahagan, B., ... Marcus, P. (2009). Recruitment methods employed in the Prostate, Lung, Colorectal, and Ovarian Cancer Screening Trial. *Clinical Trials, 6*, 52–59. doi:10.1177/1740774508100974

Gul, R.B., & Ali, P.A. (2010). Clinical trials: The challenge of recruitment and retention of participants. *Journal of Clinical Nursing, 19*, 227–233. doi:10.1111/j.1365-2702.2009.03041.x

Holmes, D.R., Major, J., Lyonga, D.E., Alleyne, R.S., & Clayton, S.M. (2012). Increasing minority patient participation in cancer clinical trials using oncology nurse navigation. *American Journal of Surgery, 203*, 415–422. doi:10.1016/j.amjsurg.2011.02.005

Joseph, G., & Dohan, D. (2009). Recruiting minorities where they receive care: Institutional barriers to cancer clinical trials recruitment in a safety-net hospital. *Contemporary Clinical Trials, 30*, 552–559. doi:10.1016/j.cct.2009.06.009

Kaur, G., Smyth, R.L., & Williamson, P. (2012). Developing a survey of barriers and facilitators to recruitment in randomized controlled trials. *Trials, 13*, 218. doi:10.1186/1745-6215-13-218

Korn, E.L., Freidlin, B., Mooney, M., & Abrams, J.S. (2010). Accrual experience of National Cancer Institute Cooperative Group phase III trials activated from 2000 to 2007. *Journal of Clinical Oncology, 28*, 5197–5201. doi:10.1200/JCO.2010.31.5382

Longbottom, M.E., Roberts, J.N., Tom, M., Hughes, S.E., Howard, V.J., Sheffet, A.J., ... Brott, T.G. (2012). Interventions to increase enrollment in a large multicenter phase 3 trial of carotid stenting vs. endarterectomy. *International Journal of Stroke, 7*, 447–453. doi:10.1111/j.1747-4949.2012.00833.x

Marcus, P.M., Lenz, S., Sammons, D., Black, W., & Garg, K. (2012). Recruitment methods employed in the National Lung Screening Trial. *Journal of Medical Screening, 19*, 94–102. doi:10.1258/jms.2012.012016

McCaskill-Stevens, W., Wilson, J.W., Cook, E.D., Edwards, C.L., Gibson, R.V., McElwain, D.L., ... Wolmark, N. (2013). National Surgical Adjuvant Breast and Bowel Project Study of Tamoxifen and Raloxifene trial: Advancing the science of recruitment and breast cancer risk assessment in minority communities. *Clinical Trials, 10*, 280–291. doi:10.1177/1740774512470315

McDonald, A.M., Treweek, S., Shakur, H., Free, C., Knight, R., Speed, C., & Campbell, M.K. (2011). Using a business model approach and marketing techniques for recruitment to clinical trials. *Trials, 12*, 74. doi:10.1186/1745-6215-12-74

McNair, A.G.K., Choh, C.T.P., Metcalfe, C., Littlejohns, D., Barham, C.P., Hollowood, A., ... Blazeby, J.M. (2008). Maximising recruitment into randomised controlled trials: The role of multidisciplinary cancer teams. *European Journal of Cancer, 44*, 2623–2626. doi:10.1016/j.ejca.2008.08.009

McSweeney, J.C., Pettey, C.M., Fischer, E.P., & Spellman, A. (2009). Going the distance: Overcoming challenges in recruitment and retention of Black and White women in a multisite, longitudinal study of predictors of coronary heart disease. *Research in Gerontological Nursing, 2*, 256–264. doi:10.3928/19404921-20090803-01

Menon, U., Gentry-Maharaj, A., Ryan, A., Sharma, A., Burnell, M., Hallett, R., ... Jacobs, I. (2008). Recruitment to multicentre trials—Lessons from UKCTOCS: Descriptive study. *BMJ, 337*, a2079. doi:10.1136/bmj.a2079

Murphy, V.H., Krumholz, H.M., & Gross, C.P. (2004). Participation in cancer clinical trials: Race-, sex-, and age-based disparities. *JAMA, 291*, 2720–2726. doi:10.1001/jama.291.22.2720

Nass, S.J., Moses, H.L., & Mendelsohn, J. (Eds.). (2010). *A national cancer clinical trials system for the 21st century: Reinvigorating the NCI Cooperative Group Program*. Retrieved from http://books.nap.edu/openbook.php?record_id=12879

National Cancer Institute. (2009). *Clinical Trial Recruitment Initiative—NCI Comprehensive Cancer Centers accrual practices: Results from three case studies*. Bethesda, MD: Office of Communications and Education. Unpublished report.

National Cancer Institute. (2010, January 1). Including clinical trials in your practice: An overview. Retrieved from http://www.cancer.gov/clinicaltrials/conducting/clinicaltrialscourse

Oncology Nursing Society. (2010). *Oncology clinical trials nurse competencies*. Retrieved from https://www.ons.org/sites/default/files/ctncompetencies.pdf

Ota, K.S., Friedman, L., Ashford, J.W., Hernandez, B., Penner, A.L., Stepp, A.M., ... Yesavage, J.A. (2006). The cost-time index: A new method for measuring the efficiencies of recruitment-resources in clinical trials. *Contemporary Clinical Trials, 27*, 494–497. doi:10.1016/j.cct.2006.05.008

Paskett, E.D., Reeves, K.W., McLaughlin, J.M., Katz, M.L., McAlearney, A.S., Ruffin, M.T., ... Gehlert, S. (2008). Recruitment of minority and underserved populations in the United States: The Centers for Population Health and Health Disparities experience. *Contemporary Clinical Trials, 29*, 847–861. doi:10.1016/j.cct.2008.07.006

Patel, Y.R., Carr, K.A., Magjuka, D., Mohammadi, Y., Dropcho, E.F., Reed, A.D., ... Hahn, N.M. (2012). Successful recruitment of healthy African American men to genomic studies from high-volume community health fairs. *Cancer, 118*, 1075–1082. doi:10.1002/cncr.26328

Penberthy, L., Brown, R., Puma, F., & Dahman, B. (2010). Automated matching software for clinical trials eligibility: Measuring efficiency and flexibility. *Contemporary Clinical Trials, 31*, 207–217. doi:10.1016/j.cct.2010.03.005

Penberthy, L.T., Dahman, B.A., Petkov, V.I., & DeShazo, J.P. (2012). Effort required in eligibility screening for clinical trials. *Journal of Oncology Practice, 8*, 365–370. doi:10.1200/JOP.2012.000646

Rooney, L.K., Bhopal, R., Halani, L., Levy, M.L., Partridge, M.R., Netuveli, G., ... Sheikh, A. (2011). Promoting recruitment of minority ethnic groups into research: Qualitative study exploring the views of South Asian people with asthma. *Journal of Public Health, 33*, 604–615. doi:10.1093/pubmed/fdq100

Schilsky, R.L. (2011). Accrual to cancer clinical trials in the era of molecular medicine. *Science Translational Medicine, 3*, 75cm9. doi:10.1126/scitranslmed.3001712

Segre, L.S., Buckwalter, K.C., & Friedemann, M.-L. (2011). Strategies to engage clinical staff in subject recruitment. *Journal of Research in Nursing, 16*, 321–332. doi:10.1177/1744987110387475

Spaar, A., Frey, M., Turk, A., Karrer, W., & Puhan, M.A. (2009). Recruitment barriers in a randomized controlled trial from the physician's perspective—A postal survey. *BMC Medical Research Methodology, 9*, 14. doi:10.1186/1471-2288-9-14

Symonds, R.P., Lord, K., Mitchell, A.J., & Raghavan, D. (2012). Recruitment of ethnic minorities into cancer clinical trials: Experience from the front lines. *British Journal of Cancer, 107*, 1017–1021. doi:10.1038/bjc.2012.240

Thadani, S.R., Weng, C., Bigger, J.T., Ennever, J.F., & Wajngurt, D. (2009). Electronic screening improves efficacy in clinical trial recruitment. *Journal of the American Medical Informatics Association, 16,* 869–873. doi:10.1197/jamia.M3119

Treweek, S., Mitchell, E., Pitkethly, M., Cook, J., Kjeldstrøm, M., Johansen, M., ... Lockhart, P. (2010). Strategies to improve recruitment to randomised controlled trials. *Cochrane Database of Systematic Reviews, 2010*(4). doi:10.1002/14651858.MR000013.pub5

Ulrich, C.M., James, J.L., Walker, E.M., Stine, S.H., Gore, E., Prestidge, B., ... Bruner, D.W. (2010). RTOG physician and research associate attitudes, beliefs and practices regarding clinical trials: Implications for improving patient recruitment. *Contemporary Clinical Trials, 31,* 221–228. doi:10.1016/j.cct.2010.03.002

Unger, J.M., Hershman, D.L., Albain, K.S., Moinpour, C.M., Petersen, J.A., Burg, K., & Crowley, J.J. (2013). Patient income level and cancer clinical trial participation. *Journal of Clinical Oncology, 31,* 536–542. doi:10.1200/JCO.2012.45.4553

Virginia Commonwealth University Massey Cancer Center. (2013). Clinical Trials Eligibility Database. Retrieved from http://www.massey.vcu.edu/research/cores/cris/cted

Wujcik, D., & Wolff, S.N. (2010). Recruitment of African Americans to national oncology clinical trials through a clinical trial shared resource. *Journal of Health Care for the Poor and Underserved, 21,* 38–50. doi:10.1353/hpu.0.0251

Chapter 25

Adherence and Retention in Clinical Trials

Lisa Francisco, BSN, RN, OCN®

Introduction

New drugs and treatment regimens provide hope for people with a cancer diagnosis. In fact, "hope for something better" is one reason some may choose to participate in a clinical trial. The U.S. Food and Drug Administration requires rigorous well-designed clinical trials to provide the evidence to approve a new drug. The National Comprehensive Cancer Network® requires a high level of evidence to recommend a treatment regimen. Novice clinical trial nurses (CTNs) may be preoccupied with the enrollment of a patient on a trial. However, experienced CTNs understand that adherence and retention of patients on a trial are even more important. Thus, ensuring participant adherence and retention on a trial provides the data needed to improve cancer care. Adherence and retention directly affect the outcome and cost of a clinical trial. Patient adherence with medical treatment is a concern on or off a clinical trial. As former U.S. Surgeon General C. Everett Koop stated, "Drugs don't work in patients who don't take them" (Koop, 1984, p. 1). Furthermore, patient nonadherence and early discontinuations on a clinical trial produce tainted data and elevate the associated costs. Retaining patients on a clinical trial for valuable follow-up and survival data is important.

Definitions of Adherence

Adherence is defined as the behavior that results from an effective relationship between the healthcare provider (HCP) and the patient (Gould & Mitty, 2010). Adherence incorporates the concept of collaboration between the patient and HCP and is an important and necessary component when discussing adherence. Ho, Bryson, and Rumsfeld (2009) referred to adherence as "the active, voluntary, and collaborative involvement of the patient in a mutually accepted course of behavior to produce a therapeutic result" (p. 3028). Initially, *adherence* and *compliance* were used synonymously until the word *compliance* started to take on a negative undertone, such as the *noncompliant patient*. *Compliance* infers the negation of the importance of a collaborative relationship between the patient and HCP. Therefore, the term *adherence* is preferred in current literature (see Table 25-1).

Nonadherence describes the patient who is inadequately complying with the agreed-upon medical or health advice. *Primary* or *intentional* nonadherence describes the patient who may have neglected to fill

Table 25-1. Comparing Compliance and Adherence

Compliance	Adherence
Clinician-centered	Patient-centered
Clinician dominance	Clinician-patient collaboration
Information is dictated	Information is exchanged
Goal: patient obedience	Goal: patient self-mastery
Activities are dictated	Activities are negotiated
Rules are dictated	Rules matched to lifestyle
Persuade, coerce	Discuss, negotiate, motivate
Resistance is not tolerated	Resistance provides information for adaptation

Note. From "Medication Adherence Is a Partnership, Medication Compliance Is Not," by E. Gould and E. Mitty, 2010, *Geriatric Nursing, 31,* p. 291. Copyright 2010 by Elsevier Mosby. Reprinted with permission.

the prescription or made a conscious decision to skip doses of a prescribed medication (Miaskowski, Shockney, & Chlebowski, 2008). The intentionally nonadherent patient hears and understands the directions but chooses not to comply for reasons such as personal health beliefs or adverse reactions. *Unintentional* nonadherence refers to the patient who is not complying with the agreed-upon medical advice because of the inability to understand the directions (Gould & Mitty, 2010). This type of nonadherence is present when the patient wants to comply but inadvertently does not. Examples are the patient who forgets to take the medication or come to an appointment or the patient who believes he or she is taking the medication as instructed but is not. The unintentionally nonadherent patient is unable to comply because of complicated instructions or simply not understanding the directions.

Factors Affecting Adherence

It is important to assess each patient for potential factors that lead to intentional and unintentional nonadherence. Studies have validated that the obvious factors such as age, gender, race, education level, socioeconomic status, disease state, and severity of the disease are not the only factors for nonadherence (Miaskowski et al., 2008). The following are factors for both intentional nonadherence and unintentional nonadherence.

Complexity of Regimen

If the medical regimen is difficult or highly disruptive to a patient's life, a greater risk exists for intentional nonadherence. An example is a medical plan that requires changes in one's lifestyle, such as smoking cessation or diet changes for weight loss, diabetes, or hypertension. The majority of newer agents are metabolized via the CYP3A4 pathway. This adds to the complexity of unintentional nonadherence. Patients must understand the potential for interactions and adhere to avoiding other medications that are either inducers or inhibitors of the CYP3A4 pathway. In addition, consuming some foods such as grapefruit also affects the prescribed regimen (Wilkes, 2011).

Clinical trials have become increasingly complex and require participants to be flexible with scheduling. Patients often are required to complete medication and side effect diaries. The time frame for obtaining tumor measurements is more rigid. Many clinical trial staff members are less willing to work around holidays for treatment schedules. These factors make following the medical regimen within the confines of a protocol more difficult for a patient to follow.

Perception of Benefit

The adage that a patient with a cancer diagnosis will strictly adhere to a prescribed treatment is false. The most robust data to dispel this notion were reported in patients with breast cancer who are prescribed endocrine therapy. Moore (2010) cited the rate of patient adherence to endocrine therapy as 53%–93% in breast cancer studies. Hershman and colleagues (2010) conducted a study of 8,769 patients with early-stage hormone-sensitive breast cancer who were prescribed tamoxifen for five years. Thirty-two percent of the participants discontinued the tamoxifen before five years. Of the 68% that continued, 28% were considered nonadherent, as they took less than 80% of the prescribed therapy (Hershman et al., 2010). In the case of endocrine therapy, patients may not believe the regimen will be helpful. Nonadherence is less likely when therapeutic benefit is experienced soon after initiation of the therapy. If a patient takes pain medication and the pain is diminished, adherence is more likely. If a physical therapy regimen is implemented in lieu of a more invasive procedure, the patient may not think this treatment regimen is aggressive enough and may not be compliant with an at-home regimen or may miss appointments.

Randomization

Randomized controlled trials are the gold standard for comparing two or more treatments. However, neither patients nor HCPs have control over the outcome of the randomization. It is imperative for patients to understand this. Patients undoubtedly have a preference before the randomization and will either be satisfied or dissatisfied with the outcome. It is important for patients to understand that treatment obtained on either arm is considered acceptable treatment and discontinuation on the trial based on the randomization result is discouraged.

Associated Costs of Treatment

Individual insurance policies and statutes vary greatly about whether clinical trial participation will be covered. Many times, it is limited to coverage of the standard of care costs *only*, and tests and exams performed outside of the standard of care are not covered. Clinical trial participants often have more office visits, which lead to more co-pays. One must also consider the travel costs that a clinical trial participant will incur for tumor measurement appointments, lab tests, and office visits. For example, the results of lab tests and radiologic studies must be known before the office visit for treatment decisions, necessitating that patients have these tests done one or two days in advance, which may incur additional co-payments.

Not all medications are provided by the study sponsor. If a portion of the treatment is already an approved medication, patients may be responsible for its cost. An example would be a randomized study in hormone receptor–positive breast cancer comparing a novel agent with exemestane versus exemestane alone. Exemestane is an approved treatment for hormone receptor–positive breast cancer. The clinical trial may not provide this medication because it is commercially available. If a patient does not have adequate drug coverage, the cost of the exemestane may be prohibitive (Moore, 2010). This is less of an issue with the passage of the Patient Protection and Affordable Care Act. CTNs must be aware of patients' financial constraints—especially before enrollment or randomization.

Adverse Effects

Adherence can be affected by the side effects experienced by a patient. CTNs are in the unique position to make sure that all side effects are minimized with appropriate interventions.

Patient Characteristics and Comorbidities

Senility, hearing loss, impaired vision, learning disabilities, poor quality of life, poor coping mechanisms, and lack of resources or support can lead to nonadherence. Older adults are less likely to take a medication as prescribed because of the aforementioned factors, as well as comorbidities that affect financial resources and increase the complexity of scheduled medications (Moore, 2010). If the patient is a child, the ability to swallow tablets cannot be assumed (Landier, 2011). Children may refuse to take medications, especially if side effects are significant. Adolescent patients may be nonadherent as, developmentally, they strive for independence and autonomy (Spano, 2004).

Provider and System Characteristics

Patients' relationships with the clinical trial staff and physicians affect patient adherence. The ability of CTNs and physicians to educate patients about the diagnosis, treatment options, and clinical trial participation affects adherence. It is important for patients to understand the options and make informed decisions. The relationship between CTNs and patients is essential. Interactions should convey knowledge, organization, and compassion (Gul & Ali, 2010). Lack of communication, disorganization, poor instructions, long wait times for testing required by the trial, uncomfortable waiting rooms, and unfriendly staff can hinder adherence and do not align with the definition of a collaborative relationship between the HCP and the patient.

Impact of Nonadherence

The average adherence rate of patients being treated for a chronic condition is approximately 40% (Cutler & Everett, 2010). Adherence in clinical trials has been diminishing. According to Tufts Center for the Study of Drug Development (2011), half of clinical trial participants completed a study in 2001. In 2010, only 25% of the participants completed a trial. Failure to recognize nonadherence in a clinical trial misleads understanding of the true clinical benefit of a treatment in the study. This is particularly true when an oral agent is being studied.

The Pharmaceutical Research and Manufacturers of America (n.d.), who represent biopharmaceutical companies, estimated these companies spent $51.1 billion in 2013 to research and develop new medicines. Nonadherence in a clinical trial affects the validity of a study. Additional subjects may need to be enrolled to complete the statistical analysis. The addition of subjects increases the cost and time to complete a study. Uncollected data as a result of missed appointments also negatively affect the study. *Attrition* refers to subjects who are lost to follow-up. The intent-to-treat analysis may need to be added to increase confidence in the validity of the findings. Intent-to-treat incorporates all patients who were randomized but were nonadherent. The reasons for attrition must be discussed in the study results (Robiner, 2005).

Nonadherence to prescribed and recommended therapy in or out of a clinical trial affects patient health. Poor adherence is associated with increased morbidity and mortality. Poor adherence is the cause of expensive hospitalizations. The cost associated with medication nonadherence in diabetes, hypertension, and dyslipidemia was estimated at $105.8 billion, or $453 per adult (Nasseh, Frazee, Vasaria, Vlahiotis, & Tian, 2012).

Assessment for Adherence

CTNs assess for adherence from recruitment until trial completion. It is essential to ascertain patient compliance in previously prescribed medical therapy. If the patient commonly missed appointments or did not take the medication as prescribed, nonadherence to the protocol is probable. Pertinent questions include (a) Can the patient come to the office for treatment and appointments? (b) Does the patient have reliable transportation and resources? and (c) Does the patient seem ambivalent about the trial? Screening for potential nonadherence risk factors minimizes problems later. CTNs should continue to assess adherence past enrollment and randomization. If a patient misses an appointment, quick follow-up is essential to intervene and keep the patient on schedule.

Determining Patient Adherence

How can patient adherence be determined? No well-controlled studies have been performed to evaluate methods that monitor oral medication adherence (Moore, 2010). Furthermore, patient adherence to clinical trials has been less studied. Indirect methods to assess adherence to oral medication include "self-report questionnaires, telephone interviews, prescription refill data, manual counting of unused medication, and electronic pill dispensers" (Miaskowski et al., 2008, p. 215). Self-reporting is not reliable because patients may omit or add information purposefully. If patients know that pills are being counted, they can simply remove pills so that the count will be correct. Electronic pill dispensers and monitoring reveal that the medication was dispensed, but not that it was taken. These devices also are expensive to employ in a study. The Hawthorne effect is impervious to self-reporting. Patients will be more adherent initially because they are aware their medication usage is being monitored (O'Carroll, Dennis, Johnston, & Sudlow, 2010). Another way to measure adherence is through collateral reports, which involve documentation of adherence by observations that can be verified by a health professional, family, friends, or caregivers (Moore, 2010).

The best method, although rarely used, is to measure adherence objectively by using pharmacologic markers, such as serum drug levels or metabolites of the medication. A high level of difficulty still exists to verify adherence through bioassays. One must consider the half-life of the medication and timing of when the patient took the medication. Using this method increases the cost of the study, adds time spent obtaining the samples, and is more unpleasant for the patient (Moore, 2010).

Why Are Patients Nonadherent?

Rosenstock (1988) created the Health Belief Model, which may be applied to problems of explaining, predicting, and influencing behaviors related to health practices. The Health Belief Model, which measures an individual's perception of his or her susceptibility to a disease, describes behaviors related to perceptions (Miaskowski et al., 2008). Gritz, DiMatteo, and Hays (1989) described a six-factor model of adherence:
- An effective communication of information must exist to ensure that the patient understands what is expected of him or her and what the patient can expect from the treatment.
- Second is the rapport that a patient has with the healthcare team; the quality of the relationship is a primary component of change. The patient must feel that the HCP exhibits behaviors such as trust, warmth, and genuine caring.
- Third, with the patient's beliefs and attitudes, which are based on the Health Belief Model, the patient must feel that negative health consequences would occur if he or she were noncompliant with a prescribed regimen.
- The patient's social climate and norms affect adherence. The sources of these beliefs and norms are family, friends, social class, and ethnicity.
- The fifth factor is behavioral intentions. This behavior is strengthened by a written contract (e.g., to lose weight, to perform breast self-exams monthly).
- The patient must have active support to decrease any barriers. For example, if the patient cannot afford medications, he or she needs financial assistance; if the patient works during the day, the clinic needs to be open later in the evening; if the patient does not have a vehicle, he or she needs a bus line or other transportation support.

Interventions to Promote Adherence

The process model of adherence intervention is based on identifying a health problem and prescribing behaviors that are supported organizationally, behaviorally, and educationally (Gould & Mitty, 2010). The informed consent form is the initial educational intervention. (See Chapter 14 for more information on the informed consent process.) The informed consent process is ongoing. Patients should be given a detailed explanation of the trial requirements, treatment, and potential side effects. This can be accomplished through a combination of verbal, written, and video presentations. The education provided should be tailored to patients' learning style. Written information should replicate the oral, and vice versa.

The first step to preventing nonadherence is the identification of risk factors and then tailoring interventions for each patient. CTNs must educate patients and caregivers about why adherence is necessary. Perhaps patients and caregivers do not understand that oral medications are just as important as IV medications. Measure the success of the education by having patients and caregivers repeat the information back. Patients must also understand why laboratory tests, radiologic tests, and examinations must be done at specific time points in the study (Moore, 2010).

Using organizational tools can assist patients whose memory skills are impaired or those who simply lack strong organizational skills. Calendars prefilled with appointments and tests can be used to prevent patients from missing important time points. Prefilled pill boxes labeled with dates and times are relatively inexpensive and help patients to remember to take medications (Moore, 2010). Patients should be provided with reminders about appointments and tests by email, telephone, postcards, or letters. Smartphone applications also can be used to promote organization. Organizational tools are also important for CTNs to minimize interruptions to patients' daily lives. It is important to attempt to schedule all tests and exams on the same day or at a time convenient for the patient, if possible, within the study guidelines. This reduces the cost of transportation, co-pays, and missed work. CTNs should minimize the time clinical trial patients wait to have laboratory tests, radiologic tests, and appointments (Robiner, 2005). Patients should have a supportive environment within the healthcare system.

CTNs should proactively manage concerns and side effects that patients experience by educating them about expected side effects and encouraging them to call when a side effect is first evident. CTNs should then contact the physician, when appropriate, for medical intervention. Patients are more likely to be adherent when side effects and concerns are efficiently addressed (Moore, 2010).

The professional relationship between patients and CTNs enhances study and medication adherence. Trial participants work closely with CTNs, which leads to trust. Each patient should have one consistent CTN. The CTN should make every effort to be present when the patient meets with the physician. Often patients do not understand what the physician says. CTNs are in a vital position to ensure all patients' questions have been answered. If patients have a scheduled test within the facility, CTNs should make a point to stop in briefly to ensure there are no problems. CTNs should convey enthusiasm about the study and appreciation to patients for their involvement. If updates about the study are available, CTNs should share that information to maintain patients' interest and subsequent adherence (Oncology Nursing Society, 2010). Patients who are on a clinical trial should feel that they are special and appreciated. CTNs can provide positive feedback whenever possible and check on perks that may be available, such as free parking, lunch vouchers, or other tokens that are given in support and appreciation. Perks are never to be used to incentivize a patient to participate in a clinical trial.

Physician/Nurse Adherence Issues

Armed with all of the knowledge and interventions, patients' chances of being nonadherent are diminished. CTNs are the hub of the wheel. Physicians, patients, and ancillary staff should work closely with CTNs who guide all through the trial. If a patient calls a physician and is given permission to change his or her next appointment or to take less than the number of pills required to maintain adherence, then the issue is lack of CTN involvement and physician education. Educating physicians regarding the protocol and protocol requirements is vital to the successful completion of a study. CTNs should make every effort to see patients with the physician to avoid errors. But, with all of the patients and multiple protocols, mistakes still occur. To prevent inadvertent physician nonadherence, patients should be taught to call their CTN if they have problems with making appointments or need to change an appointment, taking the prescribed treatment, or with any other aspect of the clinical trial.

CTNs should make physicians aware of required laboratory tests and scans and ensure they are ordered appropriately. Chemotherapy orders are written or entered in the electronic medical record by CTNs at some institutions and reviewed and signed by a physician. This provides a "double-check" mechanism to ensure that the treatment dosages and modifications, if required, are correct. CTNs should see each on-treatment patient to ensure that medications, performance status, and side effects are documented and that patients are monitored closely following institutional guidelines.

CTNs may be nonadherent to the protocol because of a lack of training and serving in multiple roles, such as a staff nurse or nurse navigator. Clinical trials are becoming increasingly complicated and require strong attention to details. Many trials have companion studies embedded within the primary study, adding to the complexity. Most studies now incorporate quality-of-life questionnaires that need to be done at specified time points. As protocols become more complex, it is important to review the components of each study. The majority of studies are opened at an institution based on the request of a physician, and this is especially true in the community setting. CTNs should be able to review the study prior to it being opened and verify that the necessary resources are available to conduct the study at that institution.

Summary

Maintaining patient adherence with a protocol provides valid data and controls the costs associated with conducting a clinical trial. CTNs are in a key position to enhance patient adherence with early assessment for adherence-related risk factors, assisting patients to overcome obstacles, and educating and working with physicians and multidisciplinary team members. Working with patients to proactively address adherence will help ensure timely and accurate completion of a clinical trial. Well-controlled studies are needed to validate the best approaches to increase adherence in clinical trials.

Key Points
- Adherence and retention directly affect the outcome and cost of a clinical trial.
- Failure to recognize nonadherence in a clinical trial misleads understanding of the true clinical benefit of a treatment in the study.
- CTNs should screen for potential nonadherence risk factors and continue to assess adherence past enrollment and randomization.

- CTNs are key in enhancing patient adherence with early assessment for adherence-related risk factors, assisting patients to overcome obstacles, and educating and working with physicians and multidisciplinary team members.

References

Cutler, D.M., & Everett, W. (2010). Thinking outside the pillbox—Medication adherence as a priority for health care reform. *New England Journal of Medicine, 362,* 1553–1555. doi:10.1056/NEJMp1002305

Gould, E.A., & Mitty, E. (2010). Medication adherence is a partnership, medication compliance is not. *Geriatric Nursing, 31,* 290–298. doi:10.1016/j.gerinurse.2010.05.004

Gritz, E.R., DiMatteo, M.R., & Hayes, R.D. (1989). Methodological issues in adherence to cancer control. *Preventive Medicine, 20,* 125–131.

Gul, R.B., & Ali, P.A. (2010). Clinical trials: The challenge of recruitment and retention of participants. *Journal of Clinical Nursing, 19,* 227–233. doi:10.1111/j.1365-2702.2009.03041.x

Hershman, D., Kushi, L., Shao, T., Buono, D., Kershenbaum, A., Tsai, W.Y., ... Neugut, A.I. (2010). Early discontinuation and nonadherence to adjuvant hormonal therapy in a cohort of 8,769 early-stage breast cancer patients. *Journal of Clinical Oncology, 28,* 4120–4128. doi:10.1200/JCO.2009.25.9655

Ho, M.P., Bryson, C.L., & Rumsfeld, J.S. (2009). Medication adherence: Its importance in cardiovascular outcomes. *Circulation, 119,* 3028–3035. doi:10.1161/CIRCULATIONAHA.108.768986

Koop, C.E. (1984, November 1). Keynote address. Improving patient compliance: Proceedings of a symposium. *National Pharmaceutical Council,* pp. 1–4.

Landier, W. (2011). Adherence to oral chemotherapy in childhood acute lymphoblastic leukemia: An evolutionary concept analysis. *Oncology Nursing Forum, 38,* 343–352. doi:10.1188/11.ONF.343-352

Miaskowski, C., Shockney, L., & Chlebowski, R.T. (2008). Adherence to oral endocrine therapy for breast cancer: A nursing perspective. *Clinical Journal of Oncology Nursing, 12,* 213–221. doi:10.1188/08.CJON.213-221

Moore, S. (2010). Nonadherence in patients with breast cancer receiving oral therapies. *Clinical Journal of Oncology Nursing, 14,* 41–47. doi:10.1188/10.CJON.41-47

Nasseh, K., Frazee, S.G., Vasaria, J., Vlahiotis, A., & Tian, Y. (2012). Cost of medication nonadherence associated with diabetes, hypertension, and dyslipidemia. *American Journal of Pharmacy Benefits, 4,* e41–e47. Retrieved from http://www.ajmc.com/articles/Cost-of-Medication-Nonadherence-Associated-With-Diabetes-Hypertension-and-Dyslipidemia

O'Carroll, R., Dennis, M., Johnston, M., & Sudlow, C. (2010). Improving adherence to medication in stroke survivors (IAMSS): A randomized controlled trial: Study protocol. *BMC Neurology, 10*(15), 1–9. Retrieved from http://www.biomedcentral.com/1471-2377/10/15

Oncology Nursing Society. (2010). *Oncology clinical trials nurse competencies.* Retrieved from http://www.ons.org/sites/defualt/files/ctncompetencies.pdf

Pharmaceutical Research and Manufacturers of America. (n.d.). About PhRMA: PhRMA members are leading the way in the search for new medicines and cures. Retrieved from http://www.phrma.org/about

Robiner, W.N. (2005). Enhancing adherence in clinical research. *Contemporary Clinical Trials, 26,* 59–77. doi:10.1016/j.cct.2004.11.015

Rosenstock, I.M. (1988). Adoption and maintenance of lifestyle modifications. *American Journal of Preventive Medicine, 15,* 349–352.

Spano, S. (2004, May). Stages of adolescent development. *Research Facts and Findings.* Retrieved from http://www.actforyouth.net/resources/rf/rf_stages_0504.pdf

Tufts Center for the Study of Drug Development. (2011, April 26). Drug developers actively improving efficiency of clinical trials. Retrieved from http://csdd.tufts.edu/news/complete_story/rd_pr_apr_2011

Wilkes, G.M. (2011). *Targeted cancer therapy.* Burlington, MA: Jones & Bartlett Learning.

Chapter 26

Clinical Trial Registries

Nina M. Trocky, DNP, RN, NE-BC, CCRA

Introduction

A *clinical trial registry* is an online repository of information. Sponsors and investigators register new trials as evidence that a trial exists. The registration process is complete when a unique identifier number is assigned to that trial. The process sets an expectation that the sponsor or investigator will publicly disseminate results making new research data available to improve health care. This type of registry is called a *results database*. This chapter explains the reasons why clinical trial registries are developed. An overview of the evolution of trial registries is presented. Examples of various trial registries and samples of national, international, and commercial registries are provided. Finally, current trends influencing registries are described.

Purpose

The World Health Organization (WHO) defines a clinical trial *register* as a "formal record of an internationally agreed minimum amount of information about a clinical trial. This record is usually stored in and managed using a database" (WHO, n.d.-b, "What is the difference between a clinical trials register and a clinical trials registry?"). A clinical trial *registry* functions as a central repository (i.e., the entity that houses the register) for information on new or ongoing clinical trials (International Federation of Pharmaceutical Manufacturers and Associations [IFPMA], 2008; WHO, n.d.-b). Complementing trial registries are trial results databases. A clinical trial results database serves as a repository for the summary data of completed clinical trials (IFPMA, 2008). Searching for information in any clinical trial registry is performed by accessing a single Internet portal and selecting a disease or condition, geographic location, and/or drug or interventional modality.

Clinical trial registries rose out of three individual yet complementary issues: (a) a desire to address the need for transparency or informing the public that a trial exists, (b) an ethical concern about data censuring or influencing the development of an accurate risk-benefit profile, and (c) concerns about scientific integrity when results were not published in the public domain.

The primary purpose of a clinical trial registry was to publicly announce that a clinical trial existed and that through this pronouncement the lay public, patients, and healthcare providers might consider enrollment options (Dickersin & Rennie, 2012). A secondary but equally important purpose was to minimize the negative consequences to advancing evidence-based practice when trial results are not disseminated (Dickersin & Rennie, 2012). All of these issues called into question the very basic premise of why trials were conducted: to develop new knowledge, to apply that knowledge to improve the health and health outcomes of the population, and to add to the body of research literature.

As early as 1986, Simes suggested that publication of clinical trial results might be influenced by the outcome of the trial. This publication bias or censorship defies the basic premise of conducting human subject research in that the data collected from those who afforded the investigator to test a hypothesis were not used to generalize new knowledge. More importantly, electing not to publish trial results inhibits the advancement of evidence-based practice and care decisions based on the best available research. The next section explains the evolution and activities that helped develop clinical trial registries and results databases. For a brief overview, see Table 26-1.

Evolution of Registries

Perhaps the National Cancer Institute (NCI) led the way in launching a single source of disease-specific

Table 26-1. Timeline of Clinical Trial Registries and Databases Initiatives

Date	Act/Initiative	Description
1977	Physician Data Query (PDQ®) (Manrow et al., 2014)	National Cancer Institute (NCI) launched PDQ, a centralized cancer information center.
1988	Health Omnibus Programs Extension of 1988	Centralized trial registry of AIDS and HIV interventional trials was created.
1989	AIDS Clinical Trial Information Service (National Institute of Allergy and Infectious Diseases [NIAID], 2002)	Telephone call-in triage and information center located in the NIAID of the National Institutes of Health (NIH) was established.
1989	CancerNet.gov (NIH, 1997)	NCI founded CancerNet, an oncology clinical trial registry.
1997	Food and Drug Administration Modernization Act (FDAMA) section 113	FDAMA mandated the first clinical trial registry. Federal law required prospective registration of U.S. Food and Drug Administration (FDA)-regulated trials for serious or life-threatening diseases and conditions.
2000	ClinicalTrials.gov (U.S. FDA, 2010)	NIH National Library of Medicine launched the ClinicalTrials.gov registry, a centralized database of federally and privately funded interventional trials testing drugs and biologics for serious or life-threatening diseases and conditions. Registry published the start and end dates of clinical trials.
2005	International Committee of Medical Journal Editors (ICMJE) position (ICMJE, 2014)	ICMJE published guidance requiring trial registration as a condition for submission of a manuscript for publication in their journals.
2005	International Federation of Pharmaceutical Manufacturers and Associations (IFPMA) position (IFPMA, 2005)	Joint position statement required prospective trial notification, publication of trials evaluating therapeutic benefit of pharmacologic agents, and member support to post trial summary results (design and methodology, results of primary and secondary outcome measures, and safety results), linking results to the published article. Guidance document suggested registration of new hypothesis-testing trials and disclosure of trial results from completed trials with products approved for marketing and commercially available in at least one country.
2006	World Health Organization (WHO) International Clinical Trials Registry Platform (WHO, 2006)	WHO established the minimum set of data required for submission with all prospective clinical trial registries and defined the 20 elements contained in the Trial Registration Data Set.
2007	Food and Drug Administration Amendments Act (FDAAA) section 801	Federal law expanded the ClinicaTrials.gov registry to include results of clinical trials.
2008	ClinicalTrials.gov results database (ClinicalTrials.gov, 2014a)	ClinicalTrials.gov added a results database to capture results on all prospectively registered trials. Results database must contain aggregate or summary-level data, not patient-level data. Trial sponsors or investigators must submit summary data, in tabular form, no later than 12 months following trial completion. Trials are linked by an identifier known as the NCT number.
2010	IFPMA (2010) revised joint position paper	This guidance document suggested that all industry-sponsored clinical trials be published in the scientific literature regardless of trial results. At a minimum, results from all phase III trials and any trial results of significant medical importance must be submitted for publication.

information when it launched the Physician Data Query (PDQ®) database in 1977 (Manrow, Beckwith, & Johnson, 2014). NCI developed PDQ to assist in the rapid dissemination of research findings, provide oncology professionals and patients with the most advanced information on cancer treatment, and facilitate recruitment into clinical trials (Manrow et al., 2014). From its inception, PDQ offered information on NCI-sponsored clinical trials. Now, it is an all-inclusive cancer database (NCI, 2013). Information offered in PDQ includes cancer information summaries, a genetic services directory, and a dictionary of cancer terms. PDQ may be accessed at www.cancer.gov/cancertopics/pdq.

Trial registration through PDQ ceased in 2010 (NCI, 2013). However, the PDQ portal allows access to the ClinicalTrials.gov registry. NCI-sponsored clinical trials can be located by accessing www.cancer.gov/clinicaltrials.

The Health Omnibus Programs Extension of 1988, often called HOPE, mandated the development of a centralized clinical trial registry specifically for AIDS and HIV interventional trials. The AIDS Clinical Trials Information Service (ACTIS) began in 1989 as a telephone call-in triage and information center located in the National

Institute of Allergy and Infectious Diseases (NIAID) of the National Institutes of Health (NIH) (NIAID, 2002). Then in 1996, ACTIS was made available as a disease-specific database and, perhaps, the first clinical trial registry. Protocol information and lists of open and enrolling NIH-funded and industry-funded trials were made available to the public (NIAID, 2002). As the AIDS call-in center was offering clinical trial information for patients and providers, NCI launched CancerNet, a registry focused on oncology clinical trials (Tse, Zarin, Williams, & Ide, 2012). Just as the HOPE legislation focused on conquering AIDS and HIV, the CancerNet registry was focused on cancer (NIH, 1997). Oncology-specific trials were published on NCI's website, making public health information available in compliance with another federal law, the National Cancer Act of 1997.

Then, in 1997, the U.S. Food and Drug Administration Modernization Act (FDAMA) established the first general clinical trial registry. Title 1, subtitle B, section 113 of FDAMA required the director of NIH to create and maintain a single repository of open and enrolling trials for serious or life-threatening diseases and conditions. This repository was the data bank (FDAMA, 1997). Moreover, section 113 mandated public acknowledgment of U.S. Food and Drug Administration (FDA)-regulated trials conducted under an investigational new drug application for serious and life-threatening conditions. Federally and privately funded clinical trials were included in this data bank.

Three years later, on February 29, 2000, the NIH National Library of Medicine released ClinicalTrials.gov (U.S. FDA, 2010). Novel in its approach, ClinicalTrials.gov was a centralized database of federally and privately funded interventional trials testing drugs and biologics for serious or life-threatening diseases and conditions. However, NIH primarily sponsored the bulk of the trials. Clinical trials were registered and published prospectively. This meant that registration was completed *before* the trial enrolled the first subject. Information posted in ClinicalTrials.gov was written in lay terminology. Required elements of trial registration were defined, called *protocol data elements*, as a method of standardizing the information such as title, study type, FDA status, and institutional review board information (ClinicalTrials.gov, 2014b). See Figure 26-1 for the ClinicalTrials.gov protocol data elements. FDAMA required sponsors to register clinical trials in ClinicalTrials.gov within 21 days following protocol approval (U.S. FDA, 2010). Trials registered in ClinicalTrials.gov are given an NCT number. Searching for trials in ClinicalTrials.gov may be performed by following the directions at http://clinicaltrials.gov/ct2/search.

The primary purpose of the repository was to offer patients, family members, and healthcare professionals a means to locate a clinical trial of interest to them. Although ClinicalTrials.gov did not include all types and phases of trials, it did offer an easily accessible and free online database of selected trials to improve public awareness and recruitment potential for sites actively enrolling subjects. The expectation was that sponsors and investigators would comply with the law, register trials, and modify information in the registry as necessary. However, compliance was less than anticipated, and oversight was limited. Still, the movement toward accountability and transparency had begun.

Figure 26-1. ClinicalTrials.gov Protocol Data Elements

1. Titles and background Information
2. Food and Drug Administration information
3. Human subjects review
4. Sponsors
5. Study description
6. Protocol review and enrollment status
7. Study design
8. Arms, groups, and interventions
9. Conditions and keywords
10. Eligibility
11. Protocol location, contact, and investigator information
12. Related information

Note. Based on information from ClinicalTrials.gov, 2014b.

In 2005, the International Committee of Medical Journal Editors (ICMJE) initiated a mandate requiring clinical trial registration as a condition for submission of a manuscript for publication in their journals. This was the first time an organization critical for influencing the body of scientific knowledge expanded the generally accepted and traditional author guidelines to include evidence of a professional obligation. These uniform requirements for manuscripts submitted to biomedical journals included a significant number of journals worldwide such as *Annals of Emergency Medicine, Clinical Drug Investigation*, and *American Journal of Nursing*. Any trial registry was, and still is, acceptable as long as the submission meets the data submission criteria established by that registry. ICMJE (2014) suggested that the clinical trials registration number be identified following the manuscript abstract. Unlike ClinicalTrials.gov, ICMJE offered a broader definition of clinical trials to include "any research project that prospectively assigns people or a group of people to an intervention, with or without concurrent comparison or control groups, to study the cause-and-effect relationship between a health-related intervention and a health outcome" (ICMJE, 2014, p. 12). Just like ClinicalTrials.gov, ICMJE considered trial registration as a repository supporting open and enrolling clinical trials, not a database for trial results. However, the ICMJE mandate advanced the goal of greater transparency and reduced the chance of selective or biased publication practices. As more attention was placed on providing assurances that the existence of clinical trials was publicly announced and researchers were bearing responsibility to conform, the lack of uniformity and standards regarding what information should be included in trial registries became evident.

In the same year, IFPMA issued its first joint position on the disclosure of clinical trial information via clinical trial registries and databases (IFPMA, 2005). IFPMA is a global nonprofit nongovernmental organization with broad membership: the European Federation of Pharmaceutical Industries and Associations, the Japan Pharmaceutical Manufacturers Association, and the Pharmaceutical Research and Manufacturers of America. Member organizations include pharmaceutical, vaccine, and biotechnology companies. As such, the potential influence to address real and sustained transparency, access to enrolling trials, and full disclosure of trial results is significant. Their global membership agreed to publish clinical trial information prospectively on all trials evaluating the therapeutic benefit of a pharmacologic agent. Members agreed to report trial summary results (design and methodology, results of primary and secondary outcome measures, and safety results) and include a link to any published article (IFPMA, 2005).

Revisions made in 2009 focused on the addition of confirmatory and exploratory trials testing pharmaceuticals in life-threatening conditions (IFPMA, 2009). On June 10, 2010, IFPMA released the *Joint Position on the Publication of Clinical Trial Results in the Scientific Literature*. This paper expressed the feelings from representatives of the pharmaceutical community that trial results must be publicly disseminated, thereby allowing healthcare practitioners and patients to benefit from knowledge generated through industry-sponsored trials. Therefore, regardless of the results, researchers should submit the results from all phase III trials, as well as clinical trial results considered medically significant, for publication in a scientific journal (IFPMA, 2010).

To address the variability among clinical trial registry information and as the number of web-accessible registries increased, WHO established the International Clinical Trials Registry Platform (ICTRP) in 2006 (WHO, 2006). A minimum set of data was identified as being necessary in a trial registry offering a "complete view" of a clinical trial so that an informed and enlightened decision may be made. From a global perspective, the need for uniformity was as important as was the responsibility to embrace trial registration as a universal scientific, ethical, and moral responsibility (WHO, n.d.-c). The initiative was focused on unifying each trial registry through a single global portal—the ICTRP—and defining the Trial Registration Data Set (TRDS), the core set of data considered acceptable to satisfy prospective registration (WHO, n.d.-a). The 20 data items in the TRDS are the minimum amount of trial information required for a fully registered trial (see www.who.int/ictrp/network/trds/en for the complete list). The WHO registry contains interventional and phase I–IV trials. Trials submitted to the WHO registry first receive a Universal Trial Number (UTN). Once a trial is fully registered by any registry, the trial is posted in the WHO portal with the UTN number listed as the secondary identifier and the registration number as the primary trial registry identification number.

WHO defined the criteria for the minimum data set in a clinical trial registry internationally. This improved the quality of information available for subjects, lay individuals, and health professionals when searching for an open trial. However, the demand for data generated from those trials was increasing. In 2007, section 801 of the Food and Drug Administration Amendments Act (FDAAA) was passed, offering an important step toward greater transparency, accountability, and publication of all trial results.

In September 2008, ClinicalTrials.gov added a results database (ClinicalTrials.gov, 2014a). For all registered trials, the results database must contain aggregate or summary-level data—not patient-level data. Trial sponsors or investigators must submit summary data, in tabular form, no later than 12 months following trial completion (ClinicalTrials.gov, 2014a). See Figure 26-2 for a description of the results data elements. In addition to publishing basic trial summary data, FDAAA required the submission of Form FDA 3674, Certification of Compliance, at the time of initial registration submission (FDAAA, 2007). A copy of this form may be found at www.fda.gov/downloads/AboutFDA/ReportsManualsForms/Forms/UCM048364.pdf. The FDAAA legislation furthered the goal of access to clinical trials, transparency, and facilitation of responsible scientific conduct through the public dissemination of basic trial results. Failure to comply would result in civil penalties and/or inability to secure future federal funding.

Federal laws mandated that sponsors and investigators must document that a clinical trial was recruiting human subjects and that all clinical trial data must be published in the public domain. However, federal law did not address the ethical imperative and responsibility that sponsors and investigators had to the participants enrolled in the clinical trials. Rather, this is addressed in the Declaration of Helsinki.

The Declaration of Helsinki is a document that defines the ethical principles guiding clinical trial con-

---

Figure 26-2. Trial Results Summary Data

- **Participant flow**—Number of participants enrolled, withdrawing, and completed; progress of participants through each stage of a study, by study arm or comparison group
- **Baseline characteristics**—Baseline data for enrolled participants by study arm; demographics, age, gender, and study-specific measures
- **Outcome measures and statistical analyses**—Summary table of outcome measures by study arm, primary and secondary outcomes, post hoc outcomes, and appropriate statistical analyses
- **Adverse events**—Summary table of all anticipated and unanticipated serious adverse events and anticipated and unanticipated other adverse events exceeding a specific frequency threshold

Note. Based on information from ClinicalTrials.gov, 2014a.

duct. Originally written in Finland in June 1964, the document continues to serve as a policy statement guiding the actions of the global medical community and those conducting human subject research (World Medical Association [WMA], n.d.). In 2008, the eighth amendment revised the document, adding the expectation that clinical trial registration in a publicly accessible database occur prior to enrollment of the first participant. Moreover, the declaration supported the ICJME position paper and set the expectation that the authors, regardless of the trial outcome, publish trial results in the public domain (e.g., peer-reviewed journal) (WMA, 2013). In 2013, WMA revised the document again, adding a new section titled "Research Registration and Publication and Dissemination of Results," which stated the ethical expectation that sponsors and researchers report and disseminate trial results (WMA, 2013). However, similar changes are not reflected in the *Ethical Guidelines for Medical Research* (Council for International Organizations of Medical Sciences [CIOMS], 2013). CIOMS has not revised its 2002 guidelines (CIOMS, 2002) to address trial registry and results publication expectations. However, a working group is reviewing the guidelines to ensure they reflect the needs of the global community of researchers and, more importantly, the rights and protections of all trial participants (CIOMS, 2013).

Ethically responsible conduct and compliance with federal laws are evident through multiple online registries housing either prospective data and/or trial results. Yet, no single point of access or single trial registry or trial results database exists that is inclusive of all open clinical trials and all trial results. Searching the Internet is necessary to locate the most appropriate trial information.

Other Registries

Foreign Registries

Following the development of the federally funded and operated ClinicalTrials.gov registry, many foreign countries and organizations developed similar free, open-access, web-based repositories for prospective trial registration. Many similarities exist among the repositories, yet each database varies, reflecting the unique needs of the lay, regulatory, and scientific communities. Most of these registries are aligned with governmental agencies and support compliance with relevant local laws. The following are examples of foreign registries.

The European Union (EU) Clinical Trials Register offers information on clinical trials maintained in the European Clinical Trials Database (EudraCT). National medicine regulatory authorities use EudraCT to comply with article 11 of Directive 2001/20/EC, but the European Medicines Agency (EMA) is accountable for maintaining EudraCT (EMA, n.d.). Beginning in March 2011, EU researchers and those working within the European Economic Area must register trials when conducting phase II–IV pharmaceutical interventional trials in adults. In addition, pediatric trials conducted in the EU, as well as trials conducted outside the EU but functioning within a collaborative pediatric investigation plan, must be registered (EMA, n.d.). Registered trials receive a EudraCT number, the unique identifier linking the protocol and trial data from inception to study termination (EMA, n.d.). All registered trials comply with the WHO ICTRP specifications. The trial registry is located at www.clinicaltrialsregister.eu.

Brazil developed a trial registry, called ReBEC, through a public-private collaboration. The Brazilian Ministry of Health, the Pan American Health Organization, and the Oswaldo Cruz Foundation designed the prospective registry to comply with the ICMJE and WHO guidelines (Brazilian Clinical Trials Registry, n.d.). All experimental and nonexperimental and phase I–IV trials must be registered. Once registered, the trial receives an RBR number. The trial registry is located at www.ensaiosclinicos.gov.br.

The German Clinical Trials Register (*Deutsches Register Klinischer Studien* [DRKS]) is a nonprofit organization that receives financial support from the Federal Ministry of Education and Research. All trials conducted in Germany require registration with DRKS prospectively and must meet both ICMJE and WHO registry guidelines (DRKS, 2014a). Trial information is available free through an open-access web portal (DRKS, 2014b). Once registered, the trial receives a DRKS-ID number. The trial registry is located at https://drks-neu.uniklinik-freiburg.de/drks_web/navigate.do?navigationId=search&reset=true.

Additional foreign-based trial registries may be found on the WHO ICTRP web portal (www.who.int/ictrp/network/primary/en/index.html). All information posted on the WHO platform is written in the English language. Registries not included in the WHO platform may or may not be available in English. See Section XI of this manual for additional information.

Pharmaceutical Registries

Pharmaceutical companies have a stake in shortening the time between trial initiation and enrollment of the first subject. More importantly, as sponsors of clinical trials, they are in a position to facilitate the data analysis and dissemination activities of responsible research conduct supporting the ethical guidelines of the Declaration of Helsinki (WMA, 2013). Some pharmaceutical companies simply support registration and entry of results in ClinicalTrials.gov. Others have developed company-specific portals that generally provide trial information on proprietary products or interventions. Trial types and phases may vary as well.

Disease Registries

Disease-specific registries focus on certain conditions or diseases. They may serve to register prospective clinical trials or offer a repository of nonexperimental trials registered in other clinical trial registries. This allows a more focused search for open and enrolling trials. One example is the Leukemia and Lymphoma Society, which supports access to trials for patients seeking information on leukemia and lymphoma. The organization does not own the disease registry. Rather, in partnership with and with partial support from Celgene Corporation and Millennium: The Takeda Oncology Company, the TrialCheck® clinical trial search service is made available on the Leukemia and Lymphoma Society website. Access to the TrialCheck registry may be found at www.lls.org/#/diseaseinformation/managingyourcancer/clinicaltrials.

NCI offers free access to thousands of open and closed oncology clinical trials via its PDQ database. Visitors may sort by cancer site, trial location, treatment preferences, trial phases, and sponsor. Cooperative group trials and research funded by a specific institute, such as the National Institute of Nursing Research, are options available to refine the search. Access to the NCI oncology clinical trials repository may be found at www.cancer.gov/clinicaltrials.

Current Trends

A tremendous amount has been accomplished over the past 25 years concerning the development of trial registries and databases. Several trends are noteworthy to identify, as they relate to improving the goals of clinical trial transparency, accessibility, standardization, results reporting, and informing evidence-based practice. For example, ClincialTrials.gov now requires registration of controlled clinical trials and trials seeking FDA approval for drugs or medical devices. Phase I trials are not included, and noncontrolled or observational and case studies may be registered but are not required to be. Therefore, true transparency has yet to be achieved, and all human subject research is not yet registered.

Next, although subject recruitment may be increased from inclusion in one or more online free registries, no single web-accessible portal exists. As a result, patients, professionals, and providers may need to search several registries using a variety of search terms and individually evaluating outputs from each before making a decision. This process may result in undue frustration and perhaps too much or not enough information. More importantly, this may present a future barrier to enrollment and recruitment efforts. Gansler et al. (2012) noted that trial matching services were influential in helping to link patients with trial information, availability, and subsequent enrollment. However, other variables, such as race, insurance, stage of disease, and performance status, must be considered during the searching process. Clinical trial matching services, which may be either web accessible or available through central call centers, offer a coordinated approach to the searching process. A sample list of trial matching services is found in Figure 26-3.

Next, the question of standardization and commonalities, for both registries and databases, is an issue. The 12 protocol data elements used in the ClinicalTrials.gov registry are slightly different from the 20 elements required by the WHO platform. This lack of standardization in the two largest registries presents a challenge. Information deemed essential might evolve over time and with input from users and the scientific community at large. Equally important would be the monitoring of registry information to ensure accuracy and completeness and the lack of gaps, omissions, or missing data.

Finally, ensuring that results are submitted within the specified period and the issue of dissemination of trial results must be addressed. Compliance with the results submission requirement may present a difficult enforcement issue for FDA. Title VIII of FDAAA (2007) clearly establishes both a responsibility and a commitment for dissemination of registered trial results. This commitment was made to the researchers, the medical community, the public at large, and, most importantly the human subjects whose participation allowed the trial to be conducted.

In February 2012, the Agency for Healthcare Research and Quality published a report calling for a central access site for all U.S.-based trial registries and databases and standardization of the data elements and information posted on the websites of the registries (Gliklich, Leavy, & Campion, 2012). Task force members conducted multiple focused interviews among care providers, the public, and federal agencies such as the Centers for Medicare and Medicaid Services. The recommendations addressed a single portal option, as well as enhancing access to open and closed trials, data standardization, and publications of scientific finding. The task force identified the following five objectives to improve the current system:

(1) to provide a searchable central listing of patient registries in the United States so as to

---

Figure 26-3. Clinical Trial Matching Services

- **American Cancer Society:** www.cancer.org/treatment/treatmentsandsideeffects/clinicaltrials/app/clinical-trials-matching-service
- **American Lung Association:** www.emergingmed.com/networks/americanlungassociation
- **Colon Cancer Alliance:** www.ccalliance.org/clinical_trials/index.html
- **EmergingMed Navigator:** www.emergingmed.com
- **Florida Cancer Trials:** http://floridacancertrials.com/en

enable interested parties to identify registries in a particular area of interest (to promote collaboration, reduce redundancy, and improve transparency); (2) to encourage and facilitate the use of common data elements and definitions in similar conditions (to improve opportunities for sharing, comparing, and linkage) through the listing and searching of such elements; (3) to provide a central repository of searchable summary results (including for registries that do not have results published in peer-reviewed literature); (4) to offer researchers a search tool to locate existing data sources (from either ongoing registries or closed registries) to request for use in new studies (secondary analyses, linkage studies); and (5) to serve as a recruitment tool for both providers and patients. (Gliklich et al., 2012, p. ES-1)

Finally, Duke University and FDA formed a unique collaborative project called the Clinical Trials Transformation Initiative (CTTI) (Sprenger, Nickerson, Meeker-O'Connell, & Morrison, 2013). More than 60 organizations have joined as paid members (CTTI, n.d.). Access to large data sets, through CTTI and ClinicalTrials.gov, may offer additional research avenues using secondary data.

As these issues are addressed, it is certain that additional needs will be identified. A collaborative effort with input from participants, the general public, and medical communities is essential.

Implications for Clinical Trial Nurses

Clinical trial nurses (CTNs) play a vital role in all aspects of the research process, including protocol development, participant recruitment, trial coordination, and results dissemination and publication. Specific responsibilities and activities of CTNs may vary among sites as well as settings. This is to be expected; however, performing effectively as a CTN requires a unique skill set. The Oncology Nursing Society (ONS) developed a basic set of core competencies that differentiate oncology nurses from oncology CTNs (ONS, 2010). The nine competencies support the intent to differentiate the contributions CTNs make to this practice specialty.

CTNs integrate information concerning trial registries and databases to develop safe, compliant, and ethical care for potential and enrolled clinical trial participants. CTNs apply knowledge concerning ethical principles, guidelines, and regulations when managing trials and during the informed consent process (ONS, 2010). Competent CTNs employ every possible strategy to support effective participant recruitment for a diverse population while using all available resources to minimize barriers to enrollment. Finally, all nine core competencies offer novice CTNs, advanced CTNs, and nurses transitioning to this practice specialty the ability to develop professionally based upon a minimum set of practice standards (ONS, 2010). The CTN core competencies recognize and differentiate the knowledge, skills, and abilities of nurses who make the commitment to educating, caring for, and protecting clinical trial participants (see Appendix 2).

Summary

A significant amount of progress has been made nationally, as well as globally, to address the original objectives of increasing clinical trial transparency and reducing data censuring and publication bias. Development of clinical trial registries offered researchers and sponsors the ability to document the existence of a clinical trial. Informing the public and medical community that a clinical trial was enrolling human subjects led to establishing an expectation and responsibility that results generated from research should be placed in the public domain for the purposes of informing and improving healthcare decision making. Perhaps now the focus is on enforcement with FDAAA (2007) and with process improvement. Concerning enforcement, FDA will develop a mechanism to monitor compliance with both registration and results, disclosure processes, and submissions mandates (Archer, 2014). Registering the appropriate trials into ClinicalTrials.gov no later than 21 days after enrollment of the first participant, as well as submitting summary results (including adverse event information) no later than one year after the trial's (primary) completion date, will require additional resources.

Submitting results to ClinicalTrials.gov is independent of publication in a peer-reviewed journal. Incentivizing responsible parties to do both may be necessary. Finally, improving access and dissemination may be further facilitated through the concerned efforts of the Agency for Healthcare Research and Quality initiative. Together, a shared commitment to patients and ethical principles, in combination with federally regulated mandates, will improve the integrity of the research process.

Key Points

- Clinical trial registries arose out of a desire for greater transparency, a need for published trial results, and an ethical need to increase the type and amount of available information to improve informed decision making.
- A clinical trial registry functions as a central repository for information on new or ongoing clinical trials.
- Clinical trial results databases expand trial registries by linking published results summaries for public review.
- ClinicalTrials.gov was the first centralized web-accessible clinical trial registry.

- FDA advanced the prospective clinical trial registration and results database requirements through the initiation of two laws (FDAMA and FDAAA).
- WHO advanced standardization of clinical trial registration elements through the initiation of the ICTRP and TRDS.
- ICMJE and IFPMA emphasized publication of all trial results as a professional expectation and requirement following prospective registration of a clinical trial.
- Many clinical trial registries are available now via pharmaceutical companies, healthcare organizations, and social media sites.

References

Archer, J. (2014, March 14). FDAAA 2007: Clinical trials disclosure—Common mistakes in compliance. Retrieved from http://www.pharmacompliancemonitor.com/fdaaa-2007-clinical-trials-disclosure-common-mistakes-compliance/6482

Brazilian Clinical Trials Registry. (n.d.). Retrieved from http://www.ensaiosclinicos.gov.br

Clinical Trials Transformation Initiative. (n.d.). Who we are. Retrieved from http://www.ctti-clinicaltrials.org/who-we-are

ClinicalTrials.gov. (2014a). About the results database. Retrieved from http://www.clinicaltrials.gov/ct2/about-site/results

ClinicalTrials.gov. (2014b, September). ClinicalTrials.gov protocol data element definitions (Draft). Retrieved from http://prsinfo.clinicaltrials.gov/definitions.html

Council for International Organizations of Medical Sciences. (2002). *International ethical guidelines for biomedical research involving human subjects.* Retrieved from http://www.cioms.ch/publications/layout_guide2002.pdf

Council for International Organizations of Medical Sciences. (2013). CIOMS Working Group on the revision of the 2002 CIOMS ethical guidelines for biomedical research. Retrieved from http://www.cioms.ch/index.php/12-newsflash/232-cioms-working-group-of-the-revision-of-the-2002-cioms-ethical-guidelines-for-biomedical-research

Deutsches Register Klinischer Studien. (2014a). FAQ: Frequently asked questions. Retrieved from https://drks-neu.uniklinik-freiburg.de/drks_web/navigate.do?navigationId=faq&messageDE=FAQ&messageEN=FAQ

Deutsches Register Klinischer Studien. (2014b). Internet portal of the German Clinical Trials Register (DRKS). Retrieved from https://drks-neu.uniklinik-freiburg.de/drks_web/navigate.do?navigationId=start&messageDE=Home&messageEN=Home

Dickersin, K., & Rennie, D. (2012). The evolution of trial registries and their use to assess the clinical trial enterprise [Editorial]. *JAMA, 307,* 1861–1864. doi:10.1001/jama.2012.4230

European Medicines Agency. (n.d.). About the EU Clinical Trials Register. Retrieved from https://www.clinicaltrialsregister.eu/about.html

Food and Drug Administration Amendments Act of 2007, Pub. L. No. 110-85, 121 Stat. 823, § 801 (2007). Retrieved from http://www.gpo.gov/fdsys/pkg/PLAW-110publ85/pdf/PLAW-110publ85.pdf

Food and Drug Administration Modernization Act of 1997, Pub. L. No. 105-115, 111 Stat. 2296 (1997). Retrieved from http://www.fda.gov/RegulatoryInformation/Legislation/FederalFoodDrugandCosmeticActFDCAct/SignificantAmendmentstotheFDCAct/FDAMA/FullTextofFDAMAlaw/default.htm#SEC

Gansler, T., Jin, M., Bauer, J. Dahlquist, K., Tis, L., Sharpe, K., ... Kepner, J. (2012). Outcomes of a cancer clinical trial matching service. *Journal of Cancer Education, 27,* 11–20. doi:10.1007/s13187-011-0296-x

Gliklich, R.E., Leavy, M.B., & Campion, D.M. (2012, February). *Developing a registry of patient registries: Options for the Agency for Healthcare Research and Quality* [Effective Health Care Program Research Report No. 34]. Retrieved from http://effectivehealthcare.ahrq.gov/ehc/products/415/963/DEcIDE34_Developing-a-registry-of-patient-registries_finalreport.pdf

Health Omnibus Programs Extension of 1988, Pub. L. No. 100-607, 102 Stat. 3048 (1988). Retrieved from http://history.nih.gov/research/downloads/PL100-607.pdf

International Committee of Medical Journal Editors. (2014, December). Recommendations for the conduct, reporting, editing, and publication of scholarly work in medical journals. Retrieved from http://www.icmje.org/icmje-recommendations.pdf

International Federation of Pharmaceutical Manufacturers and Associations. (2005, January 6). Global industry position on disclosure of information about clinical trials [Press release]. Retrieved from http://www.lillytrials.com/docs/ifpma_news_releases.pdf

International Federation of Pharmaceutical Manufacturers and Associations. (2008, November). *Joint position on the disclosure of clinical trial information via clinical trial registries and databases.* Geneva, Switzerland: Author.

International Federation of Pharmaceutical Manufacturers and Associations. (2009, November 10). *New joint industry clinical trials transparency position requires companies to disclose all clinical trials in patients.* Geneva, Switzerland: Author.

International Federation of Pharmaceutical Manufacturers and Associations. (2010, June 10). *Joint position on the publication of clinical trial results in the scientific literature.* Geneva, Switzerland: Author.

Manrow, R.E., Beckwith, M., & Johnson, L.E. (2014). NCI's Physician Data Query (PDQ®) cancer information summaries: History, editorial processes, influence, and reach. *Journal of Cancer Education, 29,* 198–205. doi:10.1007/s13187-013-0536-3

National Cancer Institute. (2013, July 24). PDQ®—NCI's comprehensive cancer database. Retrieved from http://www.cancer.gov/cancertopics/pdq

National Institute of Allergy and Infectious Diseases. (2002, November 27). Revamped AIDS Web site tailored to diverse users [Press release]. Retrieved from http://www.niaid.nih.gov/news/newsreleases/Archive/2002/Pages/aidswebsite.aspx

National Institutes of Health. (1997, March 26). The 1971 National Cancer Act: Investment in the future [Press release]. Retrieved from http://www.nih.gov/news/pr/mar97/nci-26c.htm

Oncology Nursing Society. (2010). *Oncology clinical trials nurse competencies.* Retrieved from https://www.ons.org/sites/default/files/ctncompetencies.pdf

Simes, R.J. (1986). Publication bias: The case for an international registry of clinical trials. *Journal of Clinical Oncology, 4,* 1529–1541. Retrieved from http://jco.ascopubs.org/content/4/10/1529.full.pdf+html

Sprenger, K., Nickerson, D., Meeker-O'Connell, A., & Morrison, B.W. (2013). Quality by design in clinical trials: A collaborative pilot with FDA. *Therapeutic Innovation and Regulatory Science, 47,* 161–166. doi:10.1177/0092861512458909

Tse, T., Zarin, D.A., Williams, R.J., & Ide, N.C. (2012). The role and importance of clinical trial registries and results databases. In J.I. Gallin & F.P. Ognibene (Eds.), *Principles and practice of clinical research* (3rd ed., pp. 171–181). London, England: Elsevier Academic Press.

U.S. Food and Drug Administration. (2010, January 7). *Historical perspective on the development of ClinicalTrials.gov, and an overview of FDA's role in supporting the success of the database, and accessibility to clinical trials information by the public: Background.* Silver Spring, MD: Author.

World Health Organization. (n.d.-a). About registries: WHO Trial Registration Data Set (Version 1.2.1). Retrieved from http://www.who.int/ictrp/network/trds/en

World Health Organization. (n.d.-b). International Clinical Trials Registry Platform (ICTRP): Frequently asked questions. Retrieved from http://www.who.int/ictrp/faq/en

World Health Organization. (n.d.-c). International Clinical Trials Registry Platform (ICTRP): Welcome to WHO ICTRP. Retrieved from http://www.who.int/ictrp/en

World Health Organization. (2006). WHO clinical trials initiative to protect the public. *Bulletin of the World Health Organization, 84,* 10–11. Retrieved from http://www.who.int/bulletin/volumes/84/1/who_news0106/en/index.html

World Medical Association. (n.d.). Handbook of declarations. Retrieved from http://www.wma.net/en/30publications/10policies/10about/index.html

World Medical Association. (2013, October). *WMA Declaration of Helsinki—Ethical principles for medical research involving human subjects* [64th General Assembly]. Retrieved from http://www.wma.net/en/30publications/10policies/b3/index.html

SECTION VI.

Clinical Trial Participants

Chapter 27

Investigational Agents: Procurement, Accountability, and Administration of Research Study Drugs

Siu-Fun Wong, PharmD, FASHP, FCSHP, Carol Anne Bales, RN, MSN, CCRP, Kathleen R. Hurtado, RPh, and Joan G. Westendorp, RN, MSN, OCN®, CCRP, CIM

Introduction

In the United States, clinical research with investigational agents is strictly regulated by the U.S. Food and Drug Administration (FDA) using the Federal Food, Drug, and Cosmetic Act and the Public Health Services Act. All parties engaged in clinical trials, including the National Cancer Institute (NCI), pharmaceutical collaborators, and investigators, are mandated to follow these laws. To ensure the safeguards for the rights and welfare of research participants, the regulations administered by the Office for Human Research Protections and U.S. Department of Health and Human Services must be practiced in addition to FDA regulations. Clinical investigators and institutions must abide by the Health Insurance Portability and Accountability Act to maintain the privacy rights of the research participants.

The process of drug discovery is extensive and costly (see Chapter 2), but measures have been developed to expedite drug availability for oncology treatment. Compliance with rules and regulations is essential to produce quality data in the most effective manner. In this chapter, the process of investigational or research study drug procurement, accountability, and safe handling guidelines provided by NCI for federally funded trials (NCI Cancer Therapy Evaluation Program [CTEP], 2014) will be addressed. The standards related to the administration of oncologic drugs are included to support effective, safe, and consistent delivery of research drugs. Proper documentation also is covered to ensure compliance with policies and procedures and maintenance of records for study audits.

Procurement of Research Study Drugs

In accordance with the Joint Commission standards (hospital accreditation standard, medical management chapter [MM.06.01.05] and patient rights chapter [RI.01.03.05]; see www.jointcommission.org), whenever possible, the pharmacy department should be responsible for drug receipt, storage, accountability, and preparation. The principal investigator (PI) should delegate this responsibility to the pharmacy personnel or other appropriate research study personnel. Research nurses may be designated as the pharmacy contact if the study site does not have a pharmacist who will be responsible for the handling of research drugs. The regulatory document called the *delegation of authority* form should contain a list of the personnel who are delegated the responsibility for documenting investigational product receipt, storage, accountability, preparation, destruction, and return or transfer.

Ordering of Research Drugs—Personnel

For research drugs provided by the NCI Pharmaceutical Management Branch (PMB), the order must be submitted by a CTEP-approved investigator or an approved designee. The order must include the investigator's NCI investigator number. Any investigator who receives and administers an investigational agent supplied by NCI must be registered with the institute by submitting his or her curriculum vitae, the supplemental investigator data form, and a financial disclosure form (available at http://ctep.cancer.gov/forms).

The PI registration must be renewed annually. If the PI number is unknown, it can be obtained by submitting a question to NCI CTEP (see http://ctep.cancer.gov/investigatorResources/investigator_registration_packet.htm). Investigational agents provided by NCI to a registered investigator are the direct responsibility of the PI. Secondary distribution to other registered investigators does not relieve the responsibility of the PI to whom the original shipment was made. Investigators may only order research study drugs for protocols in which their institution or group participates. See the Cancer Trials Support Unit Help Desk (www.ctsu.org/Public/CTSU contact.aspx).

For non-NCI protocols (e.g., pharmaceutical-sponsored), the research site must submit all required regulatory documents, sign a study contract, and submit a signed Form FDA 1572 before research drugs can be sent to the study site. For research drugs directly provided by the pharmaceutical company sponsor, the order must be submitted by the designated investigators approved by the sponsor. The study team should always refer to the protocol or the study's pharmacy manual for specific instructions.

In protocols where commercially available agents are being used for the study, acquisition of the drugs can be handled as it is for other nonprotocol drugs. However, researchers should always refer to the protocol or check with the study coordinator to determine whether a drug accountability form should be kept for tracking the commercially available drugs used for the protocol patients.

Ordering of Research Drugs—Procedures

Depending on the sponsor of the study protocol, research study drugs may be ordered from NCI PMB or directly from the pharmaceutical sponsor. For research drugs supplied by a pharmaceutical company sponsor, clinicians should always refer to the protocol under the drug information section for specific instructions and forms to use. The information provided in the rest of this section applies to research drugs that are supplied by NCI.

For research drugs that are supplied by NCI's Division of Cancer Treatment and Diagnosis (DCTD) through PMB, the investigators or designees *must* submit agent requests through the PMB online agent order processing application (https://eapps-ctep.nci.nih.gov/OAOP/pages/login.jspx). Access to the online agent order processing application requires establishing an NCI CTEP Identity and Access Management account (https://eapps-ctep.nci.nih.gov/iam) and maintaining an active account status and a current password. Submitters will receive a confirmation email of each successful order submission. Order status may be viewed at any time through the online agent order processing application. Normal PMB processing time for routine orders is two working days. Orders are shipped by U.S. Postal Service Priority Mail or another ground service. Agents that have special storage conditions (e.g., thermolabile agents that require refrigeration or freezing [$-20°C$ or $-70°C$]) or shipping requirements (e.g., dangerous goods, infectious substances) are shipped Monday through Thursday for next-day delivery. Please see the information that follows for emergency supply of research drugs.

Best practices are to ship to the address where drugs will be stored (e.g., central or control pharmacy). This address must match the shipping address that the investigator provided on the supplemental investigator data form. For online order submissions, a confirmation email including the order details and tracking information will be sent upon shipment. The person responsible for ordering the drug will use similar procedures for reordering, keeping in mind the processing time and appropriate amount to reorder according to the protocol accrual rate to avoid shortage of drug supply.

For emergency (overnight) supply of research drugs, orders must be submitted through the online agent ordering program by 2 pm eastern time for next-day delivery. The form should be completed with all the information as previously indicated, including the requirements for next-day delivery and an express courier name and account number. An email will be sent to confirm successful placement of the order. Urgent drug orders should only be made in emergency situations, such as starter supplies or if the current drug supply becomes unexpectedly low. Because of the additional processing of blinded agents supplied by NCI, blinded agents cannot be shipped overnight but can be expedited for two-day delivery.

In some protocols where the drug supply is limited or slow patient accrual is expected, a starter supply of the drug may not be available. Upon enrollment of a patient, staff should use the procedure for emergency supply of research drugs to order drugs or refer to the drug transfer procedures later in this chapter if the circumstances do not allow for timely delivery of the drugs via the emergency ordering procedure.

Initial drug orders for blinded studies are usually provided automatically following randomization of the patients. Staff should always consult the protocol for details.

Accountability for Research Study Drugs

Receipt of Research Drugs

Research drug shipments are accompanied by a shipment receipt. This document should be reviewed and verified with the shipment to confirm the name of the drug and dosage form, appropriate protocol number, quantity, and appropriate shipping conditions. The supplier must be contacted by phone if the shipment is incorrect or damaged to allow for replacement of the drug in a timely manner as necessary. Drug shipment receipts should always be filed so that they are readily accessible for site audits. For some studies, the drug supplier may require that a copy of the shipment receipt be faxed or mailed to the supplier to indicate acknowledgment of receipt. Study staff should refer to the protocol or shipping materials for instructions on proper handling.

Check-In of Research Drugs

For each drug supplied for a study, an NCI Investigational Agent Accountability Record, or equivalent form provided by the study sponsor, must be maintained. This form is available on the CTEP website (http://ctep.cancer.gov/forms). Other equivalent forms usually are provided by the study sponsor. These forms are designed to account for drug inventories and usage in clinical trials. A separate accountability form must be used for each protocol and each research drug. If more than one strength or dosage form of a drug is used for the same protocol, a separate drug accountability form is required for each drug product. Electronic drug accountability forms are allowed, provided that a print version of the log process is identical to the existing drug accountability form.

For blinded drug supplied by NCI or study sponsor, the investigator or a responsible party designated by the investigator must maintain a careful record of the receipt, disposition, and return of all drugs received from PMB, using the NCI Investigational Agent Accountability Record available on the CTEP website. A separate NCI Investigational Agent Accountability Record must be maintained for each patient ID number on the protocol.

When completing the drug accountability form, keep the following in mind:
- All drug supplies received must be entered into the drug log (i.e., drug received from NCI or other study sponsor).
- If the supply is patient-specific/blinded, an Investigational Agent Accountability Record is required for each patient on the study (see the protocol for details).
- Central or control pharmacy records must reflect returns from satellite locations.
- All shipping, return, and transfer receipts must be maintained for audit purposes.

To start a new Investigational Agent Accountability Record, complete the upper portion of the form with the following information.
1. Page No.: Record the page number consecutively on the forms for each drug used on the protocol.
2. Control Record: Check this box if the record is being used to account for research drug stored at the central or control pharmacy.
3. Satellite Record: Check this box if the record is being used to account for research drug at a satellite pharmacy.
4. Name of Institution: Provide the name of the location to which the drug is shipped from NCI.
5. NCI Protocol No.: Enter the NCI protocol number; may add the institutional protocol number if necessary.
6. Agent Name
7. Dose Form and Strength
8. Protocol Title: Provide the title, using abbreviations if necessary.
9. Dispensing Area: Provide the location where the drug is dispensed (e.g., infusion center pharmacy, satellite location, central pharmacy).
10. Investigator Name: This is the investigator in whose name the drug is ordered from NCI.
11. CTEP Investigator ID
12. Balance Forward: Enter "0" if the current page is the first page, or bring the balance forward from the previous page.

Upon receiving a drug shipment, enter the following information in the appropriate columns to make an entry on an existing drug accountability record form.
1. Date: Enter the date the drug is received, including year.
2. Patient's Initials and Patient's ID No.: Enter "Rec'd from [name of the study sponsor]".
3. Dose: Leave blank.
4. Quantity Dispensed or Received: Enter "+" followed by the number of vials, ampoules, tablets, or kits received.
5. Balance: Enter new total obtained by adding the new quantity received.
6. Manufacturer and Lot No.: Provide the lot number and expiration/preparation date; if the drug shipment contains more than one lot number, make separate entries for each lot number for optimal record keeping.
7. Recorder's Initials

Storage of Research Drugs

Research drugs must be stored separately by protocol and have separate drug accountability forms. Because many protocols use the same agent, consider labeling the agent container with the drug name, dosage form, and protocol number; each study also should have its own drug accountability form. The investigational agents must be kept in a secure (locked) storage area with limited access and stored under the recommended conditions. Investigational agents should be stored separately from any commercial supplies of medications. The drug storage containers should be labeled with the drug name, strength, and protocol number.

Quality assurance for drug storage should be maintained at all times. A daily temperature log must be kept for the refrigerator and the freezer used for storing research drugs and should be readily available for audit inspection. Institutional policy needs to address how to handle temperature checks if the clinic or center is not open on the weekend. Room-temperature storage control should be maintained at all times to avoid excessive heating of the drugs. Light-sensitive products should be kept in their original container prior to administration, or an amber light-protection bag should be used to provide the protection required.

Dispensing of Research Drugs

Central/Control Pharmacy

For drugs that are being prepared or dispensed at the control pharmacy, enter the following information in the Investigational Agent Accountability Record.
1. Date: The date of dispensing/preparation, including year.
2. Patient's Initials: Use the same initials as for the protocol registration.
3. Patient's ID No.: Enter the patient's study number.
4. Dose: Record the actual dose administered.
5. Quantity Dispensed: Enter "–" followed by the number of vials, ampoules, tablets, or kits dispensed.
6. Balance: Enter the new total obtained when subtracting the number dispensed.
7. Manufacturer and Lot No.: Provide the lot number(s) and expiration date(s) of the drugs; if more than one lot number is being used, make separate entries for optimal record keeping.
8. Recorder's Initials

The container of all drugs dispensed must be labeled per federal law requirements. Identification of the investigational drug or agent by the statement "Caution: New Drug—Limited by federal (or U.S.) law to investigational use" on the medication label is required.

Satellite Pharmacy

Satellite pharmacies are limited to institutions that are located on the same campus as the central/control pharmacy or near where transportation of the research drugs can be conducted by an institution employee. Mailing of research drugs to satellite pharmacies by a commercial carrier or overnight delivery service is **not** permitted. A satellite pharmacy is permitted to use only the research drug supplies received by the central/control pharmacy. The central/control pharmacy and the satellite pharmacy must be tied through affiliation agreements, and the professional staff must be shared or have joint appointments. Satellite pharmacies must follow the same procedures for research drug accountability, preparation, and dispensing as the central/control pharmacy.

Institutions that are separated geographically by greater distances (e.g., different cities or states) are not considered satellites and generally are referred to as *affiliates*. Affiliates must order the research drug from the drug supplier, and the research drugs must be shipped directly to these sites. Affiliates must follow the same procedures for drug preparation and dispensing, as well as the documentation required for the central/control pharmacy.

Dispensing of Research Drugs to Satellite Institutions

Central/Control Pharmacy

If the research drug is to be prepared at a satellite location, the drug needs to be dispensed to the satellite location. Enter the following information in the Investigational Agent Accountability Record of the central/control pharmacy.
1. Date: Enter the date, including year.
2. Patient's Initials and Patient's ID No.: Enter "dispensed to [name of satellite location]".
3. Dose: Leave blank.
4. Quantity Dispensed or Received: Enter "–" followed by the number of vials, ampoules, tablets, or kits dispensed.
5. Balance: Enter the new total obtained when subtracting the number dispensed.
6. Manufacturer and Lot No.: Enter the lot number(s) and expiration dates(s) of the drugs; if more than one lot number is being used, make separate entries for optimal record keeping.
7. Recorder's Initials

Label the package with the drug name, protocol number, patient's name (optional), and storage condition.

Satellite Pharmacy

Upon receiving the drugs, the satellite pharmacist designated to handle the research drugs should enter the following information in the Investigational Agent Accountability Record.
1. Date: Enter the date, including year.
2. Patient's Initials and Patient's ID No.: Enter "Received from [name of central/control pharmacy]".
3. Dose: Leave blank.
4. Quantity Received: Enter "+" followed by the number received.
5. Balance: Enter the new balance obtained when adding the number received.
6. Manufacturer and Lot No.: Enter the lot number(s) and expiration date(s) of the drugs; if more than one lot number is being used, make separate entries for optimal record keeping.

Documentation of Returned Drugs by Patients

For protocols that require accountability of drugs returned by patients (especially for oral medications for which adherence checks are required), a separate drug accountability log for each patient should be maintained. Drug returned from a patient should not be logged on the master drug accountability form except for double-blinded studies where a protocol-specific drug accountability form is provided to capture the information. It is highly encouraged that clinical trial nurses should confirm the proper administration of the study medications with the patients/caregivers and review the medication diaries completed by the patients, if appropriate, to ensure medication adherence and improve persistence.

Return of Research Drugs to the Supplier

For NCI-provided research drugs, investigators are required to return unused drugs under the following conditions.
- The study is completed or terminated and the research drugs cannot be transferred to another DCTD-sponsored trial.
- The research drug is outdated.
- The research drug is damaged (e.g., loss of refrigeration). Do **not** return broken vials. They should be destroyed on-site according to the institutional standard operating procedures, accompanied by proper documentation.

Research drugs should be returned within 90 days of study closure or last patient activity, although outdated or damaged drugs should be removed from the inventory immediately. For a pharmaceutical-sponsored study, refer to the protocol for specific instructions on handling of returned or unused research drugs.

To return unused research drugs to NCI or the study sponsor, complete the Return Investigational Agent Form (http://ctep.cancer.gov/forms) or forms provided by the study sponsor, respectively. Make an entry on the drug accountability form, subtracting the amount returned from the balance. A copy of the return drug form should be kept on file with the drug accountability form for audit purposes. For NCI-provided drugs, send the original Return Investigational Agent Form to the NCI Clinical Repository at the address indicated on the form. For other sponsored studies, send the drugs to the designated location as instructed by the sponsor.

All returned research drugs must be packaged securely to prevent breakage. All drugs can be returned and shipped at room temperature using standard mail because they will be disposed of thereafter. For NCI-provided drugs, do **not** use collect (known as *collect on delivery*, or *COD*) shipping.

Research drugs that have been dispensed to patients, opened, or partially used are usually destroyed on-site according to institutional procedures after proper documentation. Some study sponsors may request that the site store these drugs until a site audit has been conducted. Study staff should always refer to the study protocol for specific instructions. The institution or its source for drug destruction services should have written policies and procedures for research drug destruction on site. In general, if the research drug is classified as biohazardous, the method of disposal should follow the recommended guidelines provided by the Occupational Safety and Health Administration.

Transfer of Research Drugs

For NCI-provided research drugs, the drugs can be transferred if the following criteria are met.
- The research drugs can only be transferred within an institution.
- The drugs can **only** be transferred from one active protocol to another DCTD-approved protocol.
- The transferring investigator must be the investigator who originally ordered the agent or the investigator to whom the agent was previously transferred (i.e., double transfer).
- The receiving investigator must be an approved investigator on the trial to which the agent is being transferred.
- The transfer can only be made between registered active NCI investigators.

For example, drug transfer may be used in the following situations.
- The protocol is closed, and another protocol at the institution uses the same agent and formulation. However, transfer of DCTD-supplied agents to non-DCTD–approved protocols is **not** permitted under DCTD, NCI, and FDA policies and regulations.
- There is excessive inventory for a protocol, and the transfer will minimize drug wastage due to outdating.
- The study drug has short dating.
- In cases of medical emergency (e.g., an urgent approval of a protocol and a very sick patient who needs to begin therapy immediately): when a drug is ordered for an individual patient via a Special Exception (compassionate) protocol, it is no longer required for an on-study patient, and there is a DCTD-approved Special Exception protocol at the institution using the same study drug for the newly identified (emergency use) patient.

Transfer of research drugs should never occur under the following circumstances.
- Transfer of research drug for commercial use. This is prohibited and illegal.
- Replacement of research drug with commercial agents. This is prohibited and illegal.
- Transfer of drugs for blinded studies between protocols.
- Borrowing of a study drug. Study drugs should not be ordered for one protocol to replace what was borrowed from another protocol.

Transfer of DCTD-supplied agents from an active protocol requires prior PMB approval by phone at 240-276-6575. PMB should be notified by phone within the next business day if emergency transfers are required during weekends or holidays or after hours. An NCI Investigational Agent Transfer Form (http://ctep.cancer.gov/forms) must be completed and submitted by fax at 240-276-7893 to the PMB for each agent transferred. Transfer forms should be submitted within 72 hours of the actual transfer. A copy must be retained for accountability and future audits.

Compassionate Use, Special Exceptions, or Emergency Use of an Investigational Agent for a Patient

In some cases, patients may enroll in nonresearch (compassionate) use of investigational agents under three mechanisms: special exception, group C, and treatment referral center protocols. Patients must be refractory to standard measures, not eligible for an ongoing research protocol, and have a cancer diagnosis for which an investigational agent has demonstrated activity to be eligible as potential candidates to receive this category of drugs (see Chapter 6).

To enroll a patient, the physician is required to call the sponsor, NCI (301-496-5725), or the pharmaceutical manufacturer of the drug to obtain approval to administer the drug to the patient. The sponsor will need to know the following information.
- Patient's age, sex, diagnosis, and date of diagnosis
- Justification for requesting the study drug
- Previous cancer therapy
- Current clinical status
- Intended dose and schedule of the requested drug
- Any proposed concomitant cancer drugs or other therapies

Upon approval, the sponsor will provide verbal or written instructions regarding other information needed to complete the application. Institutional review board (IRB) approval must be obtained prior to initiation of treatment. It is pertinent to contact the IRB to ensure timely processing. Study staff will follow the same drug procurement and accountability procedure, with the exception that the recording will be patient specific.

Administration of Research Drugs

Protocol treatment is a pivotal point in a patient's clinical trial participation. All study procedures are intended to be a guide for consistent, safe, and effective administration of the investigational treatment. Pre-entry laboratory work and data obtained before protocol treatment serve as a baseline against which to compare participants' clinical response to the study treatment. Because of the critical nature of protocol agent administration, the nurse must understand the conditions under which the treatment is administered. This section will address the areas of drug dosing and monitoring of critical laboratory values.

Treatment Drug Dosing

Body surface area (BSA) is a mathematical calculation of height and weight to allow for extrapolation of drug dosing from lower mammals to humans. BSA-based dosing eventually became the requirement for FDA-approved labeling. Subsequent generations of oncologists viewed BSA-based dosing as a standard training for the safe and effective administration of cytotoxic chemotherapy.

The use of ideal versus actual body weight in determining BSA, especially in obese patients, remains controversial. Numerous published studies over the past two decades continue to support that actual body weight in dosing chemotherapy for obese patients (defined as body mass index [BMI] of 30 kg/m^2 or greater), especially in the adjuvant setting, does not have poorer prognosis, and no increased toxicity was observed (Barrett et al., 2008; Georgiadis, Steinberg, Hankins, Ihde, & Johnson, 1995; Meyerhardt et al., 2004; Rosner et al., 1996). A review article by Hunter et al. (2009), a pharmacokinetic study by Sparreboom et al. (2007), and an editorial by Gurney and Shaw (2007) strongly discouraged the use of capped BSA in the dosing of chemotherapy drugs in obese patients. Considering the variation in the dosing of chemotherapy in overweight and obese individuals with cancer, an American Society of Clinical Oncology guideline published in April 2012 provided the first consensus practice guideline on chemotherapy dosing for obese adult patients with cancer (Griggs et al., 2012). The panel recommended that full weight–based cytotoxic chemotherapy doses be used to treat obese patients with cancer, particularly when the goal of treatment is cure. Based on the data evaluated, the following recommendations can be considered for BSA-based drug dosing in research participants to reinforce consistency in the calculation if there is no protocol-specific dosing guideline.

For initial dosing, actual body weight of a patient should always be used to calculate the body surface area for drug dosing. BSA can be determined from weight and height by using a nomogram, found in most standard references, or the Mosteller equation, as indicated in the following formula.

$$BSA\ (m^2) = \sqrt{\frac{(height\ in\ cm) \times (weight\ in\ kg)}{3,600}}$$

In a severely obese patient where the actual body weight of the patient is more than two times the ideal body weight (IBW), that patient should only be considered for the protocol at the discretion of the treating physician.

Formulas for calculation of IBW are as follows.

Males: IBW = 50 kg + (2.3 kg × number of inches > 60 inches)
Females: IBW = 45.5 kg + (2.3 kg × number of inches > 60 inches)

Calculators for BSA, BMI, and IBW are available online (e.g., www.mdcalc.com, www.globalrph.com/bsa.htm). These tools calculate the subject's specific parameters (not laboratory study parameters) and help to decrease potential human error.

For dose modification during treatment, subsequent doses should be escalated or reduced based on toxicity. The dose modification should be based on a percentage escalation or reduction as indicated in the protocol. Patients should be weighed prior to initiation of a new cycle of treatment. Dose recalculation based on weight change should be done if the patient experiences weight gain or weight loss of 10% or more from the last dosing weight.

Laboratory Studies

Studies have shown that kidneys are the major route of drug excretion and clearance for many chemotherapy agents. Renal function tests are common baseline data for most studies involving investigational agents. Platinum-based chemotherapy can cause permanent changes in the glomerular filtration rate (GFR). Patients with renal dysfunction or those who have received previous chemotherapy have been shown to exhibit slower carboplatin clearance (Egorin et al., 1985). Creatinine clearance (CrCl) is a measure of kidney function that is based on serum and urine creatinine values and urine volume as indicated in the following formula, with the standard urine collection time at 24 hours. Shorter periods have been shown to be equally accurate (Baumann, Staddon, Horst, & Bivins, 1987).

$$CrCl = \frac{urine\ creatinine}{serum\ creatinine} \times \frac{urine\ volume\ (ml)}{time\ (minutes)}$$

Because of the general consensus that 24-hour urine collection to determine the GFR is difficult to obtain, resulting in inaccurate measurement, a calculated CrCl using patient characteristics of age, weight, sex, and serum creatinine as surrogates for the clearance-defined GFR is substituted. The Cockcroft and Gault (1976) method has been the most commonly used for adult and pediatric patients (Anderson, Knoben, & Troutman, 2002), as shown in the following formulas.

Males: $CrCl = \frac{(140 - age\ [years]) \times lean\ body\ weight\ (kg)}{serum\ creatinine \times 72}$

Females: CrCl = 0.85 × creatinine clearance

Pediatric patients: $CrCl = \frac{0.48 \times height\ (cm) \times BSA}{serum\ creatinine \times 1.73}$

Controversy exists surrounding the limits of the variables (body weight and serum creatinine) used in these equations and the capping of the estimated CrCl value. In general, actual body weight should be used to calculate CrCl for non-obese and cachectic patients. However, for obese patients (BMI of 30 kg/m² or greater), adjusted body weight is recommended to calculate CrCl. Adjusted body weight is most commonly determined by the following equation.

Adjusted body weight = IBW + [0.4 × (actual body weight − IBW)]

Because of the mathematical complexity of defining who is an obese patient and the lack of precision in determining adjusted body weight, some research groups, such as SWOG (2014), have elected to use actual body weight up to 140% of IBW to calculate CrCl for consistency of calculations and to minimize risks of errors.

With the introduction of the isotope dilution mass spectrometry (IDMS)-measured serum creatinine in many clinical laboratories nationwide, the values are 5%–20% lower than previously reported non–IDMS-measured serum creatinine (Miller et al., 2005). Furthermore, many patients with cancer have low serum creatinine levels (below 0.7 mg/dl), causing overestimation of CrCl, which can potentially lead to an increased risk of drug toxicity. For the purpose of consistency, many clinicians agree to use the minimum value of 0.8 mg/dl for non–IDMS-measured serum creatinine and 0.7 mg/dl for IDMS-measured serum creatinine.

Figure 27-1 summarizes the process of calculating estimated CrCl using the Cockcroft and Gault (1976) method.

Figure 27-1. Calculation of Estimated Creatinine Clearance

$$estCrCl = \frac{(140 - age) \times wt.\ in\ kg^* \times 1.00\ (male)\ OR \times 0.85\ (female)}{72 \times serum\ creatinine^\dagger}$$

* The kilogram weight is the patient weight with an upper limit of 140% of the IBW.

† Actual laboratory serum creatinine value with a minimum of 0.8 mg/dl for non–IDMS-measured serum creatinine or 0.7 mg/dl for IDMS-measured serum creatinine.

IBW—ideal body weight; IDMS—isotope dilution mass spectrometry

Note. Based on information from Cockcroft & Gault, 1976.

If the estimated CrCl will be used for area under the time-versus-concentration curve (AUC) carboplatin dosing calculations, according to a 2010 NCI action letter, the **maximum** CrCl (GFR) that can be used is 125 ml/min using the Calvert formula, which is as follows.

Carboplatin dose (mg) = target AUC (mg/min/ml) × (GFR ml/min + 25)

Although online calculators are available to aid in the determination of CrCl, many of these do not take into account the recommended adjustments of the patient parameters. The use of an online calculator is strongly discouraged for laboratory parameters.

Most cytotoxic agents cause myelosuppression in varying degrees. This side effect is a common variable that calls for subsequent dose modifications. The measurement of myelosuppression is primarily determined by complete blood count (CBC) and occasionally includes other hematologic factors. A decrease in the blood counts usually occurs within five to seven days after the therapy is started. The day the blood counts were the lowest is called the *nadir*. Other factors that contribute to myelosuppression are the patient's age, nutritional status, and overall health. The stem cells in the bone marrow, which divide rapidly, are more affected by chemotherapy than the mature cells in circulation. Most protocols specify that the white blood cell (WBC) count, absolute neutrophil count (ANC), hemoglobin (Hgb) level, and platelet count must be at a certain level prior to dosing.

WBCs comprise five cell lines (neutrophils, lymphocytes, monocytes, basophils, and eosinophils). The ANC measures the amount of segmented neutrophils (mature neutrophils) and bands (immature neutrophils) in the WBCs or leukocytes. Neutrophils provide the first line of defense against bacterial infections. The following formula is used to compute the ANC.

ANC = (% segmented neutrophils + % band neutrophils) × WBC (cells/mm^3)

Absolute granulocyte count (AGC) is also used to measure myelosuppression when a three-part differential method is used to report WBC. AGC equates to the combination of ANC, basophils, and eosinophils. Therefore, AGC is typically 5%–10% more than ANC. Neutropenia is defined by ANC less than 1,800/mm^3. Continuation of chemotherapy usually requires ANC of 1,500/mm^3 or greater. If ANC is below 1,000/mm^3, the patient is at risk for infection. ANC calculators are available online (e.g., www.mdcalc.com/absolute-neutrophil-count-anc, www.globalrph.com/anc.htm). These tools calculate the subject's ANC, thus decreasing the possibility of human error.

Red blood cells (RBCs) and platelets also can be depleted by chemotherapy. Hgb or hematocrit levels are used to measure RBC suppression and are components of the CBC. Patients are considered to be anemic when their Hgb is less than 12 g/dl and become symptomatic when Hgb is less than 10 g/dl. Thrombocytopenia is defined by platelet counts less than 150,000/mm^3. Platelet levels below 50,000/mm^3 predispose patients to petechiae and bruising. Gastrointestinal bleeding and central nervous system bleeding can occur if platelet levels fall below 20,000/mm^3 (Doyle, 1995). Clinical trial nurses will evaluate both platelet and RBC values before administering each dose of a protocol agent. They also assess blood counts any time that evidence of infection, anemia, or bleeding is present.

Documentation

As soon as treatment is administered, documentation of patient response begins. The protocol may require accurate documentation of the start and stop times for each IV fluid and chemotherapy infusion, as well as premedications given to prevent adverse effects.

Documentation during the administration of the protocol agent is very important to evaluate administration-related side effects. Therefore, baseline patient observations as defined by the clinical trial must be made prior to dosing with study agents. Next, prophylactic medications should be administered to prevent expected treatment-related side effects, such as nausea and vomiting. With the patient's cooperation, the nurse should identify and record a follow-up plan in a format that the patient can easily understand. The patient should receive written follow-up guidance, including the name of the study coordinator or nurse assigned to the patient. The study file should include the patient's correct address and telephone number in addition to an emergency contact. Monitoring the patient after administration of the protocol agent (e.g., calling the patient a day or two following the protocol therapy) helps to ensure patient safety as well as protocol compliance. If chemotherapy is administered in a location other than the research office, copies of the chemotherapy administration records and any updates to the patient contact information need to be sent to the study's PI or study coordinator (Cohen et al., 1996).

Complete and accurate treatment data are essential in clinical research. Therefore, thorough documentation before, during, and after drug administration is critical. In preparation for auditing, the medical record should include all of the information required by the protocol. Flow sheets and study-specific worksheets further enhance the documentation of treatment. Many times, these tools can be developed by the nurse and can be used as source documentation if the information is not already provided in the medical record. Such study tools should be shared with the sponsor prior to their use as source documents, and approval of the tools should be documented in a note to file, letter, or email message that is kept in the site's regulatory binder.

Guidelines

The American Society of Clinical Oncology and Oncology Nursing Society (Neuss et al., 2013) have developed the following guidelines in an effort to ensure that protocol treatment proceeds in a safe and orderly fashion.

- Always double-check the dosage calculations with another chemotherapy-competent nurse, as well as with the research pharmacist.
- If the study drug is to be administered via IV infusion using an IV pump, the settings of the pump should be double-checked by a second nurse to ensure that the proper dose is given within the time frame specified by the protocol.
- Prepare treatment packets in advance that contain patient education materials regarding side effects of the protocol agent, adherence tools (e.g., calendars, diaries), and instructions regarding the reporting of side effects.
- Provide in-service education to nursing and pharmacy staff to enhance team performance. If possible, be present during the initial dose calculations and administration of protocol agents. This support of patients and nursing staff allows potential problems to be identified and corrected before a protocol deviation occurs.
- Remain in close contact with the PI for each patient. Notify the physician if any toxicities or adverse events occur, especially those that require dose modification, discontinuation, or interruption of the drug infusion.
- Before each treatment, assess and affirm the patient's desire to continue on the protocol (see Chapter 14). Patients have the right to withdraw at any time when participating in clinical research. If the patient declines further participation in the trial, the study coordinator should be contacted so that the study sponsor can be notified appropriately.
- The study sponsor and/or the sponsor's representative can be a resource and ally in the clinical research process. Discuss problems and concerns with the sponsor's representative. Experiences occurring at other study sites may be significant to provide evolving information not previously known.
- Sign, date, and note the time on all sources of information to provide source documents.

Role of Clinical Trial Nurses

A growing number of Oncology Nursing Society members identify clinical research as their primary job focus. With the dominant influence of clinical research in oncology, it is understandable that clinical trials nursing has developed a mainstream standing in oncology, perhaps more so than in other disease areas. Deininger (2008) noted that "while oncology nursing has its origins rooted in pursuit of the magic bullet, clinical trials nursing also is grounded in the pursuit of inquiry" (p. 353). Today's oncology nurse clinicians have insight into the clinical trial process as it pertains to the study participants in whose care they may be involved. Those same clinicians may decide to enter the research subspecialty of oncology and impart added value to the research team by applying the basic nursing tenets of clinical and critical-thinking skills, bedside experience, interpersonal skills, and patient advocacy (Oncology Nursing Society, 2010). Considering the large numbers of oncology nurses who are involved in such roles, it is essential to have standards, policies, and procedures to guide their practice.

The American Society of Clinical Oncology published a policy statement in 2003 on the oversight of clinical research (American Society of Clinical Oncology, 2003). The purpose of the policy was to improve public trust of investigational/research drug development and testing. In recent years, public interest in the safety of clinical trials has been increasing, along with interest in the safety of newly developed drugs approved by FDA.

FDA published *Guidance for Industry: Investigator Responsibilities—Protecting the Rights, Safety, and Welfare of Study Subjects* in October 2009 (U.S. FDA, 2009). This guidance stipulates that the investigator is responsible for (a) personally conducting or supervising the study, (b) providing adequate training and supervision to those individuals (i.e., nurses, pharmacists) to whom investigator tasks have been delegated, and (c) at all times protecting the rights, safety, and welfare of study participants (U.S. FDA, 2009).

The Oncology Nursing Society publishes the *Chemotherapy and Biotherapy Guidelines and Recommendations for Practice* (Polovich, Olsen, & LeFebvre, 2014), which has become the standard reference for the administration of chemotherapy and biologic therapy. It includes detailed information about the preparation, administration, and disposal of hazardous drugs, as well as personal protection strategies for oncology nurses in a clinical setting. Individual online training is available through the Oncology Nursing Society. The *Infusion Nursing Standards of Practice* (Infusion Nurses Society, 2011) includes a chapter titled "Administration of Parenteral Investigational Drugs." Infusion nurses who administer investigational products in the setting of clinical trials should take the time to refer to their institution's policies, as well as to these national policies and procedures (Infusion Nurses Society, 2011; Neuss et al., 2013; Polovich et al., 2014).

Summary

Sponsoring agencies have recognized that research drug accountability continues to be a common problem observed in study audits. With NCI's leadership, the major research cooperative groups are dedicated to educating their members on the proper handling and documentation of research study drugs. Various guidelines and educational tools are being developed to achieve this goal.

This chapter presented a concise step-by-step guide for research drug handling and accountability. Investigators should take ownership in obtaining and managing research study drugs efficiently. Accurate documentation is critical in the conduct of clinical trials. Becoming familiar with these requirements will allow investigators to move one step closer to the execution of clinical trials of the highest quality.

Clinical research provides a unique opportunity to improve the care that patients with cancer receive. It holds hope for the development of less toxic and more effective treatment and increased comfort for people with cancer. Nursing roles in clinical research provide job satisfaction and the opportunity to become a ready resource to patients and colleagues alike.

Key Points

- All study personnel must review the study protocol and be ready to retrieve and confirm information in a timely manner as needs arise.
- Investigator personnel must be familiar with the process of research drug handling and administration to support drug development studies.
- All study personnel must maintain updated knowledge in research drug handling policy and procedures using *A Handbook for Clinical Investigators Conducting Therapeutic Clinical Trials Supported by CTEP, DCTD, NCI* (NCI CTEP, 2014).
- The fundamental principle of research drug handling is that every single study drug dose must be accounted for and documented.
- All study personnel involved in the care of research participants must review physician orders prior to dispensing study drugs to ensure the correct dosage and timing of doses, using a double-check system with a pharmacist or designated research nurse.
- Administration of research drugs must be performed consistently to promote quality data.
- Research nurses and pharmacists can positively influence participants' adherence to a study drug schedule through frequent communication and careful listening to participants' complaints of symptoms that may be attributed to the study drug.
- Nurses and pharmacists should work very closely with the PI to ensure that all adverse events are documented in medical records and case reports of all participants.

References

American Society of Clinical Oncology. (2003). American Society of Clinical Oncology policy statement: Oversight of clinical research. *Journal of Clinical Oncology, 21,* 2377–2386. doi:10.1200/JCO.2003.04.026

Anderson, P.O., Knoben, J.E., & Troutman, W.G. (Eds.). (2002). *Handbook of clinical drug data* (10th ed.). Kansas City, MO: Marion Merrell Dow.

Barrett, S.V., Paul, J., Hay, A., Vasey, P.A., Kaye, S.B., & Glasspool, R.M. (2008). Does body mass index affect progression-free or overall survival in patients with ovarian cancer? Results from SCOTROC I trial. *Annals of Oncology, 19,* 898–902. doi:10.1093/annonc/mdm606

Baumann, T.J., Staddon, J.E., Horst, H.M., & Bivins, B.A. (1987). Minimum urine collection periods for accurate determination of creatinine clearance in critically ill patients. *Clinical Pharmacy, 6,* 393–398.

Cockcroft, D.W., & Gault, M.H. (1976). Prediction of creatinine clearance from serum creatinine. *Nephron, 16,* 31–41. doi:10.1159/000180580

Cohen, M.R., Anderson, R.W., Attilio, R.M., Green, L., Muller, R.J., & Pruemer, J.M. (1996). Preventing medication errors in cancer chemotherapy. *American Journal of Health-System Pharmacy, 53,* 737–746.

Deininger, H.E. (2008). Specialization in clinical trials nursing. In A.D. Klimaszewski, M. Bacon, H.E. Deininger, B.A. Ford, & J.G. Westendorp (Eds.), *Manual for clinical trials nursing* (2nd ed., pp. 353–356). Pittsburgh, PA: Oncology Nursing Society.

Doyle, M.A. (1995). *Oncologic therapy.* Philadelphia, PA: Elsevier Saunders.

Egorin, M.J., Van Echo, D.A., Olman, E.A., Whitacre, M.Y., Forrest, A., & Aisner, J. (1985). Prospective validation of a pharmacologically based dosing scheme for the *cis*-diamminedichloroplatinum(II) analogue diamminecyclobutanedicarboxylatoplatinum. *Cancer Research, 45*(12, Pt. 1), 6502–6506. Retrieved from http://cancerres.aacrjournals.org/content/45/12_Part_1/6502.long

Georgiadis, M.S., Steinberg, S.M., Hankins, L.A., Ihde, D.C., & Johnson, B.E. (1995). Obesity and therapy-related toxicity in patients treated for small-cell lung cancer. *Journal of the National Cancer Institute, 87,* 361–366. doi:10.1093/jnci/87.5.361

Griggs, J.J., Mangu, P.B., Anderson, H., Balaban, E.P., Dignam, J.J., Hryniuk, W.M., ... Lyman, G.H. (2012). Appropriate chemotherapy dosing for obese adult patients with cancer: American Society of Clinical Oncology clinical practice guideline. *Journal of Clinical Oncology, 30,* 1553–1561. doi:10.1200/JCO.2011.39.9436

Gurney, H., & Shaw, R. (2007). Obesity in dose calculation: A mouse or an elephant? [Editorial]. *Journal of Clinical Oncology, 25,* 4703–4704. doi:10.1200/JCO.2007.13.1078

Hunter, R.J., Navo, M.A., Thaker, P.H., Bodurka, D.C., Wolf, J.K., & Smith, J.A. (2009). Dosing chemotherapy in obese patients: Actual versus assigned body surface area (BSA). *Cancer Treatment Reviews, 35,* 69–78. doi:10.1016/j.ctrv.2008.07.005

Infusion Nurses Society. (2011). *Infusion nursing standards of practice.* Norwood, MA: Author.

Meyerhardt, J.A., Tepper, J.E., Niedzwiecki, D., Hollis, D.R., McCollum, A.D., Brady, D., ... Fuchs, C.S. (2004). Impact of body mass index on outcomes and treatment-related toxicity in patients with stage II and III rectal cancer: Findings from Intergroup Trial 0114. *Journal of Clinical Oncology, 22,* 648–657. doi:10.1200/JCO.2004.07.121

Miller, W.G., Myers, G.L., Ashwood, E.R., Killeen, A.A., Wang, E., Thienpont, L.M., & Siekmann, L. (2005). Creatinine measurement: State of the art in accuracy and interlaboratory harmonization. *Archives of Pathology and Laboratory Medicine, 129,* 297–304.

National Cancer Institute. (2010, October 22). Follow-up for information letter regarding AUC-based dosing of carboplatin. Retrieved from http://ctep.cancer.gov/content/docs/Carboplatin_Information_Letter.pdf

National Cancer Institute Cancer Therapy Evaluation Program. (2014). *A handbook for clinical investigators conducting therapeutic clinical trials supported by CTEP, DCTD, NCI* [Version 1.2]. Retrieved from http://ctep.cancer.gov/investigatorResources/docs/InvestigatorHandbook.pdf

Neuss, M.N., Polovich, M., McNiff, K., Esper, P., Gilmore, T.R., LeFebvre, K.B., ... Jacobson, J.O. (2013). 2013 updated American Society of Clinical Oncology/Oncology Nursing Society chemotherapy administration safety standards including standards for the safe administration and management of oral chemotherapy. *Journal of Oncology Practice, 9*(Suppl. 2), 5s–13s. doi:10.1200/JOP.2013.000874

Oncology Nursing Society. (2010). *Oncology clinical trials nurse competencies.* Retrieved from https://www.ons.org/sites/default/files/ctncompetencies.pdf

Polovich, M., Olsen, M., & LeFebvre, K.B. (Eds.). (2014). *Chemotherapy and biotherapy guidelines and recommendations for practice* (4th ed.). Pittsburgh, PA: Oncology Nursing Society.

Rosner, G.L., Hargis, J.B., Hollis, D.R., Budman, D.R., Weiss, R.B., Henderson, I.C., & Schilsky, R.L. (1996). Relationship between toxicity and obesity in women receiving adjuvant chemotherapy for breast cancer: Results from Cancer and Leukemia Group B Study 8541. *Journal of Clinical Oncology, 14,* 3000–3008. Retrieved from http://jco.ascopubs.org/content/14/11/3000.abstract

Sparreboom, A., Wolff, A.C., Mathijssen, R.H.J., Chatelut, E., Rowinsky, E.K., Verweij, J., & Baker, S.D. (2007). Evaluation of alternate size descriptors for dose calculation of anticancer drugs in the obese. *Journal of Clinical Oncology, 25,* 4707–4713. doi:10.1200/JCO.2007.11.2938

SWOG. (2014, May). Dosing principles for patients on clinical trials (Policy Memorandum No. 38). Retrieved from http://swog.org/Visitors/Download/Policies/Policy38.pdf

U.S. Food and Drug Administration. (2009, October). *Guidance for industry: Investigator responsibilities—Protecting the rights, safety, and welfare of study subjects.* Retrieved from http://www.regulations.gov/#!documentDetail;D=FDA-2007-D-0307-0004

Chapter 28

Adverse Events

Elizabeth Ness, RN, MS, and Ann M. Lau Clark, RN, MSN, CCRC, CCRP

Introduction

Identifying and monitoring adverse events (AEs) is critical to protect research participants and ensure data integrity. Assessment of AEs and timely documentation are crucial to research participant safety and critical components of good clinical practice (GCP). The purposes of AE surveillance, especially those events related to the study intervention, include (Trotti, Colevas, Setser, & Basch, 2007)
- Identifying events that may have an immediate effect on the safety of the patient
- Informing regulators, investigators, and others of new and important information about events that occur on a clinical trial
- Providing a summary of adverse experiences in order to develop the drug or regimen toxicity profile.

Clinical trial nurses (CTNs) are responsible for education, protection, and safety of patients enrolled in clinical trials (Badalucco & Reed, 2011). This chapter will focus on the assessment, documentation, recording, and reporting of AEs, unanticipated problems (UPs), and the role of CTNs.

Definitions

An *adverse event* is any unwanted sign, symptom, or disease that was not seen before an individual's research participation or a worsening of a baseline symptom, regardless of expectedness of the event or relationship of the event to the research. *Toxicity, side effect*, and related terms (e.g., *adverse drug reaction, adverse drug event, acute or late effect, complication*) imply a relationship of the event to an intervention. There are many other definitions associated with AEs (e.g., serious, unexpected, suspected adverse reaction). Table 28-1 provides definitions associated with AEs from the Office for Human Research Protections (OHRP), the U.S. Food and Drug Administration (FDA), and the International Conference on Harmonisation of Technical Requirements for Registration of Pharmaceuticals for Human Use (ICH) *ICH Harmonised Tripartite Guideline: Guideline for Good Clinical Practice* (GCP). Understanding the various definitions is the first step in understanding AEs.

Adverse Event Assessment

The principal investigator (PI) or other individuals on the research team delegated to by the PI (e.g., physician subinvestigators) conducts the AE assessment, which consists of (Ness, 2013)
- Selecting the correct AE term
- Identifying the expectedness of the event (i.e., known to occur with the intervention)
- Assessing the severity of the event
- Determining the attribution of the event.

Understanding how to collect and solicit information about AEs is crucial. CTNs are well positioned to assist with AE assessment, often being the patient participant's first point of contact.

Event Terminology

It is vital that CTNs understand the importance of using appropriate terminology when assessing an AE. Using controlled vocabularies to represent clinical concepts is the best way to describe AEs. Medical Dictionary for Regulatory Activities (MedDRA®) and Systematized Nomenclature of Medicine—Clinical Terms (SNOMED

The authors would like to acknowledge Laura S. Wood, RN, MSN, OCN®, for her contribution to this chapter that remains unchanged from the previous edition of this book.

Terminology	U.S. Office for Human Research Protections	U.S. Food and Drug Administration	International Conference on Harmonisation
Adverse event (AE)	Any untoward or unfavorable medical occurrence in a human subject, including any abnormal sign (for example, abnormal physical exam or laboratory finding), symptom, or disease, temporally associated with the subject's participation in the research, whether or not considered related to the subject's participation in the research (modified from the definition of AEs in the 1996 International Conference on Harmonisation E6 guidelines for good clinical practice). AEs encompass physical and psychological harms. They occur most commonly in the context of biomedical research, although they can occur in the context of social and behavioral research.	Any untoward medical occurrence associated with the use of a drug in humans, whether or not considered drug related	Any untoward medical occurrence in a patient or clinical investigation subject administered a pharmaceutical product, which does not necessarily have a causal relationship with this treatment. An AE can, therefore, be any unfavorable and unintended sign (including an abnormal laboratory finding), symptom, or disease temporally associated with the use of a medicinal (investigational) product, whether or not related to the medicinal (investigational) product.
Life threatening	An AE that places the subject at immediate risk of death from the event as it occurred	An AE or suspected adverse reaction is considered life threatening if, in the view of either the investigator or sponsor, its occurrence places the patient or subject at immediate risk of death. It does not include an AE or suspected AE that, had it occurred in a more severe form, might have caused death.	An event in which the patient was at risk of death at the time of the event
Suspected adverse reaction	N/A	Any AE for which there is a reasonable possibility that the drug caused the AE. For the purposes of IND safety reporting, "reasonable possibility" means there is evidence to suggest a causal relationship between the drug and the AE. *Suspected adverse reaction* implies a lesser degree of certainty about causality than *adverse reaction*, which means any AE caused by a drug.	N/A
Serious	N/A	An AE or suspected adverse reaction is considered serious if, in the view of either the investigator or sponsor, it results in any of the following outcomes: death, a life-threatening AE, inpatient hospitalization or prolongation of existing hospitalization, a persistent or significant incapacity or substantial disruption of the ability to conduct normal life functions, or a congenital anomaly or birth defect. Important medical events that may not result in death, be life threatening, or require hospitalization may be considered serious when, based upon appropriate medical judgment, they may jeopardize the patient or subject and may require medical or surgical intervention to prevent one of the outcomes listed in this definition.	Any untoward medical occurrence that at any dose • Results in death • Is life threatening • Requires inpatient hospitalization or prolongation of existing hospitalization • Results in persistent or significant disability/incapacity • Is a congenital anomaly/birth defect.

(Continued on next page)

Table 28-1. Comparison of Adverse Event Terminology Among Regulatory Bodies *(Continued)*

Terminology	U.S. Office for Human Research Protections	U.S. Food and Drug Administration	International Conference on Harmonisation
Unanticipated adverse device effect	N/A	Any serious adverse effect on health or safety or any life-threatening problem or death caused by, or associated with, a device, if that effect, problem, or death was not previously identified in nature, severity, or degree of incidence in the investigational plan or application (including a supplementary plan or application), or any other unanticipated serious problem associated with a device that relates to the rights, safety, or welfare of subjects.	N/A

Unanticipated problem	Any incident, experience, or outcome that meets **all** of the following criteria:
	• Unexpected (in terms of nature, severity, or frequency) given
	  – The research procedures that are described in the protocol-related documents, such as the institutional review board (IRB)-approved research protocol and informed consent document;
	  – The characteristics of the subject population being studied
	• Related or possibly related to participation in the research (in this guidance document, *possibly related* means there is a reasonable possibility that the incident, experience, or outcome may have been caused by the procedures involved in the research)
	• Suggests that the research places subjects or others at a greater risk of harm (including physical, psychological, economic, or social harm) than was previously known or recognized.
		AE observed during the conduct of a study should be considered an unanticipated problem involving risk to human subjects, and reported to the IRB, only if it was unexpected and serious and would have implications for the conduct of the study (e.g., requiring a significant, and usually safety-related change in the protocol such as revising inclusion/exclusion criteria or including a new monitoring requirement, informed consent, or investigator's brochure).	N/A

Unexpected	Any AE occurring in one or more participants in a research protocol, the nature, severity, or frequency of which is not consistent with either
	• The known or foreseeable risk of AEs associated with the procedures involved in the research that are described in
	  – The protocol-related documents, such as the IRB-approved research protocol, any applicable investigator's brochure, and the current IRB-approved informed consent document
	  – Other relevant sources of information, such as product labeling and package inserts
	• The expected natural progression of any underlying disease, disorder, or condition of the participants experiencing the AE and the participants' predisposing risk factor profile for the AE.
		An AE or suspected adverse reaction is considered unexpected if it is not listed in the investigator's brochure or is not listed at the specificity or severity that has been observed; or, if an investigator's brochure is not required or available, is not consistent with the risk information described in the general investigational plan or elsewhere in the current application, as amended.	An adverse reaction, the nature or severity of which is not consistent with the applicable product information (e.g., investigator's brochure for an unapproved investigational product or package insert/summary of product characteristics for an approved product)

Note. Based on information from IND Safety Reporting, 2014; International Conference on Harmonisation of Technical Requirements for Registration of Pharmaceuticals for Human Use, 1996; Investigational Device Exemptions, 2014; Office for Human Research Protections, 2007; U.S. Food and Drug Administration, 2009a.

CT) are the two most common sources for terminology. MedDRA is widely used in clinical trials, whereas SNOMED CT is used for clinical care data (Richesson, Fung, & Krischer, 2008).

MedDRA is a clinically validated international medical terminology dictionary with each term having a unique code or what is referred to as a concept ID. Developed in 1994 by ICH to facilitate sharing of regulatory information internationally, MedDRA is used by the biopharmaceutical industry and regulatory authorities for AE classification. MedDRA has five hierarchal levels:

- System Organ Class (SOC): Highest level of the terminology and distinguished by anatomic or physiologic system, etiology, or purpose
- High Level Group Term (HLGT): Subordinate to SOC
- High Level Term (HLT): Subordinate to HLGT
- Preferred Term (PT): Represents a single medical concept
- Lowest Level Term (LLT): Lowest level of the terminology, related to a single PT as a synonym, lexical variant, or quasi-synonym (MedDRA Maintenance and Support Services Organization [MSSO], 2013).

See Figure 28-1 for an example of the hierarchical structure for the AE term *fatigue*.

MedDRA trademark is owned by the International Federation of Pharmaceutical Manufacturers and Associations, which functions as a trustee for ICH and is managed by MSSO. MedDRA is available in several languages including Chinese, Czech, Dutch, English, German, French, Italian, Japanese, Portuguese, and Spanish. Currently, the use of MedDRA is mandated in Europe and Japan for AE safety reporting, and FDA has adopted MedDRA terminology for its web-based Adverse Event Reporting System (AERS). MedDRA is reviewed twice a year with a major release once a year, usually in the spring, and a smaller release with additional new terms in the fall. To learn more, visit www.meddra.org (MedDRA MSSO, 2013).

Severity Rating Scales

In clinical trials, rating scales are used to measure the severity of an AE (see Table 28-2). The severity of an AE often determines if dosing interruptions, modifications, or discontinuations need to be implemented according to the protocol. Rating scales can even be used for eligibility criteria (e.g., exclusion criteria to include no grade 2 or greater peripheral sensory neuropathy). The protocol should include how the severity of AEs is to be measured, even if only providing descriptions for mild, moderate, and severe. In oncology, the standard rating scale is actually a combination of an AE term and severity rating scale, the Common Terminology Criteria for Adverse Events (CTCAE).

Common Terminology Criteria for Adverse Events

The National Cancer Institute Cancer Therapy Evaluation Program (NCI CTEP) developed the original Common Toxicity Criteria (CTC) in 1983 to aid in the recognition and assessing severity (i.e., grading) of adverse effects of chemotherapy. Since CTC version 1.0, the tool has been expanded, adapted internationally by the oncology community, renamed, and with the release of version 4.0 in May 2009, harmonized with MedDRA terminology (see Table 28-3). The CTCAE is a subset of MedDRA terms that are pertinent to the AEs seen in oncology clinical trials (Chen et al., 2012; Trotti et al., 2003, 2007).

The CTCAE is an agreed-upon terminology by experts in the oncology community for the designation, reporting, and grading of AEs that occur in oncology clinical trials. The grading or severity rating scale (a) promotes consistency among clinical researchers, (b) facilitates a common understanding of AE data shared among academic, commercial, and regulatory entities, and (c) provides a framework to compare AEs across different studies. The CTCAE has not been tested for validity or reliability (Trotti et al., 2007).

Several versions of the CTCAE are found on CTEP's website (http://ctep.cancer.gov/protocolDevelopment/electronic_applications/ctc.htm), including other related documents (e.g., mapping CTCAE version 3.0 to version 4.0). CTNs should be aware of the CTCAE version that is used. Older protocols may use a lower version of the CTCAE. The protocol will make reference to what version is to be used along with the website. It is best to go to CTEP's website, as noted above, to access the protocol-appropriate and current version of the CTCAE (NCI CTEP, 2010). The CTCAE is maintained by CTEP and will continue to be harmonized with MedDRA terminology. At the time of this writing, CTEP has solicited suggestions for CTCAE version 5.0, which ideally will incorporate the use of patient-reported data (Basch, Bennett, & Pietanza, 2011; NCI CTEP, 2013a).

How to Read the CTCAE

The CTCAE is set up in a table format with 26 MedDRA SOCs listed alphabetically (see Figure 28-2). Within each SOC, AEs are listed alphabetically. Each AE is defined and assigned a numeric grade (grades 1–5), which provides description of the event that pertains to that term (see Table 28-4). Within the description of the grade, a semicolon (;) is read as an "or" statement and an em dash (—) indicates that grade is not available for the specific AE term. Each SOC has an *Other, specify* option for reporting events not listed in CTCAE. Use the general guidelines when assessing the severity of an AE that is not currently available (see Table 28-5).

Figure 28-1. MedDRA® Fatigue Hierarchy

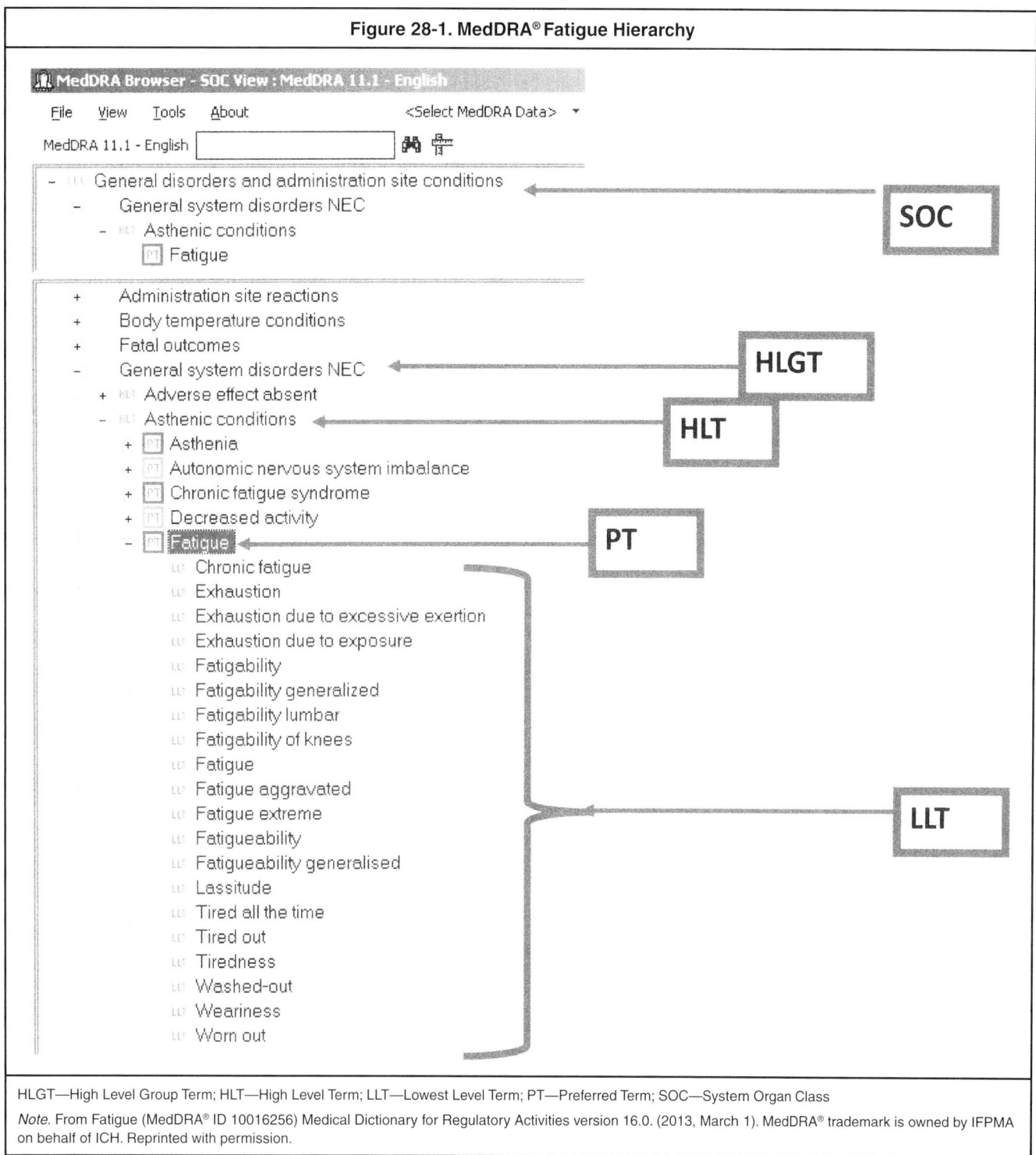

HLGT—High Level Group Term; HLT—High Level Term; LLT—Lowest Level Term; PT—Preferred Term; SOC—System Organ Class

Note. From Fatigue (MedDRA® ID 10016256) Medical Dictionary for Regulatory Activities version 16.0. (2013, March 1). MedDRA® trademark is owned by IFPMA on behalf of ICH. Reprinted with permission.

Patient-Reported Outcomes Version of the CTCAE

Many of the AE terms found in the CTCAE (approximately 10%) are actually symptoms or subjective assessments requiring the provider and research team to translate what the patient is describing to an appropriate CTCAE term (Basch et al., 2011). These types of AEs are often referred to as *patient-reported outcomes* (PROs) and are best rated by the patient participant, allowing for serious events to be reported sooner than an assessment done solely by a provider. Combining patient-reported symptoms with provider assessment can lead to improved safety (Basch et al., 2011).

FDA is encouraging drug developers to incorporate the patient perspective in the drug development process and has developed various approaches to assist with this goal (e.g., development of guidance document when using PROs in drug development and collaborating to develop a PRO Consortium) (Basch, 2013). As defined by FDA (2009b), a PRO is

> any report of the status of a patient's health condition that comes directly from the patient, without interpretation of the patient's response by a clinician or anyone else. The outcome can be measured in absolute terms (e.g., severity of a symptom, sign, or state of a disease) or as a change from a previous measure. In clinical trials, a PRO instrument can be used to measure the effect of a medical intervention on one or more concepts (i.e., the thing being measured, such as a symptom or group of symptoms, effects on a particular function or group of functions, or a group of symptoms or functions shown to measure the severity of a health condition). (p. 2)

In 2008, NCI's PRO-CTCAE project began with the goal of developing a valid, reliable, feasible, and clinically usefully patient version of the CTCAE, specifically, an electronic system for patient self-reporting of symptom AEs. As of May 2013, 81 symptoms in the CTCAE (version 4) have been identified as appropriate for patient reporting. There are 126 questions that assess various attributes of the 81 symptoms, including presence, frequency, severity, and interference with activities of daily living. The symptoms used in PRO-CTCAE are MedDRA compliant (NCI CTEP, 2013c). To learn more about PRO-CTCAE and for the most current information about the project, visit NCI's website (http://outcomes.cancer.gov/tools/pro-ctcae.html).

Determining Attribution

Once the severity of the event is established, the next step is to find the cause, or attribution, of the event. *Attribution* is the relationship or association between the research and the AE, though for any AE, a cause should be determined. In clinical trials, there can be many challenges when assessing AEs. Protocols are complex and often involve multiple drugs. Patients' prior therapies, concomitant medications, or comorbid diseases may make it difficult to determine the cause of an AE (Ness, 2013). CTNs are typically responsible for gathering initial information about the AE, discussing this with the investigator, and collaborating on further assessments to determine the severity of the AE and its attribution to the research. Determining the attribution is done by the investigator with input from the research team, including CTNs (Ness, 2013). Figure 28-3 provides a list of

Table 28-2. Types of Severity Rating Scales

Scale	Description

Common Terminology Criteria for Adverse Events	• Developed in 1983 by the National Cancer Institute Cancer Therapy Evaluation Program to aid in the recognition and grading severity of adverse effects of chemotherapy
	• Originally called the Common Toxicity Criteria
	• Grading scale
	  – Grade 1 (mild)
	  – Grade 2 (moderate)
	  – Grade 3 (severe)
	  – Grade 4 (life threatening)
	  – Grade 5 (death)

U.S. Food and Drug Administration Toxicity Grading Scale Tables	• Clinical and laboratory abnormalities
	  – Mild (grade 1)
	  – Moderate (grade 2)
	  – Severe (grade 3)
	  – Potentially life threatening (grade 4)

Note. Based on information from National Cancer Institute Cancer Therapy Evaluation Program, 2010; U.S. Food and Drug Administration, 2007.

Table 28-3. Historical Timeline of the Common Terminology Criteria for Adverse Events

Year and Version	Name	Number of Categories	Number of Terms
1983 Version 1.0	Common Toxicity Criteria	18	49
1998 Version 2.0	Common Toxicity Criteria	24	295
2003 Version 3.0	Common Terminology Criteria for Adverse Events	28	> 900
2010 Version 4.03	Common Terminology Criteria for Adverse Events	26 (Categories replaced with MedDRA® SOC)	790 (AE terms replaced with MedDRA® LLT)

LLT—Lowest Level Term; MedDRA®—Medical Dictionary for Regulatory Affairs; SOC—System Organ Class
Note. Based on information from Chen et al., 2012; Trotti et al., 2003.

questions for the PI and research team to consider when determining the attribution of the event.

An AE may be considered by the investigator to be *unrelated* or *unlikely* to be related to the study treatment. However, if enough evidence supports a causal relationship between the AE and the research, then the attribution is described as either *possibly*, *probably*, or *definitely* related. Figure 28-4 describes two approaches for determining the causal relationship between the research and an AE, the attributions, and the degree of certainty of the causality.

Figure 28-2. System Organ Class Titles Used in the Common Terminology Criteria for Adverse Events

- Blood and lymphatic system disorders
- Cardiac disorders
- Congenital, familial, and genetic disorders
- Ear and labyrinth disorders
- Endocrine disorders
- Eye disorders
- Gastrointestinal disorders
- General disorders and administration site conditions
- Hepatobiliary disorders
- Immune system disorders
- Infections and infestations
- Injury, poisoning, and procedural complications
- Investigations
- Metabolism and nutrition disorders
- Musculoskeletal and connective tissue disorders
- Neoplasms benign, malignant, and unspecified (including cysts and polyps)
- Nervous system disorders
- Pregnancy, puerperium, and perinatal conditions
- Psychiatric disorders
- Renal and urinary disorders
- Reproductive system and breast disorders
- Respiratory, thoracic, and mediastinal disorders
- Skin and subcutaneous tissue disorders
- Social circumstances
- Surgical and medical procedures
- Vascular disorders

Note. Based on information from National Cancer Institute Cancer Therapy Evaluation Program, 2010.

Table 28-4. Common Terminology Criteria for Adverse Events (Version 4.03) for Anemia

System Organ Class (SOC): Blood and lymphatic system disorders

Adverse Event	Grade 1	Grade 2	Grade 3	Grade 4	Grade 5
Anemia	Hemoglobin (Hgb) < LLN–10.0 g/dl; < LLN–6.2 mmol/L; < LLN–100 g/L	Hgb < 10.0–8.0 g/dl; < 6.2–4.9 mmol/L; < 100–80 g/L	Hgb < 8.0 g/dl; < 4.9 mmol/L; < 80 g/L; transfusion indicated	Life-threatening consequences; urgent intervention indicated	Death

Definition: A disorder characterized by a reduction in the amount of hemoglobin in 100 ml of blood. Signs and symptoms of anemia may include pallor of the skin and mucous membranes, shortness of breath, palpitations of the heart, soft systolic murmurs, lethargy, and fatigability.

LLN—lower limit of normal

Note. From *Common Terminology Criteria for Adverse Events* [v.4.03], by National Cancer Institute Cancer Therapy Evaluation Program, 2010. Retrieved from http://evs.nci.nih.gov/ftp1/CTCAE/About.html.

Table 28-5. Common Terminology Criteria for Adverse Events: Other Adverse Event Terminology

Grade	Description
1	Mild; asymptomatic or mild symptoms; clinical or diagnostic observations only; intervention not indicated.
2	Moderate; minimal, local or noninvasive intervention indicated; limiting age-appropriate instrumental ADL*.
3	Severe or medically significant but not immediately life-threatening; hospitalization or prolongation of hospitalization indicated; disabling; limiting self-care ADL**.
4	Life-threatening consequences; urgent intervention indicated.
5	Death related to AE.

*Instrumental ADL refers to preparing meals, shopping for groceries or clothes, using the telephone, managing money, etc.
**Self-care ADL refers to bathing, dressing and undressing, feeding self, using the toilet, taking medications, and not bedridden.
ADL—activities of daily living; AE—adverse event

Note. From *Common Terminology Criteria for Adverse Events* [v.4.03], by National Cancer Institute Cancer Therapy Evaluation Program, 2010. Retrieved from http://evs.nci.nih.gov/ftp1/CTCAE/About.html.

Figure 28-3. Questions to Assist in Determining Adverse Event (AE) Attribution

- What is already known about the drug, therapy, or classification of drug?
- What is the temporal relationship of the AE to the study therapy?
- Does the AE improve or disappear when drug or therapy is stopped?
- If rechallenged with the drug or therapy, does the AE reappear? Does it recur at the same severity and at the same time point?
- Is the AE a result of an existing disease or condition's signs and symptoms?
- Is the AE a worsening of baseline symptoms?
- Is the AE a result of an underlying concurrent medical condition or concurrent medication?

Figure 28-4. Two Approaches for Adverse Event (AE) Attributions

5 Attributions
- Unrelated: The AE is clearly NOT related to the intervention
- Unlikely related: The AE is doubtfully related to the intervention
- Possibly related: The AE may be related to the intervention
- Probably related: The AE is likely related to the intervention
- Definitely related: The AE is clearly related to the intervention

2 Attributions: A Dichotomous Approach
- Unrelated: The AE is clearly NOT or doubtfully related to the intervention
- Related: The AE may be or is clearly related to the intervention

The IRB and OHRP look for relatedness to the research. FDA looks for relatedness to the IND/IDE. The IBC and OBA look for relatedness to gene therapy.

FDA—U.S. Food and Drug Administration; IBC—institutional biosafety committee; IDE—investigational device exemption; IND—investigational new drug; IRB—institutional review board; OBA—Office of Biotechnology Activities; OHRP—Office for Human Research Protections

Note. From *NCI Guidelines for Investigators: Adverse Event Reporting Requirements for DCTD (CTEP and CIP) and DCP INDs and IDEs,* by National Cancer Institute, 2013, pp. 5, 12. Retrieved from http://ctep.cancer.gov/protocolDevelopment/electronic_applications/docs/aeguidelines.pdf.

Adverse Event Collection

The assessment of AEs comes from the review of participants' symptoms, physical exam, and laboratory and radiology results. Before a patient starts a clinical trial, a good baseline assessment needs to be conducted, including a physical exam noting any abnormal findings, current signs or symptoms the patient is experiencing at the time the trial begins, prior medical history, and current medications. This information is helpful in providing a baseline assessment from which an AE is identified, or it is used to help assign an attribution.

Collection of AE information begins at the initiation of a study intervention. AE information should be collected from the start of a placebo lead-in period or other observational period intended to establish a baseline status for the patient. The collection period and the data to be collected must be specified in the clinical protocol. AEs should be followed to resolution or stabilization. Follow-up is required for AEs that cause interruption or discontinuation of the study drug, or those that are present at the end of study treatment as appropriate.

In order to prevent bias collection of AEs, patients should not be questioned regarding specific events that might be anticipated while on the study. Ideally, AEs should be spontaneously reported or elicited from a research participant (a) during open-ended questioning, (b) during examination, or (c) during evaluation. Sometimes AEs may need to be collected from a family member or significant other who observes a change in the participant. This may be necessary with some pediatric participants or those with cognitive impairment.

A crucial role of CTNs is to assess the patient prior to, during, and following treatment on a protocol. CTNs, working in collaboration with other members of the healthcare team, observe, assess, evaluate, and document patients' treatment- and disease-related symptoms. Study documentation and completed case report forms (CRFs) are audited by monitors, sponsors, and FDA to ensure that toxicity assessments are accurate and that protocol treatment modifications are followed.

Patients sometimes have difficulty accurately remembering the onset, severity, and duration of symptoms experienced while on therapy. One tool that is often used is the patient diary (see Figure 28-5). Collection of AE information is just one use for a diary. A patient diary can also collect information about usage of the study medication to measure compliance, use of concomitant medications, and disease episodes on a daily basis.

The traditional approach when using a diary is to employ a paper format that contains directions, uses a large enough font for the patient to read, and has enough space for the patient to record the data. Recently, electronic methods have been used, such as dial-in phone numbers with interactive voice response systems and handheld devices (e.g., e-diaries) that have menu-driven prompts and alarms to guide the patient. The protocol should identify the purpose of the diary, the type of diary to be used, how frequently entries are to be made, surrogate completion, and how to handle missing data. For symptom-specific diaries, a PRO tool should be considered.

The use of diaries should be addressed in the informed consent document and reviewed during the informed consent discussion. CTNs play a critical role in educating patients on the use of the diary. Patients may need to be reminded to return their diaries at an appointment or to input the data if using an electronic system. Diaries should be reviewed with patients and their family members or caregivers at their visit.

If a patient is seen or hospitalized at an outside institution, the CTN will need to obtain the medical records for review or for completing a serious adverse event (SAE) report. The patient may sign a release of information; however, if the patient is unable to or is deceased when

Figure 28-5. Side Effect Diary Sheet				
Date	Time	Temperature	Side Effect	Medication Taken to Treat Side Effect

the records are sought, the Code of Federal Regulations governs the release of information. The Health Insurance Portability and Accountability Act Privacy Rule permits certain disclosures of protected health information under 45 C.F.R. § 164.512 as long as it is for research purposes. Accessing information on a deceased patient falls under the same regulation; however, the request must state that the patient is deceased and that the information is to be used for research purposes only (NCI CTEP, 2013b).

Adverse Event Documentation

It is important for all healthcare providers caring for patients on a clinical trial to document AEs (e.g., physical exam findings, review of systems). All AEs should be documented in the patients' medical records, including any workup or treatment needed. Good progress notes documenting an AE will contain both GCP documentation and good clinical research practice documentation. Therefore, a good progress note documenting an AE will contain (Ness, 2013)
- Date the AE began, including the time with infusion reaction
- Description of the event
- Treatment for the AE
- Attribution of the AE
- Dates the AE improved or worsened (i.e., grade changed)
- Date the AE resolved.

Keeping track of AEs can be an overwhelming task at times; however, it is crucial for patient safety. Reviewing and seeing trends of AEs in a patient population may alert the PI or sponsor to serious safety concerns. Capturing timely and concise information is vital to the management of data. Sponsors may provide study logs as a tool to be used to facilitate the capture and overall review of the events. These logs can be used as source documentation and require the date of review and signature of the PI. AE logs (see Figure 28-6) should be maintained on a regular basis and reviewed by the PI and sponsor monitor. However, for patients, all AE-related information should be in the medical record so that all healthcare providers are aware of what is happening with the patient.

Adverse Event Recording

Recording the AEs (i.e., data extraction or abstraction) onto a CRF is dependent on the protocol. For some protocols, such as phase I studies, all AEs will be recorded. For others, maybe only grade 2–5 events will be recorded. The protocol should clearly outline what types of AEs will be recorded. Although AE CRFs vary from sponsor to sponsor, most forms contain the following common elements: (a) description of the event, (b) AE term (e.g., CTCAE, MedDRA), (c) date the AE began, (d) treatment for the AE, (e) attribution of the AE, and (f) date the AE resolved. Always refer to the protocol for recording exceptions and the CRF completion for additional information on AE recording (Ness, 2013).

Adverse Event Reporting

The two types of AE reporting to regulatory oversight groups that impact the research team are routine and expedited. The regulatory groups include the institutional review board (IRB), sponsor, FDA, institutional biosafety committee (IBC), and the National Institutes of Health (NIH) Office of Biotechnology Activities (OBA). Events to be reported in an expedited manner ideally should be defined in the protocol, including the timeline and mechanism (e.g., form, database) for reporting.

Routine Adverse Event Reporting

Reporting to the Institutional Review Board
At the time of a continuing review, the PI will provide the IRB with information about AEs. It is important for CTNs to know which AEs need to be reported to the IRB at the time of the continuing review (e.g., all grade 2 and higher AEs with a possible, probable, or definite attribution to the research) and how the IRB wants to receive the AE information. Some IRBs may want a table format summarizing the events since the last continuing review and total number of events (see Figure 28-7) or a brief statement that AEs have occurred at the expected level of severity and frequency

Figure 28-6. Adverse Event Log

Name: _____ Study: _____ PI: _____

Event Name	Onset Date	End Date	NCI Grade	Related (R) Unrelated (UR)	Outcome	PI Initials/Date	Comments

Outcome: R = recovered/resolved; NR = not resolved; RS = resolved with sequelae; D = death; U = unknown

Figure 28-7. Sample Institutional Review Board Continuing Review Adverse Event Summary

Common Terminology Criteria for Adverse Events Term	Grade	Number of Events Since Last Continuing Review	Total Number of Events	Attribution to Research	Serious?	Unexpected?

that is expected per the protocol, informed consent, and product information (e.g., investigator's brochure). The method of presentation should provide the IRB with the information necessary to clearly identify risks to participants and determine if the previous risk determinations are still appropriate (OHRP, 2007, 2010).

Reporting to the Sponsor

The research team provides the sponsor with AE data routinely, whenever CRFs are collected. *Collection* may be done using electronic data capture, so in almost real time, or if using paper CRFs, when the monitor is at the site for a monitoring visit. Per the FDA regulations (21 C.F.R. § 312.62), the timeline for reporting of nonserious AEs should be specified in the protocol (Investigator Recordkeeping and Record Retention, 2014).

Reporting to the U.S. Food and Drug Administration

The sponsor (i.e., the investigational new drug application [IND] or investigational device exemption [IDE] holder) is responsible for providing FDA with routine AE information at the time of the annual report. Unless the research site or an investigator is the sponsor, CTNs will have no involvement with routine AE reporting to FDA. However, if CTNs are involved in assisting with the annual report, FDA does require that a summary (either tabular or narrative) be included that shows the most frequent and serious AEs by body system (Investigational Device Exemptions Definitions, 2014; Investigator Recordkeeping and Record Retention, 2014).

Reporting to the Institutional Biosafety Committee and the Office of Biotechnology Activities

The PI is responsible for reporting routine AEs to OBA in a summary fashion in the annual report. The OBA guidelines require

> information obtained during the previous year's clinical and nonclinical investigations, including 1) a narrative or tabular summary showing the most frequent and most serious adverse experiences by body system; 2) a summary of all serious AEs submitted during the past year; 3) a summary of serious AEs that were expected or considered to have causes not associated with the use of the gene transfer product such as disease progression or concurrent medications; and 4) if any deaths have occurred, the number of participants who died during participation in the investigation and causes of death. (NIH OBA, 2013, pp. 103–104)

It is important for CTNs to know the IBC's policy on routine AE reporting, which may be the same as OBA's policy (i.e., they want a copy of the annual report).

Expedited Adverse Event Reporting

A subset of AEs must be reported more quickly to regulatory groups (i.e., sooner than a continuing review or annual report). This reporting includes new and unexpected AEs that impact safety (i.e., risk) and may lead to a revision in the protocol, investigator's brochure, and/or informed consent. To understand which types of AEs need to be reported, it is important to understand the definitions of *suspected adverse reaction* (SAR), *serious adverse event* (SAE), and *unexpected event* (see Table 28-1). These definitions, plus the attribution, will drive the expedited reporting requirements for regulatory groups. CTNs should become familiar with these definitions because they are usually delegated the responsibility for the reporting of AEs. All expedited reports and any response information from the regulatory/oversight group is to be placed in the regulatory file (see Chapter 39).

Reporting to the Institutional Review Board

OHRP regulations do not specifically address AE reporting to the IRB but rather the requirement for UPs involving risks to research participants to be reported to the IRB (Protection of Human Subjects, 2009). FDA regulations support the investigator reporting AEs that are UPs that have implications for the study (Institutional Review Boards, 2014; Investigator Recordkeeping and Record Retention, 2014; U.S. FDA 2009a). Some UPs are AEs; see the UP section for more details. Specific to devices, the investigator is to report unanticipated adverse device effects (UADEs) to the IRB within 10 working days after the investigator first learns of the effect (Investigational Device Exemptions, 2014; U.S. FDA, 2009a). ICH (1996) GCP guidelines defer to the local regulatory requirements for reporting of unexpected AEs that are serious and related to the drug.

To meet these requirements, IRBs develop criteria for the reporting of AEs. Some IRBs want all SAEs to be reported, whereas others only want AEs that are also UPs to be reported. It is important for CTNs to know which AEs need to be reported to the IRB in an expedited manner, the time frame, and the format. The time frame can range from 24 hours to 7 days. Some IRBs want an initial phone call or secure email with a written report submitted as follow-up; other IRBs may just require a written report. Each IRB designates the reporting system with either a specific paper form or an electronic application to capture this data.

Reporting to the Sponsor

FDA IND regulations and GCP guidelines require the investigator to report all SAEs to the sponsor, unless identified in the protocol as not needing immediate (i.e., expedited) reporting (ICH, 1996; Investigator Recordkeeping and Record Retention, 2014). Under the IND regulations, the investigator is to immediately report study endpoints that are SAEs with a relationship between the drug and the event (e.g., death from anaphylaxis versus a death from progressive disease) (Investigator Recordkeeping and Record Retention, 2014). For IDE studies, the investigator reporting requirements to the sponsor are the same as to the IRB: UADEs must be reported to the sponsor within 10 working days after the investigator first learned of the effect (Investigational Device Exemptions, 2014). Each sponsor will have either a form or database application for reporting expedited AEs. Often these are referred to as an *SAE form*. CTNs will need to be familiar with each sponsor's requirements and report forms.

Sometimes study staff will have only limited information to work with. Often the CTN or investigator will receive a phone message indicating that a trial participant was hospitalized or died. To meet the investigator's reporting requirements to the sponsor, the CTN or investigator can

- Contact the treating physician/institution and document all conversations in the medical record
- Submit what is known, including
  - Most recent clinical evaluations, baseline history, and physical
  - A summary of the event and treatment to date
  - A plan for obtaining information
- Request medical records.

When additional information becomes available, the report is to be amended.

Reporting to the U.S. Food and Drug Administration

As with routine reporting, the sponsor is responsible for expedited reporting to FDA. Per FDA IND regulations,

> The sponsor must promptly review all information relevant to the safety of the drug obtained or otherwise received by the sponsor from foreign or domestic sources, including information derived from any clinical or epidemiological investigations, animal or in vitro studies, reports in the scientific literature, and unpublished scientific papers, as well as reports from foreign regulatory authorities and reports of foreign commercial marketing experience for drugs that are not marketed in the United States. (IND Safety Reporting, 2014, para. 6)

The sponsor is to notify FDA and all participating investigators (i.e., all investigators to whom the sponsor is providing drugs or biologics under its INDs or under any investigator-held IND) in writing of potential serious risks from clinical trials or any other source as soon as possible, but no later than 15 calendar days. These reports are referred to as *IND safety reports* (ISRs) (see Table 28-6) (Investigator Recordkeeping and Record Retention, 2014; U.S. FDA, 2009a).

In addition to the ISR, the sponsor must notify FDA of any *unexpected fatal* or *life-threatening* SAR as soon as possible, but no later than seven calendar days after the sponsor's initial receipt of the information. The initial contact is by phone or email with a written follow-up report. Upon request from FDA, the sponsor must submit any additional data or information that the agency deems necessary as soon as possible, but no later than 15 calendar days after receiving the request (U.S. FDA, 2012a).

The FDA allows for various formats for the written report, including

- General narrative summary for ISRs that include overall findings or pooled analyses from published and unpublished in vitro, animal, epidemiologic, or clinical studies
- MedWatch Form FDA 3500A, mandatory reporting form, which is the most common format, located on the FDA forms website (www.fda.gov/AboutFDA/ReportsManualsForms/Forms/default.htm)
- Council for International Organizations of Medical Sciences I Form, which is used with international studies
- FDA Safety Reporting Portal, which is for drugs and biologics.

The sponsor's report to FDA will include all previously submitted ISRs for similar SARs and analyze the significance of the SAR in light of previous similar reports or any other relevant information (Investigator Recordkeeping and Record Retention, 2014). Many sponsors will send many SAE reports that do not meet the criteria to be an ISR; however, a true ISR will result in a protocol

---

Table 28-6. Investigational New Drug Application Safety Reports

Type	Sponsor Responsibilities

Unexpected and suspected serious adverse reaction (SAR)	• Sponsor must report any SAR that is both serious and unexpected.
	• Sponsor must also report an adverse event (AE) as an SAR only if evidence suggests a causal relationship between the drug and the AE, such as
	  – Single occurrence of an event that is uncommon and known to be strongly associated with drug exposure
	  – One or more occurrences of an event that is not commonly associated with drug exposure but is otherwise uncommon in the population exposed to the drug
	  – Aggregate analysis of specific events observed in a clinical trial that indicates those events occur more frequently in the drug treatment group than in a concurrent or historical control group.

Findings from other studies	• Sponsor must report any findings from clinical, epidemiologic, or pooled analysis of multiple studies or any findings from animal or in vitro testing that suggest a significant risk in humans exposed to the drug. • Reports are required for studies from any source, regardless of whether they are conducted under the investigational new drug application or by the sponsor.
Findings from animal or in vitro testing	• Sponsor must report any findings from animal or in vitro testing, whether or not conducted by the sponsor, that suggest a significant risk in humans exposed to the drug, such as reports of mutagenicity, teratogenicity, or carcinogenicity, or reports of significant organ toxicity at or near the expected human exposure. Ordinarily, any such findings would result in a safety-related change in the protocol, informed consent, investigator's brochure (excluding routine updates of these documents), or other aspects of the overall conduct of the clinical investigation.
Increased rate of occurrence of suspected SAR	• Sponsor must report any clinically important increase in the rate of a suspected SAR over that listed in the protocol or investigator's brochure.

Note. Based on information from IND Safety Reporting, 2014.

amendment. Figure 28-8 describes what the investigator should do with an ISR.

For IDE studies, the sponsor needs to immediately conduct an evaluation of any UADEs, determine if there is an unreasonable risk to research participants, and terminate all investigations or parts of investigations presenting that risk as soon as possible. Termination shall occur no later than 5 working days after the sponsor makes this determination and no later than 15 working days after the sponsor first received notice of the effect (Investigational Device Exemptions, 2014). The report is written in a narrative format.

Reporting to the Institutional Biosafety Committee and the Office of Biotechnology Activities

The PI must submit a written safety report for
- Any SAE that is both unexpected and associated with the use of a gene transfer product (i.e., a reasonable possibility exists that the event may have been caused by the use of the product; investigators should not await definitive proof of association before reporting such events)
- Any finding from tests in laboratory animals that suggests a significant risk for human research participants, including reports of mutagenicity, teratogenicity, or carcinogenicity.

Per NIH OBA (2013), the safety report must include, but need not be limited to,

> 1) the date of the event; 2) designation of the report as an initial report or a follow-up report, identification of all safety reports previously filed for the clinical protocol concerning a similar AE, and an analysis of the significance of the AE in light of previous similar reports; 3) clinical site; 4) the PI; 5) NIH Protocol number; 6) FDA's Investigational New Drug (IND) Application number; 7) vector type, e.g., adenovirus; 8) vector subtype, e.g., type 5, relevant deletions; 9) gene delivery method, e.g., *in vivo, ex vivo*

Figure 28-8. Site Processing of an Investigational New Drug Safety Report

- Principal investigator (PI) reviews the safety report.
- PI sends to subinvestigators and clinical trial nurses (CTNs).
- PI assesses need to amend protocol and consent documents.
- Safety report is submitted to institutional review board (IRB) per local IRB policy.
- All safety reprots are placed in regulatory binder, including IRB review and comments.
- PI amends protocol and consent documents as needed.
- PI or CTNs inform currently enrolled patients *immediately* (i.e., by phone) of new potential risk and *document* conversation and patients' willingness to continue on study in medical record.
- PI or CTNs reconsent patients as guided by IRB or sponsor.

---

transduction; 10) route of administration, e.g., intratumoral, intravenous; 11) dosing schedule; 12) a complete description of the event; 13) relevant clinical observations; 14) relevant clinical history; 15) relevant tests that were or are planned to be conducted; 16) date of any treatment of the event; and 17) the suspected cause of the event. (p. 104)

The written report can be in any of the following formats:
- OBA Adverse Event Reporting Template (available at http://oba.od.nih.gov/rdna/adverse_event_oba.html)
- FDA MedWatch form
- NIH/FDA Genetic Modification Clinical Research Information System with prior approval (see http://oba.od.nih.gov/rdna/oba_gemcris_pi.html)
- Other means provided that all of the above elements are specifically included.

Report Forms

Regardless of the regulatory group to which CTNs are reporting, each report form will have similar elements, including reporter information, participant demographics, study agent or intervention information (e.g., dates given, dose, route of administration), events, attribution, and narrative summary. The narrative summary is the most important part of the report. The individual or group that is receiving the report typically does not know anything about the patient. The summary provides the background information necessary to assess the event and support the investigator's attribution. When describing the event, the reporter should provide information that puts it in perspective, including relevant patient history (i.e., underlying medical conditions, prior surgeries or procedures, family history, recent events that may be a contributing factor, concomitant medications).

Some sponsors may require other CRFs (e.g., medical history, AE) to be submitted along with the expedited report, but this is less common with an electronic reporting system. It can be beneficial to send related source documentation (e.g., discharge summary, radiology report) with the expedited report. These can help to explain the event and treatment and to support the differential diagnosis and/or investigator's attribution. CTNs should be aware of what the sponsor's and other regulatory groups' processes are for submitting additional information.

Voluntary Postmarketing Reporting

AEs that are not listed in the current labeling of the product or an SAE can be reported voluntarily by either patients or healthcare professionals as part of MedWatch, FDA's Safety Information and Adverse Event Reporting Program. CTNs can visit the website to learn more, access a report form, and submit a report: www.fda.gov/Safety/MedWatch/default.htm.

National Cancer Institute–Sponsored Clinical Trials and Adverse Events

Protocols that are sponsored by NCI are required to follow the *NCI Guidelines for Investigators: Adverse Event Reporting Requirements for DCTD (CTEP and CIP) and DCP INDs and IDEs*. The guidelines describe criteria for routine and expedited AE reporting, how to report, and how to handle persistent and recurrent AEs (see Figure 28-9 for a sample of reporting criteria). The PI has the primary responsibility for AE identification, documentation, grading, and assignment of attribution and will provide medical documentation needed to support the expedited AE report. As with IND and IDE requirements previously reviewed, the PI must report any SAE to the NCI sponsor by following the NCI expedited reporting guidelines. The protocol will include the reporting requirement outline in the guidelines.

Adverse Event Reporting System

Expedited AEs are submitted through the CTEP-AERS (NCI CTEP, 2014), formerly NCI Adverse Event Expedited Reporting System (AdEERS). In 2000, NCI began using AdEERS for electronic expedited AE reporting. Effective May 2014, AdEERS was retired and CTEP-AERS was implemented. CTEP-AERS is a more user-friendly system. Information about CTEP-AERS and how to subscribe to the distribution list is available at http://ctep.cancer.gov/protocolDevelopment/electronic_applications/adverse_events.htm.

Comprehensive Adverse Events and Potential Risks List

In August 2004, NCI introduced the Comprehensive Adverse Events and Potential Risks (CAEPR) list. This is an NCI-generated list of reported and potential AEs associated with an agent currently under an NCI IND or IDE. Information contained in the CAEPR is compiled from
- Investigator's brochures
- Package inserts (for investigational agents that are available commercially)
- Instructions for use (for a device)
- Company safety reports
- AEs submitted through CTEP-AERS
- Peer-reviewed publications that have safety information not included in the current investigator's brochure or package insert.

Initially, the CAEPR list will not show a frequency for the events (i.e., likely [> 20%], less likely [≤ 20%], rare but serious [< 3%]), but as enough AE information is collected, the CAEPR list will be updated to contain AE frequency. This can be helpful to the PI and CTN when developing the informed consent document. The list is set up as a table and follows the CTCAE in structure (see Figure 28-10). NCI requires the inclusion of a CAEPR list in the following studies though other studies may use the CAEPR list: all studies conducted under an NCI IND and all studies reviewed by CTEP or the NCI Cancer Imaging Program that include investigational agents and interventions for which NCI has a CAEPR.

The last column in the CAEPR list is a subset list known as the Specific Protocol Exceptions to Expedited Reporting (SPEER). The SPEER is specific to the protocol and provides guidelines on what is considered a reportable or expedited AE to report (NCI CTEP, 2013b). Report AEs on the SPEER only if they exceed the grade noted in parentheses next to the AE in the SPEER. If a drug specific-CAEPR is part of a combination protocol using multiple investigational agents and has an AE listed on different SPEERs, the *lower* of the grades should be used to determine if expedited reporting is required. When the CAEPR list is updated, the SPEER is also revised. The revisions are sent to all PIs registered to NCI-approved studies using the agent or agents.

Commercial agents are agents that are available to the general public and are not provided under an IND. Commercial agents may be investigational agents when the indication for use is not FDA-approved. Protocols may contain a combination of an investigational agent and a commercial agent. When an AE occurs with a commercial agent, it may or may not be reported in CTEP-AERS and may be reported voluntarily through commercial reporting of MedWatch. When a protocol uses a commercial drug and investigational drug in a treatment arm, expedited reporting is required (NCI CTEP, 2013b).

Unanticipated Problems

UPs are incidents, experiences, or outcomes that meet *all* of the following criteria (Protection of Human Subjects, 2009).
- Unexpected (in terms of nature, severity, or frequency) given the research described in the IRB-approved protocol and informed consent documents or the investigator's brochure and the characteristics of the subject population being studied
- Related or possibly related to participation in the research
- Suggests the research may place the subjects or others at a greater risk of harm (physical, psychological, economic, or social) than previously recognized

Some UPs will include AEs, but not all UPs are AEs (see Figure 28-11). The investigator can take several

Figure 28-9. National Cancer Institute Cancer Therapy Evaluation Program Phase 1 and Early Phase 2 Adverse Event Reporting[1,2]

FDA Reporting Requirements for Serious Adverse Events (21 C.F.R. Part 312)
NOTE: Investigators MUST immediately report to the sponsor (NCI) ANY Serious Adverse Events, whether or not they are considered related to the investigational agent(s)/intervention (21 C.F.R. § 312.64)
An adverse event is considered serious if it results in **any** of the following outcomes:
1) Death
2) A life-threatening adverse event
3) An adverse event that results in inpatient hospitalization or prolongation of existing hospitalization for ≥ 24 hours
4) A persistent or significant incapacity or substantial disruption of the ability to conduct normal life functions
5) A congenital anomaly or birth defect
6) Important Medical Events that may not result in death, be life threatening, or require hospitalization may be considered serious when, based upon medical judgment, they may jeopardize the patient or subject and may require medical or surgical intervention to prevent one of the outcomes listed in this definition (FDA, 21 C.F.R. § 312.32; ICH E2A and ICH E6).

All serious adverse events that meet the above criteria MUST be immediately reported to the NCI via CTEP-AERS within the timeframes detailed in the table below.

Hospitalization	Grade 1 and Grade 2 Timeframes	Grade 3–5 Timeframes
Resulting in Hospitalization ≥ 24 hrs	10 Calendar Days	24-Hour 5 Calendar Days
Not resulting in Hospitalization ≥ 24 hrs	Not required	

Note. Protocol-specific exceptions to expedited reporting of serious adverse events are found in the Specific Protocol Exceptions to Expedited Reporting (SPEER) portion of the CAEPR.
Expedited AE reporting timelines are defined as:
- "24-Hour; 5 Calendar Days"—The AE must initially be reported via CTEP-AERS within 24 hours of learning of the AE, followed by a complete expedited report within 5 calendar days of the initial 24-hour report.
- "10 Calendar Days"—A complete expedited report on the AE must be submitted within 10 calendar days of learning of the AE.

[1] Serious adverse events that occur more than 30 days after the last administration of investigational agent/intervention and have an attribution of possible, probable, or definite require reporting as follows:
Expedited 24-hour notification followed by complete report within 5 calendar days for:
- All Grade 3, 4, and 5 AEs
Expedited 10 calendar day reports for:
- Grade 2 AEs resulting in hospitalization or prolongation of hospitalization

[2] For studies using PET or SPECT IND agents, the AE reporting period is limited to 10 radioactive half-lives, rounded UP to the nearest whole day after the agent/intervention was last administered. Footnote "1" above applies after this reporting period.
Effective Date: May 5, 2011

AE—adverse event; CAEPR—Comprehensive Adverse Events and Potential Risks List; CTEP-AERS—Cancer Therapy Evaluation Program Adverse Event Reporting System; FDA—U.S. Food and Drug Administration; ICH—International Conference on Harmonisation of Technical Requirements for Registration of Pharmaceuticals for Human Use; IND—investigational new drug; NCI—National Cancer Institute; PET—positron-emission tomography; SPECT—single photon emission computed tomography

Note. From *NCI Guidelines for Investigators: Adverse Event Reporting Requirements for DCTD (CTEP and CIP) and DCP INDs and IDEs* (p. 25), by National Cancer Institute, 2013. Retrieved from http://ctep.cancer.gov/protocolDevelopment/electronic_applications/docs/aeguidelines.pdf.

---

steps to identify if the incident, experience, or outcome is actually a UP (see Figure 28-12). FDA considers AEs as UPs only if the AE was unexpected and serious and would have implications for the conduct of the study (e.g., change in protocol or investigator's brochure), in others words, an event that would be included in an ISR.

Once a UP is identified, the next steps include developing a corrective action plan and reporting to the IRB and other institutional officials. A corrective action plan can include any of the following activities.
- Revise protocol (e.g., modify inclusion or exclusion criteria to mitigate the newly identified risks or implement additional procedures for monitoring subjects)
- Suspend enrollment of new subjects
- Revise the informed consent document (e.g., provide additional information about newly recognized risks to previously enrolled subjects and inform enrolled participants)
- Increase monitoring activities
- Provide staff training or retraining
- Work with appropriate institutional officials to correct problem

OHRP regulations state that the investigator should promptly report all UPs to the IRB; however, *prompt* is not defined. OHRP (2007) recommends the following.
- A UP that is also an SAE should be reported to the IRB within seven days of the investigator's notification of the event because it could have a direct impact on the

Figure 28-10. Sample Comprehensive Adverse Event and Potential Risks (CAEPR) List			
Adverse Events with Possible Relationship to Drug X (CTCAE 4.0 Term) [n = 1141]			Specific Protocol Exceptions to Expedited Reporting (SPEER)
Likely (>20%)	Less Likely (<=20%)	Rare but Serious (<3%)	
BLOOD AND LYMPHATIC SYSTEM DISORDERS			
Anemia			Anemia (Gr 4)
	Disseminated intravascular coagulation		Disseminated intravascular coagulation (Gr 4)
	Febrile neutropenia		Febrile neutropenia (Gr 4)
	Hemolysis		Hemolysis (Gr 1)
CARDIAC DISORDERS			
	Atrial fibrillation		Atrial fibrillation (Gr 4)
	Atrial flutter		Atrial flutter (Gr 1)
	Paroxysmal atrial tachycardia		Paroxysmal atrial tachycardia (Gr 2)
	Sinus bradycardia		Sinus bradycardia (Gr 3)
	Sinus tachycardia		Sinus tachycardia (Gr 3)
	Supraventricular tachycardia		Supraventricular tachycardia (Gr 4)
	Ventricular arrhythmia		Ventricular arrhythmia (Gr 4)
	Ventricular fibrillation		Ventricular fibrillation (Gr 4)

Note. From *NCI Guidelines for Investigators: Adverse Event Reporting Requirements for DCTD (CTEP and CIP) and DCP INDs and IDEs* (p. 34), by National Cancer Institute, 2013. Retrieved from http://ctep.cancer.gov/protocolDevelopment/electronic_applications/docs/aeguidelines.pdf.

protocol's risk assessment and other research participants.
- All other UPs are to be reported to the IRB within 14 days.
- All UPs need to be reported to appropriate institutional officials (as required by an institution's written procedures), the supporting agency head or designee, and OHRP within one month of the IRB's receipt of the UP report from the investigator.

FDA defers to the IRB's process, and ICH GCP guidelines reference prompt reporting of unexpected, serious AEs related to the product (ICH, 1996; Institutional Review Boards, 2014). The UP report should include a detailed description of the UP, an explanation of the basis for determining that the event is a UP, and a description of any changes to the protocol or other corrective actions that have been taken or are proposed in response to the UP. CTNs should know how to report UPs to the various IRBs that they encounter.

Summary

Understanding AEs and UPs takes time. There are many terms to learn and regulations to understand. Each AE may have multiple regulatory groups with their own reporting requirements. CTNs play a pivotal role in the comprehensive assessment and reporting of AEs and UPs that occur during a clinical trial. A quick way to learn about or refresh knowledge about AEs and UPs is to read the OHRP (2007) and U.S. FDA (2009a) guidance documents. CTNs working on NCI-sponsored trials should also read the NCI CTEP (2013b) guidelines. Vigilant AE assessment, monitoring, and reporting ultimately ensures the protection of research participants; CTNs are in the best position to play a pivotal role in this process.

Key Points
- An AE is any unwanted sign, symptom, or disease that was not seen before an individual's research participation, or a worsening of a baseline symptom, regardless of expectedness of the event or relationship of the event to the research.
- AE assessment consists of selecting the correct AE term, identifying the expectedness of the event, assessing the severity of the event, and determining the attribution of the event.
- Understanding how to collect and solicit information about AEs is crucial. CTNs are well positioned to assist

Figure 28-11. Steps to Determine if an Event Is an Unanticipated Problem

Determine if the event or incident is an adverse event (AE) or non-AE.
- AE: Any untoward medical occurrence, including any abnormal sign, symptom, or disease, associated with the subject's participation in research (e.g., an abnormal physical exam or laboratory finding).
- Non-AE: Nonmedical events that may involve social or economic harm rather than physical or psychological harm (e.g., breach of privacy that leads to stigma or loss of insurance coverage, false HIV+ testing). This can include protocol deviations and noncompliance.

Determine if the event is serious or nonserious.
- Serious: Event results in death, hospitalization, significant disability, or is life threatening, or requires immediate action by the principal investigator to protect the rights, safety, or well-being of the participants or others (e.g., admission to the intensive care unit, reporting a confidentiality breach).
- Nonserious: Event suggests that the subject or others may be placed at an increased risk of harm, but the event was not serious or the subject did not suffer harm. However, as a result, substantive changes to the protocol, consent, conduct of the study, or other corrective actions are required to protect subjects or others. This could include a series of AEs that occurred at a greater frequency or severity than was previously known.

Determine if the event is related to the research.
- The event is a result of participation in research (e.g., research procedures, interventions, investigational or approved drugs/devices used for a new indication or a new method of delivery) and may affect participant providers as well.

Determine if the event is expected.
- If it is listed as a risk in the protocol, consent, or investigator's brochure.

Note. Based on information from Office for Human Research Protections, 2007.

Figure 28-12. Examples of Unanticipated Problems That Must Be Reported Under the U.S. Department of Health and Human Services Regulations (45 C.F.R. Part 46)

Adverse Event
1. A subject with chronic gastroesophageal reflux disease enrolls in a randomized, placebo-controlled, double-blind, phase III clinical trial evaluating a new investigational agent that blocks acid release in the stomach. Two weeks after being randomized and started on the study intervention, the subject develops acute kidney failure as evidenced by an increase in serum creatinine from 1 mg/dl prerandomization to 5 mg/dl. The known risk profile of the investigational agent does not include renal toxicity, and the institutional review board (IRB)-approved protocol and informed consent document for the study do not identify kidney damage as a risk of the research. Evaluation of the subject reveals no other obvious cause for acute renal failure. The investigator concludes that the episode of acute renal failure probably was due to the investigational agent. This is an example of an unanticipated problem that must be reported because the subject's acute renal failure was (a) unexpected in nature, (b) related to participation in the research, and (c) serious.
2. The fifth subject enrolled in a phase II, open-label, uncontrolled clinical study evaluating the safety and efficacy of a new oral agent administered daily for treatment of severe psoriasis unresponsive to U.S. Food and Drug Adminstration–approved treatments develops severe hepatic failure complicated by encephalopathy one month after starting the oral agent. The known risk profile of the new oral agent prior to this event included mild elevation of serum liver enzymes in 10% of subjects receiving the agent during previous clinical studies, but there was no other history of subjects developing clinically significant liver disease. The IRB-approved protocol and informed consent document for the study identify mild liver injury as a risk of the research. The investigators identify no other etiology for the liver failure in this subject and attribute it to the study agent. This is an example of an unanticipated problem that must be reported because although the risk of mild liver injury was foreseen, severe liver injury resulting in hepatic failure was (a) unexpected in severity, (b) possibly related to participation in the research, and (c) serious.

Non–Adverse Event
1. Subjects with cancer are enrolled in a phase II clinical trial evaluating an investigational biologic product derived from human sera. After several subjects are enrolled and receive the investigational product, a study audit reveals that the investigational product administered to subjects was obtained from donors who were not appropriately screened and tested for several potential viral contaminants, including the human immunodeficiency virus and the hepatitis B virus. This constitutes an unanticipated problem that must be reported because the incident (a) was unexpected, (b) was related to participation in the research, and (c) placed subjects and others at a greater risk of physical harm than was previously known or recognized.
2. An investigator conducting behavioral research collects individually identifiable sensitive information about illicit drug use and other illegal behaviors by surveying college students. The data are stored on a laptop computer without encryption, and the laptop computer is stolen from the investigator's car on the way home from work. This is an unanticipated problem that must be reported because the incident (a) was unexpected (i.e., the investigators did not anticipate the theft), (b) was related to participation in the research, and (c) placed the subjects at a greater risk of psychological and social harm from the breach in confidentiality of the study data than was previously known or recognized.
For more examples, see the guidance document found in the reference below.

Note. Based on information from Office for Human Research Protections, 2007.

with AE assessment and are often the patient participants' first point of contact.
- The CTCAE is an agreed-upon terminology by experts in the oncology community for the designation, reporting, and grading of AEs that occur in oncology clinical trials.
- Refer to the protocol for the version of the CTCAE that is being used.
- There are two types of AE reporting: *routine* and *expedited*. The regulatory groups CTNs may send reports to include the IRB, sponsor, FDA, IBC, and OBA.
- Events to be reported in an expedited manner ideally should be defined in the protocol, including the timeline and mechanism for reporting.
- Protocols sponsored by NCI are required to follow *NCI Guidelines for Investigators: Adverse Event Reporting Requirements for DCTD (CTEP and CIP) and DCP INDs and IDEs.*
- A UP is an incident, experience, or outcome that meets *all* of the following criteria: (a) unexpected (in terms of nature, severity, or frequency) given the research described in the IRB-approved protocol, informed consent document(s), the investigator's brochures, and the characteristics of the subject population being studied, (b) related or possibly related to participation in the research, and (c) suggests the research may place the subject or others at a greater risk of harm (e.g., physical, psychological, economic, or social harm).

References

Badalucco, S., & Reed, K.K. (2011). Supporting quality and patient safety in cancer clinical trials. *Clinical Journal of Oncology Nursing, 15,* 263–265. doi:10.1188/11.CJON.263-265

Basch, E. (2013). Toward patient-centered drug development in oncology. *New England Journal of Medicine, 369,* 397–400. doi:10.1056/NEJMp1114649

Basch, E., Bennett, A., & Pietanza, M.C. (2011). Use of patient-reported outcomes to improve the predictive accuracy of clinician-reported adverse events. *Journal of the National Cancer Institute, 103,* 1808–1810. doi:10.1093/jnci/djr493

Chen, A.P., Setser, A., Anadkat, M.J., Cotliar, J., Olsen, E.A., Garden, B.C., & Lacouture, M.E. (2012). Grading dermatologic adverse events of cancer treatments: The Common Terminology Criteria for Adverse Events Version 4.0. *Journal of the American Academy of Dermatology, 67,* 1025–1039. doi:10.1016/j.jaad.2012.02.010

IND Safety Reporting, 21 C.F.R. § 312.32 (2014). Retrieved from http://www.accessdata.fda.gov/scripts/cdrh/cfdocs/cfcfr/CFRSearch.cfm?fr=312.32

Institutional Review Boards, 21 C.F.R. pt. 56 (2014). Retrieved from http://www.accessdata.fda.gov/scripts/cdrh/cfdocs/cfcfr/CFRSearch.cfm?CFRPart=56&showFR=1

International Conference on Harmonisation of Technical Requirements for Registration of Pharmaceuticals for Human Use. (1996, June 10). *ICH harmonised tripartite guideline: Guideline for good clinical practice, E6(R1).* Retrieved from http://www.ich.org/fileadmin/Public_Web_Site/ICH_Products/Guidelines/Efficacy/E6/E6_R1_Guideline.pdf

Investigational Device Exemptions, 21 C.F.R. pt. 812 (2014). Retrieved from http://www.accessdata.fda.gov/scripts/cdrh/cfdocs/cfcfr/CFRSearch.cfm?fr=812.3

Investigator Recordkeeping and Record Retention, 21 C.F.R. § 312.62 (2014). Retrieved from http://www.accessdata.fda.gov/scripts/cdrh/cfdocs/cfcfr/CFRSearch.cfm?fr=312.62

Medical Dictionary for Regulatory Activities Maintenance and Support Services Organization Maintenance and Support Services Organization (MedDRA® MSSO). (2013, April 3). Frequently asked questions—MedDRA®. Retrieved from http://www.meddra.org/faq

National Cancer Institute Cancer Therapy Evaluation Program. (2010, June 14). *Common terminology criteria for adverse events* [v.4.03]. Retrieved from http://evs.nci.nih.gov/ftp1/CTCAE/About.html

National Cancer Institute Cancer Therapy Evaluation Program. (2013a, March 20). CTCAE v4.0 open comment period. Retrieved from http://ctep.cancer.gov/protocolDevelopment/electronic_applications/ctc.htm

National Cancer Institute Cancer Therapy Evaluation Program. (2013b, September 16). *NCI guidelines for investigators: Adverse event reporting requirements for DCTD (CTEP and CIP) and DCP INDs and IDEs.* Retrieved from http://ctep.cancer.gov/protocolDevelopment/electronic_applications/docs/aeguidelines.pdf

National Cancer Institute Cancer Therapy Evaluation Program. (2013c, May). Patient-reported outcomes version of the Common Terminology Criteria for Adverse Events (PRO-CTCAE). Retrieved from http://outcomes.cancer.gov/tools/pro-ctcae_fact_sheet.pdf

National Cancer Institute Cancer Therapy Evaluation Program. (2014, January 28). Cancer Therapy Evaluation Program Adverse Event Reporting System (CTEP-AERS). Retrieved from http://ctep.cancer.gov/protocolDevelopment/electronic_applications/adverse_events.htm

National Institutes of Health Office of Biotechnology Activities. (2013, November). *NIH guidelines for research involving recombinant or synthetic nucleic acid molecules.* Retrieved from http://osp.od.nih.gov/sites/default/files/NIH_Guidelines_0.pdf

Ness, E. (2013, November). *Adverse events and unanticipated problems* [PowerPoint presentation]. Retrieved from https://ccrod.cancer.gov/confluence/download/attachments/83530280/AEs%20and%20UPs.pdf?version=1&modificationDate=1385485391037&api=v2

Office for Human Research Protections. (2007, January 15). Guidance on reviewing and reporting unanticipated problems involving risks to subjects or others and adverse events. Retrieved from http://www.hhs.gov/ohrp/policy/advevntguid.html

Office for Human Research Protections. (2010, November 10). Guidance on IRB continuing review of research. Retrieved from http://www.hhs.gov/ohrp/policy/continuingreview2010.pdf

Protection of Human Subjects, 45 C.F.R. pt. 46 (2009). Retrieved from http://www.hhs.gov/ohrp/humansubjects/guidance/45cfr46.html

Richesson, R.L., Fung, K.W., & Krischer, J.P. (2008). Heterogeneous but "standard" coding systems for adverse events: Issues in achieving interoperability between apples and oranges. *Contemporary Clinical Trials, 29,* 635–645. doi:10.1016/j.cct.2008.02.004

Trotti, A., Colevas, A.D., Setser, A., & Basch, E. (2007). Patient-reported outcomes and the evolution of adverse event reporting in oncology. *Journal of Clinical Oncology, 25,* 5121–5127. doi:10.1200/JCO.2007.12.4784

Trotti, A., Colevas, A.D., Setser, A., Rusch, V., Jaques, D., Budach, V., ... Rubin, P. (2003). CTCAE v3.0: Development of a comprehensive grading system for the adverse effects of cancer treatment. *Seminars in Radiation Oncology, 13,* 175–181. doi:10.1016/S1053-4296(03)00031-6

U.S. Food and Drug Administration. (2007, September). *Guidance for industry: Toxicity grading scale for healthy adult and adolescent volunteers enrolled in preventive vaccine clinical trials.* Retrieved from http://

www.fda.gov/downloads/BiologicsBloodVaccines/GuidanceComplianceRegulatoryInformation/Guidances/Vaccines/ucm091977.pdf

U.S. Food and Drug Administration. (2009a, January). *Guidance for clinical investigators, sponsors, and IRBs: Adverse event reporting to IRBs—Improving human subject protection.* Retrieved from http://www.fda.gov/downloads/RegulatoryInformation/Guidances/UCM126572.pdf

U.S. Food and Drug Administration. (2009b, December). *Guidance for industry: Patient-reported outcome measures: Use in medical product development to support labeling claims.* Retrieved from http://www.fda.gov/downloads/Drugs/Guidances/UCM193282.pdf

Chapter 29

Patient and Family Education

Geri L. Schmotzer, RN, MSN, MPH, PhD

Introduction

Assessment of patient and family education needs is a vital process regardless of whether a patient chooses to participate in a clinical trial. The Oncology Nursing Society's *Standards of Oncology Education: Patient/Significant Other and Public* (Blecher, 2004) provides guidelines for developing, implementing, and evaluating patient education programs and can serve as a model for educating patients who are contemplating entering a clinical trial. Figure 29-1 lists the five standards that are used as a resource for achieving quality patient education.

Patient education is defined as "a planned learning experience using a combination of methods such as teaching, counseling, and behavior modification techniques to influence patients' knowledge and health behavior" (Bartlett, 1985, p. 323). The goal of patient education is to improve the patient's quality of life (Feudtner, 2001). Figure 29-2 shows a model to assist in determining the objectives of patient education.

Figure 29-1. Oncology Patient Education Standards

- Standard I. The oncology nurse at both the generalist and advanced practice level is responsible for education of the patient/significant others related to cancer.
- Standard II. Adequate resources to achieve the objectives of patient/significant other education related to cancer care are available and appropriate.
- Standard III. Knowledge, skills, and attitudes related to the management of human responses to cancer are reflected in the educational activity for the patient and significant others experiencing cancer.
- Standard IV. Teaching-learning theories are applied to the development, implementation, and evaluation of learning experiences related to cancer care.
- Standard V. The patient and/or significant other apply knowledge, skills, and attitudes to management of actual or potential human responses to the cancer experience.

Note. From *Standards of Oncology Education: Patient/Significant Other and Public* (3rd ed., pp. 3–8), by C.S. Blecher (Ed.), 2004, Pittsburgh, PA: Oncology Nursing Society. Copyright 2004 by Oncology Nursing Society. Reprinted with permission.

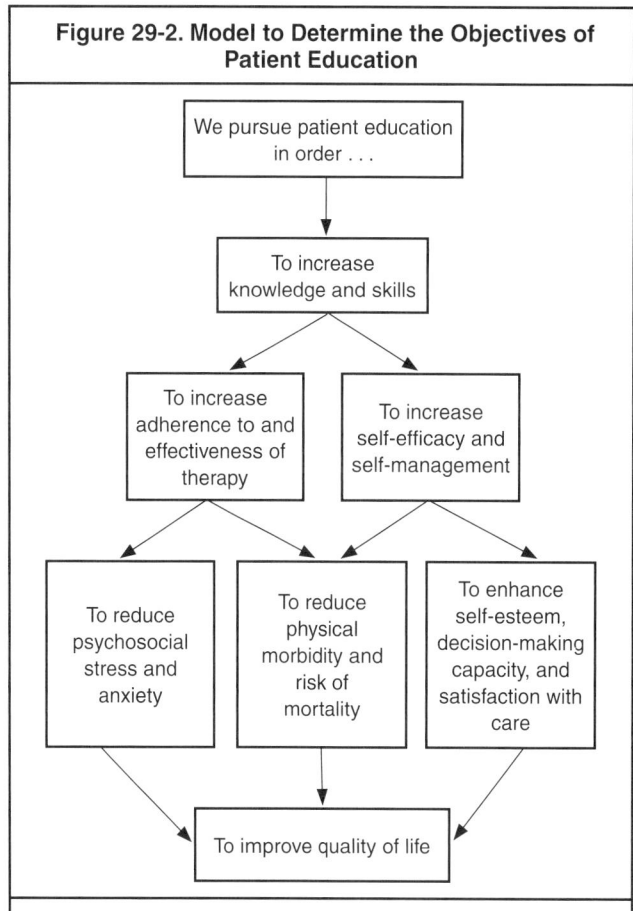

Note. From "What Are the Goals of Patient Education?" by C. Feudtner, 2001, *Western Journal of Medicine, 174*, p. 174. doi:10.1136/ewjm.174.3.173. Copyright 2001 by BMJ Publishing Group, Ltd. Reprinted with permission.

The author would like to acknowledge Kimberly Power, RN, MSN, for her contribution to this chapter that remains unchanged from the first edition of this book.

The process of developing or planning for patient education has several steps, including determining effective health communication, identifying specific information needs, and providing clear and effective communication.

Effective Patient Education Messages

The keys to a coordinator's successful teaching are understanding a patient's needs and providing clear, effective health communication. Assessment provides vital information about the patient and his or her support network. Understanding the patient's needs, concerns, preferences, and readiness to learn is critical for effective communication. Conducting this assessment allows the nurse to individualize the information for each patient.

Learning Needs

To determine a patient's learning needs, the nurse must first assess the actual level of a patient's knowledge, skill, behavior, and attitude and compare them to the desired level. A *learning need* is a gap between the actual and desired level or an absence of the knowledge, skills, behaviors, or attitudes required by a patient to self-manage his or her care, maintain current health, or progress to a more healthy condition. Although the focus is on assessment during the first few meetings with the patient, the process should be part of each patient encounter. Some considerations in assessing learning needs are (The Ohio State University [OSU] Area Health Education Center [AHEC] Clear Health Communication Program, 2007)
- The knowledge and skills the patient needs and wants
- The patient's current knowledge and skill set
- The patient's ability and willingness to learn
- The patient's priorities and expectations
- Barriers that would prevent learning.

Table 29-1 lists assessment categories, questions to ask, and observations to make.

Readiness to Learn

While caring for or talking with a patient with cancer, opportunities are available to assess the patient's readiness to learn. Learning readiness is characterized by being both willing and able to make use of instruction. It includes both emotional readiness and experiential readiness (OSU AHEC Clear Health Communication Program, 2007).

Emotional readiness is putting forth the essential effort to learn. This is often influenced by an individual's personal level of motivation. Motivation increases when the person feels the health information is pertinent to his or her life and helps him or her fulfill a perceived need or solve a problem (Inott & Kennedy, 2011; OSU AHEC Clear Health Communication Program, 2007).

A person's psychosocial adaptation to his or her health condition may also affect his or her emotional readiness to learn. If an individual has high anxiety or stress levels or is in denial, that person is often not ready to learn. It is essential to give the person a chance to express how he or she is feeling about his or her condition and what is expected of him or her.

Experiential readiness is those factors that affect a person's capacity to learn or the way he or she learns. Aspects that need to be considered include (OSU AHEC Clear Health Communication Program, 2007)
- Previous knowledge, skills, and attitudes
- Present and past experiences
- Physical capability: size, strength, coordination/dexterity, intact senses, energy level, and comfort
- Intellectual capability: reading, math, verbal, and problem-solving skills
- Health beliefs (cultural/religious)
- Language
- Support people/relationships
- Learning style.

A patient's interest and energy level determine how and when learning takes place. Everyone has different motivating factors for wanting to acquire information, and the nurse needs to be cognizant of the patient's goals. When talking to patients and families about clinical trials, understanding their motivation for entering a study may provide insight into family dynamics and potential compliance issues that may arise in the future (Jones et al., 2007). Patients and their significant others may differ in their willingness and capacity to learn.

Learning Style

Assessing patient learning style within the context in which learning occurs allows for an individualized approach that incorporates teaching modalities to maximize patient learning (Dewing, 2010). A person's learning style is his or her preferred way to receive and process information.

Patients develop their learning style as children when they discover what works best for their individual learning. Effective assessment of the patient may indicate he or she has more than one learning style that will aid in comprehension. Learning patterns include visual, auditory, and kinesthetic (Russell, 2006). Table 29-2 describes learning styles, methods, and teaching strategies to encourage patient education.

Adult Learners

To educate patients effectively, nurses must have a basic understanding of the principles of adult learning.

Table 29-1. Learning Assessment Questions and Observations

Category	Questions/Observations
Previous Health Instruction and Experience in Health Care	• Please tell me about your health problem (illness). How can I help? • What do you know about ____? • What have you been told about your condition? • What have you been doing for your condition (illness) in the past? Now? • What are you most interested in learning now? What would you like to learn first? • What do you need to know before you do ____? (self-care) • How have you and your family been dealing with your condition? • How should a person be treated for this condition? • What questions do you have?
Learning Needs/Readiness to Learn	• What do you want to know more about? • What does your health problem do to you? How does it work? • Why do you think it started when it did? • How severe is your health problem? • How long do you think it will last? • What do you think will be the major effects of your health problem on you and your family? • What have you been doing for yourself to care for your condition? • What kinds of problems do you have when doing this care? • What things will help or hinder your care at home?
Health Beliefs and Cultural Practices	• What do you think caused your health problem? • What bothers or concerns you most about your health problem? • What issues have your health problem caused you? • What do you fear most about your health problem? • What does your health problem mean to you? • What kind of treatment do you think you should receive? • What are the most important results you hope to get from this treatment? • Who in the family/community gives you health advice? How does your family help?
Comprehension and Application of Health Information	• What don't you understand as well as you would like to? • Do you usually follow directions as given or do you change them to suit yourself? • What helps you understand and remember what you have read or learned? • Once you understand something, to what extent do you try to use the information or apply it to everyday situations? • What do you think would happen if ____? • What would you do if ____? • How would you know if ____? • Who would you call if ____? • How would you explain your condition and treatment to ____? • How confident are you, on a scale of 1 to 10, that you can ____? • How confident are you, on a scale of 1 to 10, that you will ____?
Performing a Skill	• How easy do you think it will be for you to learn how to do this skill? • How do you ____? (fill in the blank with the required skill) • How would you describe your ability to learn this skill? • How would you describe your reaction to doing this skill? • How would you describe your physical ability to do this skill? • How much practice do you usually need to learn a new skill? • Show me how you would ____.
Adherence	• How did you ____? (fill in blanks with a self-care activity, such as taking medication) • Many people find it difficult to remember or do ____. How did it go for you? • When are you most likely to forget to ____? How will you handle this problem next time? • What do you think is the hardest part about ____? • Most people find changing a behavior is difficult. What problems do you think you might have? • What will you do differently next time? • Who can help you with this? • What would help you manage ____? • Describe what you are going to do.
Financial and Other Resources	• Do you have a need for financial assistance for your treatments? • Do you have the necessary equipment? • Do you need any community resources?

Note. From "Learning Assessment: Questions and Observations," by The Ohio State University Area Health Education Center (AHEC) Clear Health Communication Program, n.d. Retrieved from http://medicine.osu.edu/sitetool/sites/pdfs/ahecpublic/Learning_Assessment.pdf. Copyright by AHEC Clear Health Communication Program. Reprinted with permission.

Malcolm Knowles was the first to study how adults learn. Knowles (1970) identified six principles of adult learning.
- Adults are internally motivated and self-directed.
- Adults bring life experiences and knowledge to learning experiences.
- Adults are goal oriented.
- Adults are relevancy oriented.
- Adults are practical.
- Adult learners like to be respected.

The five characteristics of the adult learner are (Smith, 2002)
- *Self-concept:* As a person matures, his or her self-concept moves from one of being a dependent personality toward one of being a self-directed human being.
- *Experience:* As a person matures, he or she accumulates a growing reservoir of experience that becomes an increasing resource for learning.
- *Readiness to learn:* As a person matures, his or her readiness to learn becomes oriented increasingly to the developmental tasks of his or her social roles.
- *Orientation to learning:* As a person matures, his or her time perspective changes from one of postponed application of knowledge to immediacy of application, and accordingly, his or her orientation toward learning shifts from subject-centeredness to problem-centeredness.
- *Motivation to learn:* As a person matures, the motivation to learn is internal.

Pediatric Learners

Historically, approximately 60% of children with cancer enter into national clinical trials, with an additional 30% being treated on local- or regional-based offshoots of national protocols (Kupst, Patenaude, Walco, & Sterling, 2003). Figure 29-3 identifies key issues for parents of children in accepting a clinical trial.

Principles used to determine the educational needs of parents of a child who has cancer are similar to those of the adult learner (National Association for the Education of Young Children, n.d.):
1. All areas of development and learning are important.
2. Learning and development follow sequences.
3. Development and learning proceed at varying rates.
4. Development and learning result from an interaction of maturation and experience.
5. Early experiences have profound effects on development and learning.
6. Development proceeds toward greater complexity, self-regulation, and symbolic or representational capacities.
7. Children develop best when they have secure relationships.
8. Development and learning occur in and are influenced by multiple social and cultural contexts.
9. Children learn in a variety of ways.
10. Play is an important vehicle for developing self-regulation and promoting language, cognition, and social competence.
11. Development and learning advance when children are challenged.
12. Children's experiences shape their motivation and approaches to learning.

The degree to which the parents play a role in decision making depends largely on the child's age and the nature of the parent-child relationship. The emotional turmoil that parents experience after learning of their child's diagnosis of cancer is a significant obstacle when trying to understand and consider the complex medical information they receive when making treatment choices for their child (Kupst et al., 2003). When providing information to children, educators should ensure that the learning is developmentally appropriate. Atherton (2013) describes Jean Piaget's four stages of cognitive development through which children must progress to develop an understanding of the world around them (see Table 29-3). Comprehending these developmental stages assists clinical trial nurses (CTNs) in formulating appropriate learning experiences for children of various ages.

Specific Informational Needs for Study Phases

Treatment decisions regarding participation in, continuation of, and completion of clinical trials are made at different points along the healthcare continuum. By identifying where the patient is on the continuum, the nurse is better able to understand the patient's educational needs and use available internal and external resources to meet those needs. For example, at the time of diagnosis, patients with localized disease may be eligible for phase III studies, which compare the standard treatment to a new experimental therapy. Other patients are diagnosed with regional or advanced disease upon the completion of their cancer workup. For others, participation in a study is contemplated at the time of recurrent or progressive disease. Figure 29-4 shows the purpose, characteristics, and patient educational needs for phase I–III studies.

Phase I Studies

The purpose of a phase I trial is to determine the safe dosage of the study drug (Lertora & Vanevski, 2012; Miller et al., 2011). Educating patients and families con-

Table 29-2. Learning Styles, Characteristics of Learners, and Suggested Teaching Strategies

Learning Style	Characteristics	Suggested Teaching Strategies
Visual	Prefers written instructions rather than verbal instructions. Prefers to have photographs and illustrations to view when receiving written or visual instructions. Prefers a timeline, calendar, or some other similar diagram to remember the sequence of events. Observes all the physical elements in the learning environment. Carefully organizes their learning materials. Remembers and understands through the use of diagrams, charts, and maps. Studies materials by reading notes and organizing it in outline form.	Provide lots of interesting visual material in a variety of formats. Make sure visual presentations are well organized. Make handouts and all other written work as visually appealing as possible, and easy to read. Make full use of a variety of technologies: computers, overhead projection, video camera, live video feeds/close circuit TV, photography, Internet, etc.
Auditory	Remembers what they say, and what others say very well. Remembers best through verbal repetition and by saying things aloud. Prefers to discuss ideas they do not immediately understand. Remembers verbal instructions well. Finds it difficult to work quietly for long periods of time. Easily distracted by noise, but also easily distracted by silence. Verbally expresses interest and enthusiasm. Enjoys group discussions.	Rephrase points and questions in several different ways to communicate intended message. Vary speed, volume, and pitch, as appropriate, to help create interesting aural textures. Write down key points or key words before providing verbal instructions to help avoid confusion due to pronunciation. Ensure auditory learners are in a position to hear well (be sure hearing aids are inserted and functional). Incorporate multimedia applications utilizing sounds, music, or speech (use tape recorders, computer sound cards/recording applications, musical instruments, etc.).
Kinesthetic	Remembers best through getting physically involved in whatever is being learned. Enjoys the opportunity to build and/or physically handle learning materials. Will take notes to keep busy but will not often use them. Enjoys using computers. Physically expresses interest and enthusiasm by getting active and excited. Has trouble staying still or in one place for a long time. Enjoys hands-on activities. Tends to want to fiddle with small objects while listening or working. Remembers what they *do*, what they experience with their hands or bodies (movement and touch). Enjoys using tools or lessons which involve active/practical participation. Can remember how to do things after doing them once (motor memory). Has good motor coordination.	Permit frequent breaks in teaching session to allow learner to move around room. Encourage learner to write down their own notes. Encourage learner to stand or move while reciting information or learning new material. Incorporate multimedia resources (computer, video camera, overhead transparencies, photography camera, etc.) into programs (teacher presentations and student presentations). Provide lots of tactile-kinesthetic activities in the class. Have product samples available for practice. Encourage return demonstration of procedures.

Note. From "An Overview of Adult-Learning Processes," by S.S. Russell, 2006, *Urologic Nursing, 26,* p. 351. Copyright 2006 by Society of Urologic Nurses and Associates. Reprinted with permission.

cerning phase I trials is difficult. Research with subjects of phase I studies indicates trial participants misunderstand the purpose of these trials, overestimate the prospect of therapeutic benefit, and enroll for personal benefit (Miller & Joffe, 2012; Pentz et al., 2012). Once the physician explains the protocol, CTNs should be available to serve as an educational resource to answer patients' questions.

For parents of a child with cancer, deciding whether to enroll the child into a phase I study is one of the most difficult decisions they will have to make. The clinician's recommendation is the most frequently cited factor that influences adolescents' and parents' decision to participate (Miller et al., 2013; Sung & Regier, 2013). In addition to the informed consent, patients should be given information that reinforces several elements about the phase I study: (a) how the research will be conducted, (b) the risks and benefits of the treatment, (c) the unproven nature of the research, (d) alternatives to participation in research, and (e) the subject's freedom to not partic-

Figure 29-3. Key Issues for Families of Children With Cancer in Accepting a Randomized Clinical Trial

- Understanding what is meant by a clinical trial
- Understanding that a trial means that their child is not being experimented on, but is being offered the best known treatment for their situation
- Understanding the questions that the trial is asking and what they mean for their child
- Understanding the relative risks of side effects and keeping these in proportion
- Being asked to involve a competent child in decision making when they might not wish to worry them about the possibility of non-cure or details of treatment side effects

Note. From "Improving Recruitment to Clinical Trials for Cancer in Childhood," by K. Pritchard-Jones, M. Dixon-Woods, M. Naafs-Wilstra, and M.G. Valsecchi, 2008, *Lancet Oncology, 9,* p. 393. doi:10.1016/S1470-2045(08)70101-3. Copyright 2008 by Elsevier. Reprinted with permission.

Table 29-3. Stages of Cognitive Development

Stage	Characterized By
Sensory-motor (Birth–2 years)	Differentiates self from objects Recognizes self as agent of action and begins to act intentionally: e.g. pulls a string to set mobile in motion or shakes a rattle to make a noise Achieves object permanence: realizes that things continue to exist even when no longer present to the sense (pace Bishop Berkeley)
Pre-operational (2–7 years)	Learns to use language and to represent objects by images and words Thinking is still egocentric: has difficulty taking the viewpoint of others Classifies objects by a single feature: e.g. groups together all the red blocks regardless of shape or all the square blocks regardless of color
Concrete operational (7–11 years)	Can think logically about objects and events Achieves conservation of number (age 6), mass (age 7), and weight (age 9) Classifies objects according to several features and can order them in series along a single dimension such as size.
Formal operational (11 years and up)	Can think logically about abstract propositions and test hypotheses systematically Becomes concerned with the hypothetical, the future, and ideological problems

Note. From "Learning and Teaching: Piaget's Developmental Theory," by J.S. Atherton, 2013. Retrieved from http://www.learningandteaching.info/learning/piaget.htm. Copyright 2011 by J.S. Atherton. Site licensed under a Creative Commons Attribution-Noncommercial-No Derivative Works 3.0 Unported License. Reprinted with permission.

ipate in the research or to withdraw at any time (Wang, Tsai, Chen, & Tsay, 2011).

One of the goals of phase I studies is to understand the toxicity profile of the therapy being administered (Lertora & Vanevski, 2012). Usually, the side effects of the investigational treatment are unknown or knowledge is limited because drug testing may have been done only with animals. For this reason, patients and their significant others need to be instructed to report all side effects, whether treatment related or not, to the healthcare team. Education may include how to document side effects in a daily diary, as well as the importance of notifying the CTN when the patient experiences an unusual symptom.

Patients need to be aware that safety, not a beneficial response, is the goal in a phase I study. *Therapeutic misconception* is common in patients enrolling in phase I studies. Most patients participate in phase I studies because they believe they will benefit (Miller & Joffe, 2012; Pentz et al., 2012). See Chapter 12 for additional information about therapeutic misconception. Pentz and colleagues (2012) found three concepts most frequently misunderstood by patients: the main purpose of the research, overestimation of personal benefit, and risks associated with the study drug.

A study by Yoder, O'Rourke, Etnyre, Spears, and Brown (1997) revealed that patients participating in phase I studies need to maintain realistic hope but must be kept informed of their current condition and response to the treatment. They found that when families receive emotional support from the healthcare team, they are better able to meet patients' psychosocial needs (Yoder et al., 1997). According to Cox and Avis (1996), patients and families receive less information from the healthcare team as protocol treatment progresses, which causes patients to feel uncertain regarding their future.

Phase II Studies

Phase II studies are done to determine the efficacy of the study drug (Lertora & Vanevski, 2012; Miller et al., 2011). In phase II studies, additional risks and toxicities are known; therefore, more information is available for patients and families. However, uncertainty as to the actual benefit of the treatment still may exist. In phase II studies, similar to phase I studies, patients' expectations may differ from the actual goal of the clinical trial (Bergenmar, Johansson, & Wilking, 2011). From the time the protocol is presented through study completion or being taken off study, patients and families continue to need educational information and emotional support.

The major endpoints of phase II studies usually are assessment of tumor shrinkage, duration of response, and the toxicity profile of the therapy (Lertora & Vanevski, 2012; Leventhal, 1988). For these reasons, patients are educated about the importance of following their ther-

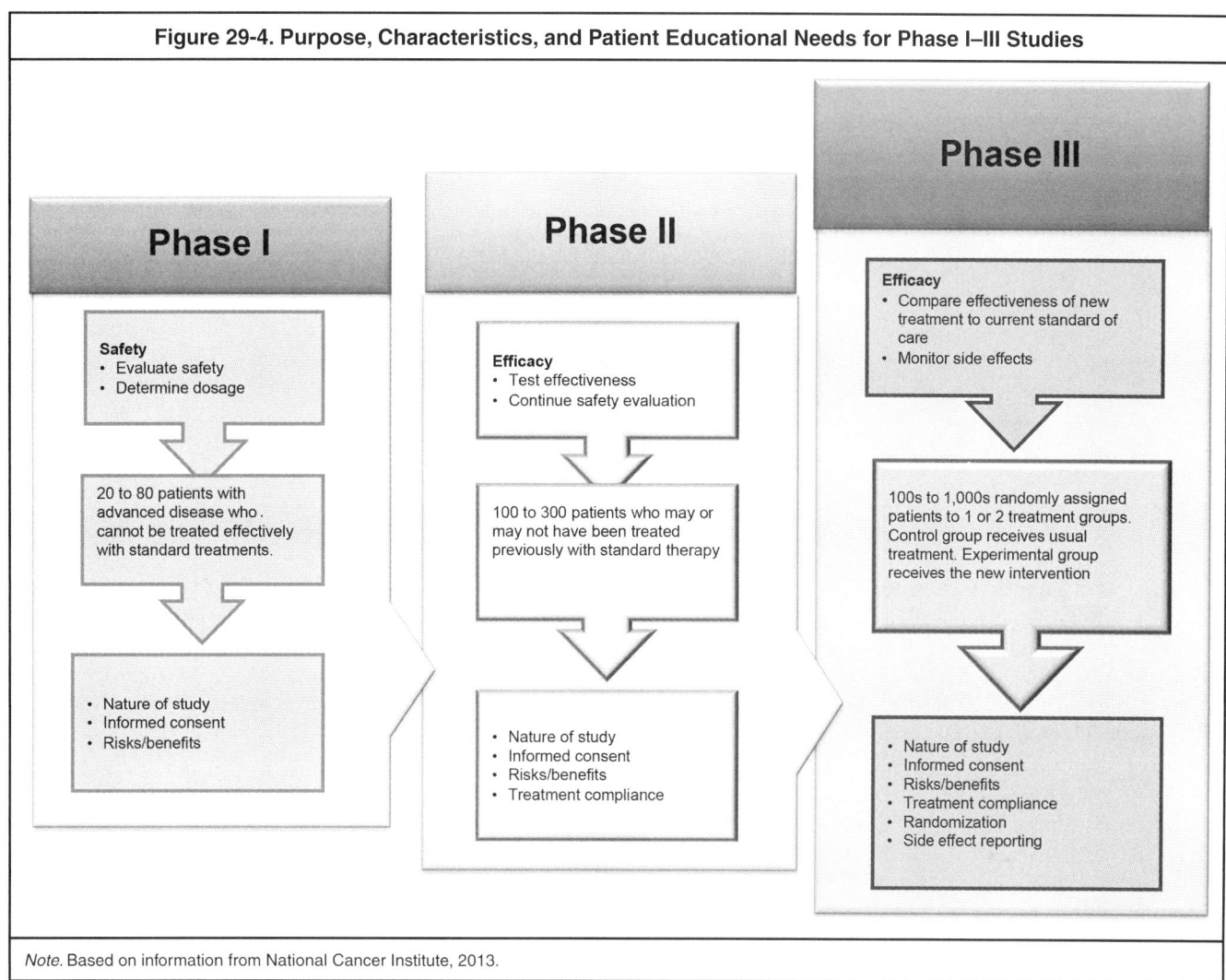

Figure 29-4. Purpose, Characteristics, and Patient Educational Needs for Phase I–III Studies

Note. Based on information from National Cancer Institute, 2013.

apy schedule as well as the testing schedule required to determine tumor response. By establishing rapport with patients, CTNs encourage protocol adherence. As with phase I studies, patients and families need instruction on the importance of reporting toxicities in a timely and comprehensive manner.

Phase III Studies

Phase III studies typically require large numbers of participants in an effort to document improvement of a new treatment over the standard therapy (Lertora & Vanevski, 2012). Patients are randomized to receive either the standard therapy for that type and stage of cancer or an investigational treatment that is thought to possibly be better. Patients and families are instructed about the different treatment arms of the study and the various potential side effects attributed to these therapies. If a patient wishes to receive a *particular* treatment, he or she should *not* be entered into a study.

The concept of randomization is difficult for patients to comprehend. Both adult study participants and parents of children participants have difficulty understanding random selection to receive a standard treatment or the study drug (Behrendt, Gölz, Roesler, Bertz, & Wünsch, 2011; Kodish et al., 2004). This is an important concept for patients to understand, and use of a metaphor such as "the flip of a coin" or "the sex of a baby" may be useful in teaching patients (Krieger, Parrott, & Nussbaum, 2010, pp. 8–9).

The treatments being administered in phase III clinical trials have documented toxicities (Lertora & Vanevski, 2012). However, researchers continue to collect toxicity information to determine any unexpected side effects or greater prevalence. Patient education focuses on the expected toxicities and interventions available to alleviate these problems. Teaching reinforces that side effects are not to be endured, but rather must be reported so that appropriate medical and nursing actions can be implemented. Locock and Smith (2011) reported that patients consent to participate in clinical trials to have access to expert staff, engage in their own health care, and receive more frequent or intensive clinical monitoring and the latest information about their condition. Additionally, Skrutkowska and Weijer (1997) found that patients who participate in clinical trials were more likely to receive follow-up telephone calls, reassurance, and patient teaching from the nursing staff than were non-protocol patients. This may be attributed to nurses and physicians wanting to maintain patient adherence and their commitment to being more accessible to patients who are entered in clinical trials.

Treatment Completion

Completion of therapy is a celebratory event; however, it also is a time of change and uncertainty for patients and families. To nurses or data managers, the end of treatment may signify that the most difficult part of the recovery process is over. To patients, the final treatment may be viewed as a departure from the support and reassurance of the healthcare team. Patients and families need to receive education at this critical time to outline expectations for the future and as a reminder that follow-up information continues to be obtained according to the protocol. Many clinical trials introduce study endpoints that include monitoring of quality of life and long-term toxicities (Pauwels, Charlier, De Bourdeaudhuij, Lechner, & Van Hoof, 2013).

Parents of children with cancer experience anxiety at the completion of their child's treatment. Fear of relapse, symptom interpretation, loss of connection to the primary oncology caregiver, and uncertainty about survivorship are some of the concerns parents have concerning their child (Hobbie et al., 2010).

Other studies examined children's perspectives upon completion of cancer therapy (Boman & Bodegard, 2004; Wu, Chin, Haase, & Chen, 2009). The researchers discovered that children need assistance in exploring the meaning of treatment completion; understanding the word *remission* and the fears that coincide with the possibility of recurrence; accepting that relationships with peers, family members, and healthcare staff are changing; and identifying life changes and the new normalcy that is to be achieved. For many children, remembering a time when life was "normal" is not possible. Their findings suggest that children with cancer should receive psychoeducational support so that they grow to become adults who are as emotionally stable as their peers (Boman & Bodegard, 2004; Wu et al., 2009).

Providing Clear and Effective Patient Education

After the patient's learning needs and readiness are determined, the information can be used as a basis for what and how the health information is provided. In order to individualize health information, CTNs should work closely with patients and families to decide what is essential, realistic, and achievable for patients. Before continuing with the teaching-learning process, CTNs should individualize the message to present relevant material. Providing patients with opportunities to ask questions and discuss concerns and outlining expectations and/or outcomes from the teaching will enhance patient teaching. Express outcomes or expectations in terms of patient behaviors or actions. A clearly defined outcome focuses on one task, and the more specific the outcome, the easier it is to observe and measure achievement in meeting the outcome (OSU AHEC Clear Health Communication Program, 2007).

Setting Priorities for Teaching

The area of clinical trials has become more complex, and the medical conditions patients experience can be more complicated. For this reason, patients may require considerable education. To organize the time more efficiently, establish the teaching priorities early. Concepts to consider are (OSU AHEC Clear Health Communication Program, 2007)
- What patients need to know
- What patients want to know
- Behaviors affecting the condition
- Important behaviors affecting patients' health status
- Behaviors that are easiest to change first
- Available resources.

What to Teach

The four things patients and their families need to know to be active partners are (1) information to make informed decisions about their health care, (2) essential self-care knowledge and skills to improve health outcomes, (3) how to recognize problems and how to respond, and (4) answers to their questions (OSU AHEC Clear Health Communication Program, 2007).

Methods for Effective Teaching

Patient teaching presents an ongoing challenge. Some patients and families are more sophisticated and knowledgeable about their healthcare and treatment choices and desire to understand and want to be involved in their treatment decisions. What a patient with cancer knows about his or her disease can affect the individual's treatment choices and how he or she copes with the illness.

To effectively provide patients with the appropriate education, CTNs should select the appropriate teaching methods and teaching tools and materials. Clarification and explanations, when given in response to questions, provide valuable information that meets a specific interest or need. Demonstration and practice are essential when teaching patients a new skill. To better prepare patients to recognize problems and respond appropriately, problem-solving and behavioral rehearsal techniques work best (OSU AHEC Clear Health Communication Program, 2007).

CTNs can provide patients with multiple ways to learn by using supplemental instruction materials and tools. A variety of creative teaching methods are available to facilitate patient learning. Easy-to-read materials, audio-recorded instructions, videos, closed-circuit TV, CDs, DVDs, interactive computer programs, models, posters, and diagrams or pictures are some tools that can facilitate patient learning (OSU AHEC Clear Health Communication Program, 2007). Patients want information that is accurate and individualized to their specific situation. Patients' needs include information about the treatment process, side effects, and how the treatment will affect their daily lives (Skalla, Bakitas, Furstenberg, Ahles, & Henderson, 2004). Table 29-2 provides recommendations for teaching strategies and method of delivery for patient education. Each teaching strategy has advantages and disadvantages. Additionally, the development of an education binder is an effective method for patient teaching. In a study conducted by Marbach and Griffie (2011), patients found the education binder "essential to their care and understanding of their disease and treatment" (p. 338).

The use of the Internet has expanded over the last 15–20 years. The Internet provides patients with large quantities of health information (Cutilli, 2010). Patients using Internet-based learning can search databases, "chat" with others, view bulletin boards, and get additional patient information. Internet sites should adhere to the Health On the Net Foundation code, which has established ethical guidelines for health-related websites (Health On the Net Foundation, 2015). The quality of health-related websites can be assessed by using the DISCERN tool (Baggott, 2011). This tool can be found at www.discern.org.uk. Figure 29-5 lists criteria for evaluating health-related online resources, while Figure 29-6 lists some reliable online resources for patient education.

Tips for Health Teaching

Prepare to give health information by being alert to one-minute teaching opportunities. Creating a positive and supportive learning environment and organizing the material prior to giving the information is essential to enhance patient learning. CTNs can do this by presenting the information in a logical manner. Limit the content to three to five of the most important points, break down complex instruction into smaller steps, and repeat the most essential points at the end of each instruction

Figure 29-5. Suggested Criteria for Evaluating Health-Related Resources Found Online

1. Author(s)
   ☐ Authors are listed.
   ☐ Credentials, educational background, and affiliations of the authors are provided.
   ☐ Author contact information is available.

2. Information
   The information is
   ☐ Accurate
   ☐ Comprehensive
   ☐ Current
   ☐ Easy to read.

3. References
   References are
   ☐ Listed
   ☐ Appropriate
   ☐ Recent.

4. Sponsor
   ☐ Sponsor is identified and is a reliable source (i.e., government agencies [.gov], medical schools [.edu], and nonprofit groups focusing on disease research and education [.org]). Commercial sites (.com) may or may not be helpful depending on whether they are providing a consumer service or trying to sell a product.

5. Electronic Media
   ☐ Links are appropriate.
   ☐ Graphics are useful.
   ☐ Web pages load quickly.
   ☐ Website is easy to navigate.

6. Privacy and Security
   ☐ Privacy statement explains clearly what it will do with any personal information it asks for. If joining a chat room or online discussion, the site states the terms of using the service.
   ☐ Security software information is evident.
   ☐ Encryption protocols are disclosed.

7. Evaluation
   ☐ Visitors are able to contact the website administrator with problems, questions, or feedback.

Note. From "The Internet: Friend or Foe When Providing Patient Education?" by A.S. Anderson and P. Klemm, 2008, *Clinical Journal of Oncology Nursing, 12,* 60. doi:10.1188/08.CJON.55-63. Copyright 2008 by Oncology Nursing Society. Reprinted with permission.

session. After giving the information, use the teach-back method to verify patient understanding (OSU AHEC Clear Health Communication Program, 2007).

Challenges to Learning

Several patient populations are identified as requiring in-depth and highly individualized assessment. These include some older adult patients; those who are blind, deaf, or mentally deficient; the illiterate; and

Figure 29-6. Online Patient Education Resources

General Health Information

Healthfinder.gov: www.healthfinder.gov
U.S. Department of Health and Human Services Web site that provides access to information from government agencies and other reliable resources

MedlinePlus®: www.medlineplus.gov
National Library of Medicine website that includes a medical encyclopedia and dictionary

NIHSeniorHealth: www.nihseniorhealth.gov
Provides tools to change text size and contrast and has audio to accommodate those with visual impairments

NOAH: New York Online Access to Health: www.noah-health.org
Provides state, local, and federal health resources for consumers; available in Spanish

Cancer-Specific Information

American Cancer Society: www.cancer.org
Provides medical information, treatment decision tools, news updates, and support resources (e.g., message boards); available in Spanish and some Asian languages

Association of Cancer Online Resources: www.acor.org
More than 100 online cancer-related groups that provide information and support; includes an overview of types of cancer, treatment options, and clinical trials

Ben's Game: www.makewish.org/ben
A video game to help kids who have cancer; provides a way to help relieve some of the stress of cancer treatment

CancerCare: www.cancercare.org
A national nonprofit group providing free professional support services, including education and financial assistance, for anyone affected by cancer; available in Spanish

Cancer Information Service: http://cis.nci.nih.gov
Provides cancer-related news, publications, resources, treatment options, information on clinical trials, genetic basis of cancer, causes, risk factors, and prevention strategies; available in Spanish

Cancer.Net: www.cancer.net
Information on cancer, clinical trials, coping, side effects, message boards, and patient support organizations; includes a "Find an Oncologist" database

CancerQuest: www.cancerquest.org
Information on the biology of cancer for the general public; includes an overview of cell structure and division, genetics, tumor biology, and cancer treatments in a video format

CaringBridge®: www.caringbridge.org
A nonprofit organization offering free web pages to patients and families to display journal entries and photographs; well-wishers visit the site to read updates and leave messages.

ClinicalTrials.gov: www.clinicaltrials.gov
Created by the National Institutes of Health and the U.S. Food and Drug Administration to provide patients, family members, and members of the public with current information about clinical research studies and clinical trials

Genetics Home Reference: http://ghr.nlm.nih.gov
National Library of Medicine's guide to genetics information for patients, families, and the general public

Look Good Feel Better: www.lookgoodfeelbetter.org
A national public service program to help women offset appearance-related changes from cancer treatment; video education and Spanish available

National Cancer Institute: www.cancer.gov
Overview of cancer treatment, prevention, causes, screening and testing, clinical trials, and statistics

OncoLink®: www.oncolink.com
Provides comprehensive cancer information and information on specific types of cancer, cancer treatments, and news about research advances; updated daily; key content available in Spanish

The Cancer Game: www.cancergame.org
Video game about fighting cancer and promoting healing through visualization; developed by a student who had undergone stem-cell rescue

Note. From "The Internet: Friend or Foe When Providing Patient Education?" by A.S. Anderson and P. Klemm, 2008, *Clinical Journal of Oncology Nursing, 12*, p. 58. doi:10.1188/08.CJON.55-63. Copyright 2008 by Oncology Nursing Society. Adapted with permission.

---

those who speak a foreign language. Some of these patients may be ineligible for clinical trials because of comorbidities or poor performance status, and for others, informed consent may be difficult, if not impossible, to obtain (Banda, St. Germain, McCaskill-Stevens, Ford, & Swain, 2012).

When presenting clinical trial information to some older adults, explanations must be simple and clear. Both a verbal and an easily understandable written explanation of the concept should be provided. For patients who are illiterate, patient education videos are useful to facilitate learning. The informed consent document must be read aloud and explained to these individuals, as well as to the blind. Sign-language interpreters and foreign-language translators are available to assist in communicating with special populations. When many individuals who speak a particular foreign language enroll in a clinical trial, a short, institutional review board–approved consent form written in the appropriate language may be used (Thomas, Saleem, & Abraham, 2005).

Summary

Providing education to patients and their families is essential to clinical trial participation. Understanding a patient's motivation for entering a study may help to provide insight into the patient's particular education needs. CTNs should assess the patient's age, cultural background, preferred method of learning, desire for information, placement on the healthcare continuum, attitudes toward health care, and other specific considerations to determine what style of teaching will be the most effective. Adult and pediatric learners have different communication needs. Social, cultural, and religious values influence patients' knowledge and attitude and must be taken into account when developing educational materials. Some populations require in-depth and individualized assessment. These include some older adults; those who are blind, deaf, or mentally deficient; the illiterate; and those who speak a foreign language.

Learning materials should be specific to the trial phase. Understanding patients' needs will assist CTNs in providing available internal and external education resources. Patients and families desire to understand their options and want to be involved in their treatment decisions. A variety of creative teaching methods are available to CTNs to facilitate patient learning. These include verbal and written information, audiovisual media, and computer-assisted learning.

Key Points

- To provide effective patient education, CTNs must assess the patients' learning needs, readiness to learn, and learning style.
- Identification of where a patient is along the healthcare continuum is essential for the assessment of teaching needs.
- CTNs should work with patients and their families to determine what and how the health information should be provided.
- The teaching material should be individualized to meet each patient's and his or her family's needs.
- CTNs should set teaching priorities, determine what to teach, and select the appropriate tools to provide effective patient education.

References

Atherton, J.S. (2013). Learning and teaching: Piaget's developmental theory. Retrieved from http://www.learningandteaching.info/learning/piaget.htm

Baggott, C. (2011). Patient education: To the internet and beyond. *Pediatric Blood and Cancer, 57,* 6–7. doi:10.1002/pbc.23123

Banda, D.B., St. Germain, D., McCaskill-Stevens, W., Ford, J.G., & Swain, S.M. (2012). A critical review of the enrollment of black patients in cancer clinical trials. *ASCO 2012 Educational Book,* pp. 153–157. Retrieved from https://meetinglibrary.asco.org/sites/meetinglibrary.asco.org/files/Educational%20Book/PDF%20Files/2012/zds00112000153.pdf

Bartlett, E.E. (1985). At last, a definition. *Patient Education and Counseling, 7,* 323–324. doi:10.1016/0738-3991(85)90041-2

Behrendt, C., Gölz, T., Roesler, C., Bertz, H., & Wünsch, A. (2011). What do our patients understand about their trial participation? Assessing patients' understanding of their informed consent consultation about randomised clinical trials. *Journal of Medical Ethics, 37,* 74–80. doi:10.1136/jme.2010.035485

Bergenmar, M., Johansson, H., & Wilking, N. (2011). Levels of knowledge and perceived understanding among participants in cancer clinical trials—Factors related to the informed consent procedure. *Clinical Trials, 8,* 77–84. doi:10.1177/1740774510384516

Blecher, C.S. (Ed.). (2004). *Standards of oncology education: Patient/significant other and public* (3rd ed.). Pittsburgh, PA: Oncology Nursing Society.

Boman, K.K.P., & Bodegard, G.M.D.P. (2004). Life after cancer in childhood: Social adjustment and educational and vocational status of young-adult survivors. *Journal of Pediatric Hematology/Oncology, 26,* 354–362.

Cox, K., & Avis, M. (1996). Psychosocial aspects of participation in early anti-cancer drug trials: Report of a pilot study. *Cancer Nursing, 19,* 177–186.

Cutilli, C.C. (2010). Seeking health information: What sources do your patients use? *Orthopaedic Nursing, 29,* 214–219.

Dewing, J. (2010). Moments of movement: Active learning and practice development. *Nurse Education in Practice, 10*(1), 22–26. doi:10.1016/j.nepr.2009.02.010

Feudtner, C. (2001). What are the goals of patient education? *Western Journal of Medicine, 174,* 173–174. doi:10.1136/ewjm.174.3.173

Health On the Net Foundation. (2015). HONcode. Retrieved from http://www.hon.ch

Hobbie, W.L., Ogle, S.K., Reilly, M., Ginsberg, J.P., Rourke, M., Ratcliffe, S., & Deatrick, J.A. (2010). Identifying the educational needs of parents at the completion of their child's cancer therapy. *Journal of Pediatric Oncology Nursing, 27,* 190–195. doi:10.1177/1043454209360778

Inott, T., & Kennedy, B.B. (2011). Assessing learning styles: Practical tips for patient education. *Nursing Clinics of North America, 46,* 313–320.

Jones, J.M., Nyhof-Young, J., Moric, J., Friedman, A., Wells, W., & Catton, P. (2007). Identifying motivations and barriers to patient participation in clinical trials. *Journal of Cancer Education, 21,* 237–242. doi:10.1080/08858190701347838

Knowles, M.S. (1970). *The modern practice of adult education: Andragogy versus pedagogy.* New York, NY: Association Press.

Kodish, E., Eder, M., Noll, R.B., Ruccione, K., Lange, B., Angiolillo, A., … Drotar, D. (2004). Communication of randomization in childhood leukemia trials. *JAMA, 291,* 470–475. doi:10.1001/jama.291.4.470

Krieger, J.L., Parrott, R.L., & Nussbaum, J.F. (2010). Metaphor use and health literacy: A pilot study of strategies to explain randomization in cancer clinical trials. *Journal of Health Communication, 16,* 3–16. doi:10.1080/10810730.2010.529494

Kupst, M.J., Patenaude, A.F., Walco, G.A., & Sterling, C. (2003). Clinical trials in pediatric cancer: Parental perspectives on informed consent. *Journal of Pediatric Hematology/Oncology, 25,* 787–790.

Lertora, J.L., & Vanevski, K. (2012). Clinical pharmacology and its role in pharmaceutical development. In J.I. Gallin & F.P. Ognibene (Eds.), *Principles and practice of clinical research* (3rd ed., pp. 627–639). Boston, MA: Academic Press. doi:10.1016/B978-0-12-382167-6.00043-6

Leventhal, B.G. (1988). An overview of clinical trials in oncology. *Seminars in Oncology, 15,* 414–422.

Locock, L., & Smith, L. (2011). Personal benefit, or benefiting others? Deciding whether to take part in clinical trials. *Clinical Trials, 8*(1), 85–93. doi:10.1177/1740774510392257

Marbach, T.J., & Griffie, J. (2011). Patient preferences concerning treatment plans, survivorship care plans, education, and supportive services. *Oncology Nursing Forum, 38*, 335–342. doi:10.1188/11.ONF.335-342

Miller, F.G., & Joffe, S. (2012). Phase 1 oncology trials and informed consent. *Journal of Medical Ethics, 39*, 761–764. doi:10.1136/medethics-2012-100832

Miller, J.D., Kotowski, M.R., Comis, R.L., Smith, S.W., Silk, K.J., Colaizzi, D.D., & Kimmel, L.G. (2011). Measuring cancer clinical trial understanding. *Health Communication, 26*(1), 82–93. doi:10.1080/10410236.2011.527624

Miller, V.A., Baker, J.N., Leek, A.C., Hizlan, S., Rheingold, S.R., Yamokoski, A.D., ... Kodish, E. (2013). Adolescent perspectives on phase I cancer research. *Pediatric Blood and Cancer, 60*, 873–878. doi:10.1002/pbc.24326

National Association for the Education of Young Children. (n.d.). 12 principles of child development and learning that inform practice. Retrieved from https://www.naeyc.org/dap/12-principles-of-child-development

National Cancer Institute. (2013, February 22). Cancer clinical trials. Retrieved from http://www.cancer.gov/cancertopics/factsheet/information/clinical-trials

The Ohio State University Area Health Education Center Clear Health Communication Program. (2007). Getting your message across: Clear and effective health communication. Retrieved from http://medicine.osu.edu/sitetool/sites/pdfs/ahecpublic/HL_Get_the_Message.pdf

Pauwels, E.E.J., Charlier, C., De Bourdeaudhuij, I., Lechner, L., & Van Hoof, E. (2013). Care needs after primary breast cancer treatment. Survivors' associated sociodemographic and medical characteristics. *Psycho-Oncology, 22*, 125–132. doi:10.1002/pon.2069

Pentz, R.D., White, M., Harvey, R.D., Farmer, Z.L., Liu, Y., Lewis, C., ... Khuri, F.R. (2012). Therapeutic misconception, misestimation, and optimism in participants enrolled in phase 1 trials. *Cancer, 118*, 4571–4578. doi:10.1002/cncr.27397

Russell, S.S. (2006). An overview of adult-learning processes. *Urologic Nursing, 26*, 349–352, 370.

Skalla, D.A., Bakitas, M., Furstenberg, C.T., Ahles, T., & Henderson, J.V. (2004). Patients' need for information about cancer therapy. *Oncology Nursing Forum, 24*, 313–319.

Skrutkowska, M., & Weijer, C. (1997). Do patients with breast cancer participating in clinical trials receive better nursing care? *Oncology Nursing Forum, 24*, 1411–1416.

Smith, M.K. (2002). Malcolm Knowles, informal adult education, self-direction and andragogy, the encyclopedia of informal education. Retrieved from http://www.infed.org/thinkers/et-knowl.htm

Sung, L., & Regier, D.A. (2013). Decision making in pediatric oncology: Evaluation and incorporation of patient and parent preferences. *Pediatric Blood and Cancer, 60*, 558–563. doi:10.1002/pbc.24450

Thomas, V.N., Saleem, T., & Abraham, R. (2005). Barriers to effective uptake of cancer screening among black and minority ethnic groups. *International Journal of Palliative Nursing, 11*, 564–571.

Wang, L.H., Tsai, Y.F., Chen, J.S., & Tsay, P.K. (2011). Intention, needs, and expectations of cancer patients participating in clinical trials. *Cancer Nursing, 34*, 117–123. doi:10.1097/NCC.0b013e3181efe1c0

Wu, L.M., Chin, C.C., Haase, J.E., & Chen, C.H. (2009). Coping experiences of adolescents with cancer: A qualitative study. *Journal of Advanced Nursing, 65*, 2358–2366. doi:10.1111/j.1365-2648.2009.05097.x

Yoder, L.H., O'Rourke, T.J., Etnyre, A., Spears, D.T., & Brown, T.D. (1997). Expectations and experiences of patient with cancer participating in phase I clinical trials. *Oncology Nursing Forum, 24*, 891–896.

Chapter 30

Psychosocial Distress

Kathy Czaplicki, RN, MSN, CCRC

Introduction

Cancer remains one of the leading causes of death worldwide, and as such, anxiety and fear rank high among the psychological predictors of distress within this patient population (Melchior et al., 2011). Psycho-oncology, a subspecialty of cancer care, has advanced and changed over the past 30 years and is a discipline that helps patients with cancer to mobilize their resources to live well with the disease (Bultz & Johansen, 2011; Spiegel, 2012). Psycho-oncology has developed into a science with standards of care and promotes the use of valid assessment tools to aid in the detection of distress within the cancer population (Holland, Watson, & Dunn, 2011). This chapter will focus on the impact that psychosocial distress may have on patients with cancer in the context of clinical trial participation and the end of treatment. Specific topics presented include (a) patient motivation for clinical trial participation, (b) distress and the meaning of distress, (c) distress related to clinical trial discontinuation, (d) tools to evaluate emotional distress, and (e) nursing implications for the patient experiencing emotional distress.

Background

Psychosocial distress is of fundamental concern when patients are confronted with the invasive nature of cancer and its treatment. For patients who exhibit effective coping mechanisms and have strong social support systems, the psychological impact of cancer may be marginally less than those without these mechanisms and systems in place. However, for the vast majority of patients, the use of psychosocial interventions can have an enormous impact on diminishing distress and improving quality of life (Nekolaichuk, Cumming, Turner, Yushchyshyn, & Sela, 2011).

Much knowledge has been gained from works addressing meaning, coping and adaptation, hope, anxiety, fear, anger, decision making, depression, and spirituality. These and other works offer insight and practical recommendations for addressing each issue. However, routine psychosocial patient assessment and intervention is still a goal—not the current standard of care—in oncology nursing. Research on the prevalence of distress has shown that cancer places excessive demands on patients and their families throughout the entire trajectory of care—beginning with diagnosis, then treatment, followed by survivorship, and concluding with end-of-life care (Bultz & Johansen, 2011). The current lack of routine psychosocial assessments and interventions may be taking a toll on the cancer population and especially on participants enrolled in clinical trials.

Patient Motivation for Clinical Trial Participation

The literature reflects an abundance of research exploring the reasons why patients decline participation in clinical trials (Biedrzycki, 2010; Schilsky, 2011). Therefore, the reader is referred elsewhere for a discussion of the barriers to clinical trial participation (see Section V).

Participation in cancer clinical trials has proved vital in bridging the gap between current knowledge of the natural progression of malignant disease and clinical practice (Kuroki et al., 2010). Clinical trials are prospective studies that have the capability of facilitating progress toward the improvement of diagnosis and treatment of disease by introducing innovative interventions and therapies (Gabriel & Mercado, 2011). Clinical trial partici-

---

The author would like to acknowledge Angela D. Klimaszewski, RN, MSN, for her contribution to this chapter that remains unchanged from the previous edition of this book.

pation can offer patients with cancer access to the latest drugs, the newest cancer therapies utilizing novel treatment options, and access to care at leading academic medical centers. The clinical trial decision-making process typically involves the physician, the patient, and the protocol (Biedrzycki, 2010; Klimaszewski, 2006). Clinical trial information is provided in the context of a protocol and a patient consent document. The process of making an informed decision to participate in a clinical trial is based upon pertinent treatment options provided by the proposed regimen, the physician's ability to successfully translate the protocol's treatment regimen and requirements to the patient, and the patient's ability to process this information into something comprehensible based upon his or her knowledge base (Biedrzycki, 2011). All three factors must fit together cohesively to ensure the best possible outcome for the patient.

Physician Factors

Klimaszewski (2006) noted, "The trust relationship between a physician and patient is generally considered sacrosanct" (p. 490), and Aungst, Haas, Ommaya, and Green (2003) ascertained that patients are willing to follow the advice of their physician, including his or her recommendation to participate in a clinical trial. This is echoed by the National Cancer Institute (NCI, 2005), which cited patients' unwillingness to go against their personal physician's wishes as a barrier to participation in trials for the general public. Patients may be more receptive to considering clinical trial participation if more clinicians were willing to propose the option and initiate a discussion of the option.

Physicians are in the unique position of making a significant impact in patient awareness of clinical trial involvement by informing them of the benefits and risks associated with clinical trial participation (Klabunde et al., 2011). According to Kuroki and colleagues (2010), a substantial increase in patient proclivity toward clinical trial participation was noted when the discussion was conducted by the physician—suggesting that physician buy-in is an important factor in accrual. Patients studied by Schutta and Burnett (2000) revealed that their physicians' interpersonal skills and positive attitude increased their own trust and confidence in a clinical trial. If a patient trusts the physician, he or she is more likely to follow the physician's advice regarding clinical trial participation. Conversely, if the patient perceives that the physician does not wholeheartedly support a clinical trial—or clinical trials in general—the patient is less likely to participate. Kuroki et al. (2010) found that when physicians initiated the conversation regarding clinical trial participation, recruitment rates were higher (45%) than when the discussion was initiated exclusively by the research staff (25%).

Patient Factors

Clinical trials can afford patients the opportunity to participate in novel and potentially efficacious treatments that may otherwise be unavailable outside the context of a clinical trial. Studies have shown that most people would be willing to participate in a clinical trial if faced with a cancer diagnosis (Aungst et al., 2003; Comis, Miller, Aldige, Krebs, & Stoval, 2003). Hope for a therapeutic benefit and a desire to live were cited as reasons to participate in any phase trial (Albrecht, Blanchard, Ruckdeschel, Coovert, & Strongbow, 1999; Schutta & Burnett, 2000).

Simon et al. (2004) questioned 319 women about participation in clinical trials. Results suggested that more women would participate if they were provided the opportunity. Furthermore, in a study of 1,000 adults aged 18 and older, 32% said they would be very willing to participate in a clinical trial, and another 38% would consider participating in a clinical trial if asked (Comis et al., 2003). An analysis conducted by the Center for Information and Study on Clinical Research Participation revealed that of the 25,855 clinical trial participants in the United States, 73.2% met eligibility criteria and were enrolled in phase I–IV trials. Within that percentage, 75.4% were participants in phase I clinical trials, 69.7% in phase II–III trials, and 93.8% in phase IV clinical trials (Center for Information and Study on Clinical Research Participation, 2008).

Two common themes continue to emerge when discussing clinical trial participation with patients: a desire for access to cutting-edge research and treatment options and a desire to make a difference, if not for themselves, then for someone else (Odo, 2012).

Phase I Trial Participation

Phase I clinical trials are largely presented to patients with advanced disease for whom standard treatment regimens have been either unsuccessful or nonexistent. These patients may also have received prior palliative treatment for disease control, or they could be treatment naïve (van der Biessen et al., 2013). As a rule, phase I clinical trials are designed to determine the safety profile of an agent, not to attain disease control or remission. For some patients, this may be the first time they have considered a clinical trial. Meadows (2000) noted, "Information on clinical trials may not be sought unless it becomes a compelling or desperate issue" (p. 54).

The strongest motivator for patients when considering participation in a phase I oncology clinical trial is the desire to aggressively fight their cancer. The primary concern in the decision-making process is not necessarily the details of the research project or the investigational agent's potential side effects but rather whether the investigational drug will kill the cancer cells. For this patient population in particular, the decision to participate in a clinical trial is not always based on the phase of study, the study design or drug administration, or the potential financial costs that may be associated with participation. These participants are typically knowledgeable of the less-than-favorable aspects of cancer treatments, having, for the most part, been exposed to prior chemotherapy regimens (van der Biessen et al., 2013).

Conversely, Meropol et al. (2003) reported that patients who enroll in phase I trials may foster a *therapeutic misconception*, meaning they perceive benefit when none is expected. They suggested the possibility that "high expectations of benefit among patients considering phase I trials may be an expression of confidence and hope for personal benefit" (p. 4659) rather than a misunderstanding of the purpose of the trial. See Chapter 12 for more information about therapeutic misconception.

Similarly, Roychowdhury (2003) questioned 106 patients with locally advanced or metastatic cancer with no prior chemotherapy or immunotherapy about participation in a phase I trial. Of the 99 patients who responded to the questionnaire, 58% indicated they would participate for personal benefit, 38% for the benefit of others, and 5% for reasons unspecified. Sixty-eight percent responded that they would participate in a phase I trial; 32% stated they would not. Additionally, 73% believed there would be physical benefit, and 62% believed they would benefit psychologically.

Participation in phase I trials may offer this patient population an effective way of coping and managing in a difficult situation in addition to offering a modicum of comfort (Agrawal et al., 2006).

Protocol Factors

Currently, only 20,000–25,000 patients are enrolled onto clinical trials each year, which may indicate that a significant number of newly diagnosed patients with cancer would be interested in enrolling in a cancer clinical trial but may not be presented with the opportunity (Comis, Miller, Colaizzi, & Kimmel, 2009). Of those patients presented with the option of clinical trial participation, some may find the lengthy and complicated protocol requirements a deterrent to participation. Age restrictions identified in the eligibility requirements, lack of protocol therapies in local treatment centers outside of academic centers, and an unwillingness to comply with randomization requirements can also contribute to an unwillingness to participate in a clinical trial. Withdrawal from clinical trials is not unusual and is typically because of the following factors: lack of drug effectiveness, intolerable adverse events, inadequate patient follow-up, nonadherence to protocol requirements, or patient desire to rescind consent (Comis et al., 2009; Gabriel & Mercado, 2011). Adequate communication among the physician, research staff, and the patient is key to improving protocol accrual and retention.

Distress

Distress in patients with cancer is widespread, with incidence rates estimated at 35%–55% involving all phases of illness (Carlson, Waller, Groff, Giese-Davis, & Bultz, 2013). The term *distress* encompasses an array of psychosocial issues, which may include any or all of the following: anxiety, depression, anger, decreased social skills, family issues, work-related issues, questioning one's significance in life, and spiritual issues (Adler & Page, 2008). Distress is common in patients with cancer, and 43% of these patients in the ambulatory setting report symptoms of distress (Deshields & Nanna, 2010). The National Comprehensive Cancer Network® (NCCN®) developed the first set of standards for psychosocial care and management of distress in patients with cancer. NCCN (2013) defined distress as

> A multifactorial unpleasant emotional experience of a psychological (cognitive, behavioral, emotional), social and/or spiritual nature that may interfere with the ability to cope effectively with cancer, its physical symptoms and its treatment. Distress extends along a continuum, ranging from common normal feelings of vulnerability, sadness, and fears to problems that can become disabling, such as depression, anxiety, panic, social isolation, and existential and spiritual crisis. (p. DIS-2)

NCCN uses the word *distress* because it does not have the same implied meaning (i.e., that one is "crazy") as the words *psychiatric, psychosocial,* or *emotional*. Rather, distress is viewed as a normal reaction and one that is socially acceptable. Additionally, distress "can be defined and measured by self-report" (NCCN, 2013, p. DIS-1).

Distress is often associated with reduced survival, poor quality of life, and dissatisfaction with care, so it is imperative to identify patients at high risk for persistent distress to enable the development of more successful and effective interventions (Carlson et al., 2013). Patient distress can range from vulnerability and despondency to incapacitating issues such as depression, panic, and social isolation (Kaplan, 2008; NCCN, 2013). Figure 30-1 identifies characteristics of patients who are at an increased risk for distress. It also identifies periods along the cancer trajectory when patients may be more vulnerable to experiencing distress. The periods of vulnerability cover a large part of the cancer continuum, from diagnosis, to awaiting treatment, through changes in treatment modality, to end of treatment because of completion or progres-

Figure 30-1. Psychosocial Distress Patient Characteristics

Patients at Increased Risk for Distress
- History of psychiatric disorder/substance abuse
- History of depression/suicide attempt
- Cognitive impairment
- Communication barriers (include language, literacy and physical barriers)
- Severe comorbid illnesses
- Social issues
  - Family/caregiver conflicts
  - Inadequate social support
  - Living alone
  - Financial problems
  - Limited access to medical care
  - Young or dependent children
  - Younger age; woman
  - History of abuse (physical, sexual)
  - Other stressors
- Spiritual/religious concerns
- Uncontrolled symptoms

Periods of Increased Vulnerability
- Finding a suspicious symptom
- During diagnostic workup
- Finding out the diagnosis
- Awaiting treatment
- Change in treatment modality
- End of treatment
- Discharge from hospital following treatment
- Transition to survivorship
- Medical follow-up and surveillance
- Treatment failure
- Recurrence/progression
- Advanced cancer
- End of life

Note. Reproduced with permission from *NCCN Clinical Practice Guidelines in Oncology (NCCN Guidelines®) for Distress Management V.2.2013.* © 2013 by the National Comprehensive Cancer Network, Inc. All rights reserved. The NCCN Guidelines® and illustrations herein may not be reproduced in any form for any purpose without the express written permission of the NCCN. To view the most recent and complete version of the NCCN Guidelines, go online to NCCN.org. NATIONAL COMPREHENSIVE CANCER NETWORK®, NCCN®, NCCN GUIDELINES®, and all other NCCN Content are trademarks owned by the National Comprehensive Cancer Network, Inc.

---

sive disease, to survivorship and end-of-life care (Bultz & Johansen, 2011).

Distress Related to Clinical Trial Discontinuation

Withdrawal from treatment is most often because of the lack of effectiveness of the drug or overwhelming or intolerable treatment side effects (Moore, Derry, & McQuay, 2008). While in the active treatment phase of a clinical trial, patients receive psychological as well as physical support from physicians and nurses (Carter, 2004). Ending treatment, or going off-study, may trigger feelings of isolation and abandonment (NCI, 2005).

The sense of security and continuity of care that patients experience when participating in a clinical trial may produce feelings of loss when trial participation ceases.

Within each of the following situations, patients may experience different stressors when they are no longer clinical trial participants: (a) when treatment is completed and the patient moves on to the follow-up phase, (b) when a treatment ends because of new research findings, (c) when a patient experiences disease recurrence or progression, (d) when a patient elects to withdraw from clinical trial participation because of personal reasons, and (e) when a patient withdraws because of family, caregiver, or transportation issues. Studies have shown that times of highest distress are often linked with the transition periods of treatment: at diagnosis, at the initiation and completion of treatment, at follow-up visits—particularly if tumor assessments were performed—and at disease recurrence. Although the completion of treatment can be a time of happiness and relief, patients may be fraught with increased anxiety and emotional distress. Feelings of abandonment by a supportive medical staff, fear of disease recurrence, persistent thoughts about illness, feelings of powerlessness, and fear of death may all lead to persevering anxiety (Kaplan, 2008; Rosedale, 2009).

Carter (2004) compiled a comprehensive list of patient feelings and experiences when treatment has ended (see Figure 30-2). In all instances, patients will experience a significant change in the frequency of clinic visits where healthcare providers have been at the forefront providing physical and emotional support, as well as continuous patient education.

Figure 30-2. End-of-Treatment Feelings and Experiences

- Isolation and abandonment
- Worry, anxiety, and panic
- Loss of support
- Self-doubt and poor self-image
- Coping with side effects of treatment (both temporary and permanent)
- Depression (mild to suicide)
- Grief and sadness due to losses
- Uncertainty and doubt about future
- Helplessness and hopelessness (loss of power)
- Fear of recurrence
- Lack of memory and concentration ("Have I lost my mind?")
- Residual fatigue up to a year
- Anger
- Family and social issues
- Workplace issues
- Financial and insurance challenges
- Search for the new definition of "normal"
- Difficulty making long-term plans
- Fear of the power and truth of statistics
- Changes to body, self, and sexual images and function

Note. From "End of Treatment: Laugh or Cry?" by S.E. Carter, 2004, *Community Oncology, 1*, p. 180. Copyright 2004 by Elsevier. Reprinted with permission.

Tools to Evaluate Distress

Bultz and Johansen (2011) recommended that emotional distress be viewed as the *sixth vital sign* that should be assessed, monitored, and treated along with temperature, pulse, respiration, blood pressure, and pain. To accomplish this, nurses need to assess distress at every visit, documenting and acting on their findings just as vital sign findings are documented.

The NCCN (2014) screening tool for measuring distress is shown in Figure 30-3. The Distress Thermometer, which has proved to be valid and reliable (Hegel et al., 2008; Jacobsen et al., 2005), is a two-part tool that uses a 0–10 scale drawn on a thermometer to assess distress experienced within the past week and a list of problems that the patient may have experienced within the past week. The problems are grouped as (NCCN, 2013)
- Practical
- Family
- Emotional
- Spiritual/religious
- Physical
- Other.

The Distress Thermometer uses a 0–10 Likert scale, making the assessment tool easy for patient use. A score of 4–5 or higher on the scale denotes a significant level of distress that may require a referral for additional psychosocial or supportive care (Swanson & Koch, 2010).

Figure 30-3. Screening Tools for Measuring Distress

SCREENING TOOLS FOR MEASURING DISTRESS

Instructions: First please circle the number (0-10) that best describes how much distress you have been experiencing in the past week including today.

Extreme distress — 10
9
8
7
6
5
4
3
2
1
No distress — 0

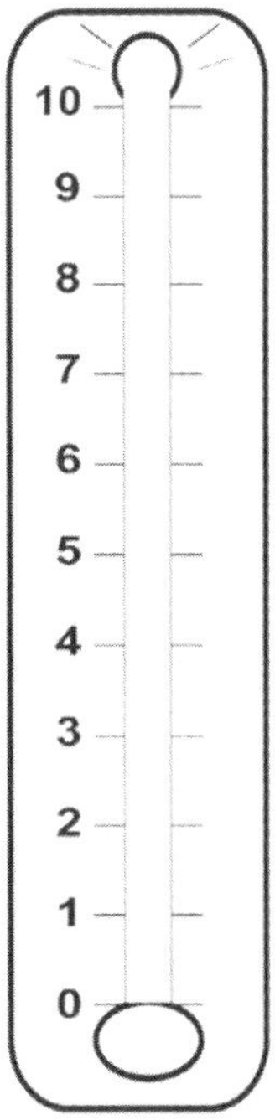

Second, please indicate if any of the following has been a problem for you in the past week including today. Be sure to check YES or NO for each.

Practical Problems (YES NO)
- Child care
- Housing
- Insurance/financial
- Transportation
- Work/school

Family Problems (YES NO)
- Dealing with children
- Dealing with partner

Emotional Problems (YES NO)
- Depression
- Fears
- Nervousness
- Sadness
- Worry
- Loss of interest in usual activities

Spiritual/religious concerns (YES NO)

Physical Problems (YES NO)
- Appearance
- Bathing/dressing
- Breathing
- Changes in urination
- Constipation
- Diarrhea
- Eating
- Fatigue
- Feeling Swollen
- Fevers
- Getting around
- Indigestion
- Memory/concentration
- Mouth sores
- Nausea
- Nose dry/congested
- Pain
- Sexual
- Skin dry/itchy
- Sleep
- Tingling in hands/feet

Other Problems: _____

Note. Reproduced with permission from *NCCN Clinical Practice Guidelines in Oncology (NCCN Guidelines®) for Distress Management V.2.2013.* © 2013 by the National Comprehensive Cancer Network, Inc. All rights reserved. The NCCN Guidelines® and illustrations herein may not be reproduced in any form for any purpose without the express written permission of the NCCN. To view the most recent and complete version of the NCCN Guidelines, go online to NCCN.org. NATIONAL COMPREHENSIVE CANCER NETWORK®, NCCN®, NCCN GUIDELINES®, and all other NCCN Content are trademarks owned by the National Comprehensive Cancer Network, Inc.

Patients are asked to mark the problem list to identify the "nature and source of their distress (whether it be physical, social, psychological, or spiritual)" (Bultz & Holland, 2006, p. 313). Patient identification of stressors is extremely useful when assessing the need for potential referrals (e.g., social work, chaplaincy services, mental health). Figure 30-4 depicts an overview of the NCCN evaluation and treatment process.

Patients and physicians found screening with the distress management tool to be satisfactory (Bultz & Holland, 2006). Bultz and Holland advised that caregivers be trained to use the screening tool routinely at each patient visit. They recommended online training for nurses utilizing the Distress Thermometer, such as the training provided by the American Psychosocial Oncology Society (www.apos-society.org).

Robbins (2007) conducted a pilot project that required the use of the NCCN tool at weeks 1 and 5 of radiation therapy. Audits of patients' charts demonstrated that the NCCN tool was used 75% of the time. Written feedback from nursing staff mentioned two reasons for not employing the tool: nurses were not always comfortable approaching patients and discussing their concerns, and physicians were not always supportive of the time the patient needed to complete the assessment. Subsequent staff in-services followed by chart audits showed an increase in use of the tool.

The Cancer Support Community published data revealing a substantial reduction in emotional distress for patients with cancer who were assessed within the framework of its distress screening program known as CancerSupportSource. The Cancer Support Community (2013) described the program as "the first comprehensive distress screening program developed for community-based hospitals, physician practices, and advocacy organizations to integrate screening, referral, and follow-up care, through a single, streamlined, program."

Patients, in any cancer care setting, complete a 25-item screening tool assessment on any computer using a standard web browser. Once the assessment is completed, CancerSupportSource furnishes the patient with a Personal Support Care Plan that includes information and

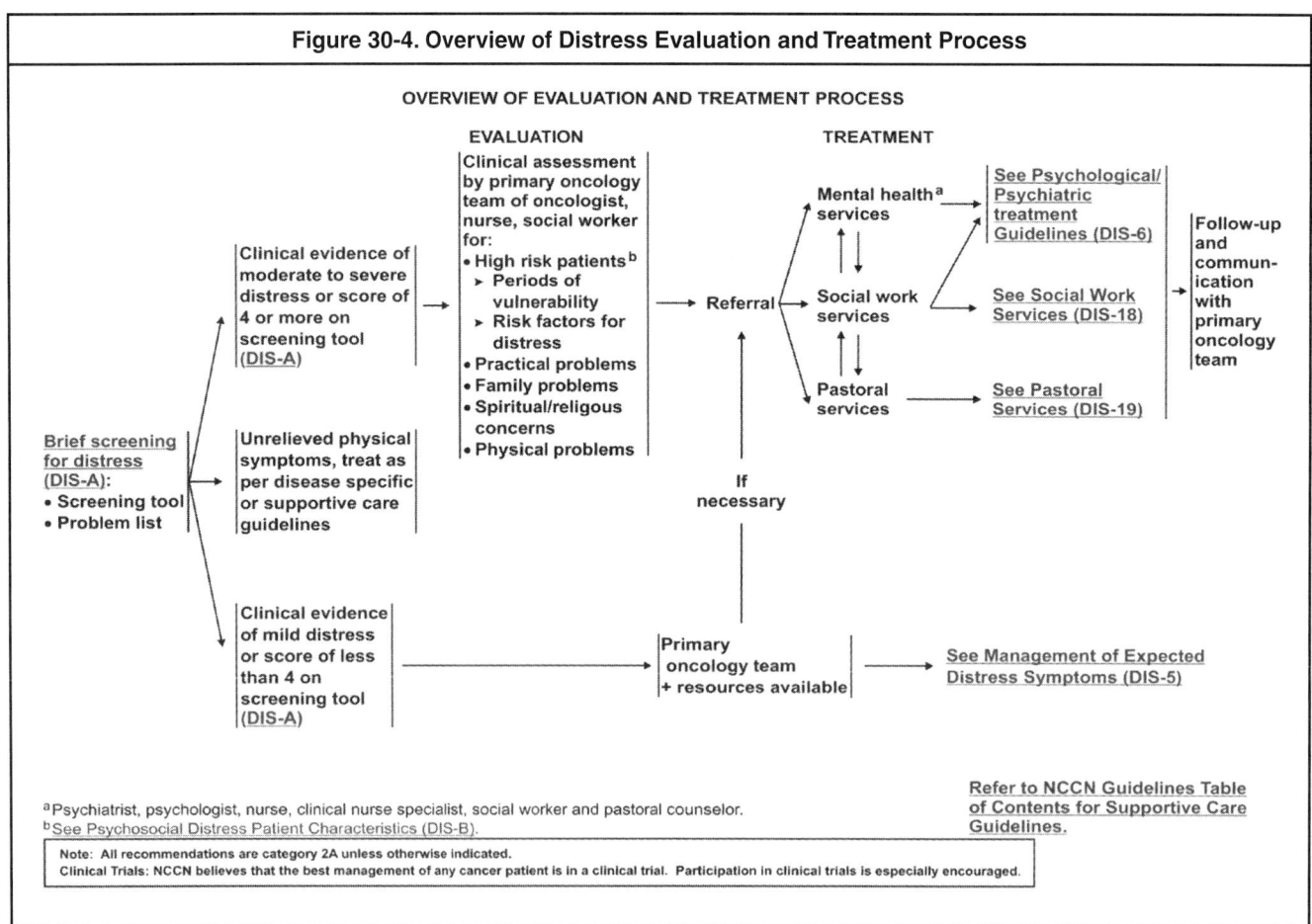

Figure 30-4. Overview of Distress Evaluation and Treatment Process

Note. Reproduced with permission from NCCN Clinical Practice Guidelines in Oncology (NCCN Guidelines®) for Distress Management V.2.2013. © 2013 by the National Comprehensive Cancer Network, Inc. All rights reserved. The NCCN Guidelines® and illustrations herein may not be reproduced in any form for any purpose without the express written permission of the NCCN. To view the most recent and complete version of the NCCN Guidelines, go online to NCCN.org. NATIONAL COMPREHENSIVE CANCER NETWORK®, NCCN®, NCCN GUIDELINES®, and all other NCCN Content are trademarks owned by the National Comprehensive Cancer Network, Inc.

referrals for support services. Physicians receive a Patient Distress Management Report—a patient summary score, which is valuable for staff triage response. CancerSupportSource is aimed toward a community practice setting, where 85% of patients with cancer are treated, and incorporates institutional and community programs to afford the necessary support resources. The goals of the program are to improve quality of care, increase patient satisfaction, and promote organizational effectiveness. This program allows healthcare providers to thoroughly assess and address the needs of patients identified as having distress.

Bruce (2007) stated, "Many healthcare providers do not look for depression or assume that depression is a normal reaction to cancer that does not warrant treatment" (p. 20). Martensson, Carlsson, and Lampic (2010) reported that discrepancies may exist between how patients and nurses perceive emotional distress. Explanations for this discrepancy may be attributed to time constraints, failure to correctly assess emotional distress because of a knowledge deficit of the patient's coping skills, and lack of emotional ability and bonding on the on the nurse's part. Madden (2006) noted that none of the reasons nurses may have for not assessing a patient's psychological distress are insurmountable. Feeling uncomfortable discussing a patient's feelings, being concerned about upsetting a patient, feeling emotionally "drained" after discussing feelings with a patient, and being under time constraints all may be addressed. Madden stated that "continuing education about psychosocial issues, discussions with peers about why nurses are reluctant to assess for distress, and an honest look inward" (p. 616) will increase a nurse's ability to routinely assess psychosocial distress.

Nursing Implications

Emotional distress can be a significant predictor of poor self-management and high healthcare costs; consequently, a targeted approach to identifying patients with poorly controlled distress may reduce medical costs. Distressed patients often present to their physicians with physical rather than emotional complaints; therefore, care coordinated jointly and in a timely and cost-effective manner can ultimately benefit patients (Fann, Ell, & Sharpe, 2012). Certainly, oncology nurses should familiarize themselves with free and low-cost behavioral psychosocial health resources, which are available in communities as well as nationally (Kaplan, 2008).

Oncology nurses should be especially perceptive to the psychosocial needs of patients during critical phases along the cancer continuum and be adept at providing assistance during these transitions with anticipatory counseling. To minimize risk and ensure individualized care, oncology nurses should meticulously and accurately validate their interpretation of their patients' needs and work with them in implementing a plan of action (Martensson et al., 2010). The Oncology Nursing Society's *Statement on the Scope and Standards of Oncology Nursing Practice: Generalist and Advanced Practice* (Brant & Wickham, 2013) addresses psychosocial distress. Specifically, oncology nurses were advised to include coping, comfort, and sexuality assessments for every patient.

Although standardized tools to assess distress in patients in clinical trials are not on the immediate horizon, the first step is to incorporate a general oncology distress assessment tool that can be incorporated into routine nursing practice. If utilization of the proposed tool is easy and can accurately identify patient psychosocial needs, perhaps a tool to specifically assess psychosocial distress in patients enrolled in clinical trials will not be necessary.

The NCCN multidisciplinary panel that developed the standards for psychosocial care and management of distress established minimal quality measures for recognizing and managing distress (Holland & Andersen, 2003). The complete NCCN standards of care for distress management are listed in Figure 30-5.

Figure 30-5. Standards of Care for Distress Management

- Distress should be recognized, monitored, documented, and treated promptly at all stages of disease and in all settings.
- Screening should identify the level and nature of the distress.
- All patients should be screened for distress at their initial visit, at appropriate intervals, and as clinically indicated, especially with changes in disease status (i.e., remission, recurrence, progression).
- Distress should be assessed and managed according to clinical practice guidelines.
- Interdisciplinary institutional committees should be formed to implement standards for distress management.
- Educational and training programs should be developed to ensure that healthcare professionals and certified chaplains have knowledge and skills in the assessment and management of distress.
- Licensed mental health professionals and certified chaplains experienced in psychosocial aspects of cancer should be readily available as staff members or by referral.
- Medical care contracts should include reimbursement for services provided by mental health professionals.
- Clinical health outcomes measurement should include assessment of the psychosocial domain (e.g., quality of life and patient and family satisfaction).
- Patients, families, and treatment teams should be informed that management of distress is an integral part of total medical care and should be provided with appropriate information about psychosocial services in the treatment center and the community.
- Quality of distress management should be included in institutional continuous quality improvement (CQI) projects.

Note. Reproduced with permission from *NCCN Clinical Practice Guidelines in Oncology (NCCN Guidelines®) for Distress Management V.2.2013.* © 2013 by the National Comprehensive Cancer Network, Inc. All rights reserved. The NCCN Guidelines® and illustrations herein may not be reproduced in any form for any purpose without the express written permission of the NCCN. To view the most recent and complete version of the NCCN Guidelines, go online to NCCN.org. NATIONAL COMPREHENSIVE CANCER NETWORK®, NCCN®, NCCN GUIDELINES®, and all other NCCN Content are trademarks owned by the National Comprehensive Cancer Network, Inc.

The implications for oncology nurses, clinical trial nurses (CTNs), and researchers are clear (see Figure 30-5). Patients must be assessed for psychological distress at each and every visit and receive an appropriate referral, if necessary. Oncology nurses are in the unique position to assess patients and their families for signs and symptoms of distress and to offer emotional support that can create an environment conducive for the sharing of psychosocial concerns (Kaplan, 2008).

Although this currently may be considered a lofty goal, the result of achieving that goal is astounding. Patients with cancer who are considering, enrolled in, or completing clinical trials may need psychosocial intervention. Nurses can help patients to cope by recognizing and focusing on the aspects of distress that may improve quality of life (Vitek, Rosenzweig, & Stollings, 2007). Distress cannot be treated if it is not identified.

CTNs are ideally knowledgeable, skilled, and compassionate. All CTNs need to introspectively assess their own sensitivity with discussing a patient's nonphysical distress and come to terms with it. Vachon (2006) noted that nurses can help patients with cancer cope with their disease and treatment by "respecting individual differences and preferences, appreciating patient perspectives, and understanding coping as a process" (p. 28). CTNs need to seek out ways to make psychosocial distress the sixth vital sign (Bultz & Johansen, 2011) and share assessment techniques with colleagues. Pilot studies, master's nursing projects, Oncology Nursing Society conference poster and podium sessions, and in-services are ways to help colleagues to appreciate what works and what does not.

The need to generalize assessments and interventions globally is apparent with the increased number of clinical trials internationally (see Section XI of this manual). The only way to achieve consistency of care worldwide is through the adoption of acceptable and effective standards. All oncology clinicians should adopt NCCN's distress management guidelines and standards as a means to that end.

Summary

Patients with cancer experience an array of personal psychological challenges as they move through the cancer treatment continuum, especially if they are part of a clinical trial. Psychosocial distress is a disconcerting consequence of oncology clinical trial participation. Evidence-based practice contributes greatly to defining the science of cancer and guiding patient care. Clinical trials promise quality of care measured by clinical effectiveness (Kelly, Ghazi, & Caldwell, 2002) and level the playing field by the implementation of novel interventions and therapies that enable the patient population to access the most current, cutting-edge treatment options (Gabriel & Mercado, 2011).

A gap exists in the routine assessment and intervention of psychological distress, which necessitates closure before oncology professionals can hope to provide truly holistic care to patients. The first step in accomplishing this goal is to adopt standards for assessment and intervention, such as the NCCN guidelines. The second step is to incorporate these standards into routine practice and ongoing research. According to Kaplan (2008), assessing and considering the psychosocial needs of patients with cancer should become standard practice. Only then will it be possible to determine whether a psychosocial distress assessment tool that is specific for clinical trial participants is required. Much work remains to be done.

Key Points

- Patients with cancer experience personal psychological challenges as they move through the cancer treatment continuum, especially if they are part of a clinical trial.
- Distress in patients with cancer is widespread, with incidence rates estimated at 35%–55% involving all phases of illness (Carlson et al., 2013).
- Distress is often associated with reduced survival, poor quality of life, and dissatisfaction with care.
- Nurses need to assess distress at every visit, documenting and acting on their findings just as vital sign findings are documented and acted upon.
- The NCCN Distress Thermometer and CancerSupportSource are two methods for assessing distress in patients with cancer.
- Whether or not a psychosocial distress assessment tool that is specific for clinical trial participants is required will only be possible to assess once routine psychosocial distress assessment of all patients with cancer is achieved.

References

Adler, N.E., & Page, A.E.K. (2008). *Cancer care for the whole patient: Meeting psychosocial health needs.* Retrieved from http://www.iom.edu/Reports/2007/Cancer-Care-for-the-Whole-Patient-Meeting-Psychosocial-Health-Needs.aspx

Agrawal, M., Grady, C., Fairclough, D.L., Meropol, N.J., Maynard, K., & Emanuel, E.J. (2006). Patients' decision-making process regarding participation in phase I oncology research. *Journal of Clinical Oncology, 24,* 4479–4484. doi:10.1200/jco.2006.06.0269

Albrecht, T.L., Blanchard, C., Ruckdeschel, J.C., Coovert, M., & Strongbow, R. (1999). Strategic physician communication and oncology clinical trials. *Journal of Clinical Oncology, 17,* 3324–3332. Retrieved from http://jco.ascopubs.org/content/17/10/3324.full

Aungst, J., Haas, A., Ommaya, A., & Green, L.W. (Eds.). (2003). *Exploring challenges, progress, and new models for engaging the public in the clinical research enterprise: Clinical Research Roundtable Workshop summary.* Retrieved from http://www.nap.edu/catalog/10757.html

Biedrzycki, B.A. (2010). Decision making for cancer clinical trial participation: A systematic review [Online exclusive]. *Oncology Nursing Forum, 37,* E387–E399. doi:10.1188/10.ONF.E387-E399

Biedrzycki, B.A. (2011). Factors and outcomes of decision making for cancer clinical trial participation. *Oncology Nursing Forum, 38,* 542–552. doi:10.1188/11.ONF.542-552

Brant, J.M., & Wickham, R.S. (Eds.). (2013). *Statement on the scope and standards of oncology nursing practice: Generalist and advanced practice*. Pittsburgh, PA: Oncology Nursing Society.

Bruce, S.D. (2007, April). Know how to assess and treat depression in patients with cancer. *ONS Connect, 22*(4), 20–21.

Bultz, B.D., & Holland, J.C. (2006). Emotional distress in patients with cancer: The sixth vital sign. *Community Oncology, 3*, 311–314.

Bultz, B.D., & Johansen, C. (2011). Screening for distress, the 6th vital sign: Where are we, and where are we going? *Psycho-Oncology, 20*, 569–571. doi:10.1002/pon.1986

Cancer Support Community. (2013). CancerSupportSource: A program of the cancer support community. Retrieved from http://www.cancersupportcommunity.org/cancersupportsource

Carlson, L.E., Waller, A., Groff, S.L., Giese-Davis, J., & Bultz, B.D. (2013). What goes up does not always come down: Patterns of distress, physical and psychosocial morbidity in people with cancer over a one-year period. *Psycho-Oncology, 22*, 168–176. doi:10.1002/pon.2068

Carter, S.E. (2004). End of treatment: Laugh or cry? *Community Oncology, 1*, 179–181. Retrieved from http://www.oncologypractice.com/co/journal/articles/0103179.pdf

Center for Information and Study on Clinical Research Participation. (2008). Clinical trials facts and figures for health professionals. Retrieved from https://www.ciscrp.org/wp-content/uploads/2014/03/ciscrp_data_archive_facts_and_figures_for_health_professionals.pdf

Comis, R.L., Miller, J.D., Aldige, C.R., Krebs, L., & Stoval, E. (2003). Public attitudes toward participation in cancer clinical trials. *Journal of Clinical Oncology, 21*, 830–835. doi:10.1200/JCO.2003.02.105

Comis, R.L., Miller, J.D., Colaizzi, D.D., & Kimmel, L.G. (2009). Physician-related factors involved in patient decisions to enroll onto cancer clinical trials. *Journal of Oncology Practice, 5*, 50–56. doi:10.1200/JOP.0922001

Deshields, T.L., & Nanna, S.K. (2010). Providing care for the "whole patient" in the cancer setting: The psycho-oncology consultation model of patient care. *Journal of Clinical Psychology in Medical Settings, 17*, 249–257. doi:10.1007/S10880-010-9208-1

Fann, J.R., Ell, K., & Sharpe, M. (2012). Integrating psychosocial care into cancer services. *Journal of Clinical Oncology, 30*, 1178–1186. doi:10.1007/S10880-010-9208-1

Gabriel, A.P., & Mercado, C.P. (2011). Data retention after a patient withdraws consent in clinical trials. *Open Access Journal of Clinical Trials, 2011*(3), 15–19. doi:10.2147/OAJCT.S13960

Hegel, M.T., Collins, E.D., Kearing, S., Gillock, K.L., Moore, C.P., & Ahles, T.A. (2008). Sensitivity and specificity of the Distress Thermometer for depression in newly diagnosed breast cancer patients. *Psycho-Oncology, 17*, 556–560. doi:10.1002/pon.1289

Holland, J.C., & Andersen, B. (2003). Distress management clinical practice guidelines in oncology. *Journal of the National Comprehensive Cancer Network, 1*, 344–374.

Holland, J.C., Watson, M., & Dunn, J. (2011). The IPOS New International Standard of Quality Cancer Care: Integrating the psychosocial domain into routine care. *Psycho-Oncology, 20*, 677–680. doi:10.1002/pon.1978

Jacobsen, P.B., Donovan, K.A., Trask, P.C., Fleishman, S.B., Zabora, J., Baker, F., & Holland, J.C. (2005). Screening for psychologic distress in ambulatory cancer patients. *Cancer, 103*, 1494–1502. doi:10.1002/cncr.20940

Kaplan, M. (2008). Cancer survivorship: Meeting psychosocial needs. *Clinical Journal of Oncology Nursing, 12*, 989–992. doi:10.1188/08.CJON.989-992

Kelly, C., Ghazi, F., & Caldwell, K. (2002). Psychological distress of cancer and clinical trial participation: A review of the literature. *European Journal of Cancer Care, 11*, 6–15. doi:10.1111/j.1365-2354.2002.00283.x

Klabunde, C.N., Keating, N.L., Potosky, A.L., Ambs, A., He, Y., Hornbrook, M.C., & Ganz, P.A. (2011). A population-based assessment of specialty physician involvement in cancer clinical trials. *Journal of the National Cancer Institute, 103*, 384–397. doi:10.1093/jnci/djq549

Klimaszewski, A.D. (2006). Psychosocial aspects of experimental therapy: Clinical trials. In R.M. Carroll-Johnson, L.M. Gorman, & N.J. Bush (Eds.), *Psychosocial nursing care along the cancer continuum* (2nd ed., pp. 489–497). Pittsburgh, PA: Oncology Nursing Society.

Kuroki, L., Stuckey, A., Hirway, P., Raker, C.A., Bandera, C.A., DiSilvesto, P.A., … Dizon, D.S. (2010). Addressing clinical trials: Can the multidisciplinary tumor board improve participation? A study from an academic women's cancer program. *Gynecologic Oncology, 116*, 295–300. doi:10.1016/j.ygyno.2009.12.005

Madden, J. (2006). The problem of distress in patients with cancer: More effective assessment. *Clinical Journal of Oncology Nursing, 10*, 615–619. doi:10.1188/06.CJON.615-619

Martensson, G., Carlsson, M., & Lampic, C. (2010). Do oncology nurses provide more care to patients with high levels of emotional distress? [Online exclusive]. *Oncology Nursing Forum, 37*, E34–E42. doi:10.1188/10.ONF.E34-E42

Meadows, B. (2000). Potential accrual base. In A.D. Klimaszewski, J.L. Aiken, M. Bacon, S.A. DiStasio, H.E. Ehrenberger, & B.A. Ford (Eds.), *Manual for clinical trials nursing* (pp. 53–55). Pittsburgh, PA: Oncology Nursing Society.

Melchior, H., Büscher, C., Thorenz, A., Grochocka, A., Koch, U., & Watzke, B. (2011). Self-efficacy and fear of cancer progression during the year following diagnosis of breast cancer. *Psycho-Oncology, 22*, 39–45. doi:10.1002/pon.2054

Meropol, N.J., Weinfurt, K.P., Burnett, C.B., Balshem, A., Benson, A.B., Castel, L., … Schulman, K.A. (2003). Perceptions of patients and physicians regarding phase I cancer clinical trials: Implications for physician-patient communication. *Journal of Clinical Oncology, 21*, 4659–4660. doi:10.1200/JCO.2003.10.072

Moore, R.A., Derry, S., & McQuay, H.J. (2008). Discontinuation rates in clinical trials in musculoskeletal pain: A meta-analysis from etoricoxib clinical trial reports. *Arthritis Research and Therapy, 10*(3), R53. doi:10.1186/ar2422

National Cancer Institute. (2005). *Cancer clinical trials: The in-depth program* [Publication No. 05-5051]. Retrieved from https://accrualnet.cancer.gov/sites/accrualnet.cancer.gov/files/InDepth_Book_m.pdf

National Comprehensive Cancer Network. (2013). *NCCN Clinical Practice Guidelines in Oncology: Distress management* [v.2.2013]. Retrieved from http://www.nccn.org/professionals/physician_gls/pdf/distress.pdf

Nekolaichuk, C.L., Cumming, C., Turner, J., Yushchyshyn, A., & Sela, R. (2011). Referral patterns and psychosocial distress in cancer patients accessing a psycho-oncology counseling service. *Psycho-Oncology, 20*, 326–332. doi:10.1002/pon.1765

Odo, R. (2012, July 6). The clinical trial debate. *Onc: The Oncology Nurse Community*. Retrieved from http://www.theonc.org/author.asp?section_id=2111&doc_id=246883

Robbins, M.A. (2007). Barriers to using the National Comprehensive Cancer Network (NCCN) distress management tool: Does it cause more stress? [Abstract 2073]. *Oncology Nursing Forum, 34*, 503. Retrieved from http://ons.metapress.com/content/8003536n87h1t836/fulltext.pdf

Rosedale, M. (2009). Survivor loneliness of women following breast cancer. *Oncology Nursing Forum, 36*, 175–183. doi:10.1188/09.ONF.175-183

Roychowdhury, D. (2003). Phase I trials: Physician and patient perceptions [Letter to the editor]. *Journal of Clinical Oncology, 21*, 4658–4659. doi:10.1200/JCO.2003.99.166

Schilsky, R.L. (2011). Accrual to cancer clinical trials in the era of molecular medicine [Commentary]. *Science Translational Medicine, 3*, 75cm9. doi:10.1126/scitranslmed.3001712

Schutta, K.M., & Burnett, C.B. (2000). Factors that influence a patient's decision to participate in a phase I cancer clinical trial. *Oncology Nursing Forum, 27*, 1435–1438.

Simon, M.S., Du, W., Flaherty, L., Philip, P.A., Lorusso, P., Miree, C., … Brown, D.R. (2004). Factors associated with breast cancer clinical trials participation and enrollment at a large academic medical center. *Journal of Clinical Oncology, 22,* 2046–2052. doi:10.1200/jco.2004.03.005

Spiegel, D. (2012). Mind matters in cancer survival. *Psycho-Oncology, 21,* 588–593. doi:10.1002/pon.3067

Swanson, J., & Koch, L. (2010). The role of the oncology nurse navigator in distress management of adult inpatients with cancer: A retrospective study. *Oncology Nursing Forum, 37,* 69–76. doi:10.1188/10.ONF.69-76

Vachon, M.A. (2006). Psychosocial distress and coping after cancer treatment. *American Journal of Nursing, 106*(Suppl. 3), 26–31. doi:10.1097/00000446-200603003-00011

van der Biessen, D.A.J., Cranendonk, M.A., Schiavon, G., van der Holt, B., Wiemer, E.A.C., Eskens, F.A.L.M., … Mathijssen, R.H.J. (2013). Evaluation of patient enrollment in oncology phase I clinical trials. *Oncologist, 18,* 323–329. doi:10.1634/theoncologist.2012-0334

Vitek, L., Rosenzweig, M.Q., & Stollings, S. (2007). Distress in patients with cancer: Definition, assessment, and suggested interventions. *Clinical Journal of Oncology Nursing, 11,* 413–418. doi:10.1188/07.cjon.413-418

SECTION VII.

Genetics and Genomics

Chapter 31

Pharmacogenetics and Pharmacogenomics

Annamalar Jeyasehar, PhD(c), MSN, RN, and Julia A. Eggert, PhD, GNP-BC, AGN-BC, AOCN®

Introduction

One of the core values of clinical trial nurses (CTNs) focuses on advancing evidence-based oncology care through the use of scientifically based research (Lubejko et al., 2011). Drug development is part of oncology care, and the goal is to develop drugs that work with maximum efficacy and minimal toxicity (Houtsma, Guchelaar, & Gelderblom, 2010; Huang & Ratain, 2009). Many drugs fail to reach the market, causing a rise in the cost of drug development (Louie & Russell, 2013). In order for a drug to become marketable, the optimum concentration needed to exert a therapeutic effect needs to be determined. This level depends on the amount of the drug administered and the amount of the drug that can be metabolized. Situations where the drug concentration is minimal or above the expected level could result in lack of drug effect or cause an adverse drug reaction (Piatkov, Jones, & McLean, 2013). To avoid unwanted toxic reactions, healthcare providers must exercise their knowledge of pharmacology and pharmacogenetics. The knowledge of pharmacogenetics not only aids in understanding the basic drug interaction process but also helps to correctly identify responders, nonresponders, and those who may be at risk to develop adverse drug reactions (Piatkov et al., 2013). CTNs must be informed about current and emerging genetic discoveries to apply the genetic information in their research practice. Not only do they need to be informed, but they also need to have working knowledge of pharmacogenomics to manage clinical trials. For treatment protocols, review cytogenetics (see Chapter 33) and tumor profiling (see Chapter 34).

The terms *pharmacogenetics* and *pharmacogenomics* describe how genetic determinants affect an individual's response to a medication. The study of these variations in a single gene is called *pharmacogenetics*. However, it is a known fact that genes interact with each other; hence, "the study of the variability of the expression of individual genes relevant to disease susceptibility as well as drug response at cellular, tissue, individual, or population level" is called *pharmacogenomics* (European Agency for the Evaluation of Medicinal Products, 2002, p. 3). These two terms are interchangeably used in the literature, and the primary difference between them is that pharmacogenomic studies look at a group of genes or the entire genome instead of a single gene (Ferraldeschi & Newman, 2011).

Many clinical trials are adding pharmacogenetics with pharmacokinetics (PK) (see Chapter 36) to determine how investigational drugs respond when people already have been diagnosed with a variety of diseases and conditions. The goal of pharmacogenetics is to personalize treatment based on an individual's genetic makeup. Some genetic information has been identified for use, but much remains unknown even though the human genome has been sequenced (Venter et al., 2001) and new technology has generated genetic information in the laboratory that continues to wait for application in the clinical setting (Huang & Ratain, 2009). As more is known regarding pharmacogenetics, CTNs need additional education and training in genetics to help their patients in clinical trials to understand the basic science of treatment (Calzone & Masny, 2004; Prows, 2011). This chapter will provide a basic foundation for understanding genetic terms, followed by a detailed discussion on pharmacogenetics. It will enable the reader to learn how metabolism of drugs is affected by an individual's genetic makeup and to describe the CTN's role in studies that incorporate pharmacogenetics.

Drug Development Process

Before the introduction of a new drug into the clinical setting, extensive preclinical testing is performed in vitro

---

The authors would like to acknowledge Carol S. Hill, BSN, RN, OCN®, Alberta Aikin, RN, BSN, CPON®, and Frank M. Balis, MD, for their contributions to this chapter that remain unchanged from the previous editions of this book.

using tumor cell lines and in vivo in animal models. A drug is first tested in the laboratory using human tumor cell lines to determine its spectrum of antitumor activity. It is administered to tumor-bearing animals to assess antitumor activity in vivo. If evidence of an antitumor effect exists, and the drug can be efficiently produced in large quantities, then the toxicology and PK are studied in several laboratory animal species (U.S. Department of Health and Human Services, 2012). PK studies play a critical role in the drug development process. The toxicology and PK studies in animals are used to determine a starting dose and schedule for the subsequent clinical trial drugs (Nomeir, 2010) (see Chapter 2).

The objectives of a phase I clinical trial are to determine the appropriate route, maximum tolerated dose, and schedule of administration; to define the spectrum of drug toxicities in healthy human subjects; and to study the PK of the new agent (U.S. Department of Health and Human Services, 2012). Because phase I trials are single-agent studies, they provide the best opportunity to identify correlations between PK parameters and the drug's pharmacodynamics (PD) (i.e., the drug's toxicity and response). The results of PK and PD studies are important components of the investigational new drug application that is submitted to the U.S. Food and Drug Administration to gain approval for commercial use of a new drug (Nomeir, 2010) (see Chapter 2).

Review of Basic Genetics

For CTNs working in the drug development area of clinical trials, understanding the genetic background can assist in education, communication, and management of the patient and family. In addition, knowledge in this evolving area of genetics will aid in communication between colleagues to ensure accurate implementation and follow-up of potentially life-threatening therapeutic drug protocols.

In clinical settings, variations in drug dose-effect and severity of adverse effects are seen among patients. One cause for interpatient variability is differences in genetic constitution (Deenen, Cats, Beijnen, & Schellens, 2011). PK and PD of a drug are influenced by proteins encoded by specific genes; variations in the constitution of these genes result in differences in drug response among individuals. Alterations in DNA sequences (by a variation in a single base pair, deletions, insertions, and gene copy number variants) contribute to genetic variability. When DNA sequences are altered, the end product (protein) of gene transcription, the protein structure, and its stability are altered. However, these changes may or may not affect the protein function depending on the location of the DNA alteration (Deenen et al., 2011).

It is well known that a gene is a molecule of DNA, which consists of four types of building blocks: adenine (A), guanine (G), cytosine (C), and thymine (T). These blocks, along with a sugar molecule and a phosphate group, are called a *nucleotide* (Lewis, 2012). For RNA, thymine (T) is replaced by uracil (U). RNA bases can be compared to an alphabet with three consecutive bases (letters) or nucleotides coding for (spelling) an amino acid. Multiple amino acids strung together create a protein. DNA remains in the nucleus of the cell and is passed to daughter cells when a cell undergoes division. The information in cellular DNA is transcribed to RNA and carried by RNA from the cell to the cytoplasm to bring about the instructions directed by the DNA (Lewis, 2012). See Figure 31-1 for an illustration.

The human genome has approximately 20,325 protein-coding genes with only a few thousand known to cause disorders or traits. Information about human disorders and traits is found in the Online Mendelian Inheritance in Man online catalog (www.omim.org). Only 1.5% of the 3.2 billion nucleotides encode proteins. The rest of the sequences may assist in protein synthesis or regulation of the function of a gene by turning them on or off. New components of DNA (e.g., microRNA) and their function are being identified, with many functions of DNA yet to be discovered (Lewis, 2012).

The collection of protein coding sequences (exons) of the genome is called an *exome*. Proteins are made up of long chains of amino acids known as *polypeptides*. To form a polypeptide, transcription occurs, enabling the RNA to enter the cytoplasm where the information is used to manufacture proteins by arranging amino acids per the instructions in RNA (translation). Through translation, the messenger RNA/mRNA is read as triplets, called codons. Each codon corresponds to an amino

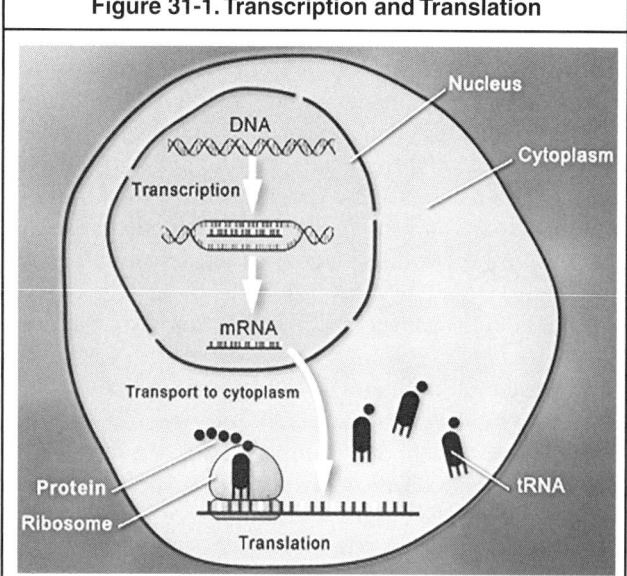

Figure 31-1. Transcription and Translation

Note. From "How Do Genes Direct the Production of Proteins?" by U.S. National Library of Medicine, n.d. Retrieved from http://ghr.nlm.nih.gov/handbook/howgeneswork/makingprotein.

acid. For example, AUG identifies methionine; UUA and UUG identify leucine. Twenty different amino acids create proteins. The amino acids are linked to each other by a chemical bond called a *peptide bond*. The protein-coding genes may differ among individuals, and the alternate forms are called *alleles*. These DNA sequence changes are caused by polymorphisms or mutations and are passed on to the daughter cells as the cell divides (Lewis, 2012). If a minor allelic variant is present in more than 1% of the population, it is called a *genetic polymorphism*, and when there is a variation in a single base pair, it is called a *single nucleotide polymorphism* (SNP) (Genetics Home Reference, n.d.). An alteration causing a disease is called a *mutation*.

To understand how alterations in DNA sequences affect protein function, a simple example with three-letter words may be used. The words have only three letters, similar to the codons (three nucleotides together and it could be any three of adenine, guanine, cytosine, or thymine). If "THE BIG FAT BOY ATE ONE EGG" corresponds to triplet coding for a protein, then a SNP in the sequence will read as "THE BIG FIT BOY ATE ONE EGG." In this example, there is meaning to the sentence in spite of a change in a single letter. Similarly, proteins may not be affected even when a single nucleotide is changed in a codon. This is called a *silent polymorphism*, as the substitution of a nucleotide does not change the amino acid and eventually has no effect on the protein (Sauna, Kimchi-Sarfaty, Ambudkar, & Gottesman, 2007). For example, AUU, AUC, AUA encodes the amino acid isoleucine. However, when there is a deletion or an insertion of a nucleotide, the reading frame shifts and the sentence makes no sense. For example, inserting a letter A in the third word results in "THE BIG FAA TBO YAT EON EEG G," or deleting a letter in the first word reads as "THB IGF ATB OYA TEO NEE GG." These two changes create an abnormal protein that causes altered function. In the *CYP2D6* gene (important in metabolism of medications), when there is a deletion of a thymine base pair at position 1707, the frameshift mutation creates a protein with no enzyme activity, causing patient problems with toxicity (Deenen et al., 2011).

A gene mutation can occur in two ways: it can be inherited or acquired. A germ-line mutation is an inherited mutation from a parent (U.S. National Library of Medicine [NLM], 2012). These mutations are passed to new generations through the DNA in the egg or sperm, so the mutations are present in every cell throughout the person's lifetime (NLM, 2012). The second type of mutation is a somatic mutation, which is acquired during a person's lifetime when changes or damage are acquired to an individual cell (NLM, 2012). Cellular changes can be a result of environmental factors, such as smoking and ultraviolet light, or can occur during DNA transcription, where a mistake is made as DNA is being copied (NLM, 2012). Somatic (acquired) mutations are not passed to future generations.

Chromosomal abnormalities are responsible for aberrations associated with metabolic problems of drugs. The two types of chromosomal aberrations are structural and numerical (Naeim, Rao, Song, & Grody, 2013). Structural aberrations are divided into four groups:
- Duplication (dup): part of the chromosome appears twice.
- Deletions (del): part of the chromosome is missing.
- Inversions (inv): a segment of chromosome is reversed.
- Translocations (t): two chromosomes exchange parts.
  Chromosome numerical changes include
- Euploidy: an increased number of the complete chromosomal sets.
- Aneuploidy: an increased or decreased number of individual chromosomes.

The International System for Human Cytogenetic Nomenclature is an international naming system to identify the chromosomes and the location of abnormalities. Chromosomes are recognized by their numbers, arms (p arm [petite arm] and q arm [q follows p]), regions, bands, and sub-bands. The total number of chromosomes, including the sex chromosomes, is separated by a comma; for example, 46, XX is a normal female, and 46, XY a normal male. Sex chromosome aberrations are usually associated by autosomal (nonsex chromosomes) aberrations. When two chromosomes have abnormalities, a comma separates the designation. For instance, [46, XY, del (7q)] is a deletion in the long arm of chromosome 7, and [47, XX, +21] is a female with trisomy 21 or Down syndrome (Shaffer, McGowan-Jordan, & Schmid, 2012).

Basic Pharmacogenomics for Clinical Trial Nurses

CTNs should understand pharmacogenetics, so terminology related to basic physiology and pharmacology will be reviewed. Prodrugs (the inactive form of drugs) are primarily metabolized in the liver to their active forms. For example, tamoxifen is a prodrug that is converted to its active metabolites in the liver. Of note, the liver is where the active metabolites are converted to inactive forms for the sake of elimination (Brauch, Mürdter, Eichelbaum, & Schwab, 2009; Golan, Tashjian, Armstrong, & Armstrong, 2012). Several enzymes and processes are involved in drug metabolism, and a superfamily among them is the cytochrome P450 enzymes, which are responsible for oxidation reactions. Well-known examples are CYP1A2, CYP2C9, CYP2C19, CYP2D6, CYP2E1, and CYP3A4 (Ingelman-Sundberg, Sim, Gomez, & Rodriguez-Antona, 2007). CYP is the root symbol for the cytochrome P450 family, followed by an Arabic number for the family, a letter to denote the subfamily, and an Arabic numeral for the individual gene (Nebert et al., 1987). The most common type of gene is denoted by an asterisk followed by number 1 (*1), and the numbers thereafter identify variations in the gene due to SNPs. The gene that encodes a particular isoenzyme follows the same nomenclature but is italicized. For example, isoenzyme CYP2C19 is a product of the gene *CYP2C19*. Populations differ in their frequency of specific alleles. In the United States, Caucasians have a high frequency of *CYP2D6*4*, and Asians have a high frequency of *CYP2D6 *10* (Teh & Bertilsson, 2012).

For an autosomal gene, every individual receives two alleles from their parents. It is possible for some genes to have several copies of an allele inherited from one parent at a particular locus in a chromosome. The common form of the gene that codes for a full functioning isoenzyme is called a *wild-type allele*. The genotype of the individual corresponds to the allele makeup for a particular gene and is reflected in the phenotype. It is important to remember that these phenotypes can be influenced by medications, herbal remedies, and food that an individual ingests (Scripture & Figg, 2006).

Phenotypically, individuals can be characterized as poor, intermediate, extensive, and ultra-rapid metabolizers. For poor metabolizers, the metabolism of the drug is significantly reduced and the drug remains in the circulation for a longer duration. Therefore, the patient experiences prolonged drug effect. If a patient is a poor metabolizer for warfarin, a prolonged drug effect can lead to severe hemorrhage (Shi, Bleavins, & de la Iglesia, 2001). At the other extreme are the ultra-rapid metabolizers, who have increased efficiency in metabolizing the drug. These individuals clear the drug from their circulation at an increased level and therefore may not receive the required drug effect, causing inadequate or no cancer treatment. Extensive metabolizers experience the drug effect to the expected level with or without minimal adverse drug reactions. The intermediate metabolizers are the heterozygotes who experience decreased drug effect and suffer from toxic drug levels. However, these individuals benefit from drugs when started in low doses and gradually increased (Prows, 2011). Read Table 31-1 to see how alleles have an impact on the metabolism of drugs and prodrugs.

Pharmacogenetics and Common Anticancer Drugs

Several well-known examples of pharmacogenetics are commonly used anticancer drugs. Although CTNs will be managing clinical trial protocols that are different from the examples that follow, these have been included so that CTNs new to research can have a better appreciation for the importance of the ability to translate molecular knowledge of pharmacogenetics into practice as it relates to potential cancer treatments.

5-Fluorouracil and Dihydropyrimidine Dehydrogenase

The dihydropyrimidine dehydrogenase (DPD) protein encoded by the *DYPD* gene is involved in metabolism of the drug 5-fluorouracil (5-FU), well known for treatment of solid tumors. Eighty percent of the 5-FU active drug is converted to inactive metabolites by the DPD enzyme. Hence, individuals who are deficient in DPD suffer from severe toxic effects (Houtsma et al., 2010). The most common variant found in DPD-deficient individuals is in an intron, *DYPD*2A* (Raida et al., 2001). This is because of a G to A mutation in the GT 5′ splice recognition site of intron 14 (here, the term *mutation* versus *polymorphism* is used, as the change in this base pair occurs in less than 1% of the population). When compared to patients with normal DPD activity, 60% of the DPD-deficient patients suffered from grade 3–4 toxicity, and 55% of them developed grade 4 neutropenia when administered 5-FU (Raida et al., 2001; van Kuilenburg et al., 2000). Pretreatment genetic screening may help identify patients who have deficient DPD activity and aid in making treatment decisions to limit toxic effects and, in some extreme cases, may save a life (Houtsma et al., 2010; Mounier-Boutoille et al., 2010). In this scenario, CTNs would be involved in completion of the consent process, education of the patient and family about pharmacogenetics and potential side effects, collection of a DNA sample, timely collection of blood and urine samples, and careful assessment and monitoring for side effects and levels of toxicity.

6-Mercaptopurine and Thiopurine S-Methyltransferase

Thiopurine S-methyltransferase (TPMT) regulates anticancer drugs such as 6-mercaptopurine (6-MP) and 6-thioguanine that are commonly used for acute lymphocytic leukemia (ALL) treatment. Because TPMT is an enzyme, its primary action is to inactivate the drug, thereby preventing toxicity from the drug (Coulthard & Hogarth, 2005). Studies have found that individuals who have low TPMT activity do not receive adequate treatment of ALL blast cells, causing escalating blast cells and higher concentrations of active 6-MP leading to toxic effects. Hence, dose regulation based on the genetic test is necessary to avoid toxicities (Lennard, Lilleyman, Van Loon, & Weinshilboum, 1990; McLeod, Relling, Liu, Pui, & Evans, 1995).

The most frequent variant alleles are *TPMT*2*, *TPMT*3A* (mostly seen in Caucasians), and *TPMT*3C* (common in Asians) and account for low or intermediate TPMT activity (Collie-Duguid et al., 1999; Hiratsuka, Inoue, Omori, Agatsuma, & Mizugaki, 2000; McLeod, Krynetski, Relling, & Evans, 2000). Individuals who carry the variant gene *TPMT*1* are wild-type

Table 31-1. Relationship Between Single Locus Genotype-Predicted Metabolizing Phenotype and Anticipated Impact on Drug			
Genotype-Predicted Phenotype	Patient's Gene Pair	Anticipated Impact on Active Drug	Anticipated Impact on Prodrug
Poor/slow metabolizer	Both members of gene pair contain variant that results in absent or non-functioning protein.	Decreased efficiency in converting active drug to inactive metabolites. Increases risk for higher levels of active drug and clinical toxicity.	Inability to convert inactive prodrug to active metabolites. If prodrug has no therapeutic properties, then patient will experience lack of efficacy despite drug dose increases.
Intermediate metabolizer	One member of gene pair consists of variant that results in absent or non-functioning protein and other member of gene pair contains variant that results in protein with reduced function -or- Pair of genes, each with variant that results in protein with reduced function -or- One member of gene pair with variant that results in protein with reduced function and other member of gene pair that has sequence consistent with full functioning protein.	Decreased efficiency in converting active drug to inactive metabolites. Increases risk for higher levels of active drug and clinical toxicity. If drug is normally dosed low and slowly titrated upward, effectiveness may be achieved sooner than in extensive metabolizers.	Decreased efficiency in converting inactive prodrug to active metabolites. Anticipate decreased effectiveness at standard maintenance doses.
Extensive metabolizer	Each member of gene pair has sequence consistent with full functioning protein.	Active drug given at standard doses metabolized to inactive components, achieving effectiveness without or with minimal adverse drug reactions (ADRs).	Prodrug converted to active metabolites achieving effectiveness without or with minimal ADRs.
Ultra-rapid metabolizer	Locus inherited from one parent has gene sequence consistent with full functioning protein, locus inherited from other parent has two or more copies of gene sequence resulting in full functioning protein. One member of gene pair has sequence consistent with full functioning protein and other member of gene pair has variant that causes increased amounts of full functioning protein to be produced.	Increased efficiency in converting active drug to inactive metabolites. Risk for decreased effectiveness at standard doses.	Increased efficiency in converting prodrug to active metabolites. Increased risk for toxicity from higher than expected levels of active metabolites.

Note. From "Infusion of Pharmacogenetics Into Cancer Care," by C.A. Prows, 2011, *Seminars in Oncology Nursing, 27,* p. 48. Copyright 2011 by Elsevier. Adapted with permission.

homozygotes and have the highest TPMT activity, followed by the heterozygotes (*1/*3) with intermediate activity, and homozygotes (*3/*3) with two variant alleles that have no or trace TPMT activity (McLeod et al., 2000). The individuals with low TPMT activity have 10–15 times the accumulation of toxic metabolites compared to those with high and intermediate TPMT activity (McLeod & Siva, 2002).

Genetic tests are available to identify the individual's *TPMT* genotype to predict enzymatic activity prior to treatment; however, these are not routinely administered outside of a clinical trial because they were not found to be cost-effective (Brownstein et al., 2012; Higgs, Gambhir, Ramsden, Poulton, & Newman, 2010; Pinto, Cohn, & Dolan, 2012; Stocco et al., 2008).

In this scenario, consent, education, DNA collection, and monitoring and management of the clinical trial protocol are extremely important. An extra addition to the monitoring would include the collection and calculation of cost measurements.

Irinotecan and UDP-Glucuronosyltransferase

Irinotecan, a prodrug commonly used in the treatment of colorectal cancers, is metabolized in the body to its active form SN-38. Conversion of active SN-38 to inactive SN-38 glucuronide is catalyzed by UGT1A1, a major isoform. This suggests that individuals who are deficient in UGT1A1 suffer from serious adverse effects when administered irinotecan (Iyer et al., 1998; Nagar & Blanchard, 2006; Palomaki, Bradley, Douglas, Kolor, & Dotson, 2009). Studies have confirmed the presence of alleles in different frequencies among different populations. The UGT1A1*28 polymorphism in the Caucasian population (because of the addition of TA to the TATA box of the UGT1A1 promoter) is the most common variant (Kaniwa et al., 2005) and is associated with a decrease in UGT1A1 expression (when homozygous). With decreased expression, the patient suffers from irinotecan toxicity (Bosma et al., 1995) such as grade 3–4 diarrhea and grade 3–4 neutropenia (Carlini et al., 2005; Innocenti et al., 2004; Massacesi et al., 2006). The allele *6 is specific is to East Asians (Araki et al., 2006; Minami et al., 2007; Sai et al., 2004). Although information about the alleles that cause toxicity is available, there currently is not enough information to dictate patient management, so pharmacogenetic testing is not required.

The need for CTNs to understand allelic nomenclature and be able to decipher and include it in communications with staff, plus to discuss it with patients and family, is obvious. Patients appreciate information that can be communicated in a simple way so they can understand how their body responds to treatments and why their response may be different than someone else's.

Drug Transporter Genes

Drug transporters are responsible for pumping out drug molecules across cell membranes. Too much or too little activity of these transporters can interfere with the efficacy of the drug. The ATP-binding Cassette (ABC) is a superfamily of transporters with one of its members encoded by the *ABCB1* gene, a P-glycoprotein (Houtsma et al., 2010; Petros & Evans, 2004). The role of P-glycoprotein is to decrease intestinal absorption and brain uptake of the drug as well as to increase the drug excretion via biliary, intestinal, or renal routes (Zhou, 2008). High P-glycoprotein levels indicate worse treatment outcomes. Low P-glycoprotein contributes to longer survival post chemotherapy (Opdam, Gelderblom, & Guchelaar, 2012). Multiple polymorphisms in the *ABCB1* gene have been identified, few with functional significance. Some are SNPs identified in exon 26 of *ABCB1* causing altered drug disposition (Cascorbi et al., 2001) and SNPs in exon 12 of *ABCB1* associated with irinotecan PKs (Mathijssen et al., 2003). When these findings from clinical trials were submitted to the U.S. Food and Drug Administration, it resulted in the requirement that the polymorphism information be incorporated into patient package inserts (Giacomini et al., 2007).

For other commonly used medications, please refer to Table 31-2 for genes, polymorphisms identified, their molecular effect, effect on drugs, and effect on therapy. This table includes examples of information that CTNs may be required to collect when managing a clinical trial protocol focusing on the use of new drugs.

Pharmacogenetic Testing

When molecular diagnostics become routinely used in clinical settings by physicians and pharmacists, the concept of standardized dosing will be replaced by individualized dosing based on patient data from genetic testing (Di Francia et al., 2012). The present barriers are the cost of the newer genetic technologies compared to the cheaper currently used ones (polymerase chain reaction [PCR]-based) and also the need for highly qualified and well-trained personnel for test result interpretation (Di Francia et al., 2012). Genotyping assays for detecting genetic polymorphisms, when compared to phenotypic assessments, have advantages such as relatively easy sample collection (small amount of peripheral blood or buccal swab) and not being compromised by drug-drug and drug-food interactions (Shi et al., 2001).

It is possible that clinical trials could utilize currently available genotyping assays. These vary from testing for (a) a single genetic variation (UGT1A1 promoter polymorphism, Mayo Medical laboratory) (Ratain, 2006), (b) a series of genes (CYP2D6 and CYP2C19 on AmpliChipCYP450 Test) (Roche Diagnostics, n.d.), (c) hundreds to thousands of genetic variants (Agilent Human Genome CGH Microarray 244A) (Agilent, n.d.), or (d) the entire human genome (23andMe, n.d.). Visit the GeneTests website (www.genetests.org) to obtain a full list of genetic tests and consultations. Note that only a fraction of them are pharmacogenetic tests (Huang & Ratain, 2009).

Phenotyping assays that can identify genetic variability are gene expression profiling and enzyme activity tests (Huang & Ratain, 2009). Prediction markers have been generated to identify chemoresistance in children with ALL (Holleman et al., 2004). Oncotype DX is currently used in breast cancer diagnosis of tumors with an estrogen influence to quantify the likelihood of recurrence and assess the benefit of chemotherapy in newly diagnosed patients (Ishibe, Schully, Freedman, & Ramsey, 2011). TPMT enzyme activity testing was the first pharmacogenomic test that has proceeded to routine use and is completed before initiation of 6-MP (Ford & Berg, 2010). These genotyping and phenotyping assays, to tumor cells, may have to be repeated in an individual before repeated treatments, but not the individual's germ-line (sex chromosome) DNA, as it remains unchanged in one's lifetime (Riegert-Johnson, Macaya, Hefferon, & Boardman, 2008).

Other methods include Taqman Allelic Discrimination Assay, a genotyping method that identifies SNPs related to drug resistance using 5′-nuclease activity of Taq polymerase during or after PCRs. These assays detect SNPs

Table 31-2. Most Significant Known Genetic Variants and Their Effect in Pharmacotherapy				
Gene*	Polymorphism (Nucleotide Translation)	Molecular Effect	Drug	Effect on Therapy
Cytochrome P450 family	Various polymorphism	Decreased enzyme activity	Various	Inter-individual variability in PK
TPMT2, 3A, 3C	Various polymorphism	Decreased enzyme activity	6-MP, thioguanine	Hematopoietic toxicity
UGT1A 28	TA repeats in 5′ promoter	Decreased enzyme activity	Irinotecan	Neutropenia toxicity
MDR1	(C3435T)	Low expression	Various	Drug resistance
TYMS	3 tandem repeats	Increased enzyme activity	5-FU, methotrexate	Drug resistance
DPYD	IVS14+1G	Decreased enzyme activity	5-FU, methotrexate	Neutropenia toxicity
DHFR	T91C	Increased enzyme activity	Methotrexate	Drug resistance
MTHFR	(C677T) (A1298C)	Decreased enzyme activity	5-FU, methotrexate	Toxicity
c-KIT	D860 N567K	Constitutive signal activation	Imatinib	Desensitizes activity in GIST
K-RAS	G12x G13D	Inhibition of the tyrosine kinase domain-binding drug	Cetuximab, panitumumab	Desensitizes activity in colon-rectum carcinoma
B-RAF	V600E	Inhibition of the tyrosine kinase domain-binding drug	Vemurafenib, gefitinib	Good response in melanomas
EGFR	L858R	Inhibition of the tyrosine kinase domain-binding drug	Erlotinib	Good response in NSCLC
BCR/ABL fusion gene	t(9;22) BCR/ABL	Constitutive signal activation	Imatinib, dasatinib, nilotinib	Good response in CML
ABL	T315I; M351T	Inhibition of the tyrosine kinase domain-binding drug	Imatinib	Drug resistance in CML
PML/RARα fusion gene	t(15;17) PML/RARα	Block of myeloid lineage cells	ATRA	Good response in AML-M3 subtypes
ADRB1, ADRB2	R389G	G-protein altered	Beta-blockers	Desensitizes activity
MHC class B 1	Several SNPs including codon K751Q	HLA-B~5701 haplotype	Abacavir	Hypersensitivity reaction
VKORC1	Many, VKORC1 haplotypes including codon G3673A	Associated with a higher/low warfarin dose	Warfarin	Variable anticoagulant effect

ABL—Abelson murine leukemia viral oncogene; ADRB—adrenergic b-receptors; AML—acute myeloid leukemia; ATRA—all-trans-retinoic acid; BCR—breakpoint cluster region; CML—chronic myeloid leukemia; DHFR—dihydrofolate reductase; DPYD—dihydropyrimidine dehydrogenase; EGFR—epidermal growth factor receptor; 5-FU—5-fluorouracil; GIST—gastrointestinal stromal tumor; HLA-B—human leukocyte antigen B; MDR1—multidrug resistance 1; MHC—major histocompatibility complex; MTHFR—5,10-methylene tetrahydrofolate reductase; NSCLC—non-small cell lung cancer; PK—pharmacokinetics; PML/RARα—promyelocytic leukemia/retinoic acid receptor alpha; 6-MP—6-mercaptopurine; SNP—single nucleotide polymorphism; TPMT—thiopurine methyltransferase; TYMS—thymidylate synthase; UGT1A1—UDP-glucuronosyltransferase 1A1; VKORC1—vitamin K epoxide reductase complex 1

* Genes are available for genotyping test or under consideration for clinical diagnostics.

Note. From "Knowledge and Skills Needs for Health Professions About Pharmacogenomics Testing Field," by R. Di Francia, D. Valente, O. Catapano, M. Rupolo, U. Tirelli, and M. Berretta, 2012, *European Review for Medical and Pharmacological Sciences, 16*, p. 783. Copyright 2012 by European Review for Medical and Pharmalogical Sciences. Reprinted with permission.

related to drug resistance and mutations such as point mutations, insertions, and large deletions (Fedick, Su, & Treff, 2012; Kamau et al., 2012). PCR with allele-specific oligonucleotide hybridization is a simple, cost-effective method used to detect a mutation. The PCR method was used in identifying extensive and poor metabolizers of CYP2D6 in the late 1990s (De Gregori et al., 2010). Quantitative real time-PCR (QRT-PCR), although expensive, is a rapid and dependable method that simultaneously amplifies and quantifies a targeted DNA molecule. It was initially used in identification of CYP2D6 alleles specific to poor metabolizers (De Gregori et al., 2010).

Currently, several hundreds of drug-metabolizing genes can be studied using commercial or custom-made chips (a microarray technology used in genetic testing). Some that are already available in the market are DMET chip (Affymetrix), VeraCode ADME chip (Illumina), and iPLEX ADME pharmacogenomics panel (Sequenom, Inc.) (Pinto et al., 2012). The DMET chip analyzes 230 drug-metabolizing genes for 1,936 SNPs, whereas the VeraCode ADME has 184 SNPs in 34 drug-metabolizing genes. In addition to these commercial chips, custom-made chips have been developed by research groups that contain specific SNPs for particular drug-metabolizing genes (Pinto et al., 2012). Cisplatin-related ototoxicity in children was studied using a custom-made chip that had 1,949 variants in 220 drug-metabolizing genes and identified TPMT and catechol-O-methyl transferase (known as COMT) enzymes to be significantly associated with ototoxicity, which was not known previously in relation to cisplatin metabolism (Ross et al., 2009).

Genome-wide association studies (GWASs) have identified significant findings related to predicting patients' risk of toxicity. A GWAS studies an entire genome for variations or SNPs (in 100s and 1,000s at the same time) that occur more often in people with a particular disease when compared to those without the disease (U.S. NLM, 2013). A GWAS newly identified an SNP that was found to be overrepresented in GRIA1, associated with hypersensitivity to asparaginase, which is used in treatment of ALL. The research looked at more than 500,000 SNPs in 485 children. This discovery would have been impossible if research was focused only on candidate genes (Chen et al., 2010).

Any of these tests, and even others in development, could potentially be used in a clinical trial. CTNs must be cognizant of the emerging technologies available for use in clinical trials and be able to explain the rationale of their use to patients.

Role of Clinical Trial Nurses

Oncology CTNs play an important role in moving the discoveries made in laboratories to the bedside. Their role in clinical trials spans the cancer continuum from conception through end-of-life care and involves research to provide an evidence base for different facets, such as risk assessment, genetic testing, prevention, profiling, pharmacogenetics, and treatments, with a need for counseling and education (Calzone & Masny, 2004). Although CTNs collect a variety of data, one of the critical role components is to obtain careful medication and food intake histories (Prows, 2011). Other medications, herbal remedies, supplements, and a variety of foods are known to interfere with anticancer drug metabolism and can lead to toxicity even if the genetic test was negative for high-risk polymorphisms (Scripture & Figg, 2006). Some clinical trials include pharmacogenetics testing to identify individuals with a high risk for toxicity of a new treatment agent being studied. This could include the need for the nurse to monitor for adverse effects and teach patients and family members to recognize or note any changes in how patients feel or react.

CTNs can adapt roles in compliance with the nine core competencies of a CTN (Lubejko et al., 2011) (see also Appendix 2). CTNs in oncology settings will need to understand pharmacogenetics to (Calzone & Masny, 2004)

- Interpret individuals' results obtained from DNA chip technology
- Perform comprehensive health assessment in relation to personal, medical, and genetic risks, as well as modifiable risk factor behaviors
- Counsel individuals about risk reduction as it relates to the clinical trial (e.g., chemoprevention using tamoxifen, referral to clinical trials)
- Educate individuals about genetic events involved in tumor initiation and progress
- Provide necessary information and assist in obtaining informed consent from individuals participating in clinical trials (see Chapter 14)
- Assess patients' knowledge about genetic terms (mutation versus polymorphism) and understanding of screening results as related to the clinical trial
- Interpret the genetic signature of the tumor to patients and families
- Explain individualized treatment recommendations based on tumor profile with education about the dose of treatment using the individual's pharmacogenetic profile
- Provide genetic profile results to physicians, assist patients to understand their personalized results involved in drug metabolism, and give details about dose recommendations based on the individual's profile.

Summary

Pharmacogenetic studies of anticancer drugs have led to evidence-based drug administration schedules that have improved patient outcomes. Patients who participate in research studies make an invaluable contribution to the knowledge base of new and conventional anticancer drugs plus diagnostics such as cytogenetics or treatment discussions using tumor profiling. CTNs play an essential role in coordinating and conducting these vital research studies that have a direct impact on the safety, effectiveness, and outcomes of anticancer drug administration. It is important that CTNs understand genetics, specifically pharmacogenetics (part of a drug clinical trial), so that they can partner with their colleagues and educate their patients to understand the important roles pharmacogenetic clinical trial studies have in the development of diagnostics and treatments in cancer care.

Key Points

- The goal of pharmacogenetics is to personalize treatment based on an individual's genetic makeup.
- The knowledge of pharmacogenetics not only aids in understanding the basic drug interaction process but also helps to rightly identify responders, nonresponders, and those who are at risk to develop adverse drug reactions.
- In clinical settings, variations in drug dose-effect and severity of adverse effects are seen among patients. Among the causes for interpatient variability is differences in genetic constitution.
- Phenotypically, individuals can be characterized as poor, intermediate, extensive, and ultra-rapid metabolizers.
- When molecular diagnostics become routinely used in clinical settings by physicians and pharmacists, the concept of standardized dosing will be replaced by individualized dosing based on patient data from genetic testing.
- CTNs play an essential role in coordinating and conducting vital research studies that have a direct impact on the safety, effectiveness, and outcomes of anticancer drug administration.

References

Agilent Technologies. (n.d.). Human genome CGH microarrays. Retrieved from http://www.genomics.agilent.com/en/product.jsp?cid=AG-PT-110&tabId=AG-PR-1079&_requestid=2731592

Araki, K., Fujita, K., Ando, Y., Nagashima, F., Yamamoto, W., Endo, H., … Sasaki, Y. (2006). Pharmacogenetic impact of polymorphisms in the coding region of the UGT1A1 gene on SN-38 glucuronidation in Japanese patients with cancer. *Cancer Science, 97*, 1255–1259. doi:10.1111/j.1349-7006.2006.00321.x

Bosma, P.J., Chowdhury, J.R., Bakker, C., Gantla, S., de Boer, A., Oostra, B.A., … Elferink, R.P.O. (1995). The genetic basis of the reduced expression of bilirubin UDP-glucuronosyltransferase 1 in Gilbert's syndrome. *New England Journal of Medicine, 333*, 1171–1175. doi:10.1056/NEJM199511023331802

Brauch, H., Mürdter, T.E., Eichelbaum, M., & Schwab, M. (2009). Pharmacogenomics of tamoxifen therapy. *Clinical Chemistry, 55*, 1770–1782.

Brownstein, C., Fusaro, V.A., Savage, S., Clinton, C., Mandl, K., Margulies, D., … Manzi, S. (2012). Integration of a standardized pharmacogenomic platform for clinical decision support at Boston Children's Hospital. *BMC Proceedings, 6*, P5. doi:10.1186/1753-6561-6-S6-P5

Calzone, K.A., & Masny, A. (2004). Genetics and oncology nursing. *Seminars in Oncology Nursing, 20*, 178–185. doi:10.1053/j.soncn.2004.04.004

Carlini, L.E., Meropol, N.J., Bever, J., Andria, M.L., Hill, T., Gold, P., … Blanchard, R.L. (2005). UGT1A7 and UGT1A9 polymorphisms predict response and toxicity in colorectal cancer patients treated with capecitabine/irinotecan. *Clinical Cancer Research, 11*, 1226–1236. Retrieved from http://clincancerres.aacrjournals.org/content/11/3/1226.full

Cascorbi, I., Gerloff, T., Johne, A., Meisel, C., Hoffmeyer, S., Schwab, M., … Roots, I. (2001). Frequency of single nucleotide polymorphisms in the P-glycoprotein drug transporter MDR1 gene in White subjects. *Clinical Pharmacology and Therapeutics, 69*, 169–174. doi:10.1067/mcp.2001.114164

Chen, S., Pei, D., Yang, W., Cheng, C., Jeha, S., Cox, N.J., … Relling, M.V. (2010). Genetic variations in GRIA1 on chromosome 5q33 related to asparaginase hypersensitivity. *Clinical Pharmacology and Therapeutics, 88*, 191–196. doi:10.1038/clpt.2010.94

Collie-Duguid, E., Pritchard, S., Powrie, R., Sludden, J., Collier, D., Li, T., & McLeod, H. (1999). The frequency and distribution of thiopurine methyltransferase alleles in Caucasian and Asian populations. *Pharmacogenetics, 9*(1), 37. doi:10.1097/00008571-199902000-00006

Coulthard, S., & Hogarth, L. (2005). The thiopurines: An update. *Investigational New Drugs, 23*, 523–532. doi:10.1007/s10637-005-4020-8

Deenen, M.J., Cats, A., Beijnen, J.H., & Schellens, J.H. (2011). Part 1: Background, methodology, and clinical adoption of pharmacogenetics. *Oncologist, 16*, 811–819. doi:10.1634/theoncologist.2010-0258

De Gregori, M., Allegri, M., De Gregori, S., Garbin, G., Tinelli, C., Regazzi, M., … Ranzani, G.N. (2010). How and why to screen for CYP2D6 interindividual variability in patients under pharmacological treatments. *Current Drug Metabolism, 11*, 276–282. doi:10.2174/138920010791196274

Di Francia, R., Valente, D., Catapano, O., Rupolo, M., Tirelli, U., & Berretta, M. (2012). Knowledge and skills needs for health professions about pharmacogenomics testing field. *European Review for Medical and Pharmacological Sciences, 16*, 781–788. Retrieved from http://www.europeanreview.org/wp/wp-content/uploads/1391.pdf

European Agency for the Evaluation of Medicinal Products. (2002, November 21). *Position paper on terminology in pharmacogenetics*. Retrieved from http://www.ema.europa.eu/docs/en_GB/document_library/Scientific_guideline/2009/09/WC500003889.pdf

Fedick, A., Su, J., & Treff, N.R. (2012). Development of TaqMan allelic discrimination based genotyping of large DNA deletions. *Genomics, 99*, 127–131. doi:10.1016/j.ygeno.2012.01.003

Ferraldeschi, R., & Newman, W.G. (2011). Pharmacogenetics and pharmacogenomics: A clinical reality. *Annals of Clinical Biochemistry, 48*, 410–417. doi:10.1258/acb.2011.011084

Ford, L., & Berg, J. (2010). Thiopurine S-methyltransferase (TPMT) assessment prior to starting thiopurine drug treatment; a pharmacogenomic test whose time has come. *Journal of Clinical Pathology, 63*, 288–295. doi:10.1136/jcp.2009.069252

Genetics Home Reference. (n.d.). Polymorphism. Retrieved from http://ghr.nlm.nih.gov/glossary=polymorphism

Giacomini, K., Brett, C., Altman, R., Benowitz, N., Dolan, M., Flockhart, D., … Krauss, R. (2007). The pharmacogenetics research network: From SNP discovery to clinical drug response. *Clinical Pharmacology and Therapeutics, 81*, 328–345. doi:10.1038/sj.clpt.6100087

Golan, D.E., Tashjian, A.H., Armstrong, E.J., & Armstrong, A.W. (2012). Drug metabolism. In C. Taniguchi & F.P. Guengerich (Eds.), *Principles of pharmacology: The pathophysiologic basis of drug therapy* (3rd ed., pp. 43–55). Philadelphia, PA: Wolters Kluwer Health/Lippincott Williams & Wilkins.

Higgs, J., Gambhir, N., Ramsden, S.C., Poulton, K., & Newman, W.G. (2010). Pharmacogenetic testing in the United Kingdom genetics and immunogenetics laboratories. *Genetic Testing and Molecular Biomarkers, 14,* 121–125. doi:10.1089/gtmb.2009.0156

Hiratsuka, M., Inoue, T., Omori, F., Agatsuma, Y., & Mizugaki, M. (2000). Genetic analysis of thiopurine methyltransferase polymorphism in a Japanese population. *Mutation Research/Fundamental and Molecular Mechanisms of Mutagenesis, 448,* 91–95. doi:10.1016/S0027-5107(00)00004-X

Holleman, A., Cheok, M.H., den Boer, M.L., Yang, W., Veerman, A.J., Kazemier, K.M., ... Relling, M.V. (2004). Gene-expression patterns in drug-resistant acute lymphoblastic leukemia cells and response to treatment. *New England Journal of Medicine, 351,* 533–542. doi:10.1056/NEJMoa033513

Houtsma, D., Guchelaar, H., & Gelderblom, H. (2010). Pharmacogenetics in oncology: A promising field. *Current Pharmaceutical Design, 16,* 155–163. doi:10.2174/138161210790112719

Huang, R.S., & Ratain, M.J. (2009). Pharmacogenetics and pharmacogenomics of anticancer agents. *CA: A Cancer Journal for Clinicians, 59,* 42–55. doi:10.3322/caac.20002

Ingelman-Sundberg, M., Sim, S.C., Gomez, A., & Rodriguez-Antona, C. (2007). Influence of cytochrome P450 polymorphisms on drug therapies: Pharmacogenetic, pharmacoepigenetic and clinical aspects. *Pharmacology and Therapeutics, 116,* 496–526. doi:10.1016/j.pharmthera.2007.09.004

Innocenti, F., Undevia, S.D., Iyer, L., Chen, P.X., Das, S., Kocherginsky, M., ... Rudin, C.M. (2004). Genetic variants in the UDP-glucuronosyltransferase 1A1 gene predict the risk of severe neutropenia of irinotecan. *Journal of Clinical Oncology, 22,* 1382–1388. doi:10.1200/JCO.2004.07.173

Ishibe, N., Schully, S., Freedman, A., & Ramsey, S.D. (2011). Use of Oncotype DX in women with node-positive breast cancer. *PLoS Currents, 3.* doi:10.1371/currents.RRN1249

Iyer, L., King, C.D., Whitington, P.F., Green, M.D., Roy, S.K., Tephly, T.R., ... Ratain, M.J. (1998). Genetic predisposition to the metabolism of irinotecan (CPT-11). Role of uridine diphosphate glucuronosyltransferase isoform 1A1 in the glucuronidation of its active metabolite (SN-38) in human liver microsomes. *Journal of Clinical Investigation, 101,* 847–854. doi:10.1172/JCI915

Kamau, E., Alemayehu, S., Feghali, K.C., Tolbert, L.S., Ogutu, B., & Ockenhouse, C.F. (2012). Development of a TaqMan allelic discrimination assay for detection of single nucleotides polymorphisms associated with anti-malarial drug resistance. *Malaria Journal, 112*(1), 23. doi:10.1186/1475-2875-11-23

Kaniwa, N., Kurose, K., Jinno, H., Tanaka-Kagawa, T., Saito, Y., Saeki, M., ... Hasegawa, R. (2005). Racial variability in haplotype frequencies of UGT1A1 and glucuronidation activity of a novel single nucleotide polymorphism 686C>T (P229L) found in an African-American. *Drug Metabolism and Disposition, 33,* 458–465. doi:10.1124/dmd.104.001800

Lennard, L., Lilleyman, J., Van Loon, J., & Weinshilboum, R. (1990). Genetic variation in response to 6-mercaptopurine for childhood acute lymphoblastic leukaemia. *Lancet, 336,* 225–229. doi:10.1016/0140-6736(90)91745-V

Lewis, R. (2012). *Human genetics: Concepts and applications* (10th ed.). New York, NY: McGraw-Hill.

Louie, S., & Russell, J. (2013). Biomarkers for safety assessment and clinical pharmacology. In H.-J. Lenz (Ed.), *Biomarkers in oncology: Prediction and prognosis* (pp. 381–400). New York, NY: Springer.

Lubejko, B., Good, M., Weiss, P., Schmieder, L., Leos, D., & Daugherty, P. (2011). Oncology clinical trials nursing: Developing competencies for the novice. *Clinical Journal of Oncology Nursing, 15,* 637–643. doi:10.1188/11.CJON.637-643

Massacesi, C., Terrazzino, S., Marcucci, F., Rocchi, M.B., Lippe, P., Bisonni, R., ... Leon, A. (2006). Uridine diphosphate glucuronosyl transferase 1A1 promoter polymorphism predicts the risk of gastrointestinal toxicity and fatigue induced by irinotecan-based chemotherapy. *Cancer, 106,* 1007–1016. doi:10.1002/cncr.21722

Mathijssen, R.H.J., Marsh, S., Karlsson, M.O., Xie, R., Baker, S.D., Verweij, J., ... McLeod, H.L. (2003). Irinotecan pathway genotype analysis to predict pharmacokinetics. *Clinical Cancer Research, 9,* 3246–3253. Retrieved from http://clincancerres.aacrjournals.org/content/9/9/3246.long

McLeod, H.L., Krynetski, E.Y., Relling, M.V., & Evans, W.E. (2000). Genetic polymorphism of thiopurine methyltransferase and its clinical relevance for childhood acute lymphoblastic leukemia. *Leukemia, 14,* 567–572. doi:10.1038/sj.leu.2401723

McLeod, H.L., Relling, M.V., Liu, Q., Pui, C.H., & Evans, W.E. (1995). Polymorphic thiopurine methyltransferase in erythrocytes is indicative of activity in leukemic blasts from children with acute lymphoblastic leukemia. *Blood, 85,* 1897–1902. Retrieved from http://www.bloodjournal.org/content/85/7/1897.long

McLeod, H.L., & Siva, C. (2002). The thiopurine S-methyltransferase gene locus-implications for clinical pharmacogenomics. *Pharmacogenomics, 3,* 89–98. doi:10.1517/14622416.3.1.89

Minami, H., Sai, K., Saeki, M., Saito, Y., Ozawa, S., Suzuki, K., ... Yamamoto, N. (2007). Irinotecan pharmacokinetics/pharmacodynamics and UGT1A genetic polymorphisms in Japanese: Roles of UGT1A1*6 and *28. *Pharmacogenetics and Genomics, 17,* 497–504. doi:10.1097/FPC.0b013e328014341f

Mounier-Boutoille, H., Boisdron-Celle, M., Cauchin, E., Galmiche, J., Morel, A., Gamelin, E., & Matysiak-Budnik, T. (2010). Lethal outcome of 5-fluorouracil infusion in a patient with a total DPD deficiency and a double DPYD and UTG1A1 gene mutation. *British Journal of Clinical Pharmacology, 70,* 280–283. doi:10.1111/j.1365-2125.2010.03686.x

Naeim, F., Rao, P.N., Song, S., & Grody, W.W. (2013). *Atlas of hematopathology: Morphology, immunophenotype, cytogenetics, and molecular approaches.* Waltham, MA: Elsevier Academic Press.

Nagar, S., & Blanchard, R.L. (2006). Pharmacogenetics of uridine diphosphoglucuronosyltransferase (UGT) 1A family members and its role in patient response to irinotecan. *Drug Metabolism Reviews, 38,* 393–409. doi:10.1080/03602530600739835

Nebert, D.W., Adnesik, M., Coon, M.J., Estabrook, R.W., Gonzalez, F.J., Guengerich, F.P., ... Levin, W. (1987). The P450 gene superfamily: Recommended nomenclature. *DNA, 6,* 1–11. doi:10.1089/dna.1987.6.1

Nomeir, A.A. (2010). Pharmacokinetics. In M.N. Cayen (Ed.), *Early drug development: Strategies and routes to first-in-human trials* (pp. 64–65). Hoboken, NJ: John Wiley & Sons.

Opdam, F.L., Gelderblom, H., & Guchelaar, H. (2012). Phenotyping drug disposition in oncology. *Cancer Treatment Reviews, 38,* 715–725. doi:10.1016/j.ctrv.2011.12.003

Palomaki, G.E., Bradley, L.A., Douglas, M.P., Kolor, K., & Dotson, W.D. (2009). Can UGT1A1 genotyping reduce morbidity and mortality in patients with metastatic colorectal cancer treated with irinotecan? An evidence-based review. *Genetics in Medicine, 11,* 21–34. doi:10.1097/GIM.0b013e31818efd77

Petros, W.P., & Evans, W.E. (2004). Pharmacogenomics in cancer therapy: Is host genome variability important? *Trends in Pharmacological Sciences, 25,* 457–464. doi:10.1016/j.tips.2004.07.007

Piatkov, I., Jones, T., & McLean, M. (2013). Drug interactions, pharmacogenomics and cardiovascular complication. In H.A. El-Shemy (Ed.), *Pharmacology, toxicology and pharmaceutical science.* doi:10.5772/48423

Pinto, N., Cohn, S.L., & Dolan, M.E. (2012). Using germ line genomics to individualize pediatric cancer treatments. *Clinical Cancer Research, 18,* 2791–2800. doi:10.1158/1078-0432.CCR-11-1938

Prows, C.A. (2011). Infusion of pharmacogenetics into cancer care. *Seminars in Oncology Nursing, 27,* 45–53. doi:10.1016/j.soncn.2010.11.006

Raida, M., Schwabe, W., Häusler, P., Van Kuilenburg, A.B., Van Gennip, A.H., Behnke, D., & Höffken, K. (2001). Prevalence of a common point mutation in the dihydropyrimidine dehydrogenase (DPD) gene within the 5′-splice donor site of intron 14 in patients with severe 5-fluorouracil (5-FU)-related toxicity compared with controls. *Clinical Cancer Research, 7,* 2832–2839. Retrieved from http://clincancerres.aacrjournals.org/content/7/9/2832.long

Ratain, M.J. (2006). From bedside to bench to bedside to clinical practice: An odyssey with irinotecan. *Clinical Cancer Research, 12,* 1658–1660. doi:10.1158/1078-0432.CCR-06-0159

Riegert-Johnson, D.L., Macaya, D., Hefferon, T.W., & Boardman, L.A. (2008). The incidence of duplicate genetic testing. *Genetics in Medicine, 10,* 114–116. doi:10.1097/GIM.0b013e31816166a7

Roche Molecular Diagnostics. (n.d.). AmpliChip CYP450 test. Retrieved from http://molecular.roche.com/assays/Pages/AmpliChipCYP450Test.aspx

Ross, C.J., Katzov-Eckert, H., Dubé, M., Brooks, B., Rassekh, S.R., Barhdadi, A., ... Rieder, M.J. (2009). Genetic variants in TPMT and COMT are associated with hearing loss in children receiving cisplatin chemotherapy. *Nature Genetics, 41,* 1345–1349. doi:10.1038/ng.478

Sai, K., Saeki, M., Saito, Y., Ozawa, S., Katori, N., Jinno, H., ... Komamura, K. (2004). UGT1A1 haplotypes associated with reduced glucuronidation and increased serum bilirubin in irinotecan-administered Japanese patients with cancer. *Clinical Pharmacology and Therapeutics, 75,* 501–515. doi:10.1016/j.clpt.2004.01.010

Sauna, Z.E., Kimchi-Sarfaty, C., Ambudkar, S.V., & Gottesman, M.M. (2007). Silent polymorphisms speak: How they affect pharmacogenomics and the treatment of cancer. *Cancer Research, 67,* 9609–9612. doi:10.1158/0008-5472.CAN-07-2377

Scripture, C.D., & Figg, W.D. (2006). Drug interactions in cancer therapy. *Nature Reviews Cancer, 6,* 546–558. doi:10.1038/nrc1887

Shaffer, L.G., McGowan-Jordan, J., & Schmid, M. (Eds.). (2012). *ISCN 2013: An international system for human cytogenetic nomenclature: Recommendations of the international standing committee on human cytogenetic nomenclature.* Basal, Switzerland: Karger.

Shi, M.M., Bleavins, M.R., & de la Iglesia, F.A. (2001). Pharmacogenetic application in drug development and clinical trials. *Drug Metabolism and Disposition, 29,* 591–595. Retrieved from http://dmd.aspetjournals.org/content/29/4/591.full

Stocco, G., Cheok, M., Crews, K., Dervieux, T., French, D., Pei, D., ... Relling, M. (2008). Genetic polymorphism of inosine triphosphate pyrophosphatase is a determinant of mercaptopurine metabolism and toxicity during treatment for acute lymphoblastic leukemia. *Clinical Pharmacology and Therapeutics, 85,* 164–172. doi:10.1038/clpt.2008.154

Teh, L.K., & Bertilsson, L. (2012). Pharmacogenomics of CYP2D6: Molecular genetics, interethnic differences and clinical importance. *Drug Metabolism and Pharmacokinetics, 27,* 55–67. doi:10.2133/dmpk.DMPK-11-RV-121

23andMe. (n.d.). Welcome. Retrieved from https://www.23andme.com

U.S. Department of Health and Human Services. (2012). The FDA's drug review process: Ensuring drugs are safe and effective. Retrieved from http://www.fda.gov/drugs/resourcesforyou/consumers/ucm143534.htm

U.S. National Library of Medicine. (2012). Genetics home reference handbook: What is a gene mutation and how do mutations occur? Retrieved from http://ghr.nlm.nih.gov/handbook/mutationsanddisorders/genemutation

U.S. National Library of Medicine. (2013). What are genome-wide association studies? Retrieved from http://ghr.nlm.nih.gov/handbook/genomicresearch/gwastudies

van Kuilenburg, A.B., Haasjes, J., Richel, D.J., Zoetekouw, L., Van Lenthe, H., De Abreu, R.A., ... van Gennip, A.H. (2000). Clinical implications of dihydropyrimidine dehydrogenase (DPD) deficiency in patients with severe 5-fluorouracil-associated toxicity: Identification of new mutations in the DPD gene. *Clinical Cancer Research, 6,* 4705–4712. Retrieved from http://clincancerres.aacrjournals.org/content/6/12/4705.long

Venter, J.C., Adams, M.D., Myers, E.W., Li, P.W., Mural, R.J., Sutton, G.G., ... Zhu, X. (2001). The sequence of the human genome. *Science, 291,* 1304–1351. doi:10.1126/science.1058040

Zhou, S. (2008). Structure, function and regulation of P-glycoprotein and its clinical relevance in drug disposition. *Xenobiotica, 38,* 802–832. doi:10.1080/00498250701867889

Chapter 32

Genetic Testing

Jacqueline M. Hale, MSN, APNC, APNG-BC, AOCN®

Introduction

With the onset of the Human Genome Project in 1990, the National Human Genome Research Institute (NHGRI) initiated concurrent research to "foster basic and applied research on the ethical, legal, and social implications of genetic and genomic research for individuals, families and communities" (NHGRI, 2013b). In 2003, the Human Genome Project was completed (NHGRI, 2013a). This was a monumental accomplishment in the scientific world, with technical, ethical, legal, and social implications (ELSI) for health care and society. Researchers raised concerns about ELSI associated with the potential use of genetic information for denial of healthcare insurance, workplace discrimination, interference with patient confidentiality, and potential violations of patients' rights (NHGRI, 2012a). Clinical trial nurses (CTNs) whose research area includes hereditary cancer syndromes, cancer predisposition testing, and use of genetic information must be familiar with ELSI, identification of genetic and genomic information associated with hereditary syndromes, and sampling and storage of genetic material and information as part of primary and ancillary trials. The conduct of research studies for screening, prevention and risk reduction, diagnosis, treatment, and survivorship in the hereditary cancer population promotes oncology care in this high-risk population. This chapter will discuss hereditary cancer predisposition testing and address the integration and utility of hereditary cancer predisposition information into oncology research protocols.

Hereditary Cancer Predisposition Testing

Genetics and Cancer Development

Cancer develops when genetic mutations accumulate and cells no longer undergo cell death at their normal rate. Mutations continue to accumulate, and the resultant aberrant cells continue to replicate. In hereditary cancer syndromes, a mutation can pass from one or both parents to a child through the sperm or ovum. This results in a predisposition, or increased risk, to develop cancer. Of all diagnosed cancers, 5%–10% are associated with a hereditary cancer syndrome (Santos et al., 2013). Most hereditary cancer syndrome mutations pass in an autosomal dominant manner. This means the offspring need to inherit the mutation from only one parent to express the trait (i.e., develop cancer) (Santos et al., 2013). *Penetrance* is "the proportion of individuals who will express a given trait, disorder, or disease, such as cancer" (Santos et al., 2013, p. 44). The mutations associated with hereditary cancer syndromes are highly penetrant, that is, very likely to cause one or more cancers in the lifetime of the individual and often at a younger age than in the general population.

Cancer risk assessment, genetic testing, and screening for cancer predisposition are valuable tools in the medical management of individuals identified with, or whose personal and family history are suggestive of, a hereditary cancer syndrome. This high-risk population has needs specific to the younger age at onset with increased screening, prevention, survivorship, treatment, and reproductive health education and support. When a cancer predisposition syndrome is suspected, further evaluation through tumor profiling, documentation of family history, and identification of any features suggestive of hereditary cancers will determine if cancer predisposition testing is appropriate. Genetic cancer predisposition testing can provide information for cancer risk management for an individual and the family. Predisposition testing provides information so that healthcare providers may tailor the treatment, screening, surveillance, prevention, and survivorship to the risks specific to the syndrome as compared to general population risks. Clinical trials, research registries for data collection, and genetic testing are sources of evidence to develop and support the unique and specific needs of this high-risk population (National Cancer Institute [NCI], 2015).

Cancer Predisposition Genetic Testing

The general population became more familiar with cancer predisposition genetic testing during the 1990s when specific genetic mutations associated with the development of cancer were identified (NCI, 2015). The mutations associated with hereditary breast and ovarian cancer are located on the *BRCA1* and *BRCA2* genes. The earliest identified mutations associated with Lynch syndrome, a colorectal and gynecologic cancer syndrome, are located on the *MLH1* and *MSH2* genes. Research demonstrated these mutations were associated with a marked increase in cancer incidence. Since the discovery of these genes, researchers have identified many more cancer predisposition mutations (NCI, 2015). Tests are available commercially for many of the common hereditary cancer syndromes. However, testing for suspected cancer syndromes that are less common may only be available in a clinical trial research setting.

Completion of the Human Genome Project and ongoing clinical trials now support identification of less penetrant genetic alterations in cancer predisposition genes. These gene variations may contribute to risk for several different types of cancer with a location adjacent to the location of disease-causative variants (Robson, Storm, Weitzel, Wollins, & Offitt, 2010). The clinical utility of testing for these less penetrant variants in clinical practice is limited, "but discoveries made through application of genomic technologies and the human genome have already had an effect on several aspects of oncologic practice and have influenced the design of clinical trials" (McDermott, Downing, & Stratton, 2011, p. 349).

Testing for inherited predisposition is now routine in the management and care of high-risk individuals (American Society of Clinical Oncology [ASCO], 2012; NCI, 2015; Robson et al., 2010). Germ-line DNA (the DNA inherited through the sperm or ovum and present in every cell) is the source for hereditary cancer predisposition testing and is obtained from blood or saliva. This differs from the DNA obtained from tumor tissue used for tumor profiling. DNA in tumor tissue has somatic or acquired mutations resulting from exposures, environment, age, and multiple cell divisions.

Hereditary Cancer Syndrome Identification

The decision to test for hereditary cancer predisposition syndromes is determined through careful assessment and consideration of how the outcome of testing will affect the patient and family and if the test will have clinical utility. At least three generations of family and personal medical history should be collected and documented. The addition of pathology reports, when available, can improve the accuracy of the recall of cancer history within a family and support identification of a hereditary cancer syndrome. A targeted physical examination should be included because some hereditary cancer syndromes have associated characteristic physical features (phenotypic traits), including benign features (Lindor, McMaster, Lindor, & Greene, 2008) (see Figure 32-1). CTNs who work with hereditary syndromes in clinical trials must be familiar with other features (often referred to as *red flags*) that suggest a hereditary cancer syndrome within a family (see Figure 32-2).

When to Test for Hereditary Cancer Syndromes: Contrasting Clinical Testing With Research Testing

Clinical utility is the primary determining factor in the decision to offer cancer predisposition testing in the clinical setting. The NCI algorithm to determine the appropriateness of testing illustrates this decision process (see Figure 32-3). This knowledge will assist CTNs to confirm the appropriateness of genetic testing, even in a clinical trial setting.

Figure 32-1. Cutaneous Features Associated With Hereditary Cancer Syndromes

- Cutaneous findings (trichilemmomas, lipomas, keratosis, café-au-lait spots, unusual freckling or pigmentation)
- Polyposis (colon or small bowel)
- Thyroid changes
- Macrocephaly (particularly if associated with autism)
- Tumor histology suggestive of a hereditary cancer (microsatellite instability, medullary thyroid cancer)

Note. Based on information from Lindor et al., 2008.

Figure 32-2. Hereditary Cancer Syndrome Red Flags

- Early onset of cancers that usually occur later in life (premenopausal breast cancer, colon cancer before age 50, endometrial cancer before age 50)
- Multiple primary cancers in a single individual (e.g., colon and endometrial, breast and ovarian, thyroid and endometrial, colon cancer more than once); may be synchronous or metachronous
- Bilateral cancer in paired organs or multifocal disease (e.g., bilateral or multifocal breast or renal cancer)
- Multiple relatives and/or multiple generations with the same type of cancer
- Male breast cancer
- Occurrence of rare or uncommon tumors (e.g., adrenocortical carcinoma, duodenal cancer, medullary thyroid cancer)
- Rare cancers associated with birth defects (e.g., Wilms tumor and genitourinary abnormalities)
- Ashkenazi heritage, which is associated with higher prevalence of *BRCA1/BRCA2* mutations

Note. Based on information from American Society of Clinical Oncology, 2012; National Cancer Institute, 2015.

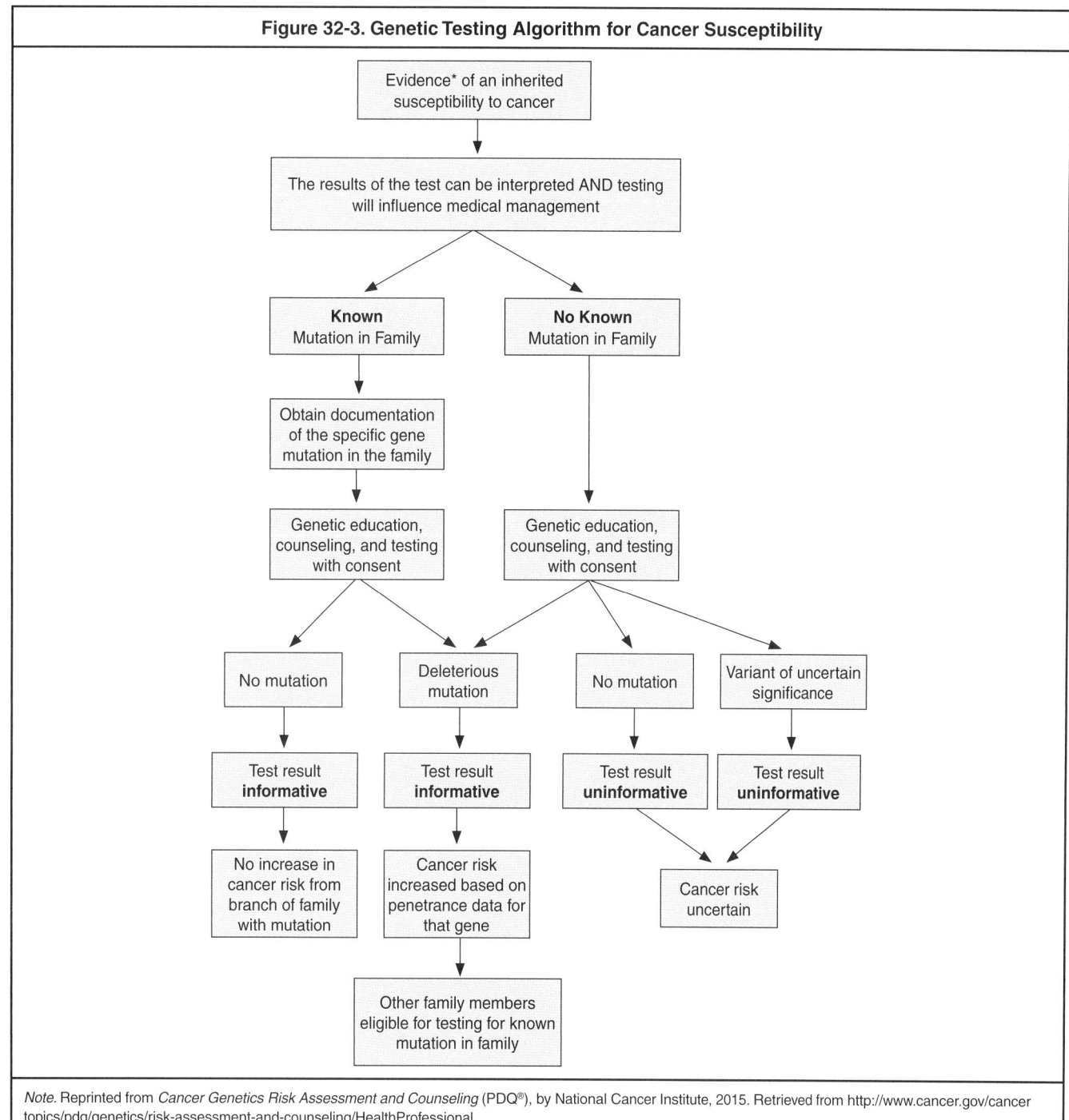

Figure 32-3. Genetic Testing Algorithm for Cancer Susceptibility

Note. Reprinted from *Cancer Genetics Risk Assessment and Counseling* (PDQ®), by National Cancer Institute, 2015. Retrieved from http://www.cancer.gov/cancertopics/pdq/genetics/risk-assessment-and-counseling/HealthProfessional.

Oncology nurses with responsibilities in research trials associated with the identification and management of hereditary cancer syndromes must understand the principles and guidelines of clinical predisposition testing (International Society of Nurses in Genetics, 2010). This essential understanding provides the foundation for educating participants in these studies. Clinical utility needs to be established through research. A 2010 ASCO position statement described the value of clinical research in cancer predisposition testing. The position noted that "prospective clinical trials, large registries, and retrospective reviews are the most accurate methods for deriving relative risks of genetic variants and measuring the response to and effectiveness of clinical interventions based on genetic cancer risk assessment" (Robson et al., 2010, p. 896). The authors encouraged research to establish evidence bases for understanding the clinical utility of genetic testing for less penetrant variants, prospective studies of genomic markers, studies of functional significance, and research to determine criteria to define the clinical utility of variants of uncertain significance. ASCO's position also encouraged research that includes behavioral and psychosocial endpoints, interactions between genetic variants (as well as with nongenetic factors), predictive accuracy, and additional psychosocial effects, as well as global and economic impact (Robson et al., 2010).

Benefits and Limitations

The physical risks for predisposition genetic testing are the same as for any blood draw via venipuncture (slight bruising, slight discomfort, low risk of infection at the venipuncture site) or buccal smear/swab or collection of saliva (potential for burning or stinging sensation if mouthwash is used). The laboratory performing the test offers instruction about the preferred or alternative collection methods. Researchers continue to investigate and evaluate the benefits and limitations of genetic tests associated with hereditary cancer syndromes, with the majority of evidence in the high-penetrance gene mutations. The existing evidence for benefits and limitations of testing for low- or intermediate-penetrance variants is limited (National Comprehensive Cancer Network®, 2015).

Identification of high-penetrance mutations can clarify risk, provide information for family members, support medical management, and more. Some individuals may not want this information or may have a negative response to a genetic test. ASCO (Robson et al., 2010), the Oncology Nursing Society (2015), and the U.S. Preventive Services Task Force (2013) recommend genetic pre- and posttest counseling. NCI (2015) supports providing counseling by a healthcare provider with genetics knowledge, noting there may be an imbalance to patient understanding of the benefits and limitations to genetic testing, resulting in an overestimation of the benefits compared to the limitations. Counseling may improve patient understanding of potential results and provide anticipatory guidance for response to results (e.g., relief, guilt, fear, anxiety). Counseling prepares patients to understand their risk for cancer when test results are uninformative or inconclusive. For example, test results are uninformative when no mutation is identified in an unaffected individual (i.e., the person has not had cancer) and no affected family member (i.e., a family member with cancer) has been tested for mutations. Test results are inconclusive when a variant of uncertain significance has been identified. Inconclusive results cannot be interpreted with confidence using existing information. Figure 32-4 lists the potential limitations and burdens of genetic testing, and Figure 32-5 lists the potential benefits.

Additional Ethical Concerns Influencing Hereditary Cancer Predisposition Testing

New discoveries, techniques, and applications of genetic and genomic information in health care, and particularly oncology care, introduced new ethical, legal, and social concerns associated with hereditary cancer syndrome testing. The World Health Organization (n.d.) stated,

> The Human Genome Project and related initiatives have introduced powerful new methods to the study of genes. Genomics has laid

---

Figure 32-4. Potential Limitations and Burdens of Genetic Testing

- Potential for uninformative result or result of uncertain significance
- May need to have other family members tested for clarification
- Lack of evidence-based guidance regarding prevention or surveillance associated with result
- Financial cost of testing and cost of increased screening or prevention measures
- Psychological distress, including anxiety, loss of self-esteem, depression
- Alteration in family communication
- Potential guilt related to transmission to children
- Survivor guilt
- Potential or perceived insurance, employment, or social discrimination (for self or extended family)
- Misunderstanding of meaning of a negative result with failure to adhere to increased screening
- Adjustment to change in expected life course
- Regret over previous decisions, such as having risk-reducing surgeries
- Family coping difficulties resulting in distress
- Identification of new information such as nonpaternity
- Feeling unprepared or not equipped to disseminate information to family
- Loss of privacy
- Failure to seek informational updates with testing advances and availability

Note. Not all instances apply to all individual situations.

Figure 32-5. Potential Benefits of Genetic Testing

- May eliminate uncertainty about inherited susceptibility
- Support for additional cancer risk management strategies, such as chemoprevention, risk-reducing surgery, or increased screening
- Opportunity to provide information to family
- Reassurance and reduction of anxiety about personal cancer risk
- Avoidance of unnecessary screening and prevention strategies
- Avoidance of aggressive interventions such as risk-reducing surgery
- Relief that children are not at increased risk
- Feeling of empowerment to obtain screening for children (in some syndromes)
- No need to rely on other family members for informative test results
- Opportunity to inform relatives about the likelihood that they have the family mutation
- Sense of overall empowerment
- Able to contribute to research
- Support for treatment decisions
- Support for family planning decisions

Note. Not all instances apply to all individual situations.

the foundations for new approaches to the diagnosis and treatment of human disease, and introduced new possibilities for reproductive choices. This progress is accompanied by important ethical and social issues. . . . Genomics is special in that gene-based approaches introduce a new language of "probability" and "susceptibility" to medical care, and furnish information about disorders that often is of great interest to third parties—be they families, governments, insurance companies, law enforcement or scientific researchers.

According to Quinn, Pal, Murphy, Vadaparampil, and Kumar (2011), genetic and genomic technology, such as prenatal diagnosis and preimplantation testing, evoke a further demand for provider-patient discussions and oncology research to investigate preimplantation genetic diagnosis for hereditary cancers. Providers and researchers, including the CTNs working face-to-face with individuals contemplating participation in a clinical trial, need to work with patients to explore knowledge and self-awareness about (a) personal choice, (b) limit setting in acceptable risk (e.g., selecting embryos based on gene mutations or variants), (c) testing of children (especially if the disorder has or is expected to have an adult-age onset), (d) testing in vulnerable populations, and (e) equal access to those with limited economic resources.

Nurses in clinical trials whose role responsibilities include provision of information about reproductive technology must be familiar with associated regulatory and policy guidelines. Katz and Schweitzer (2010) identified concerns specific to healthcare provision, policy, reproductive technology, and quality assurance, specifically (a) diffusion of genetic testing and its impact on medical practices, (b) tension between confidentiality and transparency related to health insurance, (c) expansion of genetic testing for embryo selection, and (d) evolution of regulatory frameworks for quality assurance of genetic tests.

The National Comprehensive Cancer Network (2015) recommended that patients of reproductive age should be advised about options for prenatal diagnosis and assisted reproduction, including preimplantation diagnosis, and the associated risks, benefits, and limitations of these approaches.

Informed Consent

Commercial or Nonresearch Setting

Informed consent is an element of the genetic testing process, regardless of whether it occurs in a research setting, research laboratory, or a commercial laboratory. Informed consent provides the opportunity for the provider and the individual presenting for the genetic testing to affirm that he or she has discussed essential elements of testing, including the benefits and limitations associated with potential results of the specific test (ASCO, 2012) (see Figure 32-6).

Additional discussion points often addressed during the informed consent process include an exploration of the decision made by the individual for testing and assurance that testing has been an informed personal choice. The decision must not be the result of miscommunication or coercion. The discussion must include concerns about genetic testing and limitations in the protection offered by the Health Insurance Portability and Accountability Act of 1996 (HIPAA) and the Genetic Information Nondiscrimination Act of 2008 (GINA) (discussed later in this chapter). The provider must offer the opportunity to discuss family implications and potential impact. This includes a discussion of the potential to reveal an unexpected genetic finding, such as nonpaternity. Exploration of the available medical management options provides the opportunity to review and consider anticipated responses and prepare for the results (U.S. Department of Health and Human Services [DHHS], 2003; U.S. Equal Employment Opportunity Commission [EEOC], 2008).

Figure 32-6. Elements of Informed Consent for Genetic Testing

- Process of testing (e.g., amount of blood to be drawn)
- Clarification of a person's increased risk status
- Elicitation and discussion of a person's expectations, beliefs, goals, and motivations
- Potential results (positive, negative or uninformative, true negative, or variant of uncertain significance)
- Benefits and limitations of testing
- Associated risks (e.g., unexpected results, genetic discrimination)
- Cancer risk assessment and management, if testing is not completed
- Options and anticipated medical management with or without testing (including prevention, risk reduction with chemoprevention and surgery, surveillance, and the risks, benefits, effectiveness, and limitations of the management strategies)
- Further decision making once genetic test results are received
- Time for results to become available and how results will be communicated
- Communication with family members and implications for other family members, including offspring
- Potential psychological responses and availability of counseling and support services
- Costs (testing and counseling)
- Accuracy of the test, including interpretation of results
- Privacy protection (and limitations to protection), release of results, confidentiality, and access to records
- Storage and potential use of DNA, such as for research
- Attainment of verbal and written informed consent or clarification of the decision to decline testing

Note. Based on information from Giarelli et al., 2006; Jenkins & Lea, 2005; National Cancer Institute, 2015; Robson et al., 2010.

Healthcare providers have developed several models for hereditary cancer predisposition testing and inclusion of genetic information in oncology care, as well as its implications for the family. A *second* informed consent process may be used before disclosure of genetic test results in case that person has changed his or her mind about receiving the results. Once disclosure of results occurs, a *third* informed consent discussion can address issues regarding sharing the genetic test result with healthcare providers and interested family members, either currently or in the future. Requiring written permission from the patient with the original test results to share the results with at-risk family members can avoid future problems in the event the original person is not be available to release the results (NCI, 2015).

Genetic information is defined in GINA (Definitions Specific to GINA, § 1635.3(c)(1)(i)–(v) [2014]) as information about
- An individual's genetic tests
- The genetic tests of that individual's family members
- The manifestation of disease or disorder in family members of the individual (family medical history)
- An individual's request for, or receipt of, genetic services, or the participation in clinical research that includes genetic services by the individual or a family member of the individual
- The genetic information of a fetus carried by an individual or by a pregnant woman who is a family member of the individual and the genetic information of any embryo legally held by the individual or family member using an assisted reproductive technology.

GINA also defines what genetic information *does not* include: "information about the sex or age of the individual, the sex or age of family members, or information about the race or ethnicity of the individual or family members that is not derived from a genetic test" (Definitions Specific to GINA, § 1635.3(c)(2) [2014]).

Genetic and Genomic Research Setting

Federal regulation protects human research subjects. The federal regulation in place in 2008 when GINA was passed was developed, implemented, and refined in the decades before completion of the Human Genome Project. Significant developments in technology and application of genetic and genomic information into healthcare research have stimulated interest in updating and refining the *Code of Federal Regulations*, particularly in areas of "identifiability and reconsent" as described by Edwards et al. (2012).

Technology increases utilization of genetic and genomic information and biorepository materials. Dressler et al. (2012) called for guidelines to ensure that research participants whose contributions result in actionable findings receive that information in a manner that they can use and understand. Beskow et al. (2012) offered recommendations for research recruitment subsequent to genotype information, such as hereditary cancer predisposition testing and other genetic research results.

CTNs must be prepared to discuss the ELSI that result from rapidly advancing genetic and genomic technology and application. CTNs may be responsible for discussions and answers to questions about ELSI that potential participants may have. Institutional review boards also may raise ethical questions about specific protocols, management of genetic and genomic information, and genetic testing. Researchers and clinicians could have concerns about competent disclosure of incidental genetic findings, significant new findings, and individual research results if provisions for such disclosure were not included in the original consent document (Simon, Shinkunas, Brandt, & Williams, 2012). Consent forms created as these concerns are recognized incorporate language to address the concerns, but this does not cover older consents (Simon et al., 2012).

The standard elements of informed consent described in Chapter 14 can include specific content to address concerns associated with genetic studies (NHGRI, 2012b). The informed consent includes discussion specific to the genetic content of the research and promoting participant understanding. The consent document clarifies the measures designed to protect the individual who is providing the genetic material and information. If samples are being collected and used for research purposes, or if samples may be associated with or linked to an individual, then informed consent must be obtained from the *donor*, unless waived by the institutional review board that oversees the research (NHGRI, 2012b). This information should be reviewed and discussed in depth with the research participant during the consent process.

Informed consent is an important aspect of any genetic test or research study. NHGRI is a strong proponent of careful counseling of patients who are receiving genetic testing (NHGRI, 2012c). Figure 32-7 includes recommended additions to the required components of informed consent for research using genetic material, information, and testing under the *Code of Federal Regulations* effective in 2012 (NHGRI, 2012c).

NHGRI (2012b) summarizes the essential elements and comprehensive purpose of the informed consent document, which include the following.
- Patients must be informed of the test's purpose, medical implications, alternatives, and possible risks and benefits.

- Patients must be given information about privacy rights, location of DNA storage, and who will have access to their personal information.
- Even after signing, patients may still opt out of the test or study.
- The informed consent document is not a contract.
- A patient signature is required.

The U.S. DHHS (2008) guidelines that give direction for the conduct of human subject research also include guidelines for research with biologic materials. Coded information that cannot be linked by the researcher to the participant is not considered human subject research. This definition applies to information (a) with no personal identifiers; (b) if coded, the researcher does not have the code; (c) if subjects are alive, the code cannot be released; and (d) policies and procedures are in place that prevent release of the code (U.S. DHHS, 2008).

Protection Against Discrimination

Historically, patients and healthcare providers alike expressed significant concern about the potential consequences of genetic testing. HIPAA and GINA have addressed many of these concerns. These acts contain significant, although not complete, protection against discrimination and against disclosure of health information without consent (U.S. DHHS, 2003; U.S. EEOC, 2008). CTNs should be familiar with the content of these acts so they can educate patients and other care providers. The essential informed consent elements explain the measures taken to protect against discrimination because of research participation. However, testing for hereditary cancer predisposition has an impact on family members as well as the tested individual. If the extended family was not included in the education, counseling, consenting, or disclosure discussions, they may not have full understanding of the protections or limitations of these acts. NHGRI (2011) suggested that further research is needed to more fully understand public perceptions, the effect of genomic research on family members, communication of results, genetic discrimination and stigmatization, and other ELSI topics.

Legislative Protection

The first federal-level legislation to address privacy concerns such as those associated with genetic testing was HIPAA in 1996. This act first required development of standards to protect against inappropriate use and disclosure of personal health information. Subsequent to this first requirement, the Privacy Rule came into effect on April 14, 2003. Genetic information is treated as all other personal health information within the Privacy Rule. The Privacy Rule did not preempt any state laws that were more stringent; some state laws prevailed over the Privacy Rule. Concerns persisted about the potential for misuse or abuse of the information that was obtained because of evolving technology. In 2008, GINA was passed. This law protects against discrimination by health insurers and employers based on genetic information. GINA does not include protection from discrimination based on genetic information in applications for life insurance, disability insurance, and long-term care insurance (see Figure 32-8). CTNs should be familiar with this significant legislation and its provisions, limitations, and implications for genetic testing in the research setting.

Figure 32-7. Informed Consent Elements Tailored to Genomic Clinical Trials Research

Language Explaining the Purpose
- Brief description of the genomic science supporting the research
- Type of any samples needed, as well as collection, storage, and length of storage
- Coding or de-identification and use of personal health information
- Access by other researchers
- Future contact provisions, if any
- Whether genome-wide association studies (GWAS) data-sharing is included

Financial Information
- Compensation
- Costs
- If compensation for any research injury is available
- If participants will receive any portion of the profit generated from a research discovery or product

Potential Benefits and Risks
- Personal versus societal benefit
- Psychological risks (may affect participant and family)
- Disclosure of information, including unintended disclosure
- The possibility of loss of privacy

Confidentiality
- Measures taken to protect confidentiality
- Potential for and circumstances of possible disclosure

Return of Results and/or Incidental Findings
- Description of the plan to release incidental findings, new relevant discoveries, findings of no or undetermined clinical utility, and significant findings
- Plan for disclosure of individual findings
- Plan for disclosure of group findings
- Potential participants' right "not to know," if that is their election

Withdrawal, Alternatives, and Voluntary Participation
- Information specifying that removal or elimination of data released and associated with individual DNA may not be possible if participant withdraws
- Destruction of data and samples, if possible
- Storage and use of specific data

Note. Based on information from National Human Genome Research Institute, 2012c.

Figure 32-8. Key Points of the Genetic Information Nondiscrimination Act of 2008

Prohibits
- Use of genetic information for decisions regarding hiring, promotion, terms of employment, compensation, or termination
- Use of genetic information to limit, segregate, or classify an employee or deprive an individual of employment opportunities
- Collection of genetic information of the individual or a family member (there are some exceptions)
- Refusal, or declining referral, of an individual for employment based on genetic information
- Use of genetic information for admission to apprenticeships or training and retraining, including on-the-job training
- Requirement of genetic information for eligibility, coverage, underwriting, or premium-setting decisions
- Use of genetic information to make either enrollment or coverage decisions
- Requirement of genetic testing for insurance purposes

Does Not
- Apply to members of the U.S. military, veterans obtaining health care through the Veterans Health Administration, the Indian Health Service, or federal employees obtaining health care through Federal Employees Health Benefits Program plans
- Apply to life, disability, or long-term care insurance
- Apply to small group insurers (less than 15 employees)
- Apply to individual manifested symptoms (regardless if genetically based)
- Override any more stringent state laws

Note. Based on information from Genetic Information Nondiscrimination Act of 2008, 29 C.F.R. pt. 1635 (2011).

Genetic Testing of Children

When families have a history of genetics-related illness, it is imperative that they consider the potential benefits versus the risks when considering genetic testing in children. This is especially true when working with hereditary cancer syndromes that increase the risk of childhood cancers, as well as those that are not expected to increase this risk. Nurses working with hereditary cancer syndromes must be thorough in completing and updating family histories. A thorough pedigree and updated history is an essential tool for assessing the family and can serve as the defining element in understanding any unusual presentation, such as unexpected childhood onset of cancer within an individual family. The American Academy of Pediatrics and the American College of Medical Genetics and Genomics released a joint policy statement in 2013 that addressed the concerns associated with genetic testing in children. The policy guidelines are not oncology specific but are applicable to hereditary cancer syndrome testing (American Academy of Pediatrics & American College of Medical Genetics and Genomics, 2013).

Key points relevant to testing for hereditary cancer syndromes in children include the following.
- Consider the best interests of the child.
- Include genetic counseling.
- Keep parents well informed and have the child assent when possible.
- Obtain diagnostic and predictive testing, if indicated.
- In instances of adult-onset illness, defer testing until adulthood, unless the best interest of the child indicates need.

Hereditary Cancer Predisposition Testing in Clinical Trials

Several types of clinical trials in oncology exist and are classified based on the study's primary purpose. Trial types include treatment, prevention, screening, diagnostic, and quality-of-life or supportive care (NCI, 2012).

Treatment Trials

Treatment trials include the use of chemotherapy, radiation therapy, surgery, vaccines, or stimulation of the immune system (NCI, 2012). Tumor (or molecular) profiling includes the evaluation of genomic, proteomic, and epigenomic expression factors (Santos et al., 2013).

Individual characteristics, such as protein expression and DNA replication errors in normal tissue and tumor tissue, can be indicators of an inherited increased risk for cancer and predictors of response to selected therapies. Researchers investigate single nucleotide polymorphisms, which are genetic variations on a single nucleotide base, to understand genetic variation among humans as well as *epigenetics*, factors that alter gene expression. This research contributed to the understanding of risk, prognosis, and responses to therapy (Santos et al., 2013).

Prevention Trials

Research to reduce the incidence of cancer in individuals with a hereditary predisposition to cancer explores many options, including risk reduction through lifestyle changes, chemoprevention, risk-reducing surgery, and increased surveillance with management (e.g., polyp removal). Many prevention studies target epigenetic factors to prevent new or recurrent cancers or precursor lesions.

Screening Trials

Red-flag features, such as earlier-age onset of cancers, bilateral occurrences in paired organs, synchronous occurrences, and the diagnosis of rare or unusual cancers, are the hallmarks of hereditary cancer syndromes. These cancers often present in organs not routinely screened for cancer in the general population. Research studies, including registries that collect data and investigate the effectiveness of screening on high-risk populations, are essential to refining risks and improving cancer risk management, survivorship, and surveillance for people at high risk for cancer (Travis et al., 2006).

Diagnostic Trials

Diagnostic trials study new tests or procedures that may help to identify or diagnose cancer more accurately. Diagnostic trials usually involve people who have signs or symptoms of cancer. Some cancers with increased incidence in hereditary cancer syndromes, such as pancreatic, fallopian tube, ovarian, and small bowel cancers, are difficult to identify and diagnose in early stages. Clinical trials designed to test and establish efficacy of diagnostic measures contribute to improved management of hereditary cancer syndromes.

Quality-of-Life or Supportive Care Trials

Quality-of-life trials focus on the comfort and quality of life of patients with cancer and cancer survivors. These trials often study new ways to decrease the number or severity of side effects of cancer or its treatment. How a specific type of cancer or its treatment affects a person's everyday life also may be studied. Ongoing studies in the development of secondary cancers, treatment effects, and psychosocial concerns associated with hereditary cancer syndromes can be included in quality-of-life and supportive care studies (Travis et al., 2006).

Commercial DNA Banking

Clinicians engaged in hereditary cancer syndrome assessment, testing, and research are increasingly discussing DNA banking outside of the research setting (Quillin, Bodurtha, Siminoff, & Smith, 2011). DNA banking is becoming common in clinical trials if a hereditary cancer syndrome is suspected but available testing has not identified a mutation. CTNs engaged in hereditary cancer syndrome testing within a clinical trial may be called on to facilitate DNA banking. See Chapter 35 for more information on storage of genetic material.

Implications for Clinical Trial Nurses

The evolution of genetics and genomics greatly affects the role of nurses in clinical trials. It is imperative that all nurses are knowledgeable about the role that genetics plays in health care. The American Nurses Association described the basic competencies in genetics and genomics for all nurses in *Essentials of Genetic and Genomic Nursing: Competencies, Curricula Guidelines, and Outcome Indicators,* first published in 2005 and updated with a second edition in 2008. In 2012, the American Nurses Association issued *Essential Genetic and Genomic Competencies for Nurses With Graduate Degrees* (Greco, Tinley, & Seibert, 2012). Oncology CTNs must have an understanding consistent with the essential competencies of genetics and how those work together with competencies established for CTNs (Oncology Nursing Society, 2010). Nurses participating in genetic testing for hereditary cancer predisposition demonstrate additional expertise.

Summary

Hereditary cancer predisposition testing is increasingly available for clinical trials research into hereditary cancer syndromes. More than 50 hereditary cancer syndromes have been identified (Lindor et al., 2008). Interest in hereditary cancer syndromes should continue to be driven by research leading to knowledge about the effects and functional impact of highly penetrant genetic mutations that are now better understood than those of less penetrant, less common variants. CTNs involved in hereditary cancer syndrome testing must have a thorough knowledge of the effect of genetic changes, patterns of inheritance, personal health information, HIPAA, GINA, red flags for hereditary cancers, and the rights of research participants, especially in management of genetic information in a time of rapidly advancing technology. To do so, CTNs must stay abreast of ELSI within the field, as well as opinions and adaptations considered for the management of information (researcher- and legislature-driven), and regulatory changes that influence researchers and participants. Nurses, including those in clinical trials, should receive specialized and advanced preparation in hereditary cancer syndrome genetics and should practice within the scope of their role preparation (Greco et al., 2012).

Key Points
- CTNs involved in the use of genetic information must be familiar with ELSI, hereditary syndromes, and sampling and storage of genetic material and information.
- Clinical trials, research registries, and genetic testing are sources of evidence to develop and support the needs of high-risk hereditary cancer predisposition populations.
- Key features (cancerous and benign) of hereditary cancer syndromes are red flag indicators to suggest patients and families for cancer predisposition genetic testing.

- Continued research is required to refine the interpretation, clinical utility, and the ethical, legal, psychosocial, global, and economic implications of genetic testing and use of genetic information.
- Patient education and counseling (pre- and post-test) are essential elements of management of hereditary cancer syndromes and associated genetic testing.
- Federal and state regulations are in place to protect human research subjects' privacy and the use of their genetic information.
- HIPAA and GINA contain significant, although not complete, protection against discrimination and disclosure of health information without consent.
- Genetic testing in children presents unique concerns and should focus on the best interests of the child.
- Genetic testing in clinical trials supports treatment, screening, prevention, diagnosis, and quality-of-life research.
- CTNs must have a basic understanding of genetics. Nurses working with genetic testing for hereditary cancer predisposition should demonstrate additional expertise and preparation.

References

American Academy of Pediatrics & American College of Medical Genetics and Genomics. (2013). Ethical and policy issues in genetic testing and screening of children. *Pediatrics, 131,* 620–622. doi:10.1542/peds.2012-3680

American Nurses Association. (2008). *Essentials of genetic and genomic nursing: Competencies, curricula guidelines, and outcome indicators* (2nd ed.). Retrieved from http://www.nursingworld.org/MainMenuCategories/EthicsStandards/Genetics-1/EssentialNursingCompetenciesandCurriculaGuidelinesforGeneticsandGenomics.pdf

American Society of Clinical Oncology. (2012, March). Genetic testing. Retrieved from http://www.cancer.net/all-about-cancer/genetics/genetic-testing

Beskow, L.M., Fullerton, S.M., Namey, E.E., Nelson, D.K., Davis, A.M., & Wilfond, B.S. (2012). Recommendations for ethical approaches to genotype-driven research recruitment. *Human Genetics, 131,* 1423–1431. doi:10.1007/s00439-012-1177-z

Definitions specific to GINA, 29 C.F.R. § 1635.3 (2014). Retrieved from http://www.ecfr.gov/cgi-bin/text-idx?SID=59748b93fd9f7038406e7a644c5c627b&node=se29.4.1635_13&rgn=div8

Dressler, L., Smolek, S., Ponsaran, R., Markey, J., Starks, H., Gerson, N., … Weisner, G. (2012). IRB perspectives on the return of individual results from genomic research. *Genetics in Medicine, 14,* 215–222. doi:10.1038/gim.2011.10

Edwards, K., Lemke, A., Trinidad, S., Lewis, S., Starks, H., Snapinn, K., … Burke, W. (2012). Genetics researchers' and IRB professionals' attitudes toward genetic research review: A comparative analysis. *Genetics in Medicine, 14,* 236–242. doi:10.1038/gim.2011.57

Genetic Information Nondiscrimination Act of 2008, 29 C.F.R. pt. 1635 (2011). Retrieved from http://www.gpo.gov/fdsys/pkg/CFR-2011-title29-vol4/xml/CFR-2011-title29-vol4-part1635.xml

Giarelli, E., Lea, D.H., Jones, S.L., & Lewis, J.A. (2006). Genetic technology: The frontiers of nursing ethics. In V.D. Lachman (Ed.), *Applied ethics in nursing* (pp. 61–80). New York, NY: Springer.

Greco, K.E., Tinley, S., & Seibert, D. (2012). *Essential genetic and genomic competencies for nurses with graduate degrees.* Retrieved from http://nursingworld.org/MainMenuCategories/EthicsStandards/Genetics-1/Essential-Genetic-and-Genomic-Competencies-for-Nurses-With-Graduate-Degrees.pdf

International Society of Nurses in Genetics. (2010). *Access to genomic healthcare: The role of the nurse.* Retrieved from http://www.isong.org/ISONG_PS_access_genomic_healthcare.php

Jenkins, J.F., & Lea, D.H. (2005). *Nursing care in the genomic era: A case-based approach.* Burlington, MA: Jones & Bartlett Learning.

Katz, G., & Schweitzer, S.O. (2010). Implications of genetic testing for health policy. *Yale Journal of Health Policy, Law, and Ethics, 10,* Article 2. Retrieved from http://digitalcommons.law.yale.edu/yjhple/vol10/iss1/2

Lindor, N.M., McMaster, M.L., Lindor, C.J., & Greene, M.H. (2008). Concise handbook of familial cancer susceptibility syndromes—second edition. *Journal of the National Cancer Institute Monographs, 2008*(38), 3–93. doi:10.1093/jncimonographs/lgn001

McDermott, U., Downing, J., & Stratton, M.R. (2011). Genomics and the continuum of cancer care. *New England Journal of Medicine, 364,* 340–350. doi:10.1056/NEJMra0907178

National Cancer Institute. (2012). Types of clinical trials. Retrieved from http://www.cancer.gov/clinicaltrials/learningabout/what-are-clinical-trials/types

National Cancer Institute. (2015, March 31). Cancer genetics risk assessment and counseling (PDQ®). Retrieved from http://www.cancer.gov/cancertopics/pdq/genetics/risk-assessment-and-counseling/HealthProfessional/page1/AllPages

National Comprehensive Cancer Network. (2015). *NCCN Clinical Practice Guidelines in Oncology (NCCN Guidelines®): Genetic/familial high-risk assessment: Breast and ovarian* [v.1.2015]. Retrieved from http://www.nccn.org/professionals/physician_gls/pdf/genetics_screening.pdf

National Human Genome Research Institute. (2011). ELSI research priorities and possible research topics. Retrieved from http://www.genome.gov/27543732

National Human Genome Research Institute. (2012a, May). ELSI planning and evaluation history. Retrieved from http://www.genome.gov/10001754

National Human Genome Research Institute. (2012b, February). Informed consent. Retrieved from http://www.genome.gov/10002332

National Human Genome Research Institute. (2012c, May). Informed consent elements tailored to genomic research. Retrieved from http://www.genome.gov/27026589

National Human Genome Research Institute. (2013a, January). All about the Human Genome Project. Retrieved from http://www.genome.gov/10001772#al-2

National Human Genome Research Institute. (2013b, April). The Ethical, Legal and Social Implications (ELSI) Research Program. Retrieved from http://www.genome.gov/10001618

Oncology Nursing Society. (2010). *Oncology clinical trials nurse competencies.* Retrieved from https://www.ons.org/sites/default/files/ctncompetencies.pdf

Oncology Nursing Society. (2015, January). Oncology nursing: The application of cancer genetics and genomics throughout the oncology care continuum. Retrieved from https://www.ons.org/advocacy-policy/positions/education/genetics

Quillin, J., Bodurtha, J., Siminoff, L., & Smith, T. (2011). Physicians' current practices and opportunities for DNA banking of dying patients with cancer. *Journal of Oncology Practice, 7,* 183–187.

Quinn, G., Pal, T., Murphy, D., Vadaparampil, S., & Kumar, A. (2011). High-risk consumers' perceptions of preimplantation genetic diagnosis for hereditary cancers: A systematic review and meta-analysis. *Genetics in Medicine, 14,* 191–200.

Robson, M., Storm, C., Weitzel, J., Wollins, D., & Offitt, K. (2010). American Society of Clinical Oncology policy statement update: Genetic and genomic testing for cancer susceptibility. *Journal of Clinical Oncology, 28,* 893–901. doi:10.1200/JCO.2009.27.0660

Santos, E.M.M., Edwards, Q.T., Floria-Santos, M., Rogatto, S.R., Achatz, M.I.W., & MacDonald, D.J. (2013). Integration of genomics in cancer care. *Journal of Nursing Scholarship, 45,* 43–51. doi:10.1111/j.1547-5069.2012.01465.x

Simon, C., Shinkunas, L.A., Brandt, D., & Williams, J.K. (2012). Individual genetic and genomic research results and the tradition of informed consent: Exploring US review board guidance. *Journal of Medical Ethics, 38,* 417–422. doi:10.1136/medethics-2011-100273

Travis, L.B., Rabkin, C.S., Brown, L.M., Allan, J.M., Alter, B.P., Ambrosone, C.B., ... Greene, M.H. (2006). Cancer survivorship—Genetic susceptibility and second primary cancers: Research strategies and recommendations. *Journal of the National Cancer Institute, 98,* 15–25. doi:10.1093/jnci/djj001

U.S. Department of Health and Human Services. (2003). Summary of the HIPAA Privacy Rule. Retrieved from http://www.hhs.gov/ocr/privacy/hipaa/understanding/summary/privacysummary.pdf

U.S. Department of Health and Human Services. (2008, October 16). Guidance on engagement of institutions in human subjects research. Retrieved from http://www.hhs.gov/ohrp/policy/engage08.html

U.S. Equal Employment Opportunity Commission. (2008). Genetic Information Nondiscrimination Act of 2008. Retrieved from http://www.eeoc.gov/laws/statutes/gina.cfm

U.S. Preventive Services Task Force. (2013, December). *BRCA*-related cancer: Risk assessment, genetic counseling, and genetic testing. Retrieved from http://www.uspreventiveservicestaskforce.org/Page/Topic/recommendation-summary/brca-related-cancer-risk-assessment-genetic-counseling-and-genetic-testing?ds=1&s=brca

World Health Organization. (n.d.). Ethical, legal and social implications (ELSI) of human genomics. Retrieved from http://www.who.int/genomics/elsi/en

Chapter 33

Cytogenetics

Sourat Darabi, PhD(c), and Julia A. Eggert, PhD, GNP-BC, AGN-BC, AOCN®

Introduction

Cytogenetics is a discipline in genetics that focuses on the study of chromosomes and their variations (Jorde, Carey, & Bamshad, 2009). Diagnostic cytogenetics was introduced to the United States by Victor McKusick, MD, into the division of medical genetics at Johns Hopkins in 1958 (Liu et al., 2012). One of the initial discoveries by Tijo and Levan in 1956 corrected the number of human diploid (N = 46) chromosomes (Dyce & O'Connor, 1998). Advances in molecular technology have led to the identification of several chromosome abnormalities and, in recent years, has been an important partner in the diagnosis of human disease, especially in hematologic oncology (Speicher & Carter, 2005). Clinical trial nurses (CTNs) are required to understand the nomenclature, apply the information to hematologic malignancy test results, and communicate the information to patients, families, and colleagues. For detailed information about genetics and chromosome abnormalities, refer to Chapter 31.

Chromosome Banding Techniques

Banding techniques determine chromosome abnormalities by analyzing the chromosome in metaphase with staining techniques (Speicher & Carter, 2005). These techniques include Giemsa banding (G-banding, named for Dr. Giemsa), quinacrine banding (Q-banding), centromeric banding (C-banding), reverse banding (R-banding), and nuclear organizing region stains (NOR stains) (Heim & Mitelman, 2011; Speicher & Carter, 2005).

The Giemsa method is widely used to detect chromosomal aberrations such as deletions, translocations, and insertions. This refers to the dark and light bands commonly seen in karyotypes. Trypsin is used in order to digest histones (proteins that fold DNA and aid with the formation of chromatin) that hold the chromosome together, which helps guanine and cytosine (GC)-rich regions in DNA relax and absorb the Giemsa stain. The order and size of bands specific to each chromosome are then visualized and can be compared to other homologous chromosomes. The G-banding method is simple, and the stained DNA can be stored for a long period of time (Sheth et al., 2014; Speicher & Carter, 2005).

Q-banding was the first banding method and requires a fluorescence microscope. Quinacrine mustard, an alkylating agent, is used for this technique. Q-banding method stains GC-rich regions on DNA (same as G-banding). One of the disadvantages of this technique is that it fades quickly and is not permanent (Snustad & Simmons, 2009; Speicher & Carter, 2005).

C-banding method is specialized in heterochromatin staining, and it uses Giemsa stain as well. First, the cell is treated with acid and then with alkali. The C-banding method is used to identify centromeres.

R-banding stains the chromosomes in the opposite way to Q and G banding and is specifically useful for staining chromosomal rearrangements at the ends of the chromosome. The cells are treated with a hot salt solution in order to denature the adenine and thymine–rich region of DNA, which then will be stained with Giemsa.

Fluorescence in situ hybridization (FISH) is a widely used technique where a single strand of DNA is labeled with a probe and hybridized to a chromosome in interphase, metaphase, or prophase because chromosomes are clearer and condensed in these stages. The probes are labeled and the chromosomes can be detected under the fluorescence microscope. FISH is used mainly to detect deletions, duplications, and chromosomal rearrangements. Multiple probes may be used in the technique to help diagnose several chromosomal abnormalities (Speicher & Carter, 2005).

Cancer Genetics

Cancer is a group of disorders resulting from gene alterations (You & Jones, 2012). The gene mutations associated with cancer are divided into three groups: (a) inherited cancer genes caused by germ-line mutations and located in each cell, (b) somatic mutations, which are acquired over time, found in some cells, and cause sporadic cancers, and (c) mutations associated with viral infections (Ellisen & Haber, 2010). The main characteristic of all cancers is abnormal cell growth (Speicher & Carter, 2005). The abnormal cell growth associated with any of the aforementioned mutations can lead to the formation of malignant tumors. The nomenclature of tumors is based on their tissue of origin: tumors derived from epithelial tissue are called *carcinomas*; *lymphomas* are from lymphatic tissue; *sarcomas* originated in connective tissue; *leukemias* are hematopoietic; and *gliomas* are derived from the neurogliacyte primarily in the central nervous system (Mitelman, Johansson, & Mertens, 2013).

Chromosome Alterations in Cancers

The 1970s was a decade of advances in molecular genetic techniques such as decoding DNA and understanding of tumorigenesis (Genome News Network, 2013). Knowledge growth in genetics and molecular signaling, especially since the completion of the sequencing of the human genome in 2003, has improved oncology care with clinical trials that focused on the prevention, early detection, diagnosis, and treatment of cancer (Heim & Mitelman, 2011). Mutations in oncogenes and tumor suppressor genes are precursors to changes in signaling pathways resulting in cancer development. The alteration of these genes by several mechanisms such as deletion, translocation, duplication, and inversion leads to chromosomal aberrations and, eventually, excessive growth and tumor formation. Several other genes are involved in cancer development, including the genes that regulate *apoptosis* (programmed cell death) and cell proliferation. Apoptosis is regulated by several cellular and biochemical processes; hence, any changes in these processes can cause interruption to the pathway and eventually manifestation of a disease (Zhivotovsky & Orrenius, 2006).

Leukemia

Leukemias are a group of cancers that develop in blood cells and manifest in children as well as adults. Simply, there are four different categories of leukemias found in the lymphocytic and myeloid cell lineages. The myeloid lineages generally are acute myeloid leukemia (AML) and chronic myeloid leukemia (CML), and the lymphoid lineages are chronic lymphocytic leukemia (CLL) and acute lymphocytic leukemia (ALL). The Philadelphia chromosome, AML, CML, and CLL are most common in adults, and ALL is mostly seen in children (Ellisen & Haber, 2010). However, there are many subtypes that require a nomenclature for chromosomes (see Table 33-1) to carefully provide markers for diagnosis and prognosis of those abnormal subtypes of growing cell populations. Careful awareness of the chromosome nomenclature will enable CTNs to discriminate among the different aberrations associated with hematologic malignancies and the variations seen within them.

Acute Myeloid Leukemia

Changes in the hematopoietic progenitor cells and the accumulation of acquired genetic alterations lead to AML. The karyotype is important to establish the genetic background for staging AML and identifying a personalized treatment as quickly as possible. A study by Mrózek Marcucci, Paschka, Whitman, and Bloomfield (2007) revealed that most patients with AML have at least one chromosomal aberration in their bone marrow. According to the World Health Organization classification of AML, several chromosomal aberrations are linked to AML (Mrózek et al., 2007):

Table 33-1. Common Cytogenetic Nomenclature	
Nomenclature	Meaning
,	Separates sections in nomenclature
( )	Surround structurally altered chromosomes and breakpoints
+	Gain of chromosome
-	Loss of chromosome
;	Separates rearranged chromosomes and breakpoints when more than one chromosome is involved
Del	Deletion
dn	New chromosomal abnormality; not inherited from parents
Dup	Duplication of a portion of a chromosome
Ins	Insertion of a portion of a chromosome
Inv	Inversion
Mar	Marker (Unidentifiable piece of chromosome)
T	Translocation
Tri	Trisomy
Trp	Triplication of a chromosome piece

Note. Table courtesy of UW Cytogenetics/Wisconsin State Laboratory of Hygiene, © Board of Regents of the University of Wisconsin System. Used with permission.

- t(8;21)(q22;q22)
- Abnormal bone marrow eosinophils and inv(16)(p13;q22) or t(16;16)(p13;q22)
- t(15;17)(q22;q12)
- 11q23 (MLL) abnormalities.

Several clinical trials study AML; different cytogenetic factors are critical for their inclusion and exclusion criteria and require CTNs to understand how to interpret bone marrow results—for example, high-risk AML in a patient with one or more risk factors, including Fms-like tyrosine kinase 3 (FLT-3) mutation, complex cytogenetics, abn(3q), -5/5q, -7/7q, abn(12p), abn(17p), and the secondary AML (Mrózek et al., 2007).

Philadelphia Chromosome

An example of translocation is seen in the cytogenetic report in patients with CML and ALL. The translocation between chromosomes 9 and 22 will result in Philadelphia (Ph) chromosome and is designated as t(9;22)(q34;q11). The translocation of the Abelson (*ABL*) gene on chromosome 9 to the B-cell receptor (*BCR*) gene located at chromosome 22 causes CML, which is a clonal myeloproliferative neoplasia (Cardama, Kantarjian, & Cortes, 2013).

Multiple Myeloma

Multiple myeloma, a proliferation of plasma cells, remains incurable. The severity of the disease can be determined by the genetic factors of the plasma cells. Cytogenetics of multiple myeloma includes several translocations, deletions, trisomies, and del17p13. Further disease diagnosis by subgroups and the appropriate treatments are based on the genetic defects of the disease (Kyrtsonis, Bartzis, & Papanikolaou, 2010).

Diagnosis Guidelines

The National Comprehensive Cancer Network® (2014a, 2014b) *Clinical Practice Guidelines in Oncology* for non-Hodgkin lymphomas and for AML are practical guidelines for the management of cancer and include recommendations for the assessment of cytogenetic abnormalities for certain tumor types, which may be useful in diagnosis, risk classification, and the treatment decision process. Table 33-2 shows the suggested recommendations for some cancer types.

Summary

Advances in the study of cytogenetics have enabled a greater understanding of diseases with growing familiarity of genetic components. Cytogenetics has added more specificity to the identification of chromosomes and their abnormalities. In particular, advancement in molecular technology has made it possible to detect abnormalities in chromosomes and the diagnosis of diseases. Scientists use many staining techniques for detection of abnormalities on chromosomes. This chapter described the basic cytogenetic concepts and techniques used to detect variations; for the researcher, the information included described how to interpret cytogenetic results, for example the *BRCA1* gene is located on band 21 of the long arm of chromosome 17 (17q21). Cytogenetics was recently used to identify more disease specificities such as high-risk or low-risk status for recurrence of diseases like multiple myeloma. The growth in cytogenetics emphasizes the role of CTNs to educate, provide informed consent about the complex and often confus-

Table 33-2. Recommendations for Evaluation of Cytogenetic Abnormalities in a Sample of Cancers

No.	Cancer Type	Cytogenetics
1	Chronic lymphocytic leukemia (CLL)/small lymphocytic leukemia	t(11;14), t(11q;v), +12, del(11q), del(13q), del(17p)
2	Follicular lymphoma	t(14;18), t(8;14)
3	Gastric mucosa-associated lymphoid tissue (MALT) lymphoma	t(11;18), t(1;14), t(14;18), t(3;14)
4	Nongastric MALT lymphoma	t(11;18), t(11;14), t(3;14), t(14;18)
5	Nodal marginal zone lymphoma	t(11;18), t(1;14), t(14;18), del(13q), del(7q)
6	Splenic marginal zone lymphoma	CLL panel, t(11;18), t(11;14), t(14;18), del(7q)
7	Mantle cell lymphoma	CLL panel, t(11;14), t(14;18)
8	Diffuse large B-cell lymphoma	t(14;18), t(3;v), t(8;14)
9	Lymphoblastic lymphoma	*MYC*, t(9;22), t(8;14) or variants
10	Acute myeloid leukemia	Better risk: inv(16), t(16;16), t(8;21), t(15;17) Intermediate risk: normal cytogenetics, +8 Poor risk: -5, 5q-, -7, 7q-, 11q23-non t(9;11), inv(3), t(3;3), t(6;9), t(9;22), complex (3 or more clonal chromosomal abnormalities), and monosomal karyotype

Note. Based on information from National Comprehensive Cancer Network®, 2014a, 2014b.

ing aberrations associated with a disease, manage clinical trials of diseases in this specialty with confidence, document cytogenetic results with the assurance that the communication is accurate, and offer clarity to colleagues, patients, and families.

Key Points

- Cytogenetics studies chromosomes and their variations.
- Chromosome banding techniques help with identification of chromosome abnormalities.
- Cancer genetics covers gene mutations and their association with cancer.
- Chromosome alterations in cancer explain the molecular mechanism of mutations and their correlation with disease, including cancer.
- CTNs need to understand and be able to use chromosomal nomenclature to adequately manage their patients in clinical trials with a hematologic malignancy protocol.

References

Cardama, A.Q., Kantarjian, H., & Cortes, J. (2013). Molecular biology and cytogenetics of chronic myeloid leukemia. In P.H. Wierrik, J.M. Goldman, J. Dutcher, & R.A. Kyle (Eds.), *Neoplastic diseases of the blood* (pp. 29–44). New York, NY: Springer.

Dyce, J.A., & O'Connor, B.P. (1998). Personality disorders and the five-factor model: A test of facet-level predictions. *Journal of Personality Disorders, 12*(1), 31–45.

Ellisen, L.W., & Haber, D.A. (2010). Basic principles of cancer genetics. In D.C. Chung & D.A. Haber (Eds.), *Principles of clinical cancer genetics* (pp. 1–22). New York, NY: Springer.

Genome News Network. (2013). Genetics and genomics timeline. Retrieved from http://www.genomenewsnetwork.org/resources/timeline

Heim, S., & Mitelman, F. (2011). *Cancer cytogenetics: Chromosomal and molecular genetic aberrations of tumor cells*. Hoboken, NJ: Wiley-Blackwell.

Jorde, L.B., Carey, J.C., & Bamshad, M.J. (2009). *Medical genetics* (4th ed.). Philadelphia, PA: Elsevier Health Sciences.

Kyrtsonis, M.C., Bartzis, V., & Papanikolaou, X. (2010). Genetic and molecular mechanisms in multiple myeloma: A route to better understand disease pathogenesis and heterogeneity. *Application of Clinical Genetics, 3*, 41–51. doi:10.2147/TACG.S7456

Liu, E.T. (2012). Clinical genomicist in the future of medical practice. In K.R. Dronamraju & C.A. Francomano (Eds.) *Victor McKusick and the history of medical genetics* (pp. 137–143). New York, NY: Springer.

Mitelman, F., Johansson, B., & Mertens, F. (Eds.), (2013). Mitelman database of chromosome aberrations and gene fusions in cancer. Retrieved from http://cgap.nci.nih.gov/Chromosomes/Mitelman

Mrózek, K., Marcucci, G., Paschka, P., Whitman, S.P., & Bloomfield, C.D. (2007). Clinical relevance of mutations and gene-expression changes in adult acute myeloid leukemia with normal cytogenetics: Are we ready for a prognostically prioritized molecular classification? *Blood, 109*, 431–448. doi:10.1182/blood-2006-06-001149

National Comprehensive Cancer Network. (2014a). *NCCN Clinical Practice Guidelines in Oncology (NCCN Guidelines®): Non-Hodgkin's lymphomas* [v.5.2014]. Retrieved from http://www.nccn.org/professionals/physician_gls/pdf/nhl.pdf

National Comprehensive Cancer Network. (2014b). *NCCN Clinical Practice Guidelines in Oncology (NCCN Guidelines®): Acute myeloid leukemia* [v.2.2014]. Retrieved from http://www.nccn.org/professionals/physician_gls/pdf/aml.pdf

Sheth, F., Sheth, H., Pritti, K., Tewari, S., Desai, M., Patel, B., & Sheth, J. (2014). Evolution of cytogenetics in disease diagnosis. *Journal of Translational Toxicology, 1*, 3–9. doi:10.1166/jtt.2014.1008

Snustad, D.P., & Simmons, M.J. (2009). *Principles of genetics*. Hoboken, NJ: Wiley.

Speicher, M.R., & Carter, N.P. (2005). The new cytogenetics: Blurring the boundaries with molecular biology. *Nature Reviews Genetics, 6*, 782–792. doi:10.1038/nrg1692

Wisconsin State Laboratory of Hygiene. (2013). Basic nomenclature for cytogenetics. Retrieved from http://www.slh.wisc.edu/clinical/cytogenetics/basics

You, J.-S., & Jones, P.A. (2012). Cancer genetics and epigenetics: Two sides of the same coin? *Cancer Cell, 22*, 9–20. doi:10.1016/j.ccr.2012.06.008

Zhivotovsky, B., & Orrenius, S. (2006). Carcinogenesis and apoptosis: Paradigms and paradoxes. *Carcinogenesis, 27*, 1939–1945. doi:10.1093/carcin/bgl035

Chapter 34

Tumor Profiling

Elizabeth Hassen, MSN, OCN®, and Julia A. Eggert, PhD, GNP-BC, AGN-BC, AOCN®

Introduction

Tumor profiling is a molecular analysis to identify alterations in DNA, RNA, and proteins (Adenoid Cystic Carcinoma Research Foundation, n.d.). Also referred to as *molecular profiling*, various techniques are used to analyze the tumor to help guide treatments and personalized cancer care. As Chu (2011) stated, "In theory, this approach should result in enhanced clinical efficacy, improved safety profile, and lower overall pharmacoeconomic costs" (p. 69). These analyses are already being used in the diagnostic and treatment guidelines for multiple cancers, including breast, lung, and colon cancers and lymphomas and leukemias. This chapter offers information that will assist clinical trial nurses (CTNs) working in oncology-specific research with a focus on solid tumors to understand tumor profiling and how these genetic tests can be interpreted for application to clinical trials.

Tumor Profiling

Tumor profiling uses molecular analysis to determine characteristics of tumors, which assists with prognostic assessment, treatment planning decisions, and the advancement of personalized medicine. Techniques for profiling include DNA microarrays, RNA sequencing, and next-generation DNA sequencing. Currently, DNA microarrays and RNA sequencing are most commonly used in tumor profiling, but as cost continues to decrease for next-generation sequencing of DNA, its use will increase (Walther & Sklar, 2011).

Tumor profiling is being used today to guide treatment plans, such as determining the use or type of chemotherapy and the use of specific targeted therapies for better prognosis and outcomes (Chu, 2011; Walther & Sklar, 2011). There has been a shift to molecular tumor profiling or analysis from testing for single alterations because of the increasing number of molecular-targeted drugs (Walther & Sklar, 2011). Molecular analysis allows tumors to be tested for an array of alterations and mutations, including base substitutions referred to as *single nucleotide polymorphisms*, and insertions and deletions in DNA. These genetic changes in DNA are discussed in Chapter 31. These various alterations can activate oncogenes, leading to alterations in the signal transduction pathways (Walther & Sklar, 2011). The alterations and mutations identified through tumor profiling can guide treatment decisions to determine an individual's likelihood of response to specific targeted therapies (Walther & Sklar, 2011).

When reading information about molecular profiling, one may see the terms *biomarker, single-gene marker*, or *multigene markers*. Biomarker is defined by the National Cancer Institute (NCI, n.d.-a) as "a biological molecule found in blood, other body fluids, or tissues that is a sign of a normal or abnormal process, or of a condition or disease. A biomarker may be used to see how well the body responds to a treatment for a disease or condition."

Single-gene markers usually refer to a single gene, protein, or other molecule that can be used to predict clinical outcomes (Galanina, Bossuyt, & Harris, 2011). These markers include receptors such as the estrogen receptor (ER), progesterone receptor (PR), or binding sites for key signaling proteins such as the epidermal growth factor receptor (EGFR) (Chu, 2011; Galanina et al., 2011).

Multigene biomarkers use one analysis to assess multiple genes found in a tumor (Galanina et al., 2011). Examples of multigene biomarker assays include Oncotype DX® and MammaPrint®. A list of currently used tumor markers can be found on the NCI fact sheet on tumor markers (NCI, 2011).

Biomarkers can be used as prognostic or predictive markers. *Prognostic* markers are used to determine the risk or likelihood of the disease recurring (NCI, n.d.-c). *Predictive* markers are used to determine if a patient will benefit from a specific treatment (NCI, n.d.-b). CTNs need to understand the source of the biomarker in the development of the tumor type and how the test is used (i.e., prognostically or predictively) to facilitate the correct interpretation.

Kaplan-Meier Survival Curve

Many researchers use Kaplan-Meier estimate curves to illustrate the benefit of a certain drug or treatment as it relates to patient survival, requiring CTNs to understand the definition, collect the necessary data for the calculation, and be able to communicate this information with other personnel working with the clinical trial (Oncology Nursing Society, 2010). A Kaplan-Meier curve plots the probability of an event occurring at a specified time; it is also referred to as a *product limit estimate* (Goel, Khanna, & Kishore, 2010). This estimate is commonly used in clinical trials to illustrate survival time after treatment. Specifically, it evaluates the number of living individuals who have survived after an intervention, such as a chemotherapy drug, over a period of time (Goel et al., 2010). To calculate this estimate, the total number of subjects living at the start of the intervention, minus the number of subjects who have died, is divided by the total of subjects living at the start, at a given point in time (Goel et al., 2010).

$$S_t = \frac{\text{Number of subjects living at the start} - \text{Number of subjects died}}{\text{Number of subjects living at the start}}$$

In a Kaplan-Meier survival curve, the *x*-axis represents time, and the *y*-axis represents the estimated probability of survival within a defined population (Vanderbilt University Department of Biostatistics, 2011). In general, a high start is seen to the left side of the graph with a decrease as the curve moves to the right of the graph (Vanderbilt University Department of Biostatistics, 2011). This can be explained by noting that as time elapses, the number of people decreases; they either died or became lost to follow-up during the trial. The Kaplan-Meier survival curve is an *estimate of survival* at a point in time, not the actual number of survivors at that point in time (Goel et al., 2010).

CTNs may be required to gather survival data for two groups of subjects, such as in comparison of standard treatment with a new treatment, so that the Kaplan-Meier curves can be compared. A survival plot would be created for each group, and it would be important to monitor any gaps between these two curves. A vertical gap indicates that one intervention, such as treatment, resulted in more subjects surviving at a specific time point compared to the other treatment group (Goel et al., 2010). A horizontal gap indicates a longer time of survival before one treatment group experienced a certain fraction of deaths (Goel et al., 2010).

Biomarkers in Specific Cancers

Breast Cancer

Breast cancer researchers use biomarkers to identify subsets of patients (grouping patients according to positive or negative receptors) with use as both predictive and prognostic markers. Currently, the presence or absence of ER, PR, and HER2 receptors is routinely used as a predictive marker to determine patient-specific treatment of breast cancer (Galanina et al., 2011). Furthermore, multigene biomarkers from the breast tumor are used as prognostic markers, predicting risk of recurrence. These prognostic markers, including Oncotype DX, MammaPrint, Breast Cancer Index, and PAM50 (Galanina et al., 2011), can help practitioners determine treatment types to use based on patients' personal recurrence risk. This approach offers each patient personalized medicine.

The Oncotype DX Breast Cancer Assay is a 21-gene assay that uses reverse transcription polymerase chain reaction technology on paraffin-embedded tumor tissue to calculate a recurrence score that correlates with the likelihood of breast cancer recurrence within 10 years of initial diagnosis (Genomic Health, n.d.-b; Paik et al., 2004). The National Surgical Adjuvant Breast and Bowel Project (NSABP) B-14 trial validated the correlation of the recurrence score as "quantifying the likelihood of distant recurrence in tamoxifen-treated patients with node-negative, estrogen-receptor-positive breast cancer" (Paik et al., 2004, p. 2817). Subsequently, in the NSABP B-20 trial, researchers assessed the chemotherapy benefit by testing the interaction between chemotherapy treatment and the recurrence score (Paik et al., 2006). The population used to validate the Oncotype DX assay was patients with early-stage breast cancer, defined as stage I or II, lymph node negative, ER positive (Paik et al., 2004).

An Oncotype DX Breast Cancer Assay report contains a recurrence score, a number between 0 and 100 that correlates to a specific likelihood of breast cancer recurrence within 10 years of initial diagnosis (Paik et al., 2004). The recurrence score is calculated from 16 cancer-related genes and 5 reference genes (reference genes are those that normalize the expression of cancer-related genes) (Paik et al., 2004; Zhang, Ding, & Sandford, 2005). The score places patients into one of three categories: low risk, defined as a score of less than 18; intermediate risk, defined as a score of 18–30; and high risk, defined as a score of 31 or higher (Paik et al., 2004). Using this score, a practitioner can determine if a type of treatment will provide a longer disease-free survival time.

For example, the NSABP B-20 study found that tamoxifen plus chemotherapy provided a significant benefit in the high-risk group (Paik et al., 2006). The low- and intermediate-risk groups did not show a significant statistical benefit with the addition of chemotherapy to the treatment with tamoxifen (Paik et al., 2004). Ongoing studies are evaluating the intermediate-risk group (Paik et al., 2006). The National Comprehensive Cancer Network® (NCCN®) and the American Society of Clinical Oncology guidelines incorporate the use of Oncotype DX for women with ER-positive, node-negative disease and tumors larger than 0.5 cm (Harris et al., 2007; NCCN, 2015a).

Genomic Health implemented further studies, including Eastern Cooperative Oncology Group 5194, which contributed to the development of a validated 12-gene algorithm to predict recurrence risk in patients with ductal carcinoma in situ (DCIS) (Genomic Health, n.d.-a; Solin et al., 2013). This report provides a DCIS score plus two additional scores: a percentage for any local event recurrence and an invasive local event recurrence score to be used to guide treatment plans, such as local excision without radiation (Genomic Health, n.d.-a; Solin et al., 2013).

MammaPrint is another prognostic multigene assay. It targets 70 genes associated with breast cancer and uses microarray technology to determine a recurrence score for early-stage breast cancer (van't Veer et al., 2002). The study focused on women with early-stage breast cancer, defined as invasive stage I or II (T1 or T2), smaller than 5 cm, and including both lymph node–positive and lymph node–negative disease (van de Vijver et al., 2002). MammaPrint stratified the results into two prognostic groups, good or poor, based on a correlation coefficient predicting recurrence during the first five years after therapy (van de Vijver et al., 2002). Other studies evaluated the predictive value of MammaPrint, concluding that chemotherapy plus endocrine therapy had a significant clinical benefit in the high-risk, poor-prognosis groups. The addition of chemotherapy was not shown to be beneficial to the good-prognosis group (Knauer et al., 2010).

Mammostrat is a third prognostic test for stage I and II, node-negative, ER-positive breast cancer. Mammostrat is a five-antibody immunohistochemistry panel targeting expression levels of the tumor proteins SLC7A5, HTF9C, p53, NDRG1, and CEACAM5 (Bartlett et al., 2010; Clarient Diagnostic Services, GE Healthcare, n.d.). An algorithm calculates a risk index score to classify patients into one of three categories based on the percentage of cancer recurrence in 10 years. The categories include low, moderate, and high risk for relapse. Women at low risk would probably not receive additional benefit from chemotherapy, but those at high risk would have long-term benefit from chemotherapy plus hormonal therapy. Validation studies have not incorporated the status of other hormone receptors, but more evidence is supported for the ER-positive ranking (Bartlett et al., 2010).

Lung Cancer

Strong evidence exists for EGFR, the 5′ endonuclease of the nucleotide excision repair complex (ERCC1), the *KRAS* oncogene, and the *ALK* fusion oncogene as prognostic and predictive markers (NCCN, 2015b). Additional biomarkers identified for predictive or prognostic value in non-small cell lung cancer (NSCLC) include the ribonucleotide reductase enzyme (RRM1) and thymidylate synthase (Andrews, Yeh, Pao, & Horn, 2011).

EGFR is a transmembrane receptor that is known to have predictive treatment benefit from EGFR tyrosine kinase inhibitor therapy with the presence of an exon 19 deletion or exon 21 L858R mutation (Miller et al., 2008; Sequist et al., 2008). *EGFR* mutation and copy number were positively correlated with a higher response rate and progression-free survival (Miller et al., 2008). Sequist et al. (2008) showed favorable clinical outcome for patients with *EGFR* mutation treated with first-line gefitinib, an *EGFR* inhibitor.

The *KRAS* oncogene has shown to be prognostic of survival. Studies have demonstrated that a *KRAS* mutation has an unfavorable prognostic value with shorter survival regardless of treatment (Mitsudomi et al., 1991; Slebos et al., 1990; Tsao et al., 2007). The *ALK* gene has been shown in studies to have predictive value of response to crizotinib, an *ALK* and *MET* tyrosine kinase inhibitor (NCCN, 2015b).

Testing for the expression of ERCC1 can provide both prognostic and predictive information. For prognostic value, a high ERCC1 expression is associated with improved outcomes in early-stage NSCLC (Olaussen et al., 2006). For predictive value, many studies have researched its ability to predict response to platinum-based therapies. Research results have shown that low expression of ERCC1 has improved overall survival with platinum-based treatment, especially in advanced disease (Andrews et al., 2011; Olaussen et al., 2006; Simon, Sharma, Cantor, Smith, & Bepler, 2005).

Another identified prognostic factor is the enzyme RRM1. Similar to ERCC1, studies have revealed that a high expression of RRM1 is associated with an increased survival in patients with early-stage NSCLC (Zheng et al., 2007). Zheng et al. (2007) divided patients into four subgroups based on the expression of the RRM1 and ERCC1 proteins: high expression of both proteins (high/high), low expression of both proteins (low/low), high RRM1 expression and low ERCC1 expression, and low RRM1 expression and high ERCC1 expression. The study concluded that high expression of both RRM1 and ERCC1 had a statistically significant increase in disease-free and overall survival (Zheng et al., 2007). In addition, several studies focused on the predictive role of RRM1, wherein patients with a high RRM1 expression are not sensitive to gemcitabine-based chemotherapy, and patients with low RRM1 expression have increased time to survival when the chemotherapy agent cisplatin is added to gemcitabine (Andrews et al., 2011). Andrews et al. (2011) suggested that a screening panel including more than one biomarker may be more reliable for prognostic purposes based on the ERCC1 and RRM1 data.

Colon Cancer

Much research is ongoing in the study of biomarkers for additional predictive values, or further explanations of response to therapy, in people with colon cancer. Currently, the *KRAS* oncogene is a biomarker with known predictive value for response to anti-EGFR monoclonal antibodies (Dienstmann, Vilar, & Tabernero, 2011). A study by Amado et al. (2008) demonstrated that *KRAS* mutations have a negative (inverse) predictive value, meaning that patients without *KRAS* tumor mutations had better outcomes after treatment with chemotherapy alone and no monoclonal antibody therapy. However, in another study, Bokemeyer et al. (2010) concluded that *KRAS* wild-type (typical gene without mutation) tumors have increased response rates to chemotherapy with the addition of a targeted agent. The conclusion from multiple clinical trials, including retrospective analyses, is that *KRAS* mutations can be used as a predictive marker for treatment with anti-EGFR monoclonal antibodies (Dienstmann et al., 2011). Additional predictive markers for anti-EGFR agents include *BRAF*, *NRAS*, and *PIK3CA* status. The loss of protein expression by *PTEN*, a tumor suppressor gene, continues to be investigated for predicting a lack of benefit to treatment with monoclonal antibodies and a negative correlation with overall survival (Er, Chen, Bujanda, & Herreros-Villanueva, 2014).

Similar to breast cancer, colon cancer has genomic profiling options to predict recurrence risk. These include Oncotype DX, ColoPrint, and ColDx. The Oncotype DX Colon Cancer Assay (Genomic Health, n.d.-c) is a 12-gene panel consisting of 7 cancer genes and 5 reference genes (Gray et al., 2011).

Another profiling approach discussed the relationship of tumor gene expression and risk of cancer recurrence in four individualized cohorts to evaluate surgery alone versus surgery plus adjuvant 5-fluorouracil (5-FU) plus leucovorin in both stage II and stage III disease (O'Connell et al., 2010). These researchers used the quantitative reverse transcription polymerase chain reaction technique to identify 48 genes associated with recurrence risk and 66 genes associated with benefit of 5-FU/leucovorin (O'Connell et al., 2010). From this, seven of the recurrence genes and six of the treatment-benefit genes were identified and are the foundation of the algorithm used to categorize patients with stage II and III colon cancer into three categories: low, intermediate, and high risk of recurrence (O'Connell et al., 2010). The development of this assay was validated and confirmed for stage II colon cancer in the QUASAR (Quick and Simple and Reliable) and the Cancer and Leukemia Group B 9581 studies. Use of the gene expression levels of the cancer genes allows for the calculation of a recurrence score. A report is generated with a colon cancer recurrence score that ranges from 0 to 100: a score less than 30 has a recurrence risk of 15% or less; a score of 30 or greater indicates a recurrence risk greater than 15%; and a recurrence score of 41 or greater indicates a recurrence risk greater than 18% that overlaps with T4 patients (Genomic Health, n.d.-c). The report also includes information on mismatch repair (MMR) status.

MMR is a conserved process during DNA replication that corrects mismatches of bases (Kunkel & Erie, 2005). A deficiency in MMR identifies a small subset of stage II colon cancer tumors with significantly lower recurrence risk compared to tumors with expression (Genomic Health, n.d.-c). A study by Gray et al. (2011) concluded that the 12-gene assay was able to validate the recurrence score for stage II colon cancer tumors treated with surgery alone but was not validated as a predictive marker for treatment with adjuvant 5-FU or folinic acid chemotherapy.

ColoPrint (Agendia, n.d.) is an assay that quantifies the expression of 18 genes and is a prognostic marker that classifies patients into two categories: low versus high recurrence risk (Salazar et al., 2011). In the development of the ColoPrint assay, 188 tumor samples consisting of stage I, II, and III colon cancers were categorized into A, B, and C groups based on mutational status of *BRAF* (Salazar et al., 2011). Then, using the B group, an 18-gene optimal assay was developed and validated using a sample of 206 subjects. In this study, researchers assessed the mutations for *BRAF*, *KRAS*, and *PI3KCA* in addition to running the 18-gene assay. Based on the ColoPrint analysis, patients were categorized as having either low or high risk of recurrence based on five-year survival. The study concluded that ColoPrint improves prognostic accuracy and was able to identify patients with stage II disease that could be managed without chemotherapy (Salazar et al., 2011).

ColDx (Almac Group Ltd., n.d.) is a DNA microarray multigene assay that uses 634 probes to stratify patients as having either high or low risk of recurrence (Kennedy et al., 2011). Kennedy et al. (2011) performed validation on a sample of 144 patients with stage II colon adenocarcinoma, categorizing them into the two groups based on recurrence risk at five years. The study also demonstrated that the insulin-like growth factor, tumor growth factor-beta, and the high mobility group B protein (HMGB1) signaling pathways were the most significant in the gene signature (Kennedy et al., 2011); each pathway was reported to promote tumor growth, invasion, and prevention of apoptosis, or programmed cell death (Nosho et al., 2004; Tsushima et al., 1996; Völp et al., 2006).

Prostate Cancer

Cooperberg et al. (2013) discussed the use of the Oncotype DX Prostate Cancer Assay to identify risk of metastasis in men recently diagnosed with early-stage prostate cancer. The Oncotype DX test reveals the activity of 17 genes and uses an algorithm to produce an individualized Genomic Prostate Score to indicate the likelihood of tumor spread to other organs or the bone (Cooperberg et al., 2013). This test is a prognostic marker that can be used to guide treatment decisions by patients (NCCN, 2015c).

Summary

This chapter summarized some of the biomarkers and gene panels used to predict treatment and prognosis in different solid cancers. Currently, tests are being developed at an amazing rate, each with more genes and better predictability. CTNs need to be aware of new literature as molecular testing availability increases for each specific tumor type. Because tumor profiling offers both predictive and prognostic information, CTNs must be knowledgeable as to which mutations are being used to profile different solid tumors and if the implications are different in the various tumor types. For CTNs, it enhances an individualized approach to health care to provide very personalized medicine to patients enrolled in clinical trials in order to offer new hope for alternative approaches to diagnosis or new treatment options for their metastatic, resistant, or recurring cancer (Chu, 2011).

The basics of genetics and molecular analysis on tumor tissue, along with pharmacogenomics and pharmacokinetics, are discussed in Chapter 31.

Key Points
- A variety of techniques are used for the molecular analysis of gene and protein alterations associated with profiling malignancies.
- Tumor profiling is used to personalize treatment plans to determine the use or type of chemotherapy or the use of specific targeted therapies for better prognosis and outcomes.
- The Kaplan-Meier curve is used in clinical trials to illustrate the benefit of a drug or treatment as it relates to patient survival.
- A variety of genes serve as biomarkers for specific cancer types, especially breast, lung, colon, and prostate, and are used to determine individualized treatment and prognosis.
- Genetic testing is being developed that can evaluate the presence of multiple genes with one assay.
- Understanding the significance of tumor profiling in oncology clinical trials is crucial to the role of CTNs in interpreting the correct treatment plan and educating patients and families.

References

Adenoid Cystic Carcinoma Research Foundation. (n.d.). Tumor profiling. Retrieved from http://www.accrf.org/treatment-options/tumor-profiling

Agendia. (n.d.). ColoPrint® 18-gene colon cancer recurrence assay. Retrieved from http://www.agendia.com/healthcare-professionals/colon-cancer

Almac Group Ltd. (n.d.). ColDx. Retrieved from http://www.almacgroup.com/coldx

Amado, R.G., Wolf, M., Peeters, M., Van Cutsem, E., Siena, S., Freeman, D.J., ... Chang, D.D. (2008). Wild-type *KRAS* is required for panitumumab efficacy in patients with metastatic colorectal cancer. *Journal of Clinical Oncology, 26*, 1626–1634. doi:10.1200/JCO.2007.14.7116

Andrews, J., Yeh, P., Pao, W., & Horn, L. (2011). Molecular predictors of response to chemotherapy in non-small cell lung cancer. *Cancer Journal, 17*, 104–113. doi:10.1097/PPO.0b013e318213f3cf

Bartlett, J.M.S., Thomas, J., Ross, D.T., Seitz, R.S., Ring, B.Z., Beck, R.A., ... Chetty, U. (2010). Mammostrat® as a tool to stratify breast cancer patients at risk of recurrence during endocrine therapy. *Breast Cancer Research, 12*, R47. doi:10.1186/bcr2604

Bokemeyer, C., Kohne, C., Rougier, P., Stroh, C., Schlichting, M., & Van Cutsem, E. (2010). Cetuximab with chemotherapy (CT) as first-line treatment for metastatic colorectal cancer (mCRC): Analysis of the CRYSTAL and OPUS studies according to *KRAS* and *BRAF* mutation status. *Journal of Clinical Oncology, 28*(Suppl. 15), Abstract 3506. Retrieved from http://meetinglibrary.asco.org/content/54275-74

Chu, E. (2011). Molecular profiling and personalized medicine [Editorial]. *Cancer Journal, 17*, 69–70. doi:10.1097/PPO.0b013e318217947e

Clarient Diagnostic Services, GE Healthcare. (n.d.). How is Mammostrat used? Retrieved from http://www.clarientinc.com/mammostrat-overview/how-is-mammostrat-used.aspx

Cooperberg, M., Simko, J., Falzarano, S., Maddala, T., Chan, J., Cowan, J., ... Carroll, P. (2013). *Development and validation of the biopsy-based genomic prostate score (GPS) as a predictor of high grade or extracapsular prostate cancer to improve patient selection for active surveillance* [Abstract 2131]. Oral presentation at American Urologic Association, San Diego, CA. Retrieved from http://www.genomichealth.com/en-US/Publications/ScientificPresentations.aspx#5

Dienstmann, R., Vilar, E., & Tabernero, J. (2011). Molecular predictors of response to chemotherapy in colorectal cancer. *Cancer Journal, 17*, 114–126. doi:10.1097/PPO.0b013e318212f844

Er, T.-K., Chen, C.-C., Bujanda, L., & Herreros-Villanueva, M. (2014). Current approaches for predicting a lack of response to anti-EGFR therapy in *KRAS* wild-type patients. *BioMed Research International, 2014*, Article 591867. doi:10.1155/2014/591867

Galanina, N., Bossuyt, V., & Harris, L.N. (2011). Molecular predictors of response to therapy for breast cancer. *Cancer Journal, 17*, 96–103. doi:10.1097/PPO.0b013e318212dee3

Genomic Health. (n.d.-a). Oncotype DX® Breast Cancer Assay DCIS. Retrieved from http://breast-cancer.oncotypedx.com/en-US/Professional-DCIS.aspx

Genomic Health. (n.d.-b). Oncotype DX® Breast Cancer Assay Invasive. Retrieved from http://breast-cancer.oncotypedx.com/en-US/Professional-Invasive.aspx

Genomic Health. (n.d.-c). Oncotype DX® Colon Cancer Assay. Retrieved from http://colon-cancer.oncotypedx.com/en-US/Professional.aspx

Goel, M.K., Khanna, P., & Kishore, J. (2010). Understanding survival analysis: Kaplan-Meier estimate. *International Journal of Ayurveda*

Research, 1, 274–278. Retrieved from http://www.ncbi.nlm.nih.gov/pmc/articles/PMC3059453

Gray, R.G., Quirke, P., Handley, K., Lopatin, M., Magill, L., Baehner, F.L., ... Kerr, D.J. (2011). Validation study of a quantitative multigene reverse transcriptase–polymerase chain reaction assay for assessment of recurrence risk in patients with stage II colon cancer. *Journal of Clinical Oncology, 29,* 4611–4619. doi:10.1200/JCO.2010.32.8732

Harris, L., Fritsche, H., Mennel, R., Norton, L., Ravdin, P., Taube, S., ... Bast, R.C., Jr. (2007). American Society of Clinical Oncology 2007 update of recommendations for the use of tumor markers in breast cancer. *Journal of Clinical Oncology, 25,* 5287–5312. doi:10.1200/JCO.2007.14.2364

Kennedy, R.D., Bylesjo, M., Kerr, P., Davison, T., Black, J.M., Kay, E.W., ... Harkin, D.P. (2011). Development and independent validation of a prognostic assay for stage II colon cancer using formalin-fixed paraffin-embedded tissue. *Journal of Clinical Oncology, 29,* 4620–4626. doi:10.1200/JCO.2011.35.4498

Knauer, M., Mook, S., Rutgers, E.J.T., Bender, R.A., Hauptmann, M., van de Vijver, M.J., ... van't Veer, L.J. (2010). The predictive value of the 70-gene signature for adjuvant chemotherapy in early breast cancer. *Breast Cancer Research and Treatment, 120,* 655–661. doi:10.1007/s10549-010-0814-2

Kunkel, T.A., & Erie, D.A. (2005). DNA mismatch repair. *Annual Review of Biochemistry, 74,* 681–710. doi:10.1146/annurev.biochem.74.082803.133243

Miller, V.A., Riely, G.J., Zakowski, M.F., Li, A.R., Patel, J.D., Heelan, R.T., ... Johnson, D.H. (2008). Molecular characteristics of bronchioloalveolar carcinoma and adenocarcinoma, bronchioloalveolar carcinoma subtype, predict response to erlotinib. *Journal of Clinical Oncology, 26,* 1472–1478. doi:10.1200/JCO.2007.13.0062

Mitsudomi, T., Steinberg, S.M., Oie, H.K., Mulshine, J.L., Phelps, R., Viallet, J., ... Gazdar, A.F. (1991). *Ras* gene mutations in non-small cell lung cancers are associated with shortened survival irrespective of treatment intent. *Cancer Research, 51,* 4999–5002. Retrieved from http://cancerres.aacrjournals.org/content/51/18/4999

National Cancer Institute. (n.d.-a). NCI dictionary of cancer terms: Biomarker. Retrieved from http://www.cancer.gov/dictionary?CdrID=45618

National Cancer Institute. (n.d.-b). NCI dictionary of cancer terms: Predictive factor. Retrieved from http://www.cancer.gov/dictionary?CdrID=44245

National Cancer Institute. (n.d.-c). NCI dictionary of cancer terms: Prognostic factor. Retrieved from http://www.cancer.gov/dictionary?CdrID=44246

National Cancer Institute. (2011, December 7). Fact sheet: Tumor markers. Retrieved from http://www.cancer.gov/cancertopics/factsheet/detection/tumor-markers

National Comprehensive Cancer Network. (2015a). *NCCN Clinical Practice Guidelines in Oncology (NCCN Guidelines®): Breast cancer* [v.2.2015]. Retrieved from http://www.nccn.org/professionals/physician_gls/pdf/breast.pdf

National Comprehensive Cancer Network. (2015b). *NCCN Clinical Practice Guidelines in Oncology (NCCN Guidelines®): Non-small cell lung cancer* [v.5.2015]. Retrieved from http://www.nccn.org/professionals/physician_gls/pdf/nscl.pdf

National Comprehensive Cancer Network. (2015c). *NCCN Clinical Practice Guidelines in Oncology (NCCN Guidelines®): Prostate cancer* [v.1.2015]. Retrieved from http://www.nccn.org/professionals/physician_gls/pdf/prostate.pdf

Nosho, K., Yamamoto, H., Taniguchi, H., Adachi, Y., Yoshida, Y., Arimura, Y., ... Imai, K. (2004). Interplay of insulin-like growth factor-II, insulin-like growth factor-I, insulin-like growth factor-I receptor, COX-2, and matrix metalloproteinase-7, play key roles in the early stage of colorectal carcinogenesis. *Clinical Cancer Research, 10,* 7950–7957. doi:10.1158/1078-0432.CCR-04-0875.

O'Connell, M.J., Lavery, I., Yothers, G., Paik, S., Clark-Langone, K.M., Lopatin, M., ... Wolmark, N. (2010). Relationship between tumor gene expression and recurrence in four independent studies of patients with stage II/III colon cancer treated with surgery alone or surgery plus adjuvant fluorouracil plus leucovorin. *Journal of Clinical Oncology, 28,* 3937–3944. doi:10.1200/JCO.2010.28.9538

Olaussen, K.A., Dunant, A., Fouret, P., Brambilla, E., André, F., Haddad, V., ... Soria, J.-C. (2006). DNA repair by ERCC1 in non–small-cell lung cancer and cisplatin-based adjuvant chemotherapy. *New England Journal of Medicine, 355,* 983–991. doi:10.1056/NEJMoa060570

Oncology Nursing Society. (2010). *Oncology clinical trials nurse competencies.* Retrieved from https://www.ons.org/sites/default/files/ctncompetencies.pdf

Paik, S., Shak, S., Tang, G., Kim, C., Baker, J., Cronin, M., ... Wolmark, N. (2004). A multigene assay to predict recurrence of tamoxifen-treated, node-negative breast cancer. *New England Journal of Medicine, 351,* 2817–2826. doi:10.1056/NEJMoa041588

Paik, S., Tang, G., Shak, S., Kim, C., Baker, J., Kim, W., ... Wolmark, N. (2006). Gene expression and benefit of chemotherapy in women with node-negative, estrogen receptor–positive breast cancer. *Journal of Clinical Oncology, 24,* 3726–3734. doi:10.1200/JCO.2005.04.7985

Salazar, R., Roepman, P., Capella, G., Moreno, V., Simon, I., Dreezen, C., ... Tollenaar, R. (2011). Gene expression signature to improve prognosis prediction of stage II and III colorectal cancer. *Journal of Clinical Oncology, 29,* 17–24. doi:10.1200/JCO.2010.30.1077

Sequist, L.V., Martins, R.G., Spigel, D., Grunberg, S.M., Spira, A., Jänne, P.A., ... Lynch, T.J. (2008). First-line gefitinib in patients with advanced non–small-cell lung cancer harboring somatic *EGFR* mutations. *Journal of Clinical Oncology, 26,* 2442–2449. doi:10.1200/JCO.2007.14.8494

Simon, G.R., Sharma, S., Cantor, A., Smith, P., & Bepler, G. (2005). ERCC1 expression is a predictor of survival in resected patients with non-small cell lung cancer. *Chest, 127,* 978–983. doi:10.1378/chest.127.3.978

Slebos, R.J.C., Kibbelaar, R.E., Dalesio, O., Kooistra, A., Stam, J., Meijer, C.J.L.M., ... Rodenhuis, S. (1990). K-*ras* oncogene activation as a prognostic marker in adenocarcinoma of the lung. *New England Journal of Medicine, 323,* 561–565. doi:10.1056/NEJM199008303230902

Solin, L.J., Gray, R., Baehner, F.L., Butler, S.M., Hughes, L.L., Yoshizawa, C., ... Badve, S. (2013). A multigene expression assay to predict local recurrence risk for ductal carcinoma in situ of the breast. *Journal of the National Cancer Institute, 105,* 701–710. doi:10.1093/jnci/djt067

Tsao, M.-S., Aviel-Ronen, S., Ding, K., Lau, D., Liu, N., Sakurada, A., ... Shepherd, F.A. (2007). Prognostic and predictive importance of p53 and RAS for adjuvant chemotherapy in non–small-cell lung cancer. *Journal of Clinical Oncology, 25,* 5240–5247. doi:10.1200/JCO.2007.12.6953

Tsushima, H., Kawata, S., Tamura, S., Ito, N., Shirai, Y., Kiso, S., ... Matsuzawa, Y. (1996). High levels of transforming growth factor beta 1 in patients with colorectal cancer: Association with disease progression. *Gastroenterology, 110,* 375–382. doi:10.1053/gast.1996.v110.pm8566583

Vanderbilt University Department of Biostatistics. (2011). Why use a Kaplan-Meier analysis? [Slide presentation]. Retrieved from http://biostat.mc.vanderbilt.edu/wiki/pub/Main/ClinStat/km.lam.pdf

van de Vijver, M.J., He, Y.D., van't Veer, L.J., Dai, H., Hart, A.A.M., Voskuil, D.W., ... Bernards, R. (2002). A gene-expression signature as a predictor of survival in breast cancer. *New England Journal of Medicine, 347,* 1999–2009. doi:10.1056/NEJMoa021967

van't Veer, L.J., Dai, H., van de Vijver, M.J., He, Y.D., Hart, A.A.M., Mao, M., ... Friend, S.H. (2002). Gene expression profiling predicts clinical outcome of breast cancer. *Nature, 415,* 530–536. doi:10.1038/415530a

Völp, K., Brezniceanu, M.-L., Bösser, S., Brabletz, T., Kirchner, T., Göttel, D., ... Zörnig, M. (2006). Increased expression of high mobility group box 1 (HMGB1) is associated with an elevated level of the antiapoptotic c-IAP2 protein in human colon carcinomas. *Gut, 55,* 234–242. doi:10.1136/gut.2004.062729

Walther, Z., & Sklar, J. (2011). Molecular tumor profiling for prediction of response to anticancer therapies. *Cancer Journal, 17,* 71–79. doi:10.1097/PPO.0b013e318212dd6d

Zhang, X., Ding, L., & Sandford, A.J. (2005). Selection of reference genes for gene expression studies in human neutrophils by real-time PCR. *BMC Molecular Biology, 6,* 4. doi:10.1186/1471-2199-6-4

Zheng, Z., Chen, T., Li, X., Haura, E., Sharma, A., & Bepler, G. (2007). DNA synthesis and repair genes *RRM1* and *ERCC1* in lung cancer. *New England Journal of Medicine, 356,* 800–808. doi:10.1056/NEJMoa065411

Chapter 35

Storage of Genetic Material

Kathy Wilkinson, RN, BSN, OCN®, and Julia A. Eggert, PhD, GNP-BC, AGN-BC, AOCN®

Introduction

Since the completion of the Human Genome Project, the request for sampling and submission of human genetic materials has rapidly expanded (Chan, Mackay, & Hegney, 2013). Research on human specimens has become key to finding ways to prevent, diagnose, and treat cancer. The practice of specimen collection is common to National Cancer Institute (NCI)- and industry-sponsored trials (Office for Human Research Protections [OHRP], 2009). Specimens may be tissue, blood, serum, cytologic preparations, and pathology specimens that contain DNA. Each type is considered personal healthcare information if it is not de-identified (National Human Genome Research Institute, 2015). Some studies may involve the collection of specimens for circulating tumor cells and biopsies done in early-phase clinical trials to look at a patient's tumor response to treatment. Finally, research biorepositories collect tissue that can identify participants who qualify for potential clinical trials (National Human Genome Research Institute, 2015). The age of personalized medicine has created many challenges for clinical trial nurses (CTNs). This chapter will focus on the many agencies and regulations involved in the protection of clinical trial participants and storage of their genetic materials.

In the United States, the Department of Health and Human Services (DHHS), including the Food and Drug Administration (FDA) and OHRP, are each in charge of specific aspects of research on human samples (Basic HHS Policy for Protection of Human Research Subjects, 2009; U.S. FDA, 2014; U.S. OHRP, 2009). Regulations for institutional review boards (IRBs), human subject protection, confidentiality requirements, financial disclosure by clinical investigators, and electronic medical records have been published by DHHS (OHRP, 2009). Medical information was regulated under the Privacy Rule while the Health Insurance Portability and Accountability Act (HIPAA) of 1996 established standards for privacy of individually identifiable health information. This act included the protection of electronic medical records to protect consumers' identifiable health information from being shared with inappropriate sources (OHRP, 2009). States may have additional regulations and laws that restrict the use of genetic materials, judicial rulings that direct informed consent, and claims related to tissue sampling (Raymond, Steinert, Escourrou, & Fourtanier, 2002). Specific statutes by state can be accessed via the National Human Genome Research Institute website. CTNs need to be aware of these state regulations and how they affect informed consent in their personal setting of genomics research.

Informed Consent

In clinical trials it is required that the research subject *voluntarily* become a participant after receiving enough information about the research activity to make a decision about participation (McGuire & Beskow, 2010). Adherence to the *Code of Federal Regulations* (45 C.F.R. pt. 46, subpt. A) with the eight required elements for informed consent (see Chapter 14) is strictly enforced by an IRB within a research facility (Basic HHS Policy for Protection of Human Research Subjects, 2009). For each of the eight required elements, an informed consent for a genomics study will include relevant information to consider in the context of genomics research (National Human Genome Research Institute, 2014). Sample language for each of the eight elements of informed consent specific to genomics research can be accessed at www.genome.gov/27559024. The NCI Office of Biorepositories and Biospecimen Research (OBBR) offers six issues and risks that should be specified (see Figure 35-1). Other aspects to consider for the informed consent of research including biospecimens can be accessed at the OBBR Best Practices website (http://biospecimens.cancer.gov/bestpractices). Different categories of informed consents may be used in specimen collection (see Table 35-1).

Acquiring informed consent for the collection, storage, and future research use of biospecimens can be difficult because the specifics of the future research may not be known at the time the biospecimen is collected. Under certain circumstances, informed consent may not be required or could be waived. These circumstances include (1) the specific human subject research is exempt from the regulations [45 C.F.R. § 46.101(b)] or (2) the research is nonexempt human subject research that has been granted a waiver by an IRB of the requirements for informed consent [45 C.F.R. § 46.116(c) or (d)] (NCI OBBR, 2011). OHRP regulations also define some situations in which an IRB can consider an exemption from obtaining informed consent for human tissue. These include (OHRP, 2009)

- The specimen has no personal identifiers.
- No interaction will occur between the investigator and the individual to whom the specimen belongs.
- The key to the code with personal identifiers is destroyed before the research begins.
- The investigator has an agreement with the key holder to the code that the information will not be released while the individual is alive.
- IRB policies and procedures are in place to prevent the release of the key to coded information.

A separate statement should be included to ask the subjects if they would permit future tests for unknown reasons on their sample, or if they can be contacted by the investigator about future research that could involve the subject's tissue sample (American College of Medical Genetics and Genomics, 2007).

Human Specimen Collection

When biospecimens are collected for research, specific requirements are outlined in the previously cited DHHS and FDA regulations (OHRP, 2009). In addition, the NCI OBBR (2011) website clearly specifies the technical and operational best practices including a detailed explanation and procedures for (a) the biospecimen resource management and operations, (b) the biospecimen collection processing, storage, retrieval, and dissemination, (c) quality management, (d) biosafety, (e) collection and management of clinical data, and (f) biospecimen resource informatics: data management and inventory control and tracking. CTNs need to be aware of and able to implement these best practices so that subsequent analysis of the biospecimens will not be compromised. For example, once tissue is removed from the human body it will immediately begin to be transformed into a nonliving biologic specimen with characteristics that may differ from a living being. In some instances, the sample is placed in paraffin. Although this preserves the sample, many laboratory procedures cannot be performed with paraffin-preserved tissue. CTNs need to be ready to intervene with the correct collection and storage information for the specific tissue or have given the requirements to the designated laboratory technician for careful follow-up of the specimen collection and storage requirements. For CTNs in smaller community settings, the best practices resource can be adapted for local or smaller repositories. Other resources that can be helpful to CTNs or principal investigators are found in Figure 35-2.

Figure 35-1. Some Informed Consent Inclusions for Biospecimens

For the benefit of human research participants, an informed consent document outlining important issues and risks in straightforward language should be developed and implemented. The informed consent document should specify the following:

- That patients have the right to refuse biospecimen donation, and that this will in no way influence their treatment or eligibility to participate in clinical trials.
- Why particular biospecimens are being sought and why human research participants are being asked to participate.
- The source of the biospecimens that will be collected for research; for example, whether the biospecimen will come from leftover tissue from a surgical procedure or from an additional procedure (e.g., an extra blood draw).
- Who will be the custodian of the biospecimens and what will be the custodian's role.
- How the obtained biospecimens will be used and whether they will be used in secondary research.
- Whether biospecimens will continue to be stored and shared as long as they are potentially useful for research, respectfully destroyed when no longer useful for research, or transferred to another established resource in accordance with the terms of the informed consent.

Note. From *NCI Best Practices for Biospecimen Resources* (p. 37), by National Cancer Institute Office of Biorepositories and Biospecimen Research, 2011. Retrieved from http://biospecimens.cancer.gov/bestpractices/2011-NCIBestPractices.pdf.

Table 35-1. Types of Informed Consent for Biospecimens With Definitions

Type of Consent	Definition
Specific	Project-specific, where patients are asked to donate a specimen for a specific research project and are re-contacted for each new use of their specimen for additional studies.
Tiered	Presents options for the patient to direct the use of their specimen for any combination of multiple options such as a specific study, future research, and non-related diseases.
Open	A one-time generic consent for unlimited use of the specimen in all types of research, future research, and time periods. The option to withdraw consent at any time is still available to the subject.
Presumed	Subjects are informed that their specimens will be used for future research unless they deny permission for the use.

Note. Based on information from Chan et al., 2013.

Figure 35-2. Resources for Best Practices of Tissue Repositories

- International Society for Biological and Environmental Repositories. (2011). *2012 best practices for repositories: Collection, storage, retrieval, and distribution of biological materials for research* (3rd ed.). Retrieved from http://c.ymcdn.com/sites/www.isber.org/resource/resmgr/Files/2012ISBERBestPractices3rdedi.pdf
- National Cancer Institute Office of Biorepositories and Biospecimen Research. (2011). *NCI best practices for biospecimen resources.* Retrieved from http://biospecimens.cancer.gov/bestpractices/2011-NCIBestPractices.pdf
- Eiseman, E., Bloom, G., Brower, J., Clancy, N., & Olmsted, S.S. (2003). *Case studies of existing human tissue repositories: "Best practices" for a biospecimen resource for the genomic and proteomic era.* Retrieved from http://www.rand.org/pubs/monographs/MG120.html
- *Report of the Public Responsibility in Medicine and Research (PRIM&R) Human Tissue/Specimen Banking Working Group: Part I Assessment and Recommendations.* (2007, March). Retrieved from http://www.primr.org/workarea/DownloadAsset.aspx?id=936
- World Health Organization International Agency for Research on Cancer Biobank. (2011). *Recommendations, protocols, and best practices on sample collection, storage, and retrieval in IARC Biobank.* Retrieved from http://ibb.iarc.fr/docs/recommendations_BRC.pdf

---

Human tissue repositories are used to collect, store, and distribute human tissue materials for research purposes. If supported by DHHS, they involve three components, each with specific regulatory components as shown in Figure 35-3. This figure also emphasizes the IRB's oversight of the process from tissue collection and storage to the recipient investigator's responsibilities (OHRP, 2009).

Collection of Biospecimens

The goal for every biospecimen should be a high-quality collection, maintenance, and dissemination to the recipient investigator for the intended research use. This means the tissue should resemble the tissue of origin as closely as possible when used in the research study so that the outcomes and analysis can be as accurate as possible, minimizing errors that could cost a company thousands—or millions—of dollars.

Certain preanalytic and analytic variables require careful attention. The physiology of the human research participant prior to the biospecimen collection needs to be carefully evaluated and data meticulously documented. The protocol will guide the preanalytic data collection, but CTNs should consider if other data might be important to include that might affect the variables considered in the study (NCI OBBR, 2011).

Uniformity in biospecimen collection practices needs to be maintained. Variations could affect the quality of the sample collections. For example, noting the collection time of a surgical sample after blood flow to the organ has ceased can help investigators consider changes in molecular profiles that might have been altered due to longer versus shorter delivery times for tissue (NCI OBBR, 2011).

Meticulous annotation of the data should be included on the tagged specimen (or its container) and in a database. This implies the importance of informatics as a resource in maintaining accurate data for genetic and genomic research (OBBR, 2011).

Different biospecimens, such as wet tissue, frozen tissue, glass slides, blood, serum, and urine, have different best practice standards to follow for high-quality results in research. Protocols should be followed as thoroughly as possible. Deviations should be reported or documented in the data collection record. Storage containers are important for each tissue type. Freezers should be monitored for their stable temperature status (NCI OBBR, 2011). Healthcare professionals responsible for managing the biospecimen collection, maintenance, and transfer need to be qualified and trained to adhere to the standard operating procedures. These personnel can include researchers, technicians, nurses, surgeons, pathologists, anesthesiologists, and assistants who are highly trained and aware of the goals of the biospecimen collection and maintenance facility (NCI OBBR, 2011). For example, a $-80°C$ freezer can damage cells if it is allowed to have a warmer temperature. If a sample is placed in liquid nitrogen, it is important to consider that the temperature at the top of the liquid nitrogen freezer is below $-140°C$ (NCI OBBR, 2011). Because of the sensitivity of the tissues to fluctuations in their storage environment, preparation for shipping will also require careful attention (NCI OBBR, n.d.). A sample material transfer agreement can be accessed at http://biospecimens.cancer.gov/bestpractices/Appendix4.pdf.

Data Sharing

One item of genomic-related research that can be an advantage as well as a concern is that tiered consents produce large datasets to be developed that can be shared with the broader research community. These datasets are useful beyond the particular aims of the study for which they were originally collected and also for different diseases that were studied in the original research project. This may increase the value of the data, but this possibility needs to be stated in the informed consent and be directed by the IRB for clarification regarding how it will be handled for future analysis (National Human Genome Research Institute, 2015).

Investigators funded by National Institutes of Health (NIH) for genome-wide association studies must adhere to a data sharing policy that requires de-identified genetic (genotypic and phenotypic) data be shared through a centralized NIH data repository. Documenta-

```
┌──────────────────────────────────────────────────────────────────────────────────────────┐
│         Figure 35-3. Components of Human Tissue Repositories and Regulatory Requirements  │
│                                                                                           │
│   Tissue Collector       Repository Storage and      Recipient Investigator │
│                                               Data Management Center                      │
│                                                                                           │
│                                                         │
│                                                                                           │
│     IRB Review                                 IRB Review                                 │
│   Informed Consent                        Sample Informed Consent          Recipient Agreement │
│   Submittal Agreement                    Certificate of Confidentiality         Local Policies │
│  Assurance of Compliance                  Assurance of Compliance                         │
│                                                                                           │
│ IRB—institutional review board                                                            │
│ Note. From "Issues to Consider in the Research Use of Stored Data or Tissues," by Office for Protection From Research Risks, U.S. Department of Health and Human Services, 1997. Retrieved from http://www.hhs.gov/ohrp/policy/reposit.html. │
└──────────────────────────────────────────────────────────────────────────────────────────┘
```

tion is required to describe how institutions have considered the interest and rights of the research participant in addition to consent compliance with 45 C.F.R. pt. 56 regulations (NIH, n.d.; University of California, San Diego Human Research Protections Program, 2012).

Genetic Information Nondiscrimination Act Protection

The Genetic Information Nondiscrimination Act of 2008 (GINA) has implications for human subjects and their family members participating in clinical research, especially if the study includes a component of genetic or genomic research. GINA is a federal law that prohibits discrimination in health insurance or employment situations based on an individual's genetic information. It prevents insurance companies or employers from discriminating against someone participating in a research study who was found to have some genetic mutation. One exception is that health insurers or group health plans engaged in research are allowed to request, but not require, individuals to undergo genetic testing. Another exception is each individual state's regulation, which specifies that although participation is voluntary, no genetic information may be used for underwriting purposes and the health insurer must notify the federal government in writing that they are conducting a study and must comply with all future conditions that the federal government may require (OHRP, 2009).

Implications for Clinical Trial Nurses

CTNs play a critical role in the informed consent process and education of the research subject participating in a biospecimen banking study (Sanner, Yu, Udtha, & Williams, 2013). As with other informed consents, factors such as culture, education, and literacy need to be considered in the consent process, and CTNs must ensure that participants understand the information contained within the consent.

Careful attention by the CTNs to the tissue needs for safe storage offers accurate research results in the future. CTNs should be aware that every piece of data can affect more than one life (Oncology Nursing Society, 2010).

Many studies now require tissue testing to determine if an individual is eligible to participate. This can cause the patient confusion at the start of treatment, anxiety about the type of treatment, and concern about the delay of treatment initiation. CTNs should note if the specimen will be retained or returned to the facility site of origin and ensure it is returned to the facility as needed (Oncology Nursing Society, 2010). As technology provides more sensitive molecular testing, having access to the original cancer tissue specimen could be an issue of cure for patients receiving cancer treatment in the future.

Being at the front line in cancer genetic and genomic research offers CTNs an opportunity to learn and comprehend molecular information that many healthcare professionals struggle to even appreciate the rationale for use in patient care. The role requires someone with a desire to attain as close to perfection of data collection as possible and a desire to be an active participant in the future (Oncology Nursing Society, 2010). NCI OBBR (n.d.) has many resources that can be helpful for those in the CTN role.

Summary

Storage of genetic materials is a rapidly expanding area needed to support genetic and genomic research in the private, academic, and industry settings. Many regulations exist to protect the rights of human subjects. CTNs need to be aware of the best practices necessary to obtain the correct informed consent and how to accurately obtain, process, and store the tissue for the most accurate analysis possible. As the era of personalized medicine continues to focus on the genetic and genomic questions for the diagnosis and treatment of disease, CTNs need to keep abreast of the state of the art of best practices in biobanking and use of tissue in research. This chapter provides an overview of content that CTNs need to be proficient in their role and able to educate their patients about what is happening to their research tissue sample.

Key Points

- The process of tissue sample collection and storage is common to research studies sponsored by NIH and pharmaceutical companies, especially since the completion of the Human Genome Project in 2003.
- Careful oversight of certain aspects of research on human tissue samples, with specific regulations, is regulated by the U.S. DHHS, including FDA and OHRP.
- The process of informed consent for individuals providing tissue samples for research involves the participants understanding what they are consenting to and being able to verbalize back their understanding of what will occur as a result of providing their consent to participate.
- CTNs are required to manage many facets of a research protocol in order to protect and care for both patients and the genetic or genomic biospecimens.

References

American College of Medical Genetics and Genomics. (2007, May 23). Statement on storage and use of genetic materials. Retrieved from https://www.acmg.net/StaticContent/StaticPages/Storage.pdf

Basic HHS Policy for Protection of Human Research Subjects, 45 C.F.R. §§ 46.101–46.124 (2009). Retrieved from http://www.hhs.gov/ohrp/humansubjects/guidance/45cfr46.html#subparta

Chan, T., Mackay, S., & Hegney, D. (2013). Patients' experience on donation of their residual biological samples and the impact of these experiences on the type of consent given for the future research use on of the tissue: A systematic review. *International Journal of Evidence-Based Healthcare, 10*, 9–26. doi:10.1111/j.1744-1609.2011.00251.x

McGuire, A., & Beskow, L. (2010). Informed consent in genomics and genetic research. *Annual Review of Genomics and Human Genetics, 11*, 361–381. doi:10.1146/annurev-genom-082509-141711

National Cancer Institute Office of Biorepositories and Biospecimen Research. (n.d.). Web resources. Retrieved from http://biospecimens.cancer.gov/bestpractices/wr/

National Cancer Institute Office of Biorepositories and Biospecimen Research. (2011). NCI best practices for biospecimen resources. Retrieved from http://biospecimens.cancer.gov/bestpractices/2011-NCIBestPractices.pdf

National Human Genome Research Institute. (2015, February 5). Informed consent for genomics research: Process and special considerations. Retrieved from http://www.genome.gov/27559020

National Institutes of Health. (n.d.). Genomic data sharing (GDS): Policy. Retrieved from http://gds.nih.gov/03policy2.html

Office for Human Research Protections. (2009, March 24). Guidance on the Genetic Information Nondiscrimination Act: Implications for investigators and institutional review boards. Retrieved from http://www.hhs.gov/ohrp/policy/gina.html

Oncology Nursing Society. (2010). *Oncology clinical trials nurse competencies.* Retrieved from http://www.ons.org/sites/default/files/ctncompetencies.pdf

Raymond, M., Steinert, R., Escourrou, J., & Fourtanier, G. (2002). Ethical, legal, and economic issues raised by the use of human tissue in postgenomic research. *Digestive Diseases, 20*, 257–265. doi:10.1159/000067677

Sanner, J.E., Yu, E., Udtha, M., & Williams, P.H. (2013). Nursing and genetic biobanks. *Nursing Clinics of North America, 48*, 637–648. doi:10.1016/j.cnur.2013.09.005

University of California, San Diego Human Research Protections Program. (2012, November 28). Research involving the use of existing data/specimens. Retrieved from http://irb.ucsd.edu/secondary-use.pdf

U.S. Food and Drug Administration. (2014, February 21). Vaccines, blood and biologics: 7341.002 Inspection of human cells, tissues, and cellular and tissue-based products (HCT/Ps). Retrieved from http://www.fda.gov/biologicsbloodvaccines/guidancecomplianceregulatoryinformation/complianceactivities/enforcement/complianceprograms/ucm095207.htm

Chapter 36

Pharmacokinetic Trials

Ashish Thakkar, MS

Introduction

Historically, the development of a new drug is considered to be a very complex and tedious process. However, over the past 50 years significant changes have occurred in the drug development and approval process with some drugs, such as anticancer drugs and antiretroviral drugs, receiving faster approval through expedited review for very rare and incurable diseases.

The main objective of phase I oncology clinical trials is to identify the adverse events and dose-related toxicities in order to determine the maximum tolerated dose and for optimal design of phase II trials (Borden & Dowlati, 2012) (see Chapter 4). The subsequent phases of clinical trials are used to identify the safety and efficacy of the drug candidate on ever-larger targeted populations of patients with different types of cancers before it receives final marketing approval.

During drug discovery and development, the major contributing factors that lead to drug failure are poor pharmacologic and toxicologic properties, as well as poor pharmacokinetic (PK) properties. Compared with other drugs, the failure rate for oncology drugs is considered very high, approximately 95% (DiMasi & Grabowski, 2010). PK trials usually occur during an early phase of the drug development process, especially a phase I trial, to determine the PK parameters. In this chapter, the details about PK trials, parameters, study design, and sample collection will be discussed. Clinical trial nurses (CTNs), with their in-depth knowledge of clinical trials, play a major role in conducting PK trials.

Role of Pharmacokinetic Trials in Oncology Drug Development

PK trials play a crucial role in defining the absorption, distribution, metabolism, and profile of the drug. Simply, *pharmacokinetics* (depicted in Figure 36-1) can be described as "what the body does to the drugs" (Undevia, Gomez-Abuin, & Ratain, 2005). Generally, the drug development process starts in a laboratory as development of a new chemical entity. During preclinical cancer drug development, a new drug is tested on laboratory animals with tumors to identify the antitumor pharmacodynamics (PD), PK effects, and toxicologic effects. Once these are determined, the drug with better PD and PK effects and least toxicity is transferred to a clinical phase of the drug development process.

The design for a phase I oncology clinical trial is different than that for other therapeutic areas because an anticancer drug is used to inhibit the growth of cancer cells (Narang & Desai, 2009). Another major difference for oncology drug development is the PK trials. During oncol-

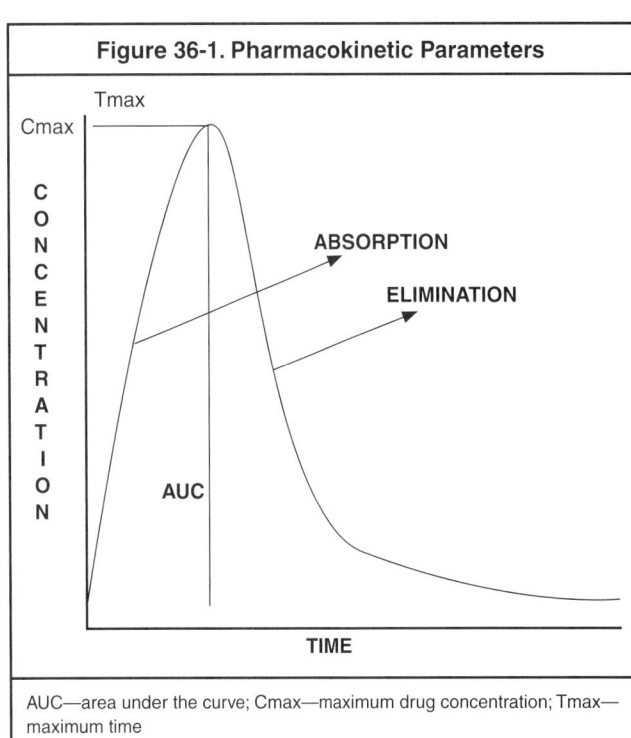

Figure 36-1. Pharmacokinetic Parameters

AUC—area under the curve; Cmax—maximum drug concentration; Tmax—maximum time

ogy drug development in the clinical setting, PK trials are carried out with patients with cancer during the phase I trial, whereas PK trials for most other drugs are done on healthy volunteers. During early-stage clinical development, different dose escalation studies are done to determine the maximum tolerated dose of the drug at a defined level of toxicity (Narang & Desai, 2009). After the dose and defined toxicity are determined, the dose is maintained throughout the later phases of clinical trials and the entire treatment period after its approval. However, if the toxicities increase during phase II or phase III clinical trials, the dose may be decreased to a tolerable dose and then maintained through the entire treatment period.

Pharmacokinetic Parameters

During dose escalation studies of oncology drugs, the PK parameters are measured at different dose levels in addition to assessing the toxicities of the studied drug. The parameters include (a) half-life of the drug, (b) maximum drug concentration, (c) bioavailability, (d) clearance, (e) area under the curve, and (f) volume of distribution. PK parameters are usually measured by collecting blood samples or other body fluids at different time intervals and recording them on a PK worksheet (see Figure 36-2). Sometimes, PK parameters are measured during phase II clinical trials to confirm the PK profile of the drug because some drugs have higher intrapatient PK variability. The PK parameters are described in Table 36-1.

Pharmacokinetic Clinical Trials Setting

U.S. Food and Drug Administration (1999) guidance requires mandatory performance of separate studies for PK analysis of a single novel agent, making the main purpose of PK studies to meet the regulatory requirement, which includes patient safety (Comets & Zohar, 2009; Gallo, 2010). A better clinical trial design gives better outcomes and saves money for the pharmaceutical company. For oncology PK trials, the optimal trial design involves (a) the study goal, (b) the number of patients included, and (c) the number of blood samples collected per patient per specified time period (Aarons & Ogungbenro, 2010). The design and sample schedule for PK trials depend on the pharmacologic effects, toxicities, and physiologic properties of a drug because these characteristics vary for each investigational drug. For oncology drug development with PK trials done as dose escalation studies, a novel drug agent is usually combined with the available standard treatment for cancer (Gustafson & Bradshaw-Pierce, 2011).

The initial dose of the study drug for a PK study should be selected from the dose obtained from the preclinical trials. Initially, the lowest dose should be administered in a limited number of patients for defined toxicity. The initial dose is a crucial consideration for PK trials. It must be carefully calculated based on available data because the outcome could cause severe toxicity and ultimately affect subsequent trials with the drug (Yap, Sandhu, Workman, & De Bone, 2010).

An appropriate method for delivering a safe and effective dose of an anticancer drug requires a narrow therapeutic index when researchers initiate the development of an anticancer drug (Gustafson & Bradshaw-Pierce, 2011). However, the PK and dosing parameters of the newer *targeted* anticancer drugs are different than those used with the conventional *cytotoxic* drugs (Gilman, 1963).

The PK parameters today are typically measured by collection of peripheral blood. During a PK trial, blood samples are collected at different time intervals that are clearly defined in the protocol, before and after the initial drug administration. A template for a PK blood collection sheet is illustrated in Figure 36-2. A typical blood sample collection schedule for a PK trial would begin prior to the administration of drug (control sample) and continue at 0.25, 0.5, 1, 2, 6, 8, 12, 24, and 48 hours after drug administration. The samples should be collected as accurately (on time) as possible. If a sample is collected late for any reason, CTNs should prepare a protocol deviation for the time variation between the target time and actual time. After collection, the samples should be processed and shipped immediately per protocol description.

CTNs play a major role in conducting PK trials beginning from patient recruitment to sample shipment. Because PK trials involve collection of more blood samples as compared to other trials, CTNs should give more attention to recording the actual time the blood samples are collected. In addition, CTNs should also be familiar with processing equipment and shipping procedures (Mais, 2006).

Basically, the two PK approaches are the standard PK approach and the population PK approach (Gao et al., 2012). The approaches differ by number of blood samples to be collected. In the standard PK approach, frequent sampling of blood is required for a small group of patients, while for the population PK approach, a limited number of blood samplings are required from larger populations.

A PK trial is quantitative; therefore, it measures the drug concentration in body fluids over period of time. Different PK models can be used to determine the PK parameters by analyzing blood samples.

Pharmacokinetic Models

Various PK models use a quantitative analysis to determine the absorption, distribution, metabolism, and exertion profiles of the drugs over a period of time.

Compartmental Model

The compartmental model is the most commonly used model to analyze blood samples from PK studies. In this approach, the body is theoretically divided into different compartments, and each is characterized as individual or a group of tissues. Although this is useful, it has some limitations, such as (a) only a limited number of drug plasma

Figure 36-2. Sample Pharmacokinetic Worksheet					
Patient Name:			**Today's Date:**		
Date of Birth:			**Dose (mg/m^2)**		
Weight (kg):			**Actual Dose (mg)**		
Height (cm):			**Dose Start Time:**		
BSA (m^2):			**Dose Completion Time:**		
Sample #	Time Post Dose	Target Time	Actual Time		Comments
1	Pre-dose				
2	5 min				
3	15 min				
4	30 min				
5	1 hr				
6	2 hr				
7	4 hr				
8	6 hr				
9	8 hr				
10	24 hr				
11	48 hr				
The Target Time in the third column of the table is calculated from the Dose Completion Time (i.e., time at the end of an IV infusion) and the Time Post Dose for each sample. For example, if an infusion ends at 9 am, then the Target Time for Sample #2 is 9:05 am.					
Note. Figure courtesy of Frank M. Balis, MD, head of the Pharmacology and Experimental Therapeutics Section, Pediatric Branch, National Cancer Institute, 2006.					

Table 36-1. Definitions of Pharmacokinetic Parameters	
Parameter	Definition
Area under the curve (AUC)	The measurement of plasma drug concentration over the period of time the drug remains inside the body
Bioavailability	The amount of drug absorbed and available to the target tissue
Drug clearance	The volume of drug cleared from the plasma per unit of time; in other words, the drug elimination rate per unit of time
Elimination half-life	The time required for drug to reduce its plasma concentration by half of the original concentration
Maximum drug concentration (Cmax)	The concentration of drug when it reaches a maximum level in plasma
Maximum time (Tmax)	Time required for drug to achieve maximum serum concentration
Metabolism	The biochemical modification of an administered drug, which leads to the activation of a prodrug inside the body
Rate of absorption	Rate of elimination
Volume of distribution	A ratio of the total amount of drug administered in the body to the total amount of blood plasma concentration of drug
Note. Based on information from DiPiro et al., 2010; Hill, 2008.	

concentrations can be analyzed, (b) variation exists based on the study population and route of drug administration, and (c) creating the proper model is difficult. This model is further classified into one-compartment and multicompartment models (www.ashp.org).

One-Compartment Model

In the one-compartment model, the body is characterized as a single central compartment after drug administration (see Figure 36-3). When drug is administered inside the body, it distributes very rapidly throughout the body, and the drug equilibrates spontaneously within tissues. In this model, the tissue drug concentration should not be considered as a drug plasma concentration (Dhillon & Kostrzewski, 2006; Gustafson & Bradshaw-Pierce, 2011).

Multicompartment Model

The body is characterized as two compartments (i.e., central compartment and peripheral compartment) (see Figure 36-4) in the multicompartment model. This model acknowledges multiple compartments; however, there is no actual division of anatomic or physiologic compartments. Some body tissues fall under the heading of a central compartment, whereas some fall under the category of the peripheral compartment. Using this model, after drug administration, the drug does not rapidly distribute throughout the body. Instead, it transfers from the central compartment to the peripheral compartment and vice versa. As a function of the multicompartment model, the drug does not spontaneously equilibrate between tissues (Dhillon & Kostrzewski, 2006; Gustafson & Bradshaw-Pierce, 2011). For instance, when drug is administered by either the oral or IV route, it is first distributed within the central compartment, then it subsequently distributes in the peripheral compartment, which indicates rapid decrease in drug concentration in the central compartment and rapid increase in drug concentration in the peripheral compartment. After some time, equilibrium is established between both compartments and the drug starts to eliminate from the central compartment.

Noncompartment Model

The noncompartment PK model defines the PK parameters between different doses of the same drug or the same drug administered at the same dose to different patients (Gustafson & Bradshaw-Pierce, 2011). This method is used mostly for calculation of data from bioequivalent trials, and the data obtained by this method

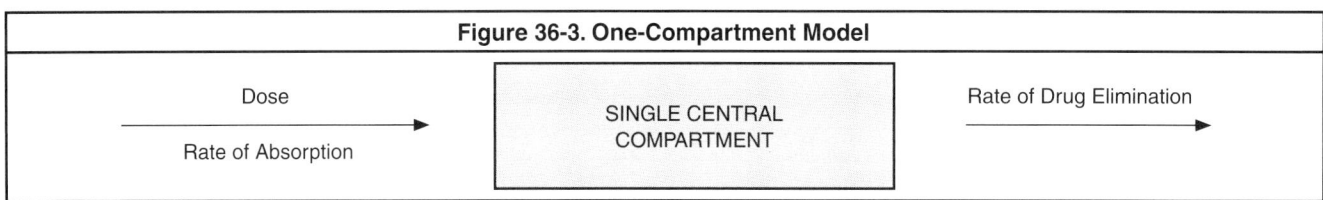

Figure 36-3. One-Compartment Model

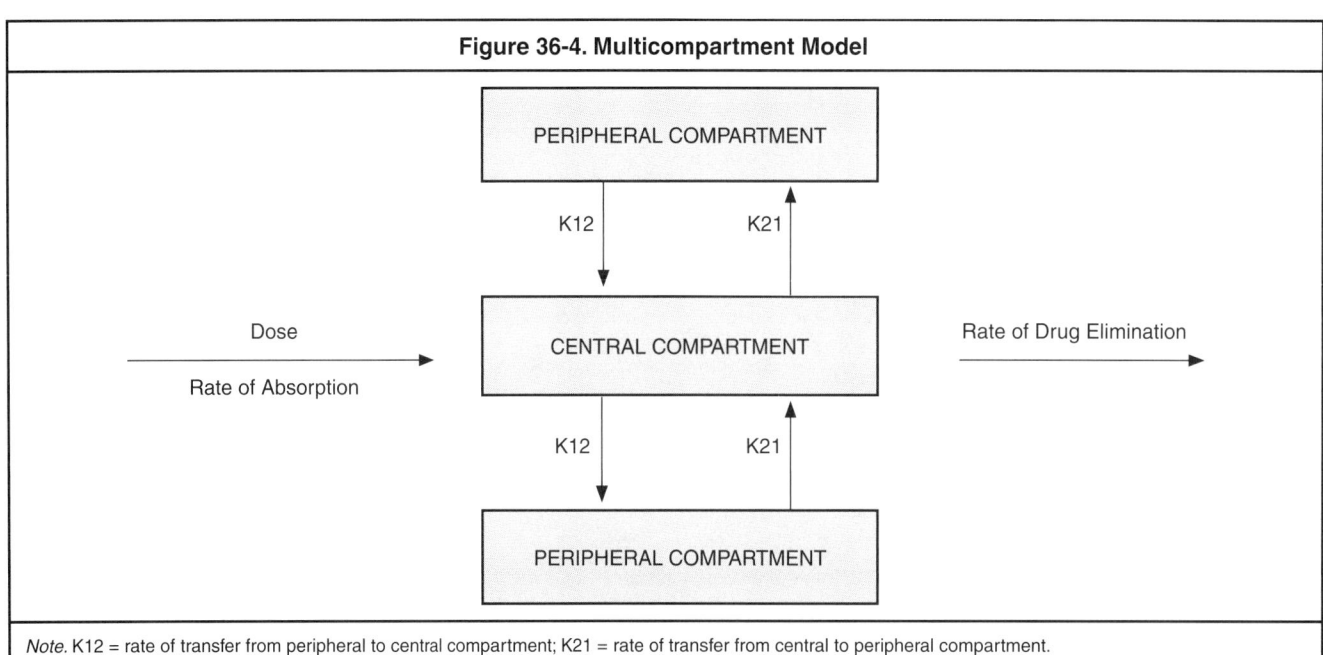

Figure 36-4. Multicompartment Model

Note. K12 = rate of transfer from peripheral to central compartment; K21 = rate of transfer from central to peripheral compartment.

are less likely to be manipulated. Although this method is not model-dependent, some authors still consider it as a model-based approach. This model requires only a few assumptions as compared to the compartmental models. For instance, if a drug is administered to patients, the PK parameters can be best described in some patients using a one-compartment model, whereas in other patients, PK parameters can be best described by a two- or multicompartment model. This model has no such compartments; therefore, it ultimately reduces the assumptions to describe the PK parameters.

Although the noncompartment model is superior to the compartmental models, it has some limitations. A study conducted for determination of PK parameters of the anti-HIV agent indinavir on animals using both compartmental and the noncompartmental analysis concluded that significant errors occurred in the analysis of terminal phase data while applying noncompartmental analysis (Hashimoto, 2009). Some of the limitations of noncompartment models are inadequate determination of nonlinear PK parameters and limited information about drug plasma concentration versus time profile.

Population Pharmacokinetic Model

The population PK model can be defined as the determination of variability in PK among special target populations by measuring plasma drug concentration in body fluids (Aarons & Ogungbenro, 2010; Hamidi, 2010). In the population PK model, small numbers of samples are collected from each individual participant with a large number of participants in the trial. This method is used for special types of populations such as pediatric or elderly patients. Because each individual patient has different demographic and physiologic characteristics, the plasma drug concentration could not be the same when the same amount of drug is administered to those patients. In this scenario, the population PK approach is a very important aspect in determining the PK variability, which ultimately helps to determine the dosing regimen for each individual patient. Furthermore, the protocol should clearly specify the appropriate number of patients and samples from each patient at appropriate time points to meet the study goals. The U.S. Food and Drug Administration (1999) described population PK as a useful tool in anticancer drug development because of the narrow therapeutic index of anticancer drugs, and the effects of the anticancer drugs depend on how drug is exposed inside the body. However, some drawbacks for this model include cost, inaccuracies in data reporting, and study design (Zandvliet, Schellens, Beijnen, & Huitema, 2007). The study design for the population PK model requires large numbers of patients to be enrolled, which ultimately increases the trial cost. Additionally, the study design is complex compared to other PK models, and the complexity may lead to inaccuracies in reporting data.

Physiologically Based Pharmacokinetic Model

The physiologically based pharmacokinetic model (PBPK) identifies the body organ or tissue that absorbed the administered drug, and then mathematically describes the drug PK by applying physiologic, chemical, and biochemical principles (Aarons & Ogungbenro, 2010; Nedelman, 2005). PBPK is usually a multicompartment model in which various body organs or tissues represent each compartment when the drug is administered inside the body; then the factors that impel the absorption, distribution, metabolism, and exertion of a drug are described in a mechanistic way. Scientists develop a PBPK model during preclinical testing to predict human PK data, and then the same model is modified during the clinical development of the drug (Khalil & Laer, 2011). The limitations of this model are the large sample size and complexity in the study design (Zhao, Rowland, & Huang, 2012).

Summary

Most of the early anticancer trials are performed to identify the safety and efficacy of a drug, and they are considered therapeutic trials because they have a direct impact on patient safety. PK trials are performed to determine the PK parameters of a drug. Because they do not have a direct effect on patient safety, they are considered nontherapeutic trials and represented to patients as optional. However, the risk associated with PK trials is minimal. These studies help in determining the absorption, distribution, metabolism, and exertion of a drug, which can be useful information in a subsequent trial. Therefore, a PK trial with an optimal design should be incorporated in early clinical drug development of an anticancer drug to maximize or improve the outcomes in subsequent trials. CTNs need to carefully complete all documents and monitor the time schedule for initiation of the drug, collection of samples, and completion of the protocol (Oncology Nursing Society, 2010).

Key Points
- PK studies play a crucial role in defining the absorption, distribution, metabolism, and exertion profile of a drug.
- During dose escalation studies of oncology drugs, the PK parameters are measured at different dose levels while assessing the toxicities of the medication targeted for study.

- A better clinical trial design provides better outcomes and can save money for the pharmaceutical company.
- The PK parameters are clearly defined in the protocol and typically measured by peripheral blood collected at different time intervals both prior to and after the initial drug administration.
- Various PK models use a quantitative analysis to determine the absorption, distribution, metabolism, and exertion profiles of the drugs over a period of time.

References

Aarons, L., & Ogungbenro, K. (2010). Optimal design of pharmacokinetics studies. *Basic and Clinical Pharmacology and Toxicology, 106,* 250–255. doi:10.1111/j.1742-7843.2009.00533.x

Borden, E.C., & Dowlati, A. (2012, December). Phase I trials of targeted anti-cancer drugs: A need to refocus. *Nature Reviews Drug Discovery, 11,* 889–890. doi:10.1038/nrd3909

Comets, E., & Zohar, S. (2009). A survey of the way pharmacokinetics are reported in published phase I clinical trials, with an emphasis on oncology. *Clinical Pharmacokinetics, 48,* 387–395. doi:10.2165/00003088-200948060-00004

Dhillon, S., & Kostrzewski, A. (2006). Basic pharmacokinetics. In S. Dhillon & A. Kostrzewski (Eds.), *Clinical pharmacokinetics* (pp. 1–44). Grayslake, IL: Pharmaceutical Press.

DiMasi, J.A., & Grabowski, H.G. (2010). Economics of new oncology drug development. *Journal of Clinical Oncology, 25,* 209–216. doi:10.1200/JCO.2006.09.0803

DiPiro, J.T., Spruill, W.J., Wade, W.E., Blouin, R.A., & Pruemer, J.M. (2010). Introduction to pharmacokinetics and pharmacodynamics. In J.T. DiPiro, W.J. Spruill, W.E., Wade, R.A. Blouin, & J.M. Pruemer (Eds.), *Concepts in clinical pharmacokinetics* (pp. 1–18). Bethesda, MD: American Society of Health-System Pharmacists.

Gallo, J. (2010). Pharmacokinetic/pharmacodynamic-driven drug development. *Mount Sinai Journal of Medicine, 77,* 381–388. doi:10.1002/msj.20193

Gao, B., Yeap, S., Clements, A., Balakrishnar, B., Wong, M., & Gurney, H. (2012, November). Evidence for therapeutic drug monitoring of targeted anticancer therapies. *Journal of Clinical Oncology, 30,* 4017–4025. doi:10.1200/JCO.2012.43.5362

Gilman, A. (1963, May). The initial clinical trial of nitrogen mustard. *American Journal of Surgery, 105,* 574–578. doi:10.1016/0002-9610(63)90232-0

Gustafson, D.L., & Bradshaw-Pierce, E.L. (2011). Fundamental concepts in clinical pharmacology, principles of anticancer drug development. In B.A. Teicher (Ed.), *Cancer drug discovery and development* (pp. 37–62). New York, NY: Springer Humana Press.

Hamidi, M. (2010). Pharmacokinetic properties of indinavir in rat: Some limitations of noncompartmental analysis. *Drug Development and Industrial Pharmacy, 36,* 355–361. doi:10.3109/03639040903173564

Hashimoto, Y. (2009). Limited sampling strategy for patient-oriented clinical pharmacokinetic trial. *Drug Metabolism and Pharmacokinetics, 24,* 199–200. doi:10.2133/dmpk.24.199

Hill, C.S. (2008). Pharmacokinetics, pharmacodynamics, and pharmacogenomics. In A.D. Klimaszewski, M. Bacon, H.E. Deininger, B.A. Ford, & J.G. Westendorp (Eds.), *Manual for clinical trials nursing* (2nd ed., pp. 235–241). Pittsburgh, PA: Oncology Nursing Society.

Khalil, F., & Laer, S. (2011). Physiologically based pharmacokinetic modeling: Methodology, application, and limitations with a focus on its role in pediatric drug development. *Journal of Biomedicine and Biotechnology, 2011,* Article ID 907461. doi:10.1155/2011/907461

Mais, K. (2006). The role of the research nurse in hospital-based oncology clinical trials. *Oncology News, 1*(3), 22–23.

Narang, A.S., & Desai, D.S. (2009). Anticancer drug development: Unique aspects of pharmaceutical development. In Y. Liu & R.I. Mahato (Eds.), *Pharmaceutical perspectives of cancer therapeutics* (pp. 49–92). New York, NY: Springer. doi:10.1007/978-1-4419-0131-6_2

Nedelman, J.R. (2005). On some "disadvantages" of population approach. *AAPS Journal, 7,* E374–E382. doi:10.1208/aapsj070238

Oncology Nursing Society. (2010). *Oncology clinical trials nurse competencies.* Retrieved from https://www.ons.org/sites/default/files/ctncompetencies.pdf

Undevia, S.D., Gomez-Abuin, G., & Ratain, M.J. (2005). Pharmacokinetic variability of anticancer agents. *Nature Reviews Cancer, 5,* 447–458. doi:10.1038/nrc1629

U.S. Food and Drug Administration. (1999). *Guidance for industry: Population pharmacokinetics.* Retrieved from http://www.fda.gov/downloads/ScienceResearch/SpecialTopics/WomensHealthResearch/UCM133184.pdf

Yap, T.A., Sandhu, S.K., Workman, P., & De Bono, J.S. (2010). Envisioning the future of early anticancer drug development. *Nature Reviews Cancer, 10,* 514–523. doi:10.1038/nrc2870

Zandvliet, A.S., Schellens, J.H., Beijnen, J.H., & Huitema, A.D. (2007). Population pharmacokinetics and pharmacodynamics for optimization in clinical oncology. *Clinical Pharmacokinetics, 47,* 487–513. doi:10.2165/00003088-200847080-00001

Zhao, P., Rowland, M., & Huang, S.-M. (2012). Best practice in the use of physiologically based pharmacokinetic kinetic modeling and simulation to address clinical pharmacology regulatory questions. *Clinical Pharmacology and Therapeutics, 92,* 17–20. doi:10.1038/clpt.2012.68

SECTION VIII.

Documentation and Data Management

Chapter 37

Documentation

Tasha D. Hall, PhD, RN

Introduction

Data generated from a clinical trial are analyzed to determine the results of the trial. The U.S. Food and Drug Administration (FDA) regulations state that it is the responsibility of the investigator to "prepare and maintain adequate and accurate case histories that record all observations and other data pertinent to the investigation on each individual administered the investigational drug or employed as a control in the investigation" (Case Histories, 2014, § 312.62(b)). Information from a patient participant's clinical record is extracted onto specific case report forms (CRFs) for the clinical trial. This extraction process may be done by clinical trial nurses (CTNs) or clinical data managers. Chapters 10 and 38 provide more information about managing data, but documentation is the first step in managing data. The basic rules of documentation in clinical practice apply for clinical trial participants with additional types of documentation needed. This chapter provides an overview of the basic rules for documentation in clinical trials and defines source documents.

Basic Rules of Documentation in a Medical Record

The basic principle underlying clinical care documentation is if it was not documented, it was not done. This includes procedures performed and discussions between the healthcare team and the patient/family. Examples of discussions that need to be documented include the informed consent process and patient education. In clinical research, it is critical to document everything that occurs as well as everything that does not occur. Each interaction that CTNs have with the study participants should be documented in the patient records. When documenting in any patient record, CTNs have to do so in a legible and legal manner. Erasing or covering mistakes is prohibited. To cross out an item, one single horizontal line should be drawn through it. Then, the writer must initial and date the crossed-out information. All documentation in patient records should be completed in ink, not pencil. Correction fluid should not be used. No abbreviations may be used on the forms for a clinical trial unless the specific protocol indicates that they are appropriate. The date and time should be recorded with each entry. Items that are observed and assessed during the interaction should be documented in the medical record. Use the patient's own words in the documentation note when describing patient-reported symptoms.

Electronic records and electronic signatures used in FDA-regulated research are covered in Title 21 C.F.R. Part 11 (Electronic Records; Electronic Signatures, 2014). Part 11 applies to records in electronic form that are created, modified, maintained, archived, or transmitted under any requirements set forth in FDA regulations. It addresses electronic CRFs, electronic patient diaries, electronic health records, software validation, and source documents. Parameters for both open and closed systems to ensure authenticity, integrity, and confidentiality of the electronic records are included in the regulation. Certification of all electronic signatures is required (U.S. FDA, 2003). For corrections in an electronic medical record, the system will retain who made the correction, when it was made, the original record, and the updated record. For more on electronic records, see Chapter 38.

Although in a research setting, CTNs are practicing under nursing licenses and need to continue to follow the state's nurse practice act, which typically will include documentation of patient participant encounters.

Source Documents

Per the International Conference on Harmonisation of Technical Requirements for Registration of

Pharmaceuticals for Human Use (ICH, 1996), *source data* are

> all information in original records and certified copies of original records of clinical findings, observations, or other activities in a clinical trial necessary for the reconstruction and evaluation of the trial. Source data are contained in source documents (original records or certified copies).

The source data entered onto CRFs are obtained from source documents. *Source documents* are

> original documents, data, and records (e.g., hospital records, clinical and office charts, laboratory notes, memoranda, subjects' diaries or evaluation checklists, pharmacy dispensing records, recorded data from automated instruments, copies or transcriptions certified after verification as being accurate copies, microfiches, photographic negatives, microfilm, or magnetic media, x-rays, subject files, and records kept at the pharmacy, at the laboratories, and at medico-technical departments involved in the clinical trial). (ICH, 1996)

Data reported on the CRF that are derived from source documents should be consistent with the source documents, and any discrepancies should be explained. Source documentation serves to substantiate the integrity of the clinical trial data, confirm observations that are recorded, and confirm the existence of study participants (Woodin, 2011). A source document is needed to support any information documented on a CRF for a clinical trial. An example would be a rating scale or questionnaire completed by the patient. The purpose of source documentation is to serve as a tool to reconstruct the clinical trial as it happened for an independent observer. The source document affirms compliance with the protocol and the integrity of the data. Accurate documentation in the source document supports the protection of subjects' safety (Bargaje, 2011). The source document also serves as an audit trail to recreate a patient's progress on a clinical trial.

Each patient participant has a medical record, either electronic or paper, and a research record. Some documents serve as source documents that are often not allowed to be placed in a medical record. However, they need to be maintained as source documents. Creating a research record allows the research team to save these types of source documents. See Figure 37-1 for examples of documents maintained in either the medical record or research record.

Many source documents for today's clinical trials are maintained electronically. Electronic record keeping ensures transferability of participant data from one clinic location to another and can be used for real-time data transfer to an electronic CRF.

Figure 37-1. Medical Record Versus Research Record

Medical Record	Research Record
(Includes all hospital records, medical charts, and clinical or office charts)	• Copy of signed informed consent document
• Physical exam findings	• Subject diaries
• Consent process	• Quality-of-life or other surveys or tools
• Diagnostic reports	• Pharmacokinetic worksheets
• Operative reports	• Eligibility checklists
• Laboratory reports	
• Data recorded from automated instruments	

Note. From *Documentation in Clinical Research* [PowerPoint Presentation], by National Cancer Institute Center for Cancer Research, n.d. Retrieved from http://clinicaltrial.vc.ons.org/file_depot/0-10000000/0-10000/3367/folder/14779/Documentation_1011.pdf.

ALCOA

The acronym ALCOA (attributable, legible, contemporaneous, original, and accurate) is synonymous with key attributes for good documentation and quality data applied throughout the drug development process (e.g., manufacturing practices and clinical trials) (Bargaje, 2011). It is referenced in the FDA guidance titled *Guidance for Industry Part 11, Electronic Records; Electronic Signatures Scope and Application.* Over time, other regulatory agencies (e.g., World Health Organization, European Medicines Agency [EMA]) have adapted ALCOA, and additional attributes have been added by EMA to include enduring, available and accessible, complete, consistent, credible, and corroborated (Bargaje, 2011). How these key attributes are used by members of the research team to document various research-specific time points are described in the next section.

Research-Specific Documentation

Documentation that is acceptable in clinical practice may need additional details when a patient, now a research participant, enters a clinical trial. Some clinical trial–specific events must be documented for research participants. CTNs do not have to provide all the documentation but should ensure that all the documentation exists.

Informed Consent Process and Eligibility Confirmation

The informed consent process should be documented with a note that the consent process occurred and the patient received a signed copy of the informed consent. The discussion of the protocol treatments, adverse events

(AEs), follow-up required, and any patient/family concerns should be included in the pretreatment notes. A note verifying eligibility needs to be made that includes the statement that the patient meets all of the inclusion criteria and has no exclusionary criteria. All results for labs, pathology, and any other procedures that are required to confirm eligibility should be in the appropriate section of the medical record (paper or electronic). The patient's past medical history and previous therapies need to be noted in a summary of the initial history and physical or in a recent one. Outside reports and records that confirm the prior therapies and pathology need to be placed in the medical record per the organization's policy (National Cancer Institute [NCI] Center for Cancer Research [CCR], n.d.).

Baseline Symptoms and Concomitant Treatments

Information about baseline symptoms and concomitant treatments (e.g., medications or other measures such as oxygen use) need to be documented in the medical record. All baseline symptoms due to either the patient's disease or prior therapies should be documented, including the start date and severity of each symptom. In addition to a list of the concomitant medications with dose and frequency given, the start date of each medication needs to be documented. Any changes to the concomitant medications, including dose adjustments and discontinuation, need to be noted. The date for concomitant medications taken prior to enrollment can be noted as month/year. Once the patient has begun study treatment, the date should also include the day in addition to month/year. The reason the patient is on the medication should also be noted. Some medications are given for indications not approved by FDA, so CTNs should not assume that the patient is taking them for the condition indicated in the package insert. This is referred to as *off-label use*. Patients may be taking over-the-counter and complementary medicines that have not been prescribed by a physician. These need to be included in the concomitant medication list because of the potential impact on the study treatment. Any new concomitant medications that the patient begins to take during the course of the study treatment need to be documented (NCI CCR, n.d.).

Protocol-Specific Activities

All protocol-related activities (e.g., clinic visits, physical exams, blood draws) need to be documented in the medical record, including when they occurred, any results, and any follow-up that may be needed. Some of the information may be on the final report (e.g., laboratory result, radiology report). Protocol-specific procedures need to be documented. Examples include pharmacokinetic blood samples being drawn and biopsies being obtained. If a scheduled visit is missed, it needs to be noted, including the reason and any follow-up that needs to occur because of the missed visit (NCI CCR, n.d.).

Any unscheduled visits (i.e., visits not per protocol) need to be documented. The location of the visit, reason for the visit, and any follow-up should be included. Examples are a patient visit for AE management at the oncology office or a visit to the emergency room. Document any telephone calls with the patient, including the reason for the call and outcome (NCI CCR, n.d.).

Adverse Events

For each AE, the following information should be documented (CCR, n.d.).
- When the AE started
- Description of the event, including how severe the event is. This information is then used to select the correct AE term and grade using the NCI Common Terminology Criteria for Adverse Events (see Chapter 28 for more detail about AEs).
- How the AE was treated, if applicable
- Attribution of the AE
- Date the severity of the AE improved or worsened if applicable
- When the AE was resolved

Study Drug Administration

All study drugs, including any pre- or post-study medications and hydration administered, must be recorded in the medical record by the licensed practitioner who gave the drugs. This documentation should include the date, time, amount, and route of administration. The time should include start and stop times for IV medications. Any missed doses and the reason the dose was missed should be noted. This documentation is typically done by the nurse who administers the medication. If a CTN is not administering the drug(s), he or she should ensure that documentation is completed in a timely manner (NCI CCR, n.d.).

Documentation of self-administered study drugs (i.e., when patients take the drug on their own) should include instructions for proper use/administration and storage, participants' adherence to regimen, and if the correct amount of drug was returned (NCI CCR, n.d.). For example, if a participant is to take 10 mg of study drug ABC123, then an entry in the medical record needs to state "the patient states she took 10 mg of ABC123 every day for the past 28 days; denies missing any doses, correct amount of drug returned." Some studies will have patient diaries that are completed and included in the research record, but a note in the medical record is still needed so as to communicate the information to other members of the healthcare team caring for the participant.

Off Treatment

When the study medication or other study intervention (e.g., radiation therapy) is discontinued, the patient comes off treatment. The reason that study intervention is discontinued and the date should be noted. The date is the day that the investigator/treating physician decided that no further treatment was warranted. This might be a result of the patient completing the planned treatment, or it might be due to disease progression, patient choice, or physician decision. Protocols routinely require ongoing follow-up after treatment is discontinued to monitor for duration of current AEs and onset of new AEs (NCI CCR, n.d.).

Off Study

A patient is considered off study when he or she has completed all study-related procedures, tests, or follow-up visits. Off-study documentation needs to include the date and reason (e.g., completed six cycles of therapy, completed follow-up, died from disease progression). For protocols that have long-term follow-up, all attempts to locate the patient should be documented before deeming the patient off study (NCI CCR, n.d.).

Discrepancy Documentation

If at any time there is conflicting documentation or discrepancies in source documents, a clarification note is required. CTNs are usually responsible for looking for these discrepancies and facilitating their resolution, which may include talking with the author(s) or writing their own note to clarify what the correct documentation is. For example, conflicting documentation can occur when two healthcare providers provide different dates or description of events. CTNs can contact the patient and ask for clarification and then document that interaction (NCI CCR, n.d.).

Challenges

Clinical trials occur over a long period of time with many members of the healthcare team documenting data in the source documents. Maintaining continuity of documentation practice over time can be difficult. Documentation for clinical research can be more extensive than what is performed as a part of routine clinical practice. Patients are treated in multiple locations, and all of these documents are considered source documents (Bargaje, 2011).

Summary

The quality of the study data is directly affected by the quality of the study documentation. CTNs frequently are responsible for ensuring that documentation is available and accurate so that CRFs are accurately completed. Although this can be viewed as a mundane task, it is vital to the success of clinical trials. Data recorded on CRFs are used, for example, to evaluate the efficacy of an investigational agent. All source documents need to be completed accurately and in a timely manner to ensure the successful completion of the study.

Key Points

- CTNs should document all patient-participant encounters per their state's nurse practice act.
- Documentation for clinical research can be more extensive than what is performed as a part of routine clinical practice.
- Source documents serve as an audit trail to recreate the research participant's progress on a clinical trial.
- The quality of the study data is directly affected by the quality of the study documentation.

References

Bargaje, C. (2011). Good documentation practice in clinical research. *Perspectives in Clinical Research, 2,* 59–63. doi:10.4103/2229-3485.80368

Case Histories, 21 C.F.R. § 312.62(b) (2014). Retrieved from http://www.accessdata.fda.gov/scripts/cdrh/cfdocs/cfcfr/CFRSearch.cfm?fr=312.62

Electronic Records; Electronic Signatures, 21 C.F.R. pt. 11 (2014). Retrieved from http://www.accessdata.fda.gov/scripts/cdrh/cfdocs/cfcfr/CFRSearch.cfm?CFRPart=11&showFR=1

International Conference on Harmonisation of Technical Requirements for Registration of Pharmaceuticals for Human Use. (1996, June 10). *ICH harmonised tripartite guideline: Guideline for good clinical practice, E6(R1).* Retrieved from http://www.ich.org/fileadmin/Public_Web_Site/ICH_Products/Guidelines/Efficacy/E6/E6_R1_Guideline.pdf

National Cancer Institute Center for Cancer Research. (n.d.). Documentation in clinical research. Retrieved from http://clinicaltrial.vc.ons.org/file_depot/0-10000000/0-10000/3367/folder/14779/Documentation_1011.pdf

U.S. Food and Drug Administration. (2003, August 28). *Guidance for industry: Part 11, Electronic records; electronic signatures—Scope and application.* Retrieved from http://www.fda.gov/downloads/RegulatoryInformation/Guidances/ucm125125.pdf

Woodin, K.E. (2011). *The CRC's guide to coordinating clinical research.* Boston, MA: Thomson CenterWatch.

Chapter 38

Data Management and Electronic Data Management Systems

Dianne M. Reeves, RN, MSN, and Anita Walden, BS, CHI

Introduction

The increasing value and sensitivity of data in clinical trials is elevating the need for careful planning and management. This chapter focuses on how clinical trial nurses (CTNs) can obtain maximum return from clinical data management plans and practices and examines the capabilities of most electronic data management systems. These systems have the ability to help CTNs manage data that are complex and typically voluminous. The need to apply rigorous processes and procedures to the handling of data requires that nurses be familiar with data management plans (DMPs) and their execution. Electronic data management systems can implement these plans to extend the reach of CTNs in data surveillance, capture, and reporting. Electronic systems have additional value over paper-based systems that must be leveraged to improve data quality and processes. Detailed information on data management practices and electronic data management systems is increasingly associated with professional-, therapeutic-, and disease-specific standards that will assist CTNs in managing time-sensitive practices and setting realistic expectations.

Clinical Data Management Practices

An important aspect of the clinical research life cycle is the collection, processing, storage, and sharing of data for analysis, which is the core of data management. There continues to be a focus on the value of data, which has highlighted the importance of quality data for study results and public safety. With growing demand to provide much-needed diagnostics, treatments, and therapies to the general public faster while managing costs, it is up to those working with data to identify technologies and methods to improve the process. Everything from cutting-edge tools to data management planning will help CTNs meet the growing demand for data to increase knowledge.

Clinical Data Management Plans

In recent years, with the implementation of new technologies and systems to capture, store, and manage data, there has been a growing awareness of the need to document the process to ensure the security, integrity, and quality of data. It is recognized that investing the time to plan the processes and activities within data management will increase the probability of meeting the intended goals of the research study while improving efficiencies and maintaining control. As a result, the development, implementation, and maintenance of DMPs has grown as good practice for conducting research and is commonplace in most organizations that handle data. Some organizations require DMPs as a condition for the funding of grants, and often sponsors or auditors will ask to review these documents along with the standard operating procedures (SOPs) (Raymond, 2011; Weaver, 2006; Woods Hole Oceanographic Institution, n.d.). In addition to compliance with regulations and requirements, the keys to a successful study are how early in the process the data planning starts, the quality of the planning, and the effectiveness of the implementation (Rondel, Varley, & Webb, 2000).

The Office of Management and Budget's Circular A-110 (2005) defines *research data* as "the recorded factual material commonly accepted in the scientific community as necessary to validate research findings, but not any of the following: preliminary analyses, drafts of scientific papers, plans for future research, peer reviews, or communications with colleagues" (p. 51881).

Data are the foundation of research, and great analysis techniques cannot make up for the lack of quality, quantity, or completeness of data needed to test a hypothesis or answer a scientific question. Regulators, sponsors, and auditors are now requesting documentation of data acquisition, curation, exchange, and sharing to provide assurances of the integrity and quality of the data (National Science Foundation, 2011, 2012).

Definition and Purpose

DMPs are living paper or electronic records that document the processes and procedures to promote consistent, efficient, and effective data management practices on an individual study (Massachusetts Institute of Technology, n.d.). It is important to provide documentation on the study level, rather than a department or program level, because each study has unique project and data requirements that should be outlined, and the documentation serves as a record of what was collected and how data were handled. The DMP should be designed to meet the needs of various types of trials, patient registries, or specific therapeutic areas. For example, community registries in which participants complete online surveys may not require a section in the DMP that describes a query process, but may have a section on validating data received through a website.

Essential aspects of the DMP provide consistent communication across the study team, promote efficient use of resources, and demonstrate a clear path to reach intended goals. It can be an effective tool to monitor progress, establish decisions, and implement changes systematically. The plan is an authoritative resource, documenting data management processes agreed upon by the stakeholders. Creating a plan at the start of the study will provide benefits such as meeting study or grant requirements, saving time and resources, and addressing potential risks that may arise.

Components of a Data Management Plan

The complexities and nature of a study can influence the DMP, but minimum standards recommended by professional clinical data management societies (e.g., Society for Clinical Data Management and the American Medical Informatics Association's data management work group) should be followed, such as (a) having a plan in place prior to the first participant being enrolled, (b) ensuring that the plan is in compliance with regulations and oversight agencies, (c) identifying and defining personnel and roles involved in decision making, data collection, data handling, and quality control, and (d) ensuring that data management processes are described and defined from study start to database lock or close.

It is important that the plan is current and versioned to document when process changes took place. The types of research (e.g., prospective, observational, registries) or therapeutic information can influence the content or design of a DMP because of the variations in requirements, types of data, and data collection methods. Usually the scope of a DMP specifies who is involved with the data handling; what deliverables, tasks, or processes are conducted; and how they are carried out.

Organizations have differing opinions on the level of detail needed in DMPs. Some place all documentation related to data management in the plan, including SOPs, whereas others may reference study files and guidelines and work instructions. What should be part of the DMP and the amount of information it should contain can depend on the role of the organization, such as who is performing the data management, and whether it is a sponsor, a contract research organization, an academic research organization, or a site. If an organization is partnering with an external group to perform data management tasks, it may require more detail in the DMP to have a complete picture of all processes and tasks and may require a list of SOPs that are followed and any deviations to those SOPs. Despite the differences across the industry, some common components are preferred (see Figure 38-1) (Society for Clinical Data Management, 2011).

Roles and Responsibilities

Maintaining a current list of all trained study team members who are working with the data on that study is important. According to the U.S. Food and Drug Administration (FDA) regulations for electronic records (21 C.F.R. § 11.10(d)), access must be limited to authorized individuals. Some guidelines recommend a list of user roles and access to security safeguards, which includes a plan for removing access (Society for Clinical Data Management, 2011). Organizations may manage this with a list of all individuals who have access to the database and the dates of access. It is strongly recommended that there is a documented record that individuals have the training or skills to perform the tasks on the trial, and some regulatory agencies require this documentation.

Figure 38-1. Components of a Data Management Plan

- Roles and responsibilities of all members who will handle data
- Description of the data that will be collected, data dictionaries, or form annotations
- List of standards or terminologies that are used along with their version
- How the data are acquired, processed, and stored
- Storage location of the data
- Data handling rules
- Data sharing or access practices/policies

Note. Based on information from Massachusetts Institute of Technology, n.d.; McFadden, 2007; Society for Clinical Data Management, 2011.

Description of Data Collected

Some organizations have a metadata file, data dictionary, or document listing the data collected for a study. This will include any data that are generated or received from sources other than paper or electronic data capture forms completed by the principal investigator, CTN or study coordinator, or study participant.

List of Standards and Terminology Dictionaries

The use of standard terminology or dictionaries usually is in reference to coding of medications and adverse events and includes research submission and exchange standards. Researchers, sponsors, and regulators want to know what standards and terminologies are used along with the versions. For long-term trials, versions may change, and it is important to document all versions. Because versions affect the data, there should be a description of how the version was implemented for the study, for example, if the entire database was versioned up or only data after a certain date. If using an autoencoder, it is important to document the workflow of how manually coded items are handled and approved.

How Data Are Collected, Processed, and Stored

Planning how data are to be collected will help ensure that they are collected in a timely manner. It is important to document whether data will be captured using electronic data capture, paper forms, directly from a participant, or downloaded from a device. For organizations using paper to collect data, the data ultimately will be entered into a database (e.g., the sponsor's database), so determining the use of single entry or double data entry is important. *Double data entry* is entering the same data twice to ensure data entry accuracy. With the increase in use of electronic tools, it should be documented what data sources are electronic. For example, some studies allow participants to enter data directly on a tablet, and the data are automatically uploaded into a database. In this case, the data uploaded are the source data, and that should be documented. Listing data transfers and how those data are processed or where they are stored once they arrive should be described.

Data Handling Rules

Written procedures should specify how data are entered and cleaned for data provenance (i.e., trace and reproduce data from the source) to ensure that changes or self-evident corrections on case report forms (CRFs) are documented, necessary, and endorsed by the investigator (Pancerella, Myers, & Rahn, 2002). Examples include conversion of units of measure, guidelines for manual queries, or correction of misspellings.

Data Sharing or Access

This component is fairly new to DMPs but is becoming increasingly more common because of regulations requiring data sharing plans to expedite translational science and increase knowledge (National Institutes of Health [NIH], 2003). Planning data sharing and access early in the study can ensure compliance with regulations and establish resources and processes that will enable effective data sharing. NIH requires a data sharing plan as part of an application for trials that meet certain criteria (NIH, 2003). See the NIH website for details (http://grants.nih.gov/grants/policy/data_sharing). The plan should help ensure that data are made publicly available in a timely manner and should describe the method used to provide access to the data.

Extensive DMPs may include
- Form design
- Edit checks
- System validation and testing
- Data flow diagrams
- Reporting and metrics
- Risk analysis
- Data exchange
- Auditing and quality control.

Maintenance and Approval of a Data Management Plan

The DMP is considered a living document that should reflect the processes and data requirements of the trial. Many changes occur during a trial because of incidents such as a protocol amendment or quality improvement, and the DMP must reflect those changes. It can be challenging to know when to modify the document because of the time it requires to keep it updated. Some organizations update the sections for major changes, whereas others may implement revisions on a cycle. A process should be created to describe when the plan should be updated, the approval process, and how the changes are communicated. The DMP often becomes the record of documentation that is referenced for responses to questions during the analysis phase.

Data Management Processes

Adherence to Regulations

Regulations are designed to maintain the privacy and security of data and improve data quality and reliability, which is to ensure the safety of the public. It is important to be familiar with the International Conference on Harmonisation of Technical Requirements for Registration of Pharmaceuticals for Human Use (ICH) E6 Guidelines for Good Clinical Practice (GCP) (1996) and the Health Insurance Portability and Accountability Act (HIPAA). If the trial uses investigational drugs, biologics, or devices, the *Code of Federal Regulations* title 21, part 11, which covers electronic data and signatures, applies (Electronic Records; Electronic Signatures, 2014).

Data Abstraction and Extraction

Original data generated from a research participant, as clinically observed or obtained directly from tests or devices, are called *source data*. Data from these sources can be entered directly into the clinical data management system (CDMS) or transcribed onto a paper CRF or study form and entered into the database at a later date. The data in the database should always match the data from the original source document; the data on a study form or CRF transcribed from the original source may not be considered the source data. If there is an intervening process from the source to the CRF (e.g., using a study form), it should be documented in the DMP. According to ICH (1996) GCP section 1.51, source data are contained in source documents (original records or certified copies).

According to U.S. FDA (2013) draft guidance, the authorized data originator can enter data obtained during a study visit directly into the electronic data capture system. The data in the electronic case report form (eCRF) are considered the source data, which will help reduce transcription errors and improve quality. FDA could still request other documents during an inspection to corroborate direct entry of a data element in an electronic data capture system. CTNs and other licensed providers need to comply with their state's licensure requirements for patient documentation.

In situations where data are abstracted from a medical record, transcribed to a paper form, and then entered into an eCRF or database, it is important that the data from the database and the source match. The source in this case would be the medical record, not the transcribed form. If data are entered into an eCRF directly from an electronic source document, such as displaying both the eCRF and the electronic medical record (EMR) on two different screens, that process should be outlined in the DMP. Most errors occur when data are transferred from sources to CRFs during medical record abstraction or transcription (Nahm, Pieper, & Cunningham, 2008). It is thought that the shift to obtaining data electronically directly from an EMR may reduce transcription errors because the data are not going through an intervening process such as data entry or copy and paste into an eCRF by a human.

Data Processing

Data are the core component of any clinical research activity, and without relevant data, the objectives will not be met. The scope of data processing, or data handling, historically began when CRFs were completed by the investigative site, but for electronic data capture studies, data processing activities start once the electronic data capture system has been designed and deployed and end with database lock or freeze. Data processing activities typically include (a) data retrieval, (b) data cleaning or validation, (c) data manipulation, which includes derivations (e.g., deriving an age using the date of birth and current date), (d) coding of events and medications, (e) data transfers, and (f) integration.

Handling Data Discrepancies and Resolving Issues

A major responsibility of data management is to provide quality data for analysis, which entails identifying and resolving discrepancies. Identification of data discrepancies can be achieved electronically or manually. Implementing an electronic process will provide consistency and reliability to review the data for possible issues. Most electronic systems include tools for communicating discrepancies for resolution, creation of standard messages, and discrepancy tracking that can inform the staff of not only which queries are open, but also the length of time the discrepancies have been unresolved. Even if an automated system for discrepancy management is in place, unique situations arise that require manual queries generated by a sponsor to a study coordinator at a site. It is important that these queries are clear and concise and do not lead the sites to give a particular response.

Once data have been entered and have met the expected level of quality, they are extracted from the CDMS into an analysis dataset using statistical software tools, such as SAS/STAT® and SPSS. Data can be transferred or views can be created to provide statisticians with access for analysis. The analysis performed on the data can sometimes identify issues that an electronic CDMS was not able to find. Many CDMSs are designed to identify discrepancies by data point; it is generally easier for analysis software to view data across patients and the study. Therefore, it is preferable that statisticians receive the data during the trial to identify issues early before trial data are locked.

Data managers usually maintain and follow instructions, known as *data handling guidelines*, on how to conduct data-related trial tasks. These instructions provide guidance on how data should be managed, including how they are entered, validated or cleaned, transferred, and coded, and how to ensure security. However, this data management activity may be part of the CTN's role.

Coding

Often, text data that are collected can be difficult to analyze unless they are standardized. Usually medications, adverse and serious adverse events, medical histories, and problem lists or diagnoses are collected using text fields. This information is classified to assess the safety of a drug or device, but it can be collected in a variety of ways. For example, one clinician may report "Fever" while another may report "Temp of 101." It is difficult to review this information electronically and determine if it is the same. Coding these terms to a single term of "Fever" will make it easier for analysis and summarization of the total occurrence of an event or medication. National or international coding dictionaries are implemented in data management systems so that once a term is entered, an autoencoder looks for similar information and codes it to a single term or identifier. If the system cannot find a match in the dictionary, the information is manually reviewed and coded. For a list of some dictionaries and terminologies used in research, see Figure 38-2.

Data Transmission and Exchange

During the course of a trial, there are data that may not come directly from the CRF or eCRF that is completed at the site but rather is generated from a different source, such as an electrocardiogram monitor or a central laboratory. These data can be transferred electronically to be placed in the CDMS or sent directly to the statistician for analysis. Data also can be transferred from the CDMS to a data coordinating center or sponsor. When receiving data electronically, it is important to understand how the data were generated, transformed (if applicable), and stored to ensure they are traceable to the source. When data are received or sent, the data transfer process should be validated to verify accurate receipt of the expected information. Steps to consider include the frequency, timing, format, and secure method of file transfer. If multiple transfers are occurring, it should be decided whether the file will contain only new data (appended) or all data, including data previously transferred (cumulative). It is recommended to perform a *test transfer* of the data. All data format changes in the database will affect the transfer file, and those changes should be communicated to the receivers so that they can make the changes on their end. Although CTNs may not be directly involved with data transfer, they should understand the overall process. They may have to perform data quality checks prior to the data being transferred or ensure that data from a patient's electronic devices have been transmitted.

Soon other types of data may be collected that may require different tools for transfer and storage. The industry is starting to include "-omic" (e.g., genomic, proteomic) data along with clinical datasets, which are very large and often referred to as "big data." Depending on the amount of data, the data transfer processes may be different from a typical exchange. As the need for integrating and accessing this type of data increases, so will the tools and skill sets.

Another consideration when transferring data is the formats that are used for exchange. The use of standards can facilitate the exchange of data between systems so that senders can communicate to receivers the data format, content, and the method of delivery (Hammond & Cimino, 2006). Data from a clinical system such as an EMR may use healthcare standards such as Health Level Seven (HL7) version 2.x or 3. Clinical research groups may use the Clinical Data Interchange Standards Consortium's (CDISC's) Operational Data Model or LAB Data Model. FDA recommends that studies submitting data to the agency for marketing approvals use the CDISC Study Data Tabulation Module format for sending their data electronically. It is helpful for technology personnel and clinicians (e.g., CTNs and investigators) to work together concerning interpretation of data or the type of study when determining the types of standards that will be used for a clinical trial.

Data Storage

The section on data management systems will cover data storage in detail, but it is important to mention that the data must be kept in a system that will ensure the data integrity and security. These systems should reside on servers that have a backup and recovery system in case of a disaster or loss of data. Many organizations are storing their data in central warehouses or data repositories so that other investigators can access the data for secondary analysis. If a study is funded by NIH, the data should meet federal record retention requirements so that the data are available under the Freedom of Information Act.

The sponsor will inform sites and other study personnel of the length of time that study forms and electronic records should be kept. According to ICH section 4.0, records should be kept for two years after the last approval of a marketing application in an ICH region or until at least two years have passed since the clinical development of the investigational product (ICH, 1996).

Figure 38-2. Examples of Dictionaries and Terminologies

- Common Terminology Criteria for Adverse Events (CTCAE): http://ctep.cancer.gov/protocolDevelopment/electronic_applications/ctc.htm
- International Classification of Diseases (ICD-10): www.cms.gov/Medicare/Coding/ICD10/index.html?redirect=/icd10
- Logical Observation Identifiers Names and Codes (LOINC®): http://loinc.org
- Medical Dictionary for Regulatory Activities (MedDRA®): www.meddra.org
- RxNorm: www.nlm.nih.gov/research/umls/rxnorm
- Systematized Nomenclature of Medicine—Clinical Terms (SNOMED CT®): www.nlm.nih.gov/research/umls/Snomed/snomed_main.html
- World Health Organization Drug Dictionary Enhanced (WHO-DRUG): www.umc-products.com/DynPage.aspx?id=2829

Because requirements may mandate that these documents and records be kept longer, the sponsor will communicate when the documents and records are no longer needed.

Data Privacy and Security

The increase in the use of technology that facilitates the ability to share information electronically has added concerns for the security and privacy of information. Clinical trials funded by federal agencies should follow Federal Information Security Management Act (FISMA) requirements to meet privacy and security standards. The act requires each federal agency to develop, document, and implement an agency-wide program to provide security for the information and information systems that support the operations and assets of the agency, including those provided or managed by another agency, contractor, or other source (National Institute of Standards and Technology, 2002). Federal agencies may require documentation to ensure that systems used to collect and store data comply with FISMA requirements. These include (a) a process for detecting, responding to, and reporting security incidents, (b) periodic assessment of risk to a system, and (c) security awareness training. A sponsor or regulatory agency may ask the research team to provide compliance documentation, which can be obtained from the information technology department.

Protected Health Information

HIPAA defines *protected health information* (PHI) as identifiable health information transmitted by electronic media, maintained in electronic media, or transmitted or maintained in any other form or medium such as information in medical records, which includes health status, provision of health care, or payment that can be linked to a specific individual (General Administrative Requirements, 2007). HIPAA pertains to health information collected and used in research studies and activities in settings related to the patient care process and covers *all humans living or dead* (Muhlbaier, 2002). Figure 38-3 contains a list of PHI identifiers. Disclosure of PHI is when information is provided to someone who is not part of the healthcare organization staff or faculty. Those who are considered a covered entity may have access to PHI as needed.

Data Quality

It is expected that the data collected for a clinical trial are reliable (i.e., have few errors) to support analysis. One way to ensure this is to measure the data quality and implement quality controls. An audit usually is conducted

Figure 38-3. Protected Health Information Identifiers

- Names
- All geographic subdivisions smaller than a state, including street address, city, county, precinct, zip code, and their equivalent geocodes
- All elements of dates (except year) for dates directly related to an individual, including birth date, admission date, discharge date, and date of death
- Telephone numbers
- Fax numbers
- Email addresses
- Social Security numbers
- Medical record numbers
- Health plan beneficiary numbers
- Account numbers
- Certificate/license numbers
- Vehicle identifiers and serial numbers, including license plate numbers
- Device identifiers and serial numbers
- Web URLs
- Internet protocol address numbers
- Biometric identifiers, including finger and voice prints
- Full-face photographic images and any comparable images
- Any other unique identifying number, characteristic, or code

Note. Based on information from U.S. Department of Health and Human Services, n.d.

at least once during the trial to evaluate the data quality and assess the control process. An audit plan describes the audit frequency, scope, criteria for passing, and a corrective action plan if the audit results do not meet the level of quality outlined in the plan. The quality control plan is designed to ensure a certain level of data quality by implementing process controls at intervals of the data life cycle. A list of quality control checks and frequency usually is part of the quality control plan. For more information on audits and inspections, see Chapter 41.

Case Report Form Design

Creation of eCRFs or paper CRFs is a critical step in data management because failure to collect the correct data will affect trial results. Forms should be created based on the study protocol, and, whenever possible, raw data versus derived data should be collected. For example, collecting the date of birth rather than age will provide more information because the age can be derived using other dates. The consequences of poorly designed forms include

- Collection of data that are not part of the study protocol
- Lack of clarity of required data
- Multiple requests for the same information (e.g., date of death)
- eCRF screens that do not display all data in a single display (i.e., a scroll bar has to be used, which results in missing data)

- Failure to collect the data needed for analysis (primary and secondary endpoints)
- Collection of data in a manner that cannot be easily analyzed
- Failure to use form or data standards
- Higher costs to develop forms.

Although data collection forms are based on the protocol, they usually contain certain categories or data modules (see Figure 38-4) along with key identifiers, such as the site identification number, protocol number, and unique patient identifier. CDISC's Clinical Data Acquisition Standards Harmonization (known as CDASH) is a standard for form development that is now widely used in clinical research. This will not only help with developing quality forms but also may enable researchers to aggregate data from other studies using the standard.

Clinical Research Standards

In recent years, more time and resources are being invested to better use technology in health care and research to improve safety and increase the availability of cutting-edge treatments. Implementing technology in isolation is not enough; there is a need to improve processes and share information across silos, such as health entities and organizations or domains, to increase knowledge that will benefit the community. This ability to collaborate across health entities will require systems and policies to work in unity and become interoperable, with a foundation in standards.

Standards are documents established by consensus and approved by a recognized body that provide, for common and repeated use, rules, guidelines, or characteristics for activities or their results, aimed at achieving the optimum degree of order in a given context (International Organization for Standardization [ISO] & International Electrotechnical Commission [IEC], 2011). Industries that have successfully implemented standards have improved data quality, increased productivity, facilitated compatibility, streamlined processes, and reduced timing of access to information. A lack of standards leads to ambiguous exchange and hinders understanding and interpretation of information within clinical research (Ewen et al., 2009; Mead, 2006).

The clinical research community is seeking the same benefits and solutions to some of their issues. Lack of access to information can result in medication errors, duplicate testing, and redundant data collection, leading to higher medical costs. Collection of the same data multiple times or from multiple sources introduces the potential for inconsistencies, which does not lead to confidence in the data. Data from multiple resources using the same term or name may have different meanings and could result in incorrect assumptions and conclusions. Standard semantic data elements, along with exchange standards, can address this issue.

Many organizations have developed their own standards, meaning they are only interoperable within their own institution and encounter challenges when engaging with other groups. Development and implementation of national or international standards will further enhance the ability for cross-functional and organizational communication. In clinical research, a number of organizations are developing standards and are involved in standards development initiatives. Some of the more well-known standards development organizations are ISO, HL7, European Committee for Standardization, and CDISC. These organizations design standards for data structure or modeling, exchange, and data semantics. Several types of standards are used in clinical research.

- Data exchange: Facilitate senders' ability to communicate with receivers on format and type of data
- Data format: Identify data (required and recommended) and outline the location of that data in a dataset
- Semantic data elements: Standardize the data element name, define the data element, and list permissible values or possible responses to questions

See Table 38-1 for an example of consensus data element standards and Table 38-2 for an example of permissible values for adverse events.

The challenge with standards is that there are many to choose from, which still presents a problem with interoperability. The healthcare and research communities are beginning to share data to increase access to information, which introduces the question of which set of standards should be used: health care or research. Gaps exist in standards (i.e., not able to cover the entire clinical research life cycle), so there is a need to continue to standardize processes and data, which requires the engagement of the clinical, clinical research, and informatics communities.

Figure 38-4. Sample Case Report Form Modules

- Demography
- Inclusion/exclusion
- Enrollment/randomization
- Medical history
- Physical examination
- Laboratory tests
- Electrocardiogram tests
- Medication history/study drug
- Treatment/intervention
- Drug accountability
- Adverse and serious adverse events
- Efficacy information
- Patient diaries
- Questionnaires
- Withdrawal, early termination, and study completion
- Approvals

Table 38-1. Example of Consensus Data Element Standards		
Data Element	**Clinical Data Definition**	**Permissible Values Set**
Date of diagnosis	Date subject diagnosed with tuberculosis or latent tuberculosis	Date
Source case sputum smear status	Whether source case had sputum that was smear positive or smear negative	Positive; negative; unknown
Underlying pulmonary disease	Underlying lung condition that puts an individual at increased risk for developing tuberculosis disease	Silicosis; chronic obstructive pulmonary disease (COPD); lung cancer; emphysema; other (specify)
Number of bacillus Calmette-Guérin (BCG) vaccinations	How many BCG vaccinations the subject has received	One; more than one

Note. Based on information from Health Level Seven International, 2009.

Table 38-2. Example of Valid Values Associated With Data Elements to Capture Adverse Event Grade		
Valid Value	**Meaning**	**Definition**
0	Absent adverse event	Grade 0 is universally defined as absence of adverse events or within normal limits or values.
1	Mild adverse event	An adverse event that is asymptomatic, involves mild or minor symptoms, is of marginal clinical relevance, consists of clinical or diagnostic observations alone, for which intervention is not indicated, or for which only nonprescription intervention is indicated
2	Moderate adverse event	An adverse event for which only minimal, local, or noninvasive intervention (e.g., packing, cautery) is indicated or that limits instrumental activities of daily living (e.g., shopping, laundry, transportation, ability to conduct finances)
3	Severe adverse event	An adverse event that is medically significant but not life threatening, for which inpatient care or prolongation of hospitalization is indicated, that is an important medical event that does not result in hospitalization but may jeopardize the patient or may require intervention either to prevent hospitalization or to prevent the adverse event from becoming life threatening or causing death, that is disabling, or that results in persistent or significant disability, incapacity, or limitation of self-care activities of daily living (e.g., getting in and out of bed, dressing, eating, getting around inside, bathing, using the toilet)
4	Life-threatening adverse event	An adverse event that has life-threatening consequences, for which urgent intervention is indicated, that puts the patient at risk of death at the time of the event if immediate intervention is not undertaken, or that causes blindness or deafness
5	Death related to adverse event	The termination of life associated with an adverse event

Note. Based on information from Health Level Seven International, 2009.

Future Considerations

The landscape of clinical research is constantly evolving, which includes integration of environmental, "-omic," and clinical data in registries and repositories to increase knowledge. The research and healthcare communities are becoming partners in data retrieval and sharing with the implementation of EMRs. Data from EMRs can be integrated into a clinical research system without the need to manually enter or recollect the data from study participants. The sharing of information from clinical EMR systems can greatly change the clinical research process, reducing the need for data entry and improving monitoring while increasing skill sets in informatics to design processes and validate data exchange software and functionality. Therefore, CTNs need to have a greater understanding of technology and its impact in clinical research.

The shift in clinical research, specifically data management, will provide new opportunities to move into a direction for developing knowledge management tools instead of focusing on data collection. Data management skills will make way for informatics skills—changing from a task focus to analysis and solution-driven roles and responsibilities. This shift helps to modernize data management and leverage the innovation that is at the heart of clinical research.

Electronic Data Management System Implications in Clinical Trials

In a guest editorial in *Applied Clinical Trials*, Robert Vogel described *remote data capture* as a "radical change" when it began to be used in clinical trials in 1983 (Vogel, 1997). Thirty years later, the use of electronic applications to capture clinical trial data has become ingrained in the operations of many organizations. Although not every corner of the clinical trial community has adopted electronic systems, considerations surrounding implementation, cost, regulatory requirements, and the best way to handle legacy operations and data deserve serious evaluation. This section will discuss the structure of an electronic data management/clinical trial management system, characteristics of electronic systems that comprise value for an organization, enhanced capabilities offered by electronic systems, and finally, a review of the state of electronic applications and their future use.

Comparison of Clinical Data Management Systems and Clinical Trial Management Systems

Confusion about the difference between a clinical data management system (CDMS) and a clinical trial management system (CTMS) is common (Laszlo, 2006). A CDMS is associated with traditional approaches to clinical trial activities; there is a heavy data management component with collection of data on paper CRFs that are then transcribed onto eCRFs. Data are cleaned and transported to various reporting and care-associated destinations. In a new paradigm, a CTMS is a means to integrate data from many systems (e.g., laboratories, genomics, adverse events), enter and clean the data in expedited steps, and store them in a repository that can serve multiple purposes over time. Key to CTMS operations is the concept of "services" or capabilities, such as the ability to handle patient randomization at the same time as adverse event reporting and creation of laboratory report alerts for clinicians.

An abundance of CDMS and CTMS systems are available from software vendors. To evaluate one of them as part of a purchase activity or to create supporting training materials or policies, CTNs need to stay focused on evaluation criteria. This includes focusing on what their organizations need in order to accomplish their missions in terms of operations, reporting, connectivity with other systems, and overall capability. The most beneficial way to evaluate electronic systems is to formulate a set of criteria *before* viewing any product demonstrations. The danger of losing sight of core requirements in the face of an appealing product is very real and potentially devastating. Weaver (2006) summarized some of the dangers in reviewing a CTMS, including the underestimation of reporting requirements and the lack of planned interoperability with other electronic systems.

Capabilities of Clinical Data Management Systems

Advances in cancer detection, prevention, treatment, and survivorship have a foundation in the data generated from clinical trials. This is a critical connection that underscores the need to guarantee the quality and validity of data that are gathered and shared. Data are the most important outcome from the conduct of clinical trials. Therefore, the need to institute systems and processes that yield the highest-quality data is paramount for any organization engaged in the conduct of clinical trials.

NIH Director Dr. Francis S. Collins (2011) noted that "medical benefits of the current revolution in biology clearly cannot be achieved without vigorous and effective translation" (p. 1). This means that processes and systems need to be examined for efficiency, costs, and overall outcomes to advance basic biomedical research to clinical applications that will benefit patients. Innovative trial designs need technology support that uses synergies between systems to create rich and dynamic data operations that reap the benefit of research for the public good. This synergy allows researchers to more clearly function in the role of domain or subject expert, identifying requirements for an electronic system but not charged with finding a solution. The creation and maintenance of a CDMS or CTMS must be a coordinated effort between information technology and the research team, reflecting a balanced relationship between humans and machines.

Scope

Multi-institutional and multicenter research consortia trials are now commonplace. What may have been unique requirements to handle data collection from disparate sites can be managed with a common data management solution. Data management teams can operate from a single point of access or from virtually anywhere a web-based portal can be accessed. By logging into one website, users can access a variety of functions based on privileges distributed by role. Based on how a person interacts with a clinical trial, the system can display customized forms, interfaces, and tools to speed workflow.

The merits of a remote entry system are extensive but must be balanced by increased security risks and concern over the data. Concerns exist as to data ownership and sharing. If one group enters data that can be shared or used by another group, policies of data governance and maintenance need to be established. Each institution or user group needs to conduct a thorough assessment of its data management needs based on projected scope, outcomes, and resources.

Scalability

CDMS and CTMS applications are designed to scale—to grow as needed without loss of function or data. This is a paramount feature because the ability to predict data management needs over time will always be limited. *Scalability* is the ability of an application or a business approach to grow without a significant loss of efficiency or effectiveness. Scalability must be considered from the inception of a project because it affects the ultimate success or failure of a data management system implementation. A system that is easy to use and easy to teach to others, completes tasks as expected in a minimum of time, and produces output reliably and efficiently is an excellent candidate for adoption by a large community of users.

In settings where performance improves even with the addition of more users, the system can be considered to be scalable. However, in the beginning phases of CDMS or CTMS implementation, it may take some time for performance improvements to surface. In one instance, electronic system solutions had the ability to produce similar data accuracy metrics as traditional paper-based approaches (Walther et al., 2011). However, adjustments in work processes and resource allocations had to be made during initiation of the system. The ability to enter data directly into an electronic system may require more up-front time but results in faster processing and availability of the data for reporting and sharing. Therefore, there is an imperative to evaluate new electronic systems realistically, allowing the time necessary for users to gain the skills and confidence they need to enter reproducible quality data. CTNs can be important members of the team who review these systems and assess the ability to meet requirements of an organization, but an even more important role is one of advocate and group support amid the changes that accompany transitions to electronic systems.

Interoperability

Interoperability is a key attribute for any successful data management system. The ability of systems to function together is part of the new approach for improved electronic systems. For example, data from a laboratory system or a registry of medical images represent a huge and valuable addition to a traditional set of clinical data. Instead of manual entry of data from one application into another, which is known to be extremely time consuming and filled with potential for error, it is more desirable to have data from these systems integrate or combine as appropriate to create a richer data flow. Data can be housed in a single repository or pulled from several sites in the form of a report or query as needed.

Interoperability is also a function of the data itself—the ability to query the content and aggregate or extract data with the same meaning. This is particularly key in the current era of big data, where sheer volumes of data affect the ability to produce reliable data in a timely manner. Quality data management systems use widely accepted external standards in which the meaning of the content being collected is documented and widely accepted. A good example is the international standard for units of measure, the Logical Observation Identifiers Names and Codes, or LOINC®, terminology. LOINC is one of the standards used in U.S. federal government systems to exchange healthcare data and is supported by the National Library of Medicine. This standard provides a universal coding system for clinical and laboratory test data that facilitates the capture, storage, aggregation, and exchange of laboratory results from multiple sites without loss of data integrity and meaning. Before 1994, no universal code system for laboratory test names existed; the LOINC standard has continued to expand and be adopted universally since its first release in 1995 (McDonald et al., 2003).

Semantic interoperability is as important as having hardware and software that function with other systems that carry clinical research data. *Semantic interoperability* focuses on the meaning of the data collected, providing a data dictionary or translation that can be used to determine meaning. Instead of a set of loosely and locally defined data points that need to be redefined with each successive trial activation, a comprehensive prospective set of comprehensive terms that can be reused and expanded over time is a much more efficient approach to the implementation of a data management system (see the later section on Semantic Interoperability).

Security and Confidentiality of Data

Confidentiality of patient data is a pivotal requirement for healthcare organizations in the United States. HIPAA mandated the adoption of federal regulations for the protection of individually identifiable health information. This means that every healthcare provider who electronically transmits health information is covered by this regulation. The use of an electronic data management system does not meet the terms and conditions of a "covered entity." It is the condition of data transmission that puts patients' data at risk for being intercepted and potentially used for other purposes. However, transactions such as healthcare claims, benefit eligibility inquiries, and referral authorization requests are covered by HIPAA requirements. This means that identifiable personal information must be stripped from a subject's healthcare information, and a standard stipulated set of codes must be substituted to safeguard a person's identity. Experts still need the ability to link events in a meaningful way to reconstruct an organization's or individual's identity. Unprotected health identifiers or nonpersonal health information data can be linked to PHI data with the appropriate password and login to access decrypted/reidentified data. When an approach such as this is used, a thorough evaluation of the process to demonstrate a lack of data intrusion or loss is required.

The sources of PHI are expanding with associated implications for security. One group has documented that large-scale sets of data containing genetic content were frequently shared and even posted on the Internet for secondary analysis without informing the study participants (Roche & Annas, 2001). Issues related to genetic and genomic research continue to challenge the current clinical research model (Lowrance & Collins, 2007; McGuire & Beskow, 2011). The issue is that genetic data are intrinsically "self-identifying," meaning that anyone intercepting this data can discover the identity of the collection source. As new sources of data emerge and are combined in an electronic system, more care must be exercised to guard against identification of subjects.

Semantic Interoperability

Semantic interoperability is the ability of a CTMS or CDMS to clearly and unambiguously define the data that are being collected, meaning that when data are shared or aggregated, they retain their full meaning. Semantic interoperability facilitates the ability of a set of data to be combined with other data, to mine the data, or to run queries appropriate for analysis, research, and reporting.

When two separate data collection systems define a data point exactly the same, the resultant data can be combined and shared without an intermediate step to transform the data in some way. This retains data integrity and reduces time and costs associated with the process. It requires that data points be defined in advance of data collection, often through the use of controlled vocabularies and clearly defined variables that come from standards or other sources. For example, a question on a CRF asks for a subject's performance status to be recorded at baseline and at mid-trial. Institution A defines this as a self-reported score, while Institution B defines this using the Karnofsky Performance Status scale. The latter results in a set of reproducible, clearly defined scores, while the former is complicated by subject bias and inconsistency. If these two groups plan to aggregate their data for a larger analysis and to reach the targeted accrual point faster, aggregation of the scores for performance status would not be possible. This is an example of a tragic loss of valuable data and the lost potential to reach trial endpoints more rapidly.

The clear definition of data points and questions creates "metadata," or descriptors that provide uniqueness and clarity for a single data point or variable. The concept of a set of descriptors for a variable is the basis for a data element (*common data element*, or CDE). A set of CDEs can be based on a collection of metadata profiles that standardize the way in which data elements/questions can be asked, collected, stored, exchanged, and reported. ISO and IEC support this idea of semantic interoperability through ISO/IEC Standard 11179, which is a specification for the creation and maintenance of data elements (ISO & IEC, 2003).

The use of CDEs as a basis for data management is a logical and efficient approach for biomedical inquiries, which change as science evolves. Metadata can be easier to revise and reuse as compared to the maintenance of multiple nonharmonized sets of CRFs and data collection instruments that each implement a different version of a set of questions. Scalability also is supported through the metadata approach in data management systems.

CDEs can support complex metadata relationships, but the creation and maintenance of these elements can be challenging. Metadata hold the key to a system's knowledge and thus must be created with great care and precision. A *curation process* that involves subject or domain experts, iterative processes to confirm that the correct descriptors have been preserved, and a careful review are all necessary. Questions need to be defined precisely and consistently to support discovery across a registry of content. Metadata registries, such as the ISO/IEC 11179–based Cancer Data Standards Registry and Repository maintained by the National Cancer Institute, provide a data element inventory at both the individual element and the CRF level (Nahm et al., 2011).

The metadata approach requires use of a governance and change-control strategy to version data elements that change, with proper reference to the actual data collected. *Code of Federal Regulations* title 21, part 11, requires preservation of all versions of CRFs/data collection instruments used in a clinical study; a natural extension of this requirement can be applied to the data elements used on CRFs and data collection instruments. Data content must be defined and tagged with descriptors to best support interoperability efforts (Covitz et al., 2003). The true foundation of a CDE is the use of standard terminology or vocabulary that can be referenced for review and reuse. The use of terminology concepts to create data elements cements their meaning across programs that reuse elements for diverse reasons. It also allows the establishment of relationships *between* data elements, ultimately supporting data sharing. Programs can match their elements to a set of commonly used concepts or terms that form a common set of variables. Although initially labor intensive, the use of CDEs or metadata is conducive to supporting very large research groups and multi-institutional research efforts.

Using Management Systems' Capabilities

Electronic systems allow individuals who are managing the data to enhance traditional data entry activities. Electronic CRFs are much more than simply a computerized paper CRF. Data are intended to be entered directly into the computer instead of abstracting it first from source documents onto a form.

One of the most popular advantages to using electronic systems is the ability to calculate information using documented and accepted algorithms, such as the derivation of body mass index from a person's height and weight. CTNs find value in a system's ability to collect the components of a calculation on one form and display the result of that operation on another. Calculations linked to laboratory test results can generate alerts, while calculations linked to subject eligibility criteria can alert providers that a patient does not meet study enrollment criteria. When calculations are used, the source of that function must be recorded. If a calculation or algorithm is used, that information must accompany collected data to support statistical analysis.

Variables that use *discrete values* use a choice list of possible responses, not a free text field, to capture valuable information. This move away from a collection of text or comment fields on CRFs can make some users uncomfortable or too constrained. However, applications that use well-defined data questions can be programmed to look for deviations or discrepancies from an acceptable set of permissible responses and flag an entry to alert a member of the research team of a needed action. Typically, the set of permissible values attached to the question is taken from a standard (such as a set of LOINC codes) or a historical set of values that have been validated. In the latter case, the list of values can expand over time to avoid adding entries as "other" in a comment field. The use of a constrained value set needs to be supplemented on a case-by-case basis by the addition of text fields to capture verbatim descriptions or subject narratives in high-priority areas. Examples of these areas include subject descriptions of adverse events or historical encounters.

Electronic systems negate the need to collect ink signatures or names of system users. Typically, CRFs include the name and date that data are entered; an electronic system captures this information based on the privileging profile of a user (see Table 38-3) and the way that each person uses the application. This information can be used in the form of an audit log to review a series of entry events that may be called into question. Personnel entering data need to be trained in how to access the audit log or request that it be accessed. Reports from the audit log can be used by the CTN, data manager, or a member of the quality assurance team to look for trends, problems in a set of questions or variables, or a set of content that generates data discrepancies at a rate higher than expected.

A number of electronic data systems have the ability to accept all entries regardless of the format or intended design. Even if an entry is not included in a constrained choice list of values, it could still be entered. However, this type of entry will generate a discrepancy that needs to be resolved. It is likely that this is one means of identifying values that need to be added to a choice list, but at the time, the user is not restricted from entering data. This is an important feature but needs to be balanced with a robust quality assurance program that reviews discrepancies for resolution and potential future actions.

Summary

The scope of data management is broad and can be complex with regulations and procedures to follow. This chapter highlighted quality data management practices and electronic data management systems that shape the transition and engagement toward a more collaborative clinical trials arena. Data management practices have evolved, and professional societies have equipped users with tools and competencies that outperform the apprentice-based approaches of years past. In addition to the creation and use of a DMP, incorporating standards, new technologies, and methodologies offers glimpses of an exciting future that will infuse data management with innovative, interoperable, and streamlined outcomes.

Electronic data management systems, CDMSs and CTMSs, are tools that enable health professionals to collect, store, exchange, and share data in increasingly efficient ways. The final determination of a successful data management system can be based upon a number of criteria, such as

- Can the system accommodate data entry from a variety of sources in a timely manner?
- Can the data from disparate groups be compiled in a meaningful way that retains their usefulness to the investigator?
- Can reports be generated for sponsors and monitoring agencies without a costly set of interim transformation steps?

Ultimately, the ability to generate metrics concerning the completeness and timeliness of these systems cannot be overemphasized. Issues of scope, scalability, interoperability, and security should be based on local and future requirements of users. Difficult decisions can be guided through the construction of realistic scenarios or use cases that illustrate the complexity and breadth of biomedical research. Careful planning with ongoing analysis is necessary to ensure a thorough evaluation of active clinical data management processes and systems.

As the landscape of data management changes, so will the need for CTNs to adapt to health care's shift toward increased use of quality standards and innovation. This shift will require awareness of industry trends and knowledge acquisition by CTNs to maintain relevance and credibility within the research communities. The momentum to integrate the healthcare industry and research community, a building block for translational research, is altering data management and the roles of those who touch data. CTNs are poised at the intersection between

Table 38-3. Sample of Role Assignments for an Electronic Data Capture System

User Role	Review User Group	Scope	Browse Manual Data	Browse Batch Data	Update Manual Data	Update Batch Data	Update Discrepancies	Verify	Approve	Lock	RDC Test Mode
Reviewer	Clinical	Project or study	Yes	Yes	No	No	No	No	No	No	All privileges
Principal investigator	Clinical	Project or study	Yes	Yes	No	No	No	Yes	No	No	All privileges
Clinical trial nurse/clinical research associate	Clinical	Project or study	Yes	Yes	Yes	Yes	Yes	Yes	No	No	All privileges
Data manager	Data management	Project or study	Yes	Yes	Yes	Yes	Yes	No	No	No	All privileges
Monitor	Clinical	Project or study	Yes	Yes	No	No	Yes	No	Yes	No	All privileges
Quality assurance	Quality assurance	Program or group	Yes	Yes	No	No	No	No	No	No	All privileges
Protocol builder	Builder	Program or group	Yes	Yes	Yes	Yes	Yes	No	No	No	All privileges

RDC—remote data capture

Note. From *Role Assignments for an EDC System*, by National Cancer Institute Center for Cancer Research, 2013, Bethesda, MD: Author.

these communities in a domain expert and, often, liaison role, with the skills and knowledge to transform potential approaches into reality.

Key Points

- DMPs are often required and are living paper or electronic records that document the processes and procedures needed to promote consistent, efficient, and effective data management practices for a study.
- Detailed information used in DMPs and electronic management systems is increasingly associated with professional and disease-specific standards that assist CTNs in managing time-sensitive activities and setting realistic expectations.
- Data are the foundation of research, but great analysis techniques cannot compensate for the lack of quality, quantity, or completeness of data required to answer a scientific question.
- Data collected in a database should always match the original source; if there are intervening processes from the source to the aggregated data, they should be documented in the DMP.
- Most errors in data occur when data are transferred from the source to a CRF or eCRF during medical record abstraction or transcription.
- Data quality is critical for a clinical trial. Audits provide valuable tools to evaluate the quality of the data and assess the level of control placed on the data.
- CDMSs are associated with the traditional approach to clinical trial data–related activities, whereas CTMSs have a means to integrate data and processes from many systems (e.g., laboratory results, adverse events, enrollment).
- The creation and maintenance of a CDMS or CTMS must be a coordinated effort between information technology and the research team, with CTNs functioning in a liaison role in many cases.
- *Interoperability* refers to the ability of systems to exchange data in ways that preserve the original meaning and intent of the data. It is a function of both the system and the data, using data and exchange standards that facilitate aggregation and sharing.
- Electronic data management systems are tools that enable health professionals to collect, store, exchange, and share data in increasingly efficient and meaningful ways.

References

Collins, F.S. (2011). Reengineering translational science: The time is right. *Science Translational Medicine, 3*, 90cm17. doi:10.1126/scitranslmed.3002747

Covitz, P.A., Hartel, F., Schaefer, C., De Coronado, S., Fragoso, G., Sahni, H., ... Buetow, K. (2003). caCORE: A common infrastructure for cancer informatics. *Bioinformatics, 19,* 2404–2412. doi:10.1093/bioinformatics/btg335

Electronic Records; Electronic Signatures, 21 C.F.R. § 11.200 (2014). Retrieved from http://www.accessdata.fda.gov/scripts/cdrh/cfdocs/cfcfr/CFRSearch.cfm?fr=11.200

Ewen, E.F., Zhao, L., Kolm, P., Jurkovitz, C., Fidan, D., White, H.D., ... Weintraub, W.S. (2009). Determining the in-hospital cost of bleeding in patients undergoing percutaneous coronary intervention. *Journal of Interventional Cardiology, 22,* 266–273. doi:10.1111/j.1540-8183.2009.00431.x

General Administrative Requirements, 45 C.F.R. pt. 160 (2007). Retrieved from http://www.gpo.gov/fdsys/pkg/CFR-2007-title45-vol1/pdf/CFR-2007-title45-vol1-part160.pdf

Hammond, W.E., & Cimino, J.J. (2006). Standards in biomedical informatics. In E.H. Shortliffe & J.J. Cimino (Eds.), *Biomedical informatics, computer applications in health care and biomedicine* (pp. 265–311). New York, NY: Springer Science + Business Media, LLC.

Health Level Seven International. (2009, February). HL7 version 3 standard: Public health; Tuberculosis domain analysis model, release 1. Retrieved from http://www.hl7.org/implement/standards/product_brief.cfm?product_id=24

International Conference on Harmonisation of Technical Requirements for Registration of Pharmaceuticals for Human Use. (1996, June 10). *ICH harmonised tripartite guideline: Guideline for good clinical practice, E6(R1).* Retrieved from http://www.ich.org/fileadmin/Public_Web_Site/ICH_Products/Guidelines/Efficacy/E6/E6_R1_Guideline.pdf

International Organization for Standardization & International Electromechanical Commission. (2003). *Information technology—Metadata registries—Part 3: Registry metamodel and basic attributes* (ISO/IEC 11179-3:2003). Geneva, Switzerland: Author.

International Organization for Standardization & International Electrotechnical Commission. (2011). *ISO/IEC directives part 2: Rules for the structure and drafting of international standards.* Retrieved from http://www.iec.ch/members_experts/refdocs/iec/isoiec-dir2%7Bed6.0%7Den.pdf

Laszlo, G. (2006, August 14). The EDC, CTMS, CDM confusion. *The Laszlo Letter.* Retrieved from http://laszloletter.typepad.com/the_laszlo_letter/2006/08/the_edc_ctms_cd.html

Lowrance, W.W., & Collins, F.S. (2007). Ethics: Identifiability in genomic research. *Science, 317,* 600–602. doi:10.1126/science.1147699

Massachusetts Institute of Technology. (n.d.). Data management. Retrieved from https://libraries.mit.edu/data-management

McDonald, C.J., Huff, S.M., Suico, J.G., Hill, G., Leavelle, D., Aller, R., ... Maloney, P. (2003). LOINC, a universal standard for identifying laboratory observations: A 5-year update. *Clinical Chemistry, 49,* 624–633. doi:10.1373/49.4.624

McFadden, E. (2007). *Management of data in clinical trials* (2nd ed.). Hoboken, NJ: Wiley.

McGuire, A.L., & Beskow, L.M. (2011). Informed consent in genomics and genetic research. *Annual Review of Genomics and Human Genetics, 11,* 361–381. doi:10.1146/annurev-genom-082509-141711

Mead, C.N. (2006). Data interchange standards in healthcare IT—Computable semantic interoperability: Now possible but still difficult, do we really need a better mousetrap? *Journal of Healthcare Information Management, 20*(1), 71–78.

Muhlbaier, L.H. (2002). *HIPAA training handbook for researchers: HIPAA and clinical trials.* Marblehead, MA: Opus Communications.

Nahm, M.L., Pieper, C.F., & Cunningham, M.M. (2008). Quantifying data quality for clinical trials using electronic data capture. *PLOS ONE, 3*(8), e3049. doi:10.1371/journal.pone.0003049

Nahm, M., Shepherd, J., Buzenberg, A., Rostami, R., Corcoran, A., McCall, J., & Pietrobon, R. (2011). Design and implementation of an institutional case report form library. *Clinical Trials, 8,* 94–102. doi:10.1177/1740774510391916

National Institute of Standards and Technology. (2002). Federal Information Security Management Act of 2002. Retrieved from http://csrc.nist.gov/groups/SMA/fisma/faqs.html

National Institutes of Health. (2003, February 26). NIH data sharing policy. Retrieved from http://grants.nih.gov/grants/policy/data_sharing

National Science Foundation. (2011, January). Grant proposal guide. Retrieved from http://www.nsf.gov/pubs/policydocs/pappguide/nsf11001/gpg_2.jsp#dmp

National Science Foundation. (2012, October). Proposal and award policies and procedures guide. Retrieved from http://www.nsf.gov/pubs/policydocs/pappguide/nsf13001/nsf13_1.pdf

Office of Management and Budget. (2005, August 31). Circular A-110. Retrieved from http://www.whitehouse.gov/sites/default/files/omb/fedreg/2005/083105_a21.pdf

Pancerella, C., Myers, J., & Rahn, L. (2002). Data provenance in the CMCS. Retrieved from http://www.ipaw.info/chicago02/papers/ProvenanceWorkshopCMCS.pdf

Raymond, L.M. (2011, April). Data management plans—The role of the library. In N. Wiest (Chair), *SAIL 2011: Into the I of the storm: Information resources undergo a sea change*. Retrieved from http://aquaticcommons.org/5127/2/319-642-1-PB-2.pdf

Roche, P.A., & Annas, G.J. (2001). Protecting genetic privacy. *Nature Reviews Genetics, 2*, 392–396.

Rondel, R.K., Varley, S.A., & Webb, C.F. (Eds.). (2000). *Clinical data management* (2nd ed.). Hoboken, NJ: Wiley.

Society for Clinical Data Management. (2011). *Good clinical data management practices*. Brussels, Belgium: Author.

U.S. Department of Health and Human Services. (n.d.). The Privacy Rule. Retrieved from http://www.hhs.gov/ocr/privacy/hipaa/administrative/privacyrule

U.S. Food and Drug Administration. (2013). *Guidance for industry: Electronic source data in clinical investigations*. Retrieved from http://www.fda.gov/downloads/Drugs/GuidanceComplianceRegulatoryInformation/Guidances/UCM328691.pdf

Vogel, R. (1997). Remote data capture: It's not about technology, it's about radical change. *Applied Clinical Trials, 6*, 36–40.

Walther, B., Hossin, S., Townend, J., Abernethy, N., Parker, D., & Jeffries, D. (2011). Comparison of electronic data capture (EDC) with the standard data capture method for clinical trial data. *PLOS ONE, 6*(9). doi:10.1371/journal.pone.0025348

Weaver, M. (2006). CTMS procurement: The seven deadly sins. *CRfocus, 17*(2), 18–20. Retrieved from http://www.clinplus.com/Portals/53286/docs/CTMS_Procurement-_The_Seven_Deadly_Sins.pdf

Woods Hole Oceanographic Institution. (n.d.). Data management and publishing. Retrieved from http://www.whoi.edu/DoR/page.do?pid=44235

SECTION IX.

Quality Assurance

Chapter 39

Creating and Maintaining a Regulatory File

Nicole Grant, RN, BSN, MPH, and Therese White, RN, MSN

Introduction

Coordinating clinical trials requires organizational skills of the highest degree, a keen eye for the smallest details, and a solid understanding of the various aspects of the trial. Even the most organized coordinators struggle with keeping track of the voluminous pages of communications, queries, approvals, and other documents associated with each trial. A key strategy for successful document management is creating and maintaining a regulatory file in which all essential protocol documents are kept. A critical step in creating the file is identifying which documents need to be saved. Every investigator who conducts a clinical trial should keep a record of all the essential documents related to the conduct of the study. The aim of this chapter is to offer a systematic approach to creating and maintaining the investigator or institution regulatory file. This chapter will not address the role of sponsors or the documents that they should maintain.

Many terms are used to describe the regulatory file, including study binder, investigator binder, administrative binder, institution regulatory file, regulatory files, and investigator's study files. Although the maintenance of regulatory files is a part of good clinical practice (GCP) guidelines and not legally binding, it has become best practice for all interventional trials to have a regulatory file, regardless of sponsorship. The U.S. Food and Drug Administration (FDA) has adopted the International Conference on Harmonisation of Technical Requirements for Registration of Pharmaceuticals for Human Use (ICH) E6 GCP as guidance (U.S. FDA, 1996). The creation and maintenance of a regulatory file may also be governed by an institution's standard operating procedures (SOPs).

Overview

A regulatory file is simply a place where essential documents are kept. ICH GCP section 8 defines essential documents as "those documents which individually and collectively permit evaluation of the conduct of a trial and the quality of the data produced. These documents serve to demonstrate the compliance of the investigator, sponsor, and monitor with the standards of good clinical practice and with all applicable regulatory requirements" (ICH, 1996, p. 41). These documents are reviewed by the sponsor and other regulatory authorities as part of the auditing or inspection process.

Contents of the Regulatory File

ICH GCP section 8 has the complete listing of the various essential documents based on the stage of the clinical trial (i.e., before, during, and after). Table 39-1 describes the various items that should be maintained in the regulatory file and organizes these documents in a format that may be useful for clinical trial nurses (CTNs) who have to develop their own file. Depending on the study, not all items may apply. The table also introduces another element that is not listed in the guidance document: training records. Institutions holding an Office for Human Research Protections (OHRP)-approved Federalwide Assurance are responsible for ensuring that their investigators conducting U.S. Department of Health and Human Services (DHHS)-supported human subject research understand and act in accordance with the DHHS regulations on the protection of human subject (OHRP, 2011). Additionally, FDA requires that investigators ensure adequate training for all staff involved in the conduct of a clinical trial (U.S. FDA, 2009). Training records such as a human subject protection course, a GCP course, sponsor meetings, protocol-specific staff meetings, or staff in-services provide documentation that the investigator and staff have been trained in human subject research and are qualified to conduct the study.

Table 39-1. Components of a Regulatory File

Title of Essential Document	Purpose of Document or Relevant Information	Helpful Tips
Investigator and Institution Information		
Form FDA 1572 from U.S. Food and Drug Administration (FDA) or investigator agreement	To document the investigator's agreement to conduct the study according to the protocol and good clinical practice. Update as investigators change and/or other pertinent information changes (e.g., address of reference lab or institutional review board [IRB]). Only clinical laboratories (not research laboratories) must be identified on Form FDA 1572. Form FDA 1572 can be found at www.fda.gov/downloads/AboutFDA/ReportsManualsForms/Forms/UCM074728.pdf. For National Cancer Institute (NCI) Cancer Therapy Evaluation Program (CTEP)-sponsored studies, use the Form FDA 1572 found on CTEP's Investigator Registration website: http://ctep.cancer.gov/investigatorResources/investigator_registration.htm. Note: Sections 6 and 7 are prepopulated for CTEP-sponsored studies.	All versions of Form FDA 1572 should be maintained. Original form should be sent to the sponsor and a copy kept in the regulatory file. For NCI CTEP–sponsored studies, maintain all MD investigators' individual Form FDA 1572 documentation provided by CTEP as part of investigator registration. **Amenable to centralization.**
Current curriculum vitae (CV) for the principal investigator (PI) and each subinvestigator	To document the investigators' qualifications to conduct the study.	Keep current and historical copies. Current version should be initialed or signed and dated within two years. **Amenable to centralization.** If CVs are filed centrally, write a signed and dated note to file indicating the location.
Copy of medical license for the PI and each MD subinvestigator	To document the investigators' qualifications to conduct the study.	**Amenable to centralization.**
Training certificates	To document that there is adequate training for all staff participating in the conduct of the study. To keep evidence of training such as human subject protection, good clinical practice, study-specific training records, and International Air Transport Association dangerous goods regulations training certificates.	This should be kept for each investigator, the clinical trial nurse or study coordinator, and other key research staff associated with the study. **Amenable to centralization.**
Study staff responsibilities and signature form	To show that the PI has delegated certain study-related tasks to others. This log should list all individuals (including signature, initials, and time span) who have been delegated study-related activities by the PI. The PI should sign the log. Revise as needed when study staff join or leave or study roles change.	Also known as a "delegation of duties/authority" log; see Chapter 10 for a sample log.
Financial disclosure/certification statements	To document that the investigators are compliant with FDA regulations in 21 C.F.R. § 312.64(d), which state: "The clinical investigator shall provide the sponsor with sufficient accurate financial information to allow an applicant to submit complete and accurate certification or disclosure statements as required under part 54 of this chapter. The clinical investigator shall promptly update this information if any relevant changes occur during the course of the investigation and for 1 year following the completion of the study."	The sponsor will often provide forms for the PI to complete. In this case, the originals should be sent to the sponsor and copies kept in the PI files.

(Continued on next page)

Table 39-1. Components of a Regulatory File *(Continued)*

Title of Essential Document	Purpose of Document or Relevant Information	Helpful Tips
Clinical trial agreement or other contract and/or legal agreements (if applicable)	A clinical trial agreement is a contractual agreement entered into between the sponsor and the institution for all industry-sponsored trials. This category could include other types of agreements such as a confidential disclosure agreement, material transfer agreement, and cooperative research and development agreements.	If this does not include an insurance or indemnification statement and data use agreement, these documents should be kept as well.
Investigator's Brochure/Device Manual		
Investigator's brochure and updates	Contains scientific information for investigational product. For U.S. FDA–approved agents, file a copy of the package insert.	Keep all versions in the investigator file.
Protocol Versions and Protocol Information		
Protocol and amendments	Contains the initial version, every protocol amendment, and a signed protocol signature page for each version, if applicable.	Save the IRB-approved protocol versions.
Study manual of procedures (MOP) and updates (if applicable)	May include the laboratory procedures manual, laboratory specimen handling instructions, test article handling and/or preparation, and protocol-specific instructions.	If this is not kept in the regulatory file, create a note to file and indicate its location. If there is no MOP, indicate this in a note to file.
Approved Informed Consent Documents and Information Given to Subjects		
Informed consent documents • Initial version • Every revised version	Includes a copy of all versions of the IRB-approved informed consent document and IRB-approved authorization for use and disclosure of protected health information (if separate from informed consent documents).	All versions should contain a version date and/or number.
Advertisements/recruitment material, participant educational material	–	These must be approved by the IRB.
IRB/Independent Ethics Committee (IEC) Documentation		
Federalwide Assurance number and expiration date	To document that the institution is registered with the Office for Human Research Protections. The information may be found by searching the following website: http://ohrp.cit.nih.gov/search.	**Amenable to centralization.**
IRB/institutional ethics committee membership roster	To document that the IRB is compliant with 45 C.F.R. § 46.107.	Membership lists should be updated as changes are made during the course of the study. Historical lists should also be maintained. **Amenable to centralization.**
IRB correspondence	21 C.F.R. § 312.66 states, "An investigator shall assure that an IRB complies with the requirements set forth in part 56 and will be responsible for the approval of the proposed clinical study at the initial submission and continuing review. The investigator shall also assure that he/she will promptly report to the IRB all changes in the research activity and all unanticipated problems involving risk to human subjects or others, and that he/she will not make any changes in the research without IRB approval, except where necessary to eliminate apparent immediate hazards to human subjects."	–

(Continued on next page)

Table 39-1. Components of a Regulatory File *(Continued)*

Title of Essential Document	Purpose of Document or Relevant Information	Helpful Tips
IRB approvals of • Initial protocol, informed consent form (ICF) • Amendments to protocol and ICF • Continuing review • Written information given to subjects (if applicable) • Advertisements for subject recruitment (if applicable) • Authorization for use and disclosure of protected health information (if separate from ICF) • Authorization to use the short form consent procedure (if applicable)	–	All correspondence regarding the approval process of the protocol, including submissions to the IRB, IRB stipulations, and the response to stipulations, should be kept. It is not necessary to keep the entire package; enough documentation should be kept to provide evidence of the approval process.
Continuing review to IRB and IRB approval for study continuation	–	Must be done at least once a year. IRB may require more frequent review.
Notification to IRB of adverse events	–	Follow institutional standard operating procedures (SOPs).
Notification to IRB of unanticipated problems involving risks to subjects and others	For U.S. Department of Health and Human Services guidance on reporting unanticipated problems, see www.hhs.gov/ohrp/policy/advevntguid.html	
Notification to IRB of protocol deviations	–	Follow institutional SOPs.
Notification to IRB of study completion and final study report	–	Follow institutional SOPs.
Safety Information		
Copy of serious adverse event (SAE) reports sent to sponsor (if applicable)	21 C.F.R. § 312.64(b) states, "An investigator must immediately report to the sponsor any serious adverse event, whether or not considered drug related, including those listed in the protocol or investigator brochure and must include an assessment of whether there is a reasonable possibility that the drug caused the event. Study endpoints that are serious adverse events (e.g., all-cause mortality) must be reported in accordance with the protocol unless there is evidence suggesting a causal relationship between the drug and the event (e.g., death from anaphylaxis). In that case, the investigator must immediately report the event to the sponsor. The investigator must record non-serious adverse events and report them to the sponsor according to the timetable for reporting specified in the protocol."	All correspondence between the sponsor or contract research organization (CRO) and the site that concerns SAE reports and any safety information should be kept.
Investigational new drug (IND) safety reports received from sponsor	–	If IRB policy is to only receive the IND safety report when an amendment is needed, still file the sponsor report in the regulatory file.
Safety and data monitoring committee reports and correspondence	–	–

(Continued on next page)

Table 39-1. Components of a Regulatory File *(Continued)*		
Title of Essential Document	**Purpose of Document or Relevant Information**	**Helpful Tips**
Other Regulatory Agency/Committee Documentation		
Approvals/authorizations of protocol, ICF, and amendments from additional regulatory agencies (if applicable)	Examples include the Radiation Safety Committee, Office of Biotechnology Activities, and Institutional Biosafety Committee.	–
Correspondence with regulatory agencies regarding safety information (if applicable)	–	–
Clinical Trial Material (CTM) Documentation		
Records of receipt of CTM and trial-related materials (if applicable)	–	–
Samples of labels attached to investigational product containers (if applicable)	–	–
Temperature log (if applicable)	Log to record the temperature of the freezer or refrigerator used to store the test article.	–
CTM dispensing/accountability records	21 C.F.R. § 312.62(a) states, "An investigator is required to maintain adequate records of the disposition of the drug, including dates, quantity, and use by subjects. If the investigation is terminated, suspended, discontinued, or completed, the investigator shall return the unused supplies of the drug to the sponsor, or otherwise provide for disposition of the unused supplies of the drug under 312.59."	If dispensing/accountability records are filed in the pharmacy, photocopies of these records should be made at study completion and inserted into the regulatory file. Create a note to file and indicate the location of the original records.
Documentation of CTM destruction if performed at site	–	–
Biologic Samples Documentation		
Copies of biologic sample transmittal forms that accompanied the shipment to the external laboratory	–	If these are not kept in the regulatory file, create a note to file and indicate the location of the records.
Correspondence regarding biologic samples	–	–
Record of retained body fluids/tissue samples (if applicable)	–	–
Laboratory Documentation		
Laboratory certification and/or accreditation	To document that specimens were processed in a lab with Clinical Laboratory Improvement Amendments or College of American Pathologists certification.	Include updates throughout the study duration and keep historical records. These must be kept for all labs used in the study and listed on Form FDA 1572. **Amenable to centralization.**
Lab normal reference ranges	To document normal values for lab tests to be performed for the clinical trial.	Keep a copy of normal ranges for all labs/tests included in the protocol. Include updates throughout the study duration. Lab results with reference ranges from a subject may be used if all personally identifiable information is redacted. **Amenable to centralization.**

(Continued on next page)

Table 39-1. Components of a Regulatory File *(Continued)*

Title of Essential Document	Purpose of Document or Relevant Information	Helpful Tips
Lab director's CV	–	Obtain for each lab used in the study. **Amenable to centralization.**
Subject Accountability Records		
Subject screening and enrollment logs	List of subjects screened for entry as well as those enrolled in the study.	This may be one document or two separate lists. Screening log should document why potential subjects were not included in the study.
Subject identification code list	List of subjects enrolled in the study and identified by a unique number.	This allows the investigator or institution to quickly identify study subjects in the case of an emergency. Note: This is a confidential list and should be maintained only at the site.
Treatment allocation and decoding documentation	Decoding procedures may be detailed in the protocol itself.	–
Blank set of case report forms (CRFs)	–	–
Signed IRB-approved ICF and authorization for use and disclosure of protected health information for each subject screened for entry into the study	–	If this is not kept in the regulatory file, create a note to file and indicate its location.
Copy of completed CRFs for each subject with any related data clarification requests (if applicable)	21 C.F.R. § 312.62(b) states, "An investigator is required to prepare and maintain adequate and accurate case histories that record all observations and other data pertinent to the investigation on each individual administered the investigational drug or employed as a control in the investigation. Case histories include the case report forms and supporting data including, for example, signed and dated consent forms and medical records including, for example, progress notes of the physician, the individual's hospital chart(s), and the nurses' notes. The case history for each individual shall document that informed consent was obtained prior to participation in the study."	If these are not kept in the regulatory file, create a note to file and indicate the location of the forms.
Copy of completed CRF transmittal forms (if applicable)	–	If this is not kept in the regulatory file, create a note to file and indicate the location of the form.
Copy of completed CRF edit logs (if applicable)	–	If this is not kept in the regulatory file, create a note to file and indicate the location of the form.
Monitoring Activities		
Site initiation visit report	–	–
Final trial closeout monitoring report	–	–
Monitoring log and reports	Log in which monitors document their visits. Site staff should initial/verify in the log that monitor was present on specific days.	–
Monitor correspondence	Contains site visit confirmation and follow-up correspondence.	–

(Continued on next page)

Table 39-1. Components of a Regulatory File *(Continued)*		
Title of Essential Document	**Purpose of Document or Relevant Information**	**Helpful Tips**
General/Sponsor Correspondence		
All correspondence between sponsor/CRO and the site concerning the study	Includes all correspondence except that concerning SAEs, safety information, and monitor correspondence, which should be filed in appropriate section.	–
Site-generated telephone contact reports or logs	–	–
Site visit letters/summaries	–	–
Clinical Study Report		
Clinical study reports	21 C.F.R. § 312.64(a) states, "The investigator shall furnish all reports to the sponsor of the drug who is responsible for collecting and evaluating the results obtained." And § 312.64(c) states, "An investigator shall provide the sponsor with an adequate report shortly after completion of the investigator's participation in the investigation."	–
Notes to File		
Notes to file (if applicable)	To provide documentation of unusual events that occur during the course of a clinical trial. Reasons to write a note to file include • When a correction was made to a document that could raise questions • When there is a change or correction to a process or policy. Improper uses of notes to file include • Noting something previously documented elsewhere • Identifying a problem with no resolution • Using in place of record keeping. In general, notes to file are used in the following instances: • To document the reason for missing, delayed, or erroneous documents in the clinical trial master file or in the PI file • To explain protocol deviations or investigator site practices that are different from the norm or from what is prescribed in the protocol.	The question to ask when writing a note is, "What are the chances that a data query, site monitor, auditor, or inspector will ask a question and find this note useful in understanding what happened in the study?" A good note to file includes • Date, author, and subject of note • What happened (who, what, where, why) • Why the incident is important • What has been or will be done to address this incident • What will be done to prevent or mitigate similar incidents in the future.
Other information felt necessary to retain but not filed elsewhere in the regulatory file	–	–

Note. Based on information from Basic HHS Policy for Protection of Human Research Subjects, 2009; Investigational New Drug Application, 2014; Investigator Recordkeeping and Record Retention, 2014; Partlo & Kirstein, 2013.

Format

Regulatory files can be found in various formats and organizational styles; they may range from paper notebooks to electronic files. DHHS states that records may be preserved in hard copy, electronic, or other media form and must be accessible for inspection and copying by authorized DHHS representatives (OHRP, 2011). Often, sponsors or institutions have a required format and organization that must be followed. Regardless of the format, the file must be organized in a manner that allows for specific documents to be found easily. An important rule of thumb with filing is consistency. The organization of the files should be easily understood by a person who is not familiar with the study. Developing a standard nomenclature model is critical for consistency and ease in finding documents for studies that are using an electronic regulatory file (e.g., protocols, amendments, financial disclosures, safety reports). Table 39-2 provides an example of standard nomenclature.

In all regulatory files, patient confidentiality should be maintained. It is important to redact all subject names and use only unique study subject identification numbers in reports (e.g., expedited adverse event reports, laboratory reference ranges). Paper files are often kept in binders that must be stored in a secure location, such as a locked file or, at minimum, a locked office. Electronic files should be kept on a secure server that is backed up daily or on a secure web-based system. At the time of monitoring visits, the electronic file can be downloaded to a secure memory device such as a thumb drive or a read-only CD and given to the monitoring personnel. Per an FDA inspector, the inspectors are willing to review electronic regulatory files on a read-only CD (personal communication, November 15, 2011).

Centralizing Essential Documents

Some essential documents may be applied to multiple studies and therefore may be centralized. For example, laboratory reference ranges, laboratory certifications (e.g., Clinical Laboratory Improvement Amendments, College of American Pathologists), curricula vitae, and medical licenses may be kept in a central file to ease the burden of duplication. If a central file is used, a note to file should be placed in each study's regulatory file indicating that centralized files exist and where they are located.

Maintenance of the Regulatory File

It is important to begin collecting essential documents before commencement of the clinical phase of the trial (at the very start of protocol development), continuing during the conduct of the trial and after completion or termination of the trial. In the ICH GCP E6 guidance, section 4.9.4 specifies that the investigator and institution should maintain the essential trial documents. The investigator and institution should take measures to prevent accidental or premature destruction of these documents. The DHHS regulations for award recipients require that research records be maintained for at least three years after completion of the research and submission of the last expenditure report (Retention and Access Requirements for Records, 2010). The FDA investigational new drug application and investigational device exemption regulations require that research records be maintained for two years following the approval/support of the marketing/premarket approval application or after the investigation is terminated or discontinued and FDA is notified (Investigational Device Exemptions, 2014; Investigational

Table 39-2. Suggestions for Standard Nomenclature for Protocol Documents When Using an Electronic Regulatory File

Document Name	File Name
Initial protocol document	Protocol number_initial protocol_date [MM-DD-YY]
Initial consent document	Protocol number_initial consent_date [MM-DD-YY]
Continuing institutional review board (IRB) review	Protocol number_CR_date [MM-DD-YY]
Investigator's brochure	Drug Name_IBversion_date [MM-DD-YY] (date = date of version) (i.e., MDX010_IBv6.2_12-10-09)
IRB approval document	Protocol number_IRB approval memo_date [MM-DD-YY]
Financial disclosure	FDA form 3455_Investigator name_date [MM-DD-YY]
Curriculum vitae	CV_investigator name_date
IRB membership roster	IRB roster_date [MM-DD-YY]
Unanticipated problem	Protocol number_event_date of event [MM-DD-YY]

New Drug Application, 2014). Sponsors are responsible for notifying the investigator and institution when documents no longer need to be retained (ICH GCP, 1996). The Health Insurance Portability and Accountability Act (HIPAA) regulations require that HIPAA-related records (e.g., authorizations, documentation of waiver approvals) be maintained for six years (Accounting of Disclosures of Protected Health Information, 2011). It is important to plan for long-term storage of these documents, either in electronic or paper forms or a combination of both, to ensure the confidentiality and availability of the records should these documents be requested by regulatory agencies, outside parties with authority, and publishers. An example of this is with a phase I clinical trial where it may take 10 or more years until the drug is approved by FDA; therefore, records need to be maintained and easily accessible if requested. The principal investigator of a study is ultimately responsible for maintenance of the regulatory file. However, this task is often delegated to other members of the research team. CTNs are most often assigned to perform this function.

Summary

Although creating regulatory files may seem like a daunting task, once created, the files become an invalu-

able resource and serve a number of important functions:
- Provide an excellent reference guide for the CTN and other members of the research team
- Greatly assist in the successful management of a trial by the investigator and sponsor
- Allow for smooth and efficient monitoring visits and audits by the sponsor and regulatory authorities as part of the process to confirm the validity of the trial conduct and the integrity of the data collected.

The most important concepts regarding these files are to know what is to be filed, file as soon as possible, ensure that the files are available at the time of an audit or inspection, and plan for long-term storage.

Key Points
- Management of essential documents and the regulatory file is not governed by regulatory agencies but is recommended per GCP guidelines and may be dictated by an institution's SOPs.
- It is important to begin collecting essential documents before the clinical phase of the trial begins, continuing throughout the life of the trial and after completion or termination of the trial.
- The various logs that are part of the regulatory file must be updated in a timely manner. To ensure accuracy, logs should be updated as soon as an event occurs.
- It is acceptable to centralize some of the documents in the regulatory file. However, the file must include a note that states where the individual elements are available.
- All regulatory files should be kept in a secure location and free of research participants' personal health information.
- Electronic regulatory files are becoming more common as the industry moves away from reliance on paper forms. Files should be kept on a secure server, and access may be granted to those involved in the trial who need access to the essential documents.
- Developing a standard nomenclature model is critical for consistency and ease in finding documents. Naming files is generally considered a challenge that is almost as difficult to tackle as remembering the name of a file that was saved (see Table 39-2).
- At the time of monitoring visits, the electronic file can be downloaded to a secure memory device and given to monitoring personnel.

References

Accounting of Disclosures of Protected Health Information, 45 C.F.R. § 164.528 (2011). Retrieved from http://www.gpo.gov/fdsys/pkg/CFR-2011-title45-vol1/xml/CFR-2011-title45-vol1-sec164-528.xml

Basic HHS Policy for Protection of Human Research Subjects, 45 C.F.R. pt. 46 (2009). Retrieved from http://www.hhs.gov/ohrp/humansubjects/guidance/45cfr46.html

International Conference on Harmonisation of Technical Requirements for Registration of Pharmaceuticals for Human Use. (1996, June 10). *ICH harmonised tripartite guideline: Guideline for good clinical practice, E6(R1)*. Retrieved from http://www.ich.org/fileadmin/Public_Web_Site/ICH_Products/Guidelines/Efficacy/E6/E6_R1_Guideline.pdf

Investigational Device Exemptions, 21 C.F.R. § 812.140 (2014). Retrieved from http://www.accessdata.fda.gov/scripts/cdrh/cfdocs/cfcfr/CFRSearch.cfm?fr=812.140

Investigational New Drug Application, 21 C.F.R. pt. 312 (2014). Retrieved from http://www.accessdata.fda.gov/scripts/cdrh/cfdocs/cfcfr/cfrsearch.cfm?cfrpart=312

Investigator Recordkeeping and Record Retention, 21 C.F.R. § 312.62 (2014). Retrieved from http://www.accessdata.fda.gov/scripts/cdrh/cfdocs/cfcfr/CFRSearch.cfm?fr=312.62

Office for Human Research Protections. (2011, January 20). Investigator responsibilities—FAQs. Retrieved from http://answers.hhs.gov/ohrp/categories/1567

Partlo, S.A., & Kirstein, T. (2013). Notes to file. *SoCRA Source*, pp. 62–68.

Retention and Access Requirements for Records, 45 C.F.R. § 74.53 (2010). Retrieved from http://www.gpo.gov/fdsys/pkg/CFR-2010-title45-vol1/xml/CFR-2010-title45-vol1-sec74-53.xml

U.S. Food and Drug Administration. (1996, April). *Guidance for industry E6 good clinical practice: Consolidated guidance*. Retrieved from http://www.fda.gov/downloads/Drugs/Guidances/ucm073122.pdf

U.S. Food and Drug Administration. (2009, October). *Guidance for industry: Investigator responsibilities—Protecting the rights, safety, and welfare of study subjects*. Retrieved from http://www.fda.gov/downloads/Drugs/GuidanceComplianceRegulatoryInformation/Guidances/UCM187772.pdf

Chapter 40

Data and Safety Monitoring Plans

Carol Anne Bales, RN, MSN, CCRP, and Gloria Adams, RN, CCRP, OCN®

Introduction

Data and safety monitoring plans (DSMPs) are an essential component to any clinical research study. They ensure that the rights and safety of research participants are protected and that the reported trial data are accurate, complete, and verifiable from source documents (Friedman & Dixon, 2012). In other words, the plans ensure that the conduct of the trial is in compliance with protocol, good clinical practice (GCP), and applicable regulatory requirements. Institutional review boards (IRBs) are charged with determining if and what type of data and safety monitoring is appropriate to ensure research participant safety. Many IRBs will require that the DSMP be part of the protocol, or at a minimum, submitted with the initial protocol application process. The need for monitoring for clinical trials is described in U.S. 45 C.F.R. § 46.111(a)(6) and 21 C.F.R. § 56.111(a)(6) (Criteria for IRB Approval of Research, 2009, 2014).

One protocol may have more than one DSMP including a description of the principal investigator's and research team's plan, the research organization's plan, or the sponsor's plan. Some studies may require a formal data monitoring committee (DMC), also known as a *data and safety monitoring board or committee* (Friedman & Dixon, 2012); for the purposes of this chapter, DMC will be used to encompass all aliases.

DSMPs should be based on (a) the study's expected risks associated with the research, (b) the population being studied, (c) the size (e.g., large enough to require multiple sites versus a single site), (d) the nature and complexity of the protocol, and (e) the population being studied. The plan should be included in the protocol to allow an IRB and other regulators to assess the plan's feasibility and rigor based on the risk. For minimal risk studies at a single site, the principal investigator and research team may be adequate to perform the monitoring functions. However, for large, multisite, complex, and high-risk studies, a monitoring group or DMC may be required. Most academic centers and government agencies have standard operating procedures (SOPs) that define the requirements for DSMPs for interventional clinical trials. The SOPs' purpose is to ensure subject safety in accordance with these regulations (Friedman & Dixon, 2012).

Clinical trial nurses (CTNs) may be involved with studies that do not require a formal DMC, but for any study, it is important to have a DSMP in place to guide the study staff in performing their duties. CTNs should be knowledgeable about the DSMP and be aware of the nature and functioning of a DMC to understand how they serve as linchpins between the study site and the analysis of the safety and risk inherent in a clinical trial. The information in this chapter will describe measures that should be undertaken to ensure the safety of study subjects regardless of whether the study includes a DMC or a simpler monitoring plan. The chapter will cover

- Selected highlights of the historical perspective of DSMPs and DMCs
- DMC guidelines, including composition, member responsibilities, operation, structure, scientific and safety review, conduct and substance of meetings, review of documentation, and consideration of impact on current study, follow-up, and ongoing business
- Benefits of such plans to the sponsor, organization, and investigator.

Background

Regulatory bodies that issue guidances and establish regulations and laws pertinent to clinical trial conduct are continually striving to improve, simplify, automate, and expedite the process of data and safety monitoring. In September 2000, Donna Shalala, PhD, former Secretary of the U.S. Department of Health and Human Services (DHHS), published an article titled "Protecting Research Subjects—What Must Be Done" (Shalala, 2000). Shalala left this important document as one of her legacies as she was completing her tenure in office. In it, she addressed four disturbing trends in the conduct of clinical trials that resulted in compromised safety of research participants. These included (Shalala, 2000)

- Researchers were not ensuring that patients were fully informed of the potential benefits and risks involved in participating in a clinical trial. In a report of an inspection by the Office of the Inspector General of the DHHS published in February 2000, sponsors and investigators were found to have coerced patients with threats if they declined participation in trials. The report described misrepresentations of the nature of trials and misleading advertisements and promotions for clinical trials.
- Many researchers were found to have deviated from standards of GCP. Instances of this trend included the enrollment of patients in clinical trials even when they did not meet the protocol eligibility criteria.
- IRBs were found to have too few resources and too little time to adequately oversee the conduct of trials.
- Potential conflicts of interest of sponsors and investigators who were conducting academic trials were not being properly managed.

As a result of these findings, several initiatives were implemented to ensure the safety of clinical trial subjects. The initiatives included (Shalala, 2000)

- The U.S. National Institutes of Health (NIH) and the U.S. Food and Drug Administration (FDA) held symposia on gene transfer safety research, including the requirement for sponsors of such research to submit monitoring plans to FDA prior to commencement of their trials.
- An improved, stronger training program sponsored by NIH and FDA provided sponsors and researchers with information on bioethics, informed consent, clinical trial audits, and provision of new information to research subjects regarding risks and safety related to the trial in which they were participating.
- A requirement that phase I and phase II clinical trial investigators submit monitoring plans to NIH along with their grant applications and to their IRBs as part of their trial submissions.
- Issuance of NIH and FDA guidance documents to clearly define and explicitly describe regulations that apply to conflicts of interest.
- Pursuance of legislation allowing FDA to issue civil monetary fines for violations of informed consent.
- The responsibilities of the Office for Protection From Research Risks were transferred to a newly renamed agency, the Office for Human Research Protections (OHRP). Dr. Edward Koski was appointed as the OHRP director. He was given the responsibility to provide leadership for 17 federal agencies that conduct human clinical trials.

The initiatives all served to strengthen the U.S. government's role in guiding the conduct of clinical trials. The third initiative will be explored further in this chapter.

U.S. Food and Drug Administration

When conducting an investigational new drug application trial, federal regulations require that the sponsor monitors the study. In March 2006, FDA published a guidance document titled *Guidance for Clinical Trial Sponsors—Establishment and Operation of Clinical Trial Data Monitoring Committees*. In addition to a DMC, the guidance also described other clinical trial oversight groups such as IRBs, clinical trial steering committees, endpoint assessment and adjudication committees, site and clinical monitoring groups, and others. Each group had established their unique SOPs used to guide their members in the performance of their individual roles (U.S. FDA, 2006). These oversight groups collaborate to ensure the safety of research participants, and the structure, purpose, function, and benefits of these collaborations are addressed in this chapter.

Because of the evolution of electronic data capture technologies, development of methods to provide confidential access to source documents and regulatory documents, and the need to cope with the increased complexity and number of clinical trials, FDA has rescinded its 1988 *Guidance on Monitoring of Clinical Investigations* and in August 2013 issued *Guidance for Industry: Oversight of Clinical Investigations—A Risk-Based Approach to Monitoring* (U.S. FDA, 2013). It states that monitoring methods need to be centralized and focused on the most critical elements of the study (e.g., remote data verification, possible fraud, serious adverse events). In fact, with more studies using electronic data capture systems and electronic medical records, centralized monitoring is increasingly used and might even be more effective in detection of data discrepancies or data gaps (U.S. FDA, 2013). This is an excellent document to assist research teams and organizations in developing a risk-based approach to monitoring.

Clinical Trials Transformation Initiative

The Clinical Trials Transformation Initiative (CTTI) established in 2007 by FDA and Duke University is a public-private partnership focused on identifying practices to improve the efficiency and quality of clinical trials. CTTI partners include academic centers, pharmaceutical industry, research organizations and societies, and government agencies involved in clinical trials (Kleppinger & Ball, 2010). A 2010 CTTI survey revealed that a broad range of practices are used for safety monitoring of human clinical trials. It also revealed that the primary method used by sponsors of such research to ensure the safety of study participants was on-site monitoring of clinical trial sites with source document verification of 100% of study data on a four- to eight-week interval schedule. However, Morrison and colleagues (2011) reported that government agencies, academic coordinating centers, and cooperative groups used this practice less often than commercial study sponsors.

International Conference on Harmonisation

In 1996, the International Conference on Harmonisation of Technical Requirements for Registration of Pharmaceuticals for Human Use (ICH) published *ICH Harmonised Tripartite Guideline: Guideline for Good Clinical Practice* (1996), which allows for alternative methods of clinical trial safety monitoring other than on-site monitoring. Within the monitoring section of the document is a description of a monitoring plan that includes limited on-site monitoring during each clinical trial: before, during, and post-trial phases. Central monitoring is suggested through the use of investigator meetings and extensive guidance documents describing how the site is expected to conduct the study and how to complete documentation.

National Institutes of Health

In 1979, NIH issued a recommendation that all clinical trials should have a provision for data and safety monitoring, which was reiterated with the June 1998 policy. The NIH policy required that each of its institutes and centers have a monitoring system in place to ensure research subject safety and the validity, integrity, and accuracy of study data for all NIH-funded or conducted human research trials (NIH, 1998). Shalala's (2000) recommendations were implemented, which broadened the NIH policy to incorporate a requirement that a DSMP be submitted to the NIH funding institutes and centers for phase I and II clinical trials and be included in the protocol. The NIH policy also included when a formal DMC is required and when one may be needed. Protocols that require a DMC include (NIH, 1998, 2000)
- Phase III clinical trials, including
  – Protocols that generate blinded/randomized data
  – Multicenter protocols presenting more than minimal risk to subjects

Protocols that may require a DMC *or* an individual independent monitor include
- Protocols using gene transfer or gene therapy methodology
- Protocols that pose more than minimal risk to the subjects
- Protocols that the sponsoring institutes and centers believe require special scrutiny because of high public interest or public perception of risk (e.g., gene transfer studies).

National Cancer Institute

The National Cancer Institute (NCI) has a policy related to data and safety monitoring that can be found in the NCI Clinical Trials Policy at http://deainfo.nci.nih.gov/grantspolicies/datasafety.pdf. Within the policy, the NCI recommendations concur with the need for various types of monitoring plans (e.g., principal investigator, independent monitoring committee, DMC) (NCI, 2014). CTNs working on NCI-sponsored trials should familiarize themselves with this policy to ensure that their protocols and institutional SOPs are in compliance.

Data and Safety Monitoring Plans

Not all research studies need to have a DSMP, but certainly all clinical trials need to have a plan (U.S. FDA, 2006) (see Figure 40-1). Since the plan will be based on the study's risk, see Chapter 16 for more information on risk assessment. Key elements of a DSMP are listed in Figure 40-2 (NCI, 2001).

Data Monitoring Committees

Historical Perspective

The history of DMCs can be traced back to the 1960s. DMCs were initially used by federal agencies (e.g., NIH, Department of Veterans Affairs) sponsoring large multi-

Figure 40-1. When a Data and Safety Monitoring Plan Is Needed
More than minimal risk research such as • Phase III clinical trials • Multisite research • Human gene transfer studies • Studies of vulnerable populations such as prisoners, pregnant women, and subjects with decisional impairments • National Institutes of Health–sponsored phase I, II, and III clinical trials (Friedman & Dixon, 2012)
Note. Based on information from Friedman & Dixon, 2012; National Cancer Institute, 2014; National Institutes of Health, 1998, 2000.

Figure 40-2. Key Elements of a Data and Safety Monitoring Plan
• Description of the monitoring processes • Who will be responsible for monitoring adherence to the protocol and the validity and integrity of the data collected • How often data will be monitored by the various individuals or groups • Process and time frame for reporting unanticipated problems, adverse events, and protocol deviations to the organization and the institutional review board (IRB) • Definition of specific events or stopping rules • Procedures and time frames for communicating outcomes of monitoring reviews to others (e.g., organization, IRB, study sponsor)
Note. Based on information from National Cancer Institute, 2001.

center randomized clinical trials to assess clinical trial participant safety. In 1967, an NIH external advisory group recommended to what was then the National Heart Institute that a formal committee, external to the research team and sponsor, be established to review data on an ongoing basis to monitor for participant safety, effectiveness, and trial conduct in an unbiased manner. Initially, DMCs were not used by industry, but recently, this has changed as a result of several factors, including

- Growing number of industry-sponsored trials with mortality and major morbidity endpoints
- Increasing collaboration between industry and government in sponsoring major clinical trials
- Heightened awareness within the scientific community of problems in clinical trial conduct and analysis possibly leading to biased or inaccurate results
- Concerns of IRBs related to monitoring and safety in multicenter trials (Friedman & Dixon, 2012; U.S. FDA, 2006).

Structure and Composition

DMCs operate under a charter that is written by the sponsor or the DMC themselves. The charter should include detailed SOPs on how the DMC will function, including member responsibilities; meeting schedule, format, and structure; and format for interim reports (U.S. FDA, 2006).

Members of a DMC must be multidisciplinary and include individuals with relevant clinical and statistical expertise. The DMC will meet at least annually depending on the activity and nature of the clinical trial being monitored. The study sponsor or a steering committee usually selects members of the DMC. The sponsor usually selects a chairperson who is knowledgeable about the study intervention and the conduct of similar clinical trials, as well as having leadership experience and objectivity (i.e., absence of conflict of interest). The appointed chairperson or the sponsor will select other DMC members. The size of the committee will depend on the characteristics and size of the study but should include at least three members. The members usually include physicians whose specialties match the medical environment from which investigators are selected. Other members may include (a) a medical statistician, (b) scientific experts in the field of study, (c) a nonscientific member representing the perspective of study participants, (d) a CTN, and (e) a research pharmacist, among other experts judged to be appropriate by the sponsor. The committee should be limited to a size that facilitates meeting arrangements, especially for global study DMCs that include members from various countries where the study is being conducted (U.S. FDA, 2006).

Responsibilities

The responsibilities of a DMC may include the following (U.S. FDA, 2006).

- Monitoring the study for effectiveness of the study intervention
- Monitoring the study for safety and risk
- Monitoring the conduct of the study, including enrollment rates, screen failure rate, noncompliance of study subjects, protocol deviations and dropout rate, data accuracy and completion within time frames agreed upon by sponsor and site, agreement of site and DMC adjudication of adverse events, and degree of balance between study treatment arms

Meetings, Follow-Up, and Ongoing Business

The initial DMC meeting is usually held prior to study initiation. Topics addressed in the initial meeting include but are not restricted to the following (U.S. FDA, 2006).

- Protocol
- Plan for analysis of study data
- Informed consent template
- Case report forms and data collection documents
- Suggestions for protocol and study plan revision
- Regulatory aspects and documents
- Plan for ongoing safety monitoring
- DMC meeting schedule
- Format of DMC interim reports
- Dissemination of safety reports to DMC membership prior to meetings
- Defining a DMC meeting quorum
- DMC meeting minutes

Ongoing meetings of DMCs are usually held on a quarterly, semiannual, or annual basis appropriate for the study phase, study size, and level of risk for adverse events. Face-to-face meetings are the norm, but if the committee served earlier-phase studies of the same investigational product or intervention, they may decide on quarterly or semiannual teleconference meetings and face-to-face annual meetings. The meetings are usually structured to include open and closed sessions with a summary session concluding the meeting. *Open* sessions allow attendance of representatives of the sponsor, the clinical research steering committee, the clinical research organization managing the study, and investigators, in addition to DMC members. Process topics and nonconfidential data are usually discussed as well as what topics will be addressed in the closed session. *Closed* session topics include those listed previously under outcome topics as well as a discussion of recommendations for continuance, revision, temporary suspension, or early termination of the study. Closed session participation is restricted to DMC members to avoid introduction of bias on the part of the study sponsor, investigators, or others who are involved in the conduct of the study (Friedman & Dixon, 2012; U.S. FDA, 2006).

Review of study outcome data includes recurring testing for statistical significance. If the data from an ongoing trial is found to have insufficient statistical power to prove or disprove the null or primary hypothesis of the protocol, the DMC may recommend early termination of the study. DMCs usually establish stopping rules that define the point at which they should recommend early study termination. This point or points may be an expression of the statistical power of the study, the percentage of subjects who experience serious adverse events, or the percentage of subjects who do or do not respond positively and significantly to the study intervention (U.S. FDA, 2006).

DMCs may consider information that stems from other trials that may affect their decisions and analysis of the trial they are analyzing. This information may involve safety concerns of the study intervention or conclusions made by DMCs for outside trials that answer the questions or prove the hypotheses of the trial they are analyzing (U.S. FDA, 2006).

DMCs can make certain decisions about their study following analysis of the data. These include (U.S. FDA, 2006)

- Continuation of the trial—the conduct of the trial and enrollment is going well and as expected
- Modification of the protocol—revision of eligibility to enhance recruitment or to restrict those participants who would be at higher risk for a particular adverse event, dropping an arm of study treatment because of high incidence of adverse events, or revision of the consent form to include new information about study design or risks involved in participation
- Early termination of the study—unexpected and overwhelming evidence of the effectiveness of the study intervention, no detectable significant difference between study treatment arms, or evidence that the amount of risk to the participants is higher than the possible benefits that could be derived from study treatment
- Extension of the study timeline—the study might benefit from additional enrollment of subjects or longer follow-up to allow for analysis of long-term results of study interventions.

The decisions made by the DMC are documented and communicated to the study sponsor in writing and in the meeting's summary session. The DMC keeps detailed minutes of each meeting for future reference. The study sponsor disseminates the DMC decisions made during each meeting to study sites, principal investigators, contract research organizations, if used, and others as appropriate (U.S. FDA, 2006).

Ongoing responsibilities of the DMC include some or all of the following.

- Review and consideration of the impact of serious unexpected study adverse reactions
- Review of unblinding of study subjects
- Review of an individual event that the investigator deems to be of major significance or interest
- Communication of significant information among study sites, the sponsor, and the DMC

Benefits of Data and Safety Monitoring Plans

Monitoring involves a primary responsibility of reviewing outcome data collected during the conduct of a research study with the objective of assuring the continued safety of study subjects, in addition to the continuing scientific merit and validity of the study. Other benefits of monitoring plans to the sponsor, organization, and investigator include enhancement of the study's scientific integrity and facilitation of the dissemination of important study results in a time frame that is quicker than if there was only data analysis after the study's conclusion.

For early-phase trials (phase I and II), unless the trial involves blinded control treatment arms, the investigator or independent monitor will benefit from reporting of serious adverse events to the central or local IRB in that the IRB will review and provide feedback to the investigator if a significant safety or integrity issue is identified. If the early-phase trial does not involve blinded control treatment arms, the investigator should strive to be objective about the data analysis done for purposes of study monitoring (Friedman & Dixon, 2012).

For late-phase trials (phase III and IV), the primary benefit derived from a DMC is to provide objective and complete analysis of study data on an interim basis during the study's conduct. The DMC, composed of members who do not have a relationship to the investigators or study participants or conflicts of interest with the study sponsor, allow investigators to avoid making prejudiced conclusions about the safety and effectiveness of study interventions (Friedman & Dixon, 2012).

Summary

CTNs help to support DSMPs through various activities outlined therein (e.g., timely and accurate reporting of adverse events) and may even be called upon to help establish a plan for each protocol. In turn, CTNs can be reassured that the cumulative evidence of safety and risk of the trial is objectively reviewed and analyzed by a group of qualified committee members. CTNs should remember that

- Use of a safety monitor, monitoring group, or DMC is necessary to ensure the safety of study participants, promote study integrity, and permit accurate statistical testing of the study data.
- NIH and FDA recommend DMCs for human clinical trials that involve possible significant risk of major morbidity or mortality to subjects and include large numbers of subjects (e.g., phase III or IV clinical trials).
- DMC decisions can result in early stopping of the study, protocol or consent form modification, dropping a study treatment arm, or early study termination.
- The primary benefit of independent DMC membership to study sponsors, study funders, and researchers is that outside experts who have no conflicts of interest relative to the study eliminate bias in decisions made with regard to the trial.

CTNs and others involved in the conduct of clinical trials should keep in mind that the clinical research environment is a constantly evolving and dynamic entity.

Key Points

- External review for more than minimal risk clinical trials is necessary to ensure the safety of study participants, to promote study integrity, and to permit accurate statistical testing of the study data.
- IRBs are charged with determining if and what type of DSM is appropriate to ensure research participant safety. Many IRBs will require that the DSMP be part of the protocol or, at a minimum, submitted with the initial protocol application process.
- The outcome of a formal DMC review can result in early stopping of the study, protocol, or consent form modification, dropping a study treatment arm, or early study termination.
- The primary benefit of DMCs to study sponsors, study funders, and researchers is that outside experts who have no conflicts of interest relative to the study eliminate bias in decisions made with regard to the trial.
- DSMPs are required for NIH-funded phase I, II, and III clinical trials, with a DMC required for phase III clinical trials.

References

Criteria for IRB Approval of Research, 45 C.F.R. § 46.111 (2009). Retrieved from http://www.hhs.gov/ohrp/humansubjects/guidance/45cfr46.html#46.111

Criteria for IRB Approval of Research, 21 C.F.R. § 56.111 (2014). Retrieved from http://www.accessdata.fda.gov/scripts/cdrh/cfdocs/cfcfr/CFRSearch.cfm?fr=56.111

Friedman, L.M., & Dixon, D.O. (2012). Data and safety monitoring. In J.I. Gallin & F.P. Ognibene (Eds.), *Principles and practice of clinical research* (3rd ed., pp. 101–108). Boston, MA: Academic Press. doi:10.1016/B978-0-12-382167-6.00009-6

International Conference on Harmonisation of Technical Requirements for Registration of Pharmaceuticals for Human Use. (1996, June 10). *ICH harmonised tripartite guideline: Guideline for good clinical practice, E6(R1)*. Retrieved from http://www.ich.org/fileadmin/Public_Web_Site/ICH_Products/Guidelines/Efficacy/E6/E6_R1_Guideline.pdf

Kleppinger, C.F., & Ball, L.K. (2010). Building quality in clinical trials with use of a quality systems approach. *Clinical Infectious Diseases, 51*(Suppl. 1), S111–S116. doi:10.1086/653058

Morrison, B.W., Cochran, C.J., White, J.G., Harley, J., Kleppinger, C.F., Liu, A., ... Neaton, J.D. (2011). Monitoring the quality of conduct of clinical trials: A survey of current practices. *Clinical Trials, 8,* 342–349. doi:10.1177/1740774511402703

National Cancer Institute. (2001, April). Essential elements of a data and safety monitoring plan for clinical trials funded by the National Cancer Institute. Retrieved from http://www.cancer.gov/clinicaltrials/conducting/dsm-guidelines/page1/AllPages

National Cancer Institute. (2014, September). National Cancer Institute clinical trials policy. Retrieved from http://deainfo.nci.nih.gov/grantspolicies/datasafety.pdf

National Institutes of Health. (1998, June 10). NIH policy for data and safety monitoring. Retrieved from http://grants.nih.gov/grants/guide/notice-files/not98-084.html

National Institutes of Health. (2000, June 5). Further guidance on a data and safety monitoring for phase I and phase II trials. Retrieved from http://grants.nih.gov/grants/guide/notice-files/NOT-OD-00-038.html

Shalala, D. (2000, 14 September). Protecting research subjects—What must be done. *New England Journal of Medicine, 343,* 808–810. doi:10.1056/NEJM200009143431112

U.S. Food and Drug Administration. (2006, March). *Guidance for clinical trial sponsors—Establishment and operation of clinical trial data monitoring committees*. Retrieved from http://www.fda.gov/downloads/Regulatoryinformation/Guidances/ucm127073.pdf

U.S. Food and Drug Administration. (2013, August). *Guidance for industry: Oversight of clinical investigations—A risk-based approach to monitoring*. Retrieved from http://www.fda.gov/downloads/Drugs/.../Guidances/UCM269919.pdf

Chapter 41

Preparing for Audits, Inspections, and Monitoring Visits

Ellen A. Patricia, MS, CIP, and Sandra A. Meadows, MPH, CIP

Introduction

Cancer researchers have an obligation to protect the rights, safety, and welfare of the participants enrolled in their studies, as well as to ensure that the data collected during the study are credible and verifiable. Good clinical practice (GCP) guidelines ideally should be followed, and data results must be properly documented. This chapter is devoted to audits, inspections, and monitoring visits, of which many types exist: federal (e.g., National Cancer Institute [NCI], U.S. Food and Drug Administration [FDA] Office for Human Research Protections), sponsor (i.e., investigational new drug application [IND] and investigational device exemption [IDE] studies), accreditation bodies (e.g., Association for the Accreditation of Human Research Protection Programs [AAHRPP]), and internal (i.e., those conducted by research sites or institutions as part of a quality management program). No matter the type, audit, inspection, or monitoring visit, preparation is essentially the same (see Figure 41-1). This chapter will provide clinical trial nurses (CTNs) with an overview of the terms and concepts associated with audits, inspections, and monitoring visits, as well as the preparation for these reviews. For ease of reference, the term *audit* will be used generically throughout this chapter, unless otherwise specified.

Purpose of an Audit

The purpose of an audit is to evaluate trial conduct and compliance with the protocol, internal standard operating procedures, GCP, and applicable regulatory requirements (federal, state, and local) (International Conference on Harmonisation of Technical Requirements for Registration of Pharmaceuticals for Human Use [ICH], 1996). Audits are necessary to assure the public and, in particular, the participants that the data generated in clinical trials are credible and that while the trial was being conducted, human subjects' rights, welfare, and safety were protected.

A clinical study site may be audited by one or all of the following entities: FDA; the study sponsor, such as a pharmaceutical company or federal sponsor (e.g., NCI, Department of Defense); or an internal auditing group, such as a compliance office or quality assurance office. Regardless of the auditing body, the goals listed in Figure 41-2 apply to all audits of clinical research.

Figure 41-1. Audit and Monitoring Definitions

Audit: A systematic review, inspection, or verification, typically conducted by an independent individual or group

Routine (not-for-cause) audit/review: An assessment or examination of research practices or procedures with the possibility or intention of instituting change if necessary

Directed (for-cause) audit/review: An audit of research and/or investigators to obtain or verify information necessary to ensure compliance with regulations, sponsor and/or institutional requirements, and institutional review board approvals, and to inform decisions about the conduct of human subject research and data validity

Monitoring visit: Performed by sponsor representatives to assess site compliance with regulations and sponsor/institutional standard operating procedures, ensure that participants are protected, and verify that data are valid

Inspection: Site visits to clinical investigators, sponsors, and institutional review boards to ensure that clinical trial participants are protected from undue hazards and to verify that research data supporting new human product approvals are reliable

Note. Based on information from The Ohio State University Office of Responsible Research Practices, 2015a.

Figure 41-2. Audit Purposes

- To determine that the rights, safety, and welfare of human participants enrolled in clinical trials are properly protected
- To ensure the integrity of scientific research and the reliability of the data generated by verifying that all data are obtained in compliance with good clinical practice
- To ensure that local, state, and federal regulatory requirements and procedures are adequately fulfilled
- To assist site personnel in the development of useful procedures to guide research endeavors
- To educate research staff and initiate follow-up mechanisms for problem resolution

Note. Based on information from International Conference on Harmonisation of Technical Requirements for Registration of Pharmaceuticals for Human Use, 1996.

U.S. Food and Drug Administration Inspections: Routine and For-Cause

FDA oversees FDA-regulated research by performing inspections of clinical investigators, sponsors, and institutional review boards (IRBs). These on-site inspections help to ensure that human subjects are protected from undue hazards and to verify that research data supporting new human product approvals are reliable (U.S. FDA, 2010).

FDA conducts inspections to determine if investigators are in compliance with FDA regulations. Inspections can be announced or unannounced. Most inspections are routinely performed (data audits) as a result of clinical data submitted to FDA in the form of an IND and the need for FDA to base important decisions on those data. Events that could trigger a for-cause inspection include a complaint made to FDA, sponsor concerns, a review division request within FDA, or current and ongoing public health issues. For-cause inspections focus primarily on the conduct of the study by the principal investigator (PI) (U.S. FDA, 2010). Because the majority of inspections are routine in nature, they will be outlined as follows.

The appropriate FDA center (e.g., Center for Drug Evaluation and Research, Center for Biologic Evaluation and Research, Center for Devices and Radiological Health) determines which clinical studies and study centers will be audited. Although the center does not release explicit details of how it goes about selecting studies and sites for audit, if a clinical trial is a pivotal trial used for the new drug application portfolio, it will likely be audited. FDA reviewers consider the number of subjects enrolled at a particular site, the number of subjects who withdrew early, and those sites with very good response rates or, conversely, very poor response rates. The reviewers will use this information to select one or several clinical sites for inspection (U.S. FDA, 2010).

FDA staff conducts on-site inspections according to FDA compliance manuals. These manuals are made available to the public to ensure transparency in what FDA expects of investigators, IRBs, and sponsors. The *Compliance Program Guidance Manual* used by FDA staff when monitoring clinical investigators can be found at www.fda.gov/downloads/ICECI/EnforcementActions/BioresearchMonitoring/ucm133773.pdf, with attention paid in particular to Part III—Inspectional. This section instructs FDA staff to assess if the investigator followed the protocol with respect to participant selection, the number of participants enrolled, required procedures and evaluations, administration of the investigational product, and frequency of observations and testing to be performed regarding participant follow-up. FDA staff verifies that the investigator followed the IRB-approved protocol and submitted amendments when necessary, reported adverse events promptly, obtained informed consent from every participant, administered study drug to only those participants enrolled onto the study, properly recorded and documented data, and reported deviations appropriately. Another helpful tool made available to FDA staff and the public is the Clinical Investigator Inspection List, which includes deficiency codes that may be used in the FDA report (see Table 41-1) (U.S. FDA, 2008).

Routine audits are scheduled in the following manner.
- The FDA center chooses a clinical site for inspection.
- The local FDA office nearest to the site is notified that a site audit must be scheduled.
- The local investigator contacts the site PI and requests an audit date, which typically is one to two weeks from the contact date.
- The local inspector arrives on the mutually agreed-upon date, presents his or her FDA credentials, and issues Form FDA 482, Notice of Inspection.

At the conclusion of the audit, typically Form FDA 483, Inspectional Observations, will be issued. The "483" is the FDA inspector's report to the site of those things that, in the opinion of the inspector, may include violations. Receiving a "483" is expected and does not represent FDA's final position on the inspection. When it is reviewed internally at FDA, the "483" may be overturned completely. The "483" is used to develop an inspectional report, which will include a more detailed description of the violations uncovered during the site inspection (if any) (U.S. FDA, 2008, 2010). This report is then reviewed at the center and the inspection results will be classified in one of three ways (U.S. FDA, 2008):
- NAI (no action indicated)
- VAI (voluntary action indicated)
- OAI (official action indicated).

Both NAI and VAI classifications result in "untitled letters." The district office has 15 working days after the inspection to submit the report to the center. The center then has 15 working days to agree or disagree. An OAI classification typically results in the issuance of a warning letter. Warning letters are issued for violations of reg-

Table 41-1. Clinical Investigator Inspection List Deficiency Codes		
Code	Deficiency	C.F.R. Reference
00	No deficiencies noted	n/a
01	Records availability	21 C.F.R. § 312.62
02	Failure to obtain and/or document subject consent	21 C.F.R. §§ 312.60, 50.20, 50.27
03	Inadequate informed consent form	21 C.F.R. § 50.25
04	Inadequate drug accountability	21 C.F.R. §§ 312.60, 312.62
05	Failure to follow investigational plan	21 C.F.R. § 312.60
06	Inadequate and inaccurate records	21 C.F.R. § 312.62
07	Unapproved concomitant therapy	21 C.F.R. § 312.60
08	Inappropriate payment to volunteers	21 C.F.R. § 50.20
09	Unapproved use of drug before IND submission	21 C.F.R. § 312.40(d)
10	Inappropriate delegation of authority	21 C.F.R. §§ 312.7, 312.61
11	Inappropriate use/commercialization of IND	21 C.F.R. §§ 312.7, 312.61
12	Failure to list additional investigators on 1572	21 C.F.R. § 312.60
13	Subjects receiving simultaneous investigational drugs	21 C.F.R. § 312.60
14	Failure to obtain or document IRB approval	21 C.F.R. §§ 312.60, 62, 66; 56.103
15	Failure to notify IRB of changes, failure to submit progress reports	21 C.F.R. § 312.66
16	Failure to report adverse drug reactions	21 C.F.R. §§ 312.64, 312.66
17	Submission of false information	21 C.F.R. § 312.70
18	Other	n/a
19*	Failure to supervise or personally conduct the clinical investigation	21 C.F.R. § 312.60
20*	Failure to protect the rights, safety, and welfare of subjects	21 C.F.R. § 312.60
21*	Failure to permit FDA access to records	21 C.F.R. § 312.68

* Codes 19, 20, and 21 became effective October 1, 2005.
C.F.R.—Code of Federal Regulations; FDA—U.S. Food and Drug Administration; IND—investigational new drug application; IRB—institutional review board
Note. From "Clinical Investigator Inspection List (CIIL) Database Codes," by U.S. Food and Drug Administration, 2009. Retrieved from http://www.fda.gov/Drugs/GuidanceComplianceRegulatoryInformation/EnforcementActivitiesbyFDA/ucm073059.htm.

ulatory significance and are available under the Freedom of Information Act at www.fda.gov/ICECI/EnforcementActions/WarningLetters/default.htm. FDA will ask the investigator to respond to the warning letter with a remedial action plan to address the compliance problems. The investigator's response must be submitted to the center within 15 working days. It will usually take the site longer to implement the plan, but FDA wants to see what is planned and will then re-inspect to assess outcome. CTNs are often an integral part of developing and implementing the corrective action plan. In extreme cases of severe noncompliance, FDA can disqualify investigators from ever conducting FDA-regulated research again, impose fines on investigators and study coordinators, and sentence the investigators and study coordinators to prison (U.S. FDA, 2008).

Investigational New Drug Application and Investigational Device Exemption Sponsors

Sponsor Audits

Sponsors sometimes conduct audits as part of quality assurance checks (e.g., ensuring quality performance of their study monitors), but most often sponsor audits are performed in preparation for an FDA inspection by a drug manufacturer/pharmaceutical sponsor audit team (ICH, 1996). The auditors assist the investigational site in preparing for the inspection. The team will ensure that source documentation is complete and well organized and may conduct further source document verification to identify potential problems. No data changes should be made after study closure. The audit team will address site concerns and questions about the pending audit and may offer tips and suggestions on how the staff should conduct itself while the audit is taking place. An audit report typically is generated as a result of this type of audit, but the report itself is exempt from FDA review. The investigational site should not make this report available to the FDA inspector.

Sponsor Visits

The study sponsor (i.e., the IND or IDE holder) may conduct a variety of visits as follows (ICH, 1996).
- Prestudy qualification visit
- Initiation visit
- Monitoring visit
- Close-out visit

Prestudy Qualification Visit

The prestudy qualification visit is conducted to determine the site's ability to conduct a clinical trial prior to commencement of the investigation (ICH, 1996). A sponsor may choose to perform this type of visit if using a new site or a site with a good reputation that might not have participated in a certain type of study previously (e.g., a phase I clinical trial). This visit allows the sponsor to meet with the site staff and inspect the facilities before placing a study at the research site. The sponsor will contact the PI, and usually the CTN will be asked to join the visit. The visits typically last about two to three hours (Ness, 2013).

Initiation Visit

The initiation visit is the first visit conducted by the sponsor after a research site has been chosen for participation and the appropriate legal agreements are in place. The visit allows the sponsor's representatives and site staff to meet and review the following (Ness, 2013).
- Roles, responsibilities, and regulatory obligations
- Protocol procedures
- Case report form (CRF) completion instructions
- Requirements for records management and retention
- Drug handling requirements
- Enrollment and consent procedures
- Adverse event reporting procedures
- Patient recruitment plan

This visit presents a time where potential problems and concerns can be identified and addressed. The PI will need to attend this visit for a portion of the time, whereas the CTN should plan to attend the entire visit, which may be as long as six hours. Recommendations on how to prepare for an initiation visit are listed in Figure 41-3. After the visit, the site may need to follow up with the sponsor on any outstanding issues (e.g., missing curricula vitae, missing supplies) and will also be sent a visit report, which should be placed in the protocol's regulatory file (see Chapter 39) (Ness, 2013).

Routine Monitoring Visit

The purpose of routine monitoring visits is to verify that the rights, safety, and welfare of clinical trial participants are protected; that the data reported to sponsors are accurate, complete, and verifiable from the source documents; and that the conduct of the trial is in compliance with the IRB-approved protocol and applicable regulatory requirements. The sponsor must ensure that trials are adequately monitored throughout the trial, and this involves on-site monitoring visits before, during, and after enrollment is complete (ICH, 1996).

The monitor will work with the investigator and staff to arrange a mutually agreed-upon date and time to conduct the monitoring visit. A room will need to be made available to the monitor in order to review records and meet with members of the research team. The staff must ensure that all requested source documents and trial-related documents are available to the monitor during the visit. Staff should remind the monitor to sign and date the site visit monitoring log at each visit (Ness, 2013).

The monitor will review and verify that each trial participant's informed consent document is properly executed, the investigator has adequate qualifications and resources to conduct the trial, investigational product is stored and maintained appropriately, investigational products are only dispensed to eligible trial subjects, the investigator and staff follow the IRB-approved protocol, records are accurate and complete, events are promptly reported to the IRB and sponsor, and CRFs are accurate and complete (ICH, 1996).

Figure 41-3. Preparing for a Sponsor Site Initiation Visit

- Review protocol and any other documents received by sponsor (i.e., case report forms, investigator's brochure).
- Become familiar with the study's procedures.
- Confirm supplies received (i.e., drug, binders, test tubes, regulatory binder, etc.).
- Write down questions for sponsor/contract research organization when reviewing documents.
- Secure room.
- Ensure staff availability for the visit.
- Clinical trial nurse can remind staff involved a few days in advance.

Note. Based on information from Ness, 2013.

The regulations do not address the timing or frequency of routine monitoring visits. The sponsor will take the following into consideration when determining the timing and frequency (ICH, 1996).
- Protocol complexity
- Disease being studied
- Rate of recruitment
- PI and staff experience
- Site performance

In 2013, FDA released *Guidance for Industry: Oversight of Clinical Investigations—A Risk-Based Approach to Monitoring*. This sponsor guidance describes various risk-based monitoring strategies focusing on critical study parameters. The guidance suggests the use of a combination of differing monitoring activities, especially encouraging greater use of centralized monitoring methods, where appropriate (U.S. FDA, 2013).

After the visit, the monitor should provide the site with a report that includes a summary of the items reviewed and statements regarding any findings and facts, deviations, deficiencies, conclusions, actions taken, and recommended actions to ensure future compliance. The report should be placed in the regulatory file (ICH, 1996).

Close-Out Visit

The purpose of the close-out visit is to perform a final review of regulatory documentation, drug accountability record forms, and record retention guidelines. The visit is conducted after the study is complete, the site's obligations are fulfilled, and all data have been retrieved and the sponsor's database locked. In some circumstances, a close-out visit occurs before a study is completed. A sponsor may decide the site had inadequate enrollment or too many protocol or regulatory violations. The PI may request that the study be terminated because the PI is leaving the research site and no other investigator is able to take over the PI responsibilities (Ness, 2013).

At the close-out visit, the monitor will
- Confirm that all original CRFs are retrieved and queries completed.
- Destroy or return all extra CRFs.
- Review the site's regulatory binder to ensure consistency with sponsor's master file.
- Ensure that all study supplies have been returned or destroyed.
- Ensure that all biologic samples have been shipped or backup samples destroyed.
- Ensure that the PI has provided the IRB with the final study report.

PIs and CTNs are typically the site staff involved in the close-out visit (Ness, 2013).

National Cancer Institute as Study Sponsor

As an IND sponsor, NCI follows the same regulations as other study sponsors, including those related to study monitoring. On-site monitoring has been active since 1982 and includes all trials conducted by the National Clinical Trials Network (formerly known as NCI's National Clinical Trials Cooperative Group Program), the NCI Community Oncology Research Program (NCORP) (which combined NCI's Community Clinical Oncology Program [CCOP] and NCI's Community Cancer Centers Program), the Cancer Trials Support Unit, and the studies conducted at cancer centers or other individual institutions that use NCI Division of Cancer Treatment and Diagnosis (DCTD)/NCI-sponsored investigational agents.

DCTD maintains policies governing the therapeutic development of new agents. The NCI Cancer Therapy Evaluation Program (CTEP) exists within DCTD and is the division responsible for the design and implementation of development plans for new agents. The Clinical Trials Monitoring Branch (CTMB) is responsible for on-site auditing of all clinical trials sponsored by CTEP and DCTD. CTMB is responsible for oversight of the Clinical Trials Monitoring Service (CTMS) and the contractor who conducts the audits (e.g., Theradex®). CTMB sets guidelines and standards for the conduct of clinical trials in order to ensure data quality and compliance with regulatory requirements for clinical research (NCI, 2011).

Cooperative groups monitor trial compliance at research sites in several ways, including central review of major elements, such as pathology, radiotherapy, surgery, and investigational agent administration; protocol chair review of CRFs; and statistical office review of subject eligibility and response. Data quality-control software is available for use by data management and statistical centers to help identify and correct or clarify inconsistencies and inaccuracies in submitted data. Cooperative groups perform their own program of on-site audits, and these are conducted by a combination of central staff and group members with direct oversight by CTMB. Typically, a CTMB staff member will attended NCI audits. On-site audits are conducted, on average, once every three years (NCI, 2014).

For early-phase CTEP studies, protocol compliance is assessed by CTMS. Research sites conducting phase 0 (exploratory IND), phase I and early phase II studies submit data to CTMS on an ongoing basis (i.e., every two weeks). CTMS reviews the data carefully for compliance with the protocol and asks for clarifications if data are missing or do not seem to flow logically. Reports are provided periodically to the investigator and to CTEP. Per the CTMS monitoring guidelines, contractors (e.g., Theradex) perform on-site visits three times per year. For more information on CTEP early-phase study monitoring, see Final Early Therapeutics Clinical Trials Network Audit Guidelines found at http://ctep.cancer.gov/branches/ctmb/clinicalTrials/monitoring.htm. Cancer centers are audited on-site by NCI or NCI-contracted auditors once every three years as part of the P30 grant mechanism (NCI, 2013).

In reporting results, NCI auditors use the ratings *Acceptable, Acceptable Needs Follow-Up,* or *Unacceptable.* For results rated less than acceptable, the institution must provide a written response, including corrective actions to ensure future compliance. Auditors have many action options when dealing with problems identified during on-site audits. In most cases, the measures are intended to be constructive and educational; however, the action options can include probation, issuance of a warning letter, suspension of patient enrollment privileges, repeat audit, removal of access to investigational agents, or termination of a grant or contract (NCI, 2013, 2014).

Internal Audits at the Investigational Site

Large research sites often have an office dedicated to clinical trial management, with an internal protocol compliance component. These offices are set up to assist investigators with regulatory submissions, data management, and study coordination and serve as a compliance safeguard for the institution. Community hospitals and private practices may decide to hire independent auditors to monitor compliance. Because a clinical study site may be audited by many entities, it makes sense to have personnel devoted to assisting with the numerous outside audits that take place every year and to perform internal audits of those trials that do not undergo routine auditing (i.e., investigator-initiated trials). The focus of such a protocol compliance group would be to educate site faculty and staff of the local, state, and federal regulations governing their clinical research. This group would also serve as the central contact when compliance questions arise. Oversight of the clinical trials office would be performed by an institutional administrator or by a medical director.

Typically, any of the research site's protocols are subject to an internal audit conducted by the protocol compliance group. An example of how a program could function is as follows: A protocol is chosen for audit, and then a representative number of subject cases are reviewed (e.g., 10% of all enrolled subjects). The associated regulatory documents also are audited. At the conclusion of the audit, an audit report is generated and distributed to study personnel and to the protocol PI. A point-by-point response to the audit report is submitted to the office and a general corrective action plan is employed to ensure that any mistakes are not repeated. Education is the key to these internal audits. Focusing on the positive aspects of the study conduct is essential, and correcting problems before they become routine is critical.

Human Research Protection Program Audits

Many IRB offices conduct routine audits of approved research protocols due in part to AAHRPP accreditation requirements. IRB staff, or a quality improvement group, work with the IRB and institutional officials to promote and maintain ethical research conduct and compliance with state and federal regulations, federal guidance, institutional policies, and best practices for human research protections (The Ohio State University [OSU] Office of Responsible Research Practices, 2015b; Schott, 2010). The staff evaluates and improves human protections and Human Research Protection Program (HRPP) activities through education, training, and monitoring.

Routine reviews of study activities and study documentation are performed at the investigator's site, and feedback is provided (e.g., written report, verbal) regarding study practices. Information is gathered through interviews, observations, and records review. Study selection for routine reviews may be random or based on particular research aspects (e.g., special populations, risk level, investigational drugs and devices) and typically draws from a list of all active protocols. Any study involving human subjects, including medical and nonmedical studies, may be selected for review (The OSU Office of Responsible Research Practices, 2015b; Schott, 2010).

Typically, the specific results of routine monitoring visits are shared only with those participating in the review. Minor concerns are addressed directly with the PI and research staff members. When necessary, IRB staff work with the PI to assist in reporting serious concerns to the IRB. Aggregate data are provided to institutional officials periodically to inform ongoing HRPP assessment and educational efforts (The OSU Office of Responsible Research Practices, 2012; Schott, 2010).

How to Prepare for an Audit

Auditors prepare for an audit by reviewing the protocol, the site's internal standard operating procedures, applicable regulations, and sponsor guidelines. These preparations are enacted to ensure an educated and efficient use of time and resources and to ensure an audit result that increases site staff knowledge and compliance. In turn, the research team must also prepare for an audit to facilitate the visit and, ideally, to achieve a positive audit outcome. Once the research team has received notification of a pending audit, the steps outlined in Figure 41-4 should be followed. To prepare for the audit, the research team should have the following items readily available.

Regulatory Files

The regulatory files will be reviewed to ensure that regulatory compliance has been properly maintained throughout the study. To facilitate review of the regulatory documents, they should be current, organized, complete, and accurate. The files should contain all versions of the protocol and consent documents, including a copy of the initially approved protocol. The file

Figure 41-4. Preparing for an Audit

- Determine the nature (i.e., for-cause, routine) and the scope of the audit. What protocols will be reviewed? How long will the auditors be on site?
- Notify all parties (as applicable) when initially contacted so that each can prepare for the visit, as necessary (e.g., the investigational pharmacy, the institutional review board, all members of the research team).
- Obtain pertinent audit information such as the number of auditors who will conduct the audit, the approximate times the auditors will work each day, whether an exit interview will take place at the conclusion of the audit, and if so, who will be required to attend.
- Follow the institution's standard operating procedures.
- Schedule a quiet room with enough space to comfortably accommodate the auditors. The room should ideally be located near a copier and restroom. A computer also should be made available for the auditors to view online medical records, x-ray and other imaging results, and online versions of the protocol, consent documents, and data forms. If more than one sponsor is auditing at the same time, it might be necessary to secure two rooms to avoid disclosing any confidentiality or proprietary information.
- Allow access to all study-related areas and subjects' medical records, including inpatient, outpatient, and physician's office records. Sites using electronic medical records will need to understand the process by which monitors access relevant records online and obtain the necessary permissions in advance or alternatively, print all desired subject records.
- Pre-review all research records (medical and regulatory) for any missing documentation.
- If time allows, perform an internal data review with assistance from the research team before the audit.

Note. Based on information from Ness, 2013.

should contain all IRB correspondence (to and from the IRB) and IRB-approved materials and associated submissions (including the initial protocol and consent, amendments, and annual continuing reviews), along with the IRB roster and meeting minutes, as applicable. The file should include adverse event reports, including evidence that adverse events were properly reported to the IRB and to the sponsor. Also contained in the file is a sponsor correspondence section (to and from the sponsor) (ICH, 1996; Ness, 2013; U.S. FDA, 2010). See Chapter 39 for more details about maintaining a regulatory file.

Informed Consent Documents

All IRB-approved consent versions will be reviewed to verify that they contain all required elements of informed consent as mandated by 45 C.F.R. § 46.116 (General Requirements for Informed Consent, 2009) and 21 C.F.R. § 50.25 (Elements of Informed Consent, 2014). The auditors will review the consent versions to ensure that they reflect the appropriate risks, tests, and procedures for each version time period. Original signed informed consent documents will be reviewed to ensure that all blanks (i.e., dates and signatures) have been properly completed and that an informed consent document exists for each participant enrolled to the study. The auditors will ask the investigator and research team questions about the consent process to ensure that participants were properly informed, such as the following (ICH, 1996; Ness, 2013; U.S. FDA, 2010).

- Were patients introduced to the concept of clinical trials and then presented all available treatment options, including research participation?
- Was consent obtained prior to the initiation of any research-related procedures?
- Was a copy of the consent given to the participant to take home?
- Was the entire consent process documented in the patient's medical record?
- Was a revised consent signed when new information became available that might affect the subject's willingness to participate in the trial?
- Was the correct version of the consent used for the appropriate time frame?

Drug Accountability Records

Accountability records for investigational agents, as well as for any other drugs supplied by the sponsor for the trial, will be subject to audit (ICH, 1996; U.S. FDA, 2010). As mentioned in Figure 41-4, the investigational pharmacist should be notified of any pending audit, as the auditors most certainly will visit the pharmacy while on site.

Drug accountability records, often referred to as *drug accountability record forms*, are compared to shipment records to ensure that the agents were properly received and logged in at the site. If products were transferred from one office to another or were shipped back to the sponsor, those records will be compared to ensure product accountability. A subject registration log should correlate with the drug dispensing records. The auditor must ensure that all enrolled subjects were dispensed the proper drug and dosage from the appropriate shipment per protocol and, conversely, that no patient other than those registered to the trial received study-supplied products. The auditor must check to see that commercial supplies versus investigational supplies were appropriately used and not interchanged.

The auditor will visit the pharmacy to ensure that the location is secure and that access to the area is restricted to authorized personnel only. If investigational products are present in the pharmacy at the time of the audit, the auditor will count the remaining drug to confirm the amount indicated on the inventory records (Ness, 2013).

Study Participant Records

The auditor will compare the data collection forms (e.g., CRFs, serious adverse event report forms) or, if using remote data entry, sponsor-supplied data printouts against the participant's medical records (both inpatient and outpatient) to verify reporting accuracy and to ensure that no omissions occurred in the reported data. This document review allows the auditor to assess how well the research staff followed the protocol requirements: Were the proper tests ordered and obtained? Were adverse events reported and in a timely fashion? Specifically, the following will be reviewed in detail (ICH, 1996; U.S. FDA, 2010).

- Subject enrollment procedures—Was the first subject enrolled after IRB approval was granted?
- Subject selection—Was each subject eligible for the trial?
- Informed consent
- Subject data
  - Inclusion and exclusion criteria
  - Protocol treatment administration records—Were treatments held or modified as required by the protocol?
  - Tumor response—Was response documented at the appropriate time points and by the methods outlined in the protocol?
  - Toxicities and adverse events—Were they reported appropriately (to the sponsor, IRB, etc.) as required by the protocol?
  - Laboratory results
  - Reasons for subject withdrawal
  - Follow-up data

Close-Out Meeting

A close-out meeting is typically held with the research team, including the protocol PI, the regulatory coordinator, the CTN or study coordinator, and the data manager. The positive audit findings should be highlighted at this meeting, and any deficiencies discovered will be discussed. It is important for the research team to take notes and write down suggestions made to later develop a meaningful and informed audit response. The auditor may suggest corrective actions at this time or may wait until obtaining input from the sponsor, IRB, or agency to include in the audit report. The auditor may also give the PI and CTN a written summary of findings or missing materials prior to leaving the site and will also send a more formal written follow-up at a later date. The PI and the research team must respond to any report that is generated by addressing all audit findings.

Summary

Audits, inspections, and monitoring visits ensure that the data generated during a clinical trial are credible, all applicable regulations governing clinical trials are followed, and participants' rights, safety, and welfare are protected. No matter what they are called or how they are classified, they should be viewed as educational tools that teach research teams the proper and ethical way to run clinical trials. Ensuring human subjects' rights to participate in clinical trials in a manner that generates meaningful data and is ethically conducted should be the ultimate goal of oncology clinical research, along with, of course, finding treatments that eventually will enhance the lives of patients with cancer and those who are at high risk for developing cancer.

Key Points

- Preparation for all visit types (e.g., audit, inspection, monitoring visit) is essentially the same.
- Multiple entities may conduct an audit, including the FDA, study sponsor, or internal auditor.
- Auditor and research team preparation in advance of the visit results in the most effective encounter.
- For-cause audit findings require that the research team provide specific responses and implement any necessary corrective actions to ensure future compliance with applicable regulations.

References

Elements of Informed Consent, 21 C.F.R. § 50.25 (2014). Retrieved from http://www.accessdata.fda.gov/scripts/cdrh/cfdocs/cfCFR/CFRSearch.cfm?fr=50.25

General Requirements for Informed Consent, 45 C.F.R. § 46.116 (2009). Retrieved from http://www.hhs.gov/ohrp/humansubjects/guidance/45cfr46.html#46.116

International Conference on Harmonisation of Technical Requirements for Registration of Pharmaceuticals for Human Use. (1996, June 10). *ICH harmonised tripartite guideline: Guideline for good clinical practice, E6(R1)*. Retrieved from http://www.ich.org/fileadmin/Public_Web_Site/ICH_Products/Guidelines/Efficacy/E6/E6_R1_Guideline.pdf

National Cancer Institute. (2011, February 10). Clinical Trials Monitoring Branch (CTMB). Retrieved from http://ctep.cancer.gov/branches/ctmb/default.htm

National Cancer Institute. (2013, January 28). *NCI guidelines for auditing of clinical trials for the Experimental Therapeutics Clinical Trials Network (ETCTN)*. Retrieved from http://ctep.cancer.gov/branches/ctmb/clinicalTrials/docs/ETCTN_Audit_Guidelines.pdf

National Cancer Institute. (2014, February). *NCI guidelines for auditing clinical trials for the NCI National Clinical Trials Network (NCTN) Program, Community Clinical Oncology Program (CCOP)/NCI Community Oncology Research Program (NCORP) and research bases*. Retrieved from http://ctep.cancer.gov/branches/ctmb/clinicalTrials/docs/ctmb_audit_guidelines.pdf

Ness, E. (2013, November). *Monitoring and auditing of clinical trials* [PowerPoint slides]. Retrieved from https://ccrod.cancer.gov/confluence/download/attachments/83530280/Monitoring%20and%20Auditing.pdf?version=1&modificationDate=1385473208587&api=v2

The Ohio State University Office of Responsible Research Practices. (2012). HRPP quality improvement activities. Retrieved from http://orrp.osu.edu/files/2012/02/HRPP-Quality-Improvement-Activities.pdf

The Ohio State University Office of Responsible Research Practices. (2015a). Investigator/staff guidance for FDA inspections. Retrieved from http://orrp.osu.edu/irb/investigator-guidance/fda-inspections

The Ohio State University Office of Responsible Research Practices. (2015b). Quality Improvement Program. Retrieved from http://orrp.osu.edu/irb/qiprogram

Schott, R. (2010). Quality assurance inspections. *SoCRA Source, 64*, 62–68.

U.S. Food and Drug Administration. (2008, December 8). *Compliance program guidance manual*. Retrieved from http://www.fda.gov/downloads/ICECI/EnforcementActions/BioresearchMonitoring/ucm133773.pdf

U.S. Food and Drug Administration. (2010, June). Information sheet guidance for IRBs, clinical investigators, and sponsors: FDA inspections of clinical investigators. Retrieved from http://www.fda.gov/downloads/RegulatoryInformation/Guidances/UCM126553.pdf

U.S. Food and Drug Administration. (2013, August). *Guidance for industry: Oversight of clinical investigations—A risk-based approach to monitoring*. Retrieved from: http://www.fda.gov/downloads/Drugs/.../Guidances/UCM269919.pdf

SECTION X.

Professional Development of Clinical Trial Nurses

Chapter 42

Clinical Trial Nurse Education

Elizabeth Ness, RN, MS

Introduction

Nurses have a professional obligation to be competent in their practice, which includes activities related to education. The American Nurses Association's (ANA's) professional performance Standard 8 states, "The registered nurse attains knowledge and competence that reflects current nursing practice" (ANA, 2010, p. 11). The 2010 report *The Future of Nursing: Leading Change, Advancing Health* from the Institute of Medicine (IOM) and the Robert Wood Johnson Foundation continues to support nurses being engaged in lifelong learning activities (IOM, 2011). The Oncology Nursing Society (ONS) Standard XIV, Professional Practice Evaluation, also supports continual evaluation of the nurse's own practice in "relation to national oncology nursing professional standards and guidelines, the state nurse practice act, relevant statewide regulatory requirements, and job-specific performance expectations" (Brant & Wickham, 2013, p. 58). It is clear that nurses, including clinical trial nurses (CTNs), are lifelong learners and need to be equipped with the skills and knowledge to competently practice.

Oncology CTNs are in a unique position. They must stay current in both oncology and clinical research; for example, they must understand the latest cancer therapies and survivorship concerns as well as trends in trial design for targeted therapies and federal laws, regulations, and guidances. In addition to ongoing participation in educational activities, the ANA (2010) education competencies address the nurse's need to identify areas for learning and personal growth needs through self-reflection, communicate experiences and ideas with peers, and maintain records to support learning activities. The measurement criteria for the ONS Professional Practice Evaluation Standard incorporates the ANA competencies, including (a) conduct formal and ongoing performance assessments to identify strengths and areas for improvement for knowledge, skills, and attitudes, (b) establish goals for further professional development, (c) acquire appropriate education and support, (d) function as a preceptor or mentor for new nurses, and (e) maintain a professional portfolio (Brant & Wickham, 2013). The ONS CTN competencies have incorporated these standards in the Professional Development competency (Oncology Nursing Society, 2010). This chapter will identify a variety of professional development activities and resources for CTNs and provide a tool for tracking educational activities.

Professional Development Activities

General

Various formal and informal learning activities are available. They can be simple (e.g., reading professional journals) or complex (e.g., preparing a manuscript for publication or completing a certificate or master's program in clinical research management or regulatory compliance). Examples of professional development activities for CTNs include

- Attending conferences, seminars, and workshops
- Completing e-learning activities
- Seeking out mentorship experiences
- Contributing to CTNs' body of knowledge through presentations and publications.

Another important activity is staying current with practice and research trends by reading the relevant literature. Recommendations for journals of interest to CTNs can be found in Figure 42-1. Each journal provides the reader with varying topics related to oncology and clinical research; whether articles are peer-reviewed depends upon the journal.

New digital technologies allow nursing professionals to tap into learning resources as never before. According to Yoder and Terhorst (2012), "There are four broad categories of technology that have profound implications for nursing professional development: 1) cloud computing, 2) e-learning, 3) mobile computing, and 4) three-dimensional virtual spaces" (p. 459), each with unique benefits (see Table 42-1). Understanding computers and how to harness information technology is a crucial skill for CTNs.

Maintaining a keen awareness of the regulatory climate is important for CTNs. In addition to e-learning activities and subscribing to various electronic mailing lists, visiting the websites of the U.S. Food and Drug Administration and the Office for Human Research Protections provides an easy way for CTNs to stay current with regulatory or guidance information in the digital age. Several agencies have developed electronic mailing lists that will deliver CTNs real-time updates of federal regulations and guidelines (see Table 42-2).

Academic and Certificate Programs

Highly trained research professionals are needed in the expanding clinical research environment. This need has led to the development of various graduate and certification programs. Some programs are offered in schools of nursing while others are offered through schools of health science. Several programs are also available outside of the United States. The best way to find a program is to perform an Internet search using the keywords *clinical research management program* and country of interest (Ness, Parreco, Galassi, & O'Mara, 2012). Most of the programs offer distance learning options with average requirements of 32–36 credits for a master's degree or 12–15 semester units for a certificate.

Professional Associations and Organizations

Oncology CTNs have numerous opportunities to attend conferences in oncology and clinical research at the local, regional, or national level. Professional oncology associations and research organizations have annual conferences with learning activities that cover a broad range of topics, in addition to regional and e-learning educational opportunities (see Table 42-3 for clinical research–specific organizations). CTNs can consider enriching the professional development experience by submitting an abstract for an oral or poster presentation for the annual conference. The conference website will provide details not only about the conference but also information related to abstract submission, including deadlines. CTNs should visit the website often to check for abstract information. For more information about abstract and poster development, see Chapter 44.

Specialty Certification

Certification is the formal recognition based on specific criteria with established parameters that reflects assessment of educational preparation and knowledge, skills, and abilities or competence developed through experience in a specialty area of practice. An examination is used most frequently to grant an individual a specialty certification. Although certification does not affect legal scope of practice, some boards of nursing are using certification as part of the requirement to grant an advanced practice license (Deininger, 2008).

Oncology CTNs have opportunities to receive certification through various professional organizations, both nursing and non-nursing (i.e., research-focused profes-

Figure 42-1. Recommended Journals

Oncology Nursing Focus
- Cancer Nursing
- Clinical Journal of Oncology Nursing
- European Journal of Oncology Nursing
- Journal of Clinical Oncology
- Journal of Gynecologic Oncology Nursing
- Journal of Pediatric Oncology Nursing
- Oncology Nursing Forum
- Seminars in Oncology Nursing

Clinical Research Focus
- Applied Clinical Trials
- Clinical and Translational Science
- Clinical Trials: Journal of the Society for Clinical Trials
- Contemporary Clinical Trials
- Journal of Clinical Research Best Practices
- The Monitor
- Research Practitioner
- SoCRA® Source

Table 42-1. Categories of Learning Technology

Type of Technology	Description
Cloud computing	Uses the Internet to access software and information without needing to store resources locally. Allows for immediate access to information. Creates ability to hyperlink information to improve cross-referencing access to information.
E-learning	Delivery of an educational activity by electronic means. Removes barriers of time and space compared to a traditional classroom setting. Improves access to on-the-job and just-in-time learning as well as formal certificate- or degree-granting educational programs. Creates a more personalized learning experience.
Mobile computing	Use of portable devices to access information and resources through wireless networking. Creates a mobile learning environment with robust impact on just-in-time learning activities.
3-D virtual spaces	Use of multiple forms of media to create an interactive learning environment. Creates experience of simulated learning that can appeal to all types of learners (i.e., visual, auditory, kinesthetic, and tactile learners).

Note. Based on information from Yoder & Terhorst, 2012.

Table 42-2. Electronic Mailing Lists	
Organization	**Description**
Office for Human Research Protections (OHRP) www.hhs.gov/ohrp/newsroom/index.html	Free email alert system. Join by sending an email to LISTSERV@LIST.NIH.GOV, with the following text message body: SUBSCRIBE OHRP-L *insert your first name followed by last name*. Email address will be automatically captured using the "From" address.
U.S. Food and Drug Administration (FDA) www.fda.gov/emaillist.html	Free email alert service to receive important FDA news and information as they become available. When signing up, you will be asked to select broad topics of interest and then select from within those topics all or some of the offerings. Some of the broad topics of interest include • Biologics • Drugs • Medical Devices • Regulations, Laws and Standards • Research.

Table 42-3. Professional Research Organizations for Clinical Trial Nurses		
Organization	**Description**	**Educational Opportunities**
Association of Clinical Research Professionals www.acrpnet.org	Established in 1976 to provide educational and networking opportunities for research nurses and others who support clinical research and development More than 18,000 members in more than 70 countries	Annual meeting in the spring Webinars E-learning courses Classroom courses Home study
International Association of Clinical Research Nurses http://iacrn.memberlodge.org	Established in 2007 to support professional development of nurses who directly or indirectly impact the care of clinical research participants More than 275 members from more than 5 countries	Annual meeting in the fall
Oncology Nursing Society (ONS) Clinical Trial Nurse Special Interest Group (CTN SIG) http://clinicaltrial.vc.ons.org	Established in 1990 to share ideas, information, and experiences with other CTNs worldwide More than 850 members	CTN SIG meeting at ONS Congress in the spring Sponsor educational sessions at Congress Virtual community with online resources including learning modules Introductory CTN online course
Society of Clinical Research Associates www.socra.org	Provides educational programs and a forum for research professionals to exchange information More than 13,700 members from several countries	Annual meeting in the fall E-learning courses Classroom courses

Note. Based on information from Association of Clinical Research Professionals, 2012; International Association of Clinical Research Nurses, 2012; Oncology Nursing Society, n.d.; Society of Clinical Research Associates, n.d.

sional organizations). For oncology nursing certification, the Oncology Nursing Certification Corporation (ONCC) (www.oncc.org) has six possible certifications: oncology certified nurse (OCN®), certified pediatric hematology oncology nurse (CPHON®), certified breast care nurse (CBCN®), advanced oncology certified nurse practitioner (AOCNP®), blood and marrow transplant certified nurse (BMTCN™), and advanced oncology certified clinical nurse specialist (AOCNS®). Currently, research certification may be obtained from non-nursing professional research organizations: certified clinical research coordinator (CCRC) from the Association of Clinical Research Professionals (2012) or certified clinical research professional (CCRP) from the Society of Clinical Research Associates (n.d.). However, the International Association of Clinical Research Nurses is developing scope and standards of practice for clinical research nurses with future plans to develop a certification through the American Nurses Credentialing Center (IACRN, 2012).

Educating Other Nurses

Sharing your knowledge and expertise with another nurse or student is the responsibility of the professional nurse (ANA, 2010). This is often done through precepting a student in an academic program or a new hire in an orientation program. Even an experienced oncology nurse who transitions to the role of a CTN will feel like a novice and in need of precepting. The new CTN should work within the organization to assist with orientation. Resources for CTN orientation are available on the ONS CTN Special Interest Group website (ONS, n.d.). Mentoring is a rich experience for both the mentor and mentee. See Chapter 43 to learn more about mentoring.

Professional Development Log

It is important for CTNs to track professional development activities to support their lifelong learning journey. A log can be used to support annual job performance reviews, identify deficit areas for learning, and support relicensure as an RN in some states. For CTNs who are certified through ONCC, the Oncology Nursing Certification Points Renewal Option (ONC-PRO) online log is required for recertification. See Figure 42-2 for a sample professional development log.

Professional Portfolio

A professional portfolio is a collection of significant information that demonstrates professional competencies and accomplishments. It provides visual support to acknowledge and assess an individual's professional skills, knowledge, and attitudes. The two types of portfolios are one that demonstrates best work (i.e., evidence of competence and expertise) or one that demonstrates growth and development (i.e., monitor and guide personal and professional goals). A portfolio needs to be succinct, clear, and dynamic; it grows as the individual's career grows and requires ongoing maintenance. A two- to three-inch three-ring binder with clear sheet protectors can be used to store materials as the professional gains experience (Shirey, 2009; Smith, 2011). Portfolios also may be maintained electronically; several software programs are available and can be found through using the keyword search terms *e-portfolio software*. Figure 42-3 provides an example of portfolio content and organization.

Summary

Becoming a lifelong learner is part of the professional development standards for nursing. Using a professional portfolio is a great way to document one's professional journey. There are increasing opportunities and venues for oncology CTNs to strengthen their oncology and clinical research knowledge and competency.

Key Points

- Nurses are lifelong learners.
- Nurses need to continually assess their learning needs and identify how to meet those needs.
- CTNs are in a unique position because they have to identify and assess learning needs in both oncology and clinical research.
- Maintaining a professional development log allows CTNs to track professional development activities that support their lifelong learning journey.
- Maintaining a professional portfolio allows CTNs to document their professional journey.

References

American Nurses Association. (2010). *Nursing: Scope and standards of practice* (2nd ed.). Silver Spring, MD: Author.

Association of Clinical Research Professionals. (2012). About ACRP. Retrieved from http://www.acrpnet.org/FunctionalMenuCategory/AboutACRP_1.aspx

Brant, J.M., & Wickham, R. (Eds.). (2013). *Statement on the scope and standards of oncology nursing practice: Generalist and advanced practice*. Pittsburgh, PA: Oncology Nursing Society.

Deininger, H.E. (2008). Specialization in clinical trials nursing. In A.D. Klimaszewski, M. Bacon, H.E. Deininger, B.A. Ford, & J.G. Westendorp (Eds.), *Manual for clinical trials nursing* (2nd ed., pp. 353–356). Pittsburgh, PA: Oncology Nursing Society.

Institute of Medicine. (2011). *The future of nursing: Leading change, advancing health*. Retrieved from http://www.iom.edu/Reports/2010/The-Future-of-Nursing-Leading-Change-Advancing-Health.aspx

International Association of Clinical Research Nurses. (2012). About us. Retrieved from http://iacrn.memberlodge.org/aboutus

Ness, E., Parreco, L.K., Galassi, A., & O'Mara, A. (2012). Consider a career in clinical research. *American Nurse Today, 7*(11), 39–42. Retrieved from http://www.americannursetoday.com/consider-a-career-in-clinical-research

Oncology Nursing Certification Corporation. (2015). 2015 oncology nursing certification renewal options. Retrieved from http://www.oncc.org/files/renewaloptionsbook_2013.pdf

Oncology Nursing Society. (n.d.). Clinical Trial Nurses SIG. Retrieved from http://clinicaltrial.vc.ons.org

Oncology Nursing Society. (2010). *Oncology clinical trials nurse competencies*. Retrieved from https://www.ons.org/sites/default/files/ctncompetencies.pdf

Shirey, M.R. (2009). The nursing professional portfolio: Leveraging your talents. *Clinical Nurse Specialist, 23*, 241–244. doi:10.1097/NUR.0b013e3181b207af

Smith, L. (2011). Showcase your talents with a career portfolio. *Nursing, 42*(7), 54–56. doi:10.1097/01.NURSE.0000398641.62631.8e

Society of Clinical Research Associates. (n.d.). Certification program overview. Retrieved from http://www.socra.org/certification/certification-program-overview/introduction

Yoder, S.L., & Terhorst, R. (2012). "Beam me up, Scotty": Designing the future of nursing professional development. *Journal of Continuing Education in Nursing, 43*, 456–462. doi:10.3928/00220124-20120904-78

Figure 42-2. Professional Development Log
January 1, 20XX–December 31, 20XX
Name: _____

Continuing Nursing Education Log

Program Date(s)	Program Title	Provider	Accrediting or Approval Organization	Contact Hours/Length of Program

Total # of hours:
Total # of contact hours awarded:
Total # of non-contact hours:

Continuing Medical Education Log

Program Date(s)	Program Title	Provider	Accrediting or Approval Organization	Contact Hours/# Credits Awarded

Total # of hours:
Total # of contact hours awarded:
Total # of non-contact hours:

Academic Education Log

Dates of Course(s)	Course Title	College or University	Final Grade Achieved	Number of Credits

Total # of hours:
Total # of contact hours awarded:
Total # of non-contact hours:

Publications Log

Date of Publication	Title of Work/Title of Publication	Type of Work (e.g., book, chapter, journal, newsletter)	Indicate if Lead Author/Editor; or Number of Co-Authors/Editors	Number of Pages or Words (for newsletters)

(Continued on next page)

Figure 42-2. Professional Development Log *(Continued)*

Presentation Log

Date(s) of Presentation	Title of Conference or Program	Title of Your Presentation(s)	Audience	Length of Your Presentation or CE Awarded for Your Part

Total # of hours:

Precepting Log

Dates of Precepting (From/To)	Name of Institution & Unit Where Precepting Completed	Name of Student's College, University or Nursing School or New Hire's Name	Number of Hours Precepting Completed

Volunteer Leadership Service Log

Dates	Organization	Name of Board/Committee/Task Force	Leadership Capacity in Which You Served (e.g., member, vice president)

Note. From *Oncology Nursing Certification Points Renewal Option (ONC-PRO)*, by Oncology Nursing Certification Corporation, n.d. Retrieved from https://oncpro.oncc.org. Copyright by Oncology Nursing Certification Corporation. Reprinted with permission.

Figure 42-3. Sample Content for a Professional Portfolio

Section One: Introduction
- Resume/curriculum vitae
- Copies of license and certifications
- Photo
- School transcripts/internships
- Career trajectories
- Mentor/mentee relationships

Section Two: Showcase Professional Accomplishments
- Evidence-based practice projects
- Research
- Sample presentations
- Sample publications
- Committee membership and activities
- Professional society memberships and accomplishments
- Professional development logs
- Awards

Section Three: Complimentary
- Accolades
- Thank-you letters
- Recommendations

Section Four: Volunteer Service
- Professional organization membership and activities
- Community service
- Photos
- News clippings

Note. Based on information from Shirey, 2009; Smith, 2011.

Chapter 43

Mentorship

Rose Ermete, RN, BSN, OCN®, CCRP

Introduction

Oncology nurses entering the arena of clinical trials assume a variety of roles and responsibilities. These functions are dependent on many variables, such as the type and size of the practice setting, patient population, and the management's and principal investigator's expectations. Nurses may be selected for this role based on their clinical expertise; however, when entering the research setting, they become novices (Benner, 2001; Cangelosi, Crocker, & Sorrell, 2009).

In many settings, clinical trial nurses (CTNs) are responsible for more than the clinical aspects of patient care. Large academic settings tend to have more resources, allowing the focus of CTNs to be more clinical. However, smaller settings tend to have fewer resources, meaning CTNs may also be responsible for many other tasks, such as data management, regulatory requirements, and budgeting (Oncology Nursing Society [ONS], 2010). This chapter will present mentorship not only as a valuable process to orient nurses and other health professionals to the subspecialty of clinical trials, but also as a foundation to mentor more seasoned CTNs to excel toward their professional goals.

Background

Clinical trials nursing is different from staff nursing and other areas of practice. New CTNs learn quickly to adapt in an environment of unfamiliar rules and regulations. Nurses evolve from being part of a team to coordinating the team (see Figure 43-1). Staff nursing tends to be task-oriented; however, in research, CTNs often provide directions and coordinate the plan of care. To function effectively, oncology CTNs need to be team leaders with a thorough knowledge of oncology, as well as the science and regulations behind the research. The focus must broaden from that of clinical issues surrounding the patient to how those issues and many others affect the study outcome, future therapy, and most importantly, patient safety (ONS, 2010). This broader focus will provide CTNs with an understanding that encompasses clinical trials.

Novice CTNs may experience significant role confusion in attempting to navigate a course toward competency. Role confusion is a result of the varying activities

Figure 43-1. The Research Nurse's Role in the Coordination of Clinical Trial Activities

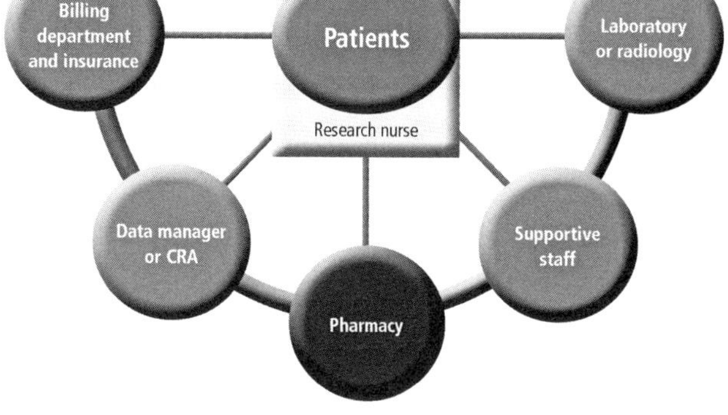

[Diagram showing Patients at center, surrounded by: Regulatory or institutional review board, Grants and contracts, Laboratory or radiology, Supportive staff, Pharmacy, Data manager or CRA, Billing department and insurance, Treatment nurse. Investigator and Research nurse labels included.]

CRA—clinical research associate

Supportive staff members include, but are not limited to, dietitians, social workers, homecare nurses, medical assistants, and scheduling personnel.

Note. From "Clinical Trials and Communicating Safely," by R.B. Ermete, 2012, *Clinical Journal of Oncology Nursing, 16,* p. 26. doi:10.1188/12.CJON.25-27. Copyright 2012 by Oncology Nursing Society. Reprinted with permission.

and responsibilities that surround the CTN profession. Coupled with increasingly complex studies, stringent regulations, and the lack of training, novice CTNs may feel completely overwhelmed. Without proper training, novices can become frustrated as they try to find their way in the dark (Cangelosi et al., 2009). This frustration could lead to the loss of potentially good CTNs. Eby and colleagues (2013) and Fox (2010) reported that mentoring new nurses increases job satisfaction and encourages retention, as well as improves patient safety. When institutions adopt a mentoring culture, time, training, and resources are provided to assist new nurses to manage challenges (Grossman, 2013; Plamondon & Canadian Coalition for Global Health Research [CCGHR], Capacity Building Task Group: Sub-Group on Mentorship, 2007). Mentorship provides novice nurses with survival skills as they transition into their new roles (Hodges, 2009; McDonald, Mohan, Jackson, Vickers, & Wilkes, 2010). These situations could be inferred to the circumstances of new CTNs. Without support, nurses may explore other areas and abandon the profession (Cottingham, Dibartolo, Battistoni, & Brown, 2011).

The current statistics surrounding the nursing shortage could possibly affect many subspecialties within nursing (American Association of Colleges of Nursing, 2012). The population of people older than age 65 will double by 2040 (U.S. Census Bureau, 2012). As nursing faculty retire, fewer nurses are entering doctoral programs, leaving a dearth of professors for nursing students. Present trends indicate that the current nursing workforce will age without a great influx of new nurses (Johnson, Billingsley, & Crichlow, 2011). This creates a problem for nursing, as it competes with other professions for students.

Nurses have a responsibility to mentor the next generation (Institute of Medicine [IOM], 2011). In today's cost-cutting environment, institutions may not see the benefit of investing money in a mentoring program. Studies demonstrate that when nurses are provided mentorship opportunities, it actually benefits the institution (see Figure 43-2). Mentorship, therefore, provides a significant return on investment (Cottingham et al., 2011; Grossman, 2013). When nurses retire, they will take their knowledge and expertise with them (McDonald et al., 2010). Experienced CTNs can create a legacy by passing their current knowledge to the next generation of CTNs. Through positive interaction with more experienced CTNs, novices will better assimilate into their new role while strengthening the subspecialty of oncology clinical trials nursing.

Mentorship Defined

The term *mentor* dates back to Greek mythology. When Odysseus left to fight in the Trojan War, he left his son, Telemachus, in the care of a trusted and wise friend, Mentor. Mentor not only raised Telemachus but also provided him with knowledge and guidance to prepare him for future responsibilities (Homer, trans. 1993).

A mentor has come to be known as a wise person who provides guidance and insight from experience. It is not the same thing as a coach or preceptor. *Coaching* generally is a top-down process that involves training toward predetermined goals that tend to revolve around the objectives of an organization. *Precepting* involves skills training that focus on assisting a novice in applying academic knowledge to function at a certain proficiency level as determined by the organization (Grossman, 2013; Kilgallon & Thompson, 2012; Thompson, Wolf, & Sabatine, 2012). In contrast, mentorship has a broader focus. It fosters a supportive environment that nurtures advancement toward self-development and professional growth. The focus is on the developmental needs and goals of the novice. Mentorship provides a reciprocal experience that empowers mentors and mentees to develop personally and professionally within a safe and collaborative environment. The mentors' roles are to challenge the mentees and offer guidance, insight, and opportunities. By being encouraged to explore outside their comfort zone, mentees can develop abilities and achieve success far beyond their original goals and dreams (Grossman, 2013; McDonald et al., 2010).

Theoretical Frameworks for Mentoring

To understand the mentorship process, it is essential to establish a theoretical framework of mentoring. Mentoring involves guiding or assisting others along a path to increased knowledge and professional growth. Several relevant learning theories exist that support this endeavor. Kilgallon and Thompson (2012) discuss Malcolm Knowles' (1990) adult learning principles and Kolb's theory on experiential learning, whereas Anderson (2011) and Grossman (2013) discuss Bloom's Taxonomy. These complementing theories support the goals of a successful mentorship program.

Knowles' (1990) theory of adult learning focuses on the needs of the adult learner. These needs are described

---

Figure 43-2. Benefits of Mentorship Programs to Institutions

- Decrease nursing turnover
- Significant decrease in cost for new hires
- Increased job satisfaction
- Increased employee productivity
- Increase in patient safety
- Increased loyalty
- Improved communication and team work within groups
- Development of future leaders

Note. Based on information from Cottingham et al., 2011; Eby et al., 2013; Fox, 2010; Grossman, 2013.

Table 43-1. The Andragogical Model	
Concept	Description
The need to know	Why do I need to know this?
The learners' self-concept	I am responsible for my own decisions. (Self-directed instead of teacher-directed)
The role of the learners' experience	I have many different types of experiences.
Readiness to learn	How does this relate to my developmental stage?
Orientation to learning	How will this help me to deal with problems I may confront in my life?
Motivation	How will this help me to achieve job satisfaction, self-esteem, and quality of life?

Note. Based on information from Kilgallon & Thompson, 2012; Knowles, 1990.

using the Andragogical Model (see Table 43-1). Adults need to know *why* they need to know something and how it will apply to their life situations. They also must be ready to learn. Learning occurs more easily if it coincides with the developmental tasks of the adult. Adult learners bring with them differences in past experiences that will affect their interpretation and internalization of what is taught. Adults generally are self-directed and motivated to learn more by internal desires than by external stimuli (Kilgallon & Thompson, 2012). This means that they will resist learning if it is perceived as enforcing the will or needs of others. These concepts need to be considered while mentoring novice and advanced beginner CTNs. Employing the Andragogical Model in mentorship allows the mentor to guide a mentee to channel energy toward his or her own professional growth and development.

Kolb's experiential learning theory focuses on the experiences of the person and how they relate to the learning milieu. Kilgallon and Thompson (2012) reviewed the four steps in Kolb's theory. The first is the *experience* itself, followed by self-reflection to understand the outcome, or *meaning of the experience*. Reflecting on the experience is of greater benefit to the learner than simply being instructed by someone else. In the next step, *generalization*, the person begins to form concepts or create generalized principles that may be utilized in similar circumstances. The last step, *active experimentation*, is when new knowledge is applied in future situations.

Bloom's theory focuses on three domains of the learner. The *cognitive* domain is the most utilized and is how we generate knowledge. The *psychomotor* domain refers to learning physical or hands-on skills. The third domain is *affective*, which involves individual values or attitudes toward learning (Anderson, 2011; Atherton, 2011).

These theories help mentors to guide the learning of mentees. Mentors can then discriminate between knowledge, comprehension, and application (Grossman, 2013). This allows the mentorship process to be focused on the mentee's needs rather than on an external entity. By allowing the new CTN to explore and problem solve with guidance and insight from a mentor, the mentee is able to build self-confidence and develop as a professional nurse.

Mentoring Competencies

Seasoned CTNs may have excellent clinical skills, but this does not necessarily make a good mentor. Mentors must have a balance of skills, attributes, and qualities. All prospective mentors should undergo training that promotes an effective mentoring experience (Plamondon & CCGHR Capacity Building Task Group: Sub-Group on Mentorship, 2009; Straus, Johnson, Marquez, & Feldman, 2013). An ineffective mentor can be deleterious to a potentially good CTN. It is important to choose mentors that do not exhibit ineffective traits (see Figure 43-3). Proper training of mentors is vital. Some preliminary competencies are described in the literature for mentors and mentees. Although there does not appear to be extensive research or agreement on these, the theoretical framework discussed previously can be applied/construed to make them of use in the mentoring process.

Plamondon and CCGHR Capacity Building Task Group: Sub-Group on Mentorship (2007) suggested an integrated conceptual model of mentor competence (see Figure 43-4). Many of the attributes or characteristics of mentors can be grouped into three domains: virtues, abilities, and competencies. These domains align well with Bloom's taxonomy of *cognitive, psychomotor,* and *affective* as well as Benner's (2001) three core concepts of *ability, support,* and *person.*

Virtues are the foundation of competence and guide one's actions. They are the strongest and most consistent positive association with all aspects of mentoring (Eby et al., 2013). The characteristics revolve around integrity, caring, and prudence (Plamondon & CCGHR Capacity Building Task Group: Sub-Group on Mentorship, 2007). Good mentors foster a professional relationship with the interest of the mentee in mind. They cre-

Figure 43-3. Toxic Mentors
• Avoidance behavior • Unapproachable or intimidating • Unreliable—don't keep promises • Dumpers—unload work or tasks on mentees that have nothing to do with their goals • Micromanagers • Undermining of individuals

Note. Based on information from Hawkins & Fontenot, 2010; Hodges, 2009.

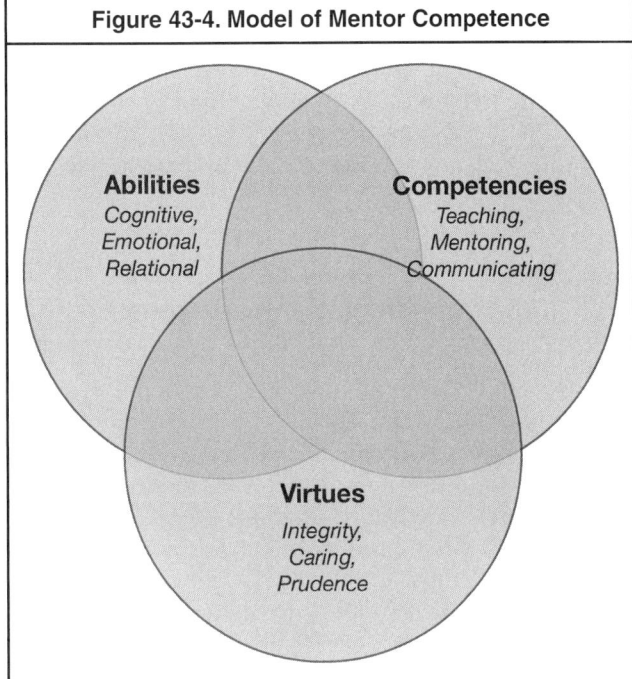

Figure 43-4. Model of Mentor Competence

Note. From *Module Two: Competency in Mentoring* (p. 8), by K. Plamondon and Canadian Coalition for Global Health Research Capacity Building Task Group: Sub-Group on Mentorship, 2007. Retrieved from http://www.ccghr.ca/wp-content/uploads/2013/05/Mentoring_Module2_Competency-in-Mentoring_e.pdf. Reprinted with permission of Canadian Coalition for Global Health Research.

ate an environment that is nonjudgmental and provides mutual respect. Their sense of integrity and prudence allows them to confront the status quo in support of what is right and just. Additional characteristics in the domain of virtues include patience, honesty, trustworthiness, reliability, accountability, supporting succession planning, credibility, passion, strong self-esteem, and political astuteness (Anderson, 2011; McCloughen, O'Brien, & Jackson, 2009; Saskatchewan Institute of Applied Science and Technology [SIAST], n.d.; Straus & Sackett, 2012b; Straus et al., 2013; Turnbull, 2010).

Abilities refer to the fundamental potential or capacity of the individual. Cognitive abilities may be demonstrated through intellectual ability and a basic foundation of knowledge of the subject matter of their discipline (Plamondon & CCGHR Capacity Building Task Group: Sub-Group on Mentorship, 2007). Mentors are approachable and promote a positive, nonthreatening relationship. They foster a safe learning environment, utilizing reflective professional practice (Fox, 2010). Emotional support is an important ability of a mentor and includes helping the mentee deal with stress, as well as encouraging life balance between work and career (Anderson, 2011; Hawkins & Fontenot, 2010; McCloughen et al., 2009; Straus et al., 2013).

Competencies refer to specific skills, knowledge, or techniques that mentors can develop through training. Mentor competencies encompass all technical aspects of mentoring: knowledge and skill in the structure and process of the mentoring relationship as well as roles and responsibilities (Plamondon & CCGHR Capacity Building Task Group: Sub-Group on Mentorship, 2007). The mentor role encourages risk taking, supporting self-improvement, and professional problem solving (Turnbull, 2010). Challenging the mentee and facilitating goal objective setting is an important competency (SIAST, n.d.). Mentors must possess strong listening and observation skills (Mead, Hopkins, & Wilson, 2011). These skills assist in the recognition of dysfunction in the relationship or communication. With these skills, a mentor can act as a guide, helping the mentee find solutions and cope with change.

The Mentoring Relationship

The success of mentoring depends on the interaction of the individuals involved. Matching individuals by age or gender does not impact on the creation of the relationship (McCloughen et al., 2009). Each person in a mentoring relationship has certain responsibilities, as well as unique qualities that he or she brings to the relationship. It is absolutely essential that the mentor and mentee understand what their responsibilities are in order to cultivate a successful relationship (see Figure 43-5). The initial meeting should be used to discuss goals and expectations of the relationship. A mentorship agreement form can aid with this discussion (see Figure 43-6).

The literature offers several models for the development of a mentoring relationship. Each model has different names, but all reflect a similar transition process.

Figure 43-5. Mentee and Mentor Responsibilities

Mentees
- Demonstrate a willingness to learn
- Identify initial learning goals
- Seek and be open to feedback
- Respect time of mentor
- Self-directed, take an active role in learning
- Active listener, reflecting critically before and after meetings
- Follow through on commitments or renegotiate appropriately

Mentors
- Have reasonable expectations of the mentee
- Help the mentee to develop an appropriate learning plan
- Facilitate professional and personal growth
- Assist in identifying resources and experiences
- Provide support and encouragement
- Provide feedback
- Allocate time and energy
- Follow through on commitments or renegotiate appropriately

Note. Based on information from Eby et al., 2013; Straus et al., 2013; Turnbull, 2010.

Figure 43-6. Sample Mentorship Agreement Template

Mentee: _____   Mentor: _____
Contacts: Contacts:
Home: _____ Work: _____   Home: _____ Work: _____
Mobile: _____ Texting ☐ Yes ☐ No   Mobile: _____ Texting ☐ Yes ☐ No
Email:_____   Email:_____
Preferred method of contact: _____   Preferred method of contact: _____

This agreement sets the parameters of the voluntary mentoring relationship. It should be completed during the first discussion to provide clarification of expectations from both parties. Both parties should sign and get a copy of the form.

Goals

1.	1.
2.	2.
3.	3.

Expectations

What will be the nature of assessments?   ☐ Self ☐ Mutual

Values, Attitudes, Interests (personal and professional)

Boundaries

How often will you meet? ☐ Weekly ☐ Monthly ☐ Other

Where will you meet?   How long will meetings be:

Who is responsible for scheduling meetings? ☐ Mentee ☐ Mentor ☐ Other:

Preferred type of meeting? ☐ face to face ☐ email ☐ video chat ☐ phone ☐ other:

If a meeting must be canceled, how should you be notified?

Are there times or days that you should not be contacted?

Mentee: Mentor:

Conflicts of Interest and Confidentiality

- This relationship is strictly confidential, and content of meetings will remain between the mentor and mentee.
- The mentor and mentee have affirmed that there are no conflicts of interest and that products, papers, projects, etc., developed through this relationship by the mentee are the intellectual property of the mentee, unless stated otherwise in this agreement.
- Both parties agree to a no-fault conclusion of the mentoring relationship.

Other Comments/Agreements:

Signature and date: Signature and date:

The first step in the process is when the two people come together. This has been called *initiation*, as well as *formation* (Hawkins & Fontenot, 2010; McCloughen et al., 2009). This is a period of getting to know each other. Identifying similar attitudes, values, beliefs, and personality traits is important in laying the foundation for a positive relationship (Eby et al., 2013). During this phase, goals and objectives are established, and boundaries are discussed. It has been suggested that a contract, formal or informal, may be helpful in laying the ground rules so that both parties understand the needs and goals of the relationship (Hodges, 2009). A lack of awareness of one's role can lead to misunderstandings and generate defective communication. Hodges (2009) stressed that differences in expectations can undermine the mentoring relationship and negatively influence the learning experience. It is important at the start of the relationship that expectations are clear (Straus et al., 2013). Figure 43-6 provides a model agreement template that can be used at the outset of the relationship.

The next phase in the relationship is where the mentoring process takes place and has been called the *middle* or *working phase* (Kilgallon & Thompson, 2012). During this phase, the mentee's professional and personal goals are addressed. The mentor provides encouragement and opportunities. The mentee gradually gains self-confidence and independence (McCloughen et al., 2009).

During the last phase, a transformation of the relationship occurs where the two become colleagues or peers. This has been called *redefinition, resolution*, and *passing the torch* (Hawkins & Fontenot, 2010). The relationship may or may not continue but would be as friends and equals. The mentee becomes part of the mentor's network and perhaps may become a mentor as well (Kilgallon & Thompson, 2012). The literature confirms that those who are mentored are more likely to mentor others, thereby continuing the legacy of lifelong learning.

Communication

Effective communication is essential to the flow and achievement of the mentoring relationship. Without effective communication, the relationship is stifled and learning and growth cannot occur. Good communication is vital to the success of any relationship (Hawkins & Fontenot, 2010). Two elements are considered basic to good communication: dialogue and listening. These two elements together provide a foundation for interpretation of the thoughts being conveyed. The mentor's role includes active listening; guidance begins with actively listening to what the mentee has to say without interjecting opinions or judgments. A mentor should never assume that he or she knows more about a stated problem than the mentee does. Effective mentors employ *active listening*, which includes paraphrasing, clarifying, summarizing, and empathy (Straus & Sackett, 2012a).

Providing feedback is another important skill in fostering professional growth. Without feedback, the mentee might not realize where improvement is needed. A supportive atmosphere that promotes growth is important when giving feedback. The mentee should feel accepted, respected, and empowered. These feelings promote communication, allowing the exploration of thoughts and feelings without fear of ridicule (Kilgallon & Thompson, 2012). These steps provide a solid framework for positive change to occur.

During the mentoring experience, conflicts can arise. The mentor must understand how to address conflict in order to maintain positive, effective interactions. Conflict, handled inappropriately, can produce negative outcomes. The mentor must keep an open mind and avoid personal judgment. When addressing problems, opinions must not be confused with facts. The mentee must have the opportunity to elucidate on the rationale without the mentor creating assumptions about what may have occurred. *I* statements should be used in place of *you* statements when confronting negative behavior. For example, the statement "*I* am concerned that the case report forms were submitted without verifying them against the medical record" is preferable to the statement "*You* did not review all the source documents before completing the case report forms." *I* statements acknowledge the thoughts and feelings behind the mentor's comments. *You* statements put the novice on the defensive (Witcomb & Witcomb, 2013). When a person is defensive, attention is diverted away from the real issues. The mentor must keep the conversation focused on the present situation, as similar past situations have no relevance to the situation at hand. By correctly addressing conflict, the mentor assists the novice in acquiring the skills necessary to manage future problems and grow professionally.

E-Mentoring

Mentoring can take place under a variety of circumstances; it can occur through a formal program or through an informal arrangement with a colleague. One barrier to mentoring that is consistently referenced in the literature is lack of time. In today's hectic workplace, it is difficult for individuals to find time for mentoring. *E-mentoring*, a mentoring relationship that is conducted via the Internet, has begun to emerge as a reasonable alternative in today's fast-paced work environment (Pietsch, 2012).

Pietsch (2012) and Faiman (2011) discussed several benefits to e-mentoring. It provides contacts far beyond one's local resources, allowing relationships to be more global. Through this process, new CTNs have access to mentors that they normally would not be able to encounter. E-mentoring is not limited by boundaries of geography, hierarchy, or time. Mentors and mentees can respond within their own time parameters, and the delay in immediate response allows time for reflection. Another advantage is the decreased likelihood of possible feelings of intimidation, discomfort, or prejudice that can sometimes occur in a one-on-one relationship.

E-mentoring can certainly present challenges of its own (see Figure 43-7). An efficient mechanism of electronic communication is required, but a personal touch needs to remain (Pietsch, 2012). With the loss of nonverbal clues and personal connection, meanings may be misinterpreted. Differences between the individual's motivation and personal characteristics can hinder continuous effective interaction. Email fatigue is also a problem with continued correspondence. If possible, an opportunity should be found to meet face to face. This could be accomplished by arranging to get together at a conference or research meeting. If meeting in person is not possible, follow-up phone calls or video chats could be employed.

To facilitate e-mentoring, mentors and mentees must have access to the Internet at both home and work, requiring availability of computers or mobile devices. Confidentiality is a concern when using the Internet; however, Pietsch (2012) found that nurses had positive attitudes toward e-mentoring, despite the drawbacks, and felt that e-mentoring is a viable option for today's workforce.

Various other mentoring programs are available to CTNs. Some of these programs are listed in the Additional Resources at the end of this chapter.

Mentorship and the Future

Mentoring benefits the mentor, the mentee, and the profession. The mentee gains valuable experience while progressing toward and attaining professional goals. Through mentoring, the mentor creates a personal legacy that positively contributes to the profession. Mentorship is important to the future of the nursing profession; CTNs must continue to nurture and encourage new and less-experienced CTNs. Experienced CTNs need to provide support and guidance for new ideas because new ideas lead to change. Without change, the subspecialty of clinical trials nursing cannot advance; therefore, no growth can occur. Without growth, the CTN role—and the nursing profession—will not survive.

Summary

CTNs work in a variety of settings and assume diverse roles. Responsibilities differ greatly from that of the traditional staff nurse. Taking on these unique responsibilities successfully can be aided by a mentoring relationship. Through mentorship, novice CTNs can assimilate into the role and grow professionally. Many opportunities for mentoring exist both locally and through various organizations. Novice nurses are best served by mentors who have good communication skills, have time for mentoring, demonstrate professionalism, and encourage professional growth and development. This would also be true for CTNs who are novices or even advanced beginners. More experienced CTNs should consider becoming mentors, not only to help guide novices but also to sustain the continued growth of the profession.

Key Points
- Mentorship fosters a supportive environment that nurtures advancement toward self-development and professional growth.
- Nurses have a responsibility to mentor the next generation.
- Mentoring provides a significant return on investment to institutions and the nursing profession.
- Proper training of potential mentors is vital to the success of the relationship.
- E-mentoring is a viable option in today's hectic work environment.

References

American Association of Colleges of Nursing. (2012, August). Nursing shortage. Retrieved from http://www.aacn.nche.edu/media-relations/fact-sheets/nursing-shortage

Anderson, L. (2011). A learning resource for developing effective mentorship in practice. *Nursing Standard, 25*(51), 48–56.

Atherton, J.S. (2011). Bloom's taxonomy. Retrieved from http://www.learningandteaching.info/learning/bloomtax.htm

Benner, P. (2001). *From novice to expert: Excellence and power in clinical nursing practice.* Upper Saddle River, NJ: Prentice Hall.

Cangelosi, P.R., Crocker, S., & Sorrell, J.M. (2009). Expert to novice: Clinicians learning new roles as clinical nurse educators. *Nursing Education Perspectives, 30,* 367–371.

Figure 43-7. Advantages and Disadvantages of E-Mentoring

Advantages	Disadvantages

• Allow more global relationships without boundaries
  – Geography
  – Hierarchy
  – Time
• Minimize bias
  – Age
  – Sex
  – Race
• Cost-effective
• Generational adaptation for younger nurses
	• Lack of nonverbal communication
	• Lacks warm human connection
	• Lack of confidentiality with Internet
	• Email fatigue
	• Older generation may not be technology savvy

Note. Based on information from Faiman, 2011; Pietsch, 2012.

Cottingham, S., Dibartolo, M.C., Battistoni, S., & Brown, T. (2011). A mentoring initiative to enhance nurse retention. *Nursing Education Perspectives, 32,* 250–255.

Eby, L.T., Allen, T.D., Hoffman, B.J., Baranik, L.E., Sauer, J.B., Baldwin, S., … Evans, S.C. (2013). An interdisciplinary meta-analysis of the potential antecedents, correlates, and consequences of protégés' perceptions of mentoring. *Psychological Bulletin, 139,* 441–476. doi:10.1037/a0029279

Faiman, B. (2011). Overview and experience of a nursing e-mentorship program. *Clinical Journal of Oncology Nursing, 15,* 418–423. doi:10.1188/11.CJON.418-423

Fox, K.C. (2010). Mentor program boosts new nurses' satisfaction and lowers turnover rate. *Journal of Continuing Education in Nursing, 41,* 311–316. doi:10.3928/00220124-20100401-04

Grossman, S.C. (2013). *Mentoring in nursing: A dynamic and collaborative process* (2nd ed.). New York, NY: Springer.

Hawkins, J.W., & Fontenot, H.B. (2010). Mentorship: The heart and soul of health care leadership. *Journal of Healthcare Leadership, 2010*(2), 31–34. doi:10.2147/JHL.S7863

Hodges, B. (2009). Factors that can influence mentorship relationships. *Paediatric Nursing, 21*(6), 32–35.

Homer. (1993). *The odyssey* (A. Cook, Trans.). New York, NY: W.W. Norton Co.

Institute of Medicine. (2011). *The future of nursing: Leading change, advancing health.* Washington, DC: National Academies Press.

Johnson, J.E., Billingsley, M., & Crichlow, T. (2011). Professional development for nurses: Mentoring along the U-shaped curve. *Nursing Administration Quarterly, 35*(2), 119–125. doi:10.1097/NAQ.0b013e31820f69c0

Kilgallon, K., & Thompson, J. (2012). *Mentoring in nursing and healthcare: A practical approach.* Chichester, West Sussex: John Wiley & Sons.

Knowles, M. (1990). *The adult learner: A neglected species* (4th ed.). Houston, TX: Gulf Publishing.

McCloughen, A., O'Brien, L., & Jackson, D. (2009). Esteemed connection: Creating a mentoring relationship for nurse leadership. *Nursing Inquiry, 16,* 326–336. doi:10.1111/j.1440-1800.2009.00451.x

McDonald, G., Mohan, S., Jackson, D., Vickers, M.H., & Wilkes, L. (2010). Continuing connections: The experiences of retired and senior working nurse mentors. *Journal of Clinical Nursing, 19,* 3547–3554. doi:10.1111/j.1365-2702.2010.03365.x

Mead, D., Hopkins, A., & Wilson, C. (2011). Views of nurse mentors about their role. *Nursing Management, 18*(6), 18–23.

Oncology Nursing Society. (2010). *Oncology clinical trials nurse competencies.* Retrieved from http://www.ons.org/sites/default/files/ctncompetencies.pdf

Pietsch, T.M. (2012). A transition to e-mentoring: Factors that influence nurse engagement. *Computers, Informatics, Nursing, 30,* 632–639. doi:10.1097/NXN.0b013e3118266cbc5

Plamondon, K., & Canadian Coalition for Global Health Research Capacity Building Task Group: Sub-Group on Mentorship. (2007). *Module two: Competency in mentoring.* Retrieved from http://www.ccghr.ca/wp-content/uploads/2013/05/Mentoring_Module2_Competency-in-Mentoring_e.pdf

Saskatchewan Institute of Applied Science and Technology. (n.d.). Mentorship competencies: Making connections—Continuing education and professional development. Retrieved from http://www.saskpolytech.ca/about/school-of-nursing/mentorship/mentorship-competencies.aspx

Straus, S.E., Johnson, M.O., Marquez, C., & Feldman, M.D. (2013). Characteristics of successful and failed mentoring relationships: A qualitative study across two academic health centers. *Academic Medicine, 88,* 82–89. doi:10.1097/ACM.0b013e31827647a0

Straus, W.E., & Sackett, D.L. (2012a). Clinical-trialist rounds: 9. Mentoring—part 3: Structure and function of effective mentoring: Advice and protection. *Clinical Trials, 9,* 272–274. doi:10.1177/1740774512436615

Straus, W.E., & Sackett, D.L. (2012b). Clinical-trialist rounds: 10. Mentoring—part 4: Attributes of an effective mentor. *Clinical Trials, 9,* 367–369. doi:10.1177/1740774512440343

Thompson, R., Wolf, D.M., & Sabatine, J.M. (2012). Mentoring and coaching: A model guiding professional nurses to executive success. *Journal of Nursing Administration, 42,* 536–541. doi:10.1097/NNA.0b013e31827144ea

Turnbull, B. (2010). Scholarship and mentoring: An essential partnership. *International Journal of Nursing Practice, 16,* 573–578. doi:10.1111/j.1440-172x.2010.01883.x

U.S. Census Bureau. (2012). Statistical abstract of the United States, 2012. Retrieved from http://www.census.gov/compendia/statab/2012/tables/12s0009.pdf

Witcomb, C.A., & Witcomb L.E. (2013). *Effective communication skills for engineers.* Hoboken, NJ: John Wiley & Sons.

Additional Resources

American Nurses Association Mentoring Resources: http://nursingworld.org/DocumentVault/NewsAnnouncements/Resources-on-Mentoring.aspx

Campaign for Nursing: www.discovernursing.com/becoming-an-advocate#.UU_CTleNAuc

International Mentoring Association: www.mentoring-association.org

Kansas City Health Careers Nurse Mentoring Toolkit: http://kchealthcareers.com/mentoring-toolkit/nurse-mentoring-toolkit

The Mentoring Group: www.mentoringgroup.com

MentorNet: www.mentornet.net

National Surgical Adjuvant Breast and Bowel Project (NSABP) Mentoring Program: https://members.nsabp.pitt.edu/Treatment_Mentor_Program.asp (Note: A password is needed to access this site. Nurses who use the NSABP will have a password.)

Oncology Nursing Society: Consult an Oncology Nursing Research Expert: www.ons.org/practice-resources/researchers

Oncology Nursing Society, CJON Writing Mentorship Program: https://cjon.ons.org/content/writing-mentorship-program

Robert Wood Johnson Foundation Mentorship Opportunities: www.newcareersinnursing.org/scholars/career-central/mentorship

Saskatchewan Institute of Applied Science and Technology (SIAST): http://saskpolytech.ca/about/school-of-nursing/mentorship/index.aspx

Sigma Theta Tau International Chiron Mentoring Program: www.nursingsociety.org/learn-grow/leadership-institute

Chapter 44

Publishing Guidance for Clinical Trial Nurses

Angela D. Klimaszewski, RN, MSN

Introduction

Clinical trials conducted with integrity move medical science forward and help to determine the most beneficial therapeutic interventions for patients. However, if the results of clinical trials are not published and shared with the medical, nursing, and lay communities, vital knowledge that could help people is lost. This chapter will discuss why clinical trial nurses (CTNs) should publish, what to write, how to write, how to receive authorship credit for writing and study coordination, and writing with integrity. Although much of the information imparted is general in nature and not specific to CTNs, wherever possible, it will be directed to CTNs' publishing needs.

Why Publish?

Nurses have many reasons to publish, including generating and disseminating evidence from their practice, improving patient care, sharing discoveries and knowledge, advancing the profession, or fulfilling a requirement for career advancement (Grech & Evans, 2012; Nicoll, 2011; Saver, 2011). However, Tumber and Dickersin (2004) may have best stated the reasons why CTNs should publish: "to provide a record of the work done, convey information to the community, and support translation of research into clinical practice" (p. 271).

CTNs have an opportunity and a responsibility to provide information about multiple aspects of clinical trials to nurses in the clinical, educational, and research settings. Possible topics that CTNs may address in publications are listed in Figure 44-1.

Figure 44-1. Possible Topics for Clinical Trial Nurses to Publish*

- Results of a clinical trial (study drug, device, randomized controlled trial)
- Insights into the use of study drug or device
- Symptom clusters identified while caring for patients receiving study drug
- Patient beliefs and misconceptions about study drug or device
- Adverse events in patients receiving study drug
- Nursing interventions to prevent and/or manage adverse events in patients receiving study drug
- Patient education required while being treated with study drug or device
- Patients' reports on adverse events during and after study drug therapy
- Study of nursing care satisfaction of patients receiving study drug
- Disease process treated with study drug or device
- Relationship of demographic age, gender, weight with an adverse effect of study drug
- Case study of a patient's experience from treatment with a study drug or device
- New black box warnings for a previously approved drug or device

* Clinical trial nurses should check their local/institutional publication policies before embarking on abstract submissions or publications.

Article, Abstract, or Poster

Once CTNs determine the topic to develop and publish and have checked for institutional policies regarding publishing, deciding if the topic would be best suited as an article, an abstract for a conference, or a poster presentation is next. Each has value and unique characteristics, as well as some that overlap.

The author would like to acknowledge Janice Phillips, PhD, RN, FAAN, Shanita Williams-Brown, PhD, MPH, APRN-BC, and Anne E. Belcher, PhD, RN, AOCN®, CNE, FAAN, ANEF, for their contribution to previous editions of the Manual for Clinical Trials Nursing.

Article

An *article* is a composite of written ideas about a topic that is communicated to a specific audience via a print or online journal. It should be written in the author's distinctive voice or style of writing; reading it out loud will help the author decide if it sounds authentic or reads as snippets of other people's words.

Each journal will have specific author guidelines that need to be followed. These typically include topics to write about; article length (e.g., word limit, page limit); use of abbreviations; reference style (e.g., American Psychological Association [APA], Harvard); use of tables, photos, and illustrations; format to be used (e.g., double-spaced, one-inch margins), and how to prepare and submit a manuscript. Often a letter of inquiry is a first step to see if the journal is interested in the topic. CTNs may visit the journal's website to locate information about a letter of inquiry and guidelines. For example, the Oncology Nursing Society's website for authors interested in submitting a manuscript to the *Oncology Nursing Forum* addresses submission, financial disclosure, and a detailed section on manuscript preparation (https://onf.ons.org/content/onf-authors). Additionally, it is important for CTNs to know that several layers or levels of review may occur once the final draft of an article or abstract is completed, especially if there is a contractual agreement with a study's sponsor. Therefore, it will be vital for CTNs to plan preparation, writing, and revision time accordingly.

There are many types of articles, some of which would not directly pertain to CTNs. To increase the likelihood of an article being accepted for publication, CTNs should select a journal that targets the audience for whom the article is written. For example, communicating implications for practice has a different focus than articles published in a research journal. Types of articles that CTNs might be interested in publishing may be found in Table 44-1.

An original journal article that is the first to document research findings is considered the *primary* source (APA, 2010; Mee, 2011). A primary source article can be identified by three features: (a) it is a report that has not been published, (b) it has been reviewed by peers, and (c) it can be accessed by readers in the future (APA, 2010).

Guidelines for Reporting Research Results

Specific reporting guidelines are available for different study designs that authors should use while writing. Many of the guidelines are specific to particular types of health research reports. Enhancing the Quality and Transparency of Health Research (EQUATOR) is a summary of all health research writing guidelines for CTNs and other authors to use (www.equator-network.org) (see Table 44-2).

Table 44-1. Types of Articles That Clinical Trial Nurses Might Publish

Article Type	Definition
Research or empirical studies	Report of an original research study including an introduction, method and analysis, results, and conclusions
Evidence based	A review and integration of knowledge and scientific evidence to improve clinical practice and patient outcomes
Clinical	A description of content applicable to clinical practice
Case study	A summary of the care of a single patient (real or hypothetical) to propose a resolution for a defined problem
Literature review	Documentation of a systematic review or meta-analysis

Note. Based on information from Alexander, 2011; American Psychological Association, 2010; Gobel & Tipton, 2009; Pierson, 2009.

CTNs may be asked to assist in manuscript preparation for studies they coordinate, such as providing demographic or adverse events data. Understanding how to use the current Consolidated Standards of Reporting Trials (CONSORT) (Schulz, Altman, & Moher, 2010) guidelines or adhering to the international standards of the Second World Conference on Research Integrity (Wager & Kleinert, 2012) will help keep CTNs on point in reporting randomized controlled trials completely, accurately, ethically, and without bias. Guidelines for reporting research results help the author to describe the research and methodology in detail, which conveys important information to readers, peers, reviewers, and editors (International Committee of Medical Journal Editors [ICMJE], 2013b). See Figure 44-2 for advice on getting research published.

Abstract

An *abstract* is the self-contained summation of a completed work (International Association of Clinical Research Nurses [IACRN], 2013). The dictionary definitions for abstract can be used to clarify the two types of abstracts CTNs would most likely be writing: an *article abstract* ("a brief written statement of the main points or facts in a longer report, speech, etc.") and a *conference abstract* ("something that summarizes or concentrates the essentials of a larger thing or several things") (Abstract, n.d.).

Article Abstract

An *article abstract* is a condensed version of an article that summarizes key points, giving readers a way to determine if they are interested in reading the full text of the arti-

Table 44-2. Examples of Reporting Guidelines for Writing Research Articles

Type of Article/Source of Guideline	Guidelines	Website
Randomized trials	CONSORT 2010	www.consort-statement.org
Systematic reviews and meta-analyses	PRISMA	www.prisma-statement.org
Observational studies	STROBE	http://strobe-statement.org
Diagnostic accuracy studies	STARD	www.stard-statement.org
Literature reviews	STARLITE	www.ncbi.nlm.nih.gov/pmc/articles/PMC1629442
Health research	EQUATOR	www.equator-network.org Lists all reporting guidelines for health research
U.S. National Library of Medicine	Research Reporting Guidelines and Initiatives by Organization	www.nlm.nih.gov/services/research_report_guide.html Lists the major biomedical research reporting guidelines as well as editorial style guides for writing research reports or other publications

CONSORT—Consolidated Standards of Reporting Trials; EQUATOR—Enhancing the Quality and Transparency of Health Research; PRISMA—Preferred Reporting Items for Systematic Reviews and Meta-Analyses; STARD—Standards for the Reporting of Diagnostic Accuracy Studies; STARLITE—Standards for Reporting Literature searches; STROBE—Strengthening the Reporting of Observational Studies in Epidemiology

Note. Based on information from Booth, 2006; Liberati et al., 2009; Moher et al., 2009; Schulz et al., 2010; U.S. National Library of Medicine, 2013.

Figure 44-2. Advice for Publishing Research

- Use a short, simple, readable title.
- Use the style of the journal.
- Follow the journal's author guidelines.
- Check that the flow of the manuscript is logical (i.e., write out and compare the first sentence of every paragraph).
- Explain methodology completely.
- Use your own words.

Note. Based on information from Gennaro, 2012; Sherman, 2011.

---

cle (Abstract, n.d.; Alexander, 2011; APA, 2010). Abstracts should be accurate, short, clear, and unbiased and will be descriptive (i.e., the statement of purpose, not the contents of the article) or informative (an overview of the contents of the article) (Alexander, 2011; APA, 2010; Rutgers Aresty Research Center for Undergraduates, 2013).

A publisher's website will have formatting procedures in its guidelines for authors that specify what is expected to be in an abstract or article. It is important to *only* include information from the article in an abstract and to adhere to other requirements of the publisher such as word count, font size, and deadlines (IACRN, 2013). Generally, an article abstract should contain a title, introduction, purpose, design, setting, subjects, measures, results, and conclusions (Alexander, 2011; Rutgers Aresty Research Center for Undergraduates, 2013).

CONSORT for Abstracts (Hopewell et al., 2008) can help CTNs construct an abstract for reporting randomized controlled trials within the constraints of a publisher. It is a 19-item checklist that can apply to a randomized controlled trial report in a journal or conference abstract. Other types of abstracts and their contents are summarized in Table 44-3.

Conference Abstract

A *conference abstract* is usually published in the conference proceedings. The focus of a conference abstract may be clinical, research, evidence-based, quality improvement, or a creative solution to a problem (IACRN, 2014). Conference abstracts may be submitted as a podium, poster, or symposium presentation and may be up to 20 minutes in length followed by a five-minute period for attendee questions (IACRN, 2014). The conference website will provide instructions that need to be followed, especially staying within the allotted word limit, which can average 350 words (IACRN, 2014). Once submitted, a conference abstract will be objectively evaluated. It is vital that CTNs have a complete understanding of the criteria for evaluation that will be used. Professional organization with conferences to which the CTN may consider submitting an abstract include the Oncology Nursing Society, Society of Clinical Research Associates, Association of Clinical Research Professionals, and IACRN, to name a few.

Sherman (2011) composed three key points for writing an abstract for a conference: target the abstract to the audience at the conference, craft a title that is "descriptive and compelling" (p. 217), and follow the guidelines available regarding sections, word count, fonts, and font sizes. To be certain that a conference abstract is a success, follow the four Cs of writing an abstract (IACRN, 2014, p. 15).

- Complete: Covers the major parts of the project.
- Concise: Contains no excess wordiness of unnecessary information.
- Clear: Readable, well organized, and not too jargon-laden.
- Cohesive: It flows smoothly between the parts.

Table 44-3. What to Include in an Abstract	
Type of Abstract	Components
Research	Problem Participants and their characteristics Features of methodology Findings including effect sizes and confidence intervals Conclusion with applications
Randomized clinical trial	Title, authors, and trial design Methods, participants, interventions, objective, outcome, randomization, and blinding Results, randomized numbers, recruitment, analyzed numbers, outcome, and harms Conclusions, trial registration, and funding
Literature review or meta-analysis	Problem Eligibility criteria Participants and their characteristics Conclusions and limitations Implications for practice
Case study	Subject and characteristics Intervention to resolve a problem Implications for clinical practice and future research
Conference	Introduction, background and purpose, and rationale Scope Methods Results Significance and implications Discussion Conclusion Focus may be clinical, research, evidence-based, quality improvement, or a creative solution to a problem.

Note. Based on information from Alexander, 2011; American Psychological Association, 2010; Hopewell et al., 2008; International Association of Clinical Research Nurses, 2014.

Before submitting a conference abstract, CTNs should confirm with their supervisor that they will be able to attend the conference, and if so, what costs the employer would assume and what costs they would need to cover. CTNs should also confirm if they will be able to use work time for any conference-related activities or if the abstract development will be on their own time.

Poster

Posters are a visual means of presenting primary research results, clinical reports, and other information at meetings or conferences. Poster sessions are usually informal, compared to an oral presentation, and consist of a display (the poster), handouts (single-page summary and business cards), and possibly a prescheduled time for a three-to-five–minute verbal presentation and interaction with conference attendees (Elghblawi, 2009; Hess, 2010). Posters tell the reader why what was done is important. Using text blocks to display an introduction, method, results, and conclusions can be effective (Blakesley & Brizee, n.d.; Hess, 2010).

Conference research posters are large, ranging in size from four feet wide by three feet tall to six feet wide by four feet tall, or may be electronic (e-poster). The poster instructions may be found on a conference website or are sent directly to the lead poster author. A poster must be easily read and understood in just a few minutes, so it needs to be comfortably readable from a distance of about six feet (Blakesley & Brizee, 2008; Elghblawi, 2009; Hess, 2010). Posters are typically read from the left to the right and from the top down, making it important to arrange text so it is pleasing to the eye, balancing text with graphics and illustrations, and limiting text blocks to 50–75 words (Blakesley & Brizee, n.d.; Hess, 2010). Limiting colors to two or three that are soft will prevent eye fatigue in the reader (Hess, 2010). It is important for CTNs to pay attention to the instructions; in some countries, posters are read top to bottom but not left to right and are often taller than wider (e.g., six feet tall by four feet wide).

The information presented in a poster must be accurate, useful, and legible; using bulleted points of text and placing related information in close proximity will help to make content flow smoothly (Blakesley & Brizee, 2008; Sherman, 2011). Make a draft of the poster on letter- or legal-size paper and have at least one peer review it and offer constructive feedback before final proofreading and construction. For a fee, copy centers can print a poster on banner material that is easy to transport in a large tube. It is important for CTNs, before submitting an abstract for a poster, to know who will be covering the costs of the poster printing and any other print material that will be at the conference. E-poster development follows the same preparatory steps listed herein.

References that may be helpful are "How to Prepare and Present a [Medical] Poster" (Volz, 2011) and "Developing and Presenting Posters" (IACRN, 2011). The first is a free one-hour video of a live presentation by Tracy Volz, PhD, from Rice University in Houston, Texas. The second is a free PowerPoint presentation endorsed by IACRN.

Creating an Article From an Abstract or Poster

An abstract or a poster for a conference may be written as an article at a later date. Use the abstract or poster as an outline, add a literature review, include tables and figures with permission for use (or create your own), and make changes based on feedback received for the abstract or poster at the conference (Elghblawi, 2009;

Sherman, 2011). The information conveyed in an abstract or poster could be made more general or specific as an article that is targeted to a particular audience for a specific journal.

To begin, use the title of the abstract or poster for the first draft of the article, adding headings and subheadings to direct the writing, making the article easy to read. Plug in main concepts from the abstract or poster and shore them up with peer-reviewed evidence-based literature. Bulleted points on a poster must be developed into lucent discussions in an article (Elghblawi, 2009). Present technical material clearly and concisely, ensuring that nontechnical readers will understand what is being conveyed (Webb, 2009). As with any writing, ask for feedback from peers who represent the target audience before finalizing and submitting the article (Osborne, 2010). This is an excellent way for CTNs to build upon work already completed.

Authorship

Authorship, or recognizing the person or people who wrote an article or abstract, is a visual way to document who made significant contributions to and accepts full accountability for an article, abstract, or poster (APA, 2010; ICMJE, 2013b). Many colleagues are comfortable with agreeing to authorship with just a handshake before embarking on a writing project. However, the way to guarantee proper authorship is to (a) discuss plans of what (articles or abstracts) should be written at the end of a project before the project begins, (b) document it in an agreement, and (c) follow the agreement.

Who gets credit for what? The ICMJE-recommended criteria for authorship for articles submitted to biomedical journals (see Figure 44-3) supports the inclusion of all people who qualify as designated authors (ICMJE, 2013b). They recommend that those listed as authors participate sufficiently and accept accountability for the work they have contributed. ICMJE requires that authors contributing to ICMJE-member journals meet the criteria. However, many national and international journals voluntarily require use of the ICMJE criteria for authorship before an article will be published (ICMJE, 2013a, 2013b).

Authorship is generally conveyed with a byline, a line usually at the beginning of an article that notes the person's or people's names and affiliations, or group authorship where many authors are credited, possibly under one group name (APA, 2010; Dulhunty, Boots, Paratz, & Lipman, 2011; ICMJE, 2013b). The *lead author* of an article or abstract is generally agreed upon before writing and may be the individual who suggested the topic, has expertise or interest in the topic, or represents a group such as the president of a special interest group in an organization.

The *corresponding author* is the person to whom all correspondence for the publication is directed. He or she deals with all editorial and publishing issues and assumes responsibility for the publication, including accuracy (data, facts), integrity, and how the contributions to the publication were determined (authorship) (Brent, 2011; ICMJE, 2013b).

The term *gift authorship* has been used to describe authorship conferred to a person who has not contributed to the research, the writing, or the revising of an article, such as a department chairperson or supervisor. Gift authorship is a false representation of authorship and is a type of plagiarism (Brent, 2011). People who are not contributors to the project and do not meet the criteria of the ICMJE for authors (see Figure 44-3) should be listed under acknowledgments instead (Graf et al., 2009; ICMJE, 2013b). For example, a nurse who recruited patients for a clinical trial but did not conduct the research, contribute to the research process or the writing and revision of an article for publication, or take public responsibility for the integrity of the research should be *acknowledged* and not cited as an author.

Order of Authors

The order of authors in a byline of an article that will be submitted for publication is often established by the authors before the project begins. It is common practice for the principal contributor (who does the most work) to be listed first, followed by the other authors according to their individual level of contribution

---

Figure 44-3. International Committee of Medical Journal Editors Author Requirements for Manuscripts Submitted to Biomedical Journals

Authorship credit should be based on
1. Substantial contributions to conception or design of the work; or the acquisition, analysis, or interpretation of data for the work; AND
2. Drafting the work or revising it critically for important intellectual content; AND
3. Final approval of the version to be published; AND
4. Agreement to be accountable for all aspects of the work in ensuring that questions related to the accuracy or integrity of any part of the work are appropriately investigated and resolved.

Note. This is a reprint of the ICMJE Recommendations for the Conduct, Reporting, Editing, and Publication of Scholarly Work in Medical Journals (2013b). The Oncology Nursing Society prepared this reprint. The ICMJE has not endorsed nor approved the contents of this reprint. The ICMJE periodically updates the Uniform Requirements, so this reprint, prepared on October 19, 2014, may not accurately represent the current official version at www.ICMJE.org. The official version of the Recommendations for the Conduct, Reporting, Editing, and Publication of Scholarly Work in Medical Journals is located at www.ICMJE.org. Users should cite this official version when citing the document.

(APA, 2010). CTNs who are the coordinator of a clinical trial should ask the principal investigator or sponsor for inclusion in the byline and writing process before the trial begins. Following up with a memorandum to the principal investigator or sponsor summarizing the discussion and agreed terms for authorship might just secure the deal.

The listing of all authors in the byline is referred to as the *conventional form of authorship* (Dulhunty et al., 2011). The written agreement should stipulate that if the principal contributor cannot make the planned contribution, the person who does the most work will then be slated as the lead author (Graf et al., 2009). Other arrangements, such as a lead author and coauthors in alphabetical order, may be agreed upon if one or more authors have published prolifically or are mentors and are content to give front position author placement to other, less experienced, authors.

Authorship in Multicenter Clinical Trials

Multicenter research has several advantages over single-center research including faster accrual rates, less scientific misconduct, and greater generalizability of the results (Dulhunty et al., 2011). Multicenter authorship, on the other hand, can be a source of conflict if a plan for authorship is not developed beforehand and a hundred or more contributors want to be recognized in the byline. All authors of multicenter trials must meet the ICMJE criteria for authorship (see Figure 44-3). No universally accepted guidelines exist, leaving researchers and sponsors to individually determine the best approach.

Authorship Agreement or Policy

Historically, the verbal agreement of a lead author or principal investigator of a research study or project lead for an evidence-based project was all that was needed to confer authorship. Today, however, a written agreement should be signed *before* a project is started to avoid misconceptions and conflict. The agreement should delineate the project tasks, workload division, tasks that earn authorship credit, and the order in which authors will be listed (APA, 2010). Although this may not be a critical issue when CTNs decide to write an article for a nursing journal about adverse events relating to a study drug, it can take on tremendous importance when one considers that the study was planned and carried out by investigators, research nurses, clinical research assistants, statisticians, pharmacists, sponsor employees or contractors, and other members of the research team (Graf et al., 2009).

Some institutions or companies have a *policy for authorship* that employees must follow. CTNs should inquire about such a policy before embarking on an endeavor that will result in a publishable manuscript (Graf et al., 2009). By doing so, they will protect their contributions to the research process.

Company-Sponsored Medical Research

Representative members of the International Society for Medical Publication Professionals developed good publication practice guidelines, version 2 (GPP2) to aid authors of research reports sponsored by companies in writing manuscripts that are ethical and unbiased (Graf et al., 2009). The GPP2 guidelines are intended to be used by authors writing articles for company-sponsored research for peer-reviewed journals and presentations for scientific meetings (Graf et al., 2009). Topics covered in the GPP2 are listed in Figure 44-4.

The GPP2 guidelines include a 19-item checklist for articles and presentations that covers areas of integrity, completeness, transparency, accountability, and responsibility, as well as an 11-item checklist of elements to be included in a written publication agreement (Graf et al., 2009). The GPP2 guidelines are important for CTNs who are coordinating a clinical trial sponsored by a company because CTNs may be involved with writing or contributing to an article or abstract for presentation at a conference. In that case, CTNs would be expected to adhere to the GPP2 guidelines, presenting their topic ethically and without bias while crediting the sponsor or company.

Although it is ideal for CTNs to document an authorship agreement in writing that describes how authorship will be determined in a single-site or multicenter clinical trial and what method will be used to assign contributors to a manuscript (Whellan et al., 2009), it may be more common for CTNs to know the publication policy of the institution or sponsor, discuss with the principal investigator writing a nursing article, and sharing nurs-

---

Figure 44-4. Topics Addressed in the Good Publication Practice Guidelines for Communicating Company-Sponsored Research

- Roles and responsibilities: Written agreement, access to data, reimbursement
- Publication steering committee
- Authors
- Contributorship and acknowledgements
- Professional medical writers: Working with authors, as authors
- Conflicts of interest
- Recommendations for specific types of articles and presentations: Primary and secondary publications, duplicate publication, presentations, review articles, and reporting standards
- Planning, registering, posting, and documenting: Publication planning, before publication, and documentation

Note. Based on information from Graf et al., 2009.

ing implications with peers. If there is no institutional or sponsor-driven policy for publication, CTNs may be wholly dependent on the professional relationship they share with the principal investigator.

Acknowledgments

Acknowledgments are used to credit all project contributors who do not meet the criteria for authorship (ICMJE, 2013a). This may include statisticians, technical personnel, department chairs, data collectors, supervisors, medical writers, sponsoring companies or agencies, funding agencies, and others (Graf et al., 2009; ICMJE, 2013b). Generally, written permission must be obtained from the people being acknowledged to confirm their understanding that readers may construe their acknowledgment as their endorsement of everything stated in the article (ICMJE, 2013b).

Acknowledgments may have predetermined placement in an article based on a journal's guidelines, usually on the front two pages or the very last page. Acknowledgments for poster presentations will usually be found in italics at the very end of the poster.

Medical Writers

Medical writers are proficient in scientific writing and editing and may work closely with authors to prepare articles, abstracts, posters, or presentations (Clemow & Drug Information Association Medical Writing Special Interest Area Community Competency Model Working Group, 2011; Graf et al., 2009). Lang (2008) differentiates medical writers from authors by describing a scientific document as content and presentation. He contends that authors create, select, and modify content, whereas medical writers organize, clarify, explain, and condense that content into words, figures, and tables.

Generally, medical writers are not granted authorship; rather, their contribution is noted in the acknowledgments. *Ghostwriting* is the term used to describe the omission from the byline or acknowledgments of the actual author; the person who wrote is not credited and the person credited for writing did not control and direct the writing (Graf et al., 2009; Mayer, Mahon, & Eaby, 2009). This is unethical and should never be allowed (Woolley, 2009).

Medical writers are employed by pharmaceutical companies and other sponsors to plan, prepare, and manage single or multiple documents; maintain templates, standards, formats, and styles; develop knowledge and skills; share knowledge and experience with clients; and more (Clemow & Drug Information Association Medical Writing Special Interest Area Community Competency Model Working Group, 2011). This may include heading a publication committee; preparing a publication plan, briefing documents, applications, investigator's brochure, and exemptions; and ensuring that regulatory and publication guidelines are met (Clemow & Drug Information Association Medical Writing Special Interest Area Community Competency Model Working Group, 2011).

If a CTN is coordinating a clinical trial sponsored by a pharmaceutical company, he or she may need to collaborate with a medical writer who is a company employee. Although the CTN would benefit from the medical writer's expertise, he or she should be aware of the company's policy regarding medical writers' authorship. For example, if a CTN collaborates with a medical writer to pen an article on managing the adverse effects of a new drug, the CTN should be sure that the journal to which the article is submitted accepts manuscripts that have a medical writer as an author. The editorial policies of *Oncology Nursing Forum* and *Clinical Journal of Oncology Nursing* allow for the inclusion of articles that have medical writer involvement. However, the exact involvement of the medical writer must be disclosed, and the article will not be eligible for continuing nursing education credit (L. McGee, personal communication, March 27, 2013).

Writing With Integrity

Writing with integrity is a moral and ethical responsibility of every author. It means taking the time and effort to produce an original work and guaranteeing the originality of that work to the publisher. It also means guaranteeing the accuracy of scientific knowledge and giving credit to others when their work is used (APA, 2010).

Plagiarism

One of many definitions of plagiarism is "taking credit for the creative, expert, or scientific work of someone else" (Klimaszewski, 2012, p. 525). There are several types of plagiarism, two of which have been discussed: gift authorship and ghostwriting. Duplicate publishing and unintentional plagiarism are equally unethical.

Duplicate publishing occurs when an article is published in a journal as original when, in fact, one similar to it has been published elsewhere in print or online and the previous article is not credited (ICMJE, 2013b). Not only are ideas and data misrepresented as being original, but available evidence is altered, and copyright violations against the author can result (APA, 2010; Brent, 2011; ICMJE, 2013b). A form of duplicate publishing is piecemeal publishing, where ideas and data from one project are divided into multiple manuscripts and presented as new findings (APA, 2010; Brent, 2011).

Plagiarism is not necessarily intentional. Unintentional plagiarism may occur as a result of something as simple as not citing, or improperly citing, a reference.

Citations

Reference citations provide readers with evidence about where in time scientific, literary, or other contributions were published (APA, 2010). When an article is cited, it implies that the author read and reflected upon the work of that person. Citations enable readers to return to the work of others that influenced or supported an author's ideas, theories, or scientific or creative work (APA, 2010). Reasons to cite references are listed in Figure 44-5.

Frequently, authors become flummoxed about whether material must have a citation. Every source must have a citation (Menager & Paulos, 2009). Information found on the Internet is either copyrighted or in the public domain. Regardless of copyright status, information from the Internet should always include attribution to the original authors similar to citations for books, journals, or any other source.

Copyrighted material is indicated by the symbol © or the word or abbreviation *Copyright* or *Copr.* along with the year of copyright and the copyright owner's name (U.S. Copyright Office, 2012a). Permission must be obtained to reprint or adapt (i.e., change) a figure or table from material that is copyrighted. Permissions must be submitted to the publisher at the time the manuscript is submitted. More detailed information about copyright may be found at www.copyright.gov.

An exception to copyright law is the *fair use doctrine*, which allows a short passage of copyrighted material (text) to be reprinted for research, scholarship, criticism and comment, teaching, and news reporting without asking permission (U.S. Copyright Office, 2012b). For example, a CTN may quote a short passage from a copyrighted work to clarify or validate an observation and will not need to request permission from the copyright owner to do so. However, the material used must have quotation marks and a proper reference citation.

Information in the *public domain* (i.e., government or government-funded publications and material for which a copyright has been lost, not renewed, or expired) may be copied word-for-word if a correct reference citation is provided (Brent, 2011). For example, if a CTN elects to use a figure from a government website or a short passage from a website without a copyright, he or she may do as long the source is cited in the text of the manuscript and the reference list or bibliography. See Table 44-4 for suggestions about how to prevent plagiarism by using citations.

Preventing Unintentional Plagiarism

Preventing plagiarism is more time consuming than complicated (Klimaszewski, 2012). Every source of ideas or information incorporated into an original manuscript must be accurately cited in the reference style format required by the publisher (Menager & Paulos, 2009). To prevent plagiarism,
- Know the reference style used by the publisher.
- Use source information correctly: paraphrasing, summarizing, or quoting the work of another.
- Accurately cite source information in the text of the article, abstract, or poster.
- Put it all together in a reference list or bibliography.

Paraphrasing

Paraphrasing is taking detailed information from the work of another and restating it in one's own words. This can be time consuming because the intent or meaning must be captured *without* using the original author's words, word sequencing, or sentence sequencing (Lipson, 2008; Menager & Paulos, 2009). Paraphrasing requires an in-text citation (adding the page number of the original work is suggested) (APA, 2010) and a full reference in the reference list or bibliography.

Summarizing

Summarizing is using one's own words to *shorten* the length of the original author's text without altering the meaning (Menager & Paulos, 2009; Neville, 2009). One way to accomplish this is to read what needs to be summarized and put it aside, returning later to jot down the key points without going into detail. The intent is to preserve, and not change, the original meaning in a shortened version and in the voice of the person writing the summary. Summarizing requires a citation in text and a full reference in the reference list or bibliography.

Quoting

Quoting is copying the words of another word-for-word (Gilmore, 2009; Menager & Paulos, 2009). Never copy

---

Figure 44-5. Reasons to Cite References

- Show respect to the original author
- Give credit for ideas, theories, words, or creations
- Stimulate critical thinking about the original work
- Provide evidence for conclusions
- Validate an argument
- Show where research being reported was obtained
- Provide the information a reader needs to go directly to the source
- Signal to the reader that text has been paraphrased or summarized
- Protect oneself from plagiarism

Note. Based on information from Martin, 2004; Menager & Paulos, 2009; Neville, 2010; Nicoll, 2011.

Table 44-4. Preventing Plagiarism With Citations

Material Used	Action
Ideas or data (print or online)	Cite the source properly in text. Add websites, date of posting or update, and digital object identifier (DOI) to reference list.
Public domain content (print or online)	Cite the source properly in text. Add websites, date of posting or update, and DOI to reference list.
Copyrighted material that qualifies as fair use (print or online)	Cite the source properly in text. Add websites, date of posting or update, and DOI to reference list.
Copyrighted material that does not qualify as fair use (print or online)	Obtain permission for use. Cite the source as directed by the copyright holder. Use quotation marks in text but not in figures and tables. Add to reference list in the form directed by the copyright holder. Submit approval for use to editor/publisher.

Note. Based on information from Brent, 2011; Gilmore, 2009; Menager & Paulos, 2009.

phrases, sentences, or paragraphs word-for-word from a journal or online source without enclosing them in quotation marks or offsetting larger passages (40 words or more) into a block quotation. Be mindful that quotation marks can be viewed as a distraction by the reader, so keep the amount of text quoted in an article to a minimum (Posner, 2007). If a page number is not available on the Internet, cite the paragraph number after the year. For example, "CTNs are vital to the development of therapeutic interventions for patients with cancer" (Smith, 2013, para. 2) (APA, 2010). Quoting requires accuracy in copying, quotation marks or block quotation format, an in-text citation with the page or paragraph number of the original passage, and a full reference in the reference list or bibliography.

Summary

CTNs have an opportunity and a responsibility to provide information about clinical trials and their unique role to nurses and others in the clinical, educational, and research settings. Writing for publication provides a vehicle to convey that information and record it for access by others in the future. Most importantly, writing can advance patient outcomes, contribute to the evidence base that currently exists in the literature, and support the translation of research into practice.

CTNs who have never published may wish to start with an abstract or poster session before embarking on an article.

Once the decision to write an article has been made, CTNs may choose to coauthor first. Many support systems exist for new and seasoned authors: guidelines, journal policies, institutional policies, and even mentorship programs such as the *Clinical Journal of Oncology Nursing* Writing Mentorship Program (see http://cjon.ons.org/content/writing-mentorship-program). The opportunity to publish is there; CTNs just need to embrace it.

Key Points
- Control and direct all actions associated with your writing.
- Write with integrity and without bias.
- Write as if speaking; read the manuscript out loud.
- Direct the publication to the target audience.
- Follow policies and guidelines when available; follow instructions on a journal or conference website.
- Cite references for anything that is not common knowledge or your original thought.
- Paraphrase content in your own words.
- Cite primary references even if you find the information in a secondary source.
- Adhere to timelines for written submissions.
- Articles, conference or article abstracts, and poster presentations all can contribute to the translation of research to clinical practice.

References

Abstract. (n.d.). In *Merriam-Webster's online dictionary.* Retrieved from http://www.merriam-webster.com/dictionary/abstract

Alexander, M. (2011). Organizing the article. In C. Saver (Ed.), *Anatomy of writing for publication for nurses* (pp. 65–82). Indianapolis, IN: Sigma Theta Tau International.

American Psychological Association. (2010). *Publication manual of the American Psychological Association* (6th ed.). Washington, DC: Author.

Blakesley, D., & Brizee, A. (n.d.). Purdue University Writing Lab Indiana Department of Transportation Workshop Series: Designing research posters. Retrieved from http://owl.english.purdue.edu/media/pdf/20080626013023_727.pdf

Booth, A. (2006). Brimful of STARLITE. *Journal of the Medical Library Association, 94,* 421–429, e205. Retrieved from http://www.ncbi.nlm.nih.gov/pmc/articles/PMC1629442

Brent, N.J. (2011). Legal and ethical issues. In C. Saver (Ed.), *Anatomy of writing for publication for nurses* (pp. 141–160). Indianapolis, IN: Sigma Theta Tau International.

Clemow, D.B., & the Drug Information Association Medical Writing Special Interest Area Community Competency Model Working Group. (2011). Pharmaceutical medical writing competency model. *AMWA Journal, 26,* 62–70. Retrieved from http://www.amwa.org/files/Journal/2011v26n2_online.pdf

Dulhunty, J.M., Boots, R.J., Paratz, J.D., & Lipman, J. (2011). Determining authorship in multicenter trials: A systematic review. *Acta Anaesthesiologica Scandinavica, 55,* 1037–1043. doi:10.1111/j.1399-6576.2011.02477.x

Elghblawi, E. (2009). Double duty: Convert your poster presentations into papers. *Nurse Author and Editor, 19*(1). Retrieved from http://nurseauthoreditor.com/article.asp?id=120

Gennaro, S. (2012). Five tips for getting research published [Editorial]. *Journal of Nursing Scholarship, 44,* 203–204. doi:10.1111/j.1547-5069.2012.01461.x

Gilmore, B. (2009). *Plagiarism: A how-not-to guide for students.* Portsmouth, NH: Heinemann.

Gobel, B.H., & Tipton, J.M. (2009). PEP up your practice: An introduction to the Oncology Nursing Society Putting Evidence Into Practice resources. In L.H. Eaton & J.M. Tipton (Eds.), *Putting evidence into practice: Improving oncology patient outcomes* (pp. 1–8). Pittsburgh, PA: Oncology Nursing Society.

Graf, C., Battisti, W.P., Bridges, D., Bruce-Winkler, V., Conaty, J.M., Ellison, J.M., ... Yarker, Y.E. (2009). Good publication practice for communicating company sponsored medical research: The GPP2 guidelines. *BMJ, 339*, b4330. doi:10.1136/bmj.b4330

Grech, C., & Evans, D. (2012). Promoting academic publishing. *Nurse Author and Editor, 22*(2). Retrieved from http://www.nurseauthoreditor.com/tocs.asp?yr=2012&num=2

Hess, G.R. (2010). Effective scientific posters: Quick reference. Retrieved from http://www.ncsu.edu/project/posters/documents/QuickReferenceV3.pdf

Hopewell, S., Clarke, M., Moher, D., Wager, E., Middleton, P., Altman, D.G., ... the CONSORT Group. (2008). CONSORT for reporting randomized controlled trials in journal and conference abstracts: Explanation and elaboration. *PLoS Medicine, 5*(1), e20. doi:10.1371/journal.pmed.0050020

International Association of Clinical Research Nurses. (2011, August). Developing and presenting posters [PowerPoint slides]. Retrieved from http://www.iacrn.memberlodge.org/Resources/Documents/2013%20Conference/Developing%20and%20Presenting%20Posters%20CE%20091611.ppsx

International Association of Clinical Research Nurses. (2014, May 15). Writing a conference abstract: Tips for success [PowerPoint slides]. Retrieved from http://iacrn.memberlodge.org/Resources/Documents/Abstract_Devel_Handout_2perpage.pdf

International Committee of Medical Journal Editors. (2013a). Journals following the ICMJE recommendations. Retrieved from http://www.icmje.org/journals-following-the-icmje-recommendations

International Committee of Medical Journal Editors. (2013b). Recommendations for the conduct, reporting, editing, and publication of scholarly work in medical journals (Updated August 2013). Retrieved from http://www.icmje.org/recommendations/archives/2013_aug_urm.pdf

Klimaszewski, A. (2012). Preventing plagiarism. *Oncology Nursing Forum, 39*, 525–527. doi:10.1188/12.ONF.525-527

Lang, T. (2008). What do you think constitutes authorship? *AMWA Journal, 23*, 65–67. Retrieved from http://www.amwa.org/files/Journal/2008v23n2.pdf

Liberati, A., Altman, D.G., Tetzlaff, J., Mulrow, C., Gøtzsche, P.C., Ioannidis, J.P., ... Moher, D. (2009). The PRISMA Statement for Reporting Systematic Reviews and Meta-Analyses of Studies That Evaluate Health Care Interventions: Explanation and elaboration. *PLoS Medicine, 6*(7), e1000100. doi:10.1371/journal.pmed.1000100

Lipson, C. (2008). *Doing honest work in college: How to prepare citations, avoid plagiarism, and achieve real academic success* (2nd ed.). Chicago, IL: University of Chicago Press.

Martin, B. (2004, February 4). Plagiarism: Policy against cheating or policy for learning? Retrieved from http://www.uow.edu.au/~bmartin/pubs/04plag.pdf

Mayer, D.K., Mahon, S.M., & Eaby, B. (2009). Writing for hire: Advice for authors (and readers) [Editorial]. *Clinical Journal of Oncology Nursing, 13*, 131–132. doi:10.1188/09.CJON.131-132

Mee, C. (2011). Writing the clinical article. In C. Saver (Ed.), *Anatomy of writing for publication for nurses* (pp. 177–192). Indianapolis, IN: Sigma Theta Tau International.

Menager, R., & Paulos, L. (2009). *Quick coach guide to avoiding plagiarism*. Boston, MA: Wadsworth Cengage Learning.

Moher, D., Liberati, A., Tetzlaff, J., Altman, D.G., & The PRISMA Group. (2009). Preferred reporting items for systematic reviews and meta-analyses: The PRISMA statement. *PLoS Medicine, 6*(7), e1000097. doi:10.1371/journal.pmed.1000097

Neville, C. (2010). *The complete guide to referencing and avoiding plagiarism* (2nd ed.). New York, NY: McGraw-Hill Open University Press.

Nicoll, L.H. (2011). Finding and documenting sources. In C. Saver (Ed.), *Anatomy of writing for publication for nurses* (pp. 51–64). Indianapolis, IN: Sigma Theta Tau International.

Osborne, H. (2010). Writing in plain language: A quick guide from start to finish. *AMWA Journal, 25*, 169–171. Retrieved from http://www.amwa.org/files/Journal/2010v25n4_online.pdf

Pierson, C.A. (2009). The PRISMA Statement: What does it mean for nurse authors, reviewers, and editors? *Nurse Author and Editor, 19*(4), 1–3. Retrieved from http://www.nurseauthoreditor.com/tocs.asp?yr=2009&num=4

Posner, R.A. (2007). *The little book of plagiarism*. New York, NY: Pantheon Books.

Rutgers Aresty Research Center for Undergraduates. (2013). How to write an abstract. Retrieved from http://aresty.rutgers.edu/sites/default/files/pdf/aresty/abstract.pdf

Saver, C. (2011). Anatomy of writing. In C. Saver (Ed.), *Anatomy of writing for publication for nurses* (pp. 3–20). Indianapolis, IN: Sigma Theta Tau International.

Schulz, K.F., Altman, D.G., & Moher, D. (2010). CONSORT 2010 statement: Updated guidelines for reporting parallel group randomized trials. *BMJ, 340*, 698–702/c332. doi:10.1136/bmj.c32

Sherman, R. (2011). Writing abstracts for podium and poster presentations. In C. Saver (Ed.), *Anatomy of writing for publication for nurses* (pp. 211–226). Indianapolis, IN: Sigma Theta Tau International.

Tumber, M.B., & Dickersin, K. (2004). Publication of clinical trials: Accountability and accessibility. *Journal of Internal Medicine, 256*, 271–283. doi:10.1111/j.1365-2796.2004.01392.x

U.S. Copyright Office. (2012a). Copyright basics (Circular 1, reviewed 5/2012). Retrieved from http://www.copyright.gov/circs/circ01.pdf

U.S. Copyright Office. (2012b). Fair use (FL-102, reviewed 6/2012). Retrieved from http://www.copyright.gov/fls/fl102.html

U.S. National Library of Medicine. (2013). Research reporting guidelines and initiatives: By organization. Retrieved from http://www.nlm.nih.gov/services/research_report_guide.html

Volz, T. (2011). Poster design and presentation skills [Webcast]. Retrieved from http://digbig.com/5betqd

Wager, E., & Kleinert, S. (2012). Responsible research publication: International standards for authors. In T. Mayer & N. Steneck (Eds.), *Promoting research integrity in a global environment* (pp. 311–318). Singapore: World Scientific Publishing.

Webb, C. (2009). Writing for publication. Retrieved from http://www.nurseauthoreditor.com/WritingforPublication2009.pdf

Whellan, D.J., Ellis, S.J., Kraus, W.E., Hawthorne, K., Piña, I.L., Keteyian, S.J., ... O'Connor, C.M. (2009). Method for establishing authorship in a multicenter clinical trial. *Annals of Internal Medicine, 151*, 414–420. doi:10.7326/0003-4819-151-6-200909150-00006

Woolley, K. (2009). Nurses, medical writers, editors, can work together ethically [Letter]. *Clinical Journal of Oncology Nursing, 13*, 261–262.

SECTION XI.

International Clinical Trials Research

Introduction to International Section

Over the 45 years since I graduated as a registered nurse, I have witnessed, as an oncology nurse and researcher, the birth and evolution of a medical field called Cancer Clinical Trials. From the earliest beginnings, which might now seem archaic, to the current global initiatives, this field has escalated almost beyond belief.

Along with the enormous benefits from evidence-based therapies being realized for the improved comfort and survival of people with cancer, there have also evolved incredible complexities in conducting cancer research. Constructive growth in the regulatory, ethical, methodologic, translational, and quality assurance "industries" has led to accompanying restrictive effects on clinical trial activities. At the same time, international buy-in of research outcomes has been enhanced by concurrent intergroup collaborations. Again, a positive but complex development.

Fortunately, these collaborations are not limited to the activity of scientific investigators but rather encompass the entire network, including clinical trial nurses, data managers, study project leaders, and others supporting the operational aspects of the research. Only with these cooperative partnerships can today's cancer clinical trials succeed.

The countries represented in the following section of this manual are all collaborators in international cancer research initiatives—some seasoned, some new, all dedicated. The authors of these chapters take great pleasure in sharing their national information and knowledge. All agree that only through recognition and understanding of the variance in standard operating procedures, rules, regulations, and requirements can partnerships successfully proceed.

I take the opportunity of this brief introduction to present a summary of operational tools, templates, and guidelines developed over the past decade by the Harmonization Committee of the Gynecologic Cancer Inter-Group (see Figure 1). Many of the authors of this International Section have contributed to these documents. Additionally, many of these tools and templates have been used by the authors and the research groups with which they are affiliated. In the hope that these materials might be of service to the reader, they are shared here.

Respectfully contributed,
Monica Bacon, RN
Oncology Nurse and Researcher
Operations Manager, Gynecologic Cancer InterGroup

Figure 1. Resources Available From Harmonization Committee of the Gynecologic Cancer InterGroup

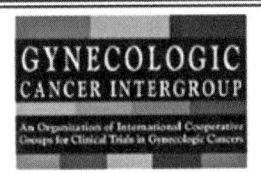

CURRENT STATUS

Harmonisation Information available at GCIG website:

Harmonisation Guidebook. What is GCIG, Practical issues, SAE, Insurance, IDMC, DM, others.
Appendix 1: Intergroup Agreement Template (Company Intellectual Property Acknowledgement and GCIG/ Roles and Responsibilities). Agreement for intergroup collaboration (general frame).
Appendix 2 : Data Monitoring Committees for GCIG Trials. Monitoring Board, mandatory for GCIG Phase III trials.
Appendix 3: Checklist for Tissue Banking Consent Form. Prevent essential information missing CF.
Appendix 4: Essential Documents Check-list. Minimal requirements for CA approvals per Group.
Harmonization Working Group, Group Contacts & Summaries. How are Groups organized.
Group Participation Summary. What are groups doing within GCIG.
Group Specific Appendix, GSA Guidelines. Special agreements for project specific issues.
Summary of EDC and archiving by GCIG Groups. EDC and archiving electronic data capability.

Other Information available at GCIG website:

Principles of independence.
Membership policy.
Governance and statutes. GCIG publication statement
GCIG meetings. Last meeting presentations. Provide information of what GCIG has done recently
Roster. Identify contact data for each group
Clinical Trials and Contacts
Groups web links. Provide groups information (including activities outside GCIG)
Events. Provide information of what is coming

Note. Figure courtesy of the Gynecologic Cancer InterGroup. Used with permission.

Chapter 45

Australia

Catherine Johnson, RN, and Kim Adler, RN

Introduction

Cancer clinical research has an established foundation in Australia; however, the period since 2008 has seen the evolution of the regulatory and ethics review system and consolidation of the Australasian Cancer Cooperative Trials Groups' capacity to conduct high-quality clinical research (Clinical Oncology Society of Australia [COSA], 2012). This chapter highlights some of the key features of conducting trials in the Australian research environment.

History and Foundation

Clinical Oncology Society of Australia

COSA is the peak national multidisciplinary society for health professionals working in cancer care and control. Formed in 1971, COSA (n.d.-c) hosts an annual scientific meeting, as well as seminars and educational activities related to current cancer issues such as cancer research, diagnosis, treatment, and care of people with cancer.

COSA is composed of a number of groups, which are either therapeutic-specific or dedicated to speciality areas in the field of cancer. Fourteen national cancer cooperative groups are affiliated with COSA, covering a broad range of solid tumor types and hematologic cancers. In addition, two groups within COSA specifically address clinical research as a discipline and the conduct of cancer clinical trials: the Cancer Biology group and the Clinical Trials Research Professionals Group (CRPG) (COSA, n.d.-a, n.d.-b).

Cancer Biology Group

The Cancer Biology group, one of the first groups established within COSA, was originally envisioned as bridging the gap between basic, laboratory-based cancer research and applied research in a clinical setting (COSA, n.d.-a). The Cancer Biology group is exploring new means to fill this role, specifically facilitating COSA collaboration with relevant research-based societies as well as with the researchers themselves. One specific area of focus has been the provision of biospecimens in collaboration with the cooperative cancer trials groups.

Clinical Trials Research Professionals Group

The COSA CRPG represents professionals involved in cancer research, including clinical trial coordinators, research nurses, clinical research managers, data managers, clinical research associates, and health information managers. CRPG is committed to achieving and promoting excellence in cancer clinical research with the professional contribution of data managers through education, information, leadership, networking, and professionalism (COSA, n.d.-b).

National Cancer Cooperative Trials Groups

The National Cancer Cooperative Trials Groups (NCCTG) established a record of conducting world-class research. Recent work with COSA through the Enabling Project accomplished significant achievements in standardizing clinical trials across Australia. The most significant achievements include the formation of the Executive Officers Network, the Umbrella Clinical Trials Insurance Scheme, and educational programs for clinical trials staff (COSA, n.d.-d). The Commonwealth Government has provided support and funding for NCCTG through Cancer Australia to assist NCCTG in building the capacity to conduct cancer clinical trials in Australia (Cancer Australia, 2013a).

Cancer Nurses Society of Australia

The Cancer Nurses Society of Australia (CNSA) is the national professional organization for cancer nurses established in 1998 and is an affiliated group of COSA. CNSA is committed to achieving and promoting excellence in cancer care through the professional contribution of nurses. CNSA offers a research grants program to support the development of cancer nursing. The purpose of the program is to provide financial assistance to facilitate research in the area of cancer nursing, which will contribute to improvements in the care of people with cancer (CNSA, n.d.).

Australasian Health and Research Data Managers Association

The Australasian Health and Research Data Managers Association (2005) is an association of health researchers, research nurses, study coordinators, and data managers working across Australia, New Zealand, and Asia. Its primary aim is to foster and promote health research and data management through the provision of professional development grants, educational opportunities, and resource materials.

Government Initiatives in Cancer Research

Cancer Australia, an initiative of the Australian federal government, has developed a number of initiatives to support the functioning of NCCTG. Cancer Australia provides a centralized high-quality national secretariat service to NCCTG. Cancer Australia established the Chair in Cancer Quality of Life to provide expert advice and support to NCCTG to initiate and incorporate quality-of-life studies into cancer clinical trials. The Health/Pharmaco-Economic Unit was established to assist NCCTG to incorporate relevant health and pharmacoeconomic analyses into trial protocols. The Psycho-Oncology Cooperative Research Group is funded to develop resources to support researchers in assessing health-related quality of life and other patient-reported outcomes in cancer (Cancer Australia, 2013b). Cancer Australia administers the Priority-Driven Collaborative Cancer Research Scheme (PDCCRS). Cancer Australia partners with other organizations to fund cancer research through PDCCRS that will reduce the impact of cancer on the community and improve outcomes for people affected by cancer (Cancer Australia, 2012).

In the state of New South Wales (NSW), the state government initiated the Cancer Institute NSW in 2003 to establish a research support program that builds research capacity and facilitates the translation of research findings into clinical practice. Improvements in recruitment, cancer research funding, trials conducted, and publication numbers are cited as key outcomes of the Cancer Institute NSW Research Program (Cancer Institute NSW, 2011).

Clinical Trials: Fundamental Information

Clinical Research Team

The clinical research team includes a variety of staff members who are relevant to the conduct of the study. Individual team members are responsible for the tasks delegated to them by the principal investigator. The principal investigator is responsible for oversight of the trial. Other team members may include doctors, nurses, social workers, psychologists, statisticians, trial coordinators, data managers, psychologists, phlebotomists, pharmacists, and other healthcare professionals.

Legal, Regulatory, and Legislative Issues

The Therapeutic Goods Administration, part of the Australian Government Department of Health and Ageing, the national regulatory authority, regulates clinical trials in Australia under two schemes: the Clinical Trial Notification scheme and the Clinical Trial Exemption scheme.

The most common scheme used is the Clinical Trial Notification scheme, which requires that all study material relating to the trial, including the protocol, scientific and background information regarding study drugs, and information provided to study participants, is submitted to an approved human research ethics committee (HREC) for review. The Therapeutic Goods Administration (n.d.) receives approximately 700 clinical trials annually. Once HREC grants approval, the completed Clinical Trial Notification form is signed by (a) the study sponsor, (b) an HREC representative (usually the chairperson), (c) a legal representative for the institution approving authority to conduct the trial (usually the hospital manager), and (d) the site investigator, and it then is submitted to the Therapeutic Goods Administration with an acknowledgment issued that the trial can commence. Phase III trials are usually conducted under the Clinical Trial Notification scheme. The research nurse is responsible for ensuring that the Clinical Trial Notification form is completed correctly and returned to the sponsor. If the trial is an investigator-initiated study, the site may submit directly to the Therapeutic Goods Administration.

Under the Therapeutic Goods legislation, HREC is responsible for monitoring the study at each associated institution. Deviations from the trial protocol and unexpected and protocol therapy–related serious adverse events (SAEs) that occur in Australian patients are required to be reported to HREC and the Therapeutic Goods Administration. However, all other SAEs that occur, including safety letters or updates from sponsors regarding events that have occurred outside Australia, are reported to HREC only. Deviations from the trial protocol and unexpected and protocol therapy-related SAEs for each site are also reported to the authorizing institution in a separate process known as *research governance* (National Health and Medical Research Council, n.d.-b).

The Clinical Trial Exemption scheme is used less frequently and is employed when a sponsor requests regulatory evaluation of an agent early in its clinical development (usually phase I or II) or for newer technologies such as gene therapy. Whether conducted under the Clinical Trial Notification or Clinical Trial Exemption scheme, all trials must be conducted in accordance with the protocol, associated documents, and the internationally accepted International Conference on Harmonisation of Technical Requirement for Registration of Pharmaceuticals for Human Use (ICH, 1996) guidance on good clinical practice, which the Therapeutic Goods Administration (2004) has adopted in principle.

Progress toward a joint Australia-New Zealand therapeutics regulatory scheme continues. A possible framework for the joint regulatory scheme has been released for comment from interested parties.

Sponsoring Agencies

The Australian Therapeutic Goods Act (1989) and subsequent amendments mandate that a national sponsor (a person, body, organization, or institution) is identified to take overall responsibility for the conduct of a clinical trial. The sponsor may initiate, organize, and support the clinical trial and usually carries the medical and legal responsibilities with the conduct of the trial. For pharmaceutical company–sponsored trials, the company affiliate will take on the role of sponsor, or it could be delegated to a contract research organization.

For investigator-initiated trials, the regulations permit the individual investigator or local institution to take on the role of sponsor. In the case of multicenter trials, the collaborative or coordinating group often acts as sponsor on behalf of many sites, whether initiated nationally or by international groups.

Defining sponsorship can be a complex component of the trial to set up, particularly if multiple parties are involved contractually in the conduct of the clinical trial. Increasingly, pharmaceutical companies, who may be providing the study drugs for the trial in investigator-initiated trials, do not accept the role of trial sponsor. Determination of which party provides clinical trial indemnity can often provide clarity about who is defined as the trial sponsor.

Intergroup Trials

Australia has a sound history of collaboration among research groups. Collaborations are frequently established between an Australian-based group or a joint Australian and New Zealand group (Australasian) and other international groups. Collaborations exist between many of the main tumor-specific NCCTGs in Australia (e.g., Australasian Gastro-Intestinal Trials Group) and established overseas groups (e.g., National Surgical Adjuvant Breast and Bowel Project [U.S.], NCIC Clinical Trials Group [Canada], European Organisation for Research and Treatment of Cancer [Belgium], Medical Research Council [United Kingdom]). International collaboration is essential to the success of clinical trials, permitting the generation of data that are generalizable across populations, as well as improved acceptance of the data for publication and changes in clinical practice (COSA, n.d.-a).

Standard Operating Procedures

ICH defines *standard operating procedures* (SOPs) as "detailed, written instructions to achieve uniformity of the performance of a specific function" (ICH, 1996, p. 8). In 2004, the COSA Clinical Research Professional Group (now known as CRPG) recognized the need for clinical units in Australia to have SOPs available when participating in clinical research. Many larger units in Australia have developed their own SOPs; however, smaller units with fewer resources experienced limited capacity to develop their own comprehensive SOPs, including a process for regular review and update of the SOPs. COSA purchased a set of Investigative Site SOPs from the Centre for Clinical Research Practice in 2004 and adapted them to the Australian Regulatory Environment. These are now available for purchase by COSA members. The advantages of these are that they are compliant with ICH good clinical practice and the U.S. Food and Drug Administration *Code of Federal Regulations*, and they are regularly reviewed and updated (COSA, n.d.-b).

Protocol Development, Review, and Approval

Informed Consent and Patient Recruitment

Patients are informed by their specialist physician of clinical trials available to them. However, increasingly, patients become aware of clinical trials through the media and Internet-based clinical trial registries and specifically seek out treatment at sites based on the institution's participation in clinical trials. State and national bodies, such as the state-based Cancer Councils, provide information about clinical trials and the benefits of participation. After the physician introduces a trial to a patient, specific information and education about the study are given both verbally and in writing. Although the format varies from site to site, all written participant information and consent forms are approved by HREC and are in accordance with elements outlined in ICH good clinical practice guidelines. All information provided to patients discusses the study treatment and other available options. Patients are advised of study results as they become available during the study period and after the conclusion of the study.

The research nurse plays a pivotal role throughout the informed consent process by acting as the primary contact for patients and communicating the study's requirements. Patients are then given time to consider participation, commensurate with the imperative to begin treatment in a timely manner as appropriate to both their condition and study protocol timelines. The informed consent process is ongoing from the initial visit until the study is concluded; however, patients are formally reconsented if adverse reactions, changes to the protocol, or interim results necessitate. This reconsent process is conducted verbally by the physician and in writing via an HREC-approved amended information and consent form.

Protocol Development and Response Assessment

In investigator-initiated trials, protocol development may occur at the site level, with the intention of running the trial as either a single institution trial or as a multicenter project. Protocols may be written by the investigator; however, the investigator may engage a number of team members to contribute to the protocol by providing their own specialist expertise (e.g., statistician, research nurse, data manager, pharmacist). A rigorous peer-review process of completed protocols is encouraged to elicit any constructive criticism and further development. Locally generated case report forms, which enable consistent data to be collected, are also developed for use with investigator-initiated trials.

For trials initiated under the auspices of an NCCTG, a central coordinating center may be designated where the protocol is developed by an operations team, usually a clinical trial manager in consultation with the principal investigator, key co-investigators, and the study statistician. Increasingly, draft proposals may be presented in a formal meeting of NCCTG members designed specifically to develop research in an efficient manner. The format of a protocol follows the elements outlined in ICH (1996) good clinical practice guidelines, with relevant SOPs followed.

Studies initiated by international groups often permit Australian contribution through an international steering committee to review the protocol before finalization. This consultation prevents initiating protocols that are not feasible because of differences in clinical practice and protocols between countries. For both local investigator–initiated and international studies, each collaborative group will scrutinize the protocol through scientific advisory committees to assess the scientific merit and feasibility of the protocol and provide feedback and commentary on the protocol design.

Protocol Considerations

Studies are considered by a site using set criteria, regardless of whether the study is investigator initiated, run by a cooperative group, or overseen by a pharmaceutical company. The protocol is reviewed by the site first to assess suitability for participation. Attention is paid to scientific rigor, patient population, eligibility criteria, competing studies, and the individual capabilities of the site to conduct and adhere to the specifics of the individual protocol and meet the required accrual target. Assessment of site resources and the trial budget are also considered before final agreement to participate is given.

With the new multicenter submission to a lead HREC, part of the assessment discussion with the sponsor when deciding to participate is the allocation of coordinating (lead) investigator/site. Once agreement to participate has been reached, the lead site prepares the HREC submission. This involves completion of a web-based National Ethics Application Form. This application form is mandatory for all multicenter research being conducted at public hospitals in Australia. Currently, the states of Queensland, NSW, and Victoria have ratified a mutual acceptance, whereby one National Ethics Application Form submission to a lead HREC covers all public sites within the states participating in the study. While this process is occurring, the non-lead sites are completing their site-specific assessment applications and preparing the regulatory documents required to finalize site governance approval.

When final HREC and site governance approval is attained and the required regulatory documentation is processed, the study may commence. The sponsor or investigator and research nurse conduct an on-site initiation. The site initiation includes communication and education about the conduct of the study to the relevant staff, including ward and outpatient direct care and treatment nurses and pharmacy, radiation therapy, laboratory, and imaging staff.

The research nurse is responsible for ensuring that the trial is conducted according to protocol. Information aids may be adapted from material provided by the sponsor or developed by the research nurse specific to the needs of the site. As the complexity of clinical trials has increased over time, a corresponding increased need to provide accurate and detailed instructions to site staff is necessary to ensure adherence to the protocol. Both site staff and protocol authors must pay specific attention to the effect of the study on the local indigenous (Aboriginal and Torres Strait Islander) population. The ways in which this population is affected vary widely, and consideration should be given to the six core values identified as being important to these communities: (a) reciprocity, (b) respect, (c) equality, (d) responsibility, (e) survival and protection, and (f) spirit and integrity (National Health and Medical Research Council [NHMRC], 2014).

Ethical Review and Site-Specific Assessment

Therapeutic Goods Administration legislation covers the ethical review of clinical trials in Australia. More than 200 HREC-based institutions and organizations across Australia are governed by the Australian Health Ethics Committee. The responsibilities of HRECs are outlined in the NHMRC National Statement on Ethical Conduct in Human Research (2014), which has also been adopted in Therapeutic Goods Administration legislation.

The ethical review process in Australia has been evolving over a number of years to streamline ethical review of multicenter research. The national approach, known as the Harmonisation of Multi-centre Ethical Review (HoMER), enables the recognition of a single ethical and scientific review of multicenter research within and across the states and territories (see Figure 45-1) (NHMRC, n.d.-a). All states and territories are at different stages of implementing their processes to accept single ethical review. The single ethical review considers if a project is scientifically and ethically acceptable and meets the requirements of the National Statement on Ethical Conduct in Human Research (NHMRC, 2014). Additionally, the process removes unnecessary duplication of ethical review for a research proposal at each participating institution (NHMRC, n.d.-b). A coordinating (lead) investigator is responsible for the preparation and submission of the research proposal and for communicating the outcome of the ethical review to other participating sites.

A second process called *site-specific assessment* has been developed in tandem to the single ethical review. The site-specific assessment application allows the public health organization to assess whether the project meets its research governance requirements. These requirements include consideration of the investigator's skills, training, and experience; availability and suitability of facilities; and available resources, such as funding, indemnity, and contractual arrangements. A site-specific assessment application must be made for each site at which the research is to be conducted; each application is assessed by the responsible Research Governance Office and considers matters pertinent to the organization rather than issues of scientific and ethical acceptability. Only when authorization to conduct the project has been received from the Research Governance Office may a project proceed. Consideration of the stage of implementation of the HoMER approach should be given to each state and territory as the process continues to roll out (NHMRC, n.d.-b).

Financial Factors

Workload Determination and Resource Allocation

Distribution of workload within a clinical trial unit is a continuing challenge for many units. Determining the level of work for a specific trial that addresses both the complexity and the frequency of specific tasks involved in a study to ensure that adequate resources are available remains a challenge. Research is limited in this area. The most promising research to date was developed by the Ontario Institute of Cancer Research. The Ontario Protocol Assessment Level (OPAL) tool provides clinical trial departments with an objective method of quantifying clinical trial activities on the basis of study protocol complexity (Smuck et al., 2011). OPAL scores can be used to provide (a) the number of cases managed per staff member, (b) the number of trials per staff member, (c) the total workload per staff member, (d) the ability to equalize or capture distribution of workload, and (e) objective data to assess the need for additional or reallocated resources. The next step would be to adapt and test this tool in the Australian environment.

Budget and Funding

During the early assessment of a new study protocol at a site, the site staff prepare a study budget based on estimated costs to conduct the study at the site. Generally, the budget provides an estimate of the accrual numbers anticipated during the life of the study and considers the complexity of study procedures and screening, as outlined in Figure 45-2.

The site must have sufficient funding and resources available to conduct and complete the study. Reimbursement of costs via per-patient payments is the usual method by which costs are recovered. Funding levels for clinical trials still vary greatly from study to study. Pharmaceutical company–supported trials generally provide sufficient funding to cover the conduct of the study at each site. However, cooperative group and investigator-initiated studies may be funded to a lesser degree. Associated costs are covered through in-kind use of resources to ensure these clinical trials are conducted

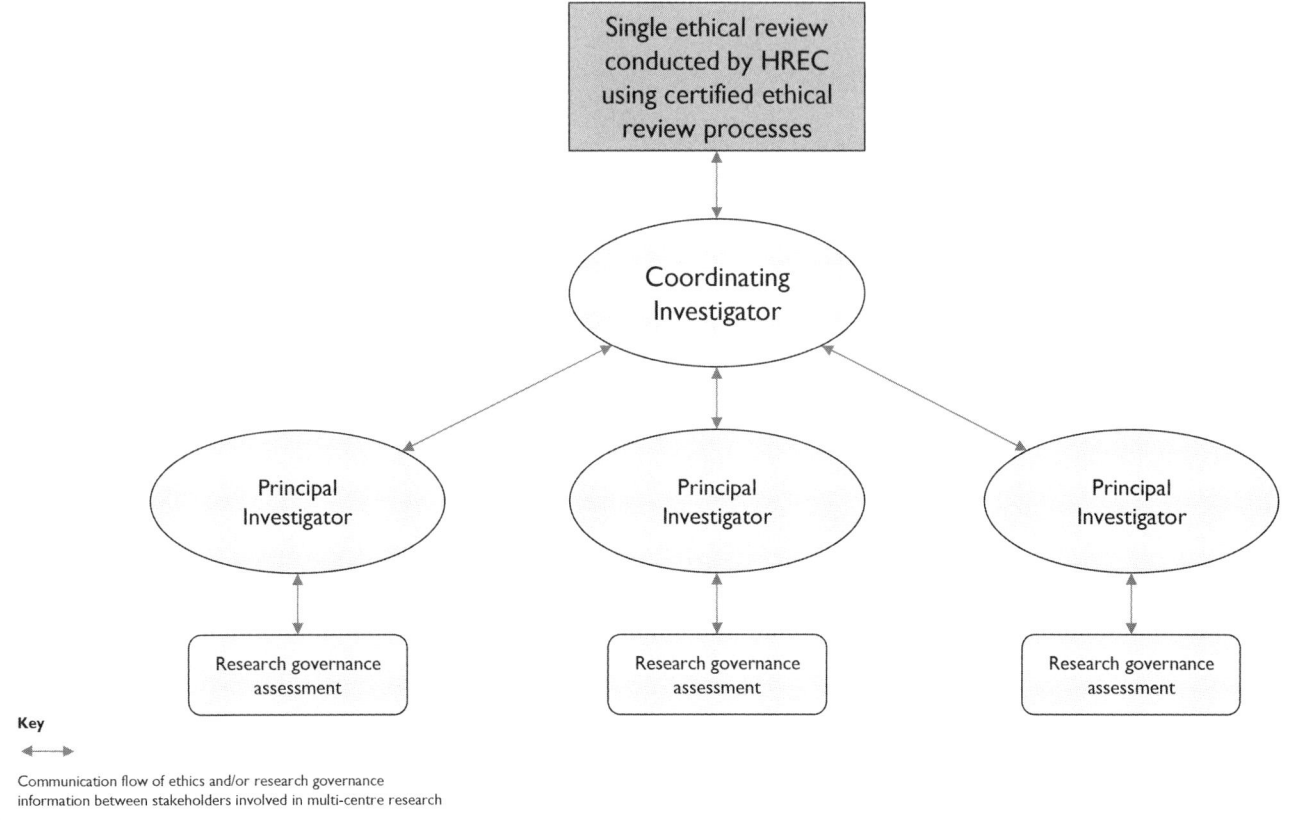

Figure 45-1. Single Ethical Review

- Coordinating Investigator (CI) submits an ethics application to one human research ethics committee (HREC) that is using certified ethical review processes.
- One HREC conducts an ethical review of the research proposal (i.e., single ethical review occurring for one research proposal).
- CI receives the response of one HREC.
- Principal investigators at each participating institution provide the outcome of the single ethical review to their respective institution.
- Each participating institution uses the outcome of the single ethical review and their site-specific research governance information to determine whether research will commence at their institution.

Key
←→ Communication flow of ethics and/or research governance information between stakeholders involved in multi-centre research

Note. From "What Is Meant by 'Single Ethical Review'?—Concept Diagram for Single Ethical Review," by National Health and Medical Research Council, n.d. Retrieved from http://hrep.nhmrc.gov.au/national-approach/single-ethical-review.

and patients gain access to a greater number of clinical trial options. With current economic constraints in health care, part of the decision whether to participate in a cooperative group– or investigator-initiated study involves the site assessing its capacity to provide these in-kind resources.

Figure 45-2. Considerations for a Clinical Trial Budget

- Actual cost of all procedures and tests
- Investigator and study coordinator time
- Additional investigator and study coordinator time if site is the lead site
- Collection and preparation of specimens for shipment to the central laboratory
- Administration costs of the study including overheads, which are payable to the hospital institution
- Other requirements as and when necessary

Studies conducted by cooperative groups usually require significantly greater funds to support the costs of the study at the central coordinating center. This ensures that study requirements are met and that the trial is run in accordance with ICH (1996) good clinical practice and local regulations. A budget is prepared based on projected costs of key trial activities such as resources and staff involved in project management, site management, data management, statistical analysis, and trial administration.

Following the development of a budget proposal, a number of factors will be considered as to where funding will be sought. For trials in which an international group or pharmaceutical company is involved, a per capita payment is often made based on patient recruitment. Pharmaceutical companies will often provide an educational grant to support the study conduct, as well as the provision of study agents, depending on the marketing status of the drug.

Where the trial has no direct involvement or relationship with external sponsors, funding is usually sought through grant funding bodies, such as NHMRC, the lead government-funded research body, or from charitable organizations. However, funding is allocated on a competitive basis against other applicants from a wide range of disciplines including basic science research. Co-funding can often be sought from funding bodies/nonprofit organizations to supplement income from sponsors or groups.

In Australia in 2010, COSA and NCCTG responded to growing concerns around the risks of conducting cancer clinical trials. COSA and NCCTG arranged an umbrella clinical trials insurance scheme for NCCTG-sponsored trials and developed the use of the Standard Clinical Trial Agreement for Collaborative (or cooperative) Research (COSA, n.d.-c).

Recruitment and Retention

Public and Patient Education

Provision of information to the public and patients about clinical trials is an important activity in which research nurses may engage. International Clinical Trials Day, celebrated on May 20 each year, provides research nurses with an opportunity to raise the profile of clinical trials in their workplace. Information for the public may include
- What a clinical trial is
- Why clinical trials are important
- Where to find information about clinical trials
- Improvements in health care generated by clinical trials
- Reasons to participate in a clinical trial.

Accrual Base, Recruitment, and Promotion Strategies

Successful clinical trial accrual depends on teamwork, open communication, and collaboration. Effective resource management is important to ensure staff is available to identify potential participants. Opportunities to identify the accrual base, enhance recruitment, and promote new and ongoing clinical trials include screening of clinic lists, participation in multidisciplinary team meetings, patient database searches, and regular research meetings. Clinical trials may be promoted in other ways depending on the nature of the HREC approval sought for advertising through a variety of media, including social media, such as Facebook.

Adherence and Retention

Research nurses and members of the research team must adequately assess potential participants for their ability to adhere to the study requirements. This may include assessing patients' capacity to adhere to clinical trial protocol procedures, such as attending the clinic for review, assessment, treatment, follow-up, and safety assessments. It should also include assessment of adherence to medication schedules. A variety of strategies, including tablet counts, questionnaires, and plasma drug levels, are frequently included in clinical trial protocols to assess participants' adherence to medication schedules (Warren et al., 2011).

The protocol usually specifies the follow-up intervals and duration. Treatment of cancer is becoming more successful with the diagnosis of cancer occurring earlier, and as such, the period of follow-up is increasing in duration. Monitoring patients over long periods of time is complex, and research nurses have an important role in participant retention by ensuring contact is maintained with patients at specified intervals and that they do not become lost to follow-up. Deteriorating levels of health and the remoteness of parts of Australia add additional challenges to maintaining patient contact during the follow-up period.

During follow-up, ensuring patients' ongoing consent to participate is important. Toxicities and side effects that occurred during treatment continue to be monitored and treated, as well as any other issues identified during the treatment period. Any SAEs continue to be reported to HREC and the sponsor, usually until 30 days following the last dose of study drug or as dictated by the protocol. Many adjuvant studies now have long-term side effects of interest, such as cardiac toxicity, that are monitored for many years after the last dose of study drug.

Clinical Trial Registries

In 2004, the International Committee of Medical Journal Editors, which includes editors of the *Medical Journal of Australia*, *Lancet*, and *The New England Journal of Medicine*, mandated the registration of clinical trials at inception in an authorized registry as a condition necessary for their review of clinical trials for publication (De Angelis et al., 2004). The World Health Organization (n.d.) International Clinical Trials Registry Platform ensures that a comprehensive overview of research is available to those involved in healthcare decision making. Registration of clinical trials is a scientific, ethical, and moral responsibility (World Health Organization, n.d.).

The Australian New Zealand Clinical Trials Registry (2007) was established in 2005 to assist patients and health practitioners with access to information about trials, covering the full range of therapeutic trials, including cancer trials. This is an important resource that assists cancer research nurses in providing patients with accurate information about ongoing and planned clinical trials. The Australian New Zealand Clinical Trials Registry (2007) is consistent with the requirements set out by

Clinical Trial Participants

Eligibility

Eligibility criteria are clearly defined within each protocol, and the research nurse, in collaboration with the physician, is responsible for patient assessment and ensuring eligibility criteria are followed. Eligibility criteria may dictate the need for specific assessments and the time frames in which they are to be conducted. The research nurse, in consultation with the patient and the physician, coordinates these assessments as required.

Patients are assessed by the research nurse for their personal capacity to manage and adhere to the often rigorous responsibilities that are associated with study participation, such as self-administration of treatments and the use of new technologies (e.g., electronic communication devices, infusion devices).

The research team and patient must consider the ability of the site and the patient to meet the study requirements, particularly in a geographically diverse country such as Australia. Patients may be required to travel great distances to receive specialized cancer treatments. Additional travel, as a consequence of participation in a clinical study, may place an undue or unnecessary burden on patients and their caregivers. This is an important consideration for patients being assessed for participation in a study involving multiple visits for pharmacokinetics or prolonged treatment periods. A number of satellite centers or regional clinics now exist with clinical trial physicians and research nurses either on-site or visiting from comprehensive cancer centers. This permits improved patient access to new medicines or therapies and ensures adequate monitoring and follow-up.

Careful planning and effective communication by the research nurse and physician with patients, site staff, and sponsors are required to ensure that eligibility criteria are met and diagnostic assessments are conducted within the limits specified in the protocol. Time zone differences and public holidays may prove to be problematic when coordinating eligibility and randomization; thus, particular care needs to be taken to consider and overcome these obstacles.

Investigational Agents: Procurement, Administration, and Accountability of Research Study Drugs

The hospital pharmacist is generally responsible for the procurement, storage, disposal, and security of investigational agents. Sophisticated systems for ensuring that sufficient investigational agents are available at the site have been developed and are generally monitored by the pharmacist. The storage of investigational agents in a secure environment is important, as is storing agents as specified in the protocol; this may include a monitored temperature-controlled environment. The pharmacist is responsible for the correct preparation of investigational cytotoxic agents and any placebos that may be used during the study. The pharmacist is also responsible for the correct documentation of the treatment in the study pharmacy manual. The treatment nurse (who in some instances may be the research nurse) is responsible for the correct administration of the treatment, as per the protocol, including appropriate monitoring of the patient before, during, and after the treatment as specified in the protocol. The research nurse is usually responsible for ensuring the treatment nurse has been trained in the administration of the new trial drug and understands the required patient monitoring for the particular protocol treatment.

Adverse Events

Adverse events or toxicities of the treatment are assessed at intervals prescribed in the protocol; however, more frequent assessment may be warranted if a patient experiences significant toxicities or an SAE occurs. Cancer protocols generally use the National Cancer Institute Cancer Therapy Evaluation Program (2010) Common Terminology Criteria for Adverse Events for the evaluation and grading of toxicities.

Appropriate baseline documentation of disease signs and symptoms and any ongoing toxicities or side effects from any prior treatments are important to clearly differentiate between new and old toxicities or side effects. Continuing patient and caregiver education promotes understanding of the importance of prompt reporting of new events, so that the appropriate toxicity intervention can be implemented.

SAEs *must* be reported to the sponsor and the HREC per local requirements within 24 hours of the site becoming aware of the event. The research nurse is responsible for ensuring the appropriate documentation is prepared and forwarded to the sponsor or local HREC.

Patient, Family, and Staff Education

Although the role of the research nurse varies among sites, three major functions are generally fulfilled:
- As a *specialist nurse* available to discuss problems and side effects with the patient, caregiver, and other team members
- As a *support nurse* for the patient, caregivers, and other team members, ensuring that the appropriate resources (physical, emotional, psychological, informational, and educational) are available throughout the duration of the study. This role extends to that of a *tele-*

phone clinic where patients are encouraged to consult the nurse between visits.
- As an *educator*, which includes educating patients about the trial in which they are to participate, including potential side effects from and the management and education of the direct care and treatment nurses on clinical research, new studies, and treatments.

Psychosocial Distress

The research nurse, in consultation with the principal investigator, is responsible for ensuring that the patient continues to be eligible to receive study treatment as dictated by the protocol. Any change in disease status or physical and psychosocial well-being of the patient should be considered within the context of the protocol, treatment modifications or delays specified, or criteria outlined for withdrawal from treatment. Psychosocial issues are increasingly assessed via a variety of validated self-reporting tools that evaluate a range of physical and psychosocial issues. The research nurse and other health professionals work together with the patient, using a variety of methods and assessments to ensure that both the physical and psychosocial needs of the patient are met (Lee, Katona, DeBono, & Lewis, 2010; NHMRC, 2012, 2014; Smuck et al., 2011).

Genetics and Genomics

Pharmacogenetics and Pharmacogenomics

Interest in incorporating pharmacogenetic and pharmacogenomic studies with cancer clinical trials is rapidly evolving. These studies include analyses of biospecimens, tissue, or blood and allow correlation of clinical outcomes with biomarkers that may predict response to treatment or provide prognostic information. Informed consent of patients participating in this type of research is important and should include specific information about protection of privacy, sample storage, sample use, and any limitations on future research (Kronenthal, Delany, & Christman, 2012).

COSA and NCCTG have been working toward a national coordinated approach to biobanking in Australia to achieve the following objectives:
- Improve the quality and efficiency of research through access to a larger bank of biospecimens, increased quality of samples, and economies of scale
- Improve availability of research funding and clinical trial activity as a consequence of improved infrastructure and research quality
- Improve economic benefits flowing from reduced expenditure on inefficient treatments and streamlined approaches to clinical trial activity.

Common issues still arise surrounding the implementation of pharmacogenetic and pharmacogenomic research. Those occurring most frequently include the following.
- Research and testing is dependent on a sufficient tissue supply available to researchers after use of available tissues has been used for diagnostic purposes.
- Collection, processing, and storage of tissue samples for use in clinical trials and subsequent retrieval of samples requires considerable research nurse effort and expertise.
- Sites undertaking this type of research require adequate resources to collect and store tissue. Resources may include centrifuge and research-specific freezers and refrigeration.
- The costs of sample collection, storage, and retrieval are not commonly factored into cost models. The cost of undertaking this type of research can be expensive with third-party providers imposing costs for the retrieval and processing of samples (COSA, 2010).

Correlative Trials

Pharmacokinetic Studies

Pharmacokinetic studies are routine in cancer clinical research. Many studies evaluating new investigational agents include a pharmacokinetic component to evaluate their absorption, distribution, metabolism, and excretion. These studies may be an optional part of the trial protocol, but increasingly, they are a mandatory part of the trial protocol. The research nurse must be familiar with the requirements for collection, processing, and storage of pharmacokinetic samples and may need to provide education to patients and other members of the trial and treatment team to ensure protocol compliance.

Companion Studies

Companion studies are increasingly included as components of clinical studies. Many clinical studies include a method of evaluating patients' quality of life during treatment. Normally, patients complete a questionnaire at regular intervals during and after the trial. However, quality-of-life components are becoming more complex, involving frequent measurements recorded by patients using devices such as a PDA that transmits data electronically from patients' homes to the site.

Patients may elect to participate in other companion protocols as an *optional extra*, which may include pharmacoeconomic protocols involving the collection of data associated with the use of health-related resources such as visits to the general practitioner or home health care. Research nurses provide patients with additional education and information to ensure that they understand the nature of the questions, can answer appropriately, and are able to use the PDA equipment as required.

Nursing companion studies may be an additional component of a clinical protocol, conducted prospectively with the main clinical trial. Types of nursing companion studies may include the evaluation of treatment effects, symptoms, cancer control, prevention, and rehabilitation. The companion study is usually developed from the main trial but seeks to answer a specific nursing question.

Documentation and Data Management

Historically, the research nurse recorded data on paper case report forms. More frequently today, however, computer- or Internet-based forms are being used as a means of recording and transmitting data in a timely and efficient fashion to the sponsor. This change is reflected in the way the site and sponsor communicate. Communicating information regarding the study, including site activation, randomization, patient treatment, and patient discontinuation, with the study sponsor via phone or post has largely been replaced by electronic methods, including interactive voice or web-based response system, email, and the Internet. Many studies provide all their safety information via dedicated web portals, further reducing the need for paper.

The research nurse is responsible for the accurate documentation of data in the case report form as acquired from the source documentation. It is important that the source documentation is comprehensive and accurately reflects the patients' experiences while they are participating in the study. The research nurse plays a vital role in ensuring that all team members understand what information is required for the study and that data are collected and documented as specified in the protocol. The research nurse is responsible for assessing, screening, monitoring, and reporting patient data throughout a trial.

Many research units in Australia now have a mixture of research nurses, clinical trial coordinators, and data managers. Depending on how the work is distributed, the nurse may be less involved in the actual case report form completion, which puts greater importance on accurate source documentation and effective communication within the research team.

Professional Development

Research is a rapidly evolving field of cancer care inclusive of advancing treatment technologies and increasing legal and ethical considerations. These developments place an imperative on the research nurse to keep abreast of changes that are integral to successful implementation of clinical studies (Wilkes, Jackson, Miranda, & Watson, 2012). Australian clinical trial nurses have a varied role, including activities related to clinical management of trial participants and protocol management.

Opportunities for professional development are important to the development of research nurses and their roles in cancer care today. The variety of professional development opportunities necessitate that the research nurses carefully select the most advantageous experience to advance and maintain their knowledge bases.

CNSA and COSA conduct annual meetings that address aspects important to the continuing education and development of research nurses in cancer care in Australia. Many other opportunities exist through tertiary courses; international avenues such as the Oncology Nursing Society, the Canadian Association of Nurses in Oncology, and the International Society of Nurses in Cancer Care; and sponsor-driven events specific to clinical studies.

Many tumor-specific cooperative groups, such as the Australian New Zealand Gynaecological Oncology Group, Australian New Zealand Breast Cancer Trial Group, and Australasian Gastro-Intestinal Trials Group, have recognized the need for ongoing education of research staff in the changing research environment and have incorporated preconference workshops as part of their annual scientific meetings to provide this education.

Research nurses are ideally placed to share and disseminate relevant information with the wider cancer care team at their institutions, ensuring that optimal conditions exist to provide the best possible outcomes for patients participating in clinical studies and for the sponsors.

Summary

Cancer clinical trials are important and integral to the care of people with cancer in Australia. Although significant change to the regulatory landscape of clinical research in Australia has occurred, research nurses continue to work closely with the research team to ensure patient safety, consent, and treatment, maintain the integrity of the protocol, and meet all regulatory requirements.

Key Points
- Australia has a vibrant cancer research community.
- Clinical research nurses are integral to cancer clinical research in Australia.
- The clinical research nurse in Australia has a key role as specialist nurse, support nurse, and educator.

- HoMER enables the recognition of a single ethical and scientific review of multicenter research within and across the states and territories of Australia.
- Clinical research nurses should be aware of the changes to the regulatory process resulting from the HoMER approach.

References

Australasian Health and Research Data Managers Association. (2005). Welcome. Retrieved from http://www.ahrdma.com.au

Australian New Zealand Clinical Trials Registry. (2007). Frequently asked questions. Retrieved from http://www.anzctr.org.au/Faq.aspx

Cancer Australia. (2012). Funding for cancer clinical trials. Retrieved from http://canceraustralia.gov.au/research-data/support-clinical-trials/funding-cancer-clinical-trials

Cancer Australia. (2013a). National cancer cooperative trials groups. Retrieved from http://canceraustralia.gov.au/research-data/support-clinical-trials/multi-site-collaborative-national-cancer-clinical

Cancer Australia. (2013b). National technical services for cooperative trials groups. Retrieved from http://canceraustralia.gov.au/research-data/support-clinical-trials/centralised-services-clinical-trials-groups

Cancer Institute NSW. (2011). NSW Cancer Research Achievements Report 2011. Retrieved from http://www.cancerinstitute.org.au/media/125925/research-achievements-report-2011.pdf

Cancer Nurses Society of Australia. (n.d.). Research committee. Retrieved from http://www.cnsa.org.au/about-us/research

Clinical Oncology Society of Australia. (n.d.-a). Cancer biology. Retrieved from https://www.cosa.org.au/groups/cancer-biology/about.aspx

Clinical Oncology Society of Australia. (n.d.-b). Clinical trials research professionals. Retrieved from https://www.cosa.org.au/groups/clinical-trials-research-professionals/about.aspx

Clinical Oncology Society of Australia. (n.d.-c). Frequently asked questions. Retrieved from https://www.cosa.org.au/about-us/faqs.aspx

Clinical Oncology Society of Australia. (n.d.-d). Select a group. Retrieved from https://www.cosa.org.au/groups.aspx

Clinical Oncology Society of Australia. (2010). Developing a nationally coordinated approach to biobanking for Cancer Clinical Trials in Australia. Retrieved from https://www.cosa.org.au/media/1050/cosa_report_developing-a-nationally-coordinated-approach-to-biobanking_2010.pdf

Clinical Oncology Society of Australia. (2012). History. Retrieved from https://www.cosa.org.au/about-us/history.aspx

De Angelis, C., Drazen, J.M., Frizelle, F.A., Haug, C., Hoey, J., Horton, F., … Van Der Weyden, M.B. (2004). Clinical trial registration: A statement from the International Committee of Medical Journal Editors. *New England Journal of Medicine, 351,* 1250–1251. doi:10.1056/NEJMe048225

International Conference on Harmonisation of Technical Requirements for Registration of Pharmaceuticals for Human Use. (1996, June 10). *ICH harmonised tripartite guideline: Guideline for good clinical practice, E6(R1).* Retrieved from http://www.ich.org/fileadmin/Public_Web_Site/ICH_Products/Guidelines/Efficacy/E6/E6_R1_Guideline.pdf

Kronenthal, C., Delaney, S.K., & Christman, M.F. (2012). Broadening research consent in the era of genome-informed medicine. *Genetics in Medicine, 14,* 432–436. doi:10.1038gim2011.76

Lee, S.J., Katona, L.J., DeBono, S.E., & Lewis, K.L. (2010). Routine screening for psychological distress on an Australian inpatient haematology and oncology ward: Impact on use of psychosocial services. *Medical Journal of Australia, 193*(Suppl. 5), S74–S78. Retrieved from https://www.mja.com.au/journal/2010/193/5/routine-screening-psychological-distress-australian-inpatient-haematology-and

National Cancer Institute Cancer Therapy Evaluation Program. (2010). *Common terminology criteria for adverse events* [v.4.03]. Retrieved from http://evs.nci.nih.gov/ftp1/CTCAE/CTCAE_4.03_2010-06-14_QuickReference_8.5x11.pdf

National Health and Medical Research Council. (n.d.-a). Concept diagram single ethical review. Retrieved from http://hrep.nhmrc.gov.au/_uploads/files/concept_diagram_single_ethical_review_0.pdf

National Health and Medical Research Council. (n.d.-b). National approach to single ethical review. Retrieved from http://www.nhmrc.gov.au/health-ethics/national-approach-single-ethical-review

National Health and Medical Research Council. (2012, January). Framework for monitoring: Guidance for the national approach to single ethical review of multi-centre research. Retrieved from http://hrep.nhmrc.gov.au/_uploads/files/Framework_for_Monitoring.pdf

National Health and Medical Research Council. (2014, March). *National statement on ethical conduct in human research.* Retrieved from http://www.nhmrc.gov.au/_files_nhmrc/publications/attachments/e72_national_statement_march_2014_140331.pdf

Smuck, B., Bettello, P., Berghout, K., Hanna, T., Kowaleski, B., Phippard, L., … Friel, K. (2011). Ontario Protocol Assessment Level: Clinical trial complexity rating tool for workload planning in oncology clinical trials. *Journal of Oncology Practice, 7,* 80–84. doi:10.1200/JOP.2010.000051

Therapeutic Goods Act of 1989, Act No. 21–62 (2014). Retrieved from http://www.comlaw.gov.au/Details/C2014C00410

Therapeutic Goods Administration. (n.d.). Clinical trials forms. Retrieved from http://www.tga.gov.au/industry/clinical-trials.htm#forms

Therapeutic Goods Administration. (2004, October 1). Access to unapproved therapeutic goods—Clinical trials in Australia. Retrieved from http://www.tga.gov.au/industry/clinical-trials-guidelines.htm#.U-PbfuNdV8E

Warren, S.R., Raisch, D.W., Campbell, H.M., Guarino, P.D., Kaufman, J.S., Petrokaitis, E., … Jamison, R.L. (2013). Medication adherence assessment in a clinical trial with centralized follow-up and direct-to-patient drug shipments. *Clinical Trials, 10,* 441–448. doi:10.1177/1740774511410331

Wilkes, L., Jackson, D., Miranda, C., & Watson, R. (2012). The role of clinical trial nurses: An Australian perspective. *Collegian, 19,* 239–246. doi:10.1016/j.colegn.2012.02.005

World Health Organization. (n.d.). International Clinical Trials Registry Platform (ICTRP). Retrieved from http://www.who.int/ictrp/en

Chapter 46

Austria

Regina Berger, PhD, SC

Introduction

In Austria, approximately 38,000 people are diagnosed with cancer per year (Zielonke, 2014). When comparing the available data from 1990 to 2011, a reduction of the risk to develop cancer as well as an increase of the survival rate can be seen. Furthermore, in 2011, the number of newly diagnosed malignancies decreased by 3% compared to 2010. However, incidences for breast and prostate cancers, the most prominent cancers in women and men in Austria, respectively, have been increasing since 1992. This is attributed mainly to better and increased screening and early detection programs ("screening effect"). The numbers of newly diagnosed patients began to decrease again in 2002 (Zielonke, 2014).

Today, many patients with cancer live longer and better. Five-year overall survival rates of patients with cancer have increased from 45% in 1987 to 61% in 2007 (Zielonke, 2010). This is a result of the improved modes of treatment and earlier detection through screening programs. Physicians now treat side effects of cancer drugs better and fight tumor growth much more efficiently than in the past. This encouraging development would not be possible without the results of clinical trials, through which new insights into tumor development, growth, and treatment are gained.

but also initiating, multicenter, multinational cancer trials to gain insight into the treatment of cancer. This is not only to serve the physicians in playing an active role in cancer research but also to increase patient survival while improving quality of life. It has been shown that patients who participate in clinical trials benefit from better therapies (Janni et al., 2005) and experience higher survival rates (du Bois, 2002; Peppercorn, Weeks, Cook, & Joffe, 2004) compared to patients not participating in clinical trials.

Austria is in the lucky position of having a very good healthcare system that guarantees healthcare services for all residents, and all treatments for patients with cancer are provided free of charge. In light of this, it is surprising that many patients are participating in clinical trials, proving that physicians and patients in Austria are aware of their importance. To aid in the conduct of these trials, several academic trial centers have been established in recent years.

In Austria, not only national trials are conducted but also many multinational, multicenter clinical trials in cooperation with international partners. For example, the AGO-Austria study group is conducting gynecologic trials in collaboration with the European Organisation for Research and Treatment of Cancer, the European Network of Gynaecological Oncology Trial Groups, and the Gynecologic Cancer InterGroup.

History and Foundation

Austria has a long history of performing clinical trials. For example, the Austrian Breast and Colorectal Cancer Study Group has conducted clinical trials in cancer for almost 30 years. In more recent years, Austrian oncology centers are not only participating in,

Clinical Trials: Fundamental Information

Only with the evidence from clinical trials is it possible to find and implement new drugs and treatment options and improve outcomes for patients with cancer. The legal basis for clinical trials in Austria is

The author would like to acknowledge Johanna Ulmer, PhD, SC, for her contribution to this chapter that remains unchanged from the previous edition of this book.

the Clinical Trials Directive 2001/20/EG (Commission Directive 2001/20/EG, 2001), which was implemented into national legislation in 2004. All trials initiated after this implementation have been performed according to Austrian pharmaceutical legislation (AMG; BGBl. Nr. 85/1983). Trials started before this implementation are allowed to be conducted according to the previously applicable regulations. Figure 46-1 lists some helpful websites that contain information regarding setting up and running a clinical trial in Austria.

Protocol Development, Review, and Approval

Any new cancer trials can be proposed by individual investigators, universities, hospitals, research groups, and pharmaceutical companies. The ideas will often arise from outcomes of previous studies or could be a novel concept, which then will be discussed internally at the individual center or within the study group. During such meetings, the scientific impact of the proposed trial will be discussed and input provided for the protocol, feasibility, and any other aspect of the trial. Any participating centers will voice their interest in participation during such meetings.

For the development of academic clinical trials, the protocol, which usually is drafted by the lead clinician, should be peer reviewed. It is recommended that study offices or clinical trial centers (CTCs) are involved in the development of the protocol itself, as well as biostatisticians, data managers, and clinical trial professionals. Because medical universities in Austria encourage physicians to further scientific progress, several CTCs have been established to support investigators in the ever-increasing complexity of the development and conduct of clinical trials.

This review process helps not only the investigator in generating a complete protocol according to the essential protocol elements as outlined in GCP but also ensures that all legal and ethical requirements are met. Furthermore, the study office or CTCs can support the investigators in grant applications, case report form development, and other trial-related issues.

Approval Processes

All clinical trials in Austria are conducted according to the Declaration of Helsinki and the International Conference on Harmonisation of Technical Requirements for Registration of Pharmaceuticals for Human Use (ICH) good clinical practice (GCP) guidelines (ICH, 1996). The legal regulations for clinical trials consist of national legislation, which includes the Austrian Pharmaceuticals Law (Arzneimittelgesetz, AMG) and the Austrian Medical Device Act (Medizinproduktegesetz, MPG). The AMG governs all fundamental prerequisites under which a clinical trial with pharmaceutical products being tested can be carried out, and the MPG regulates clinical study pertaining to medicinal products.

Data protection is regulated through national law (Datenschutzgesetz 2000), which is in parallel to the medical confidentiality ordinance through which patient information can only be collected and recorded in an anonymized form. Locally, the conduct of a clinical trial is regulated through the Krankenanstaltengesetz, the legislature pertaining to medical institutions.

Internationally, the ICH GCP guidelines govern the standardized conduct of clinical trials, consisting of standard operating procedures for the planning, conduct, and evaluation of clinical trials. Each clinical trial has to undergo several approval processes in Austria.

An approval from an ethics committee (EC) has to be obtained for every clinical trial. Austria has 27 ECs, which all have about the same requirements for documents but differ in the submission guidelines. Some accept online or digital submissions, whereas others still require multiple printed copies of documents. The requirements can be found on the websites of most ECs.

According to the AMG, a lead EC can grant approval in multicenter trials (see Figure 46-2). The lead EC is usually the committee responsible for the institution of the coordinating investigator for the trial in Austria. All

---

Figure 46-1. Useful Websites

Austrian Agency for Health and Food Safety: www.ages.at/en/startseite
Austrian Federal Office for Safety in Health Care: www.basg.gv.at/en/basg-austrian-federal-office-for-safety-in-health-care
Austrian Research Promotion Agency (FFG): www.ffg.at/en
European Medicines Agency (ICH-GCP Guidelines, regulatory information, documents): www.emea.europa.eu/ema/
Forum of Austrian Ethics Committees: www.ethikkommissionen.at
Forum Study Nurses and Coordinators in Austria: www.studynurses.at
Legal information System of the Republic of Austria; Bundesgesetzblaetter: www.ris.bka.gv.at
Medical University Graz: www.medunigraz.at
Medical University Innsbruck: www.i-med.ac.at/mypoint
Medical University Vienna: www.meduniwien.ac.at/homepage

Figure 46-2. Ethics Committees in Austria as Lead Ethics Committees
Ethics Committee of the City of Vienna: www.wien.gv.at/gesundheit/strukturen/ethikkommission **Ethics Committee of the County of Niederöesterreich:** www.noel.gv.at/ethikkommission **Ethics Committee of the County of Oberöesterreich:** http://ooe-ethikkommission.at **Ethics Committee of the County of Salzburg:** www.salzburg.gv.at/ethikkommission **Ethics Committee of the Medical University of Graz:** www.medunigraz.at/ethikkommission/Graz **Ethics Committee of the Medical University of Innsbruck:** www.i-med.ac.at/ethikkommission **Ethics Committee of the Medical University of Vienna:** http://ethikkommission.meduniwien.ac.at **Forum Ethics Commissions in Austria:** www.ethikkommissionen.at

other relevant ECs are informed of submissions to the lead EC; however, this application should be simultaneous, with ample time (usually three weeks) for communication between the lead and all other ECs. An approval by the lead EC is valid for all other participating trial center ECs.

If a clinical trial is regulated under the AMG, a submission for approval at the competent authority, the Austrian Federal Office for Safety in Health Care (BASG), is required. This can only be done after a EudraCT number has been obtained and the application to the EC has been submitted. A list of the required documents can be found on the BASG website. If no further notification or query is issued by the BASG within 35 days after submission of the required documents, the application is considered approved.

Clinical trials with medicinal products need to be entered into the Eudamed Database by the competent authority, which in Austria is the BASG. In order for the competent authority to be able to do so, the trial has to be reported to BASG by the principal investigator or sponsor using the provided and required documents.

Before initiation of a trial at a clinic or hospital, the institution has to be notified and the trial reported. Unfortunately, the report procedures are not standardized throughout Austria and are different for each institution. One medical directorate board might need only an informal document, whereas others require specific documents. Some institutions are informed directly through the ECs and do not require further actions through the sponsor or investigator.

Furthermore, all three Medical Universities of Austria require the approval of the university legal and financial departments. Only after a favorable approval has been obtained from all responsible bodies may a clinical trial be initiated at a participating trial center.

Financial Factors

Clinical trials are becoming more expensive, in part due to the increased administrative burden. It is almost unfeasible for an investigator alone to conduct an investigator-driven trial at his or her center, although some small centers in Austria are still participating in clinical trials without any support from a study nurse or study coordinator. The author believes that help of a student or at least a part-time study nurse is required for proper documentation of the trial and to ensure qualitative high-quality results. However, most medical centers are reducing staff in order to save money and more hospitals are starting to collect an overhead of incoming money for the conduct of trials. This often results in limited financial resources for the investigator conducting a clinical trial.

The investigator is responsible for ensuring a trial will have adequate funding for proper conduct. A financial plan is needed, and all necessary contracts should be drawn up before the start of any trial. When conducting a trial through a pharmaceutical company, all involved departments will collect money for any study-specific duties. These earned overheads are intended to support academic clinical trials and investigator-driven trials by covering the resulting costs, although the institution usually does not charge administrative fees.

For academic clinical trials, financial support can be provided by pharmaceutical companies or funded by government-supported grants and funding (e.g., Fond zur Förderung der wissenschaftlichen Forschung, Forschungsförderung Gesellschaft, Österreichische National Bank). However, the chances of grant approval in Austria are rather low because of the large number of applications.

Recruitment and Retention

Clinical trials are promoted mostly through investigators and delegates of clinical trial groups who are informed during local and international meetings, conferences, and congresses. Patient recruitment, on the other hand, is almost never done through advertisement but mostly through information by the treating physician or investigator.

On the local level, the larger hospitals in Austria have tumor boards where patients with newly diagnosed or recurrent cancer will be discussed by an interdisciplinary panel of oncology specialists. In such board meetings, usually a representative of the clinical trial study team, including study nurses and physicians, will be present and can suggest specific trials that are open for recruitment at the center. If the patient meets all eligibility criteria, he or she can then be informed about possible participation in a trial by an authorized and trained trials physician. In hospitals where no tumors boards are in place, it is the responsibility of the individual physicians and clinical trial personnel to know about clinical trials open for recruitment and of possible patients to be included in the studies. In any case, cancer trial groups will inform all members of ongoing, opened, or planned trials in newsletters and during conferences, congresses, or meetings.

Patient retention in the study is a joint effort of the physician and the clinical trial staff at each participating site. Usually, the patient will be informed of future visits or examination dates during the current visit. Because control visits for illnesses are covered by public health insurance in Austria, usually the financial aspect is not a problem in losing patients to follow-up. In order for physicians to remember about trials in the follow-up phase, a clinical trials office or the clinical trials group might support and prompt the centers by sending frequent newsletters and reminders.

Clinical Trial Participants

Depending on the trial and the participating center, the clinical trial study team usually consists of at least a principal investigator, subinvestigator(s), and ideally, a study nurse. Depending on the setup, a study coordinator, research nurse, pharmacist, laboratory personnel, radiologist, pathologist, and other specialists also may be needed. All members of the team should have in-depth knowledge of the clinical trial and certified training in GCP.

The core clinical trial team usually has the following tasks and obligations:
- The *principal investigator* designates the subinvestigators and defines which responsibilities are allowed to be carried out by the individual study team members. The principal investigator is responsible for the entire conduct of the trial, including assessment of adverse events and the safety of the study participants in general. In noncommercial clinical trials, the principal investigator is also responsible for sponsor-related duties as defined in ICH GCP guidelines.
- *Medical students* are often part of the clinical trial team. They usually aid in data entry and other duties that are not in direct patient contact. This gives investigators the opportunity to receive help from educated individuals, and students can obtain firsthand experiences in clinical research.
- *Study coordinators* and administrative assistants assist the principal investigator in all administrative duties, including contract negotiations, financial plan development, monitoring visits, data collection, and, if applicable, submissions to regulatory authority, competent authority, and EC; these might be responsibilities

for study nurses as well. Detailed knowledge of rules and regulations pertaining to clinical trials, participation in national and international meetings, and constant retraining are requirements for successful work in clinical trials.

Genetics and Genomics

Since predictive genetic diagnostics has been proved to be an important factor in the treatment and diagnosis of certain cancer entities (e.g., *BRCA1* and *BRCA2* for breast cancer [Maxwell & Domchek, 2012]), it is becoming increasingly important to account for genetic research in clinical trials to identify possible new directions for cancer prevention (Umar, Dunn, & Greenwald, 2012).

The future of cancer research and treatment is hypothesized to be in personalized medicine (Yusuf, Wittes, Probstfield, & Tyroler, 1991; Ziegler, Koch, Krockenberger, & Großhennig, 2012). But to enable such research, it is important that during prospective trials patients' biologic samples are collected. This is an issue enthusiastically discussed within the scientific community of Austria. Many hospitals have started to establish biobanks in order to be able to meet the demand for clinical samples for genetic and genomic testing.

Legally, genetic testing and genomics are regulated in Austria in the Gentechnikgesetz 73/1988. Any manipulation of the DNA or genes in germ-line cells is prohibited (§ 9 Abs. 2 Fortpflanzungsgesetz). Genetic analysis of predisposition for any malignancy can only be done after approval of the EC and signing of an informed consent by the patient. Retrospective analysis can be performed only on anonymized samples. Several kinds of predictive testing are possible (see Figure 46-3).

Correlative Trials

Clinical trials not only provide the opportunity to answer questions about the effectiveness of new treat-

---

Figure 46-3. Predisposition Testing

Predictive testing: to diagnose a predisposition for a malignancy long before the actual outbreak of the disease
- Heterozygote testing/screening program: Testing for inherited diseases
- Pharmacogenetic testing: Tolerability and compatibility of certain medications
- Susceptibility testing: Genetic predisposition for drug compatibility
- Screening: Where larger populations are tested for genetic variations or changes

ment options but also the opportunity for additional companion research. Such additional research studies, also called *substudies*, usually involve the collection of biologic samples such as blood, serum, urine, tumor cells, or other tissue specimens before, during, or after treatment of the clinical trial participant. The molecular characteristics of tumor specimens collected during a trial will then be analyzed to see if a relationship exists between the presence of a certain gene mutation or the amount of a specific protein. It is also possible that an evaluation of trial participants' responses to the treatment they received will be done by measuring the amount of the expression of certain genes.

Information obtained from these types of studies could lead to more accurate predictions about how individual patients will respond to cancer treatments. It can improve methods of detecting cancer earlier or establish new methods of identifying people who have an increased risk of cancer, as well as find new approaches in cancer prevention. However, often only larger centers have the resources and equipment necessary to be able to participate in such additional studies.

Other noninvasive substudies, such as quality-of-life (QOL) or patient-reported outcome questionnaires, examine issues that affect patients' well-being and day-to-day living. In Austria, QOL questionnaires from the European Organisation for Research and Treatment of Cancer are frequently used to assess the QOL of patients with cancer because the questionnaires are validated, translated, and provided free of charge for academic clinical trials.

As with genetic and genomic testing, all clinical trial participants must give their permission before any additional studies are conducted or samples are collected and evaluated. Often a separate signed informed consent will be required, and the participation is usually optional.

Documentation and Data Management

Many trials in Austria are still paper based, meaning that patients' data are recorded on paper case report forms and transferred into some sort of digital database later. However, this is becoming replaced by electronic case report forms. By omitting the step of collecting the data on paper first, the workload is reduced, transcription errors can be decreased or avoided, and data checks can be conducted more frequently. The number of academic clinical trials that are using Internet-based or digital databases for data entry is steadily increasing. The study nurse usually inputs the data, with information gathered from source documents in paper or digital form. Also, patient randomization is done either through electronic systems or via fax.

Most clinical trial centers have outsourced the data management per se to specialized companies because this is a highly specialized and time-consuming part of a clinical trial. However, the medical universities of Austria are aware of the financial aspect of this outsourcing and are in the process of developing a platform that noncommercial clinical trials, with no or little financial support, can use for data entry and management. The legal implications of this development are a major concern for legislature and ECs because patient anonymity and data safekeeping must be ensured.

Quality Assurance

Any clinical trial has to follow regulatory standards and national law and cannot run without proper submission and approval of the study. During the approval process, the trial will be assessed as to the safety of the participants, as well as production of good quality data. The aspects of a trial that are investigated by ECs as well as EC compositions are listed in Figure 46-4.

All clinical trial groups in Austria recommend that their participating centers use ICH (1996) GCP guidelines and develop standard operating procedures to ensure high-quality and uniform conduct of all trials. Most investigators are becoming more aware of the importance of GCP training for all clinical trial team

---

Figure 46-4. Ethics Committee Duties and Constitution

Ethics committees are independent boards whose duties are to advise investigators on the conduct of clinical trials and give positive or negative votes regarding a clinical trial or study project.
- The following are considered:
  - Relevancy of the study and the concept
  - Gain versus risk evaluation
  - Protocol evaluation
  - Informed consent: adequateness, appropriateness, and completeness
  - Patient insurance and indemnity for damages
  - Compensation of patients and investigators
  - Patient selection (inclusion and exclusion criteria)
- Composition of the board includes at least one member of each of the following groups:
  - Physician, who is certified in Austria but is not the investigator
  - Physician, who can evaluate the proposed trial (specialist in that field)
  - Representative of the upper grade of civil service of the healthcare system
  - Lawyer
  - Pharmacist
  - Patient's representative
  - Representative of a challenged person organization
  - Representative who can aid in counseling or ethical considerations

members and encourage them to participate in such trainings. However, GCP training is not yet required by the regulatory authority, competent authority, or ECs in order to conduct a trial in Austria.

For the duration of the study, data will be verified through monitoring visits of the sites, which includes source data verification and checking of general conduct of the trial. Some trial groups perform internal audits of their centers at irregular intervals to ensure proper study conduct. Acting for the BASG, the Austrian Agency for Health and Food Safety performs audits and inspections of clinical trial sites in Austria on a regular basis. In doing so, they might inspect a specific trial or the center in general.

Professional Development

It is understood that only well-educated clinical trial team members can produce high-quality clinical trial outcomes. Nothing is more expensive than conducting a clinical trial and, at the end, not being able to evaluate any results because of negligence or inadequate data. Therefore, increasingly, more emphasis is being placed on the development of adequate education of research nurses.

In Austria, nurses' responsibilities are defined in the national legislation through the BGBl Nr. 108/1997; Gesundheits und Krankenpflegegesetz, 2004. However, hospitals often have individual contracts with nurses that define their conduct and participation in clinical trials. These duties are often performed in addition to their regular work and usually encompass the support of the physician in the care of the patient and data entry. Only in recent years has the development of specific research nurse educational programs been seen in Austria. Because most study-related documents are in English and most nurses in Austria do not speak English fluently, only a few work full time as study nurses or study coordinators.

A specific education program for clinical trial professionals has been offered in Austria recently. A platform was founded by a group of study nurses that now is offering basic courses for interested study personnel, and some higher education campuses are offering in-depth courses. Communication among study nurses is being supported by study nurse organizations, which also provide regular meetings, an online platform, and an educational program (see Figure 46-1).

The importance of GCP trainings is being more widely understood, and clinical trial groups are beginning to provide high-quality training courses for all of their members.

Investigators are encouraged to attend regular meetings, not only of the study group but also internationally. Some groups have delegates who attend international congresses and share the gathered information with the other group members at local meetings.

International Clinical Trials Research

International cooperations are not only important for clinical trials to be able to reach the necessary patient numbers but also to account for national or regional variations (Fox, Goodman, Bigonzi, LeLouer, & Cohen, 2000; Kim, Johnson, & Derendorf, 2004). Only if a trial, which applies a standardized treatment plan for all participating centers, has included a large enough, randomized population will it be possible to use the information gained to change cancer therapies in the future.

Summary

For several decades, clinical trials have been performed in Austria. Until the mid-1980s, the regulations for conducting clinical trials in Austria were limited. Finally, in 1984 the Austrian Medicines Act was passed. This federal law was the first to outline the legal requirements for conducting clinical trials. This law—and several other federal laws that followed—guided the way for a very productive history of clinical research in Austria.

But still, the willingness or potential of physicians to conduct or participate in clinical trials varies widely because of the ever-increasing demand of the administrative effort. More complex clinical trials are usually only conducted in larger hospitals, especially those that are affiliated with a university. In recent years, many of these institutions have incorporated academic clinical trial centers, which support the clinical trial staff at the facility and coordinate clinical trials on a national or international level. In addition, the specializations and number of the clinical trial staff is ever increasing and adding to the acceptance and reputation of the clinical trial healthcare professionals in Austria.

Key Points
- Current legal regulations guide cancer clinical trial activities in Austria.
- Mandatory roles of Austrian regulatory bodies such as ECs and competent authority are essential to the clinical trial process.
- Tumor boards are a critical part of patient care and incorporate patient recruitment strategies in Austria.
- The educational tasks and functions of Austrian clinical trial staff have a substantial effect on patient participation and compliance.
- Austria is developing new approaches in personalized cancer treatment.

References

Commission directive 2001/20/EC of the European Parliament and of the council of 4 April 2001 on the approximation of the laws, regulations and administrative provisions of the member states relating to the implementation of good clinical practice in the conduct of clinical trials on medicinal products for human use. (2001). *Official Journal of the European Union, 44*(L 121), 34–44.

du Bois, A. (2002). Klinische studien und ihr einfluss auf die versorgungsqualität. *GynSpektrum, 10*, 3–5.

Fox, K.A.A., Goodman, S., Bigonzi, F., LeLouer, V., & Cohen, M. (2000). Inter-regional differences and outcome in unstable angina: Analysis of the International ESSENCE trial. *European Heart Journal, 21*, 1433–1439. doi:10.1053/euhj.1999.1983

International Conference on Harmonisation of Technical Requirements for Registration of Pharmaceuticals for Human Use. (1996, June 10). *ICH harmonised tripartite guideline: Guideline for good clinical practice, E6(R1)*. Retrieved from http://www.ich.org/fileadmin/Public_Web_Site/ICH_Products/Guidelines/Efficacy/E6/E6_R1_Guideline.pdf

Janni, W., Kiechle, M., Sommer, S., Rack, B., Gauger, K., Heinrigs, M., ... Dian, D. (2005). Studienteilnahme verbessert Therapiestrategien und individuelle Patientenversorgung in teilnehmenden Zentren. *Geburtshilfe und Frauenheilkunde, 65*, 966–973. doi:10.1055/s-2005-872874

Kim, K., Johnson, J.A., & Derendorf, H. (2004). Differences in drug pharmacokinetics between East Asians and Caucasians and the role of genetic polymorphisms. *Journal of Clinical Pharmacology, 44*, 1083–1105. doi:10.1177/0091270004268128

Maxwell, K.N., & Domchek, S.M. (2012). Cancer treatment according to *BRCA1* and *BRCA2* mutations. *Nature Reviews Clinical Oncology, 9*, 520–528. doi:10.1038/nrclinonc.2012.123

Peppercorn, J.M., Weeks, J.C., Cook, E.F., & Joffe, S. (2004). Comparison of outcomes in cancer patients treated within and outside clinical trials: Conceptual framework and structured review. *Lancet, 363*, 263–270. doi:10.1016/S0140-6736(03)15383-4

Umar, A., Dunn, B.K., & Greenwald, P. (2012). Future directions in cancer prevention. *Nature Reviews Cancer, 12*, 835–848. doi:10.1038/nrc3397

Yusuf, S., Wittes, J., Probstfield, J., & Tyroler, H.A. (1991). Analysis and interpretation of treatment effects in subgroups of patients in randomized controlled trials. *JAMA, 266*, 93–98. doi:10.1001/jama.1991.03470010097038

Ziegler, A., Koch, A., Krockenberger, K., & Großhennig, A. (2012). Personalized medicine using DNA biomarkers: A review. *Human Genetics, 131*, 1627–1638. doi:10.1007/s00439-012-1188-9

Zielonke, N. (2014). *Krebsinzidenz und krebsmortalität in Österreich*. Retrieved from http://www.statistik.at/web_de/statistiken/gesundheit/krebserkrankungen

Chapter 47

Belarus

Volha Matylevich, MD, PhD, Sviatlana Alimpiyeva, MD, and Sergey Mavrichev, MD, PhD

Introduction

Belarus is one of the countries of the former Soviet Union that achieved independence in 1991 and is now a member of the Commonwealth of Independent States (CIS). It is located in Central Europe and borders with Russia, Ukraine, Poland, Lithuania, and Latvia. According to official statistics, the population is about 9.5 million, and the average life expectancy is 72.6 years (67.3 years for men and 77.9 years for women) (National Statistical Committee of the Republic of Belarus, n.d., 2014). Belarus has one of the World Health Organization Euro Region's lowest levels for healthy life expectancy for men, largely due to premature adult deaths and disabilities. Over the past decade, both the population growth rate and the total population have decreased. In the past 10 years, cancer rates have increased by one-third. Increases in cancer incidence may stem from the aftereffects of the Chernobyl nuclear accident, although it is difficult to confirm whether there is a direct link (Okeanov, Moiseev, & Levin, 2012).

The delivery of health care, its structure, and its organization in Belarus have not evolved much since the Declaration of Sovereignty and the establishment of an independent nation. All citizens of Belarus have free access to government-financed health care; however, lack of available resources and funding remains a significant problem for optimal care. Total annual health expenditures per capita total less than $1,000 ($793 in 2011) (Richardson, Malakhova, Novik, & Famenka, 2013). Most sophisticated medical services are not readily available in the rural areas. Although medical care in Belarus lags behind most Western European countries and the United States, it is more easily accessible compared to other countries of the former Soviet Union.

History and Foundation

Belarus is an attractive market for clinical research in Eastern Europe. Numerous factors make the Belarusian clinical trial market desirable, including a population of nearly 10 million people with an ethnic similarity to those in North America and Europe. In addition to significant cost reductions and high recruitment rates, the market drivers include (a) centralized healthcare systems, (b) broad disease spectrum, (c) large pools of treatment-naïve populations, (d) good patient compliance, and (e) low number of dropouts (Stefanov, 2008; Varshavsky, 2002). According to some analysts, the pharmaceutical industry currently uses only 15% of the clinical study enrollment potential in Eastern Europe (Anokhina & Meshkov, 2007; Dobbin, 2008). Reports of clinical research organizations (CROs) and industry experts confirm the growth of clinical activity in this region for the past 15 years and predict that this trend will continue (Dobbin, 2008; Synergy Research Group, 2009).

Clinical Trials: Fundamental Information

Regulatory Background

Harmonization of clinical trials (both ethical and clinical approaches) is the cornerstone of mutual recognition of the results obtained in different countries. In Belarus, state regulatory principles of clinical trial conduct are as close to the International Conference on Harmonisation of Technical Requirements for Registration of Pharmaceuticals for Human Use Good Clinical Practice Guidelines (ICH GCP, 1996) as is possible, based on local economic and political circumstances. Harmonization was initiated in 1999 when the order of the Ministry of Health of the Republic of Belarus (MH RB) No. 254 On Approval of Clinical Trials of Medicinal Products was introduced (MH RB, 2007b). This document was a Russian translation of ICH GCP. In January 2009, this document became a national standard for GCP (MH RB, 2009a).

Legislative Documents

Currently, clinical research in Belarus is regulated by the following legislative documents.
- Law on Healthcare No. 2435-XII of 18 Jun 1993 with amendments (National Assembly, 1993)
- Law on Medicines No. 161-Z of 20 Jul 2006 with amendments (National Assembly, 2006) describes procedures on preclinical and clinical studies, import and export of medicinal products, and rights and responsibilities of study subjects.
- Resolution of the Ministry of Health No. 50 of 7 May 2009 on conduct of clinical trials of medicines (MH RB, 2009c) describes regulatory requirements for submission for approval for clinical trials of therapeutic drugs.
- Guideline on Ethics Committees No. 57-0004 of 21 April 2000 (MH RB, 2009b) provides guidelines on structure and operational activities of local ethics committees.
- Resolution of the Ministry of Health No. 57-0004 of 24 April 2000 on ethics Ccommittee (MH RB, 2007a) provides a description of principles and procedures of ethics committees, including clinical trial authorization, review of amendments, and inspections. The resolution outlines required content of the informed consent form, application form, and clinical trial report.

The following documents represent national standards for academic and industry sponsors conducting clinical trials in Belarus, as well as for all participants, including the clinical trial team members and subjects:
- Good Clinical Practice (GCP), Technical Code TKP 184-2009 (02040) of 8 January 2009 (MH RB, 2009a)
- Good Laboratory Practice (GLP), Technical Code 125-2008 (029040) of 5 January 2008 (MH RB, 2008b).

Regulatory Bodies

The competent authorities responsible for approval and supervision of clinical studies are the Commission on Medicines of the Ministry of Health and the Republican Center for Expertise and Clinical Trials in Healthcare (RCECTH) within the Ministry of Health (Council of Ministers of the Republic of Belarus, 2012). The decision of a clinical trial approval is made by the Commission on Medicines of the Ministry of Health based on the results of the expert review of submitted documents and the results of the quality control of the investigative drug.

Ethics Committees

Ethical review of clinical trials is carried out by the local ethics committees established at all healthcare organizations accredited to conduct such studies—hospitals, medical research institutions, medical schools, and polyclinics (i.e., primary care units). The first local ethics committees in Belarus were created in 1999 when the legislative and regulatory framework for biomedical research was introduced in accordance with the Ministry of Health Order No. 254 On Approval of Clinical Trials of Medicinal Products (MH RB, 2007b). The activities of local ethics committees are outlined in the Guidelines of the Ministry of Health on the Organization and Work of the Ethics Committees (MH RB, 2009b) and Instructions for Accreditation and Certification of Healthcare Professionals for Conducting Clinical Trials of Drugs, Medical Equipment and Medical Products (MH RB, 2004).

Local ethics committees usually consist of 5–12 members, including medical specialists experienced in clinical research and members with expertise outside of medicine and natural sciences. Decision on the clinical trial authorization can be made only in the presence of a minimum of two-thirds of the ethics committee members with constituents including at least one nonscientist. The decision is adopted by a majority of the votes. In the latter case, the opinion of the minority voters is documented and communicated to the sponsor and investigator together with the adopted decision (MH RB, 2009b).

Procedural guidelines (MH RB, 2000) stipulate that review of clinical study documentation and constant assessment of risk-benefit ratio during the study conduct is as important as the initial study approval. The ethics committee reviews (a) investigators' reports on recruitment rates, (b) adverse drug events and adverse drug reactions, (c) subject disenrollment from the study, (d) protocol amendments, (e) new data on investigational drug safety, and (f) possible protocol violations.

Although more than 50 local ethics committees were organized in the first few years following their establishment in 1999 (Voronov, 2006), it was not until 2006 when the Ministry of Health attempted to introduce some degree of centralization, coordination, and oversight into the system of local ethics committees by establishing the National Bioethics Committee. It has a status of an advisory body to the Ministry of Health and performs public control over compliance with ethical standards and rules for the conduct of clinical and preclinical trials (Famenka, 2011; Protect Life, 2013). Nevertheless, currently local ethics committees are still accountable to no one. No procedures of audit and monitoring of ethics committees are in place, and local ethics committees are not required to report results of their work to relevant bodies or inform the public about activities.

With all of the progress made in the development of bioethics in Belarus, problems still need to be solved, such as (a) further development of legal regulations, (b) ethical and legal education of the medical community and patients, (c) overwhelming bureaucracy of local ethics committees even for approval of small and safe studies, and (d) reluctances of the local ethics committee to embark on new studies (Kubar, 2007).

Clinical Trial Approval and Review

The clinical trial approval procedure is outlined in resolution No. 50 (MH RB, 2009c) and consists of the following steps (graphically depicted in Figure 47-1).
- The sponsor submits to RCECTH the application form, study protocol, investigator's brochure, informed consent form, advertising materials, certificate of analysis of the investigational drug, good manufacturing practice certificate, list of the study sites, clinical trial agreement, health insurance policy, and administrative fee.
  - RCECTH verifies regulatory compliance of submitted documents.
  - The scientific evaluation of the study by the clinical experts of the Commission on Medicines of the Ministry of Health is completed.
  - The approval process takes 35–60 days.
  - Final decision on protocol approval and clinical site designation is made by the Ministry of Health.
- The applicant (principal investigator/sponsor) submits the following items to the local ethics committee: application form, study protocol, investigator's brochure, informed consent form, advertisements for subject recruitment, diaries, questionnaires for study subjects, compensation to study subjects, curriculum vitae of investigators, and any previous resolutions of ethics committees if applicable.
  - The local ethics committee's opinion is sent to the applicant within 30 days.
  - Results of the ethics committee review are forwarded to the sponsor.

Ethical evaluation of every clinical trial authorization in Belarus is done by the local ethics committee at the health facility concerned. The chairperson determines the date of the meeting, which should be no later than 30 days after the receipt of the application. The ethics committee provides its opinion to the investigator within five days following the meeting, and it may reject the clinical trial application, approve it as is, or request certain amendments to the protocol. If the study is approved, the ethics committee sets a time frame for the approval, how often study documentation will be reviewed, the date of the first inspection, and the responsibilities of the principal investigator regarding notification of the ethics committee about protocol amendments, termination of the study, submission of the study results, or any decisions made regarding the study at other trial sites. The clinical trial may begin if approved by the local ethics committee and the Commission on Medicines of the Ministry of Health. According to Davis-Bruno, Carleer, Silva Lima, and Tas-sinari (2013), Belarus has one of the shortest clinical trial approval times in Eastern Europe (4–12 weeks, compared to 33 weeks in Russia).

Clinical Trial Sites

According to the State Law #161-Z (Chapter 3, article 15) (National Assembly, 2006), only state clinical organizations are eligible to serve as clinical trial sites, and they must be certified by the Ministry of Health. To be eligible for certification, clinical organizations must have a State Medical License and possess sufficient financial and clinical resources, including GCP-trained personnel and satisfactory medical equipment and facilities. The clinical organization must have a local ethics committee, which operates according to the state law and regulations. Certified clinical trial sites must have an approved set of standard operating procedures, which govern training of new personnel, subject recruitment practices, logistics of the interaction among clinical trial team members, and the management of structural units and personnel (MH RB, 2004).

As of the time of this writing, 57 clinical sites were certified by the Ministry of Health to conduct clinical trials, including 8 oncology units. A complete list of certified clinical organizations can be found at the RCECTH website (www.rceth.by).

Clinical Trials in Belarus

The first multinational, multicenter clinical trial (MMCT) in Belarus was conducted in 1998 (Kubar, 2007). The number of clinical trials conducted by domestic and foreign pharmaceutical companies in Belarus has grown steadily over the past 10 years.

Between January 2004 and January 2013, 280 clinical trials were completed in Belarus. Figure 47-2 represents the number of MMCTs completed in Belarus every year between 2004 and 2012 that were sponsored by domestic and foreign sponsors. The increase in the number of MMCTs in 2006 was attributable to the establishment of five CROs in Belarus. The next noticeable increase in 2010 was because of the introduction of ICH GCP as the national standard for the conduct of clinical trials in 2009 (MH RB, 2009a).

The market of cancer therapies has been expanding over the past few years, and this affected Belarus. Over the years, up to 60% of all MMCTs approved to be conducted in Belarus are studies of cancer therapies. Figure 47-3 shows that in January 2013, 21 out of 62 actively conducted clinical trials were oncologic studies. Between January 2008 and December 2012, 66 clinical trials of cancer therapies were approved in Belarus, including 30 MMCTs (45.5%) (Alimpieva, 2013).

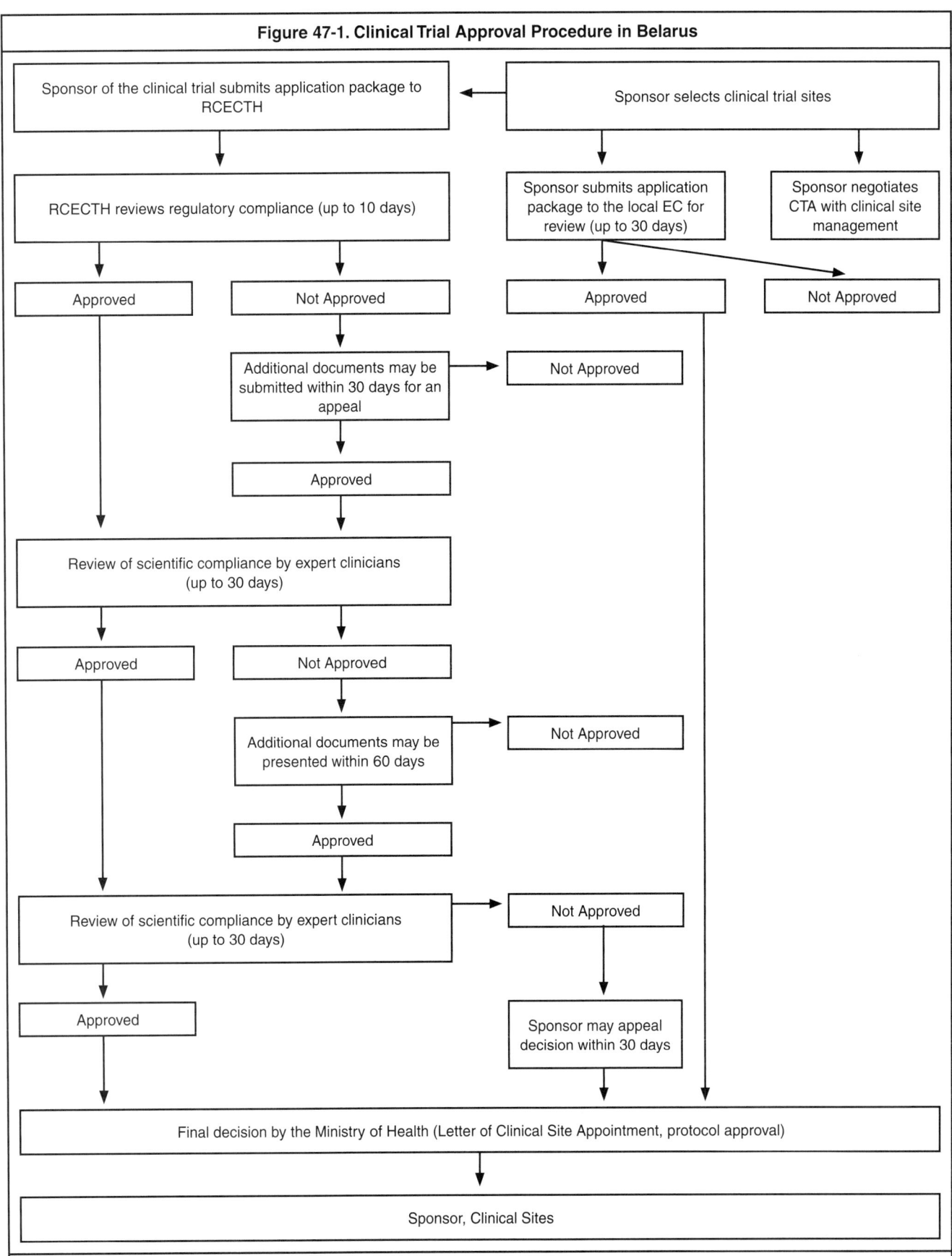

Figure 47-1. Clinical Trial Approval Procedure in Belarus

CTA—clinical trial authorization; EC—ethics committee; RCECTH—Republican Center for Expertise and Clinical Trials in Healthcare, Ministry of Health

Note. From "Good Clinical Practice (GCP), Techinical Code TKP 184-2009 (02040) of 8 January 2009," by Ministry of Health of the Republic of Belarus, 2009. Retrieved from http://tnpa.by/ViewFileText.php?UrlRid=72443&UrlOnd=ТКП. Reprinted with permission.

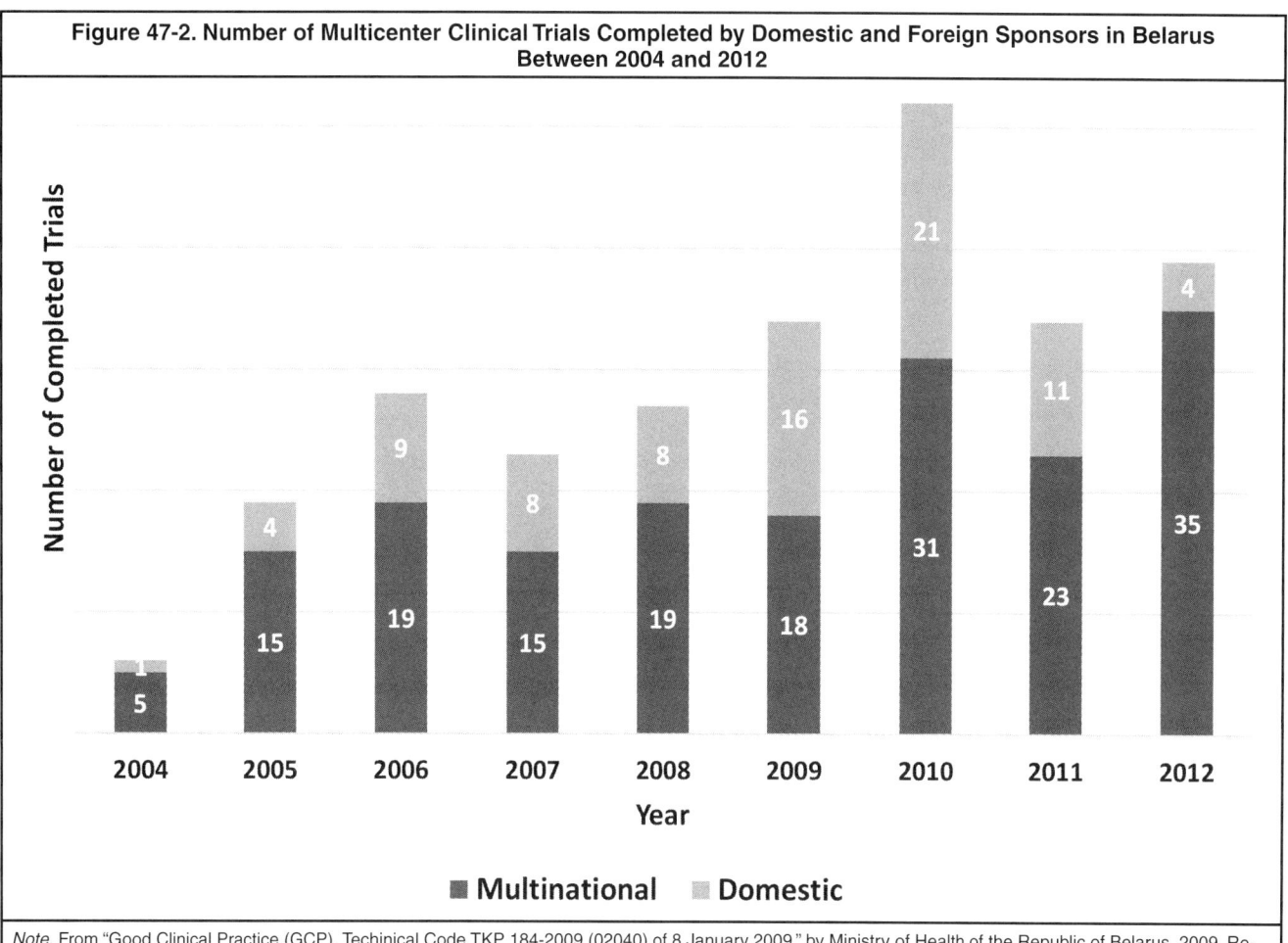

Figure 47-2. Number of Multicenter Clinical Trials Completed by Domestic and Foreign Sponsors in Belarus Between 2004 and 2012

Note. From "Good Clinical Practice (GCP), Techinical Code TKP 184-2009 (02040) of 8 January 2009," by Ministry of Health of the Republic of Belarus, 2009. Retrieved from http://tnpa.by/ViewFileText.php?UrlRid=72443&UrlOnd=ТКП. Reprinted with permission.

Protocol Development, Review, and Approval

Clinical studies in Belarus can be conducted for the following purposes: (a) to discover or verify clinical effects of the investigational medical product, (b) to identify adverse events, and (c) to study absorption, distribution, and excretion of medicinal products. The overwhelming majority of clinical studies in Belarus are initiated by drug manufacturers. As a rule, sponsors outsource clinical trial conduct (and in some instances, protocol development) to CROs. State medical research entities do initiate clinical trials, which are predominantly post-registration studies that are demographic and pathophysiologic in nature. The sponsor is responsible for seeking a trial site best suited to the needs of a particular trial. However, the choice is limited by the scope of the register of accredited organizations (institutions) hosting local ethics committees. In Belarus, the procedure of so-called *single opinion* for multicenter clinical trials has not been introduced into practice; therefore, in the case of multiclinical research, involvement of all of the local ethics committees in protocol review is required.

All participation in clinical trials is voluntary, and an informed consent procedure and form are mandatory for clinical trial approval and conduct. According to the procedural guidance on ethics committees, informed consent of the study participants is not required (a) when a person is in a life-threatening condition, (b) all conventional therapeutic methods have no effect or their efficacy is not proven, and (c) an overall amount of available information, including data from randomized placebo-controlled trials, is sufficient to estimate safety and efficacy of planning an intervention.

Clinical trials in Belarus cannot be conducted on
- Orphans and children left without parental care
- Pregnant or breast-feeding women, except when the following conditions are met: (a) the investigative drug is being developed for use in pregnant and/or breast-feeding women, (b) there is no other way to obtain the necessary information except with a clinical study, and (c) all necessary measures are taken to eliminate the risk for woman, fetus, or child.
- Armed forces personnel (to remove the influence of military commanders over participation by subordinates)
- People in detention
- Adults incapable of giving informed consent.

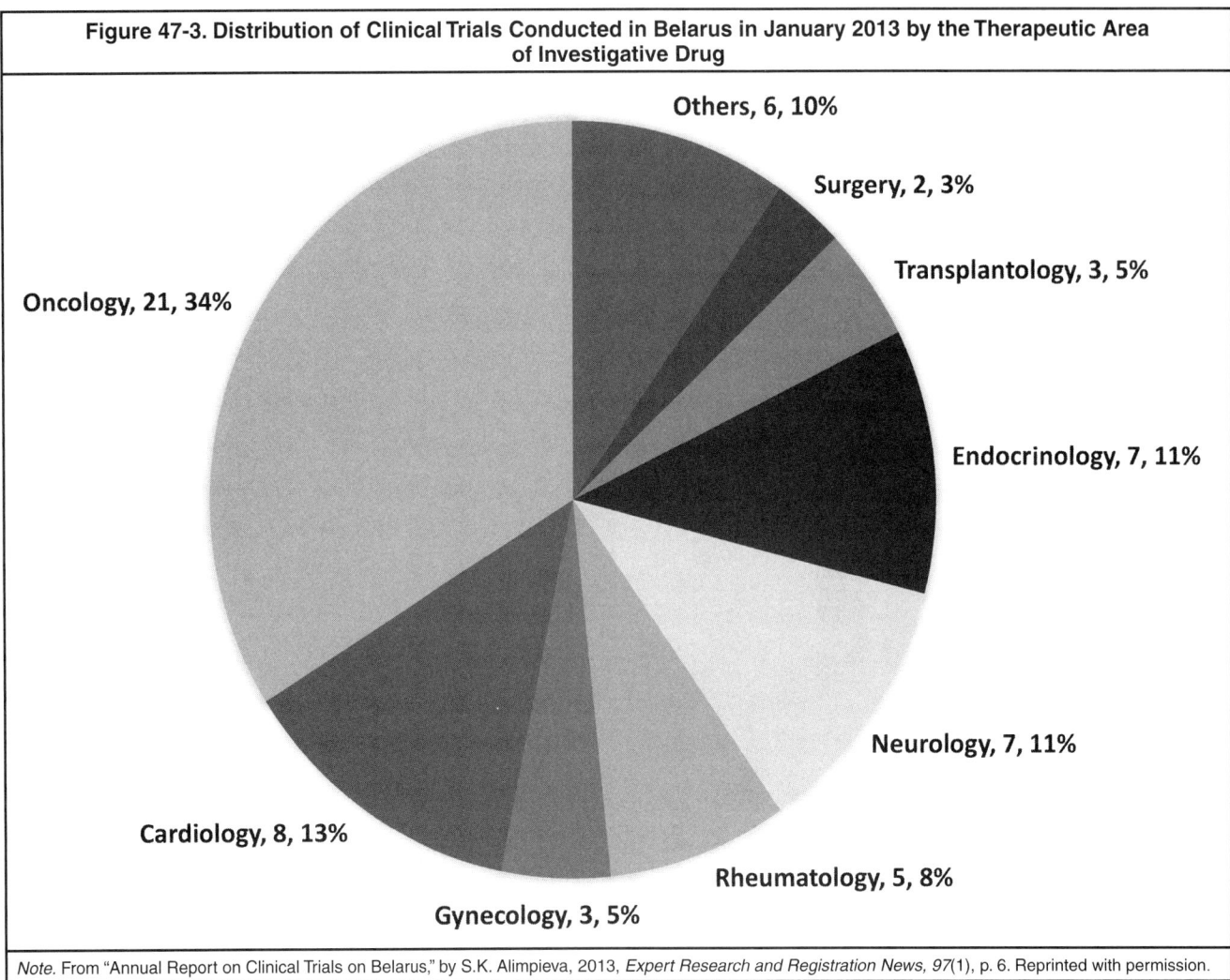

Figure 47-3. Distribution of Clinical Trials Conducted in Belarus in January 2013 by the Therapeutic Area of Investigative Drug

Note. From "Annual Report on Clinical Trials on Belarus," by S.K. Alimpieva, 2013, Expert Research and Registration News, 97(1), p. 6. Reprinted with permission.

Incapacitated adults with mental diseases can be included in the clinical study when the investigative medicine product is developed for treatment of mental diseases. The agreement of the legal representative is mandatory. Belarus requires proper justification for inclusion of patients with incurable diseases, people in retirement homes, unemployed or low-income population groups, and many more. Ethical principles on clinical research are compliant with ICH GCP and the Declaration of Helsinki.

Financial Factors

Sponsors of clinical trials bear complete responsibility for study financial support, including the purchase of health insurance policies for participants and, in some instances, malpractice insurance for clinical trial team members. The issues of insurance or indemnification to cover sponsor responsibilities, as well as payments and rewards offered and given to the participants, are within the scope of the local research ethics committee's review during the clinical trial approval process. Belarusian legislation does not have mandatory requirements for indemnity and malpractice insurance during the conduct of clinical trials. However, local ethics committees typically will not approve studies where such protection of participants is not insured. Private local insurance companies offer these services to sponsors.

As a result, the overwhelming majority of clinical trials in Belarus provide life and health insurance to participants, as well as insurance of civil liability of the investigators who carry out the study to ensure an important additional guarantee of protection of subjects' interests.

Recruitment and Retention

Patient recruitment is one of the essential parts in clinical trials that can determine the success of a particular study. It is one of the toughest features of clinical trials, especially for research involving elderly subjects. Successful patient recruitment involves more than just enrollment. In Belarus, participation in a clinical study often provides a much better standard of care for patients than the national healthcare system because it provides not only a potentially effective study medication that is usually safe and tested but also a full set of healthcare services, including free laboratory testing; diagnostics such as x-rays, computed tomography, and magnetic resonance imaging; thorough medical examination; and inpatient care in many cases. As with so many other countries around the world with very limited healthcare resources, for many people in Belarus, participation in global clinical trials may be the only way to get modern diagnostic procedures and potentially effective modern treatment and the only chance to receive lifesaving therapy. With patient recruitment rates up to 20 times faster than the West, the biopharmaceutical industry is embracing the undeniable benefits of conducting clinical trials in emerging markets such as Belarus.

Clinical sites of Belarus are large multifield hospitals allowing the quick enrollment of the necessary number of patients meeting the research criteria. Thanks to the existing public health system, strict statistical records on morbidity are kept in the republic; comprehensive databases of patients with different pathologies have been created. Generally, Belarusian patients have a positive attitude about participating in clinical trials.

When healthy volunteers are recruited for phase I studies or patients are recruited for bioequivalence studies of generic drugs, flyers are distributed in public places and doctors' offices. All promotional materials must be approved by regulatory bodies and verified for ethics, truthfulness, and reliability of content.

Clinical Trial Participants

Recruitment into studies is mainly conducted through the large clinical centers. Belarus has a concentrated population, centralized healthcare system, and large therapeutic hospitals. Most clinical centers are located in the capital of Minsk with 1.8 million people in its urban center. Studies are also conducted in Gomel, Vitebsk, Mogilev, Brest, and Grodno, where more than 2 million citizens are concentrated. Patient eligibility, screening, and enrollment are performed only by the physician investigators. During the enrollment process, investigators use printed advertising materials developed by the study sponsor and approved by the ethics committees. Currently, positions for research nurses are virtually nonexistent.

Because of the limited financial resources in the Belarusian healthcare system, any treatment that deviates from standard treatment protocols approved by the Ministry of Health must by subsidized by the study sponsor, including diagnostic testing and imaging, and study and control drugs. Treatment administration is usually conducted by the appropriate medical personnel and is always monitored by the physician investigator.

Adverse events and serious adverse events that are not outlined as potential side effects in the study protocol must be reported immediately to the sponsor and reported by fax or regular mail within three days to the local ethics committee and RCECTH and include all information that pertains to each case according to the regulations found in MH RB (2008a). In the case of death of a trial participant during the clinical trial, all patient medical records must be presented upon request to the regulatory authorities.

Genetics and Genomics

Belarusian legislation does not regulate the collection of human tissue specimens for research. However, the collection process and storage of specimens is strictly voluntarily. The reason for such sampling and the procedure itself must be outlined in the informed consent form and explained to participants during the informed consent process. It requires approval by the local ethics committee as a part of the clinical trial approval process. Genetic multicenter international studies target cardiologic conditions and blood and endocrine disorders in children and adults. Tissue collection is a part of all oncologic clinical trials where samples are shipped to international tissue banks.

Correlative Trials

A number of international multicenter studies use quality of life as one of the study end results. These studies include oncology trials, such as CANVAS (The CANcer VAccine Study for epithelial ovarian cancer) by Prima BioMed (ClinicalTrials.gov, 2013a), studies of chronic inflammatory diseases such as rheumatoid arthritis (Worldwide Clinical Trials, 2011), urologic studies such as the STAR clinical trial of the treatment options for overactive bladder syndrome (Chapple et al., 2005), and gynecologic studies as the DIVA study of endometriosis (ClinicalTrials.gov, 2013b).

Documentation and Data Management

Access to patient clinical records is limited to the hospital staff involved in patient treatment, and contents are strictly confidential. All information related to a clinical trial is presented to the sponsor in the form of paper or electronic case report forms or both. Study monitors do have access to primary patient records pertaining to the study for the purpose of data monitoring.

Quality Assurance

When conducting clinical trials in Belarus, sponsors bear full responsibility for quality assurance of the studies, including compliance with study protocol, standard operating procedures, GCP, and state regulations. All sponsors of multicenter clinical studies typically outsource trial approval, organization, conduct, and monitoring to reputable international CROs. Audits are typically performed by sponsors, quality assurance departments of CROs, and independent auditors. To date, the U.S. Food and Drug Administration has not conducted audits of clinical sites in Belarus as it has in Russia and Ukraine.

Professional Development

Although nurses in Belarus are well educated and all of them have at least an associate degree in nursing, the role of clinical trial nurses (CTNs) in Belarus is rather new. Because of the relatively low volume of clinical trials in Belarus, most of the clinical treatment, data collection, and monitoring are performed by the physicians. Nevertheless, the role of CTNs in oncology studies is rapidly developing. Oncology CTNs are being involved now not only in patient care but also in patient education and advocacy, patient monitoring, and data collection. Development of standard operating procedures for CTNs is in progress at every clinical trial site. Training of CTNs in all aspects of clinical trial conduct (i.e., protocol development, evaluation of potential study subjects, patient enrollment, data collection) may not only increase effectiveness of clinical trial performance but also open the door to CTNs to take on the roles of data manager, study coordinator, and study monitor, which are currently performed by the physicians in Belarus. Currently, nurses are being certified in GCP and trained to comply with standard operating procedures of trial protocols on demand as new clinical trials are being approved.

Summary

Belarus is an attractive market for clinical research in Eastern Europe. Factors that make it attractive for clinical research include (a) a large treatment-naïve population, (b) a centralized healthcare system, (c) one of the shortest clinical trial approval timelines, (d) significant cost reductions and high recruitment rates, and (e) good patient compliance and low number of patient withdrawals. The regulatory system is in place and ensures compliance with international standards of GCP. Since its establishment, RCECTH has trained and certified 1,439 medical professionals, including nurses, who are now eligible to conduct clinical trials according ICH GCP (Alimpieva, 2013). The number of multicenter international clinical trials has rapidly grown in the past 15 years, including studies in oncology, cardiology, and endocrinology. Clinical research nursing is currently only implemented in some of the oncology studies and is focused on the care of research participants. However, in addition to providing and coordinating clinical care, their role is expanding to include (a) ensuring participant safety, (b) ongoing maintenance of informed consent, (c) integrity of protocol implementation, (d) accuracy of data collection, (e) data recording, and (f) follow-up.

Key Points

- Belarus is considered one of the favorable emerging markets for outsourcing of clinical trials, along with other Eastern European countries, with rapid growth of the number of industry-sponsored multinational clinical studies.
- The regulatory climate is on par with international standards, and GCP is fully implemented.
- Although most of the research activities are conducted by physician investigators, the role of CTNs is rapidly growing in oncology clinical studies.

The authors would like to acknowledge Natalia Matylevich, PhD, MS, for her assistance with writing this chapter.

References

Alimpieva, S.K. (2013). Annual report on clinical trials on Belarus. *Expert Research and Registration News, 97*(1), 5–7.

Anokhina, A., & Meshkov, D. (2007). Going further east in CEE. *International Clinical Trials, 13*(1), 24–29. Retrieved from http://www.samedanltd.com/magazine/13/issue/81/article/1845

Chapple, C.R., Martinez-Garcia, R., Selvaggi, L., Toozs-Hobson, P., Warnack, W., Drogendijk, T., ... Bolodeoku, J. (2005). A comparison of the efficacy and tolerability of solifenacin succinate and extended release tolterodine at treating overactive bladder syndrome: Results of the STAR trial. *European Urology, 48,* 464–470. doi:10.1016/j.eururo.2005.05.015

ClinicalTrials.gov. (2013a). CVAC as maintenance treatment in patients with EOC in complete remission following first-line chemotherapy (CANVAS). Retrieved from http://clinicaltrials.gov/show/NCT01521143

ClinicalTrials.gov. (2013b). Daily practice treatment and influence of visanne on the patient assessment of quality of life. Retrieved from http://clinicaltrials.gov/ct2/show/NCT01595724

Council of Ministers of the Republic of Belarus. (2012, March 2). Resolution of the Council of Ministers of the Republic of Belarus No. 156. Retrieved from http://rceth.by/Documents/2sm2po20120217N156e_1v.rtf

Davis-Bruno, K., Carleer, J., Silva Lima, B., & Tassinari, M.S. (2013). A global regulatory perspective. In A.E. Mulberg, D. Murphy, J. Dunne, & L.L. Mathis (Eds.), *Pediatric drug development* (2nd ed., pp. 246–256). New York, NY: Wiley-Blackwell.

Dobbin, S. (2008). Clinical trials in Central and South Eastern Europe. *Future Pharmaceuticals*. Retrieved from http://www.argintinternational.com/images/pdf/CT_Argint.pdf

Famenka, A. (2011). Ethical review of biomedical research in Belarus: Current status, problems and perspectives. *Revista Română de Bioetică*, *9*, 74–83. Retrieved from http://www.ncbi.nlm.nih.gov/pmc/articles/PMC3372927

International Conference on Harmonisation of Technical Requirements for Registration of Pharmaceuticals for Human Use. (1996, June 10). *ICH harmonised tripartite guideline: Guideline for good clinical practice, E6(R1)*. Retrieved from http://www.ich.org/fileadmin/Public_Web_Site/ICH_Products/Guidelines/Efficacy/E6/E6_R1_Guideline.pdf

Kubar, O. (Ed.). (2007). *Ethical review of biomedical research in the CIS countries: Social and cultural aspects*. Retrieved from http://www.unesco.org/new/fileadmin/MULTIMEDIA/FIELD/Moscow/pdf/ethical_review_cis_book_kubar_english.pdf

Ministry of Health of the Republic of Belarus. (2004). Instruction of the Ministry of Health of the Republic of Belarus of 07.05.2004 No. 50-0504: "Guide accreditation of health facilities and certification of personnel for conducting clinical trials of medicines, medical equipment and health care products." Retrieved from http://belarus.news-city.info/docs/2004by/crfxfnm-tcgkfnyj41078.htm

Ministry of Health of the Republic of Belarus. (2007a, March 30). Guidelines of the Ministry of Health of the Republic of Belarus of 24 April 2000 No. 57-0004: "Guidelines: The organization and work of the ethics committee." Retrieved from http://www.levonevski.net/pravo/temy/tema04/glav/docm0951.html

Ministry of Health of the Republic of Belarus. (2007b, March 28). On approval of clinical trials of medicinal products, No. 254, August 13, 1999. Retrieved from http://pravo.levonevsky.org/bazaby/org337/basic/text0497.htm

Ministry of Health of the Republic of Belarus. (2008a). Decree of the Ministry of Health of the Republic of Belarus of 20.03.2008 No. 52: "On approval of the instruction on how to submit information about the identified adverse reactions to drugs and monitoring of adverse reactions to drugs." Retrieved from http://www.levonevski.net/pravo/norm2009/num05/d05793.html

Ministry of Health of the Republic of Belarus. (2008b). Good laboratory practice (GLP). Technical code 125-2008 (029040) of 5 January 2008. Retrieved from http://tnpa.by/ViewFileText.php?UrlRid=51849&UrlOnd=ТКП

Ministry of Health of the Republic of Belarus. (2009a). Good clinical practice (GCP), Technical Code TKP 184-2009 (02040) of 8 January 2009. Retrieved from http://tnpa.by/ViewFileText.php?UrlRid=72443&UrlOnd=ТКП

Ministry of Health of the Republic of Belarus. (2009b, July 10). Guidelines of the Ministry of Health of the Republic of Belarus of 21.04.2000 N 57-0004: "The organization and work of the Ethics Committee." Retrieved from http://www.levonevski.net/pravo/norm2009/num35/d35896.html

Ministry of Health of the Republic of Belarus. (2009c, May 7). On conduct of clinical trials of medicines, the Resolution of the Ministry of Health No. 50 of 7 May 2009—Good Clinical Practice of Belarus. Retrieved from http://www.rceth.by/en/Documents/Rcpl

National Assembly. (1993). Law of the Republic of Belarus of 18 Jun 1993 No. 2435-XII: About health care. Retrieved from http://cis-legislation.com/document.fwx?rgn=2010

National Assembly. (2006). Law of the Republic of Belarus from July 20, 2006 of No. 161-Z: About medicines. Retrieved from http://cis-legislation.com/document.fwx?rgn=13989

National Statistical Committee of the Republic of Belarus. (n.d.). Life expectancy at birth. Retrieved from http://belstat.gov.by/en/ofitsialnaya-statistika/otrasli-statistiki/naselenie/demografiya_2/osnovnye-pokazateli-za-period-s-__-po-____gody_3/life-expectancy-at-birth

National Statistical Committee of the Republic of Belarus. (2014, January 1). Demographic situation in January–December 2013. Retrieved from http://belstat.gov.by/en/ofitsialnaya-statistika/otrasli-statistiki/naselenie/demografiya_2/current-data/demographic-situation-in-january-december-2013

Okeanov, A.E., Moiseev, P.J., & Levin, L.F. (2012). *Statistics of cancer diseases in the Republic of Belarus (2002–2011)*. Minsk, Belarus: NN Alexandrov National Cancer Center.

Protect Life. (2013). Information on the activities of the national bioethics committee of the Republic of Belarus. Retrieved from http://protectlife.pp.ru/index.php/2010-11-14-08-52-05/2010-11-14-08-52-35/283-2010-11-14-16-52-39

Richardson, E., Malakhova, I., Novik, I., & Famenka, A. (2013). Belarus: Health system review. *Health Systems in Transistion*, *15*, 1–118. Retrieved from http://www.euro.who.int/__data/assets/pdf_file/0005/232835/HiT-Belarus.pdf

Stefanov, I. (2008). RussianTrojka: Speed, cost, quality. *Journal for Clinical Studies*, *15*(9), 20–23.

Synergy Research Group. (2009). *Clinical trials in Russia, year 2009*. Orange paper. 2010 Feb. Retrieved from http://www.synrg-pharm.com/modules/news/article.php?storyid=62

Varshavsky, S. (2002, March). Discover Russia for conducting clinical research. *Applied Clinical Trials*. Retrieved from http://appliedclinicaltrialsonline.findpharma.com/appliedclinicaltrials/data/articlestandard//appliedclinicaltrials/092002/10576/article.pdf

Voronov, G. (2006). *The experience of Central and Eastern Europe*. Proceedings of International Conferences on Bioethics National and Local Bioethics Committees (pp. 48–52). Minsk, Belarus.

Worldwide Clinical Trials. (2011). *Approaches in clinical development for chronic inflammatory diseases: A case study in rheumatoid arthritis* [White paper]. Retrieved from http://www.wwctrials.com/uploads/tx_wctpostersandpresentations/RA_Clinical_Development_White_Paper_WCT__03-11_.pdf

Chapter 48

Canada

Lisa Tinker, RN, BScN, MHM, Valerie Bowering, RN, CONC, and Chantale Blattler, HonBSc, CCRP

Introduction

The Canada Health Act (1985) ensures all Canadians have access to quality health care regardless of their ability to pay. This access is in the form of provincial and territorial health insurance plans that cover medically necessary hospital and physician services. Although the federal government of Canada supports these plans, the provincial and territorial governments administer and deliver these to their residents. Some provinces and territories publicly cover all cancer treatment, whereas others have adopted a combination of public and private coverage to meet the healthcare demands of their residents (Turner & Associates Inc., 2008).

Cancer will touch the lives of nearly all Canadians at some point, either directly or indirectly. In 2009, the prevalence of cancer in Canada was 2.4%, or 1 out of every 41 Canadians (Canadian Cancer Society, 2014). The Canadian Cancer Society (2014) estimated that 41% of Canadian women and 45% of Canadian men will develop cancer in their lifetime and that 191,300 new cases of cancer would be diagnosed in 2014. Despite advances in cancer treatment, cancer remains the leading cause of death of Canadians since 2009, with an estimated one in four dying from cancer in their lifetime (Canadian Cancer Society, 2014). In 2007, the federal government launched the Canadian Partnership Against Cancer, a national independent organization mandated to implement a national cancer control strategy (Canadian Partnership Against Cancer, 2011). Today, five-year survival rates are upwards of 63%, compared to about 25% in the 1940s (Canadian Cancer Society, 2013, 2014). This dramatic improvement in survival stems from advances made through research. Ongoing participation in clinical trials is crucial to the continued improvement in cancer survival in Canada and internationally (Canadian Cancer Society, 2013; Intercultural Cancer Council, 2012; Treweek et al., 2010).

History and Foundation

Health Canada

Health Canada is the division of government that oversees public health on a national level. It consists of several branches and agencies, but the Health Products and Food Branch contains the two directorates that are ultimately responsible for federally regulating clinical trials in Canada (see Figure 48-1). Health Canada's framework and policies are the result of more than a century's worth of key legislative developments in drug regulation that

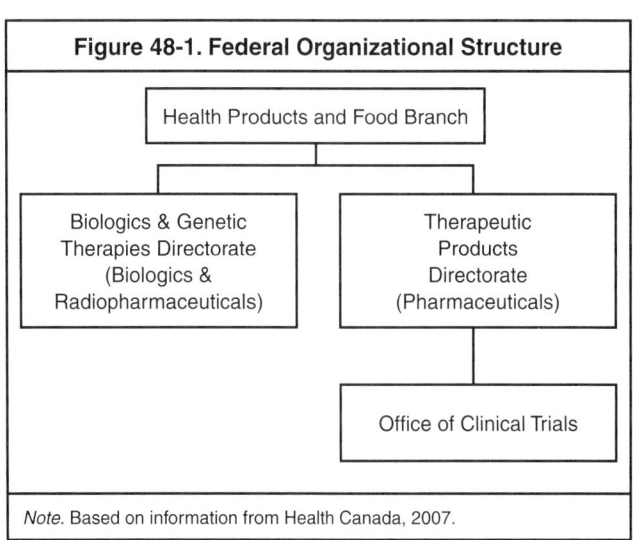

Figure 48-1. Federal Organizational Structure

Health Products and Food Branch
├── Biologics & Genetic Therapies Directorate (Biologics & Radiopharmaceuticals)
└── Therapeutic Products Directorate (Pharmaceuticals)
    └── Office of Clinical Trials

Note. Based on information from Health Canada, 2007.

The authors would like to acknowledge Monica Bacon, RN, for her contribution to this chapter that remains unchanged from the previous edition of this book.

are currently focused on premarket activities (see Figure 48-2) (Health Canada, 2007).

Oversight of food and drugs in Canada began before confederation but was limited to assurances that foods and drugs were not altered or tampered with from their original state. The legislative release of the Proprietary or Patent Medicine Act was the first policy designed to protect the public. The subsequent Food and Drugs Act further developed drug licensing requirements, which, following the 1960s thalidomide calamity, advanced regulations to require efficacy data with submissions (Health Canada, 2007). In 2001, an amendment to clinical trial regulations (part C, division 5 of the Food and Drug Regulations—Drugs for Clinical Trials Involving Human Subjects) outlined two all-encompassing objectives: (a) increase the protection for human participants of research and (b) increase the investment of research and development in clinical trials (Health Canada, 2008).

Drug Development Process

Oncology drug approval in Canada requires drugs to go through a somewhat linear development process, similar to that of the United States and internationally, involving preclinical and clinical testing before becoming available to Canadians. Once the preclinical and clinical testing is completed, the drug approval process starts with the drug's sponsor filing a new drug submission with the Therapeutic Products Directorate (TPD) of Health Canada. TPD is the national authority responsible for evaluating, regulating, and monitoring all therapeutic and diagnostic products in Canada. The process of approval through Health Canada takes approximately 18 months and is only one step in achieving access to oncology drugs in Canada (Health Canada, 2001).

Provincial and territorial Ministries of Health are responsible for making individual drug funding decisions in their respective provinces and territories as to whether the approved drugs will be publicly funded. To guide these decisions, the Pan-Canadian Oncology Drug Review (pCODR), a national review body, makes recommendations for drug funding decisions to the provinces and territories based on clinical evidence and cost-effectiveness. This review process takes approximately five to eight months and is designed to run parallel to the TPD review (pCODR, n.d.).

Expanded Access

Canadian patients with cancer may receive access to drugs currently not approved in Canada through TPD's Special Access Program. This program allows physicians to prescribe these drugs to patients when standard therapies have failed or are deemed inappropriate. TPD grants access following a physician application and review process (Health Canada, 2001).

Clinical Trials: Fundamental Information

The Interdisciplinary Clinical Team

The implementation, process, and follow-up of clinical trials is a complex undertaking requiring an interdisciplinary approach to ensure that scientific and ethical integrity is maintained. Regardless of whether the team consists of a small or large number of professionals, the

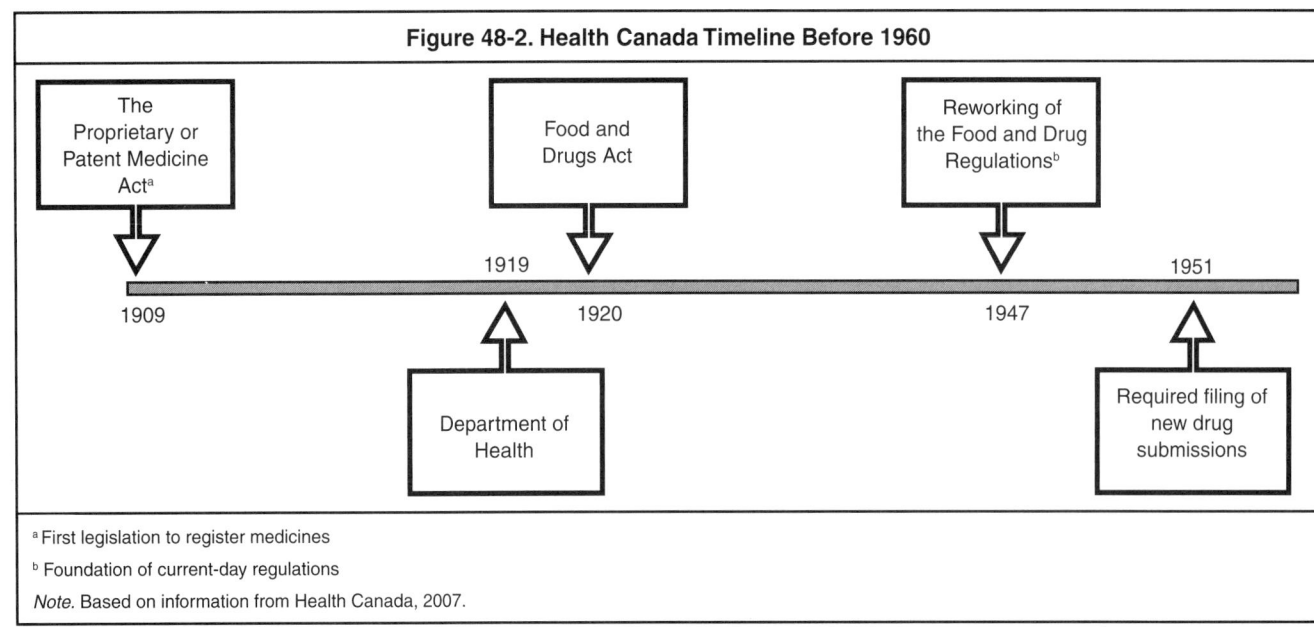

Figure 48-2. Health Canada Timeline Before 1960

[a] First legislation to register medicines
[b] Foundation of current-day regulations
Note. Based on information from Health Canada, 2007.

foundation of the team is usually the same and comprises the following.
- The *principal investigator* is responsible and accountable for the conduct of the clinical trial but has the ability to delegate responsibilities to other members of the team (Health Canada, 1997).
- *Co-investigators* are qualified members of the team trained in the protocol and clinical trials and share the responsibility of the conduct of the study.
- The *pharmacist and the pharmacy staff* play a key role as members of the interdisciplinary team and provide oversight of the investigational product.
- *Clinical research associates* may be nurses or non-nurses, with the title and the role varying across Canada.
- The *clinical trial nurse* (CTN), also known as the *clinical research coordinator*, has duties that range from regulatory submissions, budget, trial implementation, informed consent process, patient care management, data management, documentation, staff education, investigational product administration, collection of biologic samples, protocol adherence, follow-up, and study completion.

The clinical trial team relies on other areas of the hospital, such as the laboratory staff and specialized oncology nurses, to perform study-related procedures or administer the study treatment. CTNs play a crucial role in maintaining communication and education between departments to ensure quality and safety in clinical trials.

Some larger sites in Canada have taken the responsibilities of the clinical research associate and created several different roles—data coordinator, data manager, clinical research coordinator, and CTN—to create a hybrid model to meet the complex, evolving demands of conducting clinical trials today. For example, Princess Margaret Cancer Centre in Toronto has created a role called the pharmacokinetic nurse, or "PK nurse." This nurse works alongside the CTN and study team with responsibilities that include administering the investigational product, obtaining blood or body fluid samples, and performing electrocardiograms. As clinical trials continue to become more complex, other innovative roles may be adopted at Canadian sites.

Legal, Regulatory, and Legislative Issues

Health Canada approval must be obtained for a clinical trial (drug development trials phases I–III and bioavailability trials) to open within Canada. The sponsor of the trial in Canada is responsible for submitting the regulatory application to Health Canada for approval. This application is in the form of a Clinical Trial Application (CTA) and CTA-Amendment (CTA-A) and makes the sponsor legally accountable for the conduct of the trial.

In 2001, the Canadian clinical trial regulations were amended with the objectives of (a) shortening application review time, (b) improving safety mechanisms, (c) increasing involvement of the regulator in trial monitoring, and (d) increasing access to innovative therapies (Health Canada, 2008). As a result, Health Canada's review time of CTAs is a *maximum* of 30 days, at which point a No Objection Letter is received for successful applications indicating that the trial can proceed. If the application was not successful, a Not-Satisfactory Notice will be sent to the sponsor. If Health Canada requests additional information during its review, a response must be submitted within two days. A seven-day expedited review is available for bioequivalence and appropriate phase I trials in healthy volunteers (Health Canada, 2013).

Pre-CTA meetings with Health Canada are available and endorsed for trials that involve a new active substance or are complex. These consultation meetings are to be requested in writing and require an information package to be submitted 30 days before the determined meeting date (Health Canada, 2013). The CTA process is outlined in Figure 48-3.

Good Clinical Practice and Standard Operating Procedures

Health Canada requires that all approved clinical trials (as well as phase IV trials) be run in accordance with the principles of good clinical practice (GCP). Furthermore, according to Food and Drug Regulations (part C, division 5), sponsor obligations extend to ensuring that systems and procedures are in place for quality assurance (Minister of Justice, 2013). The qualified investigator subsequently needs to ensure that all individuals involved in the conduct of a trial at a site comply with the regulations and GCP. Although Health Canada (2006) is not specific about a full complement of required standard operating procedures (SOPs), it has identified three essential processes that should be documented therein: (a) informed consent process, (b) adverse event reporting, and (c) drug accountability. Many healthcare institutions and corresponding cooperative groups have developed SOPs for their clinical trials. Fonds de Recherche du Québec–Santé (FRQS), a funding agency for research institutions in the province of Quebec, along with the government of Quebec, several Quebec universities, and FRQS-funded institutions, has created a comprehensive set of SOPs designed to be tailored by the end users for their institution (FRQS, 2007). For centers across Canada that have not developed their own SOPs, Network of Networks (N2), a nonprofit incorporated organization, has developed a full complement of SOPs that are available to their members across the country (N2, n.d.).

Ethics and Clinical Trials

Currently, Canada does not have a nationally centralized research ethics board (REB), harmonized national

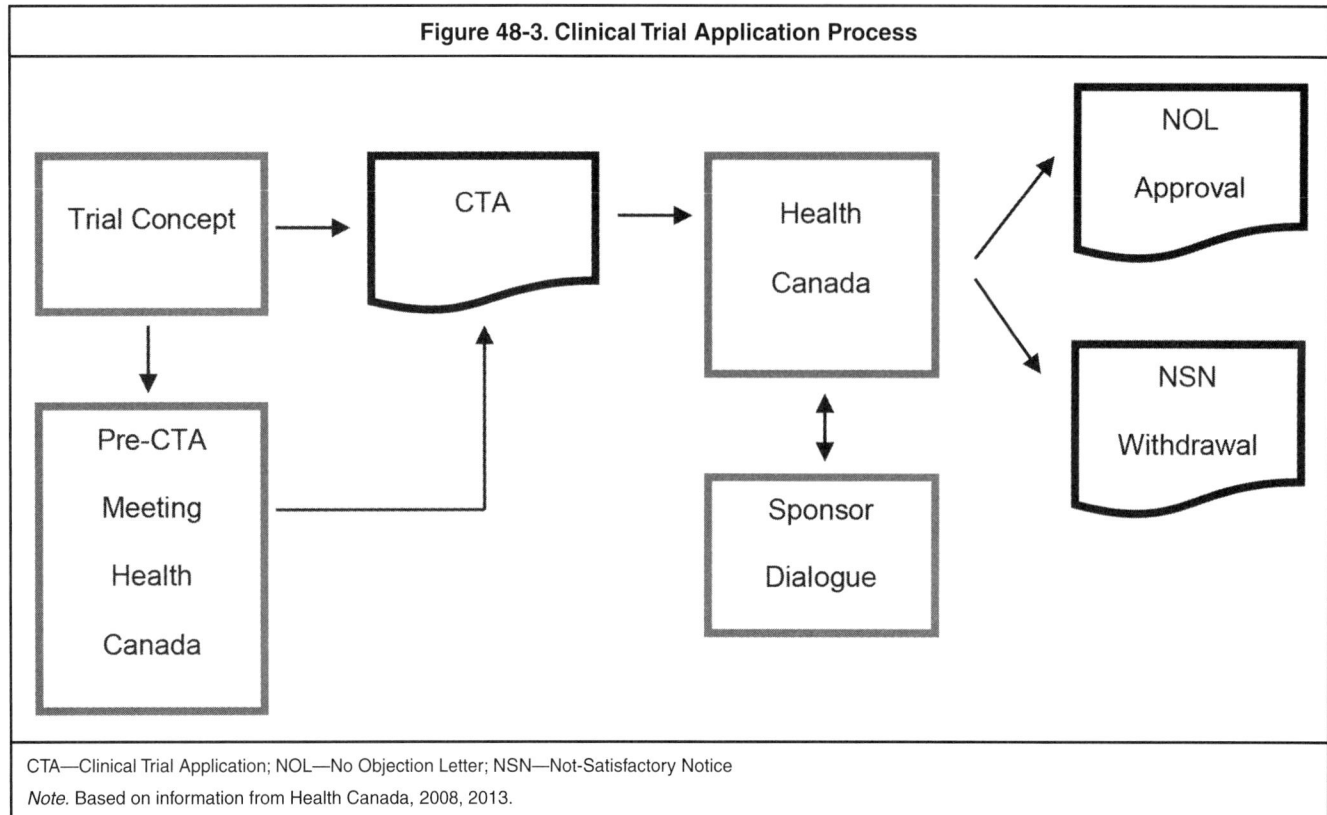

Figure 48-3. Clinical Trial Application Process

CTA—Clinical Trial Application; NOL—No Objection Letter; NSN—Not-Satisfactory Notice
Note. Based on information from Health Canada, 2008, 2013.

standards for REBs reviewing clinical trials, or an accreditation process for REBs. Although an institution can establish an REB and operate under its own principles and guidelines (Ogilvie & Eggleton, 2012), in the past decade, several provinces have developed centralized ethics review in an effort to standardize and streamline REB processes.

- In 2003, the Ontario Cancer Research Ethics Board (OCREB) was established from the Ontario Institute for Cancer Research as a centralized REB for multicenter trials. By centralizing the application process, OCREB aims to reduce workload, eliminate duplication, and accelerate trial initiation for multicenter trials across the province of Ontario (Ontario Institute for Cancer Research, 2013a).
- In 2009, the six recognized health REBs in the province of Alberta agreed to increase alignment and coordination of REBs in a provincial research ethics review system. The goal is to have an established harmonized system in place, which would include a common consent form, coordinated processes, reciprocity agreements among the institutions, and compatible operational platforms among the REBs (Magnan et al., 2010).
- In 2011, legislation was passed in the province of Newfoundland and Labrador for the Health Research Ethics Authority Act. The act states that the ethical review of all new research must be overseen by the Health Research Ethics Authority through the Health Research Ethics Board (Health Research Ethics Authority, n.d.).

Protocol Development, Review, and Approval

International Conference on Harmonisation of Technical Requirements for Registration of Pharmaceuticals for Human Use (ICH) GCP provides guidance for protocol development, review, and approval in Canada. Required protocol elements in Canada are consistent with those outlined in ICH GCP (ICH, 1996). The required elements of the informed consent document, informed consent process, and consent documentation in Canada also are consistent with those outlined in ICH GCP (ICH, 1996).

Informed Consent Process

The informed consent process in Canada is similar to that in other countries that have adopted the use of ICH GCP as their guidance document for the conduct of clinical trials. Although CTNs often play a key role in the informed consent process, all members of the research team are responsible for ensuring that patients are making informed decisions and that their decisions to participate are voluntary. This has become challenging in the past few years with the addition of multiple optional consent forms for genetic, genomic, and correlative studies in conjunction with the main study consent. Human rights in clinical trials can be protected only when informed consent is approached as a process (National Commission for the Protection of Human Subjects of Biomedical and Behavioral Research, 1979); therefore, adherence to ICH GCP is essential for the proper conduct of clinical trials in Canada.

Protocol Development and Approval

Protocol concepts can develop from many different sources: an individual idea, the result of collaboration, or the results of a previous clinical trial. Whether the concept is developed by an individual physician, an industry partner (pharmaceutical company), a collaborative network (National Cancer Institute of Canada [NCIC] Clinical Trials Group [CTG]), the Princess Margaret Hospital Consortium (PMHC), or a combination of these, it has the capability to develop into a protocol.

The process in which a protocol is authored or approved varies based on individual institutional, consortium, cooperative group, or industry policies. Most require a proposal to be drafted and peer-reviewed either formally or informally by a trial committee or disease group to determine if the scientific rationale is strong and if it could develop into a clinical trial that could be supported. In the case of investigator-initiated designs with industry support, both parties may be involved in the design and approval process, but the conduct of the study has to be performed by the investigator/sponsoring center and at arm's length from the industry supporter.

Many research groups and organizations have standardized protocol templates that highlight required protocol sections, reflect current policies, and provide authors with some structure and expectations for the required content.

Most successful clinical trial designs are those in which the various protocol drafts are reviewed by peers and study teams (e.g., data managers, pharmacists, correlative personnel, nurses) internally and at centers across the country. Reviews such as these can highlight potential difficulties that a clinical trial could experience as a result of institutional limitations or policies (e.g., resource allocation, peer buy-in) or provincial restrictions (e.g., variations in drug access, standard of care differences).

Once the protocol content is finalized, the sponsor is required to submit a CTA to Health Canada for review and approval prior to the trial being conducted in Canada. In addition to federal approval from Health Canada, investigators are required to receive local REB approval to conduct the trial at their individual site (Health Canada, 2013).

Financial Factors

Clinical trials involving investigational agents are funded in Canada through a variety of sources, including (a) pharmaceutical or biotechnology companies, (b) cooperative groups, (c) peer-reviewed granting agencies, or (d) a combination of these. Investigator-initiated trials being conducted without the support of pharmaceutical or biotechnology companies can be a costly and potentially debilitating endeavor for physician investigators and clinical research sites. Several avenues are available for the funding of such trials in Canada. Some of the pan-Canadian funding agencies and cooperative groups operating in Canada and supporting investigator-initiated trials are described in the following sections.

Canadian Institutes of Health Research

The Canadian Institutes of Health Research (CIHR) is the federal funding agency responsible for investing in Canadian health research. The agency was developed in 2000, consists of 13 virtual institutes, supports 14,100 researchers and trainees, and reports directly to the Minister of Health. Funding opportunities are available within biomedical, clinical, health system services, social, cultural, environmental, and population health research. Upwards of 80% of clinical research in Canada is funded through CIHR. Its mission is to strengthen Canadian health care and health services through new scientific information in targeted priority areas (CIHR, n.d.; Ogilvie & Eggleton, 2012).

Princess Margaret Hospital Consortium

The Princess Margaret Cancer Centre is home to PMHC, the only non-U.S. site funded through the National Institutes of Health. Since its inception in 2001, PMHC has been responsible for 100 phase I and II clinical trials with novel agents, with enrollment surpassing 2,000 patients on PMHC-led trials. Trials are designed and written by physicians across the consortium, providing them the opportunity to lead multicenter trials. PMHC has been critical of the rapid enrollment of patients and to leveraging disease-specific expertise across sites, which has significantly improved the productivity of clinical trials. The group has long-standing expertise in running and managing clinical trials across Canada.

National Cancer Institute of Canada Clinical Trials Group

NCIC was founded in 1947 to conduct cancer research programs on behalf of the Canadian Cancer Society and to provide funding for Canadian cancer research. Clinical trials supported by NCIC began in the early 1970s, and an independent CTG was created in 1977. Today, NCIC CTG is a national program and network of the Canadian Cancer Society Research Institute, the research funding program of the Canadian Cancer Society, which supports programs such as NCIC CTG through grant funding and is the largest national charitable funder of cancer research in Canada (Canadian Cancer Society, 2013). As a national cooperative group, NCIC CTG supports clinical trials nationally and internationally in cancer therapy, supportive care, and prevention. Its mission is "to develop and conduct clinical trials aimed at improving the treatment and prevention of cancer with the ultimate goal of reducing morbidity and mortality from this disease" (NCIC CTG, n.d.).

Recruitment and Retention

Enrollment in clinical trials in Canada varies across provinces. In 2009, the national average for enrollment of adults in clinical trials in cancer centers across Canada was 7%, with a range from as low as 2% in the Atlantic provinces to nearly 11% in Alberta (Dent & Yurichuk, 2011). Figure 48-4 shows the distribution of accrual by province across Canada. This same variation exists for enrollment in pediatric cancer clinical trials, where the national average for enrollment in 2009 was 37% with a range from as low as 15% in Saskatchewan to as high as 40% in Ontario (Dent & Yurichuk, 2011).

Oncology clinical trial accrual shares similar variation across the provinces and territories as well as across centers. The Province of Ontario requires reporting of accrual to oncology clinical trials from cancer centers and community hospitals. In 2011, the provincial average for enrollment in oncology clinical trials was 6.4% for cancer centers and 2.4% for community hospitals. The Princess Margaret Cancer Centre in Toronto leads accrual across Ontario, with a reported accrual rate of 18.8% for 2011 (Ontario Institute for Cancer Research, 2013b).

Canadian strategies for promotion and recruitment to clinical trials are geared more toward the medical community than directly toward patients. Family physicians, nurse practitioners, and general oncologists are able to refer patients to centers that conduct clinical trials. Patients who are given the option to participate in clinical trials as part of their treatment are assured of having health care available should they decline the offer of clinical trial participation. This assurance is one way in which Canadian strategies may differ from those used by countries where universal health care is not available.

Clinical Trial Registries

Strategies to improve recruitment into clinical trials aim to reduce either patient barriers to participation or physician/investigator barriers to patient referral. Improving transparency of clinical trials through searchable clinical trial registries is one strategy that may reach both target audiences (Moseley, 2009; Perner, 2008).

Currently, no federal regulatory requirements for clinical trial registration exist in Canada (Health Canada, 2012). However, clinical trials that are conducted in Canada under U.S. Food and Drug Administration regulations are required to be registered with ClinicalTrials.gov, a web-based resource for patients, healthcare professionals, and researchers (ClinicalTrials.gov, 2012). Clinical trials that receive funding from CIHR require registration in a public domain. This requirement does not specify which registry must be used (Ogilvie & Eggleton, 2012). Some of the searchable clinical trial registries available to patients and physicians/investigators that include Canadian trials are listed in Figure 48-5.

Public and Patient Education

In the age of ever-growing technology, some patients are arriving in physicians' offices more informed than ever before. Patients who have researched their disease and are interested in clinical trials will contact centers directly regarding participating in a specific clinical trial. CTNs in Canada may be the primary contact listed for clinical trials and therefore play a fundamental role in early education of patients regarding clinical trial processes, including eligibility. This may pose a challenge for CTNs, as patients may be disappointed to discover they are not eligible for a clinical trial that they had hoped for because inclusion or exclusion criteria not listed in the registry preclude them from participation.

Numerous publicly available resources are available to patients with cancer and healthcare providers across Canada that cover a broad spectrum of cancer-related topics, including clinical trials. Free web-based and paper-based resources are available to patients and healthcare providers through the Canadian Cancer Society and most provincial cancer agencies. CTNs play a fundamental role in the recruitment and retention

---

Figure 48-4. Adult Enrollment in Clinical Trials in Cancer Centers Across Canada, 2009

- Alberta: 10.7%
- Ontario: 8.1%
- British Columbia: 5.1%
- Manitoba: 4.5%
- New Brunswick: 2.4%
- Nova Scotia: 2.3%
- Prince Edward Island: 2.2%
- Saskatchewan: 2.1%
- Newfoundland and Labrador: 1.8%

Note. Based on information from Dent & Yurichuk, 2011.

Figure 48-5. Clinical Trial Registries Websites

- CanadaTrials.com database: www.canadatrials.com
- Canadian Partnership Against Cancer: www.canadiancancer trials.ca
- International Standard Randomised Controlled Trial Number Registry: www.isrctn.com
- U.S. National Cancer Institute clinical trial search: www.cancer.gov/clinicaltrials/search
- U.S. National Institutes of Health ClinicalTrials.gov registry and results database: www.clinicaltrials.gov
---

of patients on clinical trials. One of the keys to recruitment and retention is communication—with patients, family members, site staff, and other members of the healthcare team. With the abundance of information now available at patients' fingertips, CTNs are at the forefront of helping patients sift through and understand the information available to truly make informed decisions regarding their care.

Clinical Trial Participants

Investigational Agents

In Canada, investigational agents are regulated under the Food and Drug Regulations. These regulations provide strict guidelines on manufacturing, administration, and accountability for investigational agents (Minister of Justice, 2013). CTNs may hold responsibilities such as administration of the investigational product, education of staff in the administration of investigational products, and accountability of oral investigational products.

Adverse Events and Unanticipated Problems

Health Canada requires sponsors of clinical trials to report in an expedited manner all adverse events that are both serious and unexpected. Events that are fatal or life threatening must be reported within seven days of the sponsor becoming aware of the event. All other serious and unexpected events are to be reported within 15 days. Adverse events that do not meet the serious and unexpected criteria require only routine reporting (Health Canada, 2013).

Investigators are required to follow the reporting requirements of the sponsor and the local REB for serious and unexpected adverse events, as well as adverse events that do not meet the serious and unexpected criteria (Health Canada, 2013). CTNs play a critical role in the identification and reporting of adverse events. They often are responsible for the education of patients and families about the potential for expected and unexpected adverse events.

Patient and Family Education

Patient and family education is key to patients' understanding of their roles and responsibilities while on a clinical trial. Patients and families will sometimes have preconceived notions about clinical trials. Some medical professionals also have biases in regard to clinical research, which may affect patients' attitudes. It is an important role of CTNs to address these notions to accurately educate and inform patients and their families about clinical trials.

Patients on clinical trials may have idealistic expectations regarding the study medication and may not disclose adverse events because of fear they will be removed from the trial (Townsley et al., 2006). Along with the trial team, CTNs play a fundamental role in educating patients and families on the importance of disclosing both expected and unexpected adverse events for their own safety, as well as the safety of other trial participants.

Psychosocial Distress

Patient-centered care "seeks an integrated understanding of the patients' world—that is, their whole person, emotional needs, and life issues" (Stewart, 2001, p. 445). Sometimes, a fine balance exists between providing patient-centered care and adhering to the protocol. It is important that CTNs assess patients' psychosocial wellness throughout the trial. Tools like the Distress Assessment and Response Tool (DART), which is used at the Princess Margaret Cancer Centre, help assess the common physical, practical, and emotional issues experienced by patients (DART, 2010). The Edmonton Symptom Assessment System (ESAS) tool can assist CTNs in assessing the seven common symptoms experienced by patients with cancer. The implementation and reporting of ESAS assessment is mandatory in cancer centers across Ontario (Cancer Care Ontario, 2005). Although these tools may be useful in the identification of psychosocial distress, they present some challenges for CTNs and investigators in correlating these self-reported ratings to the National Cancer Institute Cancer Therapy Evaluation Program's Common Terminology Criteria for Adverse Events grading for clinical trial reporting.

Genetics and Genomics

Genetic Testing

With the global move toward personalized medicine, clinical trial participants are facing increasing requests for both mandatory and optional genetic testing in collaboration with participation in the primary clinical trial (Panel on Research Ethics, 2014). Although participation in such research has the promise of advancing cancer care, it is not without potential legal and ethical issues. One such issue facing Canadians is the possibility of discrimination based on genetic status. Although Canada has many regulations guiding the conduct of genetic research, currently no legislation exists preventing the use of genetic information for non-health and non-research purposes, such as insurability (The Canadian Encyclopedia, 2012).

Researchers in Canada are subject to the guidelines of the "Tri-Council Policy Statement: Ethical Conduct for Research Involving Humans" (TCPS 2) and, therefore, are required to develop and submit to the REB a plan for the management and safeguarding of information received through the use of genetic testing. If researchers plan to share the results of genetic testing with participants, they are responsible for ensuring that participants have the opportunity for informed decision making regarding whether they wish to receive or share the results with family. CTNs play a significant role in the education of patients and families regarding both optional and mandatory genetic research, particularly when patients have the opportunity to be informed of the results. Although they may not provide genetic counseling themselves, CTNs are responsible, along with the researcher, for ensuring that participants are provided with appropriate counseling as to the meaning and potential implications of the genetic results (Panel on Research Ethics, 2014).

Storage of Genetic Material

The collection and storage of genetic material in biobanks has become increasingly more common in today's healthcare environment, offering a rich resource for researchers. Access to and use of genetic material housed in biobanks in Canada is subject to the guidance set out in the TCPS 2 (Panel on Research Ethics, 2014). As such, researchers who have not received prior consent for the use of genetic material for future research are restricted to conducting research that satisfies the REB of the following requirements set out in the TCPS 2.

- Identifiable human biological materials are essential to the research
- The use of identifiable human biological materials without the participant's consent is unlikely to adversely affect the welfare of individuals from whom the materials were collected
- The researchers will take appropriate measures to protect the privacy of individuals and to safeguard the identifiable human biological materials
- The researchers will comply with any known preferences previously expressed by individuals about any use of their biological materials
- It is impossible or impracticable to seek consent from individuals from whom the materials were collected
- The researchers have obtained any other necessary permission for secondary use of human biological materials for research purposes. (Panel on Research Ethics, 2014, p. 179)

Correlative Trials

As valued members of the multidisciplinary team working on investigator-initiated studies, CTNs have a unique opportunity to create, lead, and participate in nursing companion studies. Such studies can provide valuable insights and opportunities for advancing nursing practice and improving the effectiveness of the care provided (Parahoo, 1997). Opportunities exist for CTNs in Canada to actively participate in the development of investigator-initiated clinical research either locally or nationally through groups such as NCIC CTG or PMHC. Involvement at this level provides a forum for CTNs to influence the design and conduct of investigator-initiated trials, as well as develop and lead nursing companion studies that may affect cancer nursing care internationally.

Documentation and Data Management

Documentation

Paper-based source documents and case report forms are increasingly being replaced by their electronic counterparts for the collection of data in clinical trials in an effort to improve efficiencies to the heavily burdened and resource-intense paper-based processes (Ene-Iordache et al., 2009). Throughout Canada and globally, this shift has required the design of electronic data capture systems to comply with local regulatory requirements. The requirements for electronic data capture for clinical trials are set out in ICH GCP guidance documents, which require sponsors to comply with the following when using electronic data capture in Canada:

- Ensure and document that the electronic data processing system(s) conforms to the sponsor's established requirements for completeness, accuracy, reliability, and consistent intended performance (i.e., validation).
- Maintain SOPs for using these systems.
- Ensure that the systems are designed to permit data changes in such a way that the data

changes are documented and that there is no deletion of entered data (i.e., maintain an audit trail, data trail, edit trail).
- Maintain a security system that prevents unauthorized access to the data.
- Maintain a list of the individuals who are authorized to make data changes.
- Maintain adequate backup of the data.
- Safeguard the blinding, if any (e.g., maintain the blinding during data entry and processing). (Health Canada, 1997, p. 29)

Maintaining a Regulatory File

As an extension of the forms and requirements that are completed in a CTA submission by sponsors to Health Canada for approval to conduct clinical trials, Health Canada also requires the completion of the following documents for Canadian sites.

Research Ethics Board Attestation

The research ethics board attestation (REBA) is to be completed by the REB that is reviewing and approving a clinical trial submission for a particular site. The original document is to be collected and maintained by the sponsor and is not submitted to Health Canada unless requested. A REBA is not required to be completed if the following statements are captured and documented in some capacity by the REB.

> In respect of the identified clinical trial, I certify, as representative of this Research Ethics Board that:
> 1. The membership of this Research Ethics Board complies with the membership requirements for Research Ethics Boards defined in Part C Division 5 of the Food and Drug Regulations;
> 2. This Research Ethics Board carries out its functions in a manner consistent with Good Clinical Practices; and
> 3. This Research Ethics Board has reviewed and approved the clinical trial protocol and informed consent form for the trial which is to be conducted by the qualified investigator named above at the specified clinical trial site. This approval and the views of this Research Ethics Board have been documented in writing. (Health Canada, 2009)

Clinical Trial Site Information

The intent of the Clinical Trial Site Information (CTSI) form is to provide information regarding the site, the site's Qualified Investigator, and the REB approval regarding a particular clinical trial. Sponsors must submit completed CTSI forms for each site to the appropriate directorate with the initial CTA or applicable CTA-As prior to implementation of the trial at that site (Health Canada, 2013).

Qualified Investigator Undertaking

For each clinical trial at a particular site, there can only be one designated qualified investigator participating in a trial. A qualified investigator undertaking form is to be completed by the qualified investigator, retained by the site, and available for inspection by Health Canada upon request.

Quality Assurance

Within Canada, there is an ongoing commitment to maintain and sustain the successful landscape of clinical research across the country. Although quality assurance practices contribute to maintaining a competitive advantage, the delicate balance between producing high-quality data at a cost that is financially feasible for sponsors, investigators, and institutions is an ongoing challenge.

It is the obligation of sponsors to develop quality assurance measures that are sustainable, while ensuring that patient safety and data integrity are maintained. Health Canada's adoption of ICH guidelines provides the framework within which all trials in Canada are to be conducted. These guidelines state that quality assurance and quality control systems must be in place and maintained to ensure that trials are conducted according to the protocol, Health Canada regulations, and GCP (Health Canada, 1997).

Many institutions across Canada have implemented quality assurance programs and measures to oversee the integrity of their research departments and initiatives. Integrating quality assurance parameters into the structure and running of a clinical trial is an effective method. Through education, SOPs, and voluntary and mandatory internal quality assurance audits, sites are able to ensure that they are conducting trials in compliance with Health Canada and institutional expectations.

Industry sponsors, and by extension, clinical research organizations, have different methodologies and practices for overseeing the integrity and quality of their trials. Everything from 100% source data verification to risk-based data monitoring plans, and various permutations of these two, is in practice. Likewise, cooperative groups have adopted quality assurance methods tailored to ensure the success of their programs. Typically, they involve some form of structured on-site monitoring similar to that of an industry sponsor. The objectives of the reviews are to verify eligibility, consent, drug accountability, study treatment, and investigations.

Health Canada requires all clinical trials conducted within Canada to follow the principles of GCP (Minister of Justice, 2013). Proof of GCP training is considered an essential document in a clinical trial's files for all members who have been delegated duties by the principal investigator (Health Canada, 2006). Although many institutions have developed their own in-house GCP training, it is rarely recognized as comparable to that required by sponsors. Until very recently, individual sponsors did not recognize each other's GCP training certification, thus creating a significant amount of redundancy in training among trials. The Collaborative Institutional Training Initiative (CITI), founded in March 2000, has recently been able to provide a centralized GCP training course that has been adopted by several pharmaceutical companies sponsoring trials in Canada as an acceptable method of GCP training (CITI, 2012). Successful completion of the CITI GCP training course eliminates repetitive GCP training among participating companies. Through an institution's affiliation with the Ontario Institute for Cancer Research and N2, online CITI clinical research training is available.

Professional Development

The Canadian Association of Nurses in Oncology/Association Canadienne des Infirmières en Oncologie (CANO/ACIO) is the national organization for oncology nurses in Canada. Its mission is "to lead nursing excellence in cancer control for Canadians" (CANO/ACIO, n.d.). The organization provides practice standards for specialized oncology nurses as well as generalist and advanced oncology nurses. The many local chapters across the country, as well as the special interest groups, offer novice to expert oncology nurses an opportunity for professional development. Since 1997, CANO/ACIO has supported certification in oncology nursing through the Canadian Nurses Association. Nurses who achieve certification are recognized with the credential CON(C) (certified in oncology nursing [Canada]), indicating that they have met the practice, continuous learning, and examination-based requirements for such designation.

Many Canadian nurses are also members of the Oncology Nursing Society (ONS), a professional organization in the United States that is devoted to enhancing oncology nursing practice. ONS offers CTNs, locally and internationally, the opportunity to be part of a special interest group dedicated to the specialty of clinical trial nursing. The ONS CTN Special Interest Group provides a forum for collaboration that supports ongoing professional development. In 2010, ONS published *Oncology Clinical Trials Nurse Competencies* to guide the practice of CTNs globally (see Appendix 2).

Aside from CANO/ACIO and ONS, provincial organizations offer professional development for CTNs working in oncology. In Ontario, the de Souza Institute is leading the way in providing ongoing educational support for nurses in developing the specialized skills essential for supporting patients and their families throughout their journey with cancer. The de Souza Institute has been in existence since 2008, partnering with Cancer Care Ontario and the University Health Network. It has recently expanded its mandate to include non-nurse healthcare professionals (de Souza Institute, n.d.).

CTNs in Canada have further opportunity for professional development in clinical research through nonnursing clinical research organizations such as the Society of Clinical Research Associates (SoCRA) and the Association of Clinical Research Professionals. Both offer certification in clinical research practice. SoCRA certification is more prevalent across Canada and offers a broader certification that encompasses various roles of clinical research professionals. Candidates who pass the certification examination are granted the credentials of CCRP (certified clinical research professional).

Summary

Health Canada provides governance and oversight for all clinical research in Canada, requiring sponsors and investigators to adhere to ICH GCP for the conduct of clinical trials. CTNs play a fundamental role in the recruitment, retention, conduct, and care of patients who are participating in clinical trials. Their collaboration with all members of the healthcare and research teams helps to ensure that the scientific and ethical integrity of trials is maintained, while providing essential support for patients throughout their cancer journey. Although cancer remains the leading cause of death in Canada, advances due to clinical research are continuing to improve the five-year survival locally and globally.

Key Points
- Canadians have access to quality health care in Canada through public healthcare plans regardless of their ability to pay.
- The Special Access Program allows Canadians the ability to access drugs not currently approved in Canada.
- Health Canada is responsible for the oversight of Canadian health.
- All clinical trials in Canada must receive Health Canada approval and follow the principles of ICH GCP.
- Ethical approval through local REBs is required, as Canada does not have a national REB.
- Sponsors are required to report adverse events that are both serious and unexpected to Health Canada in an expedited manner.

- Canadian strategies for promotion and recruitment of clinical trials are geared more toward the medical community than directly toward patients.

References

Canada Health Act RSC 1985 c C-6. (1985). Retrieved from http://canlii.ca/t/hzd6

Canadian Association of Nurses in Oncology/Association Canadienne des Infirmières en Oncologie. (n.d.). Retrieved from http://www.cano-acio.ca

Canadian Cancer Society. (2013). About our research. Retrieved from http://www.cancer.ca/en/about-us/our-research/?region=on

Canadian Cancer Society. (2014). *Canadian cancer statistics 2014.* Retrieved from http://www.cancer.ca/~/media/cancer.ca/CW/cancer%20information/cancer%20101/Canadian%20cancer%20statistics/Canadian-Cancer-Statistics-2014-EN.pdf

The Canadian Encyclopedia. (2012). Genetics, ethics and the law. Retrieved from http://www.thecanadianencyclopedia.ca

Canadian Institutes of Health Research. (n.d.). Canadian Institutes of Health Research. Retrieved from http://www.cihr.ca

Canadian Partnership Against Cancer. (2011). Partnership history. Retrieved from http://www.partnershipagainstcancer.ca/who-we-are/partnership-overview

Cancer Care Ontario. (2005). ESAS-Edmonton Symptom Assessment System—Description. Retrieved from https://www.cancercare.on.ca/toolbox/symptools

ClinicalTrials.gov. (2012, December). FDAAA801 requirements. Retrieved from http://clinicaltrials.gov/ct2/manage-recs/fdaaa

Collaborative Institutional Training Initiative. (2012). Good clinical practice. Retrieved from https://www.citiprogram.org

Dent, S.F., & Yurichuk, S. (2011). For cancer patients in Canada: Should clinical trials be considered part of "standard of care"? Retrieved from http://www.canceradvocacy.ca/reportcard/2010/Should%20Clinical%20Trials%20be%20Considered%20Part%20of%20Standard%20of%20Care.pdf

de Souza Institute. (n.d.). The "de Souze Difference": Where we are today. Retrieved from http://www.desouzainstitute.com/blog/%E2%80%9Cde-souza-difference%E2%80%9D-where-we-are-today

Distress Assessment and Response Tool. (2010). Patient and family education: About the UHN Patient and Family Education Program. Retrieved from http://www.uhnpatienteducation.ca

Ene-Iordache, B., Carminati, S., Antiga, L., Rubis, N., Ruggenenti, P., Remuzzi, G., & Remuzzi, A. (2009). Developing regulatory-compliant electronic case report forms for clinical trials: Experience with the DEMAND trial. *Journal of the American Medical Informatics Association, 16,* 404–408. doi:10.1197/jamia.M2787

Fonds de Recherche du Québec–Santé. (2007). Standard operating procedures (SOP) to ensure good clinical practice at clinical research sites. Retrieved from http://www.frqs.gouv.qc.ca/en/financement/SOP.shtml#01

Health Canada. (1997). Guidance for industry: Good clinical practice consolidated guideline. ICH topic E6. Retrieved from http://www.hc-sc.gc.ca/dhp-mps/alt_formats/hpfb-dgpsa/pdf/prodpharma/e6-eng.pdf

Health Canada. (2001, August). How drugs are reviewed in Canada. Retrieved from http://www.hc-sc.gc.ca/dhp-mps/prodpharma/activit/fs-fi/reviewfs_examenfd-eng.php

Health Canada. (2006, June). Guidance for records related to clinical trials (GUIDE-0068). Retrieved from http://www.hc-sc.gc.ca/dhp-mps/compli-conform/clini-pract-prat/docs/gui_68_tc-tm-eng.pdf

Health Canada. (2007, April). Brief history of drug regulation in Canada. Retrieved from http://www.hc-sc.gc.ca/dhp-mps/homologation-licensing/info-renseign/hist-eng.php

Health Canada. (2008). Review of the regulatory framework for clinical trials. Retrieved from http://www.hc-sc.gc.ca/dhp-mps/prodpharma/activit/consultation/clini-rev-exam/ctrf_dd_eccr_dt_2007-03-26-eng.php

Health Canada. (2009, October). Research ethics board attestation. Retrieved from http://www.hc-sc.gc.ca/dhp-mps/prodpharma/applic-demande/form/reba_acdr-eng.php

Health Canada. (2012, October). Harper government takes steps to bring clinical trial information home: Plans underway for first Canadian list of authorized clinical trials. Retrieved from http://www.hc-sc.gc.ca/ahc-asc/media/nr-cp/_2012/2012-155-eng.php

Health Canada. (2013). Guidance document for clinical trial sponsors: Clinical trial applications. Retrieved from http://www.hc-sc.gc.ca/dhp-mps/prodpharma/applic-demande/guide-ld/clini/ctdcta_ctddec-eng.php

Health Research Ethics Authority. (n.d). Health Research Ethics Authority. Retrieved from http://www.hrea.ca/Home.aspx

Intercultural Cancer Council. (2012). *Cancer facts: Cancer clinical trials: Participation by underrepresented populations.* Retrieved from http://iccnetwork.org/cancerfacts/ICC-CFS11.pdf

International Conference on Harmonisation of Technical Requirements for Registration of Pharmaceuticals for Human Use. (1996, June 10). *ICH harmonised tripartite guideline: Guideline for good clinical practice, E6(R1).* Retrieved from http://www.ich.org/fileadmin/Public_Web_Site/ICH_Products/Guidelines/Efficacy/E6/E6_R1_Guideline.pdf

Magnan, J., Trimbee, A., Pavlich, G., Libben, G., Brown, L., Tonge, A., … Barber, K. (2010, June). *Alberta Research Ethics harmonization: Executive Sponsors Joint Communique.* Alberta Health Services. Retrieved from http://www.albertahealthservices.ca/Researchers/if-res-alberta-research-ethics-executive-sponsors-communique.pdf

Minister of Justice. (2013, January). Food and Drug Regulations. Retrieved from http://laws-lois.justice.gc.ca/eng/regulations/C.R.C.,_c._870/index.html

Moseley, G.B. (2009). *Managing health care business strategy.* Burlington, MA: Jones & Bartlett Learning.

National Commission for the Protection of Human Subjects of Biomedical and Behavioral Research. (1979, April 18). *The Belmont report: Ethical principles and guidelines for the protection of human subjects of research.* Retrieved from http://www.hhs.gov/ohrp/humansubjects/guidance/belmont.html

NCIC Clinical Trials Group. (n.d.). About us. Retrieved from http://www.ctg.queensu.ca

Network of Networks. (n.d.). Resources: N2 SOPs. Retrieved from http://n2canada.ca/category/resources/n2-sops

Ogilvie, K.K., & Eggleton, A. (2012). Canada's clinical trial infrastructure: A prescription for improved access to new medicines. Standing Senate Committee on Social Affairs, Science and Technology. Retrieved from http://www.parl.gc.ca/Content/SEN/Committee/411/soci/dpk/01nov12/reports-e.htm

Ontario Institute for Cancer Research. (2013a). Ontario Cancer Research Ethics Board: About OCREB. Retrieved from http://oicr.on.ca/oicr-programs-and-platforms/ontario-cancer-research-ethics-board

Ontario Institute for Cancer Research. (2013b). Participation in clinical trials in Ontario. Retrieved from http://oicr.on.ca/high-impact-clinical-trials-program/clinical-trials-support-services/participation-clinical-trials-ontario

Pan-Canadian Oncology Drug Review. (n.d.). About the pan-Canadian Oncology Drug Review (pCODR). Retrieved from https://www.cadth.ca/pcodr/about-pcodr

Panel on Research Ethics. (2014). *Tri-council policy statement: Ethical conduct for research involving humans.* Retrieved from http://www.ethics.gc.ca/pdf/eng/tcps2-2014/TCPS_2_FINAL_Web.pdf

Parahoo, K. (1997). *Nursing research: Principles, process, and issues.* London, England: Macmillan.

Perner, L. (2008). Introduction to Marketing. University of Southern California. 1999–2008. Retrieved from http://www.consumerpsychologist.com/marketing_introduction.html

Stewart, M. (2001). Towards a global definition of patient centred care. *BMJ, 322,* 444–445. doi:10.1136/bmj.322.7284.444

Townsley, C.A., Chan, K.K., Pond, G.R., Marquez, C., Siu, L.L., & Straus, S.E. (2006). Understanding the attitudes of the elderly towards enrolment into cancer clinical trials. *BMC Cancer, 6,* 34. doi:10.1186/1471-2407-6-34

Treweek, S., Mitchell, E., Pitkethly, M., Cook, J., Kjeldstrøm, M., Johansen, M., ... Lockhart, P. (2010). Strategies to improve recruitment to randomised controlled trials. *Cochrane Database of Systematic Reviews, 2010*(4). doi:10.1002/14651858.MR000013.pub5

Turner & Associates Inc. (2008, April). *Issues of access to cancer drugs in Canada: A report for the Canadian Cancer Action Network.* Retrieved from http://www.ccanceraction.ca/wp-content/uploads/2014/12/3-CCAN-Pharma-Report-Final-PDF.pdf

Chapter 49

China

Yanfei Liu, MN, Ting Chang, MN, and Yuting Luan, RN

Introduction

China has accelerated clinical trial development since 2000. International multicenter clinical trials have become common throughout the country. At this rate of rapid development, learning from the experiences of developed countries in terms of clinical trial management is critical. However, national initiatives are already underway to improve systems within China's central government and local health authorities in all aspects of support. China, as a vast populous, has encountered many problems throughout the development process. For instance, clinical trials in various regions have varying degrees of attention and different levels of acceptance from different research sites. Furthermore, the current levels of constraint (e.g., infrastructure, qualified staff) cause imbalances in the development of this industry in China. However, the national plan from the central government and the Chinese Food and Drug Administration (CFDA) precisely states the support and attention for this field. Over the past 20 years, some relatively developed regions, such as Beijing and Shanghai, have gradually formed a complete system of clinical trials from phase I to phase IV. These relatively mature models promote and guide clinical trial development in the less-developed regions, such as Qinghai Province and Tibet.

History and Foundation

With the growth of clinical trial development throughout the world, increasing numbers of clinical trial centers in China gradually participated in multicenter and international studies. The course of history in this industry in China has been continuous but tortuous since the 1960s. The first formal regulation in China was issued in the early 1960s from the Ministry of Health of the People's Republic of China. However, clinical trials were administered by local or provincial Drug Regulatory Agencies. Several regulations have been developed in an effort to better manage clinical trials in China since 1970. Huge changes were taking place to daily life in China after the late 1980s, and meanwhile, more regulations were proposed according to International Conference on Harmonisation of Technical Requirements for Registration of Pharmaceuticals for Human Use (ICH, 1996) good clinical practice (GCP) guidelines as introduced to China. The supervision of all aspects of clinical trials was the key responsibility for CFDA, which was reestablished from the State Drug Administration and supervised by the Ministry of Health of the People's Republic of China from 2003 (CFDA, 2004).

In China, the Accreditation of Drug Clinical Trial Agency regulates and defines the qualified hospitals and study sites, including hospital facilities, qualification of doctors or other study staff, and clinical trial experiences. Only medical institutes officially CFDA-certified as National Institutes of Pharmaceutical Clinical Trials may conduct pharmaceutical clinical trials. Currently, affiliated hospitals of medical universities, some large public hospitals, and some special hospitals with unique features can obtain certification. Approximately 405 medical institutions from all over China possess licenses to conduct clinical trials, and 201 medical institutions passed the required recertification (every three years). Oncology trials in China are conducted in tier-I and tier-II cities where more hospitals meet the standards to be Drug Clinical Trial Agencies. The latest Drug Registration Regulation, which was enacted in 2007, is to standardize the procedures of new drug registry in China.

Clinical Trial Procedures in China

Within 10 years, ICH GCP guidelines have been embedded into China. Because of the huge potential market, a large number of global pharmaceutical companies target this area. The quantity of global and multicenter clinical trials (including oncology trials) launched has been increasing every year. All procedures are strictly conducted according to ICH GCP, Chinese GCP, and state and local regulations.

Because more than 80% of investigators prioritize their standard daily practices at hospitals, they have limited time to participate in clinical trials; therefore, clinical trial nurses or study nurses are considered important in the conduct of trials in China. However, the nursing workload is overburdened because oncology trials are more complicated than standard practice, and part-time study nurses have responsibility for more than five ongoing studies at each site. A full-time study nurse is a rarity in China.

The idea of trial management is changing. Sponsors and principal investigators (PIs) realized that the lack of manpower during study conduct is critical. Since 2005, they have applied for assigned study nurses to support trials on site, or hiring clinical research coordinators (CRCs) to manage the site in China. Another organization arising is the Site Management Organization, which is the professional organization that trains, educates, and manages CRCs for sites in China.

Ethics Committees

Ethics committees (ECs) are affiliated with each hospital. However, the main duty of ECs is similar to that in other countries and conforms to ICH GCP. A centralized EC, which is usually the EC from the lead PI's site, is acceptable for drug clinical trial agencies (agencies accept the EC's opinions).

Study nurses or CRCs update all trial documents submitted to the EC, such as the protocol, protocol amendments, informed consent forms, safety reports, serious adverse event reports, and advertising. The schedule of EC meetings is important as information provided to the site and sponsor.

Protocol Development, Review, and Approval

The types of studies in China include pharmaceutical company–sponsored and investigator-initiated. If the study includes investigational agents that are unapproved products, the sponsor or investigator must edit or develop the concept of the protocol. This must be approved by CFDA according to the Drug Registration Regulation. In response to any concerns (any processes within the protocol found to be unsecure or not beneficial for study subjects' health) from CFDA, sponsors or investigators must review and revise the protocol accordingly. Once the approval is received, trials are allowed to be initiated at the site level.

Informed Consent

All versions of the informed consent form must be approved by the local EC. Informed consent of patients is voluntary and may be withdrawn. Investigators explain the study clearly to study patients with easily understood language and answer all their questions. The site study nurse or CRC may inform patients of study details (e.g., the background of investigation drugs, details of insurance, emergency contact information); however, neither study nurses nor CRCs are currently allowed to obtain signed informed consent from the patients.

Financial Factors

The level of medical practice and requirements from trial staff are continuously greater than expected. The field of health and medical care is assigned importance by the Central Government, such that from 2011 to 2015, the total fund is estimated at 40 billion RMB (approximately $6.4 billion U.S. dollars) (Central People's Government of the People's Republic of China, 2011). PIs or experts in the biomedical industry use this fund to support their studies. For any investigator-initiated study, the pharmaceutical company, hospital, or academic institution could be the sponsor (singly or jointly). For pharmaceutical company–sponsored studies, the majority of supplies (e.g., study drugs, central lab kits, wireless card, fax machines) must be provided before the study begins. The key responsibility of study nurses or CRCs is coordination with investigators in order to update any information promptly. Insurance should cover the compensation of any incident resulting from having the study treatment. However, investigators emphasize to patients that all conditions will be handled on a case-by-case basis.

Recruitment and Retention

Project Recruitment

When China is chosen to participate in global clinical studies, a 10-fold ratio of recruitment is expected (related to other countries) because of the huge population. However, the process has not been as smooth and positive as expected. A significant factor is the time-consuming clinical trial assessment from CFDA, which can take from eight weeks to six months to complete. The accuracy of medical histories for trial patients has been another concern from the U.S. Food and Drug Administration and foreign pharmaceutical companies. Because patients are enrolled from everywhere in China, including remote areas, the medical histories might not be complete. However, this situation is improving as site investigators realize this as a compulsory factor. In cities that are tier I (such as Beijing, Shanghai, or Guangzhou) or tier II (other less-developed provincial capital cities, such as Lhasa and Tibet), where the facilities and systems of medical care are relatively advanced, all medical history will be tracked by integrated circuit cards (known simply as *IC cards*). These computerized record cards, similar to a credit card, are carried by individuals to all medical appointments. They will soon be more widely available nationally. Patients' medical histories are archived, because most of them were diagnosed and treated in hospitals.

Study nurses or CRCs collect the related medical history source documents and keep the hard copies in patients' files. They then support investigators to double-check the protocol inclusion and exclusion criteria. They update the PI about the recruitment status and inform him or her of the difficulties and contraindications when screening patients, such as lack of patients or professional resources.

Patient Compliance

Investigators communicate with patients to obtain information (e.g., education level, family) to evaluate whether the trial will provide benefit versus harm or burden.

Patients from remote regions who participate in trials, regardless of education, often have poor patient compliance, and this may become a major obstacle to the quality of the study. Economic concerns are foremost, such as covering costs of treatments, transportation, accommodation, and other expenses.

Once patients are screened successfully and enrolled into the study, they are reminded about strictly abiding by the requirements by the investigator. Despite drug diaries and other tools, mistakes in following protocol processes are not uncommon. Trial staff remain vigilant in their teaching and oversight as this is a primary concern to study nurses.

The study nurse or CRC will inform and remind patients regularly about the scheduled visits. Study coordinators will contact subjects regularly and inquire about their disease and encourage them to ask any questions. However, GCP in China does not allow study nurses to perform tasks deemed "medical judgments," so their functions are restricted.

Clinical Trial Participants

Human Resources at Trial Sites

According to ICH (1996) GCP and core regulations in China, trial sites must be Drug Clinical Trial Agencies. The PI must be a qualified professor in this field, which includes a medical degree and certification as well as working and research experience. The PI at each site is responsible for managing clinical trials, staff, and facilities of his or her specialty.

Considering the complexity of the trial, the PI makes the assignments and designations of enough and reasonable manpower as is done elsewhere; in China, the CRC or study nurse is not yet a compulsory practitioner included in trial activities.

With regard to oncology studies, more and more Drug Clinical Trial Agencies have their own study nurse teams. Their main roles are (a) coordination with the sponsor and local ethics committee, (b) management of investigational drugs and supplies, (c) study patients and visits management, and (d) data management. Otherwise, doctors or investigators take care of all medical or logistic trial tasks.

Investigational Product Management

Because the development of clinical trials in China has been unbalanced, the methods of managing investigational drugs differ among sites. The main pharmacy at a site for clinical trials is administered by pharmacists. Investigational drugs are locked at the site by investigators or nurses who are delegated by the PI. If CRCs are involved, they will support investigators to manage study agents, including (a) monitoring the storage temperatures, (b) tracking the drug inventory logs and accountability forms, (c) dispensing and receiving drugs for patients, and (d) returning or destroying drugs.

Adverse Events

Investigators assess adverse events according to their clinical experience and grade the events using the National Cancer Institute Cancer Therapy Evaluation Program (2010) Common Terminology Criteria for Adverse Events. All information for serious adverse events should be reported to CFDA within 24 hours. This requirement is in accord with GCP and sponsor requirements. Serious adverse events require follow-up reporting. Study coordinators collect the related information, inform investigators, and transfer the information to the case report form/electronic data capture (CRF/EDC) accordingly.

Genetics and Genomics

The CFDA or local EC examines and verifies the role of specimen collections in studies. If detection of genes from clinical trial patients is without any other expected benefits, CFDA or EC could ban or delete the test from the protocol.

Correlative Trials

Increasingly, studies have ancillary components that are part of the main protocol. These may include quality-of-life and patient-reported outcomes, as well as others. Many of these use internationally validated tools, such as the European Organisation for Research and Treatment of Cancer Quality-of-Life Questionnaire (commonly known as EORTC QLQ-C30). Research nurses provide patients with additional education and information to ensure that they understand the questions and can answer appropriately.

Moreover, pharmaceutical evaluation is embraced in more and more clinical trials. This plays an important role in China regardless of which type of clinical trial a patient participates in. Evaluations can provide decision-making reference information about whether the new drug research and development projects should continue. Most of the time, the study nurse or CRC will collect and summarize all related information according to the protocol.

Documentation and Data Management

Similar to in other countries, EDC systems are used by the majority of industry studies; however, for investigator-initiated studies, paper CRFs are still used because of limited budgets. All delegated staff are trained and accredited before the first patient is randomized. In order to ensure the source of EDC/CRF data, the CRC or study nurse must double-check the integrity of the medical records before transcribing data. Data managers from the sponsor or another professional company will manage and authenticate the database. Patients in oncology studies must cooperate with the long-term follow-up visits. Site investigators assess progression-free survival/overall survival and report the data.

Quality Assurance

The clinical trials center of the site should have GCP quality assurance systems that are certified by CFDA. Quality control and quality assurance are exerted over all trials conducted at the site. These checks ensure the qualifications of the investigators and facility, compliance with the protocol, GCP certification, and applicable regulatory requirements. Sites undergo sponsor monitoring and auditing and CFDA inspections regularly.

Professional Development

The development of CRCs or study nurses started in 2005. Sites and Site Management Organizations have continuing education programs for study nurses or CRCs. Unfortunately, many nursing administrators still consider study nurses as "not attending to proper work or duties." Meanwhile, the mentorship and promotion for clinical trial nurses and CRCs fall behind those of developed countries.

Summary

Because of the unbalanced clinical trial development in China, technically, the standard for Drug Clinical Trial Agencies is just in the early stages. The ability of investigators and related study staff to keep pace with the times is needed. It is indeed a huge challenge to improve the quality of clinical trials (i.e., protocol compliance). Manpower at sites and the general attitude for clinical trials are changing gradually. The Chinese experiences of clinical trials and the opportunities to learn from Western countries are both increasing. The careers of study nurses and CRCs are in their initial stage. The bright future for the career development of study nurses and CRCs is one of hope and determination.

Key Points
- Advancement of international clinical trials will be enhanced if nurses further the understanding of the history and foundation of clinical trials in China.
- Understanding the current status of clinical trials in China increases the education of clinical trial nurses worldwide.
- Nurses in China are encouraged to foster awareness of the problems and issues, as well as some of the solutions and obstacles to resolution, when developing clinical trials in China.
- It is important to promote recognition of both the similarities and differences to other countries in advancing the process and systems for clinical trials in China.

References

Central People's Government of the People's Republic of China. (2011). *The 12th five-year plan of national medicine in China*. Retrieved from http://www.gov.cn/gzdt/att/att/site1/20120119/782bcb8889ab1081f51901.pdf

Chinese Food and Drug Administration. (2004, February 19). On the issuance of "drug clinical trials accreditation agency (trial)" in State Food and Drug Safety [2004] No. 44. Retrieved from http://www.sda.gov.cn/WS01/CL0058/9346.html

International Conference on Harmonisation of Technical Requirements for Registration of Pharmaceuticals for Human Use. (1996, June 10). *ICH harmonised tripartite guideline: Guideline for good clinical practice, E6(R1)*. Retrieved from http://www.ich.org/fileadmin/Public_Web_Site/ICH_Products/Guidelines/Efficacy/E6/E6_R1_Guideline.pdf

National Cancer Institute Cancer Therapy Evaluation Program. (2010). *Common terminology criteria for adverse events* [v.4.03]. Retrieved from http://evs.nci.nih.gov/ftp1/CTCAE/CTCAE_4.03_2010-06-14_QuickReference_5x7.pdf

Chapter 50

European Union Directives

Jane Bryce, MSN, AOCNS®, and Gabriele Elser, RN

Introduction

The European Union (EU) provides guidance, legislation, and oversight of clinical trials on medicinal products conducted within its member states. Member states as of the time of this writing are listed in Figure 50-1. The European Medicines Agency (n.d.) is a decentralized body of the EU that is responsible for the scientific evaluation of medicines developed by pharmaceutical companies for use in the EU.

EU member states agree to conduct clinical trials according to good clinical practice (GCP). Since 1965, the European Commission has provided guidance and standards on the authorization for marketing of medicinal products and the conduct of clinical trials (Council Directive 65/65/EEC of 26 January 1965; Council Directive 75/318/EEC of 20 May 1975). The European Commission introduced the International Conference on Harmonisation of Technical Requirements for Registration of Pharmaceuticals for Human Use (ICH) in 1996.

Currently, requirements for the conduct of clinical trials in the EU are stated in Commission Directive 2001/20/EC (the Clinical Trials Directive [CTD]).

CTD 2001/20/EC was passed by the EU in order to harmonize European practices in clinical medicinal research. A principal objective of the directive is the *protection of human subjects* according to the Declaration of Helsinki and the ICH GCP guidelines. A second objective is to *reduce the delays in activating clinical trials* in member states through the simplification and harmonization of administrative procedures while reducing the duplication of processes. Member states were to have implemented the CTD 2001/20/EC by May 1, 2004. The key points regarding the CTD are listed in Figure 50-2.

Each member state develops its own system of registering and authorizing ethics committees (ECs). The EC considerations for rendering an opinion on a clinical trial are outlined in Figure 50-3. A single favorable opinion of the EC is required for each member state. Each must also designate its *competent authority*, the national regulatory authority that provides oversight of clinical trials on medicinal products. Guidance is provided for the evaluation of clinical trials on minors and on incapacitated adults not able to give informed legal consent, with specific restrictions outlined for each case (Commission Directive 2001/20/EC).

Figure 50-1. Member States of the European Union

- Austria
- Belgium
- Bulgaria
- Croatia
- Cyprus
- Czech Republic
- Denmark
- Estonia
- Finland
- France
- Germany
- Greece
- Hungary
- Ireland
- Italy
- Latvia
- Lithuania
- Luxembourg
- Malta
- Netherlands
- Poland
- Portugal
- Romania
- Slovakia
- Slovenia
- Spain
- Sweden
- United Kingdom

Note. Based on information from European Union, n.d.

Figure 50-2. Key Points of European Union Clinical Trials Directive Implemented in 2004

- The protection of clinical trial subjects
- The creation of an European Clinical Trials Database (EudraCT) for the registration of clinical trials and for safety reporting (EudraVigilance)
- Defining sponsor, investigator, and ethics committee responsibilities
- Compliance with good clinical practice and good manufacturing practice guidelines
- Standardized labeling of investigational medicinal products
- The requirement of both a favorable opinion by the ethics committee and the authorization by the "competent authority" of each participating member state
- The provision of study drugs to subjects free of charge
- Clinical trial insurance for indemnity or compensation for injury

Note. Based on information from Commission Directive 2001/20/EC.

> **Figure 50-3. European Union Ethics Committees, Considerations for Rendering an Opinion**
>
> - Protocol relevance, design, risks and benefits
> - Suitability of the investigator(s) and facilities
> - The investigator's brochure
> - Protection of trial subjects
> - The adequacy and completeness of the informed consent document and procedures
> - Provisions for indemnity or compensation for injury and any insurance coverage
> - Agreements between the sponsor and the facility conducting the trial
> - Arrangements for the recruitment of subjects
>
> *Note.* Based on information from Commission Directive 2001/20/EC.

> **Figure 50-4. Clinical Trial Information in EudraCT Required by Each Member State**
>
> - Request for authorization
> - Any amendments to the request
> - Any substantial protocol amendments
> - A favorable opinion by the ethics committee
> - The declaration of the end of the clinical trial
> - A reference to any good clinical practice–related inspections

The European Commission has published detailed guidelines regarding clinical trial regulations in Volume 10 of *EudraLex—The Rules Governing Medicinal Products in the European Union* (http://ec.europa.eu/health/documents/eudralex/vol-10/index_en.htm). Detailed guidance is provided in the following areas.

- The clinical trial application process and application form
- Safety reporting
- Quality of investigational medicinal product
- Inspections

The sponsor may not start a clinical trial until the EC has issued a favorable opinion and the competent authority of the member states concerned has not informed the sponsor of any grounds for nonacceptance. The procedures to reach these decisions can be parallel or not, depending on the sponsor and on national procedures. The required documentation and procedures are listed in "Detailed Guidance on the Request for Authorisation of a Clinical Trial on a Medicinal Product for Human Use," in EudraLex Volume 10 (European Commission, n.d.).

All clinical trials conducted in Europe must be registered in the EudraCT, a European database of all ongoing or completed clinical trials. This database permits communication among competent authorities of member states, the European Medicines Agency, and the European Commission. The sponsor must obtain a EudraCT number, the procedures for which are available at https://eudract.ema.europa.eu. Figure 50-4 summarizes clinical trial information in EudraCT required by each member state.

In accordance with Commission Directive 2001/20/EC, once a sponsor has submitted a protocol for opinion to the EC, the EC has 60 days within which to render its decision and to communicate such to the sponsor and competent authority. There is an automatic 30-day extension for trials with gene therapy, somatic cell therapy, and medicinal products containing genetically modified organisms, with the possibility of an additional 90-day extension if further consultation or committee review is needed. No time limit is imposed for the review of clinical trials of xenogeneic cell therapy.

The EC may make a single request for additional information from the sponsor, during which time the 60-day clock is suspended. In the case of an unfavorable opinion by the EC, a sponsor has only one opportunity to resubmit the protocol after amending the content, taking into account the reasons given for nonacceptance.

A sponsor may submit an application for a clinical trial to different European countries in parallel. A single favorable EC opinion is required for each member state. The sponsor is responsible for providing various language versions of the clinical trial documents as per national requirements.

The sponsor is responsible for obtaining authorization for the import of the investigational medicinal product in accordance with good manufacturing practices and EU regulations. The directive outlines required labeling for the investigational medicinal product, including the use of the official languages of the member state on the outer packaging.

The CTD requires investigators to immediately report serious adverse events (SAEs) to the sponsor and to report adverse events, laboratory evaluations, and any safety reporting to the sponsor as stipulated by the protocol. The sponsor is responsible for maintaining detailed records of reported adverse events.

The sponsor is responsible for reporting all relevant information about suspected unexpected serious adverse reactions (SUSARs) to the competent authorities in all the member states concerned, and to the ECs (see European Commission, 2011, for reporting guidelines). A SUSAR that is life threatening or results in death must be reported within seven days of the sponsor's knowledge of the event and within 15 days for all other cases. The sponsor must inform all investigators of *any* SUSAR. Each member state must register SUSARs that are brought to its attention, and all SUSARs are entered into EudraVigilance database. The EudraVigilance Clinical Trial Module (http://eudravigilance.ema.europa.eu) facilitates the electronic reporting of SUSARs. The sponsor must also provide an annual safety report listing all suspected serious adverse reactions that have occurred, along with a report of the subjects' safety. ICH guideline E2F (available at www.ema.europa.eu/docs/en) provides details on the required elements of the report and information about transmission to regulatory authorities.

Finally, the 2001 CTD requires that inspections be carried out to verify compliance with good clinical and manufacturing practices. Competent authorities of member states appoint inspectors and the inspections are carried out on behalf of the European Community, with mutual recognition among member states.

Several implementation and practical issues were identified soon after the issue of Commission Directive 2001/20/EC. Much of the discussion centered on (a) the increased clinical trial costs for the nonprofit sponsor related to insurance policies, (b) provision of all medicines in the clinical trial, and (c) monitoring activities to ensure GCP (Crawley, 2004; Habeck, 2003; Meunier, Dubois, Negrouk, & Rea, 2003; Meunier & Lacombe, 2003; Perrone et al., 2004; Watson, 2003). The increased costs and bureaucracy created concern that academic clinical trials in the EU could be jeopardized by a lack of competitiveness with non-EU trials. A subsequent CTD was issued in 2005 to address some of these issues, as well as to provide further guidance on the 2001 directive. Commission Directive 2005/28/EC addresses the issues summarized in Figure 50-5. Member states were to implement this directive by January 29, 2006. The directive clarifies that member states can introduce modalities to take into account noncommercial clinical trials (nonprofit-sponsored trials often referred to as academic trials) while still applying the principles of GCP.

Further, the provision and labeling of already licensed medicinal products may be simplified according to good manufacturing practices. Import authorization is outlined and must be provided by the competent authority within 90 days.

The directive outlines minimal educational requirements for inspectors and establishes that GCP inspections may take place at any time before, during, or after the conduct of a clinical trial and during or after the marketing authorization process. Member states must establish the framework for GCP inspectors and inspections such as providing adequate resources and procedures.

Figure 50-5. Key Issues of Clinical Trials Directive 2005/28/EC

- The principles of good clinical practice referred to in the 2001 directive with specific consideration to noncommercial trials
- The requirements for the authorization of the manufacture or importation of investigational medical products as foreseen in directive 2001/20/EC
- Guidelines on the documentation related to clinical trials and its archiving
- Qualifications of inspectors and inspection procedures in accordance with directive 2001/20/EC

Note. Based on information from Commission Directive 2005/28/EC.

It foresees joint training and inspections by the commission and agency and the provision of guidance documents for inspections.

Proposed Clinical Trials Regulation

In July 2012, the European Commission adopted a Proposal for a Regulation of the European Parliament and of the Council on Clinical Trials on Medicinal Products for Human Use, and Repealing Directive 2001/20/EC. When published, it is expected to address many of the issues that had been identified by stakeholders in the member states and by the commission as barriers to fully achieving the goals of harmonization set out in the CTD it will replace. The following are some of the expected changes (European Commission, 2012).

- Coordinated assessment procedures (by member states) through a single portal for clinical trial application
- Streamlined and modernized safety reporting rules for investigators, and for sponsors through interaction with EudraVigilance
- Introduction of the concept of *cosponsorship* of clinical trials for research networks
- Introduction of low-intervention clinical trials, which may be subject to shorter approval times, less stringent rules, and insurance coverage
- Clear rules regarding informed consent in emergency situations
- Recommendations for member states to establish a national indemnification mechanism to cover compensation for damages successfully claimed by clinical trial subjects

Resources for European Clinical Trial Nurses

The European Oncology Nursing Society (EONS) is an organization of professional nurses throughout Europe dedicated to the care of patients with cancer. EONS collaborates with national oncology nursing societies, individual nurses, and professional, political, and patient advocacy organizations across Europe. Its mission is to work in partnership to develop and promote excellence in cancer nursing practice through education, research, and leadership and support to cancer nurses across Europe (EONS, 2013).

The *European Journal of Oncology Nursing* is the official journal of EONS and publishes research relevant to patient care, education, management, and policy development. In addition, EONS newsletters are published monthly. EONS participates in the biannual European

Cancer Congress with a scientific nursing program, as well as its own biannual congress. EONS develops and promotes many research and educational projects. Membership and other information is available at www.cancernurse.eu.

The European School of Oncology (ESO) was established in 1982 as a nonprofit organization that seeks to increase the knowledge of healthcare professionals in cancer care (ESO, 2013). ESO provides nursing, physician, and multidisciplinary continuing education and specialization courses in cancer care. The courses are available in English and other national languages in Europe, Russia, the Balkans, the Middle East, and Latin America. ESO courses are clinically oriented and place a special focus on patient advocacy. A wide range of both basic and advanced courses is offered across many topics. ESO sponsors a Course for Clinical Trial Nurses, based on a European curriculum, and was first offered in 2005. Information about ESO events, publications, fellowships, and other activities is available at www.cancerworld.org. ESO and EONS have collaborated to conduct advanced nursing courses, Master Classes in Oncology Nursing, since 2007.

The European Organisation for the Research and Treatment of Cancer (EORTC), founded in 1962, is an international organization that aims to develop, conduct, coordinate, and stimulate translational and clinical research to improve cancer care. It is a private, nonprofit organization. Its core activity is conducting clinical trials that develop new treatments or define new standards (EORTC, 2013). Clinical trials are international, multidisciplinary, and independent. EORTC aims to provide a European platform to develop and conduct quality research, to facilitate collaboration across countries, and to promote clinically oriented research through education and policy (EORTC, 2013).

EORTC has a network of more than 200 institutions from more than 30 countries. The EORTC clinical research division is composed of many tumor site–specific research groups as well as radiotherapy and quality-of-life groups. The EORTC quality-of-life questionnaires are available in many languages and are widely used in European clinical trials. EORTC offers multidisciplinary educational courses on the topic of clinical research. Information regarding EORTC protocols, groups, publications, educational offerings, and other topics can be found at www.eortc.be.

Summary

The European Clinical Trials Directives 2001/20/EC and subsequent 2005/28/EC were aimed at harmonizing clinical research practices in Europe and protecting clinical trial participants. Although still in effect at the time of this publication, these directives will likely be replaced by more comprehensive clinical trial regulations proposed by the European Commission with widespread support of the stakeholders in clinical trials.

Key Points

- Requirements for the conduct of clinical trials in the EU are set out by the European Commission. Reference and support documents are accessible in EudraLex Volume 10.
- Clinical trials conducted in Europe are identified and registered within a European platform and share a common electronic clinical trial application process and safety reporting procedures that are managed via a national portal for each member state.

References

Commission Directive 2001/20/EC of the European Parliament and of the Council of 4 April 2001 on the approximation of the laws, regulations and administrative provisions of the member states relating to the implementation of good clinical practice in the conduct of clinical trials on medicinal products for human use. *Official Journal of the European Union, 1.5.2001*, L 121, 34–44.

Commission Directive 2005/28/EC of 9 April 2005 laying down principles and detailed guidelines for good clinical practice as regards investigational medicinal products for human use, as well as the requirements for authorisation of the manufacturing or importation of such products. *Official Journal of the European Union*, L91, 13–19.

Crawley, F.P. (2004). New European clinical trials directive: Is European research possible? *BMJ, 328*, 522.

European Commission. (n.d.). *EudraLex Volume 10*. Retrieved from http://ec.europa.eu/health/documents/eudralex/vol-10/EudraLex

European Commission. (2011). Detailed guidance on the collection, verification and presentation of adverse event/reaction reports arising from clinical trials on medicinal products for human use (2011/C 172/01). *Official Journal of the European Union*, C172, 1–13.

European Commission. (2012). Proposal for a regulation of the European Parliament and of the council on clinical trials on medicinal products for human use, and repealing Directive 2001/20/EC. Retrieved from http://ec.europa.eu/health/files/clinicaltrials/2012_07/proposal/2012_07_proposal_en.pdf

European Medicines Agency. (n.d.). About us. Retrieved from http://www.ema.europa.eu/ema/index.jsp?curl=pages/about_us/general/general_content_000235.jsp&mid

European Oncology Nursing Society. (2013). EONS mission statement. Retrieved from http://www.cancernurse.eu

European Organisation for Research and Treatment of Cancer. (2006). EORTC aims and mission. Retrieved from http://www.eortc.be

European School of Oncology. (2013). Mission statement. Retrieved from http://www.nurse.eu

European Union. (n.d.). List of countries. Retrieved from http://europa.eu/about-eu/countries/index_en.htm

Habeck, M. (2003). Gloomy prospects for European cancer research. *Lancet Oncology, 4*, 66. doi:10.1016/S1470-2045(03)00991-4

International Conference on Harmonisation of Technical Requirements for Registration of Pharmaceuticals for Human Use. (1996, June 10). *ICH harmonised tripartite guideline: Guideline for good clinical practice, E6(R1)*. Retrieved from http://www.ich.org/fileadmin/Public_Web_Site/ICH_Products/Guidelines/Efficacy/E6/E6_R1_Guideline.pdf

Meunier, F., Dubois, N., Negrouk, A., & Rea, L.A. (2003). Throwing a wrench in the works? *Lancet Oncology, 4,* 717–719. doi:10.1016/S1470-2045(03)01299-3

Meunier, F., & Lacombe, D. (2003). European Organisation for the Research and Treatment of Cancer's point of view. *Lancet, 362,* 663. doi:10.1016/S0140-6736(03)14163-3

Perrone, F., Marangolo, M., Di Costanzo, F., Colucci, G., Repeto, L., Merlano, M., ... Gallo, C. (2004). Insurance for independent cancer trials. *Annals of Oncology, 15,* 1722–1723. doi:10.1093/annonc/mdh444

Watson, R. (2003). EU legislation threatens clinical trials. *BMJ, 326,* 1348. doi:10.1136/bmj.326.7403.1348-a

Chapter 51

France

Bénédicte Votan, MSc, Post Graduate, and Nathalie Le Fur, PhD

Introduction

Since the implementation of the European Directive 2001/20/CE in 2004 (Loi No. 2004-806, 2004), many oncology trials have been launched. Although this directive has introduced some complexities and slowness in the implementation of clinical trials in France, the number of clinical trials in oncology is quite significant in comparison with other specialties.

History and Foundation

In 2003, former French Republic President Jacques Chirac initiated a plan to fight cancer. This cancer plan has been renewed since then, and challenges and objectives are reviewed every five years. Based on five areas of focus (research, observation, prevention and screening, care, and life during and after cancer), the 2009–2013 cancer plan included 30 measures and represented a significant financial investment of nearly €2 billion over five years (Institut du National Cancer [INCa], 2013). This is a sign that the fight against cancer is a top priority in France. As part of this plan, a government institution responsible for coordinating actions in this fight called the French National Cancer Institute (INCa) was created by the public health law of August 2004 and formed in July 2005. This agency has a steering and monitoring role in implementing the cancer plan. The cancer plan was updated for 2014–2019 and includes 17 objectives based on the four major ambitions of the plan, which are to heal sick people, preserve the continuity and quality of life, invest in prevention and research, and optimize management and organization (INCa, 2014a).

In its annual report, INCa stated that the cancer incidence has been rising over the past decades while mortality has been decreasing (INCa, 2012). In 2011, 365,500 new cancers were diagnosed (207,000 in the male population and 158,500 in the female population, which represent 383 cases per 100,000 men and 268.5 per 100,000 women). The mortality reached 147,500 (84,500 men and 63,000 women), with lung cancer being the leading cause of cancer death in men and breast cancer being the leading cause of cancer death in women (INCa, 2012).

More than 10% of the patients (35,000–40,000) are enrolled in cancer clinical trials based on the cancer incidence (the aim of the cancer plan is to enroll 20% of patients in clinical trials). The majority of the trials are conducted on hematologic, breast, and respiratory system cancers, and nearly 70% of them are testing drugs. Academic trials represent 80% of the oncology clinical trials in France, with approximately 40% of patients included in university hospitals and 40% in centers specifically dedicated to combatting cancer.

Oncology center staff members are well versed in performing clinical trials, and most of the larger centers are structured with a clinical trial department, clinical research associates, and study nurses.

Clinical Trials: Fundamental Information

All clinical trials are subject to the regulations of La Loi Huriet, as has been the code of biomedical research ethics in France since 1988 (Loi No. 88-1138, 1988). In 2004, this regulation was updated to the Loi de Santé Publique (Loi No. 2004-806, 2004). The key points of this revision are the integration of the new European Directive 2001/20/CE and its direct application in France, including the new pharmacovigilance safety measures. Furthermore, it attributes a new role to the French agency in that the previous process of simply notifying the agency of the commencement of a clinical trial was changed to require prior approval from the agency, thus moving from a notification process to an approval process. This law defines in greater detail the role of the parties involved in a clinical research study (e.g., investigators, sponsors, study coordinators). Responsibilities of each member of the clinical research study team are shown in Table 51-1.

Clinical studies may be sponsored by pharmaceutical companies, nonprofit organizations, or cancer centers. In France, all clinical trial protocols that involve testing drugs on humans are submitted to a national ethics committee (EC). A total of 40 ECs exist throughout the French Territory (Nouvelles Règles de la Recherche Biomédicale, n.d.). ECs are independent from the competent authorities (CAs); they have no ties to or relationship with one another. The Minister of Health oversees the proper functioning of the activities of ECs and authorizes them to pursue their operations.

Although ECs generally are attached to a hospital or a clinic, some are completely independent from any institution. By design, all ECs function in the same required manner, with the same number of members and responsibilities. Study sponsors previously could submit dossiers to whichever EC they prefer, but upon the new legal frame set forth in 2014, sponsors have to submit their dossiers to a national panel that will choose the most relevant EC.

Each EC is made of 28 members grouped in two colleges, including medical professionals, pharmacists, laypeople, and nurses. The EC reviews and approves the protocol, patient information, informed consent form, and all documents that will be presented to patients (such as quality-of-life questionnaires). It verifies the suitability of sites and investigators to perform clinical trials and that the sponsor has arranged for appropriate trial insurance. The EC has 35 days to provide its notification.

The protocol must be forwarded to the CA, the French National Agency for Medicines and Health Products Safety (Agence Nationale de Sécurité du Médicament et des Produits de Santé [ANSM]), to obtain national approval (ANSM, 2006). With the new European directive, the ethics application and the CA application may be submitted simultaneously. A clinical trial may not begin until it has obtained authorizations from both the EC and the French CA. The CA shall respond to the sponsor in a maximum of 60 days. According to the latest report activity of ANSM published in 2012, clinical trial authorization was given in an average of 41 days (ANSM, 2012).

A clinical trial can occur in one center, known as a monocenter trial, or in several centers, known as a multicenter trial.

Informed consent is accepted as a process by patients and doctors. In France, only a medical doctor involved with a given trial is permitted to review the information contained in the informed consent form with the patient (Loi No. 88-1138, 1988). Eligible patients are approached to assess their interest and opinion regarding trial participation. The doctor reviews all of the essential medical information contained in the informed consent form, as well as the benefits and possible adverse events. Patients take the form home and are asked to review it at their leisure and to return it at the next appointment with a list of questions related to the study or their conditions. Then, if the patient is satisfied with the answers to all queries and is willing to participate, both the doctor and the

Table 51-1. Responsibilities of Personnel Actively Involved in Clinical Trials in France		
Role	Description/Legal Obligations	Restrictions
Sponsor	Oversees the setup, conduct, and finances of the study and the results published Must ensure adequate clinical trial indemnity throughout the duration of study Submits to local ethics committees (ECs) and authorities to obtain approval before commencing the study Obtains insurance to cover any risks related to the trial	May not have any direct interactions with patients participating in the study
Study coordinator	An investigator selected by the sponsor to act as a representative of the study in a multicenter trial Often writes the final publications of the study	May not have any direct interactions with the health authorities with respect to the study
Investigator	A physician participating in the trial who is responsible for a given center and its staff	May not have any direct interactions with the EC or the authorities with respect to the study
Co-investigator	Synonymous with *subinvestigator* in the United States and Canada; always a physician	May not perform any tasks other than those delegated by the investigator
Study nurse	None at present	May not present the informed consent document to a patient May not prescribe any medications

patient sign the consent form, and a copy is given to the patient.

Financial Factors

In France, the money for financing a clinical trial comes either from a pharmaceutical company or, for academic trials where there is no investigational drug (like a surgery trial), INCa. In case of clinical trials in rare tumors, specific European programs may give access to European funding.

Recruitment and Retention

In France, INCa maintains a database with all clinical trials that is accessible to everybody and where patients can become aware of clinical trials (INCa, 2014b). Also, physicians play a significant role in referring and enrolling patients in clinical trials through the network of regional clinicians, along with patient advocacy groups.

Clinical Trial Participants

Eligibility

Eligibility criteria are clearly stated in all protocols, and the investigators are responsible for checking all of the criteria before including a patient. Informed consent, as approved by the EC, must always be obtained prior to the first trial-related procedures. Laboratory, x-ray, and other baseline tests must be obtained within the protocol-stated time frames and within specified acceptable limits.

Active Treatment

A pharmaceutical company supplies investigational agents, which are shipped to the pharmacy of each center. The center's pharmacy is responsible for storing, preparing, handling, dispensing, and accounting for the trial drugs. The pharmacy must receive the protocol and other trial-related documents that direct the pharmacy in the trial. In some trials, treatment can be blinded by using a placebo with the same appearance and management as the investigational drug.

During treatment, patients are assessed for adverse reactions. All adverse reactions/events and serious adverse events must be reported to the EC and CA. The clinical trial team in the hospital must ensure that accurate details of the patient's toxicities and side effects are recorded in the case report forms (CRFs). It is important to record symptoms and assess their relationship to the treatment.

Tumor response assessments are performed per protocol. Most trials will seek disease-free survival at a minimum, but many will challenge for a response. Because there are many trials in oncology, the study endpoints and goals will vary from study to study. For trials that require radiology response assessments, computed tomography is used most extensively, but positron-emission tomography also can be used in specific cases.

Follow-Up

In general, patients are evaluated until deceased, independent of the objectives of the trial (e.g., response rate or progression-free survival). Centers are asked to make every effort to fulfill the follow-up reporting required to complete the analyses. Unfortunately, no national database currently exists to locate patients who have moved out of the area or are deemed lost to follow-up. Centers can, however, contact the local town hall where a patient originally lived to obtain survival information or date of death.

Genetics and Genomics

One of the main objectives of the French national cancer plan is to develop research on the understanding of biologic mechanisms (INCa, 2013). The national objective is to associate translational research to the biomedical research of each protocol to analyze and define subsets of patients who will benefit the most from treatments.

Correlative Trials and Ancillary Studies

Most clinical studies include a patient-reported outcome (patient's quality-of-life [QOL] evaluation), as it is well known that the QOL balance is very important for patients with cancer. The most common QOL tools used in France are the European Organisation for Research and Treatment of Cancer general and disease-specific assessments (Fayers et al., 2001), followed by the Functional Assessment of Chronic Illness Therapy FACIT.org, n.d.). These questionnaires are administered as part of the original investigations. Nurses in France conduct very few nursing-oriented companion studies. Patients are referred to a psycho-oncologist at the time of their initial diagnosis and as needed, but rarely more than once or twice during treatment.

Documentation and Data Management

Per the reviewed legislation currently applicable in France, two new information systems became effective in 2007. The first is a directory (available at https://icrepec.ansm.sante.fr/public) for patients and their families of all trials conducted that provides basic details on eligibility criteria, primary endpoints, and investigator contact information.

The second is the Clinical Trials in Cancer Registry (Registre des Essais Cliniques en Cancérologie), which is a national registry of all patients participating in a clinical trial in oncology. This registry serves as a tool for investigators and clinical study and is available at www.e-cancer.fr/recherche/recherche-clinique/registre-des-essais-cliniques (INCa, 2014b).

Quality Assurance

All clinical trials and personnel involved must adhere to the International Conference on Harmonisation of Technical Requirements for Registration of Pharmaceuticals for Human Use (ICH) good clinical practice (GCP) guidelines (ICH, 1996). Clinical studies, whether industry sponsored or not, are monitored by clinical research associates. They determine if the study personnel followed GCP by verifying the integrity of the data and ensuring the patients' rights. This is done via a full review of the source documents and the information in the CRFs. Electronic CRFs and trial master files are gaining popularity in France, as they substantially decrease the heavy trial-associated paperwork. The frequency of monitoring depends on the terms of the study.

Audits from the quality assurance department of the pharmaceutical companies or from the national CA can occur at any time. Centers are expected to archive all study patients' records and documentation for a minimum of 15 years after the results have been published and the study considered officially closed.

Professional Development

In France, nurses follow a minimum curriculum of three years and have a variety of professional role possibilities from which to choose, including the field of clinical research. No official nursing society exists, and there is no requirement to update credentials after graduation from the basic nursing program. The titles of study nurse and coordinator just recently have been recognized in France, as a result of the ever-increasing number of clinical trials in the hospital and private settings. Although creation of a specific training program for study nurses has been discussed, no organization has undertaken this project.

Specifically, the study nurse's role is to act as the communication liaison between doctors and patients. Investigators rely on study nurses to review the required protocol procedures, and patients will refer to the nurses for questions or problems concerning treatment or other study-related issues. The role of oncology study nurses within the hospital setting often features an array of activities, including bedside care, treatment administration, and toxicity assessments. Oncology nurses working in cancer centers will carry out those same tasks but with a smaller number of patients, thus allowing them to have more time to complete CRFs and perform other trial-related functions. The support function of study nurses is key in the successful recruitment and conduct of a study at a given research center. Furthermore, academic trials designed with study nurses' collaboration often yield a smoother process throughout the duration of the study, as nurses tend to have more practical approaches to logistical issues.

Summary

Centers that use study nurses for trials yield fewer study deviations. Study nurses can positively affect a center by being more acquainted with the specifics of trials where the data generated (source documents and CRFs) are of higher quality. Patients appreciate the availability of study nurses, as they are almost always present during their treatment and are a readily available contact for questions and answers. Study nurses do not replace the medical oncologist in a trial; however, given the complexity of today's trials, they are a definite advantage to have in a clinical trial team.

Key Points
- Oncology clinical trials in France must be approved by both the EC and CA before initiation.
- All clinical trials and personnel involved must adhere to ICH GCP.
- A clinical trial may not begin until it has obtained authorizations from *both* the EC and the French CA.

References

Agence Nationale de Sécurité du Médicament et des Produits de Santé. (2006, May 24). Arrêté du 24 mai 2006 fixant le contenu, le format et les modalités de présentation à l'Agence française de sécurité sanitaire des produits de santé du dossier de demande d'autorisation de recherche biomédicale portant sur un médicament à usage humain, article 3 [Decree of 24 May 2006 fixing the content, format and method of presentation to the French Agency for Safety of Health Products of biomedical research authorization application file on a human drug]. *French Official Gazette, 124,* 8042. Retrieved from http://www.legifrance.gouv.fr/affichTexte.do;jsessionid=6DFE297364948FC4C10FF2B9DF724735.tpdjo14v_1?cidTexte=JORFTEXT000000457818&dateTexte=20060530

Agence Nationale de Sécurité du Médicament et des Produits de Santé. (2012, April). Clinical trials for medicines (not including cell gene therapy or treatment) activity statement. Retrieved from http://ansm.sante.fr

Fayers, P.M., Aaronson, N.K., Bjordal, K., Groenvold, M., Curran, D., & Bottomley, A. (2001). *EORTC QLQ-C30 scoring manual* (3rd ed.). Brussels, Belgium: European Organisation for Research and Treatment of Cancer.

Functional Assessment of Chronic Illness Therapy. (n.d.). Questionnaires. Retrieved from http://www.facit.org/FACITOrg/Questionnaires

Institut National du Cancer. (2012, June). *Activity report, 2011*. Retrieved from http://www.e-cancer.fr/linstitut-national-du-cancer

Institut National du Cancer. (2013). Les plans cancer de 2003 à 2013 [Cancer Plan 2003–2013]. Retrieved from http://www.e-cancer.fr/en/le-plan-cancer/les-plans-cancer-de-2003-a-2013

Institut National du Cancer. (2014a, February). *Plan cancer 2014–2019: Priorités et objectifs [Cancer plan 2014–2019: Priorities and objectives]*. Retrieved from http://www.e-cancer.fr/le-plan-cancer/plan-cancer-2014-2019-priorites-et-objectifs

Institut National du Cancer. (2014b, January). Registre des essais cliniques en cancérologie. Bilan 2007–2012 [Registry of clinical trials in oncology: Balance 2007–2012]. Retrieved from https://www.e-cancer.fr/publications/59-recherche/756-registre-des-essais-cliniques-en-cancerologie-bilan-2007-2012

International Conference on Harmonisation of Technical Requirements for Registration of Pharmaceuticals for Human Use. (1996, June 10). *ICH harmonised tripartite guideline: Guideline for good clinical practice, E6(R1)*. Retrieved from http://www.ich.org/fileadmin/Public_Web_Site/ICH_Products/Guidelines/Efficacy/E6/E6_R1_Guideline.pdf

Loi No. 2004-806 du 9 août 2004 relative à la politique de santé publique [Law No. 2004-806 of 9 August 2004 on public health policy]. (2004). *Journal Officiel de la République Française, 185*, 14277.

Loi No. 88-1138 du 20 décembre 1988 relative à la protection des personnes qui se prêtent à des recherches biomédicales [Law No. 88-1138 of 20 December 1988 on the protection of persons participating in biomedical research]. Retrieved from http://legifrance.gouv.fr/affichTexte.do?cidTexte=JORFTEXT000000508831

Nouvelles Règles de la Recherche Biomédicale. (n.d.). Comités de protection des personnes. Retrieved from http://www.recherche-biomedicale.sante.gouv.fr/pro/comites/coordonnees.htm

Chapter 52

Germany

Gabriele Elser, RN, and Belinda Chung Yee Borrmann, RN

Introduction

Clinical oncologic research in Germany is based on the oldest and largest scientific association in oncology, the German Cancer Society, known as *Deutsche Krebsgesellschaft e.V.*, which began around 1900. Detailed information about the German Cancer Society is available at www.deutsche-krebsgesellschaft.de. The society is split into 23 working groups and 6 interdisciplinary working groups. Members include physicians, scientists, medical technicians, nurses, psychologists, and other professionals working in oncology; all are searching to identify the basic mechanisms of cancer, develop new diagnostic and therapeutic methods, and prevent and follow malignant diseases.

History and Foundation

Several independent academic research organizations (academic study groups) were established that specialize in different tumor entities (e.g., the AGO Study Group [gynecologic tumors], the NOGGO [North-East German Society for Gynecological Oncology, gynecologic tumors], the GBG [German Breast Group], the WSG [Women's Health Care Study Group, breast cancer]). Networks that focus on various tumor types also were established, such as the Competence Network/Malignant Lymphomas. The scientific study group Deutsches Krebsforschungszentrum (German Cancer Research Center), found at www.dkfz.de, systematically investigates the mechanisms of cancer development and works on the identification of cancer risk factors. Most of the academic research organizations are supported by the pharmaceutical industry or receive subsidies from different institutions and contributors.

Drug Development Process and Investigational New Drug Process

The drug development and investigational new drug processes are performed by the pharmaceutical industry, often in cooperation with academic-based study groups. A clear definition of tasks and responsibilities for each party is the basis of the quality of such collaboration and is fixed in individual agreements depending on the specific project.

Types of Clinical Research

Clinical trials are widely spread, and research is undertaken with medicinal products in phases I–III, such as medical devices, surgery, radiotherapy, transplantation, psychotherapy, diagnostics, nutrition, imaging, and other areas of interest. Furthermore, epidemiologic studies and meta-analyses are common methods of research. One aspect is patient-oriented research, which is supported by an initiative of the German Research Association (*Deutsche Forschungsgemeinschaft*, or DFG) (www.dfg.de/en). Most parts of trials with medicinal products and medical devices are conducted in a prospective, randomized setting. Observational studies are mostly linked to phase III clinical trials.

Expanded Access to Investigational Drugs

The compassionate use program (known as *Arzneimittel-Härtefall-Verordnung*) is regulated by section 80 of the Medicinal Products Act (*Arzneimittelgesetz*, or AMG). With respect to these specific regulations, patients now can be treated with new drugs that are not already registered.

The authors would like to acknowledge Heike Busse, RN, for her contribution to this chapter that remains unchanged from the previous edition of this book.

Sponsoring Agencies

Agency involvement in clinical trials depends on the nature of the study. Most agencies run international registration studies with a new drug. These trials are centrally activated by the company and involve several oncology sites. The trials are organized using a high level of experience and manpower of the involved sponsoring team. Conversely, local staff organizes local investigator-sponsored trials (known as ISTs or IITs) and have the same obligations when acting as sponsor of a clinical trial. Directive 2001/20/EC and national law (Medicinal Products Act; Ordinance on the Implementation of Good Clinical Practice in the Conduct of Clinical Trials on Medicinal Products for Use in Humans [GCP-V]) have to be respected.

Clinical Trials: Fundamental Information

The Clinical Research Team/ Interdisciplinary Team

The clinical research team typically consists of the *Prüfer* (equalized with principal investigator [PI]), *Stellvertreter* (deputy PI), *ärztliche Mitglieder der Prüfgruppe* (equalized with co-investigator[s]), *nicht-ärztliche Mitglieder der Prüfgruppe* (equalized with nurses, a pharmacist, and laboratory personnel), and, depending on the clinical trial, additional physicians and specialized staff.

Prior to starting the clinical trial, the PI delegates the responsibilities for the specific study, including obtaining patient consent, administering treatment, assessing toxicity, documenting, reporting, and much more. This will be documented on a signature list where every involved person has to sign in. The sponsor or monitor usually conducts the training program for the clinical research team during the initiation visit.

Legal, Regulatory, and Legislative Issues

Clinical trials are subject to conditions of regulatory and ethical requirements such as the European Union (EU) Directive, national and international laws and guidelines, good clinical practice (GCP), and the Declaration of Helsinki. The most relevant law is the Medicinal Products Act, which has new regulations enforced on October 12, 2012, and the GCP-V.

Good Clinical Practice

All staff involved in clinical trials must have a high level of knowledge of oncology respective of their area of expertise and GCP. This must be demonstrated and documented according to the Medicinal Products Act, §§ 4(25) and 40(1a), enforced since October 12, 2012, and GCP-V § 7(3)(6).

Standard Operating Procedures

All parties involved in clinical trial conduct should have training according to standard operating procedures. These may vary depending on the role each person or team plays in the specific trial. Training also varies by the definition of roles and responsibilities established for each project.

Ethics and Clinical Trials

The ethics committee (EC) is comparable to the institutional review board. Every clinical research site has a local EC that governs and monitors the researchers that are linked to them. Regarding the latest Medicinal Products Act and GCP directive, the lead EC's approval (the lead EC who is responsible at the coordinating investigators site) must be respected. A clinical trial may not start until the EC has issued a favorable opinion and the legal sponsor has not been informed of nonacceptance by the competent authority for any reason.

Protocol Development, Review, and Approval

Elements of a Protocol

Based on the nature of a protocol (e.g., national trial; international collaboration, including EU and non-EU collaboration; pharmaceutical company trial), the elements will be written according to international scientific standards. Statistical considerations are based on the nature of a protocol and must be carefully checked.

Informed Consent Process

The informed consent document contains specific, required information about the clinical trial. It is a legal document and must be reviewed and approved by the EC. The informed consent document must be written for laypeople in understandable language.

All trial-related examinations and procedures can begin only if the patient understands the implications of the clinical trial and has given written informed consent. The consent is effective as long as the patient does not withdraw from the clinical trial. The investigator may delegate obtaining informed consent to a designee who is also a physician. Special consideration must be taken for children in clinical trials; the consent of their legal representative is required. The consent of a legal representative or authorized representative also is required for adult patients who are not able to understand the nature, impact, and consequences of a clinical trial. Every clinical trial has specific requirements for who can and cannot participate. Inclusion and exclusion criteria are used to protect participant safety during a clinical trial.

To participate in a clinical trial, participants must meet certain standards that are mainly related to
- Age (older than 18 years; special criteria for trials with children must be requested)
- Gender (for AGO Study Group trials, only female patients are permitted)
- Type and stage of a disease
- Previous or current medications
- Existing medical conditions
- Recent participation in a clinical trial.

Protocol Development and Response Assessment

Response assessment is dependent on the objectives of the clinical trial. In most oncologic trials, response assessment is based on the Response Evaluation Criteria in Solid Tumors (RECIST) (Eisenhauer et al., 2009; Schwartz et al., 2009). (See Chapter 15 for more information about RECIST.)

Protocol Review and Approval Process

The legal sponsor and coordinating investigator check the protocol for formal, scientific, and statistical aspects, as well as for feasibility. After final signature of each, the protocol is approved and can be submitted for obtaining regulatory approvals. After favorable approval, the investigator and co-investigators at the participating sites need to sign off on the protocol after having read and understood it.

Financial Factors

Workload Determination and Resource Allocation

Determining trial manageability takes into account the workload for documentation (paper, electronic), patient examinations (physical, imaging, special examinations), preparation of tumor samples or blood samples (who is involved), determination of treating units' availability (unit census), and patient compliance. Overall, GCP criteria must be achieved, and staffing is adjusted accordingly.

Billing, Budget, and Funding

Based on the nature of a protocol, costs are assessed according to the study requirements. Calculations must be made to ascertain that the trial is sufficiently equipped. Additional financial support may be needed for documentation materials and staff; additional examinations for imaging, laboratory, or other tests that will not be covered as standard of care by the health insurance; and fees for the ethical review board, the federal health authority, and trial insurance. Negotiations with the various partners must be done prior to agreements to ensure that the trial can be opened at all applicable centers. A trial needs to have a well-balanced financial structure that covers all items and is sufficient to achieve the expected study quality.

Contracting

A signed investigator's agreement/contract needs to be in place between the legal sponsor and the participating PI and the PI's administrative department prior to site initiation. The agreement should include paragraphs on the roles and responsibilities of each party.

Financial Risk Assessment and Monitoring

The sites need to evaluate the complexity of a clinical trial with consideration of the number and kind of examinations, external experts that need to be involved, treatment duration and follow-up, and, finally, the number of patients that should be enrolled. Site feasibility questionnaires can help to evaluate a protocol prior to the final decision of participating.

The terms of GCP principles must be followed: "The rights, safety, and well-being of the trial subjects are the most important considerations and should prevail over interests of science and society" (International Conference on Harmonisation of Technical Requirements for Registration of Pharmaceuticals for Human Use, 1996, p. 13). Centers are advised to avoid having more than one active clinical trial in the same population set.

Financial Conflict of Interest

Each investigator involved in a clinical trial must disclose the presence of a conflict of interest on financial issues. This is also requested and must be available as part of the protocol submission process to the EC (GCP-V, § 7(3)(7)).

Recruitment and Retention

Public and Patient Education

The German Cancer Society offers several programs for the public, including nutrition education, smoking cessation programs, and early cancer detection programs. Selected information regarding clinical trials for a specific kind of cancer is offered to the public community. The Cancer Information Service (*Krebsinformationsdienst*, www.krebsinformationsdienst.de) of the German Cancer Research Center develops the bulk of all patient education materials related to clinical trials. More and more, the industry sponsors prepare informational material that can be distributed by nurses at clinical trial sites. Medical physicians and clinical trial investigators approve all patient education materials.

The German government developed a national cancer plan (*Nationaler Krebsplan*) in 2008 (Federal Ministry of Health, n.d.; German Cancer Society, n.d.). The plan consists of 13 major goals and corresponding recommendations for achieving them (Federal Ministry of Health, n.d.). The five goals most important for patients were

- Fair and rapid access to innovative treatments
- High-quality patient information
- Interdisciplinary patient care
- Informed decision making
- Psychosocial oncology care.

Accrual Base, Recruitment, and Promotion

Recruitment strategies are based on the nature of the clinical trial. The majority of patients in oncology trials are seen in clinical departments and hospitals specialized according to the tumor being treated. The available patient medical records are screened to select eligible patients.

The recruitment base in oncology trials is broad because patients want the best treatment for their cancer. On the other hand, not all sites have the capability to take part in a clinical trial because of a lack of manpower, trained staff, or support of their administration regarding department issues (Sehouli, Kostromitskaia, Stengel, & du Bois, 2005). The investigator exerts an important influence on the recruitment of patients (Harter et al., 2005). Thus, the investigator is the most important person in conducting a clinical trial. The investigator oversees the number of eligible patients in the institution and has the ability, together with the clinical staff, to educate all potential patients. More and more, patients are obtaining information about clinical trials from online sources.

Of concern is whether older adult patients can take part in clinical trials, as most studies have a cutoff of 75–80 years of age. When planning clinical trials, researchers should consider rethinking the view of limiting older adult participation.

Adherence and Retention

The more the patient and family are involved in the activities of the clinical trial, the better the patient compliance will be. However, the clinical staff that is taking care of a patient is responsible to ensure this involvement. With lengthy treatments, especially in oncology maintenance trials, it becomes a challenge for the trial team to convince patients to maintain adherence and participation for the long treatment period.

Clinical Trial Registries

"The purpose of a clinical trials registry is to promote the public good by ensuring that everyone can find key information about every clinical trial whose principal aim is to shape medical decision making" (De Angelis et al., 2005, p. 2928). According to the Declaration of Helsinki, the registration of a trial in a publicly available register should be completed prior to enrolling patients.

According to the recommendations of the International Committee of Medical Journal Editors (De Angelis et al., 2005), clinical trials should be listed on accepted registries. A list of those registries can be found at International Clinical Trials Registry Platform of the World Health Organization (www.who.int/ictrp/en). The most widely used international registry is ClinicalTrials.gov (www.clinicaltrials.gov), which is free of charge. Another commonly used database is the ISRCTN registry (www.isrctn.com).

Clinical Trial Participants

Educating Staff

The majority of nurses caring for patients with cancer are associates in the Conference on Oncological and Pediatric Oncological Care (*Konferenz Onkologischer Kranken- und Kinderkrankenpflege*, or KOK), the national society for oncology nurses in Germany. More information is available at www.kok-krebsgesellschaft.de. A variety of educational offerings from institutions and companies with different learning content about clinical research are available. One of these is the study assistant training offered by the German Cancer Society together with clinical trial centers.

The Network of the Coordinating Centres for Clinical Trials (*Koordinierungszentren für Klinische Studien*, or KKS Network) is a network for clinical trials consolidated in 2005. The network originally included 12 German universities but has since grown (Bruns, Maier-Lenz, & Wolff, 2009) (see Table 52-1). Their aim is to encourage cooperation among university disciplines, maintenance units, and the pharmaceutical and medicine-technological industry, as well as to provide educational training to investigators and study site staff (Bruns et al., 2009).

Investigators are obliged to have a certificate on GCP training including training on national law (Medicinal Products Act and GCP-V) when conducting clinical trials.

Investigational Agents: Procurement, Administration, and Accountability of Research Study Drugs

Physicians prescribe study drugs according to the clinical trial protocol. Drug dosages have to be calculated and recalculated according to the protocol-specific guidelines. Compliance with described formulas for dose calculation should be documented in the patient record. Research professionals, mostly physicians and pharmacists, need to recheck the calculations. All guidelines for dose reduction and dose interruption must be followed.

The specific laboratory or physical values and any reported side effects must be evaluated prior to each calculation and scheduling of the study treatment. The pharmacist prepares most cytotoxic agents. The treating staff must be trained in administration of the drugs and observation of the patient during treatment. For documentation purposes, all treatment data should be kept in the medical record.

Depending on the drug and the study, the site's pharmacy department is responsible for drug receipt, storage, accountability, and preparation. The study assistants order the drugs for patients from the trial-specific distributor. Pharmacy department staff must agree with the documentation of received, dispensed, and destroyed drugs, as well as the balance, charge documentation, and expiration dates that are reported on the study-specific documentation.

Finally, the storage resources need to be checked from time to time, for example, ensuring sufficient storage capacity and proper storage conditions for different drugs, such as temperature and responding equipment.

Adverse Events and Unanticipated Problems

Before starting the study treatment, patients are informed about specific side effects and instructed in the handling of these effects. Patients are informed about examinations during the treatment interval (e.g., weekly blood draws). Additionally, the use of supporting agents, such as antiemetics or growth factors, is explained to patients. A patient diary can be helpful for recording and reporting symptoms. Symptoms must be recorded in the trial documentation according to the protocol guidelines.

Adverse events (AEs) experienced by a patient in a clinical trial should be reported according to the protocol-specific assessment scales. The recent toxicity criteria of the U.S. National Cancer Institute (NCI), the Common Terminology Criteria for Adverse Events (NCI Cancer Therapy Evaluation Program, 2010), currently are used for grading and reporting toxicities in clinical trials.

The specific definitions for adverse events of special interest (AESIs), serious adverse events (SAEs), and suspected unexpected serious adverse reactions (SUSARs) have to be taken into consideration. The investigator or designee must report AESIs, SAEs, and SUSARs to the sponsor within 24 hours after becoming aware of them. Also, follow-up reports are requested in cases of initially

Table 52-1. Network of the Coordinating Centres for Clinical Trials (KKS Network) Locations in Germany

City	Website
Berlin	www.kks.charite.de
Bonn	www.studienzentrum-bonn.de
Cologne	www.zks-koeln.de
Dresden	www.kksdresden.de
Düsseldorf	www.uniklinik-duesseldorf.de/kks
Essen	www.zkse.de
Freiburg	www.studienzentrum.uniklinik-freiburg.de
Halle	www.kks-netzwerk.de/en/network/members/kks-halle.html
Hannover	www.clinical-trial-center.de
Heidelberg	www.kks-hd.de
Jena	www.zks.uniklinikum-jena.de
Leipzig	www.zks.uni-leipzig.de
Lübeck	www.zks-luebeck.de
Mainz	www.izks-mainz.de
Marburg	www.kks-mr.de
Munich	www.muenchner-studienzentrum.me.tum.de
Münster	http://campus.uni-muenster.de/zks.html
Regensburg	www.uniklinikum-regensburg.de/zentren/zentrum-fuer-klinische-studien
Witten/Herdecke	www.uni-wh.de/gesundheit/forschung-gesundheit/forschungszentren/zks-uwh

Note. Based on information from KKS Network, n.d.

unresolved SAEs. All further obligations regarding the reporting and recording of any AEs have to be respected by the trial's sponsor.

Patient and Family Education

The investigator, along with the trial staff at the treating institution, informs the patient and the patient's relatives about expected discomforts or complaints during the study treatment, as well as how to deal with them. Verbal and written instructions regarding medications (if the patient has to take medication at home) should be given to the patient. Communication with the general practitioner is a great help to the patient during treatment and follow-up. Therefore, it is important for the clinical trial investigator to confer with the patient's general practitioner throughout the patient's time in the study. After the study results are made public, patients should be informed about the outcome.

Psychosocial Distress

The psychosocial aspect is an important factor that often is underrepresented. At the time of protocol treatment completion, patients have follow-up examinations. Comprehensive cancer centers provide psychosocial support for their patients. For example, patients with breast cancer are offered psycho-oncologic support from the time of first diagnosis until departure from the hospital. After treatment completion, self-care groups generally continue the program. The establishment of a breast cancer nurse position and pelvic care nurse who supports patients has come into force during the past years.

Genetics and Genomics

Pharmacogenetics and Pharmacogenomics

The evaluation of pharmacokinetics and genetics in clinical trials in Germany is planned carefully with consideration given to time and effort. Ethics and data protection, which is governed by the Federal Data Protection Act (*Bundesdatenschutzgesetz*, or BDSG), must be taken into serious consideration and respected. Study site personnel assist the investigators in sample preparation and processing. Even the technical requirements (e.g., dry ice, liquid nitrogen) and logistics (e.g., shipping procedures) have to be confirmed with the investigating and laboratory staff to ensure compliance (International Air Transport Association, n.d.).

Further special attention needs to be given to genetic testing in patients with gynecologic malignancies and/ or *BRCA1* or *BRCA2* hereditary disposition. Germ-line mutations in a number of genes involved in the recombinational repair of DNA double-strand breaks have been associated with predisposition to breast and ovarian cancer. The German Consortium for Familial Breast and Ovarian Cancer is obliged to follow very strict regulations, and only specialized centers are allowed to counsel those patients and their families (BRCA Network, n.d.; German Cancer Aid, n.d.).

Furthermore, the Genetic Diagnostics Act (*Gendiagnostikgesetz*, or GenDG) must be adhered to as well.

Genetic Testing

Genetic testing and storage usually is possible at sites located in university hospitals. If clinical trials are being performed in smaller institutions, the equipment needs to be checked prior to initiation of the trial. Whenever genetic testing and storage are completed, the process for transportation should be clearly defined and a checklist should be available.

Correlative Trials

Nursing Companion Studies

In Germany, the culture of nursing companion studies needs to be improved. An ongoing project called Health Services Research Germany has the aim of getting more information on examples of best practice models and facilitating the exchange of research results (Grenz-Farenholtz, Schmidt, Zach, Verheyen, & Pfaff, 2011).

Translational Research and Biologic Studies

Translational research has become part of most clinical trials. Systems for human material collection and archiving are going to be established, and many university hospitals are running biomaterial banks. In cases where participants gave their separate informed consent, samples will be stored in a separate space and can be linked to clinical data. Biomarker-driven studies will be the future and can help to improve the establishment of targeted therapy.

Economic Questions

Economic questions are becoming popular, especially to obtain information on costs during and after completion of drug treatment. Also, lifestyle information on over-the-counter drugs can be obtained with such questions.

Sub-Studies

Depending on the nature of the clinical trials, sub-studies can be part of the trial itself or can be done as separate analyses after publication of the primary endpoint.

Documentation and Data Management

Documentation

When participating in clinical trials, the clinical trial team is responsible for data entry using either paper case report forms (CRFs) or electronic CRFs (e-CRFs). They are required to follow the guidelines given for each specific protocol. Training starts with initiation visits with the monitoring team and is ongoing. Regarding e-CRFs, different systems may be used depending on the sponsor. Knowledge and experience in technical and software skills are required.

The site/hospital internal systems must be compatible with the study system (for example, too restrictive firewalls can be a major hurdle, and information technology staff needs to be involved before setting up a system). Online training sessions are provided and noted in an education record for each participant. Study assistants should learn the steps for the reporting of data, changing of data entries, and query processing.

Even in intergroup trials, the coordinating (or lead) group is responsible for establishing the set of master CRFs, which are used by all groups and adapted for international conditions. As done in the Gynecologic Cancer Intergroup, the definition of common data elements should be recommended and instructions for data collection established.

Clinical Trial Management Systems

Clinical trial management systems are helpful instruments for storing and retrieving all relevant trial information.

Maintaining a Regulatory File

Maintaining a trial master file (commonly known as a TMF) is the sole task and responsibility of the legal sponsor and should be organized according to existing standard operating procedures. All relevant documentation must be archived with respect to national guidelines (compulsory archiving). Both the sponsor and site should ensure sufficient space for archiving or seek alternatives such as electronic file systems.

Quality Assurance

Data and Safety Monitoring Plans

With regard to data management, adequate plans should exist in-house for performing plausibility checks and detecting deviations. Also, plans for corrective actions for when systematic errors are detected need to be available. Defining key quality indicators is of great help.

Clinical trial quality requires consistent adherence to measurable and verifiable standards to achieve uniformity of output that satisfies specific customer or user requirements. Key quality indicators to document during the conduct of clinical research include, but are not limited to
- Patient eligibility criteria
- Informed consent process
- SAE and AE ascertainment and management
- Scheduled tests and procedures
- Missed visits, tests, and procedures
- Recording of concomitant medications
- Use of prohibited medications
- Study drug or device administration.

For data monitoring, it is helpful to draft a monitoring plan as a guide. Nowadays, risk-adapted monitoring is increasingly being used in clinical trials.

Finally, it is recommended to set up a data monitoring committee (DMC), which can evaluate the integrity and safety of the trial. Commonly used quality management definitions are published on the Clinical Research Resource Hub (2011).

Monitoring and Audit Preparation

The criteria for auditing and monitoring must be described in the German language as a separate section of the protocol. Monitoring encompasses the routine source data verification and checking of protocol compliance. It may include checking the investigator's site files, informed consent documents, and drug accountability documentation. Personnel of the trial's study sponsor conduct the study closure visit. Depending on the protocol and the monitoring plan, these visits can take place routinely, such as at 8–12-month intervals.

An audit is the review by authorized sponsor personnel of the entire study documentation, including the investigator's site files, informed consent form, institutional review board regulatory files, and drug accountability records. Occasionally, audits are initiated upon the authority of the Ministry of Health competent authority. A U.S. Food and Drug Administration inspection, or inspection conditional upon the local regulatory body, may be initiated for international trials.

Monitoring and audit visits are arranged with the investigator and study team to ensure that all involved people are available.

Professional Development and Clinical Trials Nursing Education

The majority of nurses caring for patients with cancer are associates in the KOK, the national society for oncology nurses in Germany. More information is available at www.kok-krebsgesellschaft.de. A variety of educational offerings from institutions and companies with different learning content about clinical research are available. One of these is the study assistant training offered by the German Cancer Society together with the coordinating centers for clinical trials.

Summary

Conducting clinical trials in Germany includes struggles with bureaucracy, regulations, and finances. The support of nonpharmaceutical-sponsored trials through public institutions should receive more appreciation. The definition of a clinical trial nurse is not as commonly established as it is in many other European and overseas countries. The more common terms of *study nurse*, *research nurse*, and *study assistant* frequently are used in Germany. Nevertheless, the nurses all work within the same broad domain of cancer research. Widely varying views on education exist. Thus, it would be preferable to establish a more structured education and culture in this professional field worldwide. Increasing specialization not only in nursing but also in technical and language skills is becoming essential.

Key Points
- Processes of protocol development and required elements are integral to national research activity in Germany.
- Assurances are mandatory per German law.
- Successful German cooperation with other study groups and participation in international intergroup trials are a source of pride.
- Public, patient, and family education related to participation and compliance in clinical trials in Germany is a valuable component of clinical trials research.
- Following the updated local medicinal law, the status of German clinical research teams and interdisciplinary teams continues to evolve.
- Psychosocial considerations are included in research in Germany.
- German clinical trial registries and resources are collaborators in research.
- Specialization in clinical research nursing is a growing field in Germany.

References

BRCA Network. (n.d.). Retrieved from http://www.brca-netzwerk.de

Bruns, I., Maier-Lenz, H., & Wolff, S. (2009). [The Coordinating Centres for Clinical Trials Network. Objectives and significance for research sites]. *Bundesgesundheitsblatt—Gesundheitsforschung—Gesundheitsschutz, 52,* 451–458. doi:10.1007/s00103-009-0828-2

Clinical Research Resource Hub. (2011). Commonly used QM definitions. Retrieved from http://hub.ucsf.edu/qm-definitions

De Angelis, C.D., Drazen, J.M., Frizelle, F.A., Haug, C., Hoey, J., Horton, R., ... Van Der Weyden, M.B. (2005). Is this clinical trial fully registered? A statement from the International Committee of Medical Journal Editors. *JAMA, 293,* 2927–2929. doi:10.1001/jama.293.23.jed50037

Directive 2001/20/EC of the European Parliament and of the Council of 4 April 2001 on the approximation of the laws, regulations and administrative provisions of the Member States relating to the implementation of good clinical practice in the conduct of clinical trials on medicinal products for human use. (2001, May 1). *Official Journal of the European Communities, L121,* 34–44. Retrieved from http://eur-lex.europa.eu/legal-content/EN/TXT/?uri=uriserv:OJ.L_.2001.121.01.0034.01.ENG

Eisenhauer, E.A., Therasse, P., Bogaerts, J., Schwartz, L.H., Sargent, D., Ford, R., ... Verweij, J. (2009). New response evaluation criteria in solid tumours: Revised RECIST guideline (version 1.1). *European Journal of Cancer, 45,* 228–247.

Federal Ministry of Health. (n.d.). National Cancer Plan. Retrieved from http://www.bundesgesundheitsministerium.de/themen/praevention/nationaler-krebsplan.html

Genetic Diagnostics Act. (2010, February). Retrieved from http://www.gesetze-im-internet.de/gendg/index.html

German Cancer Aid. (n.d.). Hereditary breast and ovarian cancer. Retrieved from http://www.krebshilfe.de/wir-helfen/adressen/familiaerer-krebs/brustkrebszentren.html

German Cancer Society. (n.d.). Health policy. Retrieved from http://www.krebsgesellschaft.de/gcs/german-cancer-society/health-policy.html

Grenz-Farenholtz, B., Schmidt, A., Zach, D., Verheyen, F., & Pfaff, H. (2011). [Project database health services research Germany]. *Gesundheitswesen, 73,* 862–864. doi:10.1055/s-0031-1295424

Harter, P., du Bois, A., Schade-Brittinger, C., Burges, A., Wollschlaeger, K., Gropp, M., ... Pfisterer, J. (2005). Non-enrolment of ovarian cancer patients in clinical trials: Reasons and backgrounds. *Annals of Oncology, 16,* 1801–1805. doi:10.1093/annonc/mdi367

International Air Transport Association. (n.d.). Dangerous goods. Retrieved from http://www.iata.org/whatwedo/cargo/dgr/Pages/index.aspx

International Conference on Harmonisation of Technical Requirements for Registration of Pharmaceuticals for Human Use. (1996, July). *Good clinical practice.* Retrieved from http://ec.europa.eu/health/files/eudralex/vol-10/3cc1aen_en.pdf

KKS Network. (n.d.). The members of the KKS Network. Retrieved from http://www.kks-netzwerk.de/en/network/members.html

Medicinal Products Act, *Federal Law Gazette,* Pt. I, p. 3394, last amended by Article 1 of the Law of 19th October 2012 (*Federal Law Gazette,* Pt. I, p. 2192). Retrieved from http://www.gesetze-im-internet.de/englisch_amg/englisch_amg.html#p0073

National Cancer Institute Cancer Therapy Evaluation Program. (2010). *Common terminology criteria for adverse events* [v.4.03]. Retrieved from http://ctep.cancer.gov/protocolDevelopment/electronic_applications/ctc.htm

Ordinance on the implementation of Good Clinical Practice in the conduct of clinical trials on medicinal products for use in humans (GCP Ordinance—GCP-V) of 9 August 2004. (2004). *Federal Law Gazette,* Pt. 1, No. 42. Retrieved from http://www.pei.de/SharedDocs/Downloads/EN/pu/clinical-trials/gcp-ordinance.pdf?__blob=publicationFile&v=1

Schwartz, L.H., Bogaerts, J., Ford, R., Shankar, L., Therasse, P., Gwyther, S., & Eisenhauer, E.A. (2009). Evaluation of lymph nodes with RECIST 1.1. *European Journal of Cancer, 45,* 261–267.

Sehouli, J., Kostromitskaia, J., Stengel, D., & du Bois, A. (2005). Why institutions do not participate in ovarian cancer trials—Results from a survey in Germany. *Onkologie, 28,* 13–17. doi:10.1159/000082183

Chapter 53

India

Saritha Shamsunder, MD, FRCOG, Bhavesh Kumari, MSc, MA, Satya Pal Kataria, MD, DM, and Vijay Zutshi, MD, FICOG

Introduction

In 2011, India's population totaled 1.21 billion, reflecting an increase of 181.5 million in 10 years (Office of the Registrar General and Census Commissioner, India, 2011). The literacy rate has increased from 65% in 2001 to 74% in 2011. Life expectancy has also increased, from 35 years in 1947 when India gained independence to approximately 65 years currently (Raina, 2005; World Bank, 2015). Globalization of cancer research has prompted many developing countries to conduct trials in India (Nundy & Gulhati, 2005). The Indian regulatory bodies therefore have updated their guidelines and protocols to facilitate smooth conduct of trials. This chapter gives an overview of the process of conducting clinical trials in India.

History and Foundation

Medicine and research in India date back to as early as 1500 BC, when the various diseases and treatments were described in the Vedic scripture *Atharva Veda* as the eight divisions of Ayurveda. The great sage Charaka described medicinal plants and their usage for treatment of ailments in his treatise, *Charaka Samhita* (Chillayah, n.d.; Life Positive, n.d.). Much later, small controlled clinical trials were carried out to satisfy regulatory requirements to market drugs in India that were already being used abroad. India became a part of international trials in the 1990s when multinational companies included the country in their international trials.

Contract research organizations are attracted to India because it has a large number of patients, low costs, and English-speaking doctors. Academic trials are conducted in which the sponsor is not from the pharmaceutical industry. There has been a 30% increase in the number of clinical trials in India over the past few years, which is almost double the global average (Bajpai, 2013; Ernst & Young India & Federation of Indian Chambers of Commerce and Industry, 2009; Pais, n.d.). A large patient pool is available because of the large numbers of participants, variety of disease conditions, and treatment-naïve patients as a result of the lack of universal health care (Ernst & Young India & Federation of Indian Chambers of Commerce and Industry, 2009; Pais, n.d.). However, as per available data, 2,242 deaths have been reported in the past five years during the conduct of clinical trials. Out of 436 serious adverse events (SAEs) and deaths during clinical trials reported in 2012, 16 were attributed directly to such research (Ministry of Health and Family Welfare, 2013a).

Cancer Scenario in India

Cancer incidence is generally much lower in India than in the developed world, with the average national age-adjusted rate being approximately 120 per 100,000 compared with more than 300 per 100,000 per year in developed countries (Indian Council of Medical Research [ICMR] National Cancer Registry Programme [NCRP], 2005; Ramnath & Nandakumar, 2011). The causes of low cancer rates have been variously attributed to underreporting, ethnic and racial factors, lifestyle, food habits, and shorter life expectancy. It is estimated that 0.44 million people died of cancer in 2011. The number is projected to be 0.5 million in 2016 and 0.6 million in 2021 (D'Souza, Murthy, & Aras, 2013).

Cancer incidence shows significant variations in individual regions, and the incidence of types and organs affected also varies widely among the different regions of India (ICMR NCRP, 2005). For example, in males, stomach cancer is the most common cancer in the south, whereas lung cancer is most common in the north. In females, cancer of the cervix is more common in the south, whereas breast cancer is more common in the north. Other common cancers are head and neck in males and gallbladder in females, both comparatively uncommon in the West. Among men and women, the incidence of breast cancer alone is expected to exceed 100,000 by 2020 (Ramnath & Nandakumar, 2011).

Clinical Trials: Fundamental Information

Cancer Research in India

The diversity and number of cancer cases in India offer a unique opportunity for sponsors to carry out different trials in various parts of the country (Nundy & Gulhati, 2005). The largest single advantage to the multinational trials has been the ability to carry out trials in a shorter period of time as a result of faster recruitment (Mani & Pai, 1997). Fortunately, benefits to India have also been immense: for the first time, good clinical practice (GCP) norms, which were virtually unheard of before 1995, have been established in many parts of the country (Central Drugs Standard Control Organization [CDSCO], 2004).

Funding through clinical trials has helped improve infrastructure in many public hospitals that are perennially poorly funded. Trial offices have been set up in some large cancer centers with state-of-the-art facilities. Standard operating procedures (SOPs) have been established, and laboratory facilities have improved (Mani & Pai, 1997).

Clinical trials conducted under the guidance of the U.S. National Cancer Institute for the treatment of childhood acute lymphoblastic leukemia and non-Hodgkin lymphoma have helped improve survival dramatically with reduced costs because of a standard treatment protocol (Sharma, 2002).

The INDOX Cancer Research Network (http://indox.org.uk) is a network of publicly funded regional cancer centers that was formed to carry out cancer studies in India. The network consisted of six centers (Delhi, Mumbai, Ahmedabad, Hyderabad, Bangalore, and Trivandrum) at its formation in 2005 and has since expanded to include 12 centers (Oxford Group, n.d.). Intense deliberations and discussions are ongoing, including visits to all centers to ascertain abilities, strengths, and weaknesses. It is hoped that the efforts of this network will accelerate the process of good regulation and governance. There are plans to regularly impart GCP training to establish quality control.

International Collaboration

ICMR established an Indo-Foreign Cell (IFC) in the early 1980s to enable collaboration in biomedical research between India and other countries and international agencies. In 2000, the IFC was upgraded to the Division of International Health (ICMR, n.d.-a). India has many bilateral agreements with other countries in areas of biomedical research (ICMR, n.d.-a).

Health Ministry's Screening Committee

Indian investigators conducting research projects involving foreign assistance or collaboration need to apply through ICMR for approval from the Government of India. The approval is granted through the Health Ministry's Screening Committee (HMSC), which has representatives from the Ministries of Health and Family Welfare, External Affairs, Finance, Department of Biotechnology, and Science and Technology, and the Directorate General of Armed Forces and Medical Services and Directorate General of Health Services. It is chaired by the Secretary of the Department of Health Research, Ministry of Health and Family Welfare (ICMR, n.d.-a). HMSC functions through the International Health Division at ICMR, which coordinates applications and organizes research meetings of HMSC.

Protocol Development, Review, and Approval

Schedule Y of the Indian Drugs and Cosmetics (IInd Amendment) Rules of 2005 defined a clinical trial as "a systematic study of new drug(s) in human subject(s) to generate data for discovering and/or verifying the clinical, pharmacological (including pharmacodynamic and pharmacokinetic) and/or adverse effects with the objective of determining safety and/or efficacy of the new drug" (Ministry of Health and Family Welfare, 2005).

Application for conducting a clinical trial has to be made on the prescribed form to the Drug Controller General of India (DCGI) after approval of the ethics committee of the institution where the trial is proposed to be carried out (Ministry of Health and Family Welfare, 2005). If the new drug was discovered in India, it has to go through phase I–III clinical trials; the permission is also granted in stages based on the data from the earlier phase or phases. For drugs discovered outside of India, permission for concurrent phase II and III trials is given only after data from phase I trials conducted outside of India have been submitted to the licensing authority (Ministry of Health and Family Welfare, 2005).

CDSCO, under DCGI, then screens the applications and refers them for review by the relevant advisory committees, which consist of experts from various clinical disciplines (CDSCO, 2004). This adds to the scientific value of the trial and gives confidence to all stakeholders, including the study participants. The experts' opinion is given within six weeks of receipt of the proposal (Jayasheel, 2012).

Regulatory Approval

Various regulatory bodies are involved in pharmaceutical trials (Jayasheel, 2010). The Government of India, via CDSCO under the Ministry of Health and Family Welfare, largely works on developing standards and regulatory measures by amending acts and rules and regulating the market authorization of new drugs in an effort to standardize clinical research in India and bring safer drugs to the market (CDSCO, 2004).

Ethics Committee

Schedule Y of the Drugs and Cosmetics Rules (amended in 2005) specifies that it is the responsibility of the ethics committee that reviews and approves a trial protocol to safeguard the rights, safety, and well-being of all trial subjects (Ministry of Health and Family Welfare, 2005). It is mandatory that all clinical trials be approved by the institutional ethics committee (IEC) in the institution where the trial will be carried out to safeguard the welfare and rights of the participants. This review for approval can be done at the same time the protocol is being reviewed by DCGI (Desai & Naik, 2011). There are also independent ethics committees functioning outside the institutions for researchers who do not have IECs. The committees are not only entrusted with the initial review of the proposed research protocols prior to the initiation of the projects but also have a continuing responsibility of regular monitoring of approved projects to oversee ethical compliance during the project. This is in accordance with the international guidelines and SOPs of the World Health Organization.

The IECs provide advice to researchers on all aspects of the welfare and safety of the research participants after ensuring the scientific soundness of the proposed research through appropriate scientific review. In institutions where it is lacking, IECs take the dual responsibility of review of the scientific content and the ethical aspects of the proposal. Small institutions could form an alliance with other IECs or approach a registered IEC (ICMR, 2006).

IECs are multidisciplinary and multispectral in composition; their independence and competence are the two hallmarks. The number of members is kept fairly small (7–11 people). The companies that conduct clinical trials have to seek registration of their IECs to deter abuses in testing of a new drug (ICMR, 2006).

IECs are required to ensure that drug trials are free of any abuse and that adverse events are reported. They must report any malpractice by any clinical trial organization and any adverse effects on human subjects undergoing the trial. IECs need to report SAEs to the drug controller and review the informed consent forms (Ministry of Health and Family Welfare, 2013a, 2013b).

Review Process

IECs provide complete and adequate review of the research proposals submitted to them. They meet periodically to review new proposals, evaluate annual reports of ongoing trials, review SAE reports, and assess final reports of all research activities involving human beings through a previously scheduled agenda, amended whenever appropriate. The ethics review is done in formal meetings, which are held every three to six months (ICMR, 2006).

Informed Consent Process

Informed consent of prospective participants is essential for all clinical trials involving human participants. If an individual is incapable of giving informed consent, consent of the legal guardian is essential (ICMR, 2006). Participants are given information about the research in a printed form in a language they can understand, and a copy of the form is given to participants. If a participant is unable to sign, a thumb impression is taken, witnessed by a person unrelated to the trial (ICMR, 2006). A legal guardian or duly authorized representative should be the witness if the participant is not competent to give written consent.

Financial Factors

Financial Assistance

ICMR, the Department of Science and Technology, and the Department of Biotechnology provide financial assistance to promote biomedical and health research. The assistance is provided by way of grants to scientists in regular employment in universities, medical colleges, postgraduate institutions, recognized research and development laboratories, and nongovernmental organizations. All the details and requirements are available in the *Guidelines for Operation of Projects for Grantees of ICMR's Extramural Research Project* (ICMR, n.d.-b).

Compensation for Participation

ICMR guidelines state that participants are to be reimbursed for the expenses incurred as a result of their participation in research. They may be compensated for the inconvenience incurred or may be provided free medical services, free auxiliary care, and referrals, if needed. All payments, reimbursement, and medical services to be provided to research participants should be approved by the IEC (ICMR, 2006).

Compensation for Accidental Injury

Patients who experience physical injury or temporary or permanent disability as a result of participation in a clinical trial need to be adequately compensated, financially or otherwise, by the sponsor, or given medical insurance coverage by the sponsor as set forth in an "a priori agreement," meaning that it is in place before the research begins. If death occurs as a result of the trial, the participant's dependents are entitled to material compensation. Sponsors need to provide compensation for unforeseen injury whenever possible (ICMR, 2006). The institution will form an arbitration committee to decide the issue of compensation on an individual case basis.

Recruitment and Retention

Clinical Trials Registry–India

The Clinical Trials Registry–India (CTRI) was launched by ICMR's National Institute of Medical Statistics and has been operational since July 20, 2007. CTRI's mission is "to encourage all clinical trials conducted in India to be prospectively registered, i.e., before the enrolment of the first participant" (CTRI, n.d., "Mission").

Since June 2009, prospective registration with CTRI has been mandatory for all trials conducted in India. CTRI is a free, online system. International trials with India as a participating country also need to be registered with CTRI, even if they have been registered in an international registry. Full details of the trial sites in India, the investigators, and sample size from India are entered (CTRI, n.d.). Regular updates by trialists on the trial status are available for public display. Registered trials are freely accessible from both the World Health Organization's International Clinical Trials Registry Platform (www.who.int/ictrp/search/en) and CTRI (http://ctri.nic.in/Clinicaltrials/advancesearchmain.php).

Selection of Special Groups as Research Participants

Special groups (e.g., pregnant and nursing women) and vulnerable populations (e.g., prisoners, students, subordinates, employees, service personnel, older adults) should not be participants in research projects or clinical trials unless the investigators provide adequate justification (ICMR, 2006).

Post-Trial Access

In its Declaration of Helsinki in 2000, the World Medical Association (WMA) stated that every study participant should have access to the best proven prophylactic, diagnostic, and therapeutic method identified by the study. The practicality of this was extensively debated. However, in 2004, WMA reaffirmed its stand and reiterated that "post-trial access arrangements or other care must be described in the study protocol so the ethical review committee may consider such arrangements during its review" (WMA, 2004, p. 6).

Genetics and Genomics

An explosion in knowledge in the field of human genetics, gene therapy, and genetic engineering has resulted in debate and guidelines regarding the potential ability to produce "designer babies" by gene therapy or genetic engineering (ICMR, 2006). ICMR prohibits germ line therapy and eugenic genetic engineering and advises against attempts to use gene therapy for enhancement of genetic characteristics (ICMR, 2006).

Genetic counseling entails discussion on reproductive options and choices, which could have far-reaching social implications. Therefore, it needs to be carried out with special care documented in research proposals and reviewed carefully by IECs. Genetic manipulations have consequences for the future, some of which are unknown. Hence, greater care toward potential dangers is necessary.

Increasing misuse of genetic tests prompted the Government of India to enact the Pre-Natal Diagnostic Techniques (Regulation and Prevention of Misuse) Act in 1994, which includes all researchers in this area. It was amended in 2003 as the Pre-Conception and Pre-Natal Diagnostic Techniques (Prohibition of Sex Selection) Act to include all preconception diagnostic techniques (ICMR, 2006).

Correlative Trials

A meta-analysis of qualitative studies in India reported on why patients in India choose to participate in clinical trials: personal health benefits, altruism, monetary benefits, and faith in government-sponsored trials. Lack of faith and fear of the healthcare system were the major reasons for mistrust in trials earlier (Shah et al., 2010).

Documentation and Data Management

All documentation and communication regarding the trial are dated, filed, and preserved, including the composition of the IEC, copies of the protocol, correspondence with IEC members and investigators, agendas and minutes of all meetings, record of premature termination of the study, if applicable, and the final report of the study. All records are maintained for at least three years after study termination or completion (ICMR, 2006).

Quality Assurance

Monitoring

The oversight mechanism of the IEC monitors approved studies. In case of adverse events or violation of human rights being reported, site visits are made and periodic status reports are requested at appropriate intervals. Sponsors are required to monitor studies per the recommendations of the Data Safety Monitoring Board (ICMR, 2006).

Conflicts of Interest

Academic institutions conducting research with industries or commercial companies need to review and probe any conflicts of interest between the scientific responsibility of researchers and business interests (ICMR, 2006). If the review committee thinks that a conflict of interest could potentially mar the scientific integrity of a project or cause harm to the research participants, the committee advises accordingly.

Investigators need to declare such conflicts of interest in applications submitted to IECs for review. Institutions and IECs have self-regulatory processes to prevent, monitor, and resolve such conflicts of interest (ICMR, 2006).

Professional Development

No specific courses in clinical trials nursing are available; however, cancer centers in India (e.g., Tata Memorial Hospital, Mumbai; Regional Cancer Centre, Thiruvananthapuram) offer short- and long-term courses in oncology nursing. The Tata Memorial Hospital in Mumbai conducts an International Oncology Nursing Fellowship program. The Oncology Nurses Association of India (https://tmc.gov.in/medical/departments/nursing.htm) enhances professional development of nurses.

Summary

India has become a hub of clinical trials sponsored by international pharmaceutical companies, with the number of global trials being conducted in India doubling in the past decade (Ernst & Young India & Federation of Indian Commerce and Industry, 2009). The prime advantage to companies was the low cost and faster speed of recruitment; as a result, the country has also benefited with improvements in infrastructure and improved standards of patient care (Raina, 2005).

Globally, concern exists regarding the ethical and scientific implications of trials in developing countries (Bhatt, 2010). However, GCP guidelines, changing patent laws, and the registration of clinical trials have helped make research in India transparent and accountable. Training of ethics committees, mandatory accreditation of all stakeholders, and regulatory and ethical supervision are essential to sustain global interest.

In an effort to improve the quality of clinical trials in India, the Government of India enacted a new rule stating that "no Ethics Committee shall review and accord its approval to a clinical trial protocol without prior registration with the Licensing Authority as defined [by the rule]" (as cited in Gaffney, 2013, Reforms section, para. 2). The registration will be valid for three years (Gaffney, 2013). The licensing authority (i.e., the DCGI) ensures that clinical trials are carried out only after permission is granted, ensures provision of medical treatment in case of injury due to the trial, ensures compensation to participants or their legal heirs, conducts regular inspection of trial sites, and ensures penalties for conducting trials without permission. Irregularities in conducting trials carry stringent punishments, which could include imprisonment (Drugs and Cosmetics [Amendment] Act, 2013).

Key Points
- India is a global hub of clinical trials because of its large patient pool, variety of diseases, and treatment-naïve patients.
- It is mandatory for all international clinical trials to follow ICMR guidelines.
- DCGI is the regulatory apex body that oversees all clinical trials.

References

Bajpai, V. (2013). Rise of clinical trials industry in India: An analysis. *ISRN Public Health, 2013,* Article ID 167059. doi:10.1155/2013/167059

Bhatt, A. (2010). Evolution of clinical research: A history before and beyond James Lind. *Perspectives in Clinical Research, 1*, 6–10.

Central Drugs Standard Control Organization. (2004). Good clinical practices for clinical research in India. Retrieved from http://www.sgpgi.ac.in/sop/GCP-%20Indian.pdf

Chillayah, M.M. (n.d.). Surgery of Susrutha Samhitha and art of treatment (vaidhiya murai). Varma Kalai. Retrieved from http://silambam.asia/varmakalai_treatment.html

Clinical Trials Registry–India. (n.d.). Clinical Trials Registry–India. Retrieved from http://ctri.nic.in/Clinicaltrials/login.php

Desai, S., & Naik, S. (2011, January). Inundation of global clinical trials. Clinical trials regulation in India. *Modern Pharmaceuticals, 4*(12), 60–62. Retrieved from http://www.siroclinpharm.com/siro_pdf/articles/MPH_Jan11_Clinical_Research.pdf

Drugs and Cosmetics (Amendment) Act, 2013, Bill No. LVIII of 2013. Retrieved from http://www.prsindia.org/uploads/media/Drugs%20and%20Cosmetics/drugs%20and%20cosmetics%20bill.pdf

D'Souza, N.D., Murthy, N.S., & Aras, R.Y. (2013). Projection of burden of cancer mortality for India, 2011–2026. *Asian Pacific Journal of Cancer Prevention, 14*, 4387–4392. Retrieved from http://www.apocpcontrol.org/paper_file/issue_abs/Volume14_No7/4387-4392%206.30%20Neevan%20D%20R%20Dsouza%20(Mortality).pdf

Ernst & Young India & Federation of Indian Chambers of Commerce and Industry. (2009). *Glorious metamorphosis: Compelling reasons for doing clinical research in India.* New Delhi, India: Ernst & Young.

Gaffney, A. (2013, February 14). India's Health Ministry releases new clinical trials requirements. *Regulatory Focus.* Retrieved from http://www.raps.org/regulatoryDetail.aspx?id=8071

Indian Council of Medical Research. (n.d.-a). Guidelines for international collaboration/research projects in health research. Retrieved from http://icmr.nic.in/guide.htm

Indian Council of Medical Research. (n.d.-b). Guidelines for operation of projects for grantees of ICMR extramural research projects. Retrieved from http://www.icmr.nic.in/forms/adhocform.doc

Indian Council of Medical Research. (2006). *Ethical guidelines for biomedical research on human participants.* Retrieved from http://icmr.nic.in/ethical_guidelines.pdf

Indian Council of Medical Research National Cancer Registry Programme. (2005). *Two-year report of the population based cancer registries 1999–2000.* Retrieved from http://icmr.nic.in/ncrp/1999-00/PBCR%20Report%201999_00.pdf

Jayasheel, B.G. (2010). Carrying out clinical trials in India. Retrieved from http://ecronacunova.com/pdf/whitepapers/RAJPharma%20June%202010_Jayasheel%20final.pdf

Jayasheel, B.G. (2012). Recent changes in regulations related to clinical trials approval in India. *PharmaTimes Magazine, 44*(5), 45. Retrieved from http://rifapharma.com/clinicaltrialapprovalIndia.pdf

Life Positive. (n.d.). History of Ayurveda in India. Retrieved from http://lifepositive.com/history-of-ayurveda-in-india

Mani, H., & Pai, S.A. (1997). Research methods in cancer: Clinical trials, epidemiology and audit, Tata Memorial Hospital, Mumbai, 28 February and 1 March 1997. *National Medical Journal of India, 10,* 249–250. Retrieved from http://nmji.in/approval/archive/Volume-10/issue-5/conferences.pdf

Ministry of Health and Family Welfare. (2005). Drugs and Cosmetics (IIND Amendment) Rules, 2005. Retrieved from http://dbtbiosafety.nic.in/act/schedule_y.pdf

Ministry of Health and Family Welfare. (2013a). Clinical trials in India: Note on clinical trials in India. Retrieved from http://www.mohfw.nic.in/index1.php?lang=1&level=5&sublinkid=4481&lid=2641

Ministry of Health and Family Welfare. (2013b, August 30). Drugs and cosmetics (Fourth Amendment) Rules, 2013. *Gazette of India.* Retrieved from http://egazette.nic.in/WriteReadData/2013/E_441_2013_024.pdf

Nundy, S., & Gulhati, C.M. (2005). A new colonialism? Conducting clinical trials in India. *New England Journal of Medicine, 352,* 1633–1636. doi:10.1056/NEJMp048361

Office of the Registrar General and Census Commissioner, India. (2011). *Census of India 2011.* Retrieved from http://censusindia.gov.in

Oxford Group. (n.d.). Welcome to the INDOX Cancer Research Network. Retrieved from http://indox.org.uk/home

Pais, P. (n.d.). Clinical trials in India: Regulatory issues. Retrieved from http://www.cannectin.ca/workfiles/sg/Pais_Slides.pdf

Raina, V. (2005). Doing cancer trials in India: Opportunities and pitfalls. *Annals of Oncology, 16,* 1567–1568. doi:10.1093/annonc/mdi315

Ramnath, T., & Nandakumar, A. (2011). Estimating the burden of cancer. *National Medical Journal of India, 24,* 69–71. Retrieved from http://nmji.in/archives/Volume-24/Issue-2/Editorial-II.pdf

Shah, J.Y., Phadtare, A., Rajgor, D., Vaghasia, M., Pradhan, S., Zelko, H., & Pietrobon, R. (2010). What leads Indians to participate in clinical trials? A meta-analysis of qualitative studies. *PLOS ONE, 5*(5), e10730. doi:10.1371/journal.pone.0010730

Sharma, D.C. (2002). Standard protocol helps improve ALL survival rates in India. *Lancet Oncology, 3,* 710. doi:10.1016/S1470-2045(02)00941-5

World Bank. (2015). Life expectancy at birth, total (years). Retrieved from http://data.worldbank.org/indicator/SP.DYN.LE00.IN

World Medical Association. (2004). Declaration of Helsinki. Retrieved from http://www.firstclinical.com/regdocs/doc/?db=INT_Declaration_of_Helsinki_2004

Chapter 54

Ireland

Deirdre McDonnell, RN, RM, Tanya O'Shea, MSc Oncology, and Kathleen Scott, PhD

Introduction

Cancer clinical research in Ireland has been established primarily through the work of the All-Ireland Cooperative Oncology Research Group (ICORG), Ireland's national clinical cancer research network. ICORG, together with local hospital sites, is widely accepted as being instrumental to the success of cancer research in Ireland. Since its inception in 1996, more than 10,000 patients have been enrolled in ICORG clinical studies. ICORG's mission is "to enable Irish patients to gain early access to new cancer treatments" (ICORG, n.d.).

Other state-based organizations, such as the Health Research Board, and independent bodies, such as the Irish Cancer Society, contribute funding to enable new and ongoing cancer clinical research activities.

The Republic of Ireland has a population of 4.5 million (Central Statistics Office, 2012). Health care in Ireland is governed by the Department of Health and is provided by the public and private sectors. Established through the Health Act 2004, the Health Service Executive (HSE) is responsible for providing health care to everyone living in the Republic of Ireland. HSE is divided into four administrative regions. In addition to the public sector, there is also a large private healthcare market in Ireland. At the end of 2012, approximately 46% of the Irish population held private health insurance (Health Insurance Authority, 2012).

Cancer and its prevention, diagnosis, and treatment are major challenges for Irish society. Approximately one in four people will die from cancer, while 60% of patients with cancer die within five years of diagnosis and an estimated 120,000 cancer survivors are living post-diagnosis and treatment (National Cancer Forum, 2006). The second national cancer strategy, *A Strategy for Cancer Control in Ireland 2006*, led to the introduction of the National Cancer Control Programme (NCCP) (National Cancer Forum, 2006). NCCP "aims to prevent cancer, cure cancer, and increase survival and quality of life for those who develop cancer, by converting the knowledge gained through research, surveillance and outcome evaluation into strategies and actions" (NCCP, n.d.-a, para. 3). As part of the program, eight specialist cancer centers were designated. Other hospitals also provide cancer services, such as chemotherapy (NCCP, n.d.-b). Oncology clinical trials are conducted within public and private hospital settings, where clinical trial patients receive investigational agents alongside patients receiving standard treatments.

History and Foundation

Historically, medically led clinical research in Ireland, either of academic or pharmaceutical origin, was dependent on enthusiastic, committed individuals rather than implementation of new policy. Oncology nurses were directly employed by principal investigators to coordinate clinical trials. A group of cancer consultants established ICORG in 1996. Following their experience of specialist training and research in the United States, they became acutely aware that no national cancer research network existed in Ireland. The introduction of ICORG led to a formal structure for cancer clinical research in Ireland, transforming it into an attractive location to international cancer research groups and the pharmaceutical industry. With the establishment of the All-Ireland Cancer Consortium in 1999, government funding directly supported clinical research in the area of cancer (National Cancer Institute [NCI], 2014).

ICORG was set up to facilitate and to provide the infrastructure within which cancer clinical trials could be conducted at all hospital sites in Ireland. At its inception, the ICORG central office consisted of only three clinical research staff based at St. Vincent's University Hospital, Dublin, and only four research staff at hospital sites. At the time of this writing, the ICORG central office is staffed by more than 35 clinical research professionals, including clinical project managers, clinical research associates, clinical trial administrators, a pharmacovigilance department, a statistics and data management department, and a quality and training department, as well as finance and administration. The wider network of research professionals working at the hospital sites exceeds more than 100 staff and consists of cancer research professionals who are 100% dedicated to cancer research (e.g., clinical research managers, clinical research nurses, site data managers, research pharmacists). ICORG investigators are clinicians based on site within the academic teaching hospitals.

The structure of ICORG comprises several committees that are responsible for the strategic and scientific direction of the group (see Figure 54-1): the ICORG Board, the Executive/Executive Management Committee (EMG), and the External Scientific Advisory Review Board. The Group Central Office (GCO) is responsible for the management and coordination of clinical trial activities at all sites. The Group's scientific structure is streamlined and delineated through trials conducted within therapeutic disease areas known as Disease Specific Sub Groups (DSSGs). There are currently 11 DSSGs: Breast, Lung, Head and Neck, Gastrointestinal, Gynaecological, Genitourinary, Paediatric, Melanoma, Translational, Central Nervous System, and Haematology and Lymphoma. Studies that are reviewed and approved by each DSSG also are reviewed and approved by the Scientific Management Group (SMG). SMG is primarily responsible for ensuring that studies are adequately funded or resourced for adoption by the group and to ensure that GCO has available resources to conduct each study. Before a study is ratified by the SMG, if a peer-review process has not already taken place, it is sent for external peer review. Finally, each study is submitted to EMG for approval. ICORG's international External Strategic Advisory Committee regularly reviews

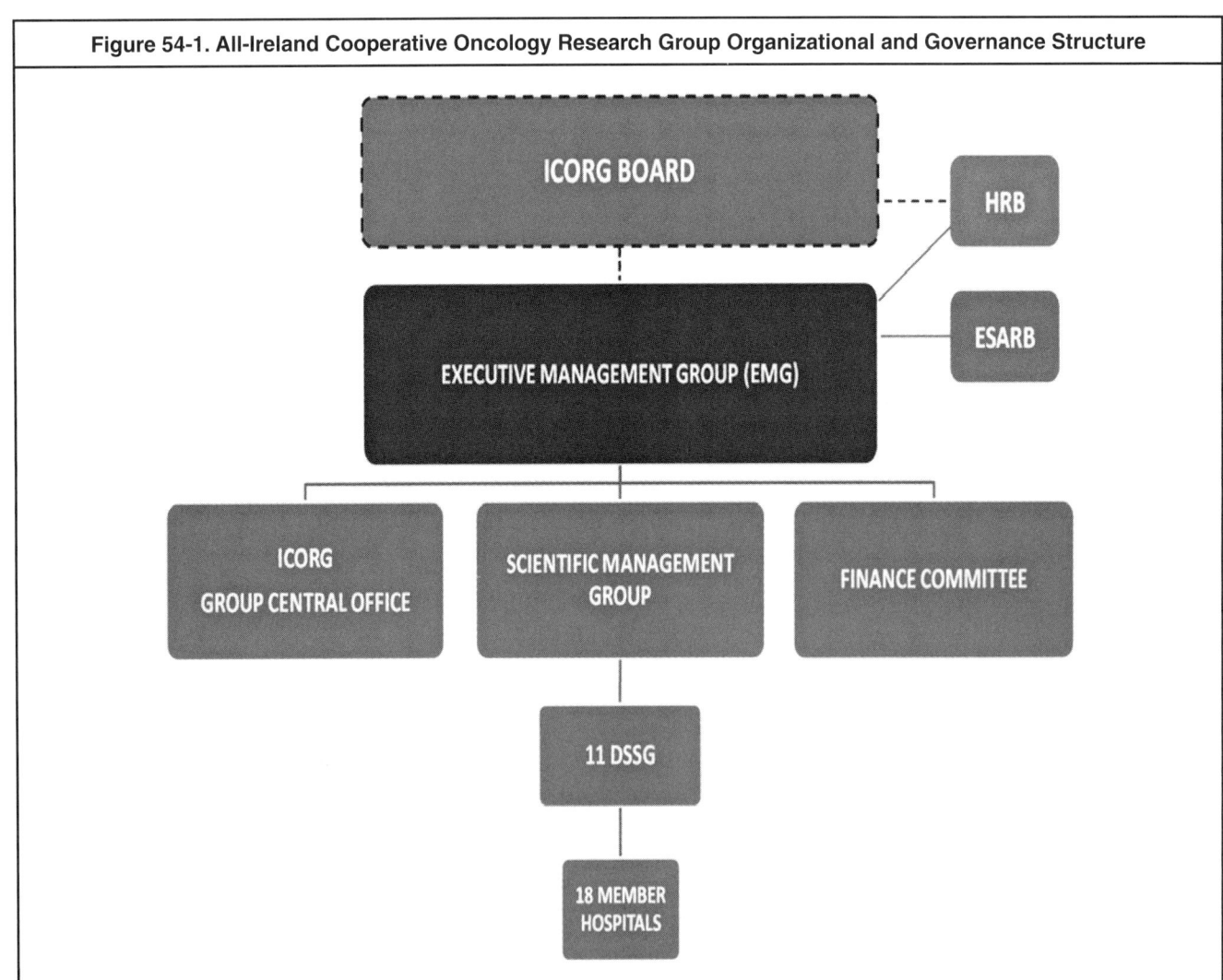

Figure 54-1. All-Ireland Cooperative Oncology Research Group Organizational and Governance Structure

DSSG—Disease Specific Sub Group; ESARB—External Scientific Advisory Review Board; HRB–Health Research Board; ICORG—All-Ireland Cooperative Oncology Research Group

Note. Figure courtesy of All-Ireland Cooperative Oncology Research Group. Used with permission.

the groups' organization and structures, trial portfolio, and research profile. This committee's role is to perform a strategic review of ICORG's operations and productivity.

Membership of ICORG exceeds 400 and includes 99% of the cancer professionals in Ireland, including medical oncologists, radiation oncologists, hematologists, surgeons, clinical research nurses, data managers, and translational research scientists, among many other groups. Through its own research portfolio and through links with industry and leading global cancer research groups, ICORG provides a unique opportunity for patients to receive treatments that are not easily accessible outside of the clinical trials arena in Ireland.

ICORG enrolled approximately 4,000 patients to trials during 2011–2013. The approximate breakdown is as follows: 1,000 patients were enrolled to international collaborative group trials, 2,000 patients to local ICORG-designed/sponsored studies, and 1,000 patients to industry-adopted studies.

Today, approximately 4,800 patients are actively being treated or are in follow-up on approximately 113 active studies (either open to enrollment or in follow-up). Through the work of the group over approximately 17 years, more than 30 different treatments have been made available to patients with cancer in Ireland, in multiple tumor sites and cancer disease areas. Although ICORG initially focused on breast cancer, its portfolio has evolved and diversified over recent years and encompasses all major disease areas in solid tumor cancers and hematology. Figure 54-2 illustrates the spread of studies across each of the disease groups. As the portfolio has expanded, the distribution of studies across disease groups has become more balanced. The group's trial portfolio encompasses all phases of clinical development (phases I–IV). The largest proportion is phase II and III studies. Multiple translational research studies are also open to accrual across many of the disease groups.

Clinical Trials: Fundamental Information

Government Initiatives in Cancer Research

The All-Ireland Cancer Consortium was established in 1999 via a memorandum of understanding signed by the Ministers for Health in Ireland and Northern Ireland and the secretary of Health and Human Services in the United States (NCI, 2014). It established collaboration to

- Identify infrastructure improvements necessary for the island of Ireland
- Formalize and facilitate interactions among the United States, Ireland, and Northern Ireland cancer control communities

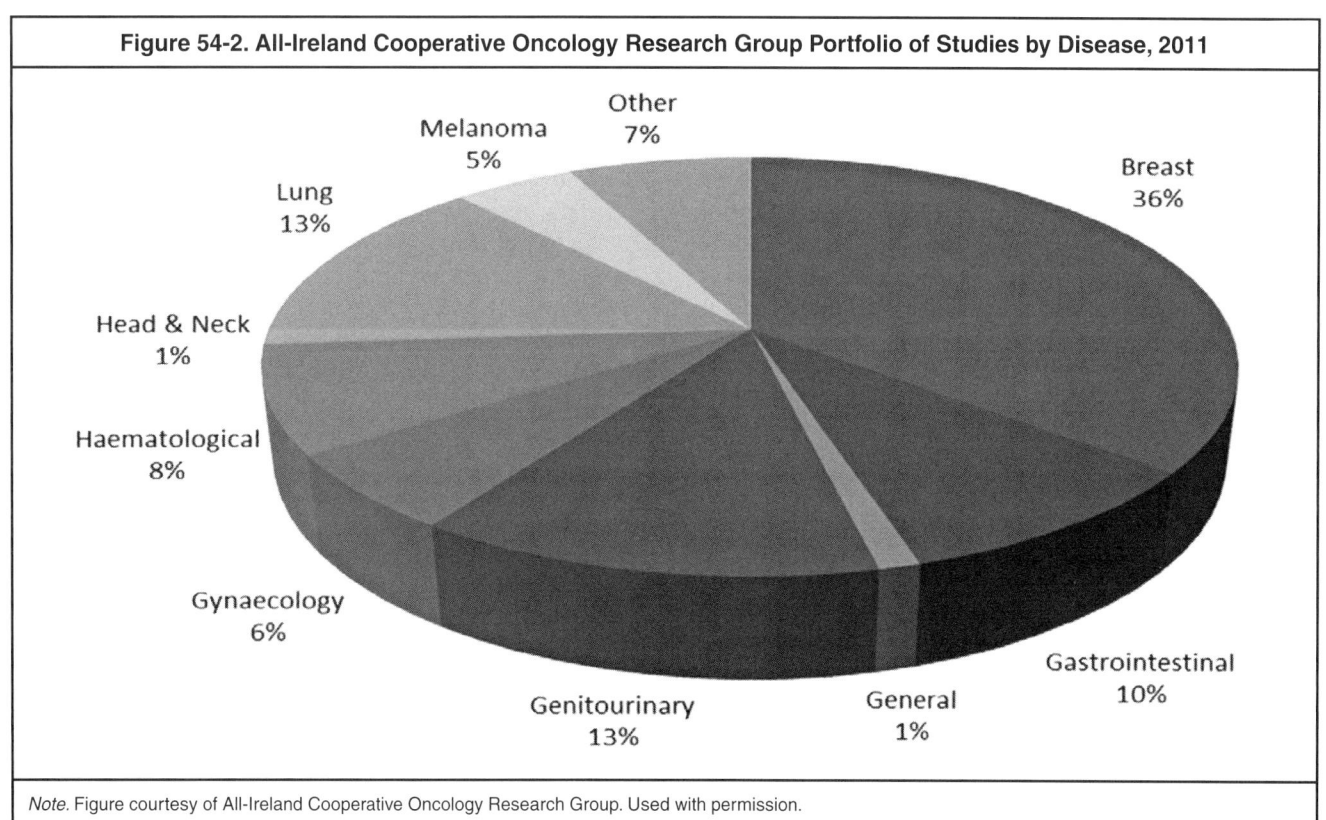

Figure 54-2. All-Ireland Cooperative Oncology Research Group Portfolio of Studies by Disease, 2011

Note. Figure courtesy of All-Ireland Cooperative Oncology Research Group. Used with permission.

- Develop joint programs that could enhance the environment for cancer control with the anticipated outcomes of improved prevention and cancer care
- Develop educational exchange programs for cancer control personnel.

Acting on behalf of their respective ministries were the Health Research Board of Ireland, the Research and Development Office of Northern Ireland, and NCI of the United States.

A number of activities have been developed under the consortium. These include ICORG conducting clinical trials in cancer and several funding schemes to access NCI expertise and build north-south collaboration in Ireland through fellowship and training programs (All-Ireland Cancer Consortium, 2011).

ICORG received initial government funding as part of this cross-border initiative, following submission of a successful Health Research Board grant by ICORG in 2001. For the first three years of funding, this took the form of a smaller project grant, evolving at subsequent grant cycles into a more comprehensive research program grant. During this period, the Irish Cancer Society provided financial support to ICORG, providing important annual funding.

The National Cancer Control Programme

The 2006 national cancer strategy recommended that cancer centers should be networked together in Managed Cancer Control Networks (National Cancer Forum, 2006). The aim was to equip each of the HSE's four regions within Ireland with broad self-sufficiency of services in relation to the more common forms of cancer such as breast, gastrointestinal, lung, genitourinary, melanoma, gynecologic, hematologic and lymphoma, central nervous system, and head and neck cancers.

Ireland's eight specialist cancer centers are now located and networked within each of the four HSE administration regions. Successful international cancer center models were examined as part of the process of designating the eight centers in Ireland. Four managed cancer control networks exist in Ireland, each with two cancer centers. The Dublin North East and Dublin Mid-Leinster network areas work very closely together and are jointly managed by NCCP. The eight cancer centers are located as outlined in Table 54-1.

National Plan for Radiation Oncology

In 2005, the Minister for Health and Children announced the government's approval for a national network for Radiation Oncology Services consisting of six centers (Department of Health, 2005). The national network consists of four large centers and two satellite centers as outlined in Table 54-1.

Table 54-1. National Cancer Control Programme (NCCP) Cancer Centers and Planned National Radiation Oncology Centers in the Republic of Ireland

NCCP Cancer Centers	Planned National Radiation Oncology Centers
NCCP East—Dublin North East Beaumont Hospital Mater Misericordiae University Hospital	Beaumont Hospital, Dublin
NCCP East—Dublin Mid-Leinster St. James's Hospital St. Vincent's University Hospital	St. James's Hospital, Dublin
NCCP South Cork University Hospital Waterford Regional Hospital	Cork University Hospital
NCCP West Mid-Western Regional Hospital, Limerick University Hospital Galway	University Hospital Galway Two integrated satellite centers: • Waterford Regional Hospital (managed by Cork University Hospital) • Mid-Western Regional Hospital (managed by University Hospital Galway)

Cancer Prevention and Screening

NCCP has established a cancer prevention working group in partnership with the Population Health Directorate of the HSE (HSE, n.d.). The terms of reference of the working group are to
- Provide guidance to the Primary Care Cancer Teams in relation to planning, prioritizing, implementing, monitoring, and evaluating cancer prevention programs in primary care, especially smoking cessation, obesity, and care in the sun
- Provide education and training materials on the use of evidence-based interventions to these primary care teams
- Develop a template for monitoring and evaluating each prevention program
- Provide education and training in relation to evidence-based approaches for smoking cessation to health personnel in general.

Cancer screening is currently provided by the National Cancer Screening Service, which encompasses two national screening programs, BreastCheck and CervicalCheck. A recently launched bowel screening program, BowelScreen, is currently being implemented on a phased basis (National Cancer Screening Service, n.d.).

ICORG has initiated work with NCCP based on a shared vision to improve the research culture across the eight major cancer centers in areas such as pharmacy and regulation for research activities, as well as communicating decisions on chosen studies and areas of priority on a regular basis.

Sponsoring Agencies

The main sponsors of cancer clinical trials in Ireland are companies within the pharmaceutical industry, ICORG itself, clinical research organizations, and collaborative and academic groups. Some single-center institutional-sponsored trials are also conducted.

European regulations require that a national sponsor (a person, body, organization, or institution) is identified to take overall responsibility for the conduct of the clinical trial (International Conference on Harmonisation of Technical Requirements for Registration of Pharmaceuticals for Human Use [ICH], 1996). The sponsor's main responsibilities are to initiate, manage, and support the clinical trial and carry the legal responsibilities for trial conduct. For pharmaceutical-sponsored trials, the company affiliate will take on the role of sponsor, or particular sponsor responsibilities could be delegated to a contract research organization. For investigator-initiated trials, regulations permit an individual investigator or local institution to act as the sponsor. In the case of multicenter trials, the collaborative or coordinating group often acts as the sponsor on behalf of many sites, whether initiated nationally or by international groups.

Defining sponsorship is a complex aspect to trial setup, particularly when multiple parties are contractually involved in a clinical trial. Typically, pharmaceutical companies, which provide the study drugs in investigator-initiated trials, do not accept the role of trial sponsor. Careful consideration of the responsibilities of each party is required, particularly which party will carry clinical trial indemnity, a factor that generally determines who is ultimately defined as the trial sponsor.

Legal and Regulatory Approval Process

Clinical trials of medicinal products in Ireland are governed by international standards, applicable local regulations, and European Union regulations, including the following.
- Good Clinical Practice (GCP) guidelines (ICH, 1996)
- Directive 2001/20/EC (European Union, 2001)
- European Union Guideline for Good Manufacturing Practice (GMP): Annex 13: Manufacture of Investigational Medicinal Products (Directive 2003/94/EC) (European Union, 2003)
- European Communities (Clinical Trials on Medicinal Products for Human Use) Regulations, 2004 to 2009 (Statutory Instrument [S.I.] No. 190 of 2004, as amended) (Department of Health, 2004b)

Ireland is a member state of the European Union; thus, clinical trials of an investigational medicinal product (IMP) are required to comply with Directive 2001/20/EC, the European Communities (Clinical Trials on Medicinal Products for Human Use) Regulations, 2004 (Department of Health, 2004b), and Directive 2005/28/EC (European Union, 2005). Trials outside the scope of the regulations are noninterventional trials and trials on nonmedicinal products (e.g., evaluations of surgical procedures, radiation oncology trials, translational research protocols).

Where ICORG or a pharmaceutical company is the trial sponsor or legal representative acting on behalf of the sponsor for an IMP trial, an application for authorization is made to the Health Products Regulatory Authority (HPRA), the national regulatory authority in Ireland. Guidelines for the completion of a clinical trial application to HPRA are based on Irish legislation: S.I. No. 190 of 2004 (Department of Health, 2004b), S.I. No. 878 of 2004 (Amendment No. 1) (Department of Health, 2004a), S.I. No. 374 of 2006 (Amendment No. 2) (Department of Health, 2006), and, for advanced therapy medicinal products, S.I. No. 1 of 2009 (Office of the Attorney General, 2009). The statutory instruments and amendments give effect to the relevant European regulations governing clinical trials of medicinal products.

According to regulation 10 of the Clinical Trials on Medicinal Products for Human Use Regulations 2004, S.I. No. 190 of 2004, a trial may only be started or conducted in Ireland if (a) the ethics committee has issued a favorable opinion, (b) HPRA has granted an authorization, and (c) the sponsor or legal representative of the sponsor is established within the European Community (Department of Health, 2004b). For trials led by external groups and sponsors, ICORG will establish the role of each respective party and who will complete the clinical trial application. For the most part, ICORG will be responsible for submission of the clinical trial application to HPRA. In the case of ICORG-led trials conducted in other countries, ICORG will either complete the clinical trial application or will support a lead center or group to complete the country-specific submission, according to the applicable regulatory requirements.

Ethics Review and Approval Process

The ethics review and approval process in Ireland complies with the European Communities (Clinical Trials on Medicinal Products for Human Use) Regulations, 2004 (Department of Health, 2004b) and the applicable regulations in Ireland. A total of 13 ethics committees, mainly based in large teaching hospitals or health areas, are recognized by the Department of Health to review and approve clinical trials of all descriptions and classes involving medicinal products (HSE Research Ethics Committees Review Group, 2008). The European Union directive and clinical trial regulations stipulate that there should be only one ethical review of a clinical trial per member state, regardless of how many sites are participating in the study (Department of Health, 2004b). Therefore, clinical trial protocols of medicinal products in multicenter trials are submitted to a nominated recognized ethics committee, which reviews the applications for all participating sites in Ireland. The standard application form (where accepted by the committee) will be completed by the sponsor or designee and, with the pre-specified supporting documents and sign-off by the chief investigator, is submitted to the committee for review. A Site-Specific Assessment (referred to as SSA) form is completed and signed for each ICORG hospital site and included in the application.

Noninterventional trials and protocols that do not involve medicinal products are considered outside the scope of the European Union directive and, therefore, the ethical review process requires the protocol to be submitted to each ethics committee at the location where the research is planned.

Protocol Development, Review, and Approval

New protocol development for ICORG investigator-initiated trials follows a clearly defined pathway from the initial trial concept phase to the final approved protocol (see Figure 54-3). A concept proposal template is used to develop a trial outline and includes critical information such as the rationale for the study, trial objectives, proposed patient population, and trial design. The principal investigator will work closely with a dedicated protocol team, which comprises a clinical project manager to provide input and expertise on trial feasibility, timelines, and resource planning and a biostatistician and data manager to determine important statistical considerations, identify key data variables to be collected, and develop case report forms (CRFs). Clinical research nurse/manager expertise is sought, particularly regarding aspects such as screening, protocol assessments, and the scheduling of visits. Broad input and review of the protocol early in its development will assist greatly in avoiding future protocol amendments.

New protocol concepts are presented and discussed at an ICORG DSSG meeting where clinicians and other professionals working in a specific area determine the scientific relevance of each proposed trial and consider the level of priority to be assigned within the group's overall trial portfolio. Following endorsement by DSSG, a new trial proposal will then undergo a peer-review process through an SMG and further internal operational review to determine the level of resources required to develop the protocol and complete funding proposals. A roles and responsibilities matrix is completed to delineate who is responsible for each core trial activity from commencement to completion.

The format of an ICORG protocol is based on the protocol elements outlined in ICH GCP guidelines (ICH, 1996) and detailed in an ICORG-specific standard operating procedure (SOP) on protocol development. Using a protocol template facilitates timely protocol development and standardizes procedures to ensure scientific quality and a high level of compliance with GCP and the applicable regulatory requirements.

The main types of protocols considered by ICORG are (a) ICORG in-house protocols, (b) cooperative group trials or academic protocols, and (c) industry-led protocols. Regardless of origin, ICORG considers new protocols according to a strict set of criteria, ensuring high ethical standards and scientific quality of each trial adopted under the ICORG trial portfolio. ICORG members will seek to identify new trials that are of high scientific interest and clinical relevance to the cancer community in Ireland, with the primary goal of adopting new studies across tumor-specific and subspecialty areas in solid tumors and hematology and to fill current gaps in treatment through clinical research studies. Maximizing opportunities to access new and innovative anticancer treatments for Irish patients with cancer through clinical trials has been a long-standing objective for ICORG since its inception.

Studies led by international groups may permit protocol review or input from ICORG prior to finalization; however, ICORG will conduct a protocol review process prior to adoption, following the pathway for adoption outlined in Figure 54-3. Likewise, industry-led trial protocols are adopted on the basis of scientific interest and opportunity for patients in Ireland to access novel treatments.

Each prospective ICORG center reviews a new protocol to assess trial feasibility and consider the availability of the patient population, study timelines, and site resources available to conduct the protocol. Confirmation of interest and capability to participate is normally documented through completion of a feasibility questionnaire or survey. Clinical research nurses play an important role throughout the feasibility process. Where possible, all ICORG centers are included in multicenter trials; however, where restrictions on the numbers of centers are necessary, referral processes are put in place to make new clinical trials available to as many ICORG investigators and their patients as possible.

Financial Factors and Trial Site Budgets

The sponsoring agency normally prepares a study budget in collaboration with the site staff based on the estimated costs to conduct the study at the site. Generally, the budget provides an estimated costing of the "outside of standard of care" procedures that are required per protocol to conduct the study correctly, and also the

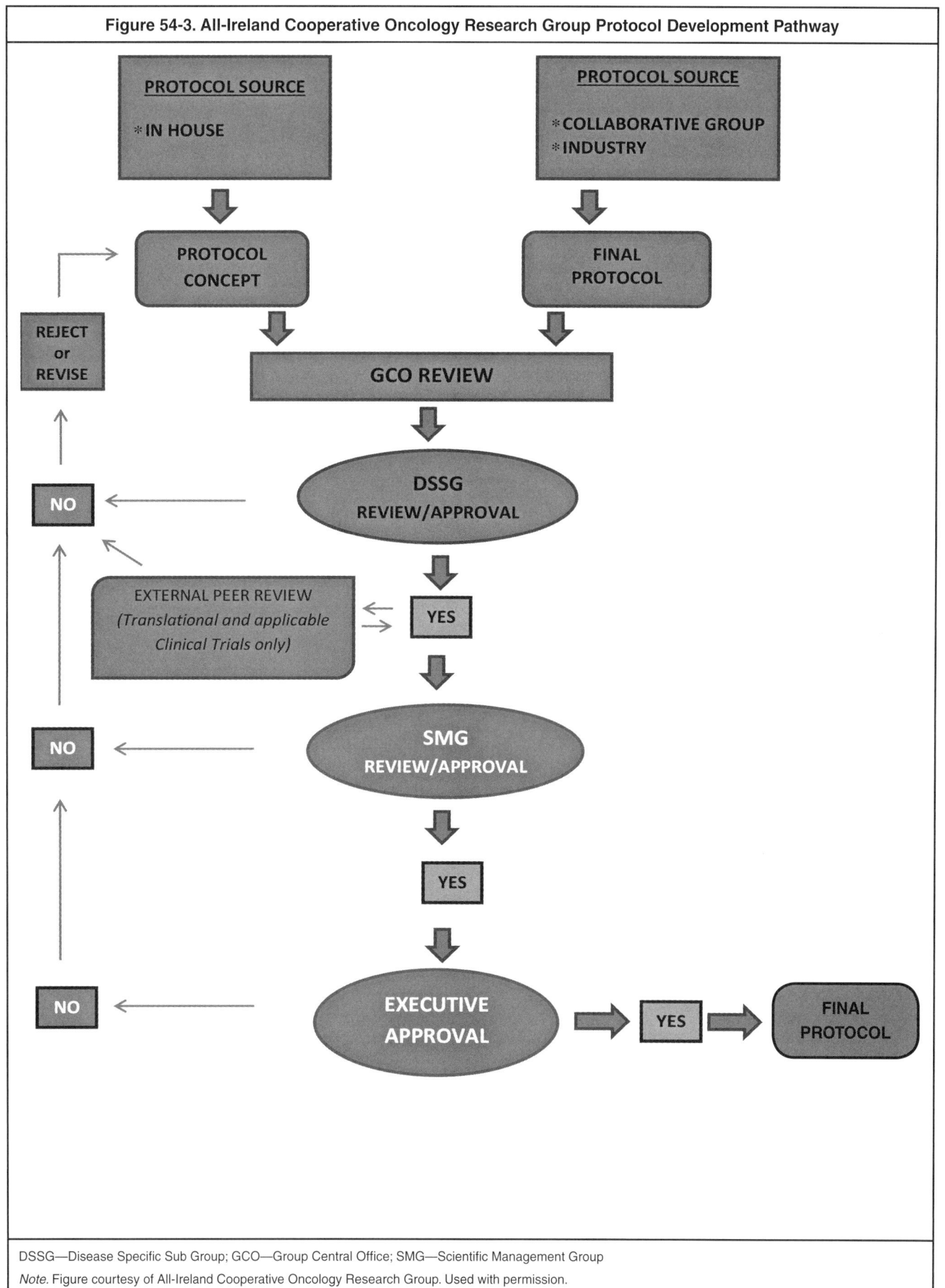

Figure 54-3. All-Ireland Cooperative Oncology Research Group Protocol Development Pathway

DSSG—Disease Specific Sub Group; GCO—Group Central Office; SMG—Scientific Management Group

Note. Figure courtesy of All-Ireland Cooperative Oncology Research Group. Used with permission.

investigator time, oncology/hematology research nurse time, and other departmental fees (e.g., pharmacy, radiology, laboratory, pathology).

Clinical trials consume considerable time and resources to ensure appropriate conduct and compliance with the protocol in accordance with international and local regulations. Each trial must be adequately funded to ensure that all study-specific procedures are carried out correctly and to minimize protocol deviations.

The funding available for clinical trials is highly variable and is generally determined by the type of trial sponsorship; for example, pharmaceutical-supported trials must always provide sufficient funding to cover the conduct of the study at each site. In contrast, site payments for cooperative group trials and investigator-initiated studies are generally much lower.

ICORG GCO prepares a budget based on the key study criteria and costs, such as project management, trial monitoring, pharmacovigilance, and data management and statistics.

Recruitment and Retention

Patients with cancer in Ireland are generally referred to one of the eight designated national cancer centers, which are based in academic teaching hospitals and offer a comprehensive range of treatment modalities, including cancer screening, diagnosis, imaging, surgery, medical and radiation oncology, and clinical trial participation. The majority of patients are referred for treatment to the local cancer center within their residential catchment area. Some patients, however, may be referred outside of their geographic area to the center acting as the national referral center for a specific disease (e.g., bone marrow transplantation, pancreatic cancer, neurology). In the private health sector, patients may select an oncologist/hematologist or private clinic known for specific disease expertise.

Cancer information resources can encourage patients to explore treatment options. The Irish Platform for Patients' Organisations, Science and Industry (IPPOSI) is one such resource. As a patient-led partnership, the platform provides a structured way of facilitating interaction between patient groups/charities, scientists, and clinicians and the industry on policy, legislation, and regulation regarding the development of new medicines, products, devices, and diagnostics for unmet medical needs in Ireland. IPPOSI is partly funded by the Health Research Board, Ireland (IPPOSI, 2013).

In 2012, IPPOSI launched a new information campaign aimed at people who have been asked to participate in a clinical trial. The campaign includes a leaflet (*So You've Been Asked to Take Part in a Clinical Trial?*) (IPPOSI, n.d.) and a website (www.clinicaltrials.ie) that provide patients with independent answers to questions related to clinical trial participation.

ICORG also provides information to the public on currently accruing clinical trials and participating sites and investigators (ICORG, n.d.).

Clinical Trial Participants

Patient Selection and Eligibility

Most patients requiring a new course of treatment and attending consultations with their oncologist/hematologist are considered potential clinical trial candidates. The research nurse may place clinical trial tools such as a study summary leaflet or posters in the clinic area, following ethics approval. During the initial consultation, the oncologist/hematologist will outline the various treatment options available, including discussion of enrollment in a clinical trial as an alternative to standard therapy.

Informed Consent Process

If patients wish to further explore the clinical trial option, they will meet with a clinical research nurse. The clinical research nurse will have received study-specific training when the trial was initiated at the site and will be familiar with the protocol in addition to having completed ICH GCP training. All patient information leaflets and informed consent forms will have been preapproved by a recognized ethics committee. The research nurse will read through the patient information leaflet and informed consent form with potential study candidates.

Patients are then given sufficient time to ask questions and to consult with other family members, friends, or their general practitioner as they consider their options. This process may require more than one visit with the investigator or study doctor.

If the patient decides to participate in the clinical trial, the investigator and the patient will sign the informed consent form prior to commencement of any study procedure. The patient is provided with a copy of the signed informed consent form. A second copy is placed in the patient's medical record, and the original is placed in the Investigator Site File. This consent process is documented in the medical record. The patient then enters the screening phase, where the clinical research nurse coordinates all assessments to evaluate the patient's eligibility for enrollment to the protocol. The patient must meet all inclusion and exclusion criteria in the study, and the investigator confirms eligibility prior to enrollment or randomization.

Long-Term Follow-Up

Long-term follow-up in cancer trials usually is essential to accurately assess the primary and secondary efficacy endpoints and to capture potential long-term safety events. Many oncology clinical trials will have expedited reporting for specific conditions that may arise during long-term follow-up, so it is critical to minimize the incidence of "lost to follow-up" participants.

Recently, NCCP encouraged patients with breast cancer to see their primary care physician, or general practitioner, for long-term follow-up after completion of treatment for early-stage breast cancer, in collaboration with the breast cancer services. This may prove challenging to clinical trial follow-up because patients may not be routinely seeing the study investigator for long-term care.

With many studies requiring follow-up for 10–20 years or until death, clinical research nurses may have to employ interpersonal skills to ensure capture of long-term follow-up data. Establishing a good relationship between the patient and the clinical trial team is essential to ensure patient adherence with follow-up assessments. Regular telephone or mail contact with patients or their general practitioner may be necessary to ensure that questionnaires, diaries, scheduled tests appointments, and survival data requirements are adhered to on a long-term basis.

Because of the small geographic size of Ireland, it normally is possible to obtain long-term follow-up data on most patients via their general practitioner. If a study candidate wishes to move to another geographic area, it may be possible to relocate to a new study site, thereby enabling the patient to remain on study follow-up. This is one of the contributing factors as to why Ireland has a low "lost to follow-up" percentage compared with many other countries.

Patient and Family Education

Clinical research nurses act as the primary advocate for patients, both prior to and throughout their participation in a research study. The research nurse's role is to educate patients and family members on the disease process, study-related procedures, and any protocol-specific instructions. Clinical trial education usually is provided by the research nurse at one of the study screening or workup visits. With increasing use of oral therapies in the oncology field, patient education regarding self-medication with investigational products is crucial. Special dietary precautions, the correct timing of ingestion (e.g., with or without food), contraindicated medicines, medications for the prevention and reduction of adverse events (AEs), dosage interruptions, and medication storage instructions are important aspects that require clear and concise explanation to patients by the research nurse.

Assessing adherence to the correct treatment dose is also essential for accurate data capture. Patients are supplied with any study tools that have been provided by the study sponsor, such as AE management guidelines or diaries, which have been preapproved by the ethics committee. The experience and skills of the research nurse group within the ICORG membership has been a major factor in the group's ability to consistently produce high-quality data and positive audit results.

Administration of Protocol Agents

In most cases, the pharmacy departments order, store, prepare, and dispense IMPs. They also complete and maintain IMP accountability logs, monitor temperature controls of storage facilities, and ensure that an aseptic environment is used as required for infusion preparations. Pharmacists receive protocol-specific training in addition to ICH GCP training. Protocol treatment prescriptions are written by delegated study investigators.

Within the Republic of Ireland, chemotherapy is administered in designated specialized units where clinical trial patients receive investigational agents alongside patients receiving standard commercial agents. While the research nurse coordinates all clinical trial–specific activities, trial education, and study assessments, nurses qualified in chemotherapy administration generally administer chemotherapy.

Adverse Events

At screening and throughout the trial, all protocol-mandated assessments are performed and patients are assessed for AEs based on a toxicity grading scale such as NCI's Common Terminology Criteria for Adverse Events (CTCAE), as specified by the protocol. A physician will perform a physical examination and full patient assessment before proceeding with protocol treatment or will implement necessary treatment delays or dose modifications as mandated by the protocol. Copies of all current clinical trial protocols are available in the clinical care area.

Serious adverse events (SAEs) are documented as required and reported via protocol-specific reporting systems, for example, the Cancer Therapy Evaluation Program Adverse Event Reporting System (CTEP-AERS) (formerly known as Adverse Event Expedited Reporting, or AdEERS) for U.S. NCI cooperative group trials. Reporting procedures are clearly defined and located in the protocol and Investigator Site File. Many clinical trials use electronic systems for capturing SAEs; however, paper-based forms are available as backup. All sites have SOPs or policies in place for SAE reporting.

It is the sponsor's responsibility to report suspected unexpected serious adverse reactions (SUSARs) to the regulatory authorities and ethics committees per local and European Union regulatory requirements. When ICORG is the trial sponsor, SAEs reported by site investigators are processed by the ICORG pharmacovigilance department and reviewed with respect to seriousness, causality, and expectedness. If the reaction is deemed to be a SUSAR, a report is submitted to the Irish competent authority and other authorities as required, according to specified regulatory reporting time frames.

Genetics and Genomics

The advent of molecular-targeted treatments for many cancers has greatly enhanced the need for high-quality, translational research to drive improvements in cancer care. Most research-focused teaching hospitals now only undertake studies that incorporate a specific translational component built into their study design. Recent trial data in cancer, regulatory decisions, and approvals of new treatments all point to the growing importance of integrated scientific and clinical research to underpin emerging cancer treatments.

ICORG includes a team dedicated to the conduct of translational cancer research and led by a translational research manager. This position has had a significant impact on Ireland's contribution to important translational-focused research questions and the development of new trials. The role of the translational research manager is to prioritize accrual to translational studies at all sites and increase the proportion of studies that incorporate translational objectives.

The clinical research nurse role has expanded with the advent of translational research. Research nurses need to be competent in processes related to the collection of biologic specimens. They coordinate the collection, preparation, storage, and shipment of whole blood, serum, plasma, tissue, urine, or stool samples as required. Many study sponsors require certification in the handling of hazardous substances (e.g., dry ice) and international shipping regulations. Research nurses also must be familiar with customs regulations when shipping material outside the European Union.

The Translational Research group of ICORG has facilitated the operation of both in-house and international research studies. The increasing focus on translational patient-oriented research in cancer, combined with improved infrastructure, has led to a steady increase in translational studies in Ireland in recent years.

Correlative Trials

Health-related quality-of-life (HRQOL) outcomes are highly important endpoints that are most commonly evaluated in phase III cancer trials. A wide array of validated HRQOL measurement instruments exist (e.g., the European Organisation for Research and Treatment of Cancer suite of HRQOL instruments and modules validated in tumor-specific settings). Trial participants are required to complete the designated HRQOL questionnaire according to the protocol. Other patient-reported outcomes measures (PROMs), for example, pain measurement scales, also may be evaluated. Paper-based questionnaires are commonly administered by research nurses and completed in the clinic by the trial participants. Some protocols may collect PROM data via a web-based interface or PDA device that the participant may be able to use at home. Research nurses play a pivotal role in educating participants as to the correct understanding of questions and ensuring that HRQOL data are collected per the protocol schedule, as this type of data cannot be retrospectively retrieved.

To evaluate the economic impact of a new drug intervention, a clinical trial protocol may include health economics endpoints. Data collected via CRFs may include healthcare resource utilization, such as the types of additional hospital visits or treatment, general practitioner visits, or community care a participant may obtain as a result of receiving protocol treatment.

At present, there is an absence of nurse companion studies within cancer clinical research in Ireland. It is hoped that with increased academic clinical research nurse education, such research will be an area for expansion in the future.

Documentation and Data Management

Trial Documentation

All sites participating in cancer research trials are required to maintain a set of essential trial documents according to ICH GCP guidelines. Essential documents, individually and collectively, permit evaluation of the conduct of a study and demonstrate compliance with GCP standards and applicable regulatory requirements (ICH, 1996). An SOP outlines which documents are required before, during, and at the close of the trial, with all required documents filed in a Project Management File at the sponsor's site for the entire project. Each site will store and maintain an Investigator Site File according to an SOP template for protocol-specific and site-specific documents. A separate Pharmacy File will be stored and maintained on site in the pharmacy department for the purposes of keeping records for IMP storage and accountability.

When ICORG is not the trial sponsor or the trial is conducted by an international group, additional documents may be required. For example, participation in U.S.-regulated trials may require a completed Form FDA 1572 from the U.S. Food and Drug Administration (FDA) for each site or an FDA financial disclosure form for each investigator.

The tracking of essential documents is vital to ensure that a current and accurate paper trail remains in place throughout the study. Trial monitors routinely collect, track, and update essential documents and other study-specific documentation as required. Tracking is normally facilitated through the use of electronic forms and spreadsheets. The project manager will ensure that all documents are collected and approvals are in place at the point of site initiation and before authorizing shipments of IMPs to sites. Clinical research nurses are the central individuals who work with the sponsor to obtain essential signed documents from the local research team. They store and maintain the Investigator Site File and therefore must be fully aware of the documentation requirements of each trial. Most clinical trial sites will have SOPs for documentation management.

Filing systems can consist of both paper-based and electronic systems. A standardized approach to filing supports adherence with GCP guidelines and the retrieval and access of documents by trial staff. All trial documents are stored securely and are only accessible to designated trial staff. Likewise, clinical research nurses are required, on behalf of the investigator, to store files in locked and secure locations.

Arrangements for archiving of trial documents at the close of the trial should be determined at the start of the trial and typically are discussed during site initiation. Because many trials are conducted over several years, archiving arrangements will help to preempt any potential issues. Sponsors and the investigators are required to retain essential trial documents in IMP trials for at least 15 years after trial completion unless otherwise specified by the sponsor. Both ICORG GCO and ICORG sites have archiving arrangements in place for the long-term storage of trial files and records to comply with GCP and regulatory requirements.

Data Management

Trials use either paper-based CRFs or electronic data capture systems for the collection of clinical trial data. For ICORG in-house trials, the ICORG data management team leader develops the CRFs in close liaison with study team members, including the clinical project manager and biostatistician. Based on the trial protocol, CRFs are generated that facilitate collection of the requisite trial data and statistical analysis. Research nurses may be consulted to ensure that CRFs are clear, feasible, and easy to use and that the CRF data fields accurately reflect the trial protocol requirements.

Data management processes comprise data review and validation, including query generation and resolution. Research nurses and data managers play a key role in working to resolve data queries on an ongoing basis and ensuring timely submission, supported throughout by study monitors. As more trials transition from paper-based data collection to electronic data capture, reduction in the time from initial data capture to availability of the data for analysis will occur, with the additional benefit of reduced query volumes, which will lead to overall time and project cost savings.

Quality Assurance

A quality management system (QMS) ensures that all trials are conducted according to ICH GCP standards and applicable regulatory requirements and underpins the quality of trial data generated. Core elements of the QMS include SOPs, training, site monitoring, and audits. A fully comprehensive set of SOPs supports each major clinical research activity undertaken by a study sponsor. New SOPs are introduced as required, and an SOP review cycle ensures that procedures remain current and in compliance with legislation and applicable guidelines. Trial staff are required to be fully familiar with core SOPs relevant to their duties.

Training in clinical trial conduct and GCP is a major activity undertaken by ICORG to ensure that all trial staff members are competent in the management and coordination of clinical trials. ICORG and hospital site staff regularly receive training updates on new information pertinent to trial conduct in Ireland and also are required to maintain training records as well as document acknowledgment of having read and understood important trial-specific and general information relevant to their role.

Site Monitoring

Sites are monitored according to ICH GCP, SOPs, and a study-specific monitoring plan. Trained monitors from sponsor organizations conduct site visits as frequently as weekly for a phase I study during active recruitment and protocol treatment phase or once every 4–12 weeks for phase II and III trials. The primary monitoring activity entails source data verification to evaluate protocol compliance and the accuracy and completeness of data reported in the patient medical records (source documents) against data reported in CRFs. An evaluation of study progress, including screening and recruitment, also is performed. Compliance with ICH GCP, including the delegation of responsibilities by the site's principal investigator, the collection and maintenance of essential documents, and investigational product accountability are activities conducted during site visits.

Monitors play a vital role in providing ongoing protocol training and support to site staff during the study. A detailed summary of monitoring activities is recorded in a report following the visit and reviewed by the designated project manager. Protocol deviations, especially significant findings, are escalated as required. Both prompt follow-up and resolution of issues identified during the visit are integral parts of the overall monitoring process.

Audits and Inspections

Audits are an integral component of the QMS. ICORG sites are audited by the ICORG quality manager according to SOPs and a study-specific audit plan. ICORG sites have been audited as part of the three-year NCI audit cycle by cooperative groups such as the National Surgical Adjuvant Breast and Bowel Project, the Eastern Cooperative Oncology Group, and the American College of Surgeons Oncology Group. Audits by study sponsors external to ICORG, as well as several regulatory inspections by HPRA and FDA, also have been conducted both at the GCO and at ICORG hospital sites.

Professional Development

Nursing Registration in Ireland

Bord Altranais agus Cnáimhseachais na hÉireann, or Nursing and Midwifery Board of Ireland (NMBI), formerly known as *An Bord Altranais*, is the statutory body that sets the standards for the education, registration, and professional conduct of nurses and midwives in Ireland. All RNs practicing in Ireland must register with NMBI annually (Bord Altranais agus Cnáimhseachais na hÉireann, n.d.).

An Bord Altranais (2007) requires nurses to demonstrate competencies in five domains of practice to be entered on the register of nurses:
- Professional/ethical practice
- Holistic approaches and integration of knowledge
- Interpersonal relationships
- Organization and management of care
- Personal and professional development.

Although these domains of competencies were developed for undergraduate programs, they also provide a useful tool for continuous professional development and for assessment of specialized practice. Nurses often maintain a professional portfolio of evidence demonstrating ongoing learning. It is the individual responsibility of research nurses to maintain and document their own professional development relevant to their clinical area or research specialty.

An Bord Altranais (2000) has presented a framework document on the scope of practice for nurses and midwives with a series of principles with which nurses can "review, outline and expand the parameters of [their] practice" (p. 1).

An Bord Altranais (2007) also issued a guidance document, *Guidance to Nurses and Midwives Regarding Ethical Conduct of Nursing and Midwifery Research*. Its purpose is to provide nurses and midwives with general guidance on ethical matters related to research and to ensure protection of the rights of research participants.

Various universities in Ireland have faculties of nursing that provide education and training toward postgraduate, third-level qualifications for oncology and hematology nurses. However, there is a scarcity of academic and postgraduate education specifically aimed at clinical research nurses. Most oncology clinical research nurses will have obtained a postgraduate oncology/hematology nursing qualification in order to specialize in their area of clinical practice.

The National Council for the Professional Development of Nursing and Midwifery issued a report in 2008 on the role of nurses in medical-led clinical research with the purpose of providing guidance in relation to career development for nurses. It reported that various titles were used, including *research nurse, research coordinator, clinical trials nurse*, and *clinical research nurse*. However, despite the best efforts of individuals to champion their role, a clear career development pathway did not exist in Ireland. The report recommended the construction of a career pathway, which should include policy, employment, and professional considerations. It also recommended that an agreed title and employment grade should be used (National Council for the Professional Development of Nursing and Midwifery, 2008).

Kehily (2009) explored the role of research nurses in Ireland through a quantitative descriptive study of 40 research nurses in Ireland and found that they were well educated both academically and in the ethical conduct of clinical trials. The research nurse role functions ranged from basic administrative tasks to those of an extended and specialized nature (Kehily, 2009).

Currently, in the Republic of Ireland, a Postgraduate Certificate in Nursing (Clinical Research) is offered at the Royal College of Surgeons in Ireland and is the only educational program available in Ireland that is specifically designed to meet the needs of clinical research nurses. The program is delivered over one academic year and includes three modules of education and practical seminars (Royal College of Surgeons in Ireland, n.d.).

Another educational initiative commenced when the All-Ireland Cancer Consortium's Nursing Workstream introduced the NCI Clinical Trials Training Program for cancer nurses. Through this program, cancer nurses from the island of Ireland spent five weeks in the United States at clinical research units and facilities learning the role of the research nurse in caring for patients in clinical trials. The consortium also organized a U.S.-based training program, the Cancer Clinical Trials Leadership and Management Programme, for cancer clinical trial nurse managers from the island of Ireland in 2010 (NCI, 2014).

ICORG is a key provider of clinical trial–specific education for staff working in oncology and hematology clinical research in Ireland. A dedicated ICORG quality and training manager is responsible for all training activities at ICORG, including face-to-face workshops for trial site staff that encompass topics such as principles of GCP, investigator responsibilities, sponsor responsibilities, ethics committees, essential documents and GCP audits/regulatory inspections; principal investigator training that entails GCP responsibilities for new investigators; and refresher GCP training, which is required every two years for all staff working on ICORG clinical trials. Additional training on site is held as required or requested.

ICORG also provides a forum for facilitating clinical research nurse leaders from all hospital sites in Ireland to meet on a quarterly basis to discuss ongoing and future work relating to their roles.

The Irish Research Nurses Network

The Irish Research Nurses Network (IRNN) was established in 2008 to support the educational and professional needs of clinical research nurses in Ireland (IRNN, n.d.). IRNN provides a forum for communication among clinical research nurses in Ireland and beyond. Its primary aims are to act as a resource for clinical research nurses by facilitating a network, providing access to shared information on a specialized website, and maintaining a contact list of research nurses in Ireland. These facilities serve as a vehicle for advertising research nurse job vacancies and career opportunities in the Irish healthcare system. IRNN holds a yearly meeting for research nurses, providing an educational opportunity relevant to the research nurse role and a networking occasion for nurses from all over Ireland.

In 2012, NCCP, in partnership with HSE, published the *Strategy and Educational Framework for Nurses Caring for People With Cancer in Ireland* (NCCP, 2012). This publication addressed nurse-led research in Ireland and suggested that lead cancer nurses could be instrumental in influencing and developing research agendas in cancer care and in promulgating research outcomes. The report recommended that separate oncology nursing research funding be made available to nurses to undertake research and that a national forum be introduced where research findings can be presented.

International Clinical Trials Research

ICORG currently maintains successful relationships with many international groups engaged in the conduct of cancer clinical trials (see Figure 54-4). Therefore, ICORG has open access to many studies in those groups' portfolios of studies.

Industry Collaborations

ICORG has established research relationships with most major pharmaceutical companies and is a part-

Figure 54-4. International Cancer Research Groups With Which All-Ireland Cooperative Oncology Research Group Conducts Collaborative Clinical Research

NSABP—National Surgical Adjuvant Breast and Bowel Project
TORI—Translational Oncology Research International
TRIO—Translational Research in Oncology
ECOG—Eastern Cooperative Oncology Group
BIG—Breast International Group
EORTC—European Organisation for Research and Treatment of Cancer
GELA—Groupe d'Etude des Lymphome de l'Adu
NCRN—National Cancer Research Network UK
CRUK—Cancer Research United Kingdom
CTRU—Clinical Trials Research Unit
MRC—Medical Research Council
NCRI—National Cancer Research Institute, UK
ACCOG—Anglo Celtic Cooperative Oncology Group
IBCSG—International Breast Cancer Study Group
ACOSOG—American College of Surgeons Oncology Group
Finnish Uro-Oncological Group
AGO-OVAR—Arbeitsgemeinschaft Gynaekologische Onkologie Ovarian Cancer Study Group
IAEA—International Atomic Energy Agency
TROG—Trans-Tasman Radiation Oncology Group
MRC Scottish Cancer Trials Breast Group—University of Edinburgh, UK
ICR—Institute of Cancer Research UK
ANZGOG—Australia and New Zealand Gynaecological Oncology Group
GCIG—Gynaecologic Cancer InterGroup
UNCCN—University of North Carolina Cancer Network
AIO—Arbeitsgemeinschaft Internistische Onkologie

Note. Figure courtesy of All-Ireland Cooperative Oncology Research Group. Used with permission.

ner in many new and innovative oncology research programs. These collaborative relationships are at various stages of development, from study start-up through follow-up, and therefore require different degrees of input from ICORG. Many of the studies are pivotal registration trials for the investigational agents involved. This work reflects the growing reputation of ICORG among its industry partners. ICORG has directly contributed to the development of a number of breakthrough cancer treatments. This has led to acknowledgment at leading international meetings and publication of ICORG investigator publications for major clinical trials in peer-reviewed journals.

Summary

Cancer clinical research is well established in the Republic of Ireland, primarily through the work of ICORG and other formal specialist networks that have built extensive collaborations with international cancer cooperative groups and pharmaceutical sponsors. Cancer clinical research nurses make a significant contribution to clinical trial participation through patient care and advocacy before and throughout a research study and will continue to play a key role in the conduct of cancer clinical research in Ireland.

Key Points

- Established in 1996, ICORG has been pivotal in the development of cancer clinical research in the Republic of Ireland.
- ICORG's mission has enabled patients with cancer and clinicians to gain early access to new cancer treatments through clinical research.
- NCCP provides a comprehensive cancer control program and network of specialist cancer centers that actively recruit patients to cancer clinical trials in Ireland.
- Recruiting more than 4,000 patients in 2011–2013, ICORG centers participate in clinical studies encompassing a broad range of tumor types and hematologic cancers.
- Cancer research nurses have gained extensive experience in the coordination of cancer trials and contribute significantly to the number of trials opened in Ireland.
- Cancer research nurses in Ireland play an integral role in protocol feasibility, informed consent, trial recruitment, patient safety, and the integrity of trial data.
- Nurses can access clinical research training opportunities in Ireland; however, few formal academic postgraduate courses are available, and the role has yet to achieve broad professional recognition and a pathway for career advancement.

The authors would like to acknowledge John Crown, Brian Moulton, Michele Cunnane, Olivia McLoughlin, Derval Kehily, and Jo Ballot for their review and comments on this chapter.

References

All-Ireland Cancer Consortium. (2011). *Ireland, Northern Ireland National Cancer Institute Cancer Consortium 2000–2011 timeline of activities.* Bethesda, MD: National Cancer Institute.

All-Ireland Cooperative Oncology Research Group. (n.d.). About us. Retrieved from http://www.icorg.ie/about-us/about-us

An Bord Altranais. (2000). *The scope of nursing and midwifery practice framework.* Dublin, Ireland: Author.

An Bord Altranais. (2007). *Guidance to nurses and midwives regarding ethical conduct of nursing and midwifery research.* Dublin, Ireland: Author.

Bord Altranais agus Cnáimhseachais na hÉireann. (n.d.). Registering to practise. Retrieved from http://www.nursingboard.ie/en/registering_to_practise.aspx

Central Statistics Office. (2012). *This is Ireland: Highlights from Census 2011, part 1.* Retrieved from http://www.cso.ie/en/census/census2011reports/census2011thisisirelandpart1

Department of Health. (2004a). The European Communities (Clinical Trials on Medicinal Products for Human Use) (Amendment) Regulations 2004 (S.I. No. 878 of 2004). Retrieved from http://health.gov.ie/wp-content/uploads/2014/04/si20040878.pdf

Department of Health. (2004b). The European Communities (Clinical Trials on Medicinal Products for Human Use) Regulations 2004 (S.I. No. 190 of 2004). Retrieved from http://health.gov.ie/wp-content/uploads/2014/04/si20040190.pdf

Department of Health. (2005, July 25). Tánaiste and Minister for Health and Children, Mary Harney, T.D. announces National Network for Radiation Oncology Services (Press release). Retrieved from http://health.gov.ie/blog/press-release/tanaiste-and-minister-for-health-and-children-mary-harney-t-d-announces-national-network-for-radiation-oncology-services

Department of Health. (2006). European Communities (Clinical Trials on Medicinal Products for Human Use) (Amendment No. 2) Regulations 2006 (S.I. No. 374 of 2006). Retrieved from http://health.gov.ie/wp-content/uploads/2014/04/si20060374.pdf

European Union. (2001). Directive 2001/20/EC of the European Parliament and of the Council of 4 April 2001 on the approximation of the laws, regulations and administrative provisions of the Member States relating to the implementation of good clinical practice in the conduct of clinical trials on medicinal products for human use. Retrieved from http://eurlex.europa.eu/LexUriServ/LexUriServ.do?uri=OJ:L:2001:121:0034:0044:EN:PDF

European Union. (2003). EU guideline for good manufacturing practice (GMP): Annex 13: Manufacture of Investigational Medicinal Products (Directive 2003/94/EC). Retrieved from http://eur-lex.europa.eu/LexUriServ/LexUriServ.do?uri=OJ:L:2003:262:0022:0026:en:PDF

European Union. (2005). Commission Directive 2005/28/EC of 8 April 2005 laying down principles and detailed guidelines for good clinical practice as regards investigational medicinal products for human use, as well as the requirements for authorisation of the manufacturing or importation of such products. Retrieved from http://eur-lex.europa.eu/LexUriServ/LexUriServ.do?uri=OJ:L:2005:091:0013:0019:en:PDF

Health Insurance Authority. (2012). *The Health Insurance Authority annual report and accounts 2012.* Retrieved from http://www.hia.ie/sites/default/files/HIA%20-%20Annual%20Report%20and%20Accounts%202012.pdf

Health Service Executive. (n.d.). Community oncology. Retrieved from http://www.hse.ie/eng/services/list/5/cancer/about/structure/Community_Oncology.html

Health Service Executive Research Ethics Committees Review Group. (2008). Review of research ethics committees and processes in Republic of Ireland. Retrieved from http://www.hse.ie/eng/services/Publications/corporate/etr/Review_of_Research_Ethics.pdf

International Conference on Harmonisation of Technical Requirements for Registration of Pharmaceuticals for Human Use. (1996, July). *Good clinical practice.* Retrieved from http://ec.europa.eu/health/files/eudralex/vol-10/3cc1aen_en.pdf

Irish Platform for Patients' Organisations, Science and Industry. (n.d.). *So you've been asked to take part in a clinical trial?* Retrieved from http://www.clinicaltrials.ie/images/leaflets/TakingPartInAClinicalTrialWebEdition.pdf

Irish Platform for Patients' Organisations, Science and Industry. (2013). About IPPOSI: Welcome to IPOSSI. Retrieved from http://www.ipposi.ie/index.php/about-ipposi-mainmenu-26

Irish Research Nurses Network. (n.d.). Welcome to the Irish Research Nurses Network (IRNN) website. Retrieved from http://irnn.ie

Kehily, D. (2009). *The role of the research nurse in clinical trials—The Irish context. An exploration of the role of the clinical research nurse in Ireland.* Submitted as part of fulfilment of the degree of MSc in Healthcare Management, School of Healthcare Management, Royal College of Surgeons in Ireland.

National Cancer Control Programme. (n.d.-a). About the National Cancer Control Programme. Retrieved from http://www.hse.ie/eng/services/list/5/cancer/about

National Cancer Control Programme. (n.d.-b). Regional cancer services. Retrieved from http://www.hse.ie/eng/services/list/5/cancer/about/services

National Cancer Control Programme. (2012). *Strategy and educational framework for nurses caring for people with cancer in Ireland.* Dublin, Ireland: Author.

National Cancer Forum. (2006). *A strategy for cancer control in Ireland.* Retrieved from http://www.hse.ie/eng/services/Publications/HealthProtection/Public_Health_/National_Cancer_Control_Strategy.pdf

National Cancer Institute. (2014). All-Ireland Cancer Consortium (AICC). Retrieved from http://www.cancer.gov/aboutnci/organization/global-health/research/aicc

National Cancer Screening Service. (n.d.). Welcome to the National Screening Service website. Retrieved from http://www.cancerscreening.ie

National Council for the Professional Development of Nursing and Midwifery. (2008). *Report on the role of the nurse or midwife in medical-led clinical research.* Dublin, Ireland: Author.

Office of the Attorney General. (2009). European Communities (Clinical Trials on Medicinal Products for Human Use) (Amendment) Regulations 2009 (S.I. No. 1 of 2009). Retrieved from http://www.irishstatutebook.ie/pdf/2009/en.si.2009.0001.pdf

Royal College of Surgeons in Ireland. (n.d.). Postgraduate Certificate in Nursing (Clinical Research). Retrieved from http://www.rcsi.ie/cat_course_detail.jsp?n=769&p=111&itemID=60

Chapter 55

Italy

Jane Bryce, MSN, AOCNS®, and Daniela Grosso, MSN

Introduction

According to the Italian Society of Medical Oncology (*Associazione Italiana di Oncologia Medica* [AIOM]) and the Italian Association of Cancer Registries (*Associazione Italiana Registri Tumori* [AIRTUM]), cancer is a significant problem in Italy, with incidence and mortality rates similar to those of other Western industrialized nations (AIOM & AIRTUM, 2013). Italy also has the additional burden of an aging population, with one of the largest and fastest-growing proportions of older adults in Europe (Statistical Office of the European Communities, 2008).

The Italian national healthcare system provides healthcare services to all residents and citizens in a system that is a mix of public and private providers (Ministero Della Salute, 2014). Several cancer institutes, which practice independently from one another, are located throughout Italy. An alliance of these institutes was formed in 2002, with one of its goals being to increase national and international oncology research collaboration (Alleanza Contro Il Cancro, 2013).

History and Foundation

Oversight of clinical research in Italy is mandated by national law and determined by the Health Ministry. Italy was one of the first member states to implement the European Directive 2001/20/EC on clinical trials of medicinal products (Decreto Legislativo, 2003). Italy had already received the European Union (EU) guidelines for good clinical practice (GCP) in medicinal clinical trials (Decreto Ministeriale, 1997) and in 1998 set guidelines for the establishment and functions of independent ethics committees (ECs) (Decreto Ministeriale, 1998). *Agenzia Italiana del Farmaco* (Italian Medicines Agency) began operating the National Monitoring Centre for Clinical Trials (*Osservatorio Nazionale della Sperimentazione Clinica* [OsSC]) in 2000. OsSC is a technical and scientific tool aimed at guaranteeing the epidemiologic surveillance of clinical trials with medicines carried out in Italy and regularly publishes reports on qualitative and quantitative trends of these trials. Furthermore, OsSC serves as a portal for clinical trial applications according to EU guidelines and for communication among sponsors, ECs, and contract research organizations. Data from OsSC are published regularly, and the following data were published in the 11th National Report of Clinical Trials of Drugs in Italy (Agenzia Italiana del Farmaco, 2012), reflecting activity from 2007 through 2011. During that period, 3,783 clinical trials were registered, the vast majority of studies being multicentered (78.6%), international (57.7%), and phase II (37.7%) or phase III (42.8%). Nonprofit sponsors promoted 38.3% of trials, whereas 61.7% were conducted by for-profit sponsors. The largest proportions of trials were conducted under the specialty of oncology, and 1,487 trials were conducted with antineoplastic and immunomodulatory drugs.

Clinical Trials: Fundamental Information

The sponsor and each single investigator are responsible for signing agreements to conduct a trial according to GCP and the governing Italian and European laws regarding clinical research and privacy. Specific assurances may be required for trials originating outside Europe. Many Italian institutions have registered their

The authors would like to acknowledge Marianna Connola, BSN, and Marzia Falanga, BSN, for their contribution to this chapter that remains unchanged from the previous edition of this book.

ECs with the U.S. Office for Human Research Protections and obtained a Federalwide Assurance to participate in U.S. federally funded trials.

Before protocol activation, a multidisciplinary team is assembled that includes physicians, nurses, pharmacists, data managers, laboratory professionals, radiologists, and other specialists depending on the institution and the type of trial. Clinical trial nurses (CTNs) and data managers have emerging roles in Italy, and although increasingly present in the multidisciplinary team, they are not yet represented in every research group.

CTNs have an important role in evaluating the protocol for its feasibility of implementation within the work environment considering patient population, staff, workload created by the protocol, additional technical and human resources that may be necessary, and any special training required by the protocol. Italian CTNs often act as research coordinators by helping establish channels of communication within the research team and collaborating in the development of a *protocol pathway* or map, which demonstrates the coordination and continuity of trial participants' care within the institution (Bryce, Bell, Colussi, De Maio, & Gini, 2004).

Protocol Development, Review, and Approval

Legal and Regulatory Issues

The procedures for gaining approval and activating a protocol are detailed in the Italian decree enacting the 2001 European Directive and its successive integrations (Decreto Legislativo, 2003). For multicenter trials, the sponsor must submit the clinical trial application to the EC of the coordinating center and the participating centers. The EC of the coordinating center issues a *single* opinion, and if favorable, the EC of each participating center may accept or refuse the opinion. The sponsor must obtain an agreement with the competent authority of the healthcare facility where the trial will be conducted, and subsequently, administrative agreements are undertaken between the coordinating center and each participating center. The sponsor must obtain special permission from the National Health Institute for all phase I studies and for clinical trials involving the use of medicinal products for gene therapy, somatic cell (including xenogeneic cell) therapy, and all medicinal products containing genetically modified organisms.

Since the activation of the 2001 Directive, a series of detailed guidance documents have been published by the European Parliament regarding (a) the modalities to request authorization from competent authorities (2005), (b) the format of the application and the documentation to be submitted for EC opinion (2006), and (c) investigational medicinal products and other medicinal products (2007). These guidelines define all the operative procedures and of required documents for a clinical trial authorization and introduce the electronic clinical trial application process. These processes were adopted in Italy in December 2007 (Decreto Ministeriale, 2007), and OsSC has become, in a single portal, a tool to edit the applications for the request of authorization for a clinical trial and to edit the opinions of the EC.

Physicians may request the compassionate use of nonregistered therapeutic agents. The pharmaceutical company (or producer of the drug) is responsible for providing the necessary documentation regarding the use of the agent (clinical motivation, efficacy and tolerability data, patient information, and plan for monitoring data relative to compassionate use). The requesting physician presents the documentation to the EC and the National Medicines Agency. After EC approval, the drug is provided free of charge. The requesting physician is responsible for providing data relative to the use of the agent; these data are used for pharmacovigilance rather than registration purposes (Decreto Ministeriale, 2003).

The framework for conducting oncology clinical trials in Italy, with independent ECs, adherence to international GCP standards, and transparent research and financial agreements, is so designed to avoid conflicts of interest among the researchers, sponsors, and institutes where clinical research is undertaken.

AIOM published recommendations to avoid conflicts of interests with the pharmaceutical industry (AIOM, 2005a) and has undertaken a study to determine oncology patients' perceptions of conflict of interest (AIOM, 2005b). Italian investigators provide financial disclosure to sponsors of investigational new drug trials as required by the U.S. Food and Drug Administration.

Italian CTNs are guided by the deontological code for nurses, which are founded on the ethical and nonprejudicial treatment of all patients (Italian National Federation of Nursing, 1999). Italian CTNs have a twofold responsibility in this regard: (a) to act as patient advocate and raise awareness of any ethical issues including potential conflicts of interest and (b) to ensure informed consent.

Proposals for new trials come from a variety of sources within oncology institutes, cooperative groups, universities, and pharmaceutical companies. Proposals are then evaluated for scientific merit and feasibility. Some groups have established scientific committees. Once a proposal is accepted, a study chair, principal investigator (PI), or steering committee is designated and a multidisciplinary writing committee is formed. The writing committee can be composed of oncology physicians and trialists, CTNs, biostatisticians, data managers, and other specialists to provide input for specific trials. The protocol is written following the essential protocol elements as outlined in GCP.

Toxicity and response criteria are based on international standards; the most often used toxicity criteria are the Common Terminology Criteria for Adverse Events (National Cancer Institute Cancer Therapy Evaluation Program, 2010), and the most often used response criteria are RECIST 1.1 (Response Evaluation Criteria in Solid Tumors, version 1.1) (Eisenhauer et al., 2009). Performance status is most often measured using the World Health Organization, Eastern Cooperative Oncology Group, and Karnofsky scales. Protocols may be written in Italian or English, and because of the high number of international trials conducted in Italy, many protocols are written directly in English. A synopsis of the protocol and the patient informed consent must be prepared in Italian.

CTNs are involved in the development and content review of the informed consent and work with the study sponsor to facilitate translation using the standard forward-backward method. This method requires translation from original language to the new language, then in a second step and by a different translator the new document is translated back to the original language. The two original language documents are then compared for semantic equivalence.

Ancillary studies are formulated concurrently with the protocol using the same review process, although members may be added to the writing committee to provide expertise according to the study objectives. Protocol amendments are written with the same process as that of the protocol.

The plan for statistical analysis is written in the protocol according to GCP. Rules for interrupting the trial and for exclusion of single subjects are detailed in the protocol and reflected in the informed consent. The statistical methodology of ancillary studies is detailed in the companion protocol.

The informed consent process begins with the first contact of patients by study staff, and the investigators or CTNs explain the study to the patients and families or caregivers. CTNs ensure that patients have adequate time to ask questions and consider whether or not to participate, documenting this process in the clinical record. Patients receive a copy of the consent and a letter for the primary care physician so that these can be reviewed and discussed before the next visit with the study team. The CTN plays an important role in enhancing patients' understanding of participation in the clinical trial through follow-up discussions with patients and families. When a patient chooses to participate in a clinical trial, the investigator and patient sign the informed consent. The informed consent process continues throughout the patient's participation in the clinical trial and can be viewed as an ongoing relationship between the patient and the research team where patient assessment and education are ongoing responsibilities of the CTN.

Financial Factors

For-profit or nonprofit sponsors cover the costs of conducting clinical trials. According to the EU Directive 2001/20/EC, the sponsor should provide an insurance policy for each clinical trial, medicines used in the trial (whether investigational or already registered), and the monitoring activities to ensure GCP compliance. This raised discussion about increased costs throughout Europe, where oncology trials are frequently promoted by nonprofit sponsors (Crawley, 2004; Habeck, 2003; Meunier, Dubbois, Negrouk, & Rea, 2003; Meunier & Lacombe, 2003; Perrone et al., 2004).

Italy issued a decree regarding noncommercial clinical trials (Decreto Ministeriale, 2004) addressing the increased burdens placed on the nonprofit sponsors. The decree innovatively defines rules for nonprofit research, in part establishing that the National Health System will cover the cost of registered drugs used in noncommercial clinical trials, the EC fees will be waived, and an institution's general insurance policy could be used to cover patients treated in clinical trials within that institute. Subsequently, minimum requisites for insurance policies were published in 2009 (Decreto Ministeriale, 2009), and the sponsor of a clinical trial in Italy must provide the local EC with a certificate that evidences insurance coverage that complies with minimal coverage as outlined in the decree, is in Italian language, is signed by the insurer, and must explicitly reference the proposed interventionist trial. The sponsor must submit all proposed financial agreements related to the conduct of the clinical research to the EC as part of the clinical trial application.

Recruitment and Retention

Clinical trial promotion is the sponsor's responsibility in terms of content and costs. Individual investigators should obtain sponsor approval of locally published or broadcasted publicity spots. Most promotional activities of clinical trials are geared toward physicians who treat the patients in a target group. Many Italian cooperative oncology groups exist, and some are united by disease site (e.g., Multicenter Italian Trials in Ovarian Cancer [MITO]; Italian Melanoma Intergroup [IMI]), or special interest (e.g., Gruppo Italiano di Oncologia Geriatrica). These groups play an important role in protocol development and promotion and enrollment into clinical trials, and CTNs are having an increasingly active role in many of these groups (AIOM, 2014; IMI, 2014; MITO, 2014).

Many Italian patients with cancer are informed protagonists in health care who actively seek information about clinical trials on the Internet and from advocacy organizations and healthcare professionals. Self-referral is becoming more common. In a survey of healthy Italians, Apolone and Mosconi (2002) reported that the public had limited knowledge in general about clinical trials and was reluctant to participate in prevention trials. Focused on healthcare professionals and patients, promotional campaigns have been successful in recruiting high-risk patients in Italian prevention and screening trials. Rotmensz, Robertson, Maisonneuve, and Boyle (1998), in reviewing the Italian Tamoxifen Breast Cancer Prevention Trial, suggested a relationship between external events, including negative media coverage, on a decrease in recruitment and problematic early voluntary withdrawal of subjects. More recently, a study of patients with advanced lung or breast cancer showed that nearly 85% of the 102 patients surveyed were willing to participate in a clinical trial (Catania et al., 2008). A review of all cases of adolescents (ages 15–19) referred to clinical trials in an Italian pediatric oncology group showed progressive improvement in referral rates (Ferrari et al., 2009).

Italian CTNs recruit potential participants in clinical trials from the institute or referring groups by evaluating the target population, examining the inclusion and exclusion criteria, and being cognizant of the timelines and protocol-specific testing that may be required. CTNs ensure that patients have signed informed consent forms before undergoing protocol-specific tests that would not have otherwise been part of standard care. Screening tools and eligibility checklists are sometimes developed with the protocol to assist in evaluating potential participants and to track the enrollment process while ensuring that eligibility requirements are met.

In this phase, CTNs consider strategies for recruitment of patients into the trial and identify potential barriers to participation. After evaluation of the protocol and development of a nursing summary, CTNs educate the appropriate staff on patient care issues and provide information to colleagues who have contacts with the accrual base so that referrals can be made. CTNs work with the PI and sponsor to organize site start-up visits and may be involved in training of other sites.

Clinical Trial Participants

Once patients' eligibility is confirmed, CTNs or data managers submit the necessary documents for enrollment. CTNs may be involved in requesting protocol waivers in particular circumstances, communicating the request to the study sponsor. CTNs inform patients of the result of the request to enroll and be randomized in the study and schedule study visits per protocol.

Active Treatment

In this phase, CTNs are engaged in administering or overseeing the administration of the experimental therapy according to the protocol. CTNs work with the pharmacist and staff nurse to ensure adequate receipt, conservation, accountability, preparation, administration, and destruction of the study drug according to the study protocol.

The pharmacist receives and dispenses the experimental drugs. Drug reconstitution is performed in the pharmacy unit (where this service is available) or by a CTN or clinical nurse. Drug dosages are physician-prescribed and confirmed by the CTN and administering nurse. Depending on the local structure, the CTN or clinical nurse administers the study drug. The CTN and the pharmacist document drug accountability and order drugs from the sponsor. Depending on the protocol requirements, the pharmacist either returns expired or unused drug to the sponsor or destroys it according to local institutional procedures.

Another key CTN responsibility during the treatment phase is patient assessment for toxicity information and the grading and reporting of adverse events. CTNs reports serious adverse events to both the sponsor and the EC. CTNs provide patient education (e.g., patient information sheets) regarding expected effects of therapy, symptom management, completion of patient diary cards, and study-specific quality-of-life evaluations. CTNs are well-positioned for early identification of patient symptoms and toxicities and for prompt intervention. Poor symptom control can affect patient adherence with therapy and willingness to continue study therapy and can lead to dose modifications or changes in the treatment plan that may have been avoidable.

Italian CTNs have an important role in coordinating the care of the patients within this phase and are the key liaison between patients and investigators. CTNs are often patients' point of contact for all study-related issues and continue to provide education and support to patients and family caregivers. CTNs ensure evaluations are scheduled according to the protocol to assess patients' response to the experimental therapy and for any other study endpoints.

Off Treatment

Long-term patient follow-up may be required by the protocol for evaluating survival, time to recurrence, and late or long-term toxicities. In Italy, CTNs continue to have an important role to not only assess and report these

data but also to provide emotional and educational support to patients who are no longer on active treatment. Patients may stop experimental therapy in a clinical trial for various reasons, including
- Conclusion of planned therapy
- Voluntary withdrawal
- Withdrawal because of disease recurrence or progression or unacceptable toxicity
- Trial interruption by the sponsor for safety or efficacy reasons (early stopping).

Patients may have different reactions and psychosocial and medical needs depending on these events, and CTNs can assist patients as they transition to the next phase of care. Patient compliance with responding to inquiries or requests for follow-up is enhanced by this ongoing nurse-patient relationship.

Genetics and Genomics

Italian CTNs have an active role in the development and conduct of ancillary studies. Studies that involve obtaining patient specimens, such as bioavailability and genetics studies, require specific informed consent. The specimen may only be used for the purposes indicated in the informed consent. Whether results of specimen evaluation will be disclosed to patients must be specified in the consent form. CTNs refer patients for genetic counseling when indicated. CTNs' responsibilities include ensuring that patients are adequately informed and have given consent (Autorità Garante Della Privacy, 2008, 2011, 2013).

CTNs must ensure adequate planning for these special studies, assessing for proper documentation tools, supplies, and coordination of sampling, shipping, and costs. CTNs provide or oversee the necessary documentation required in the clinical record and study forms and ensure tracking of specimens from collection to storage and shipping, according to protocol specifications and within national and international safety standards. Specimens are generally shipped via courier, and Italy adheres to international standards for safety of biologic and infectious materials. Dates in Italy are expressed in the day-month-year format, and time is documented using the 24-hour clock. It is Italian practice and the sponsor's responsibility to request special permission from the Health Ministry for the importation and exportation of biologic materials.

Correlative Trials

Quality-of-life studies are conducted using validated Italian language instruments. The European Organisation for Research and Treatment of Cancer QLC-C30 and subinstruments are often used. CTNs may contribute to the validation of translated instruments (e.g., Catania et al., 2013) and have long been involved in the design and implementation of quality-of-life and companion studies (e.g., Italian Group for the Study of Survival After Infarct—Nursing, 1995, 1996). Nursing companion studies and independent nursing research are growing in Italy with increased attention to multicenter nursing intervention trials promoted by nursing networks and within oncology cooperative groups.

Documentation and Data Management

Case report forms (CRFs) are developed concurrently with the protocol, and most sponsors are now using remote data capture systems that may incorporate electronic CRFs, imaging upload for centralized radiology and pathology review, and electronic patient-reported outcome questionnaires. The CRFs are developed by the sponsor and may be integrated into an existing commercial electronic data capture platform or part of an in-house system of the sponsor.

CTNs evaluate the adequacy of source documents to capture required data and work within the institution's standards to facilitate complete documentation within patients' medical records. CTNs often collaborate in the development of paper or electronic charting systems that permit more complete and accurate documentation in both the inpatient and outpatient settings. Patient education materials are reviewed by the PI and approved by the EC. Additionally, specific testing such as pharmacokinetics is addressed with the development of appropriate documentation tools for such testing and includes shipping and handling information.

CTNs are often the communication link between the sponsor and the investigator. CTNs maintain source documentation, provide for CRF completion and transmission, monitor data, and coordinate monitor visits. CTNs provide updates regarding study progress to the EC and the clinical staff and help coordinate and implement amendments to the protocol.

CTNs document within the patient medical record and provide via CRF relevant follow-up data to the study sponsor. CTNs participate in data query resolution, study closure, and audits. Patient clinical records are maintained permanently and indefinitely within the healthcare institution in which the patient participates in the trial. Clinical trial documents are the responsibility of the PI and the sponsor, and essential documents must be maintained for a minimum of seven years after the completion of the trial (Decreto Legislativo, 2007).

In Italy, CTNs participate in communicating the study results to the patients who participated in the trial (e.g., Bryce et al., 2006; D'Aiuto et al., 2003), to the EC, and to the primary care physicians. CTNs also participate in coauthoring the scientific publication of study results and have the responsibility to help patients understand information about clinical trials and research results (World Medical Association, 2008).

Data Management and Clinical Trial Units

Data management strategies are described in the protocol and include the method, timing, and mode. Source data documentation and protocol data entry occur distinctly and separately. CTNs are responsible for ensuring complete and accurate source documentation. Data managers or CTNs, depending on the local structure, transcribe, verify, and transmit data.

The role of the data manager is being defined in Italy (Italian Data Manager Group, 2005). Local data managers may be involved in transcribing and reporting source data and resolving queries, as well as administrative, supportive, or coordinative functions relative to the clinical trial. Central data managers collaborate with protocol planning and are involved with CRF development, database design, and data entry, validation, and analysis. Central data managers create standard operating procedures for paper or web-based data collection, transmit data to OsSC, and provide training to the individual research sites.

Some institutes have clinical trial units dedicated to the support of clinical trials. These units are generally composed of physicians, biostatisticians, central data managers, CTNs, pharmacists, monitors, and informatics specialists, who are involved in all aspects of the clinical trial (see Figure 55-1).

Quality Assurance

Ensuring adherence to GCP and Italian law is both the PI's and study sponsor's responsibility. On a practical level, this is ensured by the collaboration of the study monitors (clinical research associate or central data manager) with the CTN and local data manager. The sponsor provides study monitoring to ensure GCP and protocol adherence, to verify data, and to assist with resolving any quality improvement issues. The 2005/28/EC directive further emphasizes the importance of quality data (accurate and verified) and the necessity of qualified personnel in the conduct of clinical trials. The investigator is responsible for assembling a qualified research team, and the sponsor provides any additional training specific to certain trials.

Sites may develop tools, such as screening tools, eligibility checklists, timelines, protocol maps, and adequate source documents, to assist in protocol adherence. The local data manager or CTN can use electronic tools, such as databases, to follow individual cases and provide an overview of all patients enrolled in the protocol, as well as evaluate study progress, trends, and deviations from protocol or other quality issues.

The research team writes local standard operating procedures that designate specific functions and activities related to research protocols within the institute, such as drug dose verification procedures. CTNs review deviations from protocol and safety issues and work with the PI and the clinical research assistant to identify and resolve any issue that affect quality.

Independent audits may be used to assess overall compliance and may be requested by the sponsor to evaluate a specific trial, or be performed as part of an overall assessment by the participating healthcare institution, oncology cooperative group, or clinical trials unit. CTNs are involved in preparing for and assisting with audits and in the engagement of an action plan to resolve any quality issues identified during the audit.

Inspections in Italy may be carried out by the National Medicines Agency, European Medicines Agency, or U.S. Food and Drug Administration before, during, or after the conduct of a clinical trial and may be part of the verification process during the application for registration. The European Directive 2005/28/EC provides guidelines for the qualification of inspectors and for inspection procedures.

Professional Development

CTNs must identify aspects of the protocol that directly affect nursing care. Italian CTNs develop a nursing summary of the research protocol to guide patient care and treatment during clinical trials (Di Giulio et al., 1996). This summary has been established as an effective collaborative tool within nursing (Gilger, Groben, & Hinds, 2002; Max et al., 2003; Price, Spencer, Mayor, & Boyler, 2003). The nursing summary is adapted from the trial protocol and describes the steps of the research process (see Figure 55-2).

Figure 55-1. Responsibilities of the Clinical Trial Unit Team*

- Protocol development and submission for approval
- Coordination of trial activity
- Data management
- Statistical analysis
- Training of sites
- Communication and publication of results
- Pharmacovigilance
- Quality assurance

*The clinical trial unit team is composed of physicians, biostatisticians, central data managers, clinical trials nurses, pharmacists, monitors, and informatics specialists.

The specialized role of the oncology nurse in clinical trials has evolved alongside the growth of clinical research in oncology. The complex and diverse responsibilities of CTNs have been well described for some time in European and North American literature (Ocker & Pawlik-Plank, 2000; Van Wijk, Batchelor, & Dubbelman, 2001). In Italy, the integration of CTNs into research teams has evolved in recent years, and the roles and responsibilities of practicing oncology CTNs have been generally categorized (see Figure 55-3). In a survey of practicing oncology CTNs, Catania and colleagues (2012) reported that the activities in which Italian CTNs were mostly involved were experimental drug management, protocol implementation, and informed consent, whereas these nurses were least active in protocol planning, subject recruitment, and data management.

The CTN title is being used within some Italian public hospitals, as the role has become more recognized and accessible to nurses from entry level through advanced practice. After acquiring the university nursing degree (bachelor), nurses may enter into postgraduate university master's programs (one to two years) in research nursing, clinical research coordination, and oncology and palliative care. Nurses who have completed the second-level specialist degree (*laurea magistrale*) can apply for admission to doctoral programs in nursing science and nursing research.

Postgraduate clinical trial nursing residential courses (four to five days) developed by the CTN Italy group and sponsored by the European School of Oncology (see www.cancerworld.org) have been available for practicing nurses new to the CTN role. A master class in clinical research and advanced oncology nursing organized by Istituto Oncologico Veneto contributed its core curriculum and suggested course format for promoting the advanced role of practicing CTNs within a national initiative of the Alleanza Contro Il Cancro and the Ministry of Health. A prototype job description for the CTN role was also proposed on a national level within this same initiative.

The national oncology nursing association in Italy (AIIAO) is a professional resource for Italian CTNs. AIIAO members are members of European Oncology Nursing Society and collaborate with the European School of Oncology, which gives Italian research nurses the opportunity to have a research fellowship abroad or to participate in the annual master class in oncology nursing.

Summary

CTNs have an increasingly more active and recognized role in Italy. CTNs are involved in all aspects of clinical research including protocol development, screening, informed consent, active treatment, study conclusion, and communication of results. CTNs are often the link between the patients, the clinical area, and the investigator and have responsibilities to patients enrolled in a clinical trial and to the research team. The primary patient responsibilities are to ensure safety and be an advocate and caregiver, which are realized through the multiple activities of CTNs throughout the continuum of clinical research. With respect to the research team, CTNs' activities along the continuum are aimed toward maintaining integrity of the protocol and quality of research data. The complex and specialized role of oncology CTNs continues to evolve alongside advances in basic and health sciences, and CTNs are key partners of the healthcare research team and with patients enrolled in clinical trials.

Key Points
- The CTN role is becoming more widespread in Italian cancer institutes as the advanced practice roles for oncology nurses continue to evolve in Italy.
- Resources for CTNs are available within national and European oncology nursing associations, nursing and oncology research networks, and university and post-professional education.
- The Italian Medicines Agency, with its National Monitoring Centre for Clinical Trials, is the access point for clinical trial information, application, and oversight.

Figure 55-2. Protocol Nursing Summary

- Background information
- Toxicity observed in preclinical research
- Goals of the trial
- Selection criteria
- Drug information (including distribution, reconstitution, stability, storage, metabolism and excretion, measures for spillage and extravasation, hypersensitivity reactions)
- Treatment administration and scheduling
- Logistics
- Toxicity checklists or tools
- Patient self-report tools
- Study testing and follow-up schema
- Nursing care plan with strategies for patient education and symptom management

Note. Based on information from Di Giulio et al., 1996.

Figure 55-3. Components of Clinical Trials Nursing Role in Italy

- Protocol development
- Patient education and advocacy
- Patient care and coordination of care
- Consultation and staff education
- Management of patient records and data
- Authorship and dissemination of study results
- Evaluation of clinical trial performance

References

Agenzia Italiana del Farmaco. (2012). *11th national report of clinical trials of drugs in Italy*. Retrieved from http://agenziafarmaco.gov.it

Alleanza Contro Il Cancro. (2013). *Il progetto ACC*. Retrieved from http://www.alleanzacontroilcancro.it

Apolone, G., & Mosconi, P. (2002). Knowledge and opinions about clinical research: A cross-sectional survey in a sample of Italian citizens. *Journal of Ambulatory Care Management, 26*, 83–87. doi:10.1097/00004479-200301000-00008

Associazione Italiana di Oncologia Medica. (2005a, October). *AIOM recommendations on the relationship between medical oncologists and the pharmaceutical industry*. Retrieved from http://www.aiom.it

Associazione Italiana di Oncologia Medica. (2005b, October). *Prospective observational study of oncology patients' perceptions of conflict of interest between physicians and the pharmaceutical industry*. Retrieved from http://www.aiom.it

Associazione Italiana di Oncologia Medica. (2014). Working group AIOM-Nursing. Retrieved from http://www.aiom.it

Associazione Italiana di Oncologia & Medica Associazione Italiana Registri Tumori. (2013). *I numeri del cancro in Italia 2013*. Milan, Italy: Authors.

Autorità Garante della Privacy. (2008). *Linee guida per i trattamenti di dati personali nell'ambito delle sperimentazioni cliniche di medicinali del 24 luglio 2008*, published in the *Official Gazette of the Italian Republic*, n. 190 on 14 agosto 2008.

Autorità Garante della Privacy. (2011). *Autorizzazione generale al trattamento dei dati genetici del 24 giugno 2011*, published in the *Official Gazette of the Italian Republic*, n. 159 dell'11 luglio 2011.

Autorità Garante della Privacy. (2013). *Autorizzazione al trattamento dei dati genetici del 13 dicembre 2012*, published in the *Official Gazette of the Italian Republic*, n. 3 del 4-1-2013.

Bryce, J., Bell, C., Colussi, A.M., De Maio, G., & Gini, S. (2004). Clinical trial nursing: Strategies for developing role competencies and role recognition in Italy. *Oncology Nursing Forum, 31*, 381.

Bryce, J., Connola, M., Salzano de Luna, A., Caracò, C., Chiofalo, M.G., & Mozzillo, N. (2006). Participating patients' reactions to early closure of a clinical trial for negative results. *Oncology Nursing Forum, 33*, 3.

Catania, C., De Pas, T., Goldhirsch, A., Radice, D., Adamoli, L., Medici, M., ... Nolè, F. (2008). Participation in clinical trials as viewed by the patients: Understanding cultural and emotional aspects which influence choice. *Oncology, 74*, 177–187. doi:10.1159/000151365

Catania, G., Bell, C., Ottonelli, S., Marchetti, M., Bryce, J., Grossi, A., & Costantini, M. (2013). Cancer-related fatigue in Italian cancer patients: Validation of the Italian Brief Fatigue Inventory. *Supportive Care in Cancer, 21*, 413–419. doi:10.1007/s00520-012-1539-z

Catania, G., Poirè, I., Bernardi, M., Bono, L., Cardinale, F., & Dozin, B. (2012). The role of the clinical trial nurse in Italy. *European Journal of Oncology Nursing, 16*, 87–93. doi:10.1016/j.ejon.2011.04.001

Commission Directive 2001/20/EC of the European Parliament and of the Council of 4 April 2001 on the approximation of the laws, regulations and administrative provisions of the Member States relating to the implementation of good clinical practice in the conduct of clinical trials on medicinal products for human use. *Official Journal of the European Union*, , L121, 34–44. Retrieved from http://eur-lex.europa.eu/LexUriServ/LexUriServ.do?uri=OJ:L:2001:121:0034:0044:en:PDF

Commission Directive 2005/28/EC of 9 April 2005 laying down principles and detailed guidelines for good clinical practice as regards investigational medicinal products for human use, as well as the requirements for authorization of the manufacturing or importation of such products. *Official Journal of the European Union*, L91, 13–19. Retrieved from http://eur-lex.europa.eu/LexUriServ/LexUriServ.do?uri=OJ:L:2005:091:0013:0019:en:PDF

Crawley, F.P. (2004). New European clinical trials directive: Is European research possible? *BMJ, 328*, 522. doi:10.1136/bmj.328.7438.522

D'Aiuto, G., Oliviero, P., & Bryce, J. (2003, May). *Results of the Italian tamoxifen breast cancer prevention study*. Meeting of the clinical trial participants Progetto Donna: Risultati and prospettive, Naples.

Decreto Legislativo (Italian Legislative Decree). (2003). Transposition of Directive 2001/20/EC relating to the implementation of good clinical practice in the conduct of clinical trials of medicinal products for clinical use. Legislative decree n. 211 of 24/06/2003 published in the *Official Gazette of the Italian Republic*, n. 184, 9/8/2003, ordinary supplement n. 130.

Decreto Legislativo (Italian Legislative Decree). (2007). Attuazione della direttiva 2005/28/CE recante principi e linee guida dettagliate per la buona pratica clinica relativa ai medicinali in fase di sperimentazione a uso umano, nonche requisiti per l'autorizzazione alla fabbricazione o importazione di tali medicinali. Legislative decree n. 200 of 6/11/2007 published in the *Official Gazette of the Italian Republic*, n. 261, 9/11/2007.

Decreto Ministeriale (Italian Ministerial Decree). (1997). Receipt of the European Union guidelines for good clinical practice in the conduct of clinical trials of medicinal products. Decreto Ministeriale 15/7/97.

Decreto Ministeriale (Italian Ministerial Decree). (1998). Guidelines for the institution and functions of independent ethics committees. Decreto Ministeriale 18/3/98 published in the *Official Gazette of the Italian Republic*, n. 122, May 28, 1998.

Decreto Ministeriale (Italian Ministerial Decree). (2003). Therapeutic use of experimental drugs. Decreto Ministeriale 8/05/2003 published in the *Official Gazette of the Italian Republic*, n. 173, July 28, 2003.

Decreto Ministeriale (Italian Ministerial Decree). (2004). Prescriptions and general conditions, relative to the conduct of medicinal clinical trials, with particular reference to those that improve clinical practice as an integral part of health and medical care. Decreto Ministeriale 17/12/2004 published in the *Official Gazette of the Italian Republic*, n. 43, Feb. 22, 2005.

Decreto Ministeriale (Italian Ministerial Decree). (2007). Modalità di inoltro della richiesta di autorizzazione all'Autorità competente, per la comunicazione di emendamenti sostanziali e la dichiarazione di conclusione della sperimentazione clinica e per la richiesta di parere al comitato etico. 2007. Supplemento ordinario alla *Gazzetta Ufficiale* n. 53 del 3/3/2008.

Decreto Ministeriale (Italian Ministerial Decree). (2009). Requisiti minimi per le polizze assicurative a tutela dei soggetti partecipanti alle sperimentazioni cliniche dei medicinali. Decreto Ministeriale 14/07/2009 published in the *Official Gazette of the Italian Republic*, n. 213, Sept. 14, 2009.

Di Giulio, P., Arrigo, C., Gall, H., Molin, C., Nieweg, R., & Strohbucker, B. (1996). Expanding the role of the nurse in clinical trials: The nursing summaries. *Cancer Nursing, 19*, 343–347. Retrieved from http://journals.lww.com/cancernursingonline/Abstract/1996/10000/Expanding_the_role_of_the_nurse_in_clinical.2.aspx

Eisenhauer, E.A., Therasse, P., Bogaerts, J., Schwartz, L.H., Sargent, D., Ford, R., ... Verweij, J. (2009). New response evaluation criteria in solid tumours: Revised RECIST guideline (version 1.1). *European Journal of Cancer, 45*, 228–247. doi:10.1016/j.ejca.2008.10.026

European Parliament. (2005). *Detailed guidance for the request for authorisation of a clinical trial on a medicinal product for human use to the competent authorities, notification of substantial amendments and declaration of the end of the trial*. Retrieved from http://ec.europa.eu/enterprise/sectors/pharmaceuticals/files/eudralex/vol-10/11_ca_14-2005_en.pdf.

European Parliament. (2006). *Detailed guidance on the application format and documentation to be submitted in an application for an Ethics Committee opinion on the clinical trial on medicinal products for human use*. Retrieved from http://ec.europa.eu/enterprise/sectors/pharmaceuticals/files/eudralex/vol-10/12_ec_guideline_20060216_en.pdf

European Parliament. (2007). *Guidance on Investigational Medicinal Products (IMPs) and other medicinal products used in Clinical Trials*. Retrieved from http://ec.europa.eu/enterprise/sectors/pharmaceuticals/files/eudralex/vol-10/guidance-on-imp_nimp_04-2007_en.pdf

Ferrari, A., Dama, E., Pession, A., Rondelli, R., Pascucci, C., Locatelli, F., ... Pastore, G. (2009). Adolescents with cancer in Italy: Entry into the National Cooperative Paediatric Oncology Group AIEOP trials. *European Journal of Cancer, 45,* 328–334. doi:10.1016/j.ejca.2008.12.003

Gilger, E.A., Groben, V.J., & Hinds, P.S. (2002). Osteosarcoma nursing care guidelines: A tool to enhance the nursing care of children and adolescents enrolled on a medical research protocol. *Journal of Pediatric Oncology Nursing, 19,* 172–181. doi:10.1016/S1043-4542(02)00010-3

Habeck, M. (2003). Gloomy prospects for European cancer research. *Lancet Oncology, 4,* 66. doi:10.1016/S1470-2045(03)00991-4

Italian Group for the Study of Survival After Infarct—Nursing. (1995). Evaluation of the perception of the quality of health of the patient with myocardial infarct. Final report of the study. *Rivista dell'Infermiere, 14,* 16–29.

Italian Group for the Study of Survival After Infarct—Nursing. (1996). Use of drugs in patients with critical leg ischemia. *Rivista dell'Infermiere, 15,* 14–21.

Italian Data Manager Group (Gruppo Italiano Data Manager). (2005). Coodinatore di ricerca clinica/data manager: Chi é? Retrieved from http://www.gidm.org

Italian Melanoma Intergroup. (2014). Data manager and research nurse. Retrieved from http://melanomaimi.it

Italian National Federation of Nursing. (1999, May). *Il codice deontologico degli infermieri.* Retrieved from http://www.ipasvi.it

Max, A., Gattuso, J., Hinds, P., Norman, G., Price, R., Whitmore-Sisco, L., & Turnage, J. (2003). Developing nursing care guidelines for children with Hodgkin's disease. *European Journal of Oncology Nursing, 7,* 253–258. doi:10.1016/S1462-3889(03)00036-X

Meunier, F., Dubbois, N., Negrouk, A., & Rea, L.-A. (2003). Throwing a wrench in the works? *Lancet Oncology, 4,* 717–719. doi:10.1016/S1470-2045(03)01299-3

Meunier, F., & Lacombe, D. (2003). The European Organisation for the Research and Treatment of Cancer's point of view [Letter to the editor]. *Lancet, 362,* 663. doi:10.1016/S0140-6736(03)14163-3

Ministero della Salute. (2014). *Il servizio sanitaria nazionale.* Retrieved from http://www.salute.gov.it

Multicenter Italian Trials in Ovarian and Gynaecologic Cancers. (2014). Data management and research nurses. Retrieved from http://www.mito-group.it

National Cancer Institute Cancer Therapy Evaluation Program. (2010). *Common terminology criteria for adverse events* [v.4.03]. Retrieved from http://evs.nci.nih.gov/ftp1/CTCAE/CTCAE_4.03_2010-06-14_QuickReference_5x7.pdf

Ocker, B., & Pawlik-Plank, D. (2000). The research nurse role in a clinic-based oncology research center. *Cancer Nursing, 23,* 286–292. doi:10.1097/00002820-200008000-00005

Perrone, F., Marangolo, M., Di Costanzo, F., Colucci, G., Repetto, L., Merlano M., ... Gallo, C. (2004). Insurance for independent cancer trials. *Annals of Oncology, 15,* 1722–1723. doi:10.1093/annonc/mdh444

Price, L., Spencer, H., Mayor, P., & Boyle, P. (2003). Using clinical research summaries to aid research nurses. *Professional Nurse, 19,* 223–226.

Rotmensz, N., Robertson, C., Maisonneuve, P., & Boyle, P. (1998, May). *The effect of external events on a large double blind chemoprevention trial.* Paper presented at the 19th Annual Meeting of the Society for Clinical Trials, Atlanta, GA.

Statistical Office of the European Communities. (2008). Ageing characterizes the demographic perspectives of European societies. Retrieved from http://epp.eurostat.cec.eu.int

Van Wijk, A., Batchelor, D., & Dubbelman, A. (Eds.). (2001). *Manual for research nurses.* Amsterdam, Netherlands: Early Clinical Studies Group Research Nurses.

World Medical Association. (2008). *Declaration of Helsinki—Ethical principles for medical research involving human subjects.* Retrieved from http://www.wma.net

Chapter 56

Japan

Eriko Aotani, RN, MSN, CCRP, and Yuko Saito, MS, RN, CCRP

Introduction

In Japan, basic science research has been actively conducted with satisfactory outcomes. However, it is said that outcomes of clinical research need further improvement in Japan. The developing infrastructure for investigator-initiated clinical research, including active involvement by nurses, is improving in terms of operational efficiency, cost management, and quality assurance.

History and Foundation

Many cancer clinical trial groups have been established since the late 1970s in Japan. Some of them are nationwide, and others are provincial. The Japan Clinical Oncology Group (JCOG) was established as a multimodality cooperative group sponsored by the Ministry of Health, Labour and Welfare (MHLW) and has been conducting multi-institutional clinical trials since 1978. JCOG is the first and only cooperative group that has been fully supported by the Japanese government's research funds. It has greatly contributed to establishing standard therapies against cancer and has served as a model for other study groups in Japan, especially for the clinical trial infrastructure and operations (Fukuda, 2010).

Throughout the 1980s and 1990s, other nationwide cooperative groups, such as the Japanese Gynecologic Oncology Group, the West Japan Oncology Group, the Japan Adult Leukemia Study Group, and the Comprehensive Support Program for Oncology Research (CSPOR), were established. In pediatric hematologic oncology, multiple trial groups were unified into the Japanese Pediatric Leukemia/Lymphoma Study Group in 2003. Figure 56-1 lists the national oncology cooperative groups in Japan. They established their own statistical data centers that have quality assurance mechanisms and have conducted many phase II and III clinical trials, as well as observational studies. These groups are nonprofit organizations or foundations supported mostly by charitable donations from pharmaceutical companies and individuals and partially by government research funds. They have conducted important clinical trials and made great contributions to the improvement of cancer care.

Figure 56-1. Japan's National Cooperative Groups

- Comprehensive Support Program for Oncology Research
- Japan Adult Leukemia Study Group
- Japan Clinical Oncology Group
- Japanese Gynecologic Oncology Group
- Japanese Pediatric Leukemia/Lymphoma Study Group
- West Japan Oncology Group

Implementation of the International Conference on Harmonisation of Technical Requirements for Registration of Pharmaceuticals for Human Use (ICH) good clinical practice (GCP) guidelines in 1997 promoted rapid growth of quality control mechanisms for industry-sponsored indication-directed trials. In 2003, the first investigator-initiated indication-directed clinical trial, which also required full GCP compliance, was conducted as the relevant regulations were implemented in Japan. However, full compliance with GCP in non–indication-directed trials is not regulated in Japan. Therefore, the study groups and participating sites have been self-regulated while trying to achieve GCP compliance.

Japanese study groups started to participate in international collaborative oncology trials around 2005. Japanese groups were only "participants" at the beginning, but the number of patients enrolled has been increasing. They have become lead groups in the conduct of international trials in some areas, such as gastrointestinal and gynecologic oncology.

Drug Development Process

The Pharmaceuticals and Medical Devices Agency (PMDA) is the Japanese counterpart to the U.S. Food and Drug Administration and is responsible for operational aspects of drug development. PMDA reviews drug application submissions and safety reports, identifies possible regulatory issues while providing possible solutions, and conducts inspections. MHLW ultimately makes the final decision for drug approval. Drug developers, either pharmaceutical companies or investigators, who initiate indication trials need to interact with both PMDA and MHLW.

Examples of the standard pathways of new cancer drug approval are as follows.
- A stand-alone phase III comparative trial showing evidence of drug efficacy and safety in Japanese patients
- A small phase I/II "bridging study" showing that the drug efficacy and safety profile in Japanese patients looks similar to that in non-Japanese patients in another large phase III trial previously conducted
- A large international phase III trial in which the drug efficacy and safety profile in Japanese patients was similar to that in non-Japanese patients
- A small single-arm phase II trial with Japanese patients showing a strong scientific rationale in an orphan indication with no standard treatment

In any pathway of clinical trials for a new indication or modification of the approved treatment route or dose, a phase I trial for pharmacokinetic and pharmacodynamic data of Japanese patients is almost mandatory. Special attention is necessary for the definition of investigational agents in cancer drug combination regimens. Although the combination drug is approved and available in Japan for a different cancer indication or it is widely used for the same cancer in regular practice, PMDA does not want to promote unapproved usage, so it becomes an investigational agent.

Clinical development has been performed outside of Japan because of an inefficient infrastructure of clinical trials associated with high trial costs nationally, even though the scientific "seeds" were found in Japan. Currently, MHLW is actively promoting early-phase clinical trials, along with translational research, at designated institutions collaborating with the pharmaceutical industry, especially for Japan-origin "seeds" for development of new drugs.

Expanded Access to Investigational Drugs

Expanded use of investigational drugs outside of studies is prohibited in principle, with the exception of those drugs that are confirmed to be effective during the study period, and then only if the pharmaceutical company agrees to provide the investigational drugs beyond the study period, complying with a strong demand from the patients in the trial. Expanded use of investigational drugs requires an approval from PMDA in advance (MHLW, 1998a). After discussion with the patient about compassionate use, a separate written informed consent is required. In the case of industry-initiated registration-directed clinical trials, pharmaceutical companies might consider this option. However, it is highly unlikely for pharmaceutical companies to provide for the compassionate use of drugs for investigator-initiated non–registration-directed trials.

MHLW recognizes the public need for expanded access to investigational cancer drugs, especially for patients who did not meet the eligibility criteria of the registration trials. Regulatory preparations have been undertaken since 2011 and include establishment of site selection criteria and preparation of guidelines for patient safety during the expanded access. In 2013, the first expanded access to an investigational cancer drug was approved as an investigator-initiated registration-directed trial, where the national health insurance was used for cancer treatment with the investigational agent. Japanese regulation for expanded access to investigational drugs is planned to be executed in 2015. Currently, no regulation exists to allow for the use of unapproved drugs outside of registration-directed trials in Japan. Patients must pay all costs for the cancer-related treatment, including sometimes importing the drugs from abroad.

Sponsoring Agencies

In Japan, registration-directed cancer trials are mostly sponsored by pharmaceutical companies. The very few exceptions are investigator-initiated registration-directed cancer trials, most of which are sponsored by MHLW and conducted by the investigators themselves to obtain approvals for different disease indications. PMDA evaluates these protocols before executing the trial.

Resources for investigator-initiated cancer trials sponsored by the government are extremely limited, so most study groups rely on donations from pharmaceutical companies or personal donations. Recently, contract-based studies between study groups and companies have been recommended, and the number of such studies is slowly increasing.

Clinical Trials: Fundamental Information

The Clinical Research Team

An interdisciplinary approach enhances all aspects of clinical trials, from protocol development to patient care. Expert opinions in distinct disciplines, such as medical oncology, radiation oncology, pathology, and nursing, are sought when preparing protocols. The degree of interdisciplinary approach varies widely among study groups.

A principal investigator (PI) is the leader of the research team and is responsible for the scientific integrity of the study and protection of research participants. Co-principal investigators can act as decision makers along with the PI for the study. Administration officers, statisticians, project managers, study coordinators, and data managers are other key members of the clinical trial team.

Site investigators implement the study and provide feedback to improve it. Clinical research coordinators (CRCs) and clinical trial nurses (CTNs) have vital roles in implementation, which are outlined in Figure 56-2. In Japan, some CRCs are not nurses but rather pharmacists or laboratory technicians. No differences currently exist in the job descriptions of CRCs and CTNs. CTNs have fundamental knowledge of the treatments and emotional support needs of patients and their families. Hence, they are central to a research team, and input from the nursing perspective is highly valued. The roles of CRCs, CTNs, local data managers, and staff nurses overlap, depending on the organizational structure. Nutritionists, social workers, ethicists, and religious representatives are not routinely part of the research team (Niimi, Aotani, Kohara, & Saito, 2010).

Legal, Regulatory, and Legislative Issues

Since the introduction of ICH GCP into Japanese GCP in 1997, greater attention has been paid to the quality of clinical trials. Clinical trials in Japan traditionally had been divided into two categories: (a) industry-sponsored registration-directed trials that must follow GCP and (b) investigator-initiated non–registration-directed trials, which are not strictly regulated. Investigator-initiated trials were not considered acceptable for drug registration purposes until 2002, when a new category became available. At that time, the Japanese government revised the regulations so that investigators could conduct registration-directed trials that may be ignored by pharmaceutical companies. The third category of clinical trials in Japan is investigator-initiated registration-directed clinical trials, for which GCP compliance is required. This reform was expected to improve the overall quality of investigator-initiated clinical trials (Ando & Fujiwara, 2005).

The Evaluation System of Investigational Medical Care was a new clinical trial system established in 2009 to evaluate treatment with unapproved or off-label drugs or medical technologies. Such clinical trials have been recategorized as clinical trials under the Advanced Medical Service System B (AMSS-B) since 2012. MHLW authorizes the use of national health insurance for patients participating in the investigator-initiated AMSS-B trials with a high-quality management mechanism. This system brought an opportunity for investigators to conduct clinical trials with unapproved or off-label drugs when obtaining the indication label is the primary purpose of the trial. This system also required the clinical trial team to execute effective operations of clinical trials. Critical issues in the management of AMSS-B trials include the limited resources for the trial operations, serious adverse event (SAE) reporting requirements that are different from the requirements for other types of trials, management of the investigational agents, and the cost-effectiveness of trial monitoring (Aotani et al., 2012).

Good Clinical Practice

The revised GCP was legislated in 1997 as a *ministerial ordinance* in response to a revision of the Pharmaceutical Affairs Law. Before this, GCP was a *notice of a bureau chief* with no legal power. It was revised based on the ICH GCP agreement and on a report from the Task Force Committee on Establishment of Pharmaceutical Safety. This task force was established after the "sorivudine incident"—a tragedy that involved the intentional underreporting of drug-related deaths with concomitant administration of fluorouracil during a herpes registration-directed trial, which led to 15 deaths soon after marketing of the drug (Nakamura, Ohmori, Kitada, & Mochida, 1994).

The 1997 GCP (Step 5, the final step of the process for the harmonization guideline for the European Union, the United States, and Japan to move to the regulatory implementation within the country) conforms to ICH GCP, and the contents are equivalent. Regulations regarding written informed consent, institutional review board (IRB) requirements, and responsibilities of the sponsor (including protocol development, monitoring, and audits) and of the investigator (including obtaining informed consent and submitting data) are all mentioned in the 1997 GCP.

The revised GCP was issued in 2003, and investigator-initiated registration-directed trials became possible. GCP currently applies only to registration-directed clinical trials in Japan, although non–registration-directed trials strive to follow the fundamental principles of ICH GCP.

Standard Operating Procedures

Figure 56-3 lists clinical trial activities for which, according to GCP, a company and an investigator who plan a registration-directed trial must prepare standard operating procedures (SOPs). SOPs for the participating

---

Figure 56-2. Clinical Trial Nurse and Clinical Research Coordinator Roles in Clinical Trial Implementation

- Patient recruitment
- Scheduling patient visits and required tests
- Developing useful tools for trial management
- Collection of relevant clinical data
- Preparation of case report forms
- Education of patients and the research team

Figure 56-3. Clinical Trial Activities That Require Standard Operating Procedures

- Protocol development
- Selection of participating institutions and investigators
- Development of investigator's brochures
- Drug accountability
- Collection of adverse drug reaction information
- Monitoring and audits
- Preparation of clinical trial reports
- Recording of source documents
- Other activities that are related to the trial

institutions also have to be developed and maintained. The responsibility for developing such SOPs belongs to the head official of the institution. CRCs at the clinical trials office within the institution usually assume the task of preparing and maintaining SOPs.

Ethics and Clinical Trials

Protection of research participants is required in all clinical research, although GCP applies only to registration-directed clinical trials in Japan. The ethical guidelines for clinical research, issued by MHLW in 2003 and revised in 2008, apply to all clinical research, including non–registration-directed clinical trials. The guidelines clearly state ethical principles such as responsibilities of investigators and institutions, requirements for IRB approval and written informed consent, and protection of privacy (MHLW, 2008, 2012). These guidelines for clinical research were revised again by MHLW, along with the Ministry of Education, Culture, Sports, Science and Technology (MEXT), in 2014. The major revision to reinforce quality control and quality assurance of clinical research for human subjects included important ethical contents such as the governance responsibilities of the head official at the clinical research site, clinical trial registration for the public, ensured function and transparency of IRBs, informed assent process for children, more detailed requirements regarding protection of personal information of patients and others, management of investigators' conflicts of interest, the maintenance requirement of clinical research records, and mandatory monitoring for all clinical research with the audit when necessary.

Protocol Development, Review, and Approval

Elements of a Protocol

The basic elements of protocols are listed in Figure 56-4. Other important information (e.g., pathology review process, surgical guidelines) is provided as appendices to the protocol or within manuals.

Informed Consent Process

The requirements and basic elements of the informed consent process are the same as in the United States. CRCs, especially CTNs, perform vital roles in this process. They provide information about the trials and other options using plain language for patients and their family members. In addition, they ensure that participation is based on patients' autonomous decisions. Preparation of the consent document for IRB review usually is the task of CRCs (Niimi et al., 2010).

Illiteracy rates in Japan are very low. According to a study of 85 patients (Sato, Watanabe, Katsumata, & Ohashi, 2005), a detailed consent form did not improve patients' understanding of their consent but significantly improved their satisfaction. In Japan, the signature of a witness is not mandatory unless the patient's comprehension ability is questionable. Genetic testing or future use of patients' specimens usually requires an additional, separate informed consent.

Protocol Development and Response Assessment

Since 1997, protocols for cancer clinical trials in Japan have been written based on ICH GCP guidelines. Protocols must be justified both scientifically and ethically. Procedures for protocol development vary among study groups. Often a protocol committee assigns a study chair and cochairs to an approved study concept; usually one or more investigators propose study concepts. A study chair typically collaborates with cochairs, statisticians, and data managers to write a protocol. Opinions from representative CRCs or research nurses of the member

Figure 56-4. Elements of a Protocol

- Background and rationale
- Objectives
- Population (inclusion criteria and exclusion criteria)
- Study treatment/modalities
- Entry/randomization procedure
- Expected adverse events and treatment
- Treatment modifications
- Stopping rules
- Study parameters, serial observations, and evaluation criteria
- Study duration (both a patient entry period and a follow-up period)
- Study monitoring and reporting procedures
- Statistical considerations
- Publication of results
- Organizational information of the study group
- Bibliography

institutions may be solicited before the protocol is finalized.

Common endpoints of cancer clinical trials are objective tumor response rate, progression-free survival, time to progression, disease-free survival, overall survival, and adverse events, sometimes accompanied with a translational research endpoint and/or quality of life (QOL) and, recently, cost-effectiveness. Nursing research questions are rarely incorporated into cooperative group trials. The independent committee evaluates these endpoints centrally.

As the standardized method for evaluation of tumor response by radiologic imaging, the Response Evaluation Criteria in Solid Tumors (referred to as *RECIST*) is most commonly used in Japan. As the standardized method for evaluation of adverse events, the National Cancer Institute Cancer Therapy Evaluation Program's Common Terminology Criteria for Adverse Events (CTCAE) is used. Both guidelines have been translated into Japanese by JCOG (www.jcog.jp) and are widely available.

Protocol Review and Approval Process

For an external review, a scientific review committee or other disease committee of the study group reviews protocols. Next, the protocol is presented to a protocol committee or ethics committee that includes individuals who have no association with the group. No approval mechanism currently exists for review of cooperative group studies by the government. The IRB holds a vital role to ensure protection of patient rights. Interdisciplinary team review of the protocol is essential to improve the quality of clinical trials. Some Japanese institutions have two different types of review committees. One discusses the scientific part of the protocol, and the other reviews ethical issues. Committee responsibilities include a systematic review of clinical trials before, during, and after each trial.

Interdisciplinary review committees usually consist of professional members, as well as lay members who can represent the perspectives of the community. It is ideal to include professional members who represent ethics, risk management, finance, hospital administration, multiple medical departments, and co-medical departments, such as nursing, laboratory, and radiology. The extent of the interdisciplinary approach to review a clinical trial varies significantly at each institution.

Finally, each protocol must have local IRB approval prior to activation (MHLW, 2008, 2012). It is a fundamental rule to obtain IRB approval before conducting a clinical trial, and the local IRB is responsible for initially reviewing the protocols and consent forms. Registration-directed clinical trials are more strictly regulated than others, as per institutional SOPs regarding IRB reporting procedures, including protocol revisions, amendments, termination, and SAE reporting. IRB approval letters are subject to audit.

Although IRBs must follow the ethical guidelines for clinical research, continuous education for board members and quality assurance mechanisms for IRBs still are in development in Japan. Many IRBs have not yet established efficient ways of evaluating annual reports from many investigator-initiated non–registration-directed trials. Several central IRBs both in academic and commercial settings have been established and have been used. Education and some sort of certification system for IRBs are necessary, and CTNs in Japan could contribute to such education.

Financial Factors

Workload Determination and Resource Allocation

Several variables must be considered when determining workloads. Institutions determine workload from variables such as the phase of the trial, whether it is inpatient or outpatient, the seriousness of the target disease, and the frequency of the required tests and specialized tests. CRCs are routinely assigned to all registration-directed clinical trials but not to investigator-initiated non–registration-directed trials. Therefore, conducting clinical trials adds to the investigator's workload. To promote active involvement of CTNs, greater resource allocation for CTNs is needed for the care of patients in clinical trials in Japan.

Budgets and Funding

In cooperative group trials, financial factors may pose obstacles to study implementation. Budgets for cooperative groups are very limited, regardless of their funding sources. Equitable reimbursement is not given to participating institutions for costs and time/effort. Many cooperative group trials have such minimal reimbursement that investigators cannot obtain any staff support.

In industry-sponsored registration trials, the financial burdens of participating institutions are greatly reduced. Institutions can calculate the cost for each study and negotiate with the sponsors. Consideration is given for the *direct* expenses of a trial, which depend on the phase of the trial, whether it is inpatient or outpatient, the seriousness of the target disease, and the frequency of the required tests. *Overhead* expenses also are included, such as those for personnel, utilities, and administration.

For cooperative group trials using government-approved agents for indication or treatment, the additional costs of tests, medications, and potentially prolonged hospitalizations associated with the trials can be covered by national health insurance. In that case, patients usually need to pay about 30% of the total medical costs.

For industry-sponsored registration trials, the sponsors normally have to carry all expenses for the study drugs, laboratory tests, or diagnostic imaging directly associated with the trial during the period when the study drug is administered. Other expenses, such as medications to treat adverse events, except for predetermined conditions with the sponsor, may be covered by national health insurance. National health insurance coverage for these certain conditions in combination with uninsured medical expenses in clinical trials is not governmentally approved, whereas for an investigator-initiated indication-directed trial, the coverage requirement for the investigator sponsor is clearly approved by the government. National health insurance will cover only the expenses of laboratory tests, diagnostic imaging, and medications other than the same sort (i.e., the same indication) as the study drugs.

Contracting

A contract needs to be in place between the sponsor and the participating sites before conducting the trial. Financial managers of the sites review the protocol with CRCs, estimate the budgets, and negotiate with the sponsor for the contract. Institutional overhead may be added for industry sponsors, but usually not for investigator sponsors.

Financial Risk Assessment and Monitoring

Financial risk assessment and monitoring is rarely done during trials in Japan. Only when unexpected additional costs are apparent, such as additional laboratory tests, is additional payment negotiated with the trial sponsor. After trial completion, the budget and the actual costs are compared for analysis. For the analysis, a workload summary for all trial staff must be recorded, and the hidden costs that were not previously estimated in the trial budget need to be listed. More detailed information regarding trial costs needs to be accumulated at each site for proper budget management.

Internal Financial Audit and Quality Assurance

Internal financial audits for each trial are rarely conducted in Japan. Only external financial audits, especially for government-funded clinical trials, have been conducted. Quality assurance of finance in clinical trials is an important goal for improvement.

Financial Conflict of Interest

Conflict-of-interest issues have recently received much attention in Japan. The pharmaceutical industry in Japan has developed a guideline for financial disclosures to make the financial relationship between the company and the research sites transparent. The companies have made the information available to the public on their websites since 2013. This information includes research funds, donations, honoraria paid to physicians as speakers or authors, consultation fees, and costs of meeting support.

Medical societies, such as the Japanese Association of Medical Sciences, the Japanese Society of Medical Oncology, and the Japan Society of Clinical Oncology, have developed guidelines regarding conflicts of interest in clinical trials. Hospitals also have developed conflict-of-interest policies, under which the investigators are required to submit disclosure forms to the committees where each study is evaluated. In past decades, personal stockholders were relatively rare in Japan, so the concerns about investigators' stock holdings did not receive attention. However, the situation is changing. All research team members, including CTNs, need to be more sensitive to this issue while considering the ethical principles in research. Disclosing personal assets and talking about monetary involvement is an uncomfortable subject for many Japanese people. Traditionally, Japanese people believe that speaking of personal wealth outside of the immediate family or showing interests in others' assets is not proper. However, CTNs need to recognize their own personal values and the ethical implications for their patients when dealing with this issue.

Recruitment and Retention

Public and Patient Education

Patient educational materials about clinical trials and diseases, such as handmade brochures or institutional advertisement videos, are mainly prepared by CRCs. For sponsor-initiated indication-directed trials, the sponsor will provide these materials. They are prepared with sensitivity to clarify information and present visual attraction.

Opportunities for providing clinical trial education to the public audience are currently limited in Japan. Public presentations related to clinical trials may be seen at medical conferences, town hall meetings, or schools, but often are provided by physicians. CTNs need to become more involved in public and patient education to guide them in proper understanding of clinical trials, as well as to ease their stress in future encounters with clinical trials as patients or family members of patients.

Accrual Base, Recruitment, and Promotion

Since 1999, pharmaceutical companies have used media such as newspapers or Internet advertisements to find patients for registration-directed trials. When patients see an advertisement, they call the coordinating center (called a *call center*), which directs them to participating medical centers. By 2011, more than 300 such advertisements had been published. However, many of the patients who applied for the trials through those advertisements did not meet the eligibility criteria. Therefore, efficiency of patient recruitment through media advertisements varies.

Advertisements (such as pamphlets or posters) for patient recruitment for a trial within an institution are relatively efficient, especially for cancer trials. This is based on the premise that eligible candidates for the trials are readily available. IRB approval is required for any kind of patient recruitment tools for trials.

Unlike in the United States, patients who visit a hospital seeking the opportunity to participate in a clinical trial are rare in Japan because so many patients seek cancer treatment within a close geographic area of their home. However, some patients will traverse the entire country to seek clinical trials with new drugs or new modalities that have already been approved in foreign countries.

CTNs need to be knowledgeable about ways to obtain accurate trial information to help patients acquire other treatment options. Ongoing registration-directed trials are disclosed on the website of the Japanese Pharmaceutical Manufacturers Association, as well as in the clinical trial registration database (described later in the Clinical Trial Registries section) on the web.

Recruitment methods for participating institutions vary for each study group. Study groups are responsible for evaluating their participating institutions regarding the number of accruals and data quality. Although it rarely happens, an institution with low evaluations can be terminated, and new institutions may be recruited after obtaining approval from the steering committee of the study group. Some study groups invite institutions to participate through advertisements of the trial at academic meetings.

Adherence and Retention in Clinical Trials

Protocol adherence and retention have improved dramatically in Japan since CRCs became involved in registration-directed clinical trials in the late 1990s. Unfortunately, this has not been the case for investigator-initiated clinical trials. Only about 8%–17% of participating institutions have CRCs available for non–registration-directed cancer cooperative group trials. This low number is the result of very limited resource allocation to institutions and the lack of an official support system for such trials within the institutions (Aotani, 2006; Tamura, 2006).

Therefore, minor deviations, such as missing data or delays in the required tests, are not rare. In the authors' opinion, many of these deviations can be prevented if responsible CRCs or CTNs are assigned.

Clinical Trial Registries

Japan has three clinical trial registries: the University Hospital Medical Information Network Clinical Trials Registry (UMIN-CTR), the Japan Pharmaceutical Information Center Clinical Trials Information (JAPIC-CTI), and the Japan Medical Association Center for Clinical Trials Clinical Trials Registry (JMACCT-CTR). UMIN, a cooperative organization of national medical schools in Japan, is sponsored by MEXT and is now the largest, most versatile academic network information center for biomedical sciences (Matsuba, Kiuchi, Tstutani, Uchida, & Ohashi, 2006). JAPIC is a public service corporation approved by the Minister of Health and Welfare to ensure proper clinical use of medicine. This is accomplished by bridging pharmaceutical manufacturers and medical societies by collecting, processing, and offering useful information from domestic and foreign sources. JMACCT is an organization within the Japan Medical Association that was established to support investigators and medical institutions in conducting investigator-initiated clinical trials under the clinical trial promotion program subsidized by MHLW.

Most academic investigator-initiated research, including clinical trials and observational studies, is registered in UMIN-CTR. Most sponsor-initiated trials are registered in JAPIC-CTI. All investigator-initiated clinical trials supported by JMACCT are registered in JMACCT-CTR. However, clinical trials conducted only in Japan are sometimes registered in ClinicalTrials.gov. Clinical trial information is provided in Japanese for the public, as well as in English for access to key elements for those in other countries. As of May 2013, the UMIN-CTR database contained 10,542 clinical research listings, the JAPIC-CTI database included 1,151 registration-directed clinical trials, and the JMACCT-CTR database contained 125 clinical research listings that were open to the public. The listings for each are available online (UMIN-CTR: www.umin.ac.jp/ctr; JAPIC-CTI: www.clinicaltrials.jp/user/cteList_e.jsp; JMACCT-CTR: www.jmacct.med.or.jp/en/ctr/ctr_list_p1.html).

Clinical Trial Participants and Nursing Components

Educating Staff

The start-up meeting of the trial usually is the first step for staff education in Japan. CRCs often identify participants and send invitations to the meeting. To take the role of the educator, the CRC needs to have knowledge of the protocol, as well as the infrastructure of the relevant departments and personnel in the hospital. At the meeting, the site investigator explains the scientific rationale and importance of the study. The CRC identifies responsibilities of each department and each staff member and any special tests or equipment necessary to conduct the trial. Special training sessions may be planned with support of the trial sponsor to ensure appropriate use of new equipment. CTNs in Japan can be a resource for staff education in clinical trials.

Investigational Agents

Investigational drugs for registration-directed trials are all distributed directly from the sponsor to participating institutions. The drugs are sent to the institution's pharmacy, where a pharmacist is appointed for the receipt, storage, preparation, handling, disposal, and accountability of the study drugs, as well as for maintenance of records of the drug log forms. The investigational agents cannot be substituted without permission from the sponsor.

Practical aspects of drug administration, such as premedications or specific procedures, are detailed in the protocol. Modification criteria, such as dose modifications, treatment delays, and discontinuation criteria, also are stated in the protocol. Usually the first dose of each protocol agent is calculated at the patient registration center and reported to the investigator. The investigators and CRCs/CTNs are responsible for confirming accurate dosing and timing thereafter.

Drug accountability is strictly enforced for investigational drugs in registration-directed trials in Japan and is subject to audit by PMDA. The institution's pharmacy usually is responsible for drug accountability. The items that the pharmacy should record on the drug accountability logbook include (a) date, dose, and lot number of drug received, (b) the patient's initials and identification number, (c) log number and quantity of drugs dispensed for the study, (d) log number and quantity of drugs returned after administration, and (e) balance of the total drug account. The procedures for handling investigational drugs are determined by SOPs.

Adverse Events and Unanticipated Problems

Adverse events for cancer trials are graded according to the Japanese version of the CTCAE in Japan, currently version 4, which was translated by JCOG (www.jcog.jp/en). Although investigators are responsible for evaluation of adverse events, CRCs/CTNs support the grading procedure by interviewing patients and reviewing laboratory tests before conferring with the physician.

Each protocol indicates a definition of SAEs. The PI of the participating institution is responsible for reporting SAEs, as well as any medically important unanticipated problems, to the institution's IRB, the director of the institution, and the sponsor of the trial according to the institution's SOPs. Because SAEs ultimately must be reported to MHLW, CRCs are starting to play a more active role in the preparation of SAE reports to keep to a reporting timeline of 7–15 days.

Patient and Family Education

Early detection and correct evaluation of adverse reactions (ARs) to the study agent is the primary purpose of patient and family education during the clinical trial. Patients and family members are given detailed information of the expected ARs of the study agent. CTNs encourage patients to report any unpleasant symptoms and the family to report any unusual signs observed in the patient. Contact information for emergencies is provided. Patient diaries are often prepared and given to patients to record the onset date, severity, and duration of the ARs, as well as the treatment received to control it. For a study with oral medication, patient diaries frequently are used to confirm adherence to the protocol treatment.

Symptom management is one aspect of important nursing education for patients and families during clinical trials. Because nurses have no authority to write prescriptions in Japan, the treating physician prescribes drugs to prevent or treat symptoms after confirming that they are not contraindicated in the protocol treatment. CTNs can contribute to symptom management in terms of prevention, observation, and education for patients and their families. CTNs usually observe symptoms such as infection or peripheral neuropathy. Special attention is paid to such symptoms for possible attribution to the study treatment. CTNs report patients' symptoms to the physician and sometimes record them directly on the medical chart. In addition, CTNs record both subjective and objective information regarding the symptoms, often in detail, with assessment and management plans on a separate nursing chart. Interventions for loss of appetite, control of bowel movements, prevention of infection, care for peripheral edema, and psychological support are common examples of nursing interventions in symptom management.

Psychosocial Distress

A study regarding stress among patients with cancer in Japan showed relatively similar results to those in Western countries, where 4%–35% of patients with cancer experienced symptoms of adjustment disorders such as anxiety, and 4%–7% developed depression (Inagaki & Uchitomi, 2001). Many of those who developed adjustment disorders were experiencing a cancer recurrence. Many Japanese still consider a cancer diagnosis to be a death sentence. When introducing a clinical trial as a treatment option, it is crucial for CTNs to observe the readiness of patients for new information and to take enough time for patients' informed acceptance of treatment.

In Japanese culture, family members play significant roles in patients' decision-making processes. In a large 1992 survey of the family members of deceased patients with cancer, 36% requested more effective communication with the physician, and 13% requested a consultation system with medical information provided to them (Saeki, 2004).

Historically in Japanese culture, an apparent paternalistic relationship has existed between physicians and their patients and patients' families. The situation is improving, but CTNs should ensure that a coordinated effort is made for effective communication with patients and their families and that continuous efforts for improvements are made.

Psychosocial issues of patients participating in clinical trials are not routinely assessed at each hospital visit. CRCs assigned for industry-sponsored trials can take considerable time interviewing patients and assessing their psychosocial status. However, very few CRCs are assigned for investigator-initiated clinical trials. For these trials, patients will be referred to psychiatrists or other specialists only when the patients or their family members express concerns or if the investigators observe signs of psychosocial problems. Psychosocial assessment is an important area of the nursing domain. The authors believe that CTNs in Japan would like to get more involved in this area for all patients, regardless of the difference in clinical trial sponsors. For that purpose, organizational innovations of job assignments for CRCs/CTNs are essential.

Genetics and Genomics

Genetic or genomic investigation has become extremely important to find predictive factors for efficacy or toxicities of experimental agents. Therefore, it is imperative to incorporate these tests into clinical trials in Japan. The study purpose for this type of investigation must be clearly written in the protocol and the IRB-approved consent forms. It often is difficult for patients to comprehend the purpose of translational research. Continuous explanations and follow-up by CTNs to ensure the patients' understanding of translational research is essential.

Pharmacogenetics and Pharmacogenomics

Pharmacogenetics refers to genetic differences in the metabolic pathway of drugs, and *pharmacogenomics* is the technology that analyses pharmacogenetics. Since the whole human genome sequence has been sequenced, the methods to search for genes implicated in disease or drug responses have changed dramatically (Kamatani, 2011). It is now possible to look at how genetic differences affect an individual's response to drugs, toxicities, or clinical effects. Examples are UGT1A1 for irinotecan toxicities, clinical efficacies of gefitinib based on the *EGFR* mutation in patients with non-small cell lung cancer (Maemondo et al., 2010), and reversed clinical effects of cetuximab in patients with *KRAS* mutation. PMDA is enthusiastic to see how different the drug response will be between the Japanese population and others, especially Caucasians (MHLW, 1998b).

Genetic Testing

Genetic testing is a rapidly evolving component of clinical trials because of the importance of investigating pharmacogenetic features in investigational agents. However, it is an extremely sensitive issue in Japanese society. When genetic testing is planned using samples obtained from patients in a study, some local IRBs may reject the study unless the component of future tissue use is eliminated. Other local IRBs require a separate informed consent from patients each time samples or tests are used for purposes beyond the initial clinical trial. Key elements of genetic testing that require particular attention when it is a component of a clinical trial are summarized in Figure 56-5.

Cytogenetics

Cytogenetics tests the gene mapping or detects chromosomal abnormalities by using techniques such as fluorescent in situ hybridization and comparative genomic hybridization. It is also a sensitive issue in Japanese insti-

---

Figure 56-5. Key Elements of Patient Protection in Genetic Testing

- Informed consent must be obtained prior to disclosure of information to others.
- Information/specimens collected for one purpose should not be used for another purpose without obtaining further consent.
- Personal information that is not relevant for the study should not be used.
- Strict protection should be adopted to minimize the release of personal information to those other than the required research team members.

tutions to test cytogenetics because many IRBs do not allow inclusion of the "future use" of tissue for these kinds of tests without specifying the target gene or genes.

Tumor Profiling

Tumor genetic profiling is another important issue. For example, it has been demonstrated that genetic profiling of clear cell carcinoma of the ovary was not similar to that of endometrial carcinoma, but it was similar to clear cell carcinoma of the kidney (Zorn et al., 2005). This finding led Japanese investigators to new clinical trials using a mammalian target of rapamycin (known as mTOR) inhibitor, which was established to be effective in renal cell carcinoma, for clear cell carcinoma of the ovary.

Recently, the nationwide genome screening program (SCRUM-Japan) has been started as the project of an academia-industry consortium using the registration trials for new molecular-targeted agents. This program will play a key role in collecting and distributing important genome information along with clinical information toward the future of precision medicine in Japan.

Storage of Genetic Materials

Storage of materials for genetic testing in Japan is heavily dependent on each institution's SOPs, especially for frozen materials. It often is difficult to provide paraffin-embedded blocks, but alternatively, unstained slides can be submitted for the trial purpose. The National Cancer Center and several universities have established tissue banks for collection and storage of tissues from their patients. A nationwide central tissue banking system for future research including genetic material needs to be established.

Pharmacokinetic Trials

Pharmacokinetic studies often are conducted in association with phase I trials. It is necessary to obtain blood and urine samples a prescribed number of times during and after drug administration. In Japan, this typically is done in an inpatient setting if multiple blood draws are required.

Correlative Trials

Nursing Companion Studies

The cooperative groups conduct cancer clinical trials that examine standard endpoints (i.e., toxicity, tumor response, and survival), sometimes along with translational research endpoints and/or QOL and cost-effectiveness. Rarely are nursing research questions incorporated into cooperative group trials.

Nursing companion studies offer nurses the opportunity to perform independent research while conducting an oncology clinical trial. It offers them benefits such as easy access to study participants compared to an independent nursing study. However, conducting a companion study is a great challenge because obtaining permission and support from the study group is difficult.

Unfortunately, none of the cancer cooperative groups in Japan currently hold a nursing committee. Thus, opportunities for nursing companion studies have not yet matured. CTNs in Japan are expected to take vital roles in promoting recognition of nursing research within the cooperative group. The first step in promoting the recognition of nursing research may be to propose a nursing research concept and make a good presentation with emphasis on the significance of the study and the scientific research methodology to cooperative group committee members. Because many investigators have little knowledge about nursing research, it is essential to introduce them to the importance of nursing research as a science for the care of patients with cancer.

Pharmacoeconomic Studies

Recently, the national budget shortage for medical expenses has become apparent. Medical treatment costs are higher, along with the costs of developing new diagnostic and therapeutic measures, such as new molecular-targeted anticancer agents. Under such circumstances, pharmacoeconomic studies have gained more attention in Japan but are not yet common.

Methodology for pharmacoeconomic studies is the same as for those conducted in the United States. The most common approach is cost-effect analysis, in which the cost of a treatment is compared in monetary terms with the effectiveness of the treatment. It usually measures the clinical outcome in terms of number of lives saved or number of toxicities prevented. Keeping personal information confidential is essential. As with other clinical trials, pharmacoeconomic studies also need to obtain IRB approval.

Quality-of-Life Studies

QOL studies are now becoming more important components of cancer trials in Japan. QOL assessment particularly is important when the primary endpoints of two arms in a randomized trial have minimal efficacy differences but large differences in toxicity profiles. The most common QOL assessment method among Japanese study groups is the Functional Assessment of Cancer Therapy

(FACT) scales because most FACT scale components have a validated Japanese version.

CRCs/CTNs can affect the future of cancer care by making important contributions to QOL studies. The authors believe that CTNs in Japan have more potential for coordinating QOL studies in which they help patients and gather timely and reliable QOL data.

Documentation and Data Management

Documentation

Since 1997, protocols for cancer clinical trials in Japan have been written based on ICH GCP guidelines. Protocols must be justified both scientifically and ethically. The elements of a protocol were described earlier in this chapter. A protocol may be revised and amended, but it always serves as the ultimate guide for the trial. CTNs in Japan must emphasize the data collection and submission schedule because delay is common, with no penalties to investigators and institutions.

Investigators are required to retain all medical records and regulatory documents of patients who enter clinical trials. Medical records include original source documents describing basic patient identification information and materials showing that each patient has met eligibility criteria, such as pathology reports, surgery reports, laboratory test data, and radiographic image films. Regulatory documents include the signed original informed consent, the protocol and its amendments, and other communications and actions pertaining to the study. These materials and documentations are subject to audit by the study group or inspection by MHLW. CRCs are responsible for ensuring that required documents are completed and kept in place.

Data Management

Accurate and prompt data submission is important for successful clinical trials. CRCs are responsible for local data management in registration-directed trials, whereas the investigators themselves often perform local data management in investigator-initiated clinical trials.

Collecting long-term follow-up data is a challenge. Data centers collect follow-up forms with patient data, such as survival, progression, and late adverse events, according to the protocols. At the time of a patient's first visit, the hospital checks the patient's national health insurance card, which includes contact information. Some cancer centers in Japan require submission of the resident's card. When a patient moves, the patient's information, such as survival information and the new address, can be tracked from the patient's legal domicile.

Data monitoring methods differ depending on the type of trial. Registration-directed trials have on-site monitoring with strict *source document verification* (SDV) by monitors, who have a contract with the sponsor. Conversely, non–registration-directed trials have only periodic central monitoring without SDV. Establishing a data management support system for participating physicians, especially including assignment of CRCs/CTNs for clinical trials, is the most urgent step that should be taken to improve the quality of clinical trials in Japan.

Many case report forms (CRFs) for clinical trials in Japan are paper based. Each study group or pharmaceutical company develops its own templates for CRFs that are partially modified according to the protocol. CRFs and other supplies, such as the CRF manual and the examination calendar, are distributed to the institutions. Usually, the institutions receive newsletters or emails with updates, tips, and reminders. Kickoff meetings normally take place just before the activation of the trials. The data centers for each study group or study-specific data center at a contract research organization take responsibility for overseeing the data management of the trials.

Most of the pharmaceutical companies and some of the study groups have their own customized electronic data capturing (EDC) systems. Most use a web-based data entry system with personal ID and password (Saito, 2006b). However, EDC systems are not popular in investigator-initiated trials because of the high cost of preparation and maintenance of the system.

CSPOR has used a USB device for remote data entry in some studies, and the Japanese Gynecologic Oncology Group has used a Medidata Rave® web-based data entry system. The cancer cooperative groups in Japan do not have a single EDC system, so they use the clinical trial management system of each group with great variations.

No governmental agency similar to the U.S. Cancer Trials Support Unit currently exists in Japan. Increasing physician and patient access to clinical trials, standardizing data collection and reporting, and reducing regulatory and administrative burden on investigators are all responsibilities of the sponsor or study group.

Maintaining a Regulatory File

All regulatory documents, both initial and revised, such as clinical trial applications to PMDA, IRB application and approval letters, the protocol and the original informed consent documents for each patient, along with any study-related documents, must be maintained during the study and retained after study completion for the period specified in the protocol. They must be accessible for inspection at a later time. The required duration of medical record retention by the Medical Service Act in Japan is five years, so special attention is necessary for clinical trial participants' medical records.

Quality Assurance

Data and Safety Monitoring Plans

The clinical trial should be watched carefully for patient safety. How safety is monitored differs by the phase, the purpose of the study, and the study group policy. Data need to be monitored externally and internally. Members of an independent data safety monitoring committee (IDMC) monitor the data periodically, usually twice a year in addition to the time of interim analysis and final analysis for phase II and III studies. The purposes of the IDMC include early detection of unacceptable toxicities and clearly ineffective—or significantly effective—treatment. If the IDMC finds any concerns with continuing the study or any need to change the contents of the protocol or the informed consent documents, the IDMC directs these recommendations to the study chair, as well as to the group chair.

Data monitoring is also performed internally at the data center, which is called *central monitoring*. The data managers of the study continuously look through all adverse events and the frequency of the events if any unexpected safety issues arise. In some studies, and mandatory for registration-directed trials, the monitors are assigned for "on-site monitoring" to visit the participating sites for SDV. The monitors review the patient records to confirm data accuracy, including all SAE reporting, patient eligibility, and appropriate conduct of the study at the site.

Audit Preparation

Audits are essential components in conducting clinical trials to ensure the quality of data obtained during the trials. Audits usually are initiated by (a) notification of the date and the patient numbers to be audited, (b) submission of the curricula vitae of the auditors to the institution, and (c) reservation of a room and necessary equipment for the audit.

The investigators are responsible for preparation of medical records, radiographic imaging films, and regulatory documents, including IRB approval letters, original informed consent documents signed by patients, and protocols and amendment records. CRCs may help with preparation for the audit.

The audit team of the sponsoring company or the contract research organization can perform audits for registration-directed trials sponsored by pharmaceutical companies. Inspections may be conducted by PMDA or MHLW, and GCP violations can be subject to penalty. Audits for investigator-initiated non–registration-directed trials are not regulated by GCP. However, cancer trial groups such as JCOG and the Japanese Gynecologic Oncology Group employ audit mechanisms in which investigators from other participating institutions can audit members for educational purposes.

Professional Development

Clinical Trial Nurse Education

In Japan, no specialization in clinical trials nursing is available. However, recognition of CRCs as clinical trial specialists gradually is increasing in research communities. The Japanese Society of Cancer Nursing established 14 special interest groups in 2006. Among those is one for CTNs, where CTNs working as CRCs at institutions can collaborate with those working as study coordinators or auditors at the data centers of cooperative groups. They exchange information and nursing skills about clinical trials at educational sessions several times a year, maintain a professional network, and may contribute to improved awareness of CTNs/CRCs as a profession. Members communicate by small group meetings and a mailing list (Niimi et al., 2010).

Oncology nurse programs that prepare nurses to be certified nurse specialists are available at 56 universities in Japan. Additionally, the Japanese Nursing Association endorses programs to produce certified nurses in five areas of oncology-related nursing: chemotherapy, pain control, palliative care, breast cancer, and radiation therapy (Japanese Nursing Association, n.d.). Several educational programs exist for CRCs. Parts of the Japanese government, such as MHLW or MEXT, support periodic CRC seminars. Cancer cooperative groups also provide seminars for their members.

Currently, no specific academic courses are designed for CTNs in Japan. Instead, several graduate programs are available that provide advanced education for CRCs.

Three organizations provide certification for CRCs in Japan: the Society of Clinical Research Associates, the Japanese Society of Clinical Pharmacology and Therapeutics, and the Japan Site Management Organization Association. They also provide continuous education and certification examinations (Niimi et al., 2010; Saito, 2006a). There are currently a few certified CRCs from the Association of Clinical Research Professionals in Japan.

Since 2012, the Japan Society of Clinical Trials and Research has provided a GCP passport for the entry level of clinical research professionals in Japan, which can be taken by CRCs or CTNs.

Mentorship

Currently, no formal mentorship program for CTNs exists in Japan. Most CTNs are educated through on-the-job training with senior CTNs as informal mentoring (Niimi et al., 2010).

Publication Issues in Clinical Trials Nursing

The authors of publications for clinical trials must have made a significant contribution to the design and/or implementation of the trial. In many cases, the PI from the institution with the largest number of patients accrued chooses either to be the first author of the manuscript or to be the presenter at a major academic meeting. The second author usually is the study chair or statistician, depending on the trial group policy. Other coauthors include study cochairs and investigators from institutions where significant numbers of patients were enrolled. CRCs and CTNs are not normally listed on publications, but sometimes their names appear in the acknowledgments section.

Implications for Nurses

The CTN role in Japanese clinical trials has increased greatly in the past decade. However, much still needs to be done to bring Japanese CTNs to an equivalent level with their foreign peers. Nurse CRCs need to gain nursing perspectives within their current roles to contribute to successful clinical trials.

It can be a challenge for Japanese CTNs to show their unique contributions to clinical trials "as a nurse." However, being involved in oncology trials as a nurse brings several advantages. Oncology trials require specialized knowledge of cancer treatment and its standardized evaluation criteria. In addition, the study participants are patients with cancer who face the fear of death, which requires ethical judgments and psychological support from CTNs. Furthermore, research teams consisting of multidisciplinary professionals surround the patients and their families. This requires effective communication and coordination skills so that principles of family nursing can be applied. Patients expect to receive advice for symptom management. The authors believe that nurses possess the educational background to fulfill those expectations. Therefore, recognition of these advantages by nursing societies and the nursing community would be important to increase the number of CTNs in Japan.

Summary

A number of improvements have occurred in the infrastructure for clinical trials in Japan with establishment of cancer cooperative groups and introduction of the team approach to protect patients' safety and the scientific integrity of the trial. Given the recent increased complexity clinical trial design, and within the context of the research sites, investigators, and other supporting entities, all with their own ongoing priorities, CTNs need to ensure good nursing care for patients throughout their cancer treatment period, regardless of whether they are in a trial.

Key Points
- The infrastructure of investigator-initiated clinical trial groups started to be established in the late 1970s in Japan. In accordance with ICH GCP, continuous efforts for quality improvement are underway.
- Japanese GCP is mandated by law for the registration-directed clinical trials. Other investigator-initiated trials must follow the ethical guidelines for clinical research published by the government.
- The Japanese government is promoting the establishment of early-stage clinical research centers to efficiently develop Japanese-made new drugs.
- For quality assurance of clinical research in Japan, especially for investigator-initiated non–registration-directed trials with limited research funds, the importance of the research team approach is now recognized. The effective methodology for the research team approach is being evaluated.

The authors would like to acknowledge the following professionals for their expert and insightful reviews: Haruhiko Fukuda, MD, Director, JCOG Data Center/National Cancer Center, Japan; Izumi Kohara, RN, PhD, CCRP, Jichi University, Japan; Keiichi Fujiwara, MD, Saitama Medical University, Japan; and Yasuo Ohashi, PhD, University of Tokyo, Japan.

References

Ando, M., & Fujiwara, Y. (2005, January). Changes to the clinical trials system in Japan. *ASCO News*, p. 35.

Aotani, E. (2006). Support for the GOG participating institutions. *Proceedings of the 4th Annual Meeting of Japanese Society of Medical Oncology, 4*(SII-5), 135.

Aotani, E., Hata, T., Kawakami, A., Tsuboi, S., Numagami, N., Ushitani, M., ... Fujiwara, K. (2012). Clinical trial coordination under the Evaluation System of Investigational Medical Care in Japan: Operational challenges in multi-center cancer clinical trials. *Japanese Pharmacology and Therapeutics, 40*(Suppl.), S67–S79.

Fukuda, H. (2010). Development of cancer cooperative groups in Japan. *Japanese Journal of Clinical Oncology, 40*, 881–890. doi:10.1093/jjco/hyq135

Inagaki, M., & Uchitomi, Y. (2001). Psychological burden after cancer diagnosis. *Igaku No Ayumi, 197*, 288–289.

Japanese Nursing Association. (n.d.). Certified nurse specialist. Retrieved from http://www.nurse.or.jp/nursing/education/nintei/index.html

Kamatani, N. (2011). [Current status of researches in genomic medicine and the guidelines for pharmacogenomics (PGx)]. *Yakugaku Zasshi, 131*, 263–268. doi:10.1248/yakushi.131.263

Maemondo, M., Inoue, A., Kobayashi, K., Sugawara, S., Oizumi, S., Isobe, H., ... Nukiwa, T. (2010). Gefitinib or chemotherapy for non–small-cell lung cancer with mutated EGFR. *New England Journal of Medicine, 362,* 2380–2388. doi:10.1056/NEJMoa0909530

Matsuba, H., Kiuchi, T., Tstutani, K., Uchida, E., & Ohashi, Y. (2006). The Japanese perspective on registries and a review of clinical trial process in Japan. In M.A. Foote (Ed.), *Clinical trial registries: A practical guide for sponsors and researchers of medicinal products* (pp. 83–106). Basel, Switzerland: Springer Birkhäuser BioSciences.

Ministry of Health, Labour and Welfare. (1998a). *Conduct of clinical trials after filing application for the drug manufacture and sales approval* (Pharmaceutical Safety Bureau, Evaluation and Licensing Division Notice No. 1061). Retrieved from http://www.japal.org/contents/19981201_1061.pdf

Ministry of Health, Labour and Welfare. (1998b). *Ethnic factors that need to be considered when using clinical data from foreign countries* (Pharmaceutical Safety Bureau, Evaluation and Licensing Division Notice No. 672). Retrieved from http://www.pmda.go.jp

Ministry of Health, Labour and Welfare. (2008). Ethical guidelines for clinical research. Retrieved from http://www.mhlw.go.jp/general/seido/kousei/i-kenkyu/rinsyo/dl/shishin.pdf

Ministry of Health, Labour and Welfare. (2012). Good clinical practice. Retrieved from http://law.e-gov.go.jp/htmldata/H09/H09F03601000028.html

Nakamura, H., Ohmori, S., Kitada, M., & Mochida, A. (1994). Preventive measures against drug-drug interaction: Lessons for pharmacists from the sorivudine side effect case. *Journal of Toxicological Sciences, 19*(3), 89–93.

Niimi, M., Aotani, E., Kohara, I., & Saito, Y. (2010). *An introduction to clinical trials for nurses.* Tokyo, Japan: Igaku-shoin.

Saeki, T. (2004). Psychosocial intervention for cancer patients and family members. *Japanese Journal of Psychosomatic Medicine, 44,* 496–501.

Saito, Y. (2006a). CRC education and future perspective in cancer clinical trials. *Rinsho Yakuri, 37,* 70–74.

Saito, Y. (2006b). *System development of connections between electronic medical chart and EDC system.* Proceedings of the SAS Users Forum 2006. Tokyo, Japan: SAS Institute Japan.

Sato, K., Watanabe, T., Katsumata, Y., & Ohashi, Y. (2005). Japanese breast cancer patients prefer detailed consent forms: A comparative study of detailed forms vs. standard forms. *Journal of Clinical Oncology, 23*(Suppl. 16), Abstract 6046. Retrieved from http://meeting.ascopubs.org/cgi/content/short/23/16_suppl/6046

Tamura, K. (2006). Infrastructure of the participating institutions for a cooperative group. *Proceedings of the 4th Annual Meeting of Japanese Society of Medical Oncology, 4*(SII-2), 132.

Zorn, K.K., Bonome, T., Gangi, L., Chandramouli, G.V.R., Awtrey, C.S., Gardner, G.J., ... Birrer, M.J. (2005). Gene expression profiles of serous, endometrioid, and clear cell subtypes of ovarian and endometrial cancer. *Clinical Cancer Research, 11,* 6422–6430. doi:10.1158/1078-0432.CCR-05-0508

Chapter 57

Mexico

Adriana Chávez-Blanco, DVM, Rosa Maria Álvarez-Gómez, MD, Patricia Cortés-Esteban, MD, Dolores Gallardo-Rincón, MD, and Abelardo Meneses-García, MD

Introduction

One of the major concerns of every nation, government, and society is health. In Mexico, the National Health System and private and academic institutions have combined their efforts in the search and implementation of better health strategic plans for the Mexican population. Research is part of such health programs generating new knowledge and facilitating, troubleshooting, and promoting technological development with contribution to achievement of a better quality of life (QOL) for the population. All parties involved in this process are working to strengthen the weak points in the system for the benefit of the country.

Within the diseases included in health and research programs, cancer is the third cause of death in Mexico. In 2009, the mortality rate due to cancer was 65 for every 100,000 people, according to the most recent figures from the National Institute of Statistics and Geography (Subsecretaría de Prevención y Promoción de la Salud, 2013).

History and Foundation

Coordinating Committee for National Health Institutions and High Specialty Hospitals

The Coordinating Committee for National Health Institutions and High Specialty Hospitals (*Comisión Coordinadora de Instituciones Nacionales de Salud y Hospitales de Alta Especialidad* [CCINSHAE], www.ccinshae.gob.mx) was created in August 1989. CCINSHAE is an administrative entity that provides support and orientation with the aim of excellent access to health services as well as infrastructure for research. Within its responsibilities is the conduct of the public politics in federal and regional research projects by creating and implementing policies, strategies, and models to achieve effectiveness and quality of management in private, social, and international funding (CCINSHAE, n.d.).

This commission promotes and provides orientation for the development and execution of research projects addressing the identification and modification of factors that determine the incidence, prevalence, and final outcomes of the main health problems in the country. It sponsors and conducts research health programs with the participation of the National Bioethics Commission, the federal public administration entities, and the state governments. It contributes to and promotes the achievement of collaborative agreements with other national and international research institutions for science and technology development.

National Cancer Institute of Mexico

The National Cancer Institute of Mexico (*Instituto Nacional de Cancerología* [INCan], www.incan.salud.gob.mx) was founded in 1946 with the purpose of attention to four basic necessities for cancer care: assistance, teaching, research, and human and financial resources. These focused on the diagnosis, treatment, rehabilitation, research, and palliation of patients with cancer.

INCan is a decentralized public organization that grants service to patients without medical insurance. Since its creation, several changes have taken place, from basic healthcare practice to the development of models of integrated health care, such as the creation of functional units, medical attention to research, and the development of the tumor bank and translational medicine.

Since 2003, INCan has implemented a wide program of work aimed to make its activities and services function more efficiently, seeking a multidisciplinary structure.

INCan is a leading organization in program design, investigation strategies, and consolidation of multi-institutional projects. The infrastructure and equipment for diagnosis and treatment have been consolidated. In the past three years, the institute has registered 88 new protocols and has been following 155 protocols that were in progress from previous years (see Figure 57-1). INCan is an MD Anderson Cancer Center Sister Institution and is currently working in association with several international multidisciplinary groups and institutions.

Figure 57-1. National Cancer Institute of Mexico Main Research Lines

- Breast cancer
- Carcinogenesis
- Cervical cancer
- Environmental pollution and cancer
- Epigenetics and cancer
- Oncogenomics
- Ovarian cancer
- Quality of life
- Translational research on lung cancer
- Viruses and cancer

State Cancer Centers Network

In 1963, a state cancer centers network (CC) was created throughout the country. Currently, 25 centers are participating within this decentralized organization with a governing council coordinated by INCan. CC gives high-quality medical attention and training for human resources in oncology with programs in clinical, basic, and translational research. Through INCan, CC promotes scientific multidisciplinary oncology research with alliances of national universities and pharmaceutical company partnerships to achieve mutual benefits. With the generation of resources for education and research activities, INCan provides the national oncology clinical and research guidelines for CC and high specialty hospitals.

Clinical Trials: Fundamental Information

In recent years, the wide experience and substantial contributions of Mexican investigators to international cancer clinical trials have led to an increase in Mexico's presence within international cancer associations, universities, and institutions and the creation of cooperative groups, such as the following.

- The Ovarian Cancer Research Group (*Grupo de Investigación en Cáncer Ginecológico de México* [GICOM], www.gicom.org.mx), the Mexican cooperative group for research in ovarian cancer, was created in 2007 and has contributed to establishing standard therapies for gynecologic cancer. Its main objective is the development of clinical, basic, and translational research within the gynecologic cancer area, working with CCs in the country. Additionally, GICOM contributes to academic activities and prevention and early detection strategies by developing alliances with national universities. Currently, GICOM has 140 oncology professionals across the country in a network for oncology research and educational work in the gynecologic cancer area.
- The Latin American Cooperative Oncology Group (LACOG, www.lacog.org.br), founded in 2008 by a group of medical oncologists interested in the development of academic clinical research, is the first multinational cooperative group in Latin America dedicated to clinical and translational research in cancer. Mexico's institutions are part of the 49 institutions of the region and together see approximately 6,000 new cases of cancer a month, about 1,000 of which are breast cancers.
- In 2010, INCan (www.incan-mexico.org) became a member of the American cooperative group SWOG (formerly the Southwest Oncology Group), one of the principal cooperative groups of clinical investigation of cancer worldwide. It has included protocols of non-small cell lung, breast, and colon cancers.

None of these cooperative groups has a nursing committee except SWOG (Nursing Program Committee). Most nurses at participating institutions are involved in clinical trials as clinical attendants.

Protocol Development, Review, and Approval

As in other countries, regardless of the trial origin (e.g., academic, existing or investigational new drug study, industry proposals), the process for carrying out the project is similar. This process must adhere to the General Health Law, the General Health Law Regulations for Health Research; the Federal Commission for the Protection Against Sanitary Risk (COFEPRIS) regulations; and the International Conference on Harmonisation of Technical Requirements for Registration of Pharmaceuticals for Human Use (ICH) good clinical practice (GCP) guidelines (ICH, 1996; *Norma Oficial Mexicana*, 2013).

Once a protocol has been reviewed by the clinical trial team, it is presented to the local institutional review board (IRB), which is composed of the ethics, research, and biosecurity committees. Depending on the review findings, the protocol will be approved by the IRB or returned to the investigator because it requires modifications or clarification or was rejected. In addition to the protocol review, all the documentation related to the study, such as the informed consent form and the patient information sheet, must be reviewed and approved by the IRB.

In the case of clinical trials originating at the site, case report forms (CRFs), informed consent forms, and additional documents are designed according to the data requirements and generated by the research team involved in the protocol. For external trials (intergroup or industry sponsored), these documents are provided by the sponsor's clinical trial team.

Preparation

Preparation for pharmaceutical-sponsored and academic clinical trials in Mexico is similar to that in other countries. The site cannot be initiated until the IRB and COFEPRIS approvals are granted, as well as import licenses for study drug and clinical supplies, if required. Thus, a well-detailed and realistic action plan should be implemented at the site to avoid any delay that could affect the study timelines.

For trials sponsored by the pharmaceutical industry, a complete team is dedicated to assist the site staff in all steps of the study processes. Once the sponsor has evaluated and approved the research site and staff, a clinical trial agreement (CTA) between the sponsor and site or investigator (two-way CTA) or sponsor, site, and investigator (three-way CTA) is executed. This CTA will include a financial attachment, in which the payment schedule and pertinent financial remarks are stated. A kick-off meeting is held with all the parties involved in the trial. Usually, action plans for regulatory issues, training needs, site staff definition, and timelines are discussed at this meeting.

Spanish versions of the study protocol and documents are required for the IRB and regulatory submissions, and these are provided to the site staff by the sponsor (see Figure 57-2).

The submission to the local IRB is performed by the site investigator, who has previously completed the site-specific template for protocol review. This template will be attached to the study protocol and documents along with a detailed letter addressed to the IRB chair explaining the nature of the clinical trial.

Following the IRB protocol approval, the preparation and completion of the regulatory dossier is accomplished by the site obtaining, from the hospital director and study staff, all required letters and curricula vitae and providing these to the sponsor, who completes and submits the materials to COFEPRIS.

Once COFEPRIS approval is granted, the sponsor performs the site initiation visit. At this visit, protocol-specific training, as well as GCP guidelines, standard operating procedures, and local regulations, is given to the site staff to ensure complete understanding of the study. During this visit, the investigator site file is provided along with other study documents and templates required for the study development. CRF completion training is also provided at this visit.

In the case of academic studies, the preparation process is similar to that of the industry-sponsored trials. The difference is that the human and material resources have to be optimized. Because these studies are unfunded or minimally funded, all the tasks performed for the sponsor are completed by the research staff. The coordinating site has the responsibility of collecting documents, completing the regulatory dossier, submitting to COFEPRIS, training, monitoring, and so on. As these activities are time consuming, frequently the lead investigator and team have insufficient time for close supervision. An external person with experience in clinical trial management may be hired for this purpose.

Ethics and Regulations

Under the provisions of article 41a in the General Health Law, every public, private, or social institution of health care belonging to the national health system will have, according to their complexity and resolution level, a hospital bioethics committee and a research ethics committee. The hospital bioethics committee is responsible for analysis, discussion, and support in decision making related to bioethical dilemmas that emerge from care delivery or teaching; for promoting the elaboration of institutional guidelines and protocols for these ends; and for promoting permanent bioethics training among its members and institutional personnel. The research ethics committee is responsible for the ethical evaluation of the research protocols on human beings. Local ethics, research, and biosecurity committees are autonomous, interdisciplinary, pluralistic, and consultative to evaluate research trials. These committees must comply with local and international regulations (*Comisión Nacional de Bioética* [National Bioethics Commission], 2012).

Protocol submission processes and timelines, with some exceptions, are similar throughout the country. A meeting schedule is set, and the investigator proceeds as previously discussed in the Preparation section. The time

---

Figure 57-2. Study Documents Required in Spanish for the Institutional Review Board and Regulatory Submissions (NOM-012-SSA3-2012, DOF)

- Study protocol
- Investigator's brochure or prescription information of the study drug
- Informed consent form
- Patient information sheet
- Quality-of-life questionnaires in their validated versions for México
- Patient diary cards or any other documents for patients

of response from the IRB usually takes two months from the submission date; however, this may vary from site to site depending on the IRB's workload.

In Mexico, any clinical trial at any stage of research (phases I–IV), for the use of health products, procedures, or experimental activities in humans or human biologic samples for completion, must conform to the provisions of the General Health Law, the General Health Law regulations on health research, ICH GCP guidelines, and other applicable provisions. All must be reflected in the research protocol and other required documents and should have COFEPRIS authorization.

COFEPRIS is a decentralized body with administrative, technical, and operational autonomy. It is headed by a federal commissioner designated by the president of Mexico, upon recommendation by the Minister of Health, because the Department of Health supervises COFEPRIS. It is also pertinent to mention that in Mexico, the IRB and regulatory process for approval is sequential: first, IRB approval has to be obtained for its inclusion in the regulatory application dossier, and second, it is submitted to COFEPRIS.

Financial Factors

Because INCan and other institutions in the National Health System provide service to patients without socially secure coverage, indifference toward or abandonment of patients has been an important problem. As a result of this, since 2006, INCan and other similar institutions have participated in the social protection program called *gastos catastróficos* ("catastrophic expenses") (www.salud.df.gob.mx/ssdf/seguro_popular/index/gastos.php). Included in the program is *seguro popular* ("popular insurance"), which incorporates some malignant neoplasias so that patients can be covered for treatment and have access to oncologic medicine and rehabilitation (www.seguro-popular.salud.gob.mx). Since 2006, patients with testicular, prostate, cervical, and breast cancers and lymphomas as well as teenagers with malignant tumors have been included. Currently, approximately 9,000 patients have been assisted by this program. In addition, since 2011, the Chamber of Deputies has supported women with ovarian cancer by granting integral treatment to them, from diagnosis to follow-up and relapse, while at the same time allowing research protocols to molecularly reclassify the ovarian tumors and perform studies of oncologic drug resistance.

Recruitment and Retention

Since 1990, pharmaceutical companies and research sites started using advertisements through the mainstream media, such as radio, television, and newspapers, as a means of patient preselection for a particular trial. Although this strategy has worked for most of the therapeutic areas, for cancer trials, it has not been an efficient method for patient recruitment.

During recent years, the use of websites for institutions and public and private hospitals and clinics, as well as pharmaceutical companies, has provided information to patients about cancer, treatment options, and clinical trials. The use of flyers or posters for patient recruitment within an institution and patient referral from other hospitals or clinical networks have also been useful for this end.

Clinical Trial Participants

Patient Selection and Eligibility

According to the eligibility criteria defined in each protocol, the investigator, co-investigators, and study coordinator are responsible for patient assessment and adherence to the inclusion and exclusion criteria. In most cases, there are specific assessments that require time, and patients must travel to the research site. This needs to be discussed between the patient and investigator before the patient signs the informed consent form.

In industry-sponsored trials, a fee for transportation and meals for the patient and a companion person is contemplated. However, in academic studies, this type of expenditure cannot be covered.

Patients should be informed in a clear manner about the study protocol, procedures, and any additional study derived from the protocol by the investigator and delegated staff. Once patients have understood and agree to participate, they must sign the informed consent form (in duplicate) in the presence of two witnesses and the investigator before any protocol procedure can be initiated (including the screening phase) (*Norma Oficial Mexicana*, 2013).

When preselected patients have met the eligibility criteria, the investigator or co-investigator proceeds to registration or randomization according to the specific protocol. If the study protocol is dose finding, the investigator determines the dose at this time.

Active Treatment and Drug Accountability

The investigational drug, concomitant medication, and clinical supplies for industry trials are provided by the sponsor to the site. The study staff receives and reviews them upon delivery to the hospital pharmacy. In academic studies, the study drug is taken from the pharmacy's stock, and the hospital provides other clinical supplies.

It is the investigator's responsibility to ensure the correct storage, handling, accountability, disposal, and destruction of the investigational drug. In common practice, the investigator delegates the supervision and accountability oversight of the drug to the study coordinator. This requires continuous communication with the pharmacist for any inconvenience related to the handling or status of the study drug. Drug accountability is the responsibility of the pharmacist, who registers the amount of drug received, dispensed, and any other pertinent information in the record books and institution pharmacy control system. In parallel, the study-delegated person for this task performs the accountability log according to the study plans after verifying physically and against pharmacy records. At the end of the active treatment period, the investigator returns the remaining study drug or empty vials to the sponsor (commercial trials) or, if it is requested, the certificate of destruction.

Before active treatment starts, the investigator and study staff, including the chemotherapy nurse who administers the treatment, review the treatment schedule based on the protocol treatment specifications, dose adjustments, dose calculations, dose modifications, treatment windows, expected side effects, treatment discontinuations, and protocol violations.

Prior to each course of treatment, the investigator or co-investigator reviews patients' assessments, evaluating the medical conditions since the previous cycle to determine which treatment and dose will be given. The chemotherapy nurse administers the treatment to the patients and records any side effect or adverse reaction (related or not to the study drug) during the treatment cycle in the medical record.

Adverse Events

The suspicion of any serious adverse events, expected or unexpected, must be reported to the sponsor within 24 hours of the site becoming aware of the event and to the IRB and the National Center of Pharmacovigilance (*Centro Nacional de Farmacovigilancia* [CNFV]) within 15 days after the site was notified of such event (Regulatory Affairs in Latin America, n.d.).

An initial report with all available information about the event is submitted to CNFV. If the event has an outcome, the investigator should indicate that the case is closed. When the first report indicates an ongoing event, follow-up reports are submitted each time new information is generated until the case is closed.

In cases where pregnancy is the serious adverse event, it is considered an ongoing event and the follow-up period will continue during six months after the *product* delivery. During this period, the investigator must inform the local IRB and CNFV on a regular basis about the patient status.

Off-Treatment Follow-Up

Currently, cancer trials have incorporated longer periods of follow-up once patients have completed their active treatment. During this period, patients should be consented for data collection. Sites continuously collect data and complete follow-up reports. Maintaining contact with patients is one of the most difficult tasks for the study site during this period when the trial is looking for survival data, especially for patients who reside outside the city where the site is located. Patients' relatives often forget to notify the site staff about changes of residence or the patient's death, resulting in the case being lost to follow-up.

Genetics and Genomics

Despite the current relevance of genetics and genomics in clinical trials, in Mexico, most of the cancer research protocols involving molecular studies and the use of genomic tools are in the preclinical phases.

Most of the universities and the national institutes of health have the necessary infrastructure for conducting translational medicine, a practice that is spreading across the country, to incorporate advances of basic research into clinical research and practice (Lavalle-Montalvo, 2012; Mas-Oliva, Ninomiya-Alarcón, & García-Carrancá, 2007). In this context, identification of targeted mutations in tumor tissue for the use of a drug-specific therapy (molecular-targeted therapy) and genotyping of polymorphisms that confer increased or decreased susceptibility to cancer treatment (personalized medicine through pharmacogenomics) or that relate to a prognostic factor are the strategies that have involved molecular analysis and genetic aspects in clinical trials.

Another study group consists of clinical trials that target cancer diagnosis as a result of germ line mutations in a single gene that confer a hereditary genetic predisposition to develop cancer throughout life (predictive test). The related protocols are conducted according to the Declaration of Helsinki, GCP, and local ethical and legal requirements.

Obtaining DNA samples from tumor or peripheral blood requires a specific protocol stating that the use of the sample needs the previous approval from the local IRBs (ethical and research committees) and COFEPRIS. This type of research is conducted in public and private institutions located in the major cities throughout the country (centralization of healthcare system), so the protocol approval process should ensure that patients were fully informed about the study and have provided written consent.

The informed consent form must explain the purpose of the study in detail and with colloquial vocabulary. It must ensure the confidentiality of information obtained and the protection of the patient's identity (*Ley General de Salud* [General Health Law], 2013). IRBs approve protocols that specify the time during which DNA samples are stored and that clarify that if the samples are used for another study, a new and separate informed consent from patients is required each time samples are used.

Correlative Trials

Quality-of-Life Studies

In recent years, QOL studies have become part of the cancer research protocol. Usually, data for these studies are collected using the European Organisation for Research and Treatment of Cancer (EORTC) QOL questionnaires (QLQs). The study coordinator instructs patients on how to complete the questionnaire after they have given their consent for this part of the trial. The study coordinator emphasizes to patients the importance of gathering this information. When QLQs are generated outside the country (i.e., EORTC QLQ 30), validated and translated versions for Mexico should be used.

Pharmacoeconomic Studies

In 2004, the Mexican College of Pharmacoeconomics and Research (COMEFAE) began collaborating with the General Health Council and, in 2006, formed an alliance with the International Society for Pharmacoeconomics and Outcomes Research. COMEFAE members belong to the public, private, pharmaceutical industry, and academic sectors, and part of their mission is that of transferring pharmacoeconomic information and health outcomes of practice, ensuring that society gets the best knowledge to allocate scarce resources for health in a sensitive, fair, and efficient manner. These alliances support pharmacoeconomic studies for cancer diseases in Mexico.

Documentation and Data Management

When participating in the coordination of a clinical trial, the study staff is trained on protocol-specific data collection and provided with the necessary study materials. Such training includes the completion of CRFs and, where applicable, patient diary cards, QLQs, and any other questionnaires.

An extensive review of the CRF completion guidelines is performed with the study team. In addition, each site has its method to ensure the correct collection of required data. Commonly, the staff will create trial-specific worksheets based on the original CRFs and protocol schedule for investigations and procedures. These worksheets are included in patients' clinical charts, which are the source data documents, and treatment schedules are given to the investigator, co-investigator, and study nurse.

In commercial trials, electronic CRFs are the more common format. Data are entered into a specific database on a laptop or via a website, which allows the sponsor to have immediate access to the data. Nevertheless, some commercial trials still use paper CRFs. For academic trials, paper CRFs are used at the sites; this format is protocol-specific and allows the study site to have an original copy of the data. In both cases, electronic and paper CRFs, the study coordinator is the team member in charge of entering the data in the CRFs. The investigator or co-investigator reviews the CRFs before data are sent to the sponsor.

Information System Resources and Patient Support

The National Health System, through its public institutions and hospitals across the country, has a wide web of education, information, and patient support on cancer and clinical research. Private hospitals and clinical trial units are contributing to expand this web, with the purposes of (a) providing information about cancer types, prevention, cancer detection, and treatment alternatives, (b) giving comprehensive information about clinical trials, and (c) having sites dedicated to cancer treatment.

INCan created the first cancer information system, INFOCÁNCER (www.infocancer.org.mx), in Mexico, which is endorsed by the American Cancer Society. It provides information about cancer in Mexico through a call center, website, and information center. Topics include prevention and detection, types of cancer and treatment, help coping with the disease, and improvement in QOL for patients and their families, as well as the population in general.

The Cancer Network (*Red Contra el Cáncer*, www.redcontraelcancer.org.mx) was created in 2000 with the aim of providing a network of social and private assistance organizations working for the Mexican population's health and QOL. It is a site of interaction and interrelation of its members and the various sectors of the Mexican population, specifically in regard to the prevention, detection, care, and control of cancer, preferably for the benefit of vulnerable, poor populations and those without social security. Currently, this network comprises more than 45 organizations that perform several activities, some of which are mentioned in Figure 57-3.

Quality Assurance

According to the *Guidelines for Compliance With Good Clinical Practices in Health Research* (COFEPRIS, 2012),

Figure 57-3. Cancer Network Activities

- Preventive actions and care for breast, cervical, and uterine cancer and women's health in general
- Attention for all types of cancer, through economic and psychological support, drugs, treatments, devices, or prostheses
- Shelters for poor patients and relatives living outside México City
- Support for transplant or hemolytic anemia and iron-overload cases
- Attention and support for patients with leukemia, non-Hodgkin lymphoma, and laryngeal, gastric, and colorectal cancers

all the parties involved in a clinical research trial must adhere to the national and international ethical standards and ICH GCP.

Within the responsibilities and obligations stated, the principal investigator (PI) has the obligation of knowing and applying the established guidelines before, during, and after the conduct of the clinical trial. The sponsor will ensure and control the quality of the investigation and compliance with the research protocol and the standard operating procedures previously established, through monitoring visits, audits, and in some cases, reports derived from inspections or verifications of regulatory authorities.

The sponsor is responsible for performing study monitoring on a continuous basis according to the trial-specific plan. The PI must ensure that all of the site study documentation is available for review during the monitoring, quality control, and audit visits, as well as access to the hospital charts, archives, and pharmacy.

For academic study trials, the research group that originated the clinical trial must ensure that the study will be monitored and that quality control, quality assurance, and site audits are performed.

groups and participation in multicenter projects with international investigators and sites.

In Mexico, clinical trial units provide trial coordinators and data managers. When the trial is conducted at a public institution, human resources are not enough. Clinical trial units, contract research organizations, and pharmaceutical companies provide courses in ICH GCP and local and international guidelines and regulations that help to develop research staff in this field. Nowadays, contract research organizations and academic, public, and private institutions have implemented diploma courses for monitoring clinical trials.

Clinical research associates (CRAs), study coordinators, and data managers are medical students, physicians, any sciences professional (BSc, DDS, DVM, Nutritionist), and nurses who have been trained in a specific clinical research activity. For academic trials, physicians working as data managers have master of science degrees or are master's students trained in statistics and epidemiology.

Oncology nursing programs are available in three universities, offering specialization to nurses in oncology and research. They have tumor-related continuing education, which has brought forth more nurses interested in training as data managers/CRAs. Nurses participate in outpatient clinics, helping patients who are enrolled in clinical trials to better understand hospital processes, clarifying doubts, scheduling appointments, and administering different questionnaires. To achieve the best therapeutic adherence of patients, these nurses remain in touch with them and are part of the research team working with the investigator and the social worker.

The Oncology Nursing Society is interested in giving support and certification to nurses trained as data managers/CRAs. They are trained in cancer research with national university programs carried out in oncology national health institutions.

Professional Development

The National School of Nursing and Obstetrics (*Escuela Nacional de Enfermería y Obstetricia* [ENEO], www.eneo.unam.mx) was created in 1907, and by 1922, the nursing schools in Mexico were incorporated to the National Autonomous University of Mexico. Nursing and obstetrics was recognized as an academic career in 1966, leading to the implementation of postgraduate studies by the late 1990s. In recent years, the specialty of oncology nursing has been implemented by the National Autonomous University of Mexico and is imparted at INCan and other institutions within the country.

Since 1997, ENEO has been recognized as a Collaborating Centre of the World Health Organization and Pan American Health Organization for the development of professional nursing and promotes research work in

Summary

Currently, the participation of oncology nurses in clinical trials has been mainly in the active treatment process of study chemotherapy administration in only a nursing capacity. As for those trial-related activities that are performed by clinical trial nurses in other countries, in Mexico, they are carried out by study staff with other academic credentials and previously trained for these tasks. Sometimes, in the off-treatment periods, the PI assigns an oncology nurse for patient follow-up, but usually this activity is performed by a social worker.

However, although it is in an early stage, the process for developing clinical trial nurses has been started within the country with academic and research development programs. It is expected that in the near future, the knowledge and contribution of clinical trial nurses will be an advantage to the achievement of clinical trial goals.

Key Points

- Research contributes to the health strategic plans for the Mexican population.
- The achievement of a better QOL for the population is the goal of healthcare research in Mexico.
- Mexico is working to strengthen weak points in its health system.

References

Comisión Coordinadora de Instituciones Nacionales de Salud y Hospitales de Alta Especialidad [Coordinating Committee for National Health Institutions and High Specialty Hospitals]. (n.d.). Acerca de la C.C.I.N.S.H.A.E. [About the C.C.I.N.S.H.A.E.]. Retrieved from http://www.ccinshae.gob.mx/2012/acercade.html

Comisión Federal para la Protección contra Riesgos Sanitarios [Federal Commission for the Protection Against Sanitary Risk]. (2012). *Lineamientos para cumplir las buenas prácticas clínicas en la investigación para la salud* [Guidelines for compliance with good clinical practices in health research]. Retrieved from http://www.cofepris.gob.mx/AS/Documents/Protocolos%20de%20Investigacion/Lineamientos%20Bioequivalencia/Lineamientos%20BPC%2031052012.pdf

Comisión Nacional de Bioética [National Bioethics Commission]. (2012). *Guía nacional para la integración y funcionamiento de los comités de ética en investigación* [National guide for integration and functioning of research ethics committees]. Retrieved from http://www.conbioetica-mexico.salud.gob.mx/descargas/pdf/registrocomites/Guia_CEI.pdf

International Conference on Harmonisation of Technical Requirements for Registration of Pharmaceuticals for Human Use. (1996, July). *Good clinical practice*. Retrieved from http://ec.europa.eu/health/files/eudralex/vol-10/3cc1aen_en.pdf

Lavalle-Montalvo, C. (2012). Science in Mexico. *Cirugia y Cirujanos, 80*, 403–405.

Ley General de Salud [General Health Law]. (2013, April 13). Últimas reformas. *Diario Oficial de la Federación*. Retrieved from https://www.diputados.gob.mx/LeyesBiblio/pdf/142pdf

Mas-Oliva, J., Ninomiya-Alarcón, J., & García-Carrancá, A. (2007). *Advances in cancer research at UNAM*. Mexico City, Mexico: Manual Moderno.

Norma Oficial Mexicana [Official Mexican Standards]. (2013, January 4). NOM-012-SSA3-2012: Que establece los criterios para la ejecución de proyectos de investigación para la salud en seres humanos. *Diario Oficial de la Federación*. Retrieved from http://www.saludzac.gob.mx/site/images/stories/ensenanza/NOM001SSA32012.pdf

Regulatory Affairs in Latin America. (n.d.). Pharmacovigilance. Retrieved from http://latampharmara.com/mexico/pharmacovigilance

Subsecretaría de Prevención y Promoción de la Salud. (2013). Los 5 tipos de cáncer que más afectan a mexicanos. Retrieved from http://www.spps.gob.mx/noticias/1445-5-tipos-cancer-mas-afectan-mexicanos.html

Chapter 58

New Zealand

Belinda Egan, RN Dip Cert.

Introduction

As noted by the Ministry of Health (2014), "Cancer is a major health issue for all New Zealanders. One in three will have some experience of cancer, either personally or through a relative or friend." Although many advances have been made in reducing mortality rates, many challenges remain. This chapter describes features of clinical trials research in New Zealand (NZ) and the important developments that have been accomplished. It highlights the contributions made to improving public health outcomes and the pivotal role that the research nurse plays in achieving these goals.

History and Foundation

In NZ, six regional oncology centers provide medical oncology, radiation oncology, and hematology services. Radiation treatment is offered at all of these centers; however, some cancer chemotherapy and surgical services are offered in most other hospitals throughout the country.

The regional oncology centers are in Auckland, Hamilton, Palmerston North, Wellington, Christchurch, and Dunedin. Each of these centers has its own research unit. Before 1990, these research units were small, with only limited numbers of phase III clinical trials being carried out. Over time, with the development of newer drugs and more innovative treatments, the research units have expanded, and they now are running phase I, II, and III studies. These are primarily pharmaceutical–company sponsored and collaborative group studies.

The Health Research Council (HRC) of NZ is the main governing body that oversees research in NZ. Set up under the Health Research Council Act of 1990, the council's functions include advising the minister of health on health research; administering funds in relation to the national health research policy; fostering the recruitment, education, training, and retention of those engaged in health research in NZ; and initiating and supporting health research (HRC of NZ, 2002). HRC administers a number of committees, which provide advice on gene technology, accredit health and disability ethics committees and institutional ethics committees, monitor the safety of large clinical trials, and review applications to use new medicines in clinical trials.

As NZ's population is just slightly over four million, the majority of oncology clinical trials being conducted are initiated in other countries. The main collaborative groups, Australia and New Zealand Gynaecological Oncology Group (ANZGOG), Australasian Gastro-Intestinal Trials Group (AGITG), Trans Tasman Radiation Oncology Group (TROG), and Australia and New Zealand Breast Cancer Trials Group (ANZBCTG), are based in Australia; a number of oncologists and research nurses from NZ play an active role within each of these groups.

In 2003, Cancer Trials New Zealand (CTNZ) was established. This is a collaborative group whose main goal is to support investigator-driven research in phase I and II trials in NZ with an emphasis on supporting studies that have particular relevance to New Zealanders. It assists with concept development, protocol writing, trial development, and central coordination where necessary. CTNZ is also investigating establishing links among, and uses for, rare tumor registries, national clinical databases, and pathology repositories.

Clinical Trials: Fundamental Information

Legal and Regulatory Issues

Before a patient can be registered into a study, the clinical site must have obtained approval for the current protocol, and the local information, and consent form from the relevant ethics committee. Before 2012, NZ had six regional ethics committees and one multiregional ethics committee where all multicenter ethics application documents were submitted. One site would take on the role of *lead site* and would liaise with the ethics committee and the other participating sites. Since July 2012, the system has been changed and all applications are processed electronically.

Once an application and accompanying documentation has been submitted online, it is forwarded to one of four ethics committees. Each committee consists of at least eight members, of which three must be laypeople and at least one must have a recognized awareness of te reo Māori (Māori language) and understanding of tikanga Māori (Māori culture). These changes to the ethics submission process have improved the efficiency, consistency, and transparency of the NZ Health and Disability Ethics Committees (n.d.) review process.

To obtain final ethics approval in NZ, the researchers must receive approval from their local hospital management to run the study at that institution and receive approval from their local Māori committee. Each ethics application is sent to the local Māori research advisory committee, which ensures that the study is conducted according to the principles set out in the Treaty of Waitangi, signed February 6, 1840. These principles include the protection, participation, and partnership of Māori. The HRC guidelines (2002) state, "Practices and beliefs of an ethnic and/or religious nature must be fully respected. Research must be undertaken in a culturally sensitive and appropriate manner, in full discussion and partnership with the research participants whatever their ethnicity or religious affiliation" (p. 21).

If an application is made for research involving the clinical trial of a preregistration drug, an approval from the Standing Committee on Therapeutic Trials (SCOTT) is required. This committee provides recommendations to the director-general of health on the scientific validity of applications for clinical trials of new medicines. Section 30 of the Medicines Act (1981) empowers the director-general of health to allow the use of medicines that have yet to receive approval for registration in NZ in clinical trials for the purpose of obtaining clinical and scientific information. Trials involving postregistration medicines do not require the approval of SCOTT but still undergo the ethics committee review process (New Zealand Medicines and Medical Devices Safety Authority, 2012).

Once a study is open, the principal investigator is responsible for online forwarding of any amendments or changes to the patient information sheet or protocol to the ethics committee for reapproval before they can be used. Ethics committees require annual progress reports of each study until study completion.

Protocol Development, Review, and Approval

The processes involved in the decision to participate in a new clinical trial vary across centers, but the principles remain the same. New clinical trials are considered when a collaborative group or pharmaceutical company approaches oncology centers or investigators. Once a confidentiality agreement is signed, a synopsis is sent and reviewed. An external feasibility assessment is then completed and returned to the group or company. If the study is considered suitable, it is discussed at a clinical trials meeting, which includes oncologists, research staff, pharmacists, radiation therapy staff, and oncology nurses. An internal feasibility assessment is then completed to look specifically at the scientific question, potential patient numbers, allocation of resources, and research staff time required. Pharmaceutical companies may also conduct a site selection visit in order to review the site's facilities.

A study start-up meeting is organized by the sponsoring organization or company either in person or by teleconference. At the meeting, study-specific procedures are discussed with all relevant staff. This ensures that the trial conforms to the NZ guidelines for good clinical practice (GCP).

The NZ GCP guidelines are based upon the European Union, United Kingdom, Nordic, Australian, World Health Organization, and the Committee for Proprietary Medicinal Products guidelines and codes for GCP. GCP guidelines ensure that clinical studies involving human participants are designed and conducted to the highest scientific and ethical standards. The first edition was legislated in September 1996, and the third, and current, edition was legislated in January 2010.

The research nurse will prepare study documentation, study diaries, and patient information folders and will ensure that all staff members are educated about the specific treatment as outlined in the protocol.

Financial Factors

As part of the ethics process, the research nurse must ensure that the regulatory documentation and approvals are completed prior to commencing patient recruitment. This includes liaising with the legal department at the relevant district health boards to ensure that the trial is being carried out in accordance with NZ law and that appropriate indemnities are in place. If the ethics committee decides that the study is not being done for the benefit of a drug manufacturer, the trial will be covered under the accident compensation laws of NZ.

The accident compensation scheme provides coverage for injuries and accidents for all NZ citizens, residents, and temporary visitors, no matter who is at fault. This includes participants in a clinical trial. In return, people forgo the right to sue for personal injury, other than for exemplary damages. It is funded by government and a premium paid by all New Zealanders and is administered by the Accident Compensation Corporation (ACC). This is considered unique to NZ (ACC, n.d.).

To date, the majority of funding to run a clinical trial in New Zealand has come from the pharmaceutical company or collaborative group conducting the trial; however, increasingly this funding is insufficient. An investigator can apply for a grant sponsored by an organization, such as the Cancer Society of NZ or the Genesis Oncology Trust, for research funding to help run the trial. Funding, however, is not guaranteed.

Patients are made aware of current clinical trials through a variety of means, including direct contact with a specialist, information provided by the Cancer Society of NZ, and Internet resources. Participants are screened for recruitment in several ways, including the research nurse reviewing all new patient referrals and analyzing the database of the existing patient population. A study will be offered to potential participants when treatment options are discussed in the clinic setting. The fact that only six main study centers exist presents a barrier to recruitment in NZ. Patients who live far from these centers, which are based in NZ's six major cities, must agree to travel for all protocol-related procedures and treatment.

All patients with cancer in NZ are, however, equally assured of having access to health care should they decline participation in a study.

Clinical Trial Participants

Eligibility and Informed Consent

Eligibility criteria for each study are clearly stated in the protocol. The research nurse and the principal investigator for each specific study carry out assessment of participant eligibility. Assessments include the histologic/cytologic diagnosis, the medical history, previous treatments, a patient's performance status, and ability to comply with all study requirements. Various tests such as computed tomography scans and blood tests are performed to confirm eligibility. Genetic testing often is carried out on a patient's specific tumor to see if they are positive for certain biomarkers. Currently, many studies are looking at targeted therapies for specific biomarkers. Throughout this process, careful planning and coordination is required to ensure compliance with time frames stated in the protocol.

Once the eligibility criteria have been met, the study is discussed with the participants, and they are provided with written information to review and discuss with family (whanau). *Whanau* is the Māori word describing the close family links a person has with not just their immediate family but also with extended family of aunts, uncles, and grandparents. Patients are encouraged to bring their whanau to clinic appointments.

Informed consent is an ongoing process from the initial visit until completion of the trial. If the patient agrees to take part in the study, the patient and investigator sign a consent form. Special emphasis is placed on the collection of human tissue in NZ, as many Māori believe that their tissue is part of their extended family; therefore, they do not have the right to consent to it being sent away. Consent forms must contain a choice as to whether the patients agree to their tissue being used for research purposes (HRC, 2005; Sporle & Koea, 2004).

Separate guidelines and consents for children exist, and children are required to give their assent to participate where possible. When obtaining consent from older adults, special consideration is given to their comorbidities. Further explanation and time may be required to ensure their full understanding. All participants are encouraged to have a support person with them. Prisoners are treated no differently than the general population (HRC, 2005).

No study-specific tests may be performed before the signing of consent; however, once consent is obtained, baseline assessments can be carried out as per protocol. Education is then given to the patient, whanau, and friends about potential side effects of proposed treatment and any interactions that may occur with other concurrent medications. They also are advised of whom to contact in an emergency. At the initial and subsequent clinic visits, patients are questioned by the investigator and research nurse on their support network, how they are coping with the treatment, and whether they need help in any areas. As required, referrals to other disciplines are made, such as dietitians, social workers, and the palliative care team (HRC, 2002; Sporle & Koea, 2004).

Administration of Protocol Agents and Assessments

Drugs are prepared in a designated cytotoxic unit, where a research oncology pharmacist takes responsibility for the preparation, storage, handling, and distribution of the drug according to study protocols (Occupational Safety and Health Service, 1997).

Once a patient is randomized, he or she is scheduled for treatment, usually in the outpatient setting. Cytotoxic-credentialed nurses administer chemotherapy in NZ, whereas biologic agents are administered by non–cytotoxic credentialed staff. The research nurse is responsible for taking pharmacokinetic and study blood samples, electrocardiograms, and other prespecified tests during treatment.

Before each administration of the study drug, the investigator and oncology research nurse will see the patient in an outpatient clinic. Study-specific requirements will be carried out, blood results reviewed, and toxicities assessed and documented. A decision based on these assessments will then be made regarding continuing, dose modifying, or delaying treatment.

Side effects of treatment are assessed using the United States' National Cancer Institute Cancer Therapy Evaluation Program (2010) Common Terminology Criteria for Adverse Events (versions 3 [2006] used for older trials). Tumor assessments are carried out according to protocol timelines and are reviewed using Response Evaluation Criteria in Solid Tumors (known as RECIST) (European Organisation for Research and Treatment of Cancer [EORTC], 2014). All of this information is recorded in source documentation, which is then used to correctly complete case report forms (CRFs). The District Health Boards and Nursing Council of NZ have strict guidelines on documentation requirements, which must be followed in detail.

Many patients come to their first visit having searched the Internet for information about their disease or possible treatments. The research nurse is responsible for providing study-specific information that includes education about chemotherapy and its side effects and written instructions regarding what to do in case of an adverse event. Patients receive printed booklets, developed in conjunction with the Cancer Society of NZ. These cover a number of areas, including general information about chemotherapy, diet, exercise, and sexuality. Patients also have access to videos on radiation therapy and its side effects. Additionally, the mental and emotional well-being of patients and their families is addressed by providing information regarding wig consultants, the Look Good Feel Better NZ (n.d.) self-esteem course, accommodations, transportation, and appropriate support groups. Where appropriate, a referral to a genetic service is made.

Long-Term Follow-Up

Follow-up for a study is determined by the protocol, stating the data to be collected at each visit. All toxicities are followed post-treatment, and if a serious adverse event should occur within 30 days after treatment, it must be reported to the company or sponsoring group. Toxicities considered to be drug-related are followed until resolution. Follow-up visits usually take place in the oncology outpatient clinic; however, if a patient is from out of town, visits may take place in an oncology satellite clinic located in smaller cities and towns in NZ.

Any new data or updates on long-term side effects must be provided to patients at their next follow-up visit. If necessary, the patient will be reconsented, ensuring that he or she has received the full information. Patients are asked to explain back to the clinical trial nurse what they understand regarding any new information received.

Genetics and Genomics

Translational research is becoming increasingly common in clinical trials as more and more studies include targeted therapies. NZ plays a role, not only in the collection of samples for genetic and genomic testing overseas, but also through a number of groups studying the link between genetics and disease and genomic data. The University of Otago Centre for Translational Cancer Research (n.d.) is one such group. Some of their work includes investigating genes in breast cancer, the inherited susceptibility of gastric cancer, and genetic predictors of capecitabine toxicity. Specimen collection usually happens at the site that is carrying out the clinical trial and is stored there until the overseas company or group requests them. NZ has a number of tissue banks and contributes to a large number of them overseas. NZ differs from other countries because of researchers' approach to the specimen collection from Māori participants. Although Māori understand the benefits of genetic research to help identify genetic trends in their whanau, they see that it is in direct conflict with their cultural beliefs. It is for this reason that many NZ trials have two patient information sheets: a main consent to the study and an optional consent for translational research (Sporle & Koea, 2004).

Ancillary Studies

Increasingly, studies have ancillary components that are part of the main protocol. These may include quality of life, resource use, and optimism questionnaires, many of which are internationally validated tools (such as the EORTC QLQ-C30 quality-of-life questionnaire). Ethnicity data are collected for most studies, which then are used to target the future delivery of services.

Documentation and Data Management

One of the research nurse's main responsibilities is the entry of accurate documentation onto CRFs. Electronic CRFs are now more commonly used in preference over paper CRFs. Sponsoring company monitors visit on a regular basis to check that data recorded on CRFs are accurate and of high quality.

Randomization of patients is accomplished either by faxing directly to the sponsor (company or group) or by using a telephone interactive voice recognition or web-based system.

Other tools used to assist in the smooth running of clinical trials are newsletters, CRF completion guidelines, data management manuals, patient study diaries, PowerPoint presentations, and prompt cards for inclusion/exclusion criteria.

Quality Assurance

As in most countries, all drug company–sponsored trials are monitored on a regular basis. This is usually done after the first patient has started treatment and is carried out by either an independent monitoring company or a clinical research associate employed by them. Because monitoring takes place at the site on a six-week to three-month basis, the research nurse must ensure all CRFs are current and the source documentation is available. The investigator and pharmacist must be available for the monitoring visit if required. Collaborative groups tend not to do on-site monitoring because of the financial costs and travel required; therefore, they will monitor the electronic CRFs remotely or have the paper CRFs sent to them. Because there is not the regular on-site monitoring, the three main groups from Australia (AGITG, ANZBCTG, and ANZGOG) that carry out trials in NZ have an auditing program in place for all sites. An audit takes place over one to two days and includes meetings with the research nurse and the principal investigator at the beginning and end of the audit. An auditor will review three to four patients on that specific trial and will review all data, source documentation, and the site file for completeness, authenticity, and adherence to GCP guidelines.

Professional Development

The NZ Nurses Organization has a long-established cancer nurses' group and a research nurses' group, both of which hold annual conferences. Both groups provide their members with regular newsletters, online discussion groups, online resources, articles of interest, and access to resources.

The majority of research conferences, study meetings, and ongoing education are held in Australia or elsewhere. However, in 1999, the NZ Haematology/Oncology Research Coordinators held its first meeting, and in 2004, the NZ Association of Clinical Research held its inaugural conference. Both of these meetings are now annual events.

Research nurses in NZ have a number of opportunities for further study. This can be at a local level with in-service education and cytotoxic credentialing or at one of the universities to complete a postgraduate certificate, diploma, and master's in oncology and hematology nursing or clinical research.

Summary

By international standards, NZ is a small country, but the goal of conducting high-quality research, thereby reducing the impact and incidence of cancer, remains the same. In the past 10 years, a number of changes have occurred in the research field including the introduction of electronic CRFs, an increase in the amount of regulatory requirements, and changes in the types of drugs from chemotherapy alone to the addition of such agents as vascular disrupting agents and anti–vascular endothelial growth factor monoclonal antibodies. In addition, the current trend is moving toward individualizing treatment based on the study of gene mutations. As a result of the ever-changing face of research, nurses must ensure they continually improve skills and are aware of new treatments available for their patients. As a result of these changes, research nurses' role continues to be very rewarding.

Key Points

- Although NZ is a small country, it plays a pivotal role in cancer research with the six NZ oncology centers working collaboratively, thereby making an international impact on research.
- By participating in clinical trials, New Zealanders gain access to treatments not necessarily available in a country of this size.
- As a result of recent significant changes to the NZ ethical and legal requirements, New Zealanders are able to initiate clinical trials in an expedited fashion.

The author would like to acknowledge and thank Anne Smith, RN, BA, CNM, for her assistance with the writing of this chapter.

References

Accident Compensation Corporation. (n.d.). About ACC. Retrieved from http://www.acc.co.nz/about-acc/index.htm

European Organisation for Research and Treatment of Cancer. (2014, July 24). RECIST: Response Evaluation Criteria in Solid Tumors. Retrieved from http://www.eortc.org/investigators-area/recist

Health Research Council of New Zealand. (2005). *Guidelines on ethics in health research*. Retrieved from http://www.hrc.govt.nz/sites/default/files/HRC%20Guidelines%20on%20Ethics%20in%20Health%20Research.pdf

Look Good Feel Better New Zealand. (n.d.). Our workshops. Retrieved from http://www.lookgoodfeelbetter.co.nz/lgfb-in-action/our-workshops

Ministry of Health. (2014, June). Cancer programme. Retrieved from http://www.moh.govt.nz/cancercontrol

National Cancer Institute Cancer Therapy Evaluation Program. (2006). *Common terminology criteria for adverse events* [v.3.0]. Bethesda, MD: National Cancer Institute.

National Cancer Institute. (2010, June 14). *Common terminology criteria for adverse events* [v.4.03]. Retrieved from http://evs.nci.nih.gov/ftp1/CTCAE/CTCAE_4.03_2010-06-14_QuickReference_5x7.pdf

New Zealand Health and Disability Ethics Committee. (n.d.). Application forms and guidelines. Retrieved from http://ethics.health.govt.nz/ethical-standards-health-and-disability-research

New Zealand Medicines and Medical Devices Safety Authority. (2012). *Guideline on the regulation of therapeutic products in New Zealand. Part 11: Clinical trials—Regulatory approval and good clinical practice requirements* (1.3 ed.). Retrieved from http://www.medsafe.govt.nz/regulatory/Guideline/GRTPNZ/part11.doc

Occupational Safety and Health Service. (1997). *Guidelines for the safe handling of cytotoxic drugs and related waste*. Retrieved from http://www.business.govt.nz/worksafe/information-guidance/all-guidance-items/cytotoxic-drugs-and-related-wastes-guidelines-for-the-safe-handling-of/cytodrug.pdf

Sporle, A., & Koea, J. (2004). Māori responsiveness in health and medical research: Key issues for researchers (Part 1). *New Zealand Medical Journal, 117,* U1199.

University of Otago Centre for Translational Cancer Research. (n.d.). Centre for Translational Cancer Research: Translating research into healthcare. Retrieved from http://www.otago.ac.nz/ctcr

Chapter 59

Romania

Adriana Placintar, RN

Introduction

Clinical trials are essential for the improvement and development of methods of prevention, detection, and treatment of diseases. The primary objective of any trial is the identification of the most effective treatment with minimal side effects for patients.

In the early stages of clinical research, both civil society and the medical world expressed certain reserves in regard to the application of experimental treatments upon human subjects. There was a general apprehension caused by the impression that the patients were being used as "lab rats," that they were not sufficiently informed, that they were taken advantage of, that their rights were disregarded, and that obscure interests governed the research programs.

It was due to the sustained effort of a handful of courageous and visionary researchers who realized the importance of scientific pursuit that the medical field was able to progress. Their work ethics and scientific activity have constituted the main arguments for the use of clinical studies and patient recruitment as a generally accepted means of medical development. Since then, the Romanian legislation has been aligned to the European and international norms of conduct, making it impossible for a clinical study to be conducted without respecting the standards and principles provided by the Declaration of Helsinki and the International Conference on Harmonisation of Technical Requirements for Registration of Pharmaceuticals for Human Use (ICH) good clinical practice (GCP) guidelines.

The Romanian hospitals have created and adopted patient care protocols and have implemented the necessary treatment technology to satisfy demands for the practice of clinical studies. Medical staff must maintain certain professional standards to be able to participate in clinical trials, including developing practical abilities and being aware of the latest technical and scientific developments.

History and Foundation

The first controlled clinical trials in Romania were conducted by Professor Valentin Stroescu, who has led the Pharmacology Department of the Medical Faculty in Bucharest since 1974 and has been considered a reformer of pharmacologic study and a promoter of clinical pharmacology.

In 1999, approximately 40 clinical trials were conducted in Romania. Because of the experience acquired over time, the volume increased, reaching a current yearly average of 250 trials. According to data from the National Agency for Medicines and Medical Devices (*Agenția Națională a Medicamentului și a Dispozitivelor Medicale* [ANMDM]), Romania is currently occupying the 14th place of 25 European Union members. Phase III trials are the most frequent, and among the variety of tested drugs, the antineoplastics are reported to be the most common.

Statistical data collected in recent years place Romania among the countries with a moderate cancer-related mortality rate. The most frequent malignancies are lung, breast, colorectal, gastric, uterine cervix, prostate, liver, bladder, pancreatic, and ovarian cancers. The cancer-related mortality rate has been slowly but progressively increasing. This tendency is explained by the process of demographic aging and the evolution of socioeconomic factors, with an especially large risk detected in highly urbanized and industrialized environments. Recent statistics have shown that pulmonary cancer has the highest mortality rate in men, followed by colorectal, prostate, stomach, and bladder cancers. In women, the most prevalent cause of cancer death is breast cancer, followed by malignant tumors of the genital tract (the uterus, the ovary), colorectal cancer, and bronchopulmonary cancer.

The number of patients who have benefited from systemic treatment (chemotherapy, hormone therapy, cytokines, and molecular-targeted therapy) subsidized through the Romanian National Program of Oncology has steadily grown from 75,000 patients in 2007 to

96,700 in 2010. Approximately 3,400 patients are treated yearly with expensive molecules, with the approval of the National Commission of Oncology.

The climate in Romanian cancer research is influenced by several factors—economic, political, and scientific—and the country has developed an increasing presence in international trials, high recruitment potential, and increasingly experienced investigators. Clinical research is vital to the development and improvement of preventive measures, as well as methods of detection and treatment.

Clinical Trials: Fundamental Information

The aim of clinical trials is to demonstrate the validity and efficiency of a medical therapy. In Romania, the clinical evaluation of drugs meant for human consumption and with therapeutic purposes can be conducted exclusively in medical units with a profile that is appropriate to the research objectives proposed to the Ministry of Health. The network of hospital units with an oncologic profile is composed of three National Oncologic Institutes that are placed within the nation's three main academic centers (Bucharest, Cluj-Napoca, and Iași), county or municipal hospital departments, and private treatment and diagnosis centers.

The Ministry of Health grants authorization for clinical studies with therapeutic benefits, at the request of the research units, after checking the following documents.

- Sanitary permit that attests to the medical units' rights to function
- The medical personnel's legal authorization to practice medicine and be involved in clinical trials
- Documents that attest to the existence of an internal system capable of evaluating and securing the quality of the clinical trials
- A list with the names of the main investigators, including confirmation of medical titles and the personnel's curricula vitae
- The existence of a competent emergency service or a contractual agreement with medical units able to offer such services

ANMDM is the competent authority in the field of pharmaceutical products intended for human consumption and, alongside other legal attributions, has the responsibility of authorizing the conduct of clinical trials and evaluating and monitoring their quality. The clinical trials that are conducted on Romanian territory are authorized by ANMDM in accordance with the 95/2006 law regarding reform in the medical field.

To obtain the authorization needed to initiate a clinical trial, ANMDM must confirm that the provisions of the Ministry of Public Health's Order No. 904/2006 regarding the norms that must be upheld during the conduct of clinical trials with the purpose of human consumption are respected. This government order is aligned to Directive 2001/20/CE approved by the European Parliament and the European Council on 4th of April, 2001, regarding the harmonization of all legislation, regulation, and administrative measures of member states referring to the implementation of norms meant to regulate the practice of clinical trials. The clinical research provisions must also be respected by the Committee for Drug Patents adopted through ANMDM Hotărârea Consiliului Științific (HCS) No. 39/2006, alongside the European legislation and directives.

From a procedural perspective, the pharmaceutical producer (the sponsor) addresses a request to ANMDM for approval to conduct clinical trials as a first step toward marketing the product. According to ANMDM HCS No. 22/Sept. 2001, the sponsor must provide the following documents.

- Letter of intention, which must contain the EudraCT number, the protocol number, and the name of the trial and must underline the special characteristics of the trial
- The request form needed to authorize a clinical trial
- The study protocol
- The pharmaceutical product's file for clinical investigation
- The file of the noninvestigated drugs used during the study

The request form must be accompanied by the form containing the qualifications of each of the main investigators and their written commitment to participate in the study.

A clinical trial may be initiated only after ANMDM has authorized it. In the case of multicenter trials, the National Ethics Commission must give its approval. In the case of single-center trials, the approval of the Institutional Ethics Commission is needed.

The National Ethics Commission is an independent organization that is composed of professionals from the medical field and individuals who are not necessarily in the medical field. The main attributions of the commission are the protection of the rights, safety, and comfort of the clinical trial participants and the reassurance of this protection to the public. This occurs by evaluating the protocol of the trial, the aptitudes of the investigators, and the quality of the facilities involved in the study, as well as the methods and documents used to inform the participants and obtain their consent and involvement.

The Institutional Ethics Commission is an independent organization formed of medical and research specialists and individuals without medical training, whose main function is to secure the protection of the rights, safety, and comfort of the subjects involved in the study. The commission evaluates, gives approval, and verifies the study's protocol and the methods and materials used in obtaining the study subjects' consent to participate.

The essential documents for undergoing a clinical study are those that, individually and collectively, permit the evaluation of the study and the quality of the obtained data. These documents are necessary to demonstrate that the investigators, the sponsor, and monitors have respected all existing legal regulations. The responsible completion of these documents can be a contributing factor to the success of the study. They are then verified by an independent agent of the sponsor and by the ANMDM as a part of the validation process.

These documents are categorized in three groups depending on the phase undergone by the clinical study: (a) before initiating the clinical phase of the study, (b) during the clinical phase of the study, and (c) after the end of the clinical study. See Figure 59-1 for documents required before initiating a study.

Protocol Development, Review, and Approval

The Research Team

Principal investigators are either doctors or individuals in a profession that is compatible with organizing a clinical study, according to the existing legislation, resulting from their scientific qualifications and experiences in the field of patient care. They are responsible for the conduct of the clinical study, and if a number of specialists are involved, they also are considered the team leader. Principal investigators must confirm that all the staff participating in the study are adequately informed regarding the protocol, investigational product, and individual tasks and functions. They ensure that the criteria regarding informed consent, inclusion and exclusion of the subjects, administration of the product, and communication with the Ethics Commission are satisfied. They are responsible for obtaining, recording and transmitting the correct information. They are obligated to allow local authorities to inspect the facilities and the proceedings, to respect the approved protocol, and to perform immediate notification regarding any adverse events as required. Investigators must ensure that the administration and handling of the investigational drug are in accordance with the provisions required by the protocol and added sources of information provided by the sponsor. Their team must contain an adequate number of qualified people, as well as the necessary technology and facilities needed for the duration of the study for it to be conducted in a safe and efficient manner.

The main investigator assigns the nurses who are working in the study and designates their individual responsibilities. The medical nurse must have the necessary qualifications, experience, and availability to manage and administer the drugs and to assess and manage the potential side effects.

Informed Consent

One of the fundamental conditions for participating in a clinical study is the informed consent of the participants. Prior to obtaining consent, the investigator must provide the patient with information regarding the study using a nontechnical and accessible language.

Figure 59-1. Documents Produced Before Initiating the Clinical Phase of a Trial

- The investigator's brochure—a compilation of clinical and nonclinical data regarding the drug that is being tested. The purpose is to showcase the importance of certain essential aspects of the protocol, such as the dosage, the frequency of the dosage, the method of administration, and the monitoring procedures.
- The signed protocol, the amendments, if there are any, and the report form model
- All information given to participants in the study, including the consent form, in all the languages it might be distributed in, and all written information and any advertisements intended for recruitment
- The financial status of the study
- Insurance documentation to confirm that participants will be compensated in case the measures taken in the study affect their health
- The signed contract between the parties involved in the study
- The approval from the Ethics Commission
- The structure of the Ethics Commission
- National Agency for Medicines and Medical Devices approval
- Any relevant documentation that will attest to the qualification of the investigators
- The normal values/limits for the procedures and tests
- The certification of the laboratory
- Samples of the drug's container with the appropriate classification on it
- Instructions for use of the drug intended for clinical study and of the materials involved in the study
- The recordings of the investigational drug and transportation of the necessary materials
- The analysis certificate for the transported investigational drug
- The decoding procedures for blinded studies
- The basic list for randomization
- The monitoring report done before initiating the study
- The monitoring report regarding the initiation of the study

The investigator must obtain a signed informed consent form from all participants or their individual legal representatives before initiating any clinical trial procedures. The form must be signed and dated personally by either the subject or the subject's legal representative and by the investigator. The written informed consent form must contain information regarding
- The nature, objective, and duration of the study
- The risks and benefits
- Alternative treatments available to the patient
- Existing legal procedures in connection to the study
- Financial compensation
- Confidentiality
- The rights of the patient
- Whom to contact in case of any unexpected event.

The investigator must make available to patients or their legal representative a copy of the consent form and additional information relevant to the study, written in a nontechnical and accessible manner. The signing of the informed consent form is confirmed by the investigator in the case report form (CRF) or electronic case report form (eCRF).

Financial Factors

In Romania, several academic grants are available where the capital to conduct clinical trials is assured by the universities, and phase I studies are usually financed by the pharmaceutical industry. Most clinical studies are international multicenter studies. Depending on the financial agreements signed prior to the initiation of the study, the sponsor often secures resources for
- The medication used during the study
- Investigations relevant to the study
- The transportation expenses of the participants
- The medical insurance for any possible damage inflicted on the participants resulting from the administration of the test drugs or any other medical procedure conducted within the study.

The drugs used in parallel to the tested drugs and medical care often are provided by the national health system.

Recruitment and Retention

No registry of clinical studies currently exists in Romania, although it has been solicited by both the Association of Federations of Cancer Patients and the general medical community. Most of the hospitals specializing in oncologic treatment have a list of ongoing clinical trials displayed on their websites, which includes the trial type, duration, and participating staff. The pharmaceutical companies that conduct clinical trials make this information available on their websites.

Generally, there is a close collaboration between medical professionals of different specializations (e.g., surgery, radiation therapy, radiodiagnostics, chemotherapy) who guide eligible patients toward appropriate trials.

Clinical Trial Participants

The clinical study nurse may be delegated assignments depending on the decision of the principal investigator (see Figure 59-2). To be considered eligible for participation in a clinical trial, patients must be able to comprehend the informed consent form and meet the basic eligibility criteria of the study, including age, prior treatment, and type of illness. It is important to note that patients retain the right to withdraw from the trial at any point.

Adverse events (AEs) are defined as unforeseen medical incidents occurring during the patient's treatment within the framework of a clinical trial. All AEs are recorded, both in the source documents as well as in the report forms, in a detailed manner using standard medical terminology. Serious adverse events (SAEs) are defined as any AE occurring during the patient's treatment that (a) justifies the initiation or extension of intensive medical care, (b) produces congenital anomalies, (c) puts the life of the patient in jeopardy, (d) may produce physical disability, or (e) leads to the death of the patient.

Investigators are responsible for informing the sponsor of all occurring SAEs. SAE forms must be completed

---

Figure 59-2. Examples of Clinical Study Nurse Assignments From the Principal Investigator

- **Observing and recording the patient's vital signs.** To do this, nurses must be able to ensure that all monitoring systems are functioning properly.
- **Obtaining, processing, and sending biologic samples to the laboratory for further study.** Study nurses must be able to perform venipuncture so that patients are neither traumatized nor disturbed; they must process the samples correctly, according to the specifications of the manual, and contain them in an adequate manner until they are sent to the laboratory. They must correctly document the requisition form to avoid creating confusion or produce erroneous results.
- **Stocking, preparing, and administering the study drug, supervising patients, and managing the side effects efficiently, respecting the norms imposed by the manufacturer.** Study nurses must follow the protocol and the indications of the investigator when preparing and administering treatment. The drug accountability log, the drug preparation log, and all of the documentation regarding the drug from the study file must be updated periodically.
- **Study nurses bear a great responsibility because of all of the members of the medical personnel, they are the closest link to patients. It is on their qualifications and communication skills that the comfort and compliance of patients depend.**

in great detail, avoiding unnecessary abbreviations and using standard medical terms.

Genetics and Genomics

According to several studies, almost one-third of reported cancer cases involve a genetic predisposition, which may be detected through familial medical history or genetic tests allowing the implementation of effective prophylactic measures. In the field of pharmacogenomics, genetic information is used to better understand why different individuals respond differently to the same medication by studying the genetic variations that produce a specific reaction to the drug. The main goals are to develop safer and more effective drugs and to improve their administration to the patients. For pharmacogenomic studies to be conducted efficiently, systematic DNA testing is necessary.

In Romania, numerous clinical studies involve genomic research. Genetic material may be collected only after patients sign an additional informed consent form expressing their approval of the procedure.

Correlative Trials

In Romania, patients entering a treatment clinical trial are frequently presented with quality-of-life (QOL) questionnaires to enable the medical staff to better assess the impact of the illness and treatment. Generally, QOL questions tend to refer to (a) mobility and independence in undergoing daily activities, (b) pain intensity, and (c) psychological state. The QOL questionnaires are attached to the CRF/eCRF documents.

Documentation and Data Management

Every patient treated and investigated for a cancer-related medical issue is the subject of a clinical observation chart, which contains the following information: identification data, case history, informed consent, past clinical investigations, height, weight, parallel symptoms and treatments, and the applied therapeutic procedures. All those involved in the investigation and care of the patient (e.g., medical nurses or doctors) have access to the clinical observation chart and must add to it the proper additional information.

The data collected from the patients are recorded in the CRFs/eCRFs. The aim is to obtain a complete record of the necessary data using standard medical language. In the case of CRFs/eCRFs, the data are recorded by those members of the medical staff who have been assigned to this task by the main investigator. The information must be transmitted to the sponsor or the designated contract research organization. It is then evaluated and processed to protect the anonymity of the subject. The investigator must ensure that the data transmitted to the sponsor do not contain any mention of the patient's name. The investigator verifies the data for accuracy and completeness before they are transmitted to the sponsor. The source documents and the CRFs/eCRFs are periodically checked by an appointed monitor. It is the duty of the investigator to preserve all relevant documentation connected to the clinical trial for 15–20 years, depending on the sponsor's demands and the internal politics of the hospital.

Quality Assurance

ANMDM grants authorization to sponsors to conduct clinical trials on a certain medical therapy. Sponsors are responsible for implementing and maintaining the system of insurance and quality control based on the standard operating procedures adopted. This guarantees that the development of the studies and the process of obtaining, recording, and reporting data are coordinated with the protocol and legal regulations. Sponsors may transfer functions to a contract research organization, but the final responsibility for the integrity and quality of the recorded data is always attributed to the sponsor. The choice of partner in such cases resides with the sponsor as an exclusive executive prerogative; ANMDM does not have any decisional power. Also, sponsors support all financial costs connected to the proceedings.

During the clinical study, any change or actualization must be added to the collection of already existing documents to prove that investigators are constantly receiving relevant information as it becomes accessible. Documentation of the following also must exist.

- The record of the monitor's visit and observations
- Other relevant contacts to underline, along with certain documentation, any essential discussion regarding the way the study is proceeding
- The consent forms, dated and signed, to prove that consent had been given before the start of the clinical study in accordance to the GCP regulation
- Source documents to prove the existence of the subject and the integrity of the data collected
- The signed and dated report form for the completed case
- The record of corrections made to the case report
- The report sent to the sponsor by the investigator regarding potential SAEs
- Information regarding the safety and well-being of the subject, transmitted by the sponsor to the investigator
- Intermediary or annual reports made to ANMDM and any other required recipients

- The table with the names of the subjects intended for the selection process
- List of the subjects' identification codes
- List of selected subjects
- Administration of the investigational drug at the designated place of study
- The record of the signature samples

After the study's conclusion, all documents must be stored with the following.

- The accountability log
- Documentation regarding the disposal of the unused investigational drug
- The list of identification codes attributed to the patients
- Audit certificate
- Report regarding the act of monitoring the closure of the study
- The investigator's final report addressed to ANMDM and any other required recipients
- The clinical report where the results of the study are recorded and interpreted

Professional Development

Today, two basic types of medical education are available for nurses in Romania: (a) postgraduate sanitary school, which is three years, and (b) medical college for nurses, which is four years. To work in the medical field, graduates of the specialized schools must have a membership certificate released by the Order of Generalist Medical Nurses, Midwives and Medical Nurses of Romania (*Ordinul Asistenților Medicali Generaliști, Moașelor și Asistenților Medicali din România* [OAMGMAMR]). The certificate is initially issued by the county representative of OAMGMAMR. It is reconfirmed yearly after the completion of the civil responsibility insurance report for potential mistakes in the individual's professional conduct and with the condition that the individual has accumulated the necessary 30 credits on a yearly basis.

In addition to the courses and the annual congress organized by OAMGMAMR, medical nurses who work in oncology have access to specialized training programs. In recent years, the Romanian Society of Radiotherapy and Medical Oncology compiled a section dedicated to nurses where informative courses are provided regarding new techniques applied in the field and GCP.

The curricula vitae of nurses applying for a position within a clinical study must contain their qualifications, professional experience, and experience in clinical studies, as well as the specialization courses attended. All of these details are confirmed by official documentation.

Summary

Clinical trial protocols are created with great care, with patient safety as an essential priority. Participants have access to the latest breakthroughs in the medical treatment of their conditions and are closely observed, often more frequently than patients receiving standard care.

Clinical trials are strictly controlled, starting from the implementation of the protocol through its duration, so as to respect participants' rights to the best medical care, as stated in the Declaration of Helsinki. Documents and clinical study procedures can be checked at any time by both national and international institutions that oversee their functioning.

Medical personnel involved in clinical studies must be professionally well prepared and apply the principles of ICH GCP. Hospitals in which studies are held must meet strict standards regarding patient care and observation of the medical study participants.

In conclusion, clinical trials have contributed to the elevation of legislative standards and treatment of patients with cancer and to the increase in scientific and professional capabilities of medical personnel in Romania.

Key Points
- Romanian hospitals have the protocols and treatment technology to conduct clinical trials.
- The Ministry of Health oversees clinical research in Romania.
- Informed consent is obtained in accordance with ICH GCP.
- Clinical trial/research nurses are only just beginning to have roles and opportunities in clinical research.

Chapter 60

Spain

Gema Piqueres Zafra, CTN, Marisa Teruel López, CTN, Irene Fernández-Bravo Del Olmo, CTN, and Susana Baviera Rincón, CTN

Introduction

A clinical trial is any experimental investigation of a substance or medicine and the study of its administration in human beings. This scientific process is used to evaluate new interventions or new indications for previously approved interventions; however, access to the intervention may be restricted to clinical trial participants (Oncology Nursing Society [ONS], 2010).

The significance of clinical investigations in Spain has increased greatly in recent decades, especially from 1979 to the present. There has been an increase from about 10 research units to more than 150 research units in different clinical hospitals sites and other health centers throughout the country. The specific types of personnel involved at individual institutions will depend on the requirements of the trials and the resources of the institution (ONS, 2010).

History and Foundation

The specialty of medical oncology was officially recognized in Spain in 1981. Thereafter, the Spanish Society of Medical Oncology (*Sociedad Española de Oncología Médica* [SEOM]) was created with support from the Ministry of Health. The legalization and legislation of certain aspects of human and animal research began in 1994 with Act No. 41/2002 of 14 November (Ley 41/2002), regulating action on patient autonomy and on the rights and obligations in matters of clinical information and documentation:

> The regulation of the right to protection of health, contained in Article 43 of the 1978 Constitution, the materialization of the rights relating to the clinical information and individual autonomy of patients in relation to their health, has been the subject of a basic regulation at the State level, by means of the General Health Act 14/1986 of 25 April.

Currently, there is global interest in cancer research because of increased cancer incidence. This research is carried out in two branches: clinical and genetic.

Clinical Trials: Fundamental Information

Spanish Medicines Agency

The Spanish Agency of Medicines and Medical Devices (*Agencia Española de Medicamentos y Productos Sanitarios* [AEMPS]) was created as an agency of the Ministry of Health and Consumer Affairs. It guarantees the quality, safety, and efficacy of medical devices marketed in Spain to the general population. AEMPS has a dual responsibility: to act as the authority that oversees Spanish public health and to act within the European Agency Network with the European Medicines Agency.

As a health authority, AEMPS undertakes the responsibilities for medicines and medical devices that the Spanish Constitution attributes to the general administration of the State. As such, in accordance with Act No. 29/2006 (Ley 29/2006), it conducts, *inter alia*,

- Authorization and inspection of pharmaceutical companies
- Authorization after checking the quality conditions of medicines and medical devices
- Surveillance of adverse reactions during the product's use
- Continuous risk-benefit assessment of marketed products
- Control of illegal or counterfeit medical devices
- Facilitation of the introduction of new effective medicines for diseases for which current drugs are inade-

quate, and the safest possible access to these medicines by patients
- Allowing the submission of electronic clinical trial applications that provide updated and follow-up data
- Transmitting necessary information at the European level
- Exchanging information with the Independent Ethics Committees (IECs) and autonomous communities and supporting the public clinical trial registry
- Scheduling inspections and pharmacovigilance of clinical trials to ensure data reliability and quality
- Streamlining processing and facilitating access to compassionate-use medicines or foreign medicines according to therapeutic needs.

AEMPS includes an IEC that harmonizes inspection procedures and criteria of good clinical practice (GCP).

Types of Clinical Research

The development of research in Spanish society occurs in several ways: intramural research, cooperative research, pharmaceutical industry research, and care research.

Intramural research is conducted at the actual site with its own funding. This type of research can sometimes include a joint sponsorship; for example, the same project may receive two or more sponsors who may be public (through grants) or private (through foundations or associations).

Cooperative research includes regional groups (of little relevance) and national cooperative groups—professional nonprofit associations that aim at promoting the study and research of certain diseases. They encourage and sponsor clinical research through GCP and the ongoing training of its members to increase the quality of the research. They also play an important role in the development and efficacy of new drugs.

Some Spanish groups with international significance are GEICO, GEICAM, GEIS, GECP, SOGUG, SOLTI (Innovative Breast Cancer Research), TTD, TCTC, and PSAMOMA, and new groups are constantly being added. SEOM works with all cooperative groups and aims at encouraging the study and research of cancer and the official approval of the various therapeutic criteria in its diagnosis. International collaboration (e.g., European Organisation for Research and Treatment of Cancer, Gynecologic Oncology Group) is necessary for the development of scientific knowledge.

Pharmaceutical industry research has a significant economic impact on clinical cancer research. Care research includes supportive treatments and palliative care.

Types of Clinical Trials

The various clinical trials can be classified according to objectives, design methodology, number of sites, and blinding. Classification based on objectives includes the following (Camps & Guillem, 2008).
- Phase I trials, which are conducted to determine the toxicity profile. There are few in Spain, but they are on the rise.
- Phase II trials, which assess the level of antitumor drug activity. Only 14% of phase II clinical trials are positive in oncology (Booth, Glassman, & Ma, 2003).
- Phase III trials, which compare a drug or drug combination with standard treatment. The result of phase III trials changes the outlook of cancer therapeutics.
- Phase IV trials, which are confirmatory studies or those with primary objectives.

Protocol Development, Review, and Approval

Protocol Approval

Clinical trials to be performed in Spain require prior authorization from the Ministry of Health and Consumer Affairs, specifically AEMPS, as stated in Royal Decree 520/1999 of 26 March, *Official State Gazette* (*Boletín Oficial del Estado*) of 31 March, approving the Charter of AEMPS: "This authorisation shall take place in the midst of the process with the qualification of the investigational medicinal product." For authorization, the accredited prior report of the IEC shall be required (Article 15 of Royal Decree 223/2004 and Article 64 of the Medicinal Products Act).

Article 8 of Royal Decree 561/1993 specifies the 12 basic sections of a clinical trial protocol: synopsis, contents, general information, rationale and objectives, type and design of clinical trial, selection of subjects, description of treatment, conduct of the trial and response assessment, adverse events, ethical considerations, practical considerations, and statistical analysis. Additional documents required include the case report form (CRF) data, the investigator's brochure, standard operating procedures, and report of analytical samples used (Ministerio de Sanidad y Consumo, 1993).

Independent Ethics Committees

The first European IECs appeared in 1975, thanks to scientific and medical groups influenced by those in the United States that alerted society of the risks of new biotechnologies used in medicine. This resulted in the formation of the National Bioethics Committees.

The term *IEC* is defined in Article 2, Chapter 1 of Royal Decree 223/2004:

> An independent body, consisting of healthcare professionals and nonmedical members, whose responsibility it is to protect the

rights, safety and well-being of human subjects involved in a trial and to provide public assurance of that protection . . . by expressing an opinion on the trial protocol, the suitability of the investigators and the adequacy of the facilities, and on the methods and documents to be used to inform trial subjects and obtain their informed consent.

For multicenter clinical trials, the IEC responsible for issuing the opinion is called the Reference Independent Ethics Committee.

IECs should have a minimum of nine members (to ensure a majority in their decisions), including a pharmacologist, a pharmacist, and a nurse, and at least one member must be independent of the sites where the research projects that require ethical review by the committee are to be carried out. The presence of at least two non–healthcare professionals is also required, one of whom must have a degree in law. They must be competent and experienced in relation to the methodologic, ethical, and legal aspects of research, pharmacology, and clinical practice.

In Spain, IECs will be accredited by the competent health authorities in each Autonomous Community. Such accreditation will be renewed periodically and reported to AEMPS and IEC coordination center.

Functions

The reference IEC and the local IECs have different roles. The reference IEC's role is to determine
- Relevance of the clinical trial, taking into account the available knowledge
- Relevance of its design to obtain reasoned conclusions with an adequate number of subjects in relation to the study objective
- Selection criteria, withdrawal of trial subjects, and equitable selection of the sample
- Justification of predictable risks and inconveniences in relation to anticipated benefits for trial subjects, other patients, and the community
- Justification of the control group (either placebo or active treatment)
- Plans for monitoring the trial
- Suitability of written information for trial subjects and the procedure for obtaining informed consent, as well as justification of research on people who are unable to give informed consent
- Insurance or financial guarantee planned for the trial
- Plan for the recruitment of subjects
- Where appropriate, planned remuneration or compensation for investigators and trial subjects
- Suitability of the investigator and subinvestigators (at the site)
- Suitability of the facilities (at the site).

The local IEC is responsible for assessing the suitability of the research team and facilities for conducting the trial. It must prepare a report for the reference IEC, assessing the following.
- Suitability of the investigator and subinvestigators: Qualification, accreditation of training in GCP standards, participation in other trials, previous inspection and audit results, experience in the type of patients who are to undergo the research, and publications in the field of the research are aspects to be considered.
- Suitability of the facilities: The local IEC will take into account the quality of the facilities necessary for the proper conduct of the clinical trial (e.g., human resources, laboratories, imaging methods), paying particular attention to the facilities required to perform procedures or follow-up different from those in routine clinical practice.
- Notifications of serious and unexpected adverse events that have occurred in Spain and any information involving a significant change in the safety profile of the investigational product: This information is forwarded to AEMPS, which is responsible for assessing it and also has access to information at the European level. As such, the local IEC may delegate the ability to alert to AEMPS.

The reference IEC is not responsible for monitoring the progress of the trial at each site, whereas the local IEC must know the progress of the trial in its area.

Conflicts of Interest

Pursuant to article 4 of Act No. 25/1990 of 20 December on Medicines (Ley 25/1990), belonging to an IEC shall be incompatible with any kind of interest arising from the manufacture and sale of medicines and medical devices (Camí, 1995). If the principal investigator (PI) has any direct personal relationship with any of the parties involved, this should be reported.

The adoption of Act and Royal Decree 561/1993 on clinical trials laid the groundwork for the normalization of economic relations between sponsors and research sites:

> All economic aspects related to the clinical trial should be reflected in a contract between each site where the trial is to be conducted and the sponsor . . . the contract shall contain the initial budget for the trial, specifying the indirect costs that apply to the site and special direct costs, considering as such expenses other than those that would have been incurred if the subject had not participated in the trial, such as additional laboratory tests and examinations, changes in the duration of care for patients, reimbursement of costs incurred by patients, purchase of equipment and compensation for trial subjects and investigators. It shall also include the terms and conditions of payments and any other secondary liability agreed

upon by both parties. (Ministerio de Sanidad y Consumo, 1993, Article 20 of Royal Decree 561/1993 of 16 April)

Financial Factors

Health care in Spain is characterized as being public health care. This means that an attempt is made to ensure the health of the entire population with the same services. An additional private health system exists, which people can access by paying for a policy.

Management and Finance Unit

The Spanish National Research and Development Plan, which is public, began in 1988. A major part of this plan is intended for cancer research. Health Research Fund grants also are available, which finance both basic and clinical research projects. Projects mainly concern the fields of epidemiology, prevention, and identification of risk factors and diagnostic methods. Pharmaceutical companies develop research projects on the therapeutic effects of their drugs in the treatment of tumors (López-Otín, 2001).

The creation of foundations opened a new avenue of funding for research on cancer and other diseases. These include the Cancer Association Foundation, the Ramón Areces Foundation, the Mutua Madrileña Foundation, and the Clinical Research Foundation of the Valencian Institute of Oncology. Foundations support economic management and the streamlining of contracts between sponsors and PIs. They are nonprofit organizations that must meet the general interest for which they were created. In this case, the interest is the development of clinical research, and its beneficiaries are generic communities of people (the beneficiaries will be selected with impartiality, nondiscrimination, and objectivity criteria according to the selection rules). Foundations are governed by state and regional legislation. See Figures 60-1 and 60-2 for information about foundations.

Insurance and Financial Guarantee

A clinical trial with investigational medicinal products can only be conducted if insurance or another financial guarantee has previously been taken out to cover any damages that may occur to study participants as a result of the trial. The sponsor is responsible for taking out liability insurance or a financial guarantee for the sponsor, PI, subinvestigators, and the hospital or site where the clinical trial will be conducted. If such insurance or financial guarantee is not taken out or does not fully cover the damages, the sponsor, PI, hospital, or site where the trial will be conducted will be held responsible. From the

Figure 60-1. Management Structure and Support of a Foundation

- Management and administration area
- Marketing and communications area
- Information technology department
- Legal department
- Quality area
- Translation unit (publication support)
- Project management and transfer office of research results

Figure 60-2. Support Department to the Foundation

- Animal experimentation and experimental surgery
- Radioisotope laboratory
- Epidemiology and methodology unit
- Genomics and proteomics unit
- Cell biology unit
- Biobanks
- Imaging unit
- Clinical trial area
- Library

year following the termination of the trial, patients are responsible for proving the relationship between the trial and the damage.

Recruitment and Retention

Patients already diagnosed with any type of cancer are treated in different oncology units of public or private hospitals, but not all hospitals have clinical trial units, nor are the same trials conducted at these units. Therefore, some patients are recruited by hospital investigators, whereas others are referred by various oncologists of other hospitals who are aware of new therapeutic lines within trials. In addition, the media (e.g., press, television, Internet) provide patients with basic information about clinical trials and new treatments that are developed in each hospital. Patients may then request additional information.

Clinical Trial Participants

In Spain, the selection of patients depends exclusively on PIs and their subinvestigators. Depending on the institution, selection can be conducted in different ways: from the clinical sessions for each condition or directly from a consultation. After selecting patients, the investigator asks them whether they would like to take part in the trial. After patients sign the informed consent form, they undergo the screening tests prescribed for each trial. Once the subject's eligibility is confirmed, the nurse/clinical trial coordinator and investigator schedule the visits and tests necessary for the conduct of the protocol.

Clinical trial nurses (CTNs) play an important role as a liaison between the investigator, sponsor, and patient. They act as support for patients and their families in achieving quality of life, giving advice on how to take the medication, and informing them about adverse effects. On some occasions, CTNs administer the study treatment; at other times, they coordinate with oncology nurses to ensure proper administration. The pharmacy department usually is responsible for the receipt, storage, and preparation of the study medication, as well as for keeping track of the actual medication.

Once patients have completed the active study treatment, they are not completely disengaged from the clinical trial unit because there are usually protocol follow-ups (e.g., quality of life, additional sampling, survival) or parallel studies (e.g., observational, financial impact).

Genetics and Genomics

CTNs are responsible for proper sampling (i.e., sampling that it is carried out accurately and at the times described in the protocol) and for the corresponding shipments (e.g., storage in dry ice or room temperature).

Practice in Spain complies with the International Air Transport Association and institutional policies for shipping and receiving biologic specimens, experimental agents, and devices (ONS, 2010).

Correlative Trials

Correlative trials in Spain commonly involve quality of life, economics, or nursing.

Documentation and Data Management

In recent years, the electronic format of the CRF has replaced the paper one, thus providing greater speed and ease in obtaining and processing data. The research team is responsible for maintaining the clinical trial documentation (investigator's file) and source documents. The clinical research assistant (CRA) supports the team with regard to maintenance and quality of the trial documentation kept at the site.

Quality Assurance

Royal Decree 223/2004 of 6 February and European Directives 2001/20/EC and 2005/28/EC laid the legal and administrative foundation for which all clinical trials and personnel involved must comply with, in addition to International Conference on Harmonisation of Technical Requirements for Registration of Pharmaceuticals for Human Use GCP guidelines. The objectives of these guidelines and ethical practices are to protect the rights and well-being of individuals and ensure data integrity and confidentiality (ONS, 2010).

Clinical trials, whether sponsored by the pharmaceutical industry or otherwise, are monitored by CRAs. They determine whether the study personnel comply with GCP and thus verify data integrity and ensure patient rights. To that end, a comprehensive review of the source documents and CRF information is conducted. The frequency of monitoring depends on the type and basis of the study. CTNs are responsible for ensuring the validity of research results through timely, accurate, and complete data documentation and the reporting of any deviations, violations, and serious adverse events (ONS, 2010).

The conduct of audits ensures the quality of the clinical data obtained. The objective is not to achieve error-free clinical trials, but to check that they are within clinically and statistically acceptable limits. Audits may be internal (carried out by the sponsor) or external (carried out by government agencies, such as AEMPS [Technical Inspection Committee], the European Medicines Agency, or the U.S. Food and Drug Administration). CTNs facilitate and participate in the preparation for and implementation of scheduled and unscheduled meetings with internal and external monitors and auditors (ONS, 2010).

Professional Development

In the clinical trials field, Spanish nursing still has a long way to go. In other countries, its formation is regulated, its role is more valued, and it has its own collective associations that increase its recognition within research teams. Courses and master's degrees in clinical research are available that are not exclusive to nursing. Thus, CTNs have a university diploma in nursing, with exclusive knowledge of and dedication to the clinical trial development. Nursing tracks unique to clinical trials are shown in Figure 60-3. All of these activities are complemented by others, and then are carried out in a nonstandardized way, for example

- Participating as investigators in epidemiologic and academic studies
- Working together with various associations and cooperative groups
- Training new professionals or preparing manuals papers
- Implementing and promoting research in nursing (nursing companion studies).

Figure 60-3. Sample Nursing Tracks Unique to Clinical Trials

- Extraction, scheduling, handling, processing, storage, and shipment of biologic samples (e.g., pharmacokinetics, pharmacogenomics)
- Quality-of-life questionnaires
- Vital signs (e.g., blood pressure, heart rate, temperature)
- Electrocardiograms
- Important health data regarding participants; medications that could interact with the investigational product, thus masking its efficacy; and additional nursing assessments
- Scheduling and supporting the investigator during patient visits
- Toxicity assessment using scales
- Keeping track of the amount of investigational product with the pharmacist
- Direct patient care (including follow-up)
- Educating patients and medical doctors on clinical trial procedures
- Dispensation and training in taking the study medication (e.g., coded systems, oral medication, patient diaries)
- Recording temperatures of refrigerators where samples and medications are stored
- Controlling the hours and administration for IV medication, which involves training in the necessary material for administration, infusion times, drug premedication, and handling and resolution of immediate side effects

Summary

Cancer is a serious health issue for Spanish society, as it is a major cause of mortality. Healthcare facilities are becoming increasingly aware that, despite the effort entailed in conducting clinical trials, they are the only way to advance new therapies and improve healthcare quality. The number of clinical trials, especially for cancer, has increased significantly in Spain over the past decade, thus giving rise to even more research units. The role of CTNs is gaining the recognition it deserves because it encompasses critical tasks within the multidisciplinary team.

Key Points

- Clinical trials in Spain are conducted by a multidisciplinary support team, in which CTNs play a key role.
- Clinical trials are funded by foundations and pharmaceutical companies, which affords hospitals the possibility of new therapeutic lines.
- To ensure the quality and reliability of data, the entire research team should follow GCP guidelines, as well as those of government agencies and ethics committees.

The authors would like to thank Federico Nepote, Andrés Poveda, and Antonio Gónzalez of the GEICO group for their help in writing this chapter.

References

Booth, B., Glassman, R., & Ma, P. (2003). Oncology's trials. *Nature Reviews Drug Discovery, 2,* 609–610.

Camí, J. (1995). Conflicto de intereses e investigación clínica. *Medicina Clínica, 105,* 174–179. Retrieved from http://www.jcami.eu/system/uploads/publication/scientific/file/32/Conflicto_de_intereses_e_investigaci_n_cl_nica._Med_Clin.pdf

Camps, C., & Guillem, V. (2008). *Metodología del ensayo clínico* (Valencia, Spain). Retrieved from http://www.ffis.es/ups/metodologia_ensayo_clinico.pdf

Directive 2001/20/EC of the European Parliament and of the Council of 4 April 2001 on the approximation of the laws, regulations and administrative provisions of the Member States relating to the implementation of good clinical practice in the conduct of clinical trials on medicinal products for human use. Retrieved from http://ec.europa.eu/health/files/eudralex/vol-1/dir_2001_20/dir_2001_20_en.pdf

Directive 2005/28/EC of 8 April 2005 laying down principles and detailed guidelines for good clinical practice as regards investigational medicinal products for human use, as well as the requirements for authorisation of the manufacturing or importation of such products. Retrieved from http://ec.europa.eu/health/files/eudralex/vol-1/dir_2005_28/dir_2005_28_en.pdf

Ley 25/1990, de 20 de Diciembre, del Medicamento [Law 25/1990 of December 20, Medicines]. Retrieved from http://www.boe.es/boe/dias/1990/12/22/pdfs/A38228-38246.pdf

Ley 29/2006, de 26 de Julio, de garantías y uso racional de los medicamentos y productos sanitarios [Law 29/2006, of 26 July, on guarantees and rational use of drugs and medical devices]. Retrieved from http://www.boe.es/buscar/pdf/2006/BOE-A-2006-13554-consolidado.pdf

Ley 41/2002, de 14 de Noviembre, básica reguladora de la autonomía del paciente y de derechos y obligaciones en materia de información y documentación clínica [Law 41/2002, of 14 November, regulating patient autonomy and rights and obligations regarding clinical information and documentation]. Retrieved from http://www.boe.es/diario_boe/txt.php?id=BOE-A-2002-22188

López-Otín, C. (2001). La investigación oncológica en España [Cancer research in Spain]. *Arbor, 168*(662), 247–253. doi:10.3989/arbor.2001.i662.834

Ministerio de Sanidad y Consumo. (1993, May 13). Real Decreto 561/1993 de 16 de Abril, por el que se establecen los requisitos para la realización de ensayos clínicos con medicamentos [Royal Decree 561/1993 of April 26, establishing the requisites concerning clinical trials on drugs]. *Boletín Oficial del Estado, 114,* 14346–14364. Retrieved from http://www.boe.es/boe/dias/1993/05/13/pdfs/A14346-14364.pdf

Oncology Nursing Society. (2010). *Oncology clinical trials nurse competencies.* Retrieved from https://www.ons.org/sites/default/files/ctncompetencies.pdf

Real Decreto 223/2004, de 6 de febrero, por el que se regulan los ensayos clínicos con medicamentos [Royal Decree 223/2004 of 6 February, that clinical drug trials are regulated]. *Boletín Oficial del Estado, 33,* 5429–5443.

Chapter 61

Thailand

Manmana Jirajarus, MSN, APN, and Suwannee Sirilerttrakul, MEd, APN

Introduction

Thailand is a developing country in Southeast Asia where medical and healthcare research has not been well established, and the cancer-related mortality rate remains high. The Ministry of Public Health (2011) reported that cancer in Thailand had one of the highest of all mortality rates from 2007 to 2011, with an expectation that the trend will increase in the future (see Figure 61-1). The top five cancers in men are colorectal, lung, liver, esophageal, and tongue cancers, while breast, cervical, colorectal, lung, and ovarian cancers are the most prevalent cancers in women (Attasara & Buasom, 2011). Healthcare professionals face a major challenge in reducing the mortality rate and increasing the quality of life (QOL) of patients with cancer. Therefore, several oncology clinical trials are being conducted, including those involving novel chemotherapy and targeted therapy. Most clinical trials conducted in Thailand are a part of collaboration with global multicenter studies.

This chapter describes clinical trials performed in Thailand by government organizations or pharmaceutical companies and the participation of research nurses.

History and Foundation

In the past, successful outcomes of cancer treatment were not met because of advanced disease stages, knowledge deficiencies, inadequate chemotherapy, and financial concerns. In the past three decades, medical oncologists who had completed training in developed countries, especially the United States, returned to Thailand. They founded the Thai Society of Clinical Oncology (TSCO) in 1996 (TSCO, n.d.). One of the objectives was to support medical oncology research and related subspecialties. For instance, the Pattern of Epidermal Growth Factor Receptor Mutations and Association to Treatment in Lung Adenocarcinoma study, initiated in 2011 and still ongoing, is one of the multicenter trials that is being conducted by TSCO.

The optimal outcome of cancer treatment is to prolong patients' lives and improve their QOL (Bacon, 2008). Therefore, innovative treatment modalities such as novel targeted therapy or immunotherapy drugs (including cancer vaccines and targeted therapies) are being rapidly developed. Clinical trials have been expanded in comprehensive cancer centers, medical schools, the National Cancer Institute, and regional branches. Generally, pharmaceutical companies have conducted and sponsored the majority of clinical trials. The remaining trials have been conducted by experienced medical oncologists in the comprehensive cancer centers. However, multicenter and multidisciplinary clinical trials are uncommon and remain challenging in Thailand.

Besides TSCO, other multidisciplinary cancer groups in Thailand include the Thai Gynecologic Cancer Society (TGCS), Thai Oncology Nurses Society, Thai Society of Therapeutic Radiology and Oncology (THASTRO), Thai Society of Hematology, and Thai Breast Disease Society. At the end of 2013, TSCO, TGCS, and THASTRO launched the first Thai collaborative cancer conference. This provided an opportunity to develop clinical trials among cancer groups to enhance treatment outcomes in the future.

International Clinical Trials Research

Thailand has been involved in conducting international clinical trials, particularly of the most common cancer sites. For instance, TGCS collaborated with the International Gynecologic Cancer Society and conducted a clinical trial of the human papillomavirus vaccine. In 2013, Thai sites joined an international Gynecologic Cancer InterGroup study in a randomized phase III clinical trial of weekly versus triweekly cisplatin-based chemoradiation in locally advanced cervical cancer

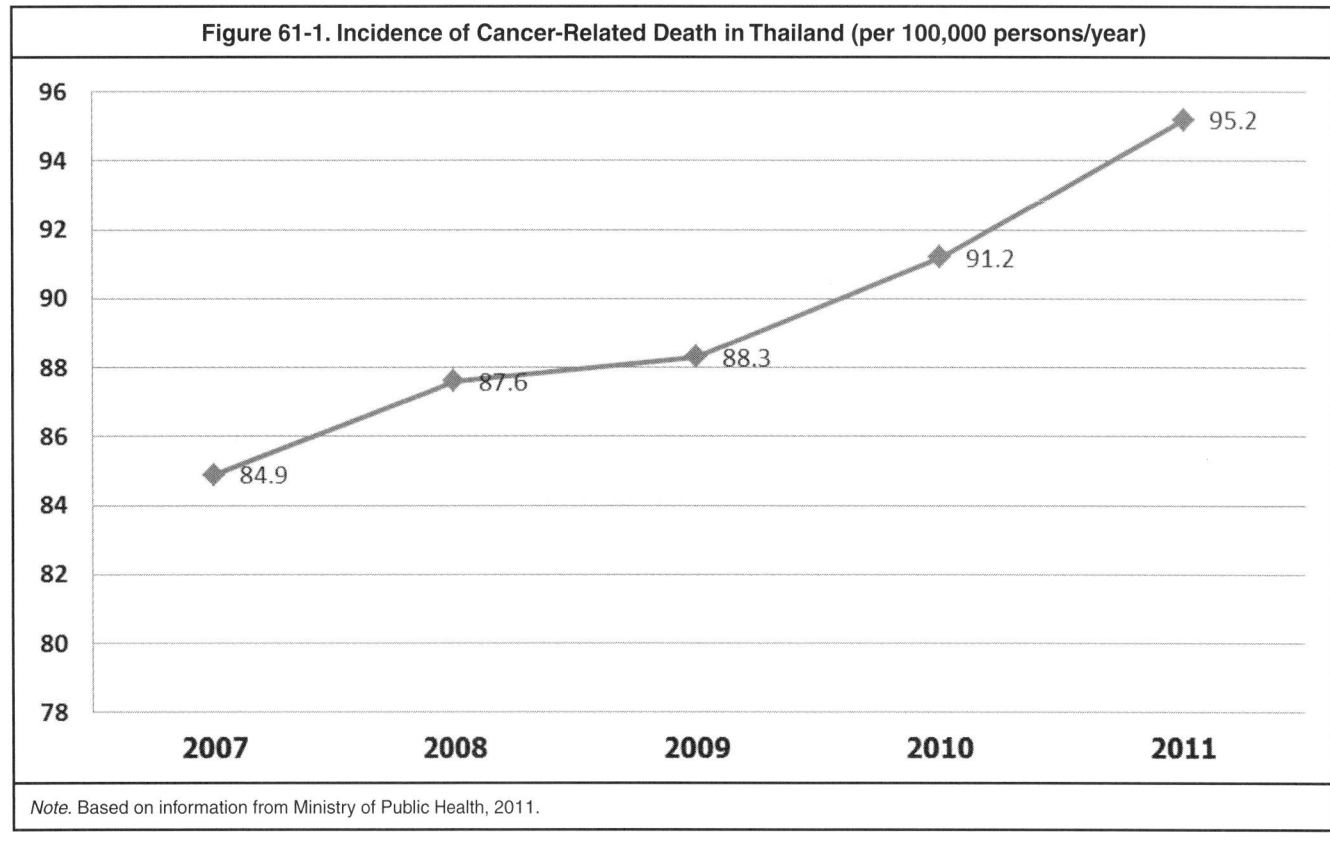

Figure 61-1. Incidence of Cancer-Related Death in Thailand (per 100,000 persons/year)

Note. Based on information from Ministry of Public Health, 2011.

(Korean Gynecologic Oncology Group & TGCS, 2012). Moreover, Thailand has collaborated with the network of colorectal cancer multidisciplinary teams in the Asia-Pacific region and participated in the international registration of colorectal cancer cases with liver metastases in 2012.

Several clinical trials have been conducted by large pharmaceutical companies in western countries and extended collaboration to other parts of the world, including Thailand. For a clinical trial that uses investigational new drugs, the import license must be obtained in advance from the Thai Food and Drug Administration (FDA), which is under the direction of the Ministry of Public Health.

Clinical Trials: Fundamental Information

Regulatory

Generally, the final review of clinical trial protocols must be approved by the local institutional review boards (IRBs), known as ethics committees (ECs). IRBs protect confidentiality and advocate for patients' rights. Subsequently, the locally approved application will be resubmitted to the Thai FDA for final approval. However, the Thai FDA has granted 10 large cancer research institutions for local IRB approval without resubmission to the Thai FDA (see Figure 61-2). This will shorten the regulatory process.

Ethics

Because most Thai patients speak Thai and are unable to understand foreign languages very well, including English, protocol consents must be written in the Thai language. Although the Thai consent is required to be comprehensible to laypeople, some patients, especially older and low-educated patients, may not be able to understand it clearly. A crucial role of research nurse coordinators and principal investigators (PIs) is to explain risks and benefits of the study to these groups of patients and ensure their understanding. Moreover, the final decision should theoretically come from the patients themselves. In Thai culture, family members may have significant influence on patients' decisions.

Protocol Development, Review, and Approval

Clinical research has been increasingly developing each year in Thailand. The majority of clinical trials are phase III studies. They are initiated by medical team

Figure 61-2. Ten Large Cancer Research Institutions for a Local Institutional Review Board Approval Without Resubmission to Thai Food and Drug Administration

- Ministry of Public Health
- Chulalongkorn University
- Ramathibodi Hospital, Mahidol University
- Siriraj Hospital, Mahidol University
- Tropical Medicine, Mahidol University
- Chiang Mai University
- Prince of Sonkhla University
- Khon Kaen University
- Phramongkutklao College of Medicine
- Institute for Development of Human Research Protection

leaders of pharmaceutical companies. Thereafter, they approach PIs at each study site to assess feasibility, such as experience of site staff and status of available facilities (e.g., laboratory, pharmacy preparation room, administration room). PIs will review and comment on the study protocol before acceptance for activation and participation.

Recently, early-phase clinical studies have been growing in Thailand. A phase I clinical trial has been recently initiated with collaboration with comprehensive cancer centers in developed countries such as the United States. Thai investigators have more input in protocol development. In addition, research nurse coordinators review an initial protocol and provide input from their perspective. PIs will receive comments from all team members and finalize the protocol. Moreover, many preclinical studies, which are initiated by Thai investigators, are ongoing in the country, focusing on common cancers in Thailand such as cholangiocarcinoma and nasopharyngeal cancer. These preclinical studies could provide a strong rationale in clinical development of novel therapy in the future.

Financial Factors and Budget

For investigator-initiated studies in Thailand, government organizations such as the Thailand Research Fund, the National Research Council of Thailand, the Thai FDA, and the Thailand Center of Excellence for Life Sciences (n.d.) provide funding for collaborative cancer groups and other specialty groups. Apart from those organizations, each medical institute or comprehensive cancer center also promotes and supports funding. Because of limited resources, investigator-initiated studies in Thailand are extremely challenging.

However, for pharmaceutical-initiated studies, which are more common in the country, the pharmaceutical company develops a protocol and approaches a PI at the potential site to participate. Most institutions will require that the pharmaceutical company be responsible for all study-related expenses.

Accordingly, pharmaceutical companies conduct clinical trials and take responsibility for all relevant expenses, including overhead expenses for a local EC, investigational drugs, premedication, imaging, drug preparation, drug administration, and subject transportation. Occasionally, PIs and local IRBs negotiate with pharmaceutical companies prior to signing an agreement in order to meet a suitable balanced budget.

Fortunately, some pharmaceutical companies have a compassionate use program for their newly approved drugs. Medical oncologists (site staff) discuss these investigational drugs with patients. If patients agree to treatment with these drugs, then minimal contact information and consent are collected for notification, in case adverse events are identified later.

Recruitment and Retention

Generally, most subjects in clinical trials are recruited from a clinical practice in each institute. Some potential candidates are referred from other institutes by personal contact with a specialist.

Many obstacles hinder the recruitment of Thai participants for clinical trials, such as

- Lack of other healthcare professionals' awareness of active studies
- Rarity of certain cancers in clinical trials, such as primitive neuroectodermal embryogenic tumors
- Unwillingness of patients to possibly receive a placebo
- Negative attitudes of patients, who feel like "guinea pigs" and decline participation.

Clinical Trial Participants

Participants' eligibility depends on inclusion and exclusion criteria. The recruitment process for clinical trials generally has four steps.

- The PI identifies a potential candidate from the clinic or referrals.
- The PI and nurse coordinator discuss the trial with the potential candidate and family and clearly inform them of the risks and benefits of participation.
- The potential candidate signs a consent before undergoing initial screening.
- The PI and the nurse coordinator check the inclusion and exclusion criteria.

Usual essential eligibility parameters in oncology trials are types of cancer, stage of disease, pathologic type, performance status, measurable and nonmeasurable lesions, comorbidity and concomitant treatment, types of prior treatment (including prior chemotherapy and targeted therapy regimens), and laboratory results. Subjects who meet all of the inclusion criteria will be enrolled in the study.

Genetics and Genomics

Since the human genome project was publicly announced in 2000, the Thai government has recognized the usefulness of life sciences and has established the Thailand Center of Excellence for Life Sciences and six other organizations to create innovative life science products to serve Thailand and the global market (Thailand Center of Excellence for Life Sciences, n.d.). Large-scale genetic and genomic research has been gradually conducted and expanded into clinical trials in Thai medical schools.

Thailand conducts genetic and genomic studies of several types of cancer that are prevalent in Thailand such as cholangiocarcinoma and esophageal, colorectal, and liver cancers. Next-generation sequencing and microarray technologies have been used to identify differential somatic alterations, including single nucleotide variations, small insertions or deletions of bases in the DNA (known as *indels*), and copy-number variations in cancer cells. Recently, a Thai cancer researcher was selected as one of the winners of the Rare Disease Science Challenge: Be HEARD (Helping Empower and Accelerate Research Discoveries) organized by the Assay Depot and the Rare Genomics Institute in the United States.

To facilitate cancer genetics and genomics research, a tumor biobanking facility containing tumor tissue and blood samples of patients with cancer has been established. Because Thailand is a developing country, it has several limitations, such as limited training programs in genetics and genomics medicine, qualified personnel, sophisticated equipment, and scientific funding. Therefore, international collaborations of genomics study are necessary.

Correlative Trials

The development of knowledge regarding tumor biology has enhanced cancer treatments and survival rates. The competition among pharmaceutical companies introducing numerous investigational new drugs in clinical trials is very high. Outcome measurements should be considered in quantity and quality dimensions. These new effective drugs have a great impact on clinical research outcomes. Traditionally, the primary endpoint focuses on quantity of life, such as survival rate, tumor response rate, and toxicities. On the other hand, nowadays, the concept of QOL is involved in clinical trials. Most of these measurements are performed as secondary endpoints. Oncology advanced practice nurses recognized the potential parameter of QOL measurements in clinical trials. Therefore, research for testing psychometric properties was conducted in 2000. Thai advanced practice nurses led this project with colleagues from different fields: medical oncologists, a psychiatrist, and a native English-speaker to translate QOL measurements. The Functional Assessment of Cancer Therapy–General (FACT-G), the European Organisation for Research and Treatment of Cancer quality-of-life questionnaire (EORTC QLQ-C30), and some specific disease modules in Thai versions were published in 2001, 2002, and 2006 (Ratanatharathorn et al., 2001; Silpakit et al., 2006; Sirisinha et al., 2002). These QOL questionnaires are considered as one parameter in many phase III clinical trials and medical research in Thailand (Wilailak et al., 2011).

Documentation and Data Management

Good clinical practice has to guide the completion of patients' files. If there is no documentation in a patient's file, it means nothing occurred. In Thailand, the research nurse coordinator plays a vital role to ensure data collection and complete source documentation that validate the integrity of the clinical trial. Therefore, all information has to be documented in each patient's file, as well as in case report forms. The essential information includes

- Patient information (e.g., patient's initials, date of birth, body weight, height, body surface area, performance status, consent form)
- Disease information (e.g., grade and stage of cancer [pathology report], date of first cancer diagnosis, comorbidities)
- Treatment and outcome information (e.g., date of recruitment, previous chemotherapy and other treatments, investigational drug names, dose, time of administration, adverse events, serious adverse events, tumor measurements).

Currently, electronic data capturing systems have been replacing paper case report forms in global trials. For confidentiality purposes, the web-based data system is designed to have an ID and password (Aotani & Saito, 2008). Furthermore, the specifically designed website can capture and transfer data from the machine (e.g., electrocardiogram) to an international research center. After the end of the study, all source documents must be kept for 20 years for auditing.

Quality Assurance

Safety of human subjects in clinical trials is crucially recognized by the study team. The quality assurance program ensures that clinical trials can be carried out within the appropriate regulatory standards. Site selection is the initiation of the quality assurance process. Site staffs such as PI, research nurse, and others who are involved in clinical trials have to be qualified and experienced. Internal monitoring by a clinical research assistant ensures that all data are valid and complete. Some clinical trials are randomly audited by an external audit team or the contract research organization to ensure that quality data are obtained (Bacon, 2008).

Clinical trials must not only meet the primary objectives but also must be reliable and follow standard good clinical practice. Therefore, valid outcomes of clinical trials are derived from quality assurance.

Professional Development

The Thai Oncology Nurses Society (n.d.) was established in 2011. One of its objectives is to promote and support nursing education and oncology nursing research. Since then, it has not conducted any oncology nursing research. However, oncology nursing research has been performed in universities in postgraduate degree programs. Generally, oncology research studies are associated with nursing issues such as symptom management, QOL, caregiver role, and stress and coping.

Clinical trials are increasing in number every year, and interdisciplinary cooperation is necessary. The oncology research nurse is a key person in a clinical trial. In the past, oncology nurses focused on direct patient care practices, such as patient education, chemotherapy administration, psychosocial support, and symptom and side effect management. Now, the oncology nurse role has developed and extended to include responsibility in clinical trials. Oncology research nurses act as study coordinators. Important roles include communication among team members (e.g., PI, sponsors, participants, ethics committee, pathologists, radiologists), participant recruitment, informed consent process, data collection, and provision of nursing care and support to participants. Therefore, research nurse coordinators must learn to apply knowledge and experience in a new environment, including taking an active role in providing direction to other healthcare team members (Lubejko et al., 2011).

The Oncology Nursing Society (ONS) developed the clinical trial nurse (CTN) competencies (see Appendix 2) because of the complexity of oncology clinical trials. ONS stated that

> the Oncology CTN Core Competencies include the fundamental knowledge, skills, and expertise required to proficiently (a) identify and care for a participants in clinical trials with a past, current, or potential diagnosis of cancer, (b) manage oncology clinical trials in diverse settings, (c) ensure protection of subjects enrolled in clinical trials, and (d) ensure that scientific integrity is maintained through data reliability and strict adherence to regulatory mandates. (ONS, 2010, p. 7)

The core values of the role require CTNs to "advocate for patient safety and trial integrity, advance evidence-based oncology care through scientifically sound research, [and] recognize the unique value that professional nurses contribute to the successful conduct and outcomes of clinical trials" (ONS, 2010, p. 7).

In Thailand in the past, RNs worked in a clinical practice, which often was task oriented, and were invited to participate in clinical research. Research coordinators enhanced their knowledge, experience, and skill in oncology and research methodology by themselves. Generally, except for comprehensive cancer centers, institutions do not define a position of a research nurse coordinator. Additionally, CTN competency is not defined by the Thai Nurse Council. Therefore, there is no certification for CTNs in Thailand. However, oncology research nurse coordinators follow ONS's CTN competencies.

The clinical research center (CRC) network was initiated by intrahospital processes to facilitate and empower clinical research methodology. Moreover, it supported the position of a research nurse coordinator. The first CRC was established in Siriraj Hospital at Mahidol University in 2003 and has been expanded to other comprehensive cancer centers. Now, the CRC of each center initiates a good clinical practice workshop to educate and certify study personnel. Ideally, in the future, the Thai nursing organizations will develop and conduct educational programs for clinical research nurses.

Cultural Aspects

The Thai family is an expanded family. Therefore, several family members might be involved in patient care (Meecharoen, Northouse, Sirapo-ngam, & Monkong, 2013). Setting up a family meeting for the discussion of clinical study participation can be challenging and time consuming. Family members may influence patients' decisions regarding participation in the clinical trial and result in delayed accrual. On the other hand, several family members may support patient care during the study. They could provide transportation according to study requirements, help in reporting adverse events and compliance (in case of oral study medications), and offer spiritual support.

Herbal and alternative medicines are widely used in Thailand. Most patients are recommended herbal or alternative medicines by their friends, family members, advertisements on public broadcasting, and the Internet. Some patients may discuss this use with their doctors and nurses beforehand, but some may not. Therefore, it is essential for research nurse coordinators and PIs to always evaluate the use of herbal and alternative medicines before accrual and during the study.

Summary

Important components for the success of clinical research in Thailand are collaboration and coordination of a study team. The research nurse is the key person responsible for most of this process. In Thailand, oncology clinical trials are growing. The national collaborative cancer organizations should initiate graduate programs for promoting research nurse core competencies in clinical research methodology, as it could improve the quality of cancer research in Thailand.

Key Points
- Thailand is quickly developing infrastructures and expertise in the field of clinical trials.
- Clinical trial nurses' competencies are slowly being created, supported, and expanded.
- Research nurse coordinators are a new type of expert in Thailand.

The authors would like to thank Associate Professor Dr. Boosakorn Vijchulata, PhD, in linguistics (U.S.) and Nuttapong Ngamphaiboon, MD, for reviewing and editing the English language in this chapter.

References

Aotani, E., & Saito, Y. (2008). Japan. In A.D. Klimaszewski, M. Bacon, H.E. Deininger, B.A. Ford, & J.G. Westendorp (Eds.), *Manual for clinical trials nursing* (2nd ed., pp. 391–401). Pittsburgh, PA: Oncology Nursing Society.

Attasara, P., & Buasom, R. (Eds.). (2011, July). Hospital based cancer registry. Retrieved from http://www.nci.go.th/th/File_download/Nci%20Cancer%20Registry/Hospitalbase2011.pdf

Bacon, M. (2008). Canada. In A.D. Klimaszewski, M. Bacon, H.E. Deininger, B.A. Ford, & J.G. Westendorp (Eds.), *Manual for clinical trials nursing* (2nd ed., pp. 383–390). Pittsburgh, PA: Oncology Nursing Society.

Korean Gynecologic Oncology Group & Thai Gynecologic Cancer Society. (2012). TACO: Tri-weekly administration of cisplatin in locally advanced cervical cancer (GCIG/KGOG 1027/THAI 2012). Retrieved from http://www.tacotrial.com

Lubejko, B., Good, M., Weiss, P., Schmeider, L., Leos, D., & Daugherty, P. (2011). Oncology clinical trials nursing: Developing competencies for the novice. *Clinical Journal of Oncology Nursing, 15,* 637–643. doi:10.1188/11.CJON.637-643

Meecharoen, W., Northouse, L.L., Sirapo-ngam, Y., & Monkong, S. (2013). Family caregivers for cancer patients in Thailand: An integrative review. *SAGE Open, 3*(3). doi:10.1177/2158244013500280

Ministry of Public Health. (2011). Number and death rates per 100,000 population of first 10 leading cause groups of death (according to ICD Mortality Tabulation List, 10th Revision). Retrieved from http://bps.ops.moph.go.th/E-book/statistic/statistic54/2.3.1_54.pdf

Oncology Nursing Society. (2010). *Oncology clinical trials nurse competencies.* Retrieved from https://www.ons.org/sites/default/files/ctncompetencies.pdf

Ratanatharathorn, V., Sirilerttrakul, S., Jirajarus, M., Silpakit, C., Maneechavakajorn, J., Sailamai, P., & Sirisinha, T. (2001). Quality of life, Functional Assessment of Cancer Therapy-General. *Journal of the Medical Association of Thailand, 84,* 1430–1442.

Silpakit, C., Sirilerttrakul, S., Jirajarus, M., Sirisinha, T., Sirachainan, E., & Ratanatharathorn, V. (2006). The European Organization for Research and Treatment of Cancer quality of life questionnaire (EORTC QLQ-C30): Validation study of the Thai version. *Quality of Life Research, 15,* 167–172. doi:10.1007/s11136-005-0449-7

Sirisinha, T., Ratanatharathorn, V., Jirajarus, M., Sirilerttrakul, S., Silpakit, C., Sirachainan, E., & Tanvetyanon, T. (2002). The European Organization for Research and Treatment of Cancer quality of life questionnaire: Translation and reliability study of the Thai version. *Journal of the Medical Association of Thailand, 85,* 1210–1219.

Thailand Center of Excellence for Life Sciences. (n.d.). Thailand Center of Excellence for Life Sciences. Retrieved from http://www.tcels.or.th/en/home/page

Thai Oncology Nurses Society. (n.d.). The Thai Oncology Nurses Society. Retrieved from http://www.nci.go.th/tons/active1.php

Thai Society of Clinical Oncology. (n.d.). Vision and mission. Retrieved from http://www.tsco.or.th/index.php/2010-12-11-15-26-35

Wilailak, S., Lertkhachonsuk, A.A., Lohacharoenvanich, N., Luengsukcharoen, S.C., Jirajaras, M., Likitanasombat, P., & Sirilerttrakul, S. (2011). Quality of life in gynecologic cancer survivors compared to healthy check-up women. *Journal of Gynecologic Oncology, 22,* 103–109. doi:10.3802/jgo.2011.22.2.103

Chapter 62

United Kingdom

Karen Carty, CCR, and Andrea Harkin, BA, CCR

Introduction

In the United Kingdom (UK), the National Health Service (NHS) was established in 1948 to provide health care to all citizens. NHS is funded by the UK taxpayers and managed by the UK Government's Department of Health in England and by the governments of the devolved nations (Scotland, Wales, and Northern Ireland). Since its foundation, NHS has seen many changes to its organizational structure and the provision of patient services.

History and Foundation

Framework for Health Research Within the United Kingdom

The National Institute for Health Research (NIHR) is a large, multifaceted, nationally distributed organization funded through the Department of Health (England) to improve the health and wealth of the nation through research. Since its establishment in April 2006, NIHR has worked with key partners involved in different elements of NHS research to transform research in NHS. It has increased the volume of applied health research for the benefit of patients and the public, driven faster translation of basic science discoveries into tangible benefits for patients and the economy, and developed and supported the people who conduct and contribute to applied health research.

NIHR provides the support and facilities NHS needs for first-class research that results in high-quality care for patients and the public. Key facilities include
- Clinical Research Networks: Disease-specific networks (cancer, stroke, mental health, diabetes, medicines for children, dementia, and neurodegenerative diseases), a Primary Care Research Network, and a Comprehensive Research Network to encourage clinical trials in all diseases
- Biomedical Research Centres
- Biomedical Research Units
- Patient Safety Research Centres
- Clinical Research Facilities for Experimental Medicine
- Healthcare Technology Cooperatives
- Collaborations for Leadership in Applied Health Research and Care
- Research Capability Funding
- Office for Clinical Research Infrastructure
- Diagnostic Evidence Cooperatives.

The NIHR equivalent organizations within the devolved nations of the UK are
- Scotland: Chief Scientist Office
- Wales: Wales Office of Research and Development for Health and Social Care
- Northern Ireland: Health and Social Care Research and Development Office.

A key NIHR partner/stakeholder is the UK Clinical Research Collaboration (UKCRC). UKCRC was established in 2004 with the aim of reengineering the clinical research environment in the UK to benefit the public and patients by improving national health and increasing national wealth. The partnership brings together the major stakeholders that influence clinical research in the UK. It includes the main UK research funding bodies; academia; NHS; regulatory bodies; the bioscience, healthcare, and pharmaceutical industries; and patients.

National Framework for Cancer Research

National Cancer Research Institute

The National Cancer Research Institute (NCRI) is a UK-wide partnership between the government, charity, and industry that promotes cooperation in cancer research among the 22 member organizations for the benefit of patients, the public, and the scientific community. NCRI was set up in 2001 to develop common plans for cancer research and to avoid unnecessary duplication of effort. Until NCRI came together, there was little joint planning or management of cancer research, and collaborations were patchy. There was no single source of information about the research being carried out, so it was difficult to assess needs for new work. The main mission of NCRI is to ensure that patients benefit from cancer research in the UK. They also promote research for cancer prevention.

In addition to funding cancer research, NCRI partners aim to make research results as widely available as possible. New knowledge can be applied in further research, and companies can use the information to develop new treatments and diagnostics. NCRI partners aim to ensure that the public is well informed about the most important discoveries.

NCRI helps with joint planning and coordination among its members. They focus on areas where progress could not be achieved by a single member organization on its own. Specifically, NCRI

- Maintains a Cancer Research Database (CaRD) and analyzes what research is being done, which informs decisions about new research
- Organizes annual cancer conferences for showcasing the best British and international cancer research
- Develops initiatives on specific topics to which a group of members will contribute
- Helps to coordinate clinical trials and experimental cancer medicine research within the networks throughout the UK
- Develops facilities and resources for research.

Clinical Studies Groups

New ideas for noncommercial clinical trials are developed by NCRI Clinical Studies Groups (CSGs). CSGs represent a central component of the framework for cancer research in the UK. There are currently 22 NCRI CSGs: 16 cancer site–specific groups, 5 generic groups (Teenage and Young Adults, Biomarkers and Imaging, Palliative and Supportive Care, Primary Care, and Psychosocial Oncology), and 1 Consumer Liaison Group.

CSGs bring together clinicians, scientists, statisticians, clinical trials staff, and lay representatives to coordinate development of a portfolio of clinical trials within the field of the CSG. Members of CSGs are competitively appointed, and each CSG meets approximately two or three times per year. Several CSGs have subgroups or working parties, which are open to individuals who are not necessarily members of the parent group.

CSGs are charged with the development of national cancer clinical trials and work toward broad but common tasks and activities. This includes overseeing existing studies, considering new research questions, developing proposals, and securing funding from NCRI members and other sources, as well as providing expert advice. The groups are funded by the major cancer charities and the Medical Research Council and are UK-wide in their scope.

National Cancer Research Institute–Accredited Clinical Trials Units

With a more strategic approach to coordination of cancer clinical trials in the UK, it was acknowledged that the clinical trials units (CTUs) have a central role in the development and successful completion of clinical trials. Prior to the establishment of NCRI, the approach to the management of these trials evolved in an ad hoc manner, with little coordination among the CTUs and with little or no strategy. One of the key recommendations of the NCRI strategic review was to identify a network of NCRI-accredited CTUs in the UK. These CTUs must display key competencies in the coordination of cancer clinical trials (see Figure 62-1).

Nine NCRI-accredited units exist in the UK: seven based in England, one in Scotland, and one in Wales. Potential benefits for cancer clinical trials in the UK will be that potential researchers and research groups will have access to and links with relevant national expertise and confidence in working with a nationally accredited unit. Good communication among the accredited units provides more general benefits, such as development of central resources and systems, discussion of information technology–related issues, sharing of expertise and working practice, and standardization of data among units.

National Cancer Research Network

In addition to the implementation of NCRI in April 2001, the National Institute for Health Research Cancer Research Network (NCRN) was established. NCRN provides researchers with the practical support they need to make cancer clinical studies happen within NHS so that more research takes place across the country and more patients take part. NCRN consists of 32 Local Research Networks (LRNs) within NHS in England. These networks coordinate and facilitate the conduct of cancer clinical research and offer researchers a range of services to support study setup and delivery.

Scotland, Wales, and Northern Ireland have their own cancer research networks: the Scottish Cancer Research Network, the Wales Cancer Trials Network, and the All-Ireland Cooperative Oncology Research Group (see Chapter 54). These networks are all partners of NCRN.

Experimental Cancer Medicines Centres Network

As part of the National Framework for Experimental Medicine, the Department of Health in England

---

Figure 62-1. Key Competencies of Clinical Trials Units in the United Kingdom

- Display a track record in the coordination of phase III multicenter trials
- Employ a core team of expert staff
- Implement quality assurance and archiving systems
- Show evidence of long-term viability
- Contribute to the national program of cancer trials

and the devolved administrations, together with Cancer Research UK (CR-UK), established the Experimental Cancer Medicines Centres (ECMC) Network in 2007. Their aim is to bring together laboratory and clinical patient-based research to speed up the development of new therapies. There are 19 individual ECMCs, and the network is supported by a small secretariat team based at CR-UK and supported by NIHR. The secretariat helps with developing links, arranging specialist meetings and workshops, and managing the governance of the network.

Medicines and Healthcare Products Regulatory Agency

Within the UK, medication licensing is regulated by the Medicines and Healthcare Products Regulatory Agency (MHRA). The agency was formed in 2003 from a merger of the previous regulatory bodies—the Medicines Control Agency and the Medical Devices Agency. MHRA is the government agency responsible for ensuring that medicines and medical devices work and are acceptably safe. They assess the safety, quality, and efficacy of medicines and authorize their sale or supply in the UK for human use. They are responsible for the regulation of clinical trials of medicines and medical devices in the UK.

Medicinal products need to have a marketing authorization granted before they can be prescribed or sold to patients. Before this is granted, clinical trials are undertaken to allow collection of data on the safety and efficacy of new products. A clinical trial authorization (CTA) is required from MHRA for a product or trial before the product can be tested on human subjects. Further information regarding the application of CTAs for clinical trials is detailed in the Ethics and Regulations section.

Clinical Trials: Fundamental Information

Legal, Regulatory, and Legislative Issues

Clinical trials in the UK must abide by several regulations, including the International Conference on Harmonisation of Technical Requirements for Registration of Pharmaceuticals for Human Use (ICH) good clinical practice (GCP) guidelines (ICH, 1996). The objective of these guidelines is to provide and maintain unified standards of care. All clinical trials within the UK and other European Union (EU) countries must be conducted according to ICH GCP standards.

Trials in the UK must also abide by EU Clinical Trials Directive (CTD) 2001/20/EC. Figure 62-2 identifies the goals of that directive, and a complete overview of the EU CTD and its impact on clinical trials in Europe appears in Chapter 50.

Figure 62-2. Goals of European Union Clinical Trials Directive 2001/20/EC

- Protect the rights, safety, and well-being of trial participants.
- Simplify and harmonize the administrative provisions governing trials.
- Establish a transparent procedure that will harmonize trial conduct in the European Union and ensure the credibility of results.

Each EU Member State (country) is responsible for implementation of the directive within its national laws. The UK regulations took effect on May 1, 2004, and all clinical trials from that point must adhere to the regulations. The directive only applies to clinical trials involving investigational medicinal products. All trials in the UK should follow the NHS Research Governance Framework. MHRA is responsible for ensuring that all clinical trials that fall under the EU CTD are conducted according to this regulatory standard.

The directive had a major effect on clinical trial activity in the UK, particularly within the academic sector. All trials must have a legal sponsor responsible for the conduct of the study and patient safety. The EU CTD defines the sponsor as "an individual, company, institution or organization which takes responsibility for the initiation, management and/or financing of a clinical trial" (Directive 2001/20/EC, article 2, paragraph (e)).

Ethics and Regulations

All clinical trials in the UK must obtain a favorable ethical opinion prior to commencement of the study. The National Research Ethics Service (NRES) provides guidance and leadership for NRES Research Ethics Committees (RECs) and the ethics system by coordinating the development of operational and infrastructure arrangements. This includes the implementation of standards to ensure national consistency and the provision of training for committee members.

In the UK, a unified set of web-based systems holds the information required to manage health and social care and community care research. This system, called the Integrated Research Application System (IRAS), is a single system for applying for permissions and approvals for health and social care and community care research in the UK. It was designed and built to make the processes of information input, retrieval, and dissemination faster and easier for everyone involved in the conduct of trials.

IRAS captures the information needed for the applications to the following review bodies in the UK.
- Administration of Radioactive Substances Advisory Committee (ARSAC)
- Gene Therapy Advisory Committee (GTAC)
- MHRA

- Ministry of Justice
- NHS/Health and Safety Commission (HSC) research and development (R&D) offices
- NRES/NHS/HSC RECs
- National Information Governance Board
- National Offender Management Service
- Social Care Research Ethics Committee

Clinical trials in the UK are conducted in accordance with the Declaration of Helsinki and ICH GCP guidelines. The purpose of RECs in the UK is to safeguard the rights, safety, dignity, and well-being of research participants. An essential aspect of any clinical trial is the informed consent process. In compliance with the recommendations of the Declaration of Helsinki, each patient must be fully informed of the aims, methods, benefits, and potential risks of the trial (World Medical Association, n.d.).

NHS RECs and clinical research in general in the UK have undergone significant changes following the introduction of the EU CTD. One of the aims of the directive was to standardize regulatory and approval procedures for the conduct of clinical trials. The requirements of the directive in relation to ethical review were

- Decisions on a valid application must be delivered within 60 days.
- One decision would be valid for the whole UK, with applicants being restricted to one written request for clarification or further information.

The chief investigator for the trial is responsible for applying for favorable ethical opinion. Once the ethics application for the trial has been completed via IRAS, the central allocation system of NRES is contacted to book the application for review. The booking service identifies and allocates applications to the appropriate REC for review, depending on the category of research.

In addition to ethical approval, any clinical trial involving an investigational medicinal product requires a CTA prior to commencement. The application for a CTA is completed via IRAS and submitted to MHRA. There are set time frames for the assessment of the application; the initial assessment will be performed within 30 days of receipt of a valid application by MHRA. A fee is charged for the CTA, which can be costly depending on the type of trial.

All clinical trials conducted in the UK require research management and governance approval, usually referred to as R&D approval, from the R&D department of each hospital participating in the trial. Applications for R&D approval are completed via IRAS. This approval is required for all research studies involving NHS patients, their tissues, or information, or studies involving NHS staff participating by virtue of their profession. The R&D approval process ensures

- An appropriate study sponsor is identified
- The scientific quality of the study (as required) is confirmed
- Favorable ethical opinion from the appropriate REC has been received
- Appropriate regulatory authorizations are in place
- Appropriate risk-benefit analysis has been conducted
- Provisions for appropriate insurance/indemnity are completed
- The financial and resource implications of the study are assessed
- Appropriate trial registration has occurred
- All researchers have substantive or honorary NHS contracts
- All researchers are adequately qualified
- Support department approval has been received
- Formal agreements or contracts with external bodies meet the requirements of the hospital.

R&D departments establish the likely impact and cost implications that participating in the trial will have on the hospital. Generally, hospitals will fund the excess treatment and service support costs of NCRN-badged trials. They receive an income for this research activity into an R&D budget from their associated government organizations.

Depending on the type of trial, additional approvals or licenses may be required before the trial can commence. An example of this is a license from ARSAC, which is required for any trial involving the administration of radioactive medicinal products to humans, such as multigated acquisition scans or bone scans. Applications for an ARSAC license are prepared via IRAS.

Trials involving the use of gene therapy require approval from GTAC. GTAC is the UK national research ethics committee for clinical trials of gene therapy, other advanced therapy medicinal products, and certain other types of research. GTAC is part of NRES. Applications to GTAC are prepared via IRAS in the same way as other applications.

Standard Operating Procedures

To meet the requirements of the EU CTD with standardized regulatory and approval procedures, standard operating procedures (SOPs) for RECs were introduced. The procedures became effective March 1, 2004. All NHS RECs in the UK are required to operate in accordance with these SOPs. Since the introduction of the EU CTD, the complexity of conducting clinical trials has increased significantly, and as a result, trials have become more expensive. Guidelines on the processes involved in setting up and managing trials under the EU CTD are clearly summarized in the toolkit developed by Medical Research Council in the UK, which can be accessed at www.ct-toolkit.ac.uk. Through the use of an interactive route map, the site provides information on best practice and outlines the current legal and practical requirements for conducting clinical trials in the UK.

Safe Handling and Workplace Safety

HSC and the Health and Safety Executive (HSE) are government advisory bodies responsible for the regulation of almost all of the risks to health and safety arising from work activity in the UK. HSE provide guidelines for complying with Control of Substances Hazardous to Health regulations (HSE, n.d.). HSE, Department of Health, and Her Majesty's Inspectorate of Pollution provide guidance on the safe handling of cytotoxic drugs, radiation therapy, radioactive substances, and specimens.

All hospitals and institutions involved in the handling of cytotoxic drugs and radiation therapy must comply with the guidelines provided by HSE and the other noted governing bodies. Each hospital will also have its own SOPs. Biologic specimens are handled according to the SOPs of the hospital. Specimens requiring shipment by air are shipped in accordance with the International Air Transport Association guidelines.

The safety and protection of staff, patients, and their relatives is essential. Staff must be fully educated on all aspects of safety to achieve a safe working environment. Education of staff is repeated and updated as required, particularly in instances where changes are made to guidelines.

Protocol Development, Review, and Approval

Trial Ideas and Concepts

As with most countries, ideas and concepts for new cancer clinical trials in the UK can be initiated by a number of sources, including industry (pharmaceutical companies), research groups (e.g., Scottish Gynaecological Cancer Trials Group or NCRI CSGs), or a single investigator at a hospital site. Ideas or concepts can be completely new, such as a feasibility study, or can be the result of a line of previous research trials.

Before the protocol is drafted, it is common for a study proposal to be put together. Investigator-led studies may be reviewed by the hospital clinical trial committee or by the study group. Investigators are encouraged to work with a CTU at an early stage to develop the protocol and grant application, if applicable. In addition, consumer input to the development of the protocol is highly encouraged and often can be mandatory depending on the peer-review body or funder. Investigator-initiated protocols from industry are often prepared in-house initially and then circulated to known experts in the field for review.

Peer Review

Peer review of clinical trials is an important aspect of protocol development in the UK. It is important for noncommercial trials to obtain support from the appropriate NCRI CSG. CSGs consist of leading investigators from across the UK who come together under the CSG chair. CSGs have a central role in the development of a balanced national portfolio and are the preferred route for the generation of noncommercial cancer clinical trials in the UK.

Cancer Research UK Clinical Trials Awards and Advisory Committee

CR-UK, as one of the leading public-sector funders of cancer trials and supporters of CTUs in the UK, developed a committee, the Clinical Trials Awards and Advisory Committee (CTAAC), to streamline and accelerate the peer-review process of cancer clinical trial proposals. Proposals to CTAAC are assessed and scored under the criteria listed in Figure 62-3. Many of the applications to CTAAC are expected to be developed or endorsed by NCRI CSG, although applications are accepted via other routes. If successful, protocols approved/endorsed by CTAAC are included in the NCRN (NIHR) portfolio and, if requested, also may be awarded grant funding.

With the growing importance of well-designed translational studies in cancer research, CR-UK has a scientific committee with a broad scope spanning basic and translational cancer research. Grant applications for funding to conduct biomarker research can be submitted for assessment by the Biomarker Expert Review Panel, a sub-panel of the Science Committee. Applications are considered that cover research in all types of biomarkers (i.e., predisposition, screening, diagnostic, prognostic, predictive, pharmacologic, and surrogate response) using invasive methods (i.e., surgical specimens or biofluids) and imaging technologies (i.e., magnetic resonance imaging, computed tomography, positron-emission tomography, single-photon emission computed tomography, other nuclear medicine methods, ultrasound, optical).

Protocol Development and Review

Protocols are normally drafted by the lead clinician for the study, known in the UK as the chief investigator.

Figure 62-3. Clinical Trials Awards and Advisory Committee Criteria to Assess and Score Proposals

- Clinical and scientific importance of the research question
- Adequacy of the background and preliminary data
- Study design and statistics
- Expected interest to patients and potential accrual
- Fit with current National Cancer Research Network trial portfolio

Most study groups and CTUs have an SOP that provides a template of the key sections to be included in the protocol and outlines the review process. Following implementation of the EU CTD, a number of items must be included in the clinical trial protocol, such as the end-of-study definition, expected adverse events, and a list of study responsibilities.

Once the chief investigator has completed the first draft of the protocol, it will be circulated for review to the trial management team. This should include the clinical trial coordinator, project manager, study statistician, quality assurance manager, pharmacovigilance manager, study sponsor representative, and any co-investigators.

Risk Assessment

Currently, in the UK, the sponsor will perform a risk assessment of the clinical trial protocol in accordance with the EU CTD. This assessment ensures that systems and procedures are in place to minimize risk to patients, the sponsor, and the quality of research. The level of monitoring required for a trial is determined by the risk assessment. The risk assessment of a clinical trial can result in changes being made to the draft protocol.

Chemotherapy and Pharmacy Advisory Service

In the UK, the Chemotherapy and Pharmacy Advisory Service (CPAS) is a multidisciplinary national team of pharmacists, research nurses, and oncologists set up by NCRN to advise chief investigators, CTUs, and CSGs on the chemotherapy and pharmacy content of protocols. CPAS offers a protocol review service, which is now mandatory for new drug trials approved by CTAAC. The aim of the service is to help trials across the entire NCRN portfolio run as smoothly and quickly as possible and to improve quality of care and management of risks in prescribing, preparing, and administering chemotherapy. Protocols are sent to CPAS for review at the final draft stage.

Protocol Approval

Once the final draft of the protocol is produced and approved by the trial management team, it must be given a version number and dated to enable version control. Although a great deal of work is put into ensuring the accuracy of the final version of the protocol, unfortunately, amendments often are inevitable. These can be simple amendments for administrative errors or changes or can be the result of new findings in relation to the study drug or regimen. Version control of the protocol thus becomes vital at this point.

Preparation

Preparation for any clinical trial, whether it is commercial (pharmaceutical/industry sponsored) or noncommercial (academic), in the UK is essentially similar. Recruitment to a clinical trial cannot begin until the necessary ethics and regulatory approvals have been granted. Beyond the ethics and regulatory approvals, a large amount of preparatory work is necessary before commencement of the trial.

For commercial trials, pharmaceutical companies often conduct visits with potential sites to assess a site's suitability to participate in the trial. The company will check the site for the necessary qualified staff, facilities, and resources to conduct the trial. When it is agreed that a site will participate in a clinical trial, financial agreements are drawn up between the site and the company (sponsor), documenting the financial aspects of the trial. In addition, a signed agreement is drawn up between each party stating their responsibility in relation to the trial.

The relevant essential documents for conducting a trial in accordance with ICH GCP guidelines are collected before commencement of the trial. These documents individually and collectively permit evaluation of the conduct of the trial and the quality of the data produced. They demonstrate the compliance of the investigator, sponsor, and monitor with the standards of GCP and with all applicable regulatory requirements (ICH, 1996). Essential documents include the curricula vitae for the staff involved in the trial, laboratory normal ranges and accreditation certificates for laboratory tests and procedures to be carried out in the trial, the site responsibility log, and necessary ethical and regulatory approvals.

It is normal practice for the sponsor to either conduct site initiation visits or provide site initiation training to the hospital research team to ensure that the staff involved understand the trial and the required procedures. At the time of the initiation visit, an investigator site master file and pharmacy file will be provided. These files house all of the required essential documents for the conduct of the trial.

The preparation for noncommercial (academic) trials is similar to the preparation for a commercial trial. These trials tend to be investigator-led and generally are in collaboration with other hospitals or research groups. For noncommercial trials, site feasibility questionnaires, as opposed to site visits, often are used to assess a site's suitability to participate in the trial. The questionnaire will ascertain if the site has the necessary qualified staff, facilities, and resources to conduct the trial. As with commercial trials, the sponsor and each participating site must prepare agreements. The coordinating CTU must collect the necessary documents from each site.

In addition to the previously mentioned documents, much preparation work goes into the design and development of paper and electronic case report forms (CRFs) for the trial to ensure it captures the required data of the protocol. CRFs and the CRF completion guidelines are reviewed and approved by the trial team.

Financial Factors

The funding arrangements for commercial trials are straightforward. NHS is required to recover, from industry, all costs over the standard NHS treatment cost. Industry costing templates have been developed to provide transparency, greater consistency, and predictability in deriving research study costs.

In comparison, the funding arrangements for noncommercial NHS research can be more complex, often involving a number of partner organizations. It is essential that both NHS and its partner organizations identify and quantify the full cost of the noncommercial research and reach a shared understanding of how these costs are recovered through appropriate funding arrangements. The AcoRD (Attributing the Costs of Health and Social Care Research and Development) guideline provides a transparent and consistent basis for attributing the costs of noncommercial NHS research (Department of Health, 2012). The attribution of costs must be performed prior to any grant funding applications to support the noncommercial trial and is part of the application process.

Recruitment and Retention

Trials often are promoted through the members of cancer trials groups, research organizations, or pharmaceutical companies if a company sponsors the trial. Depending on the size of the trial, this could be at the local, national, or international level. The trial may be presented at trial group meetings to generate interest or presented at international conferences to encourage collaboration from other trial groups. Alternatively, investigators who have previously participated in trials of trial groups or pharmaceutical companies may be approached directly.

Promotion of cancer trials in the UK tends to be aimed at investigators and research groups rather than patients. However, patients have access to clinical trial information via various websites from organizations such as CR-UK and Macmillan Cancer Support. Macmillan Cancer Support is a cancer information charity that provides up-to-date cancer information and practical, medical, and financial support for patients with cancer and their families and caregivers. CR-UK's website provides easy-to-understand patient information and also allows (where possible) patients to see what research and trials are being carried out in different hospitals throughout the UK. Figure 62-4 provides a list of websites that offer support and information to patients about cancer, treatments for cancer, and clinical trials.

Recruitment to trials is performed at the local level in cancer centers and smaller associated cancer units within the networks. The type of trials undertaken is dependent on the population covered by the network and its local strategy.

Staff multidisciplinary teams hold meetings, often on a weekly basis, in their region to make decisions regarding the diagnosis and treatment of individual patients. These teams include surgical, medical/clinical oncology, pathology, radiology, and nursing staff, as well as clinical trial staff, who can advise on any current trials that may be appropriate for patients.

Off-Treatment Follow-Up

Trial protocols will provide clear guidance for when patients are considered to be off protocol treatment, as well as follow-up intervals and their duration. The duration of the follow-up period depends on the phase of the trial. Follow-up for phase I trials tends to be relatively short, whereas phase III trials, which look for survival data, may require patients to be followed until death. Patients' continued consent to collect data in this period is required. If patients withdraw their consent for the trial, no further data would be collected. Sometimes patients are lost to follow-up. This can happen for a variety of reasons, such as when patients move or continue follow-up at a local hospital. Every effort is made to collect follow-up data on patients. It may be possible to obtain informa-

---

Figure 62-4. Useful Websites in the United Kingdom

Patient Support Websites
- Bowel Cancer UK: www.bowelcanceruk.org.uk
- Breakthrough Breast Cancer: www.breakthrough.org.uk
- Cancer Research UK: www.cancerresearchuk.org
- Macmillan Cancer Support: www.macmillan.org.uk
- Ovacome (ovarian cancer support charity): www.ovacome.org.uk

Regulatory Websites
- Clinical Trials Unit Glasgow, Cancer Research UK: www.glasgowctu.org
- Medical Research Council Clinical Trials Toolkit: www.ct-toolkit.ac.uk
- Medicine and Healthcare Products Regulatory Agency, Department of Health: www.gov.uk/mhra
- National Cancer Research Institute: www.ncri.org.uk

Professional Websites
- Institute of Clinical Research: www.icr-global.org
- Royal College of Nursing: www.rcn.org.uk
- United Kingdom Oncology Nursing Society: www.ukons.org

tion from patients' general practitioners or via the Medical Research Information Service, although this incurs a cost.

Clinical Trial Participants

Eligibility

Protocols for any clinical trial conducted in the UK clearly state the eligibility criteria for the trial, outlining the inclusion and exclusion criteria. The eligibility criteria are an important aspect of the protocol. Many factors need to be taken into account when considering a patient for a trial. Written informed consent must be obtained for all patients, and this must be done prior to commencement of any trial-specific procedures. Informed consent generally is taken by the local principal investigator or co-investigator for the study. On occasions, this duty may be delegated to a research nurse, depending on the type of study. Patients' understanding of the clinical trial information sheet and consent form is ascertained by verbal questioning.

The majority of protocols have a table of investigations that summarizes the investigations and procedures and required time points. Before patients can be registered or randomized to the trial, the required baseline investigations, as dictated in the protocol, must be carried out.

The principal investigator or a delegated member of the research team is responsible for taking written informed consent from patients, assessing patients' eligibility for the trial, and ensuring completion of the necessary investigations. A registration or randomization form is completed at this point, confirming patients' eligibility for the trial. If a research nurse or data manager is assigned to the trial, this person may complete the registration or randomization form, but it ultimately is the principal investigator or co-investigator who checks patients' eligibility for the trial and signs the registration or randomization form.

The study sponsor or coordinating CTU will complete the registration or randomization by telephone, fax, or Internet. Patients are given a unique trial identifier. If the trial is a randomized trial, patients are assigned to a treatment arm. If the purpose of the trial is dose-finding, the dose is determined at this point.

The use of waivers in trials to allow entry of patients who are otherwise ineligible for the trial is strictly prohibited.

Active Treatment

The investigational agents used in clinical trials are either supplied by the pharmaceutical company sponsor to the hospital pharmacy of each participating site or, as may be the case in noncommercial trials, taken from the hospital pharmacy's own stock.

When the investigational agent is received on site, the hospital pharmacy is responsible for ensuring the correct storage, preparation, handling, accountability, disposal, and destruction of the agent. The majority of hospital pharmacies now have clinical trial pharmacists and technicians dedicated to work on clinical trials. It is essential for these staff to be involved in the trial from an early stage. This ensures that any practical issues related to the dispensing of the investigational agent are addressed prior to commencement of the trial. Often, the premedication, hydration, or antiemetic regimens specified in the protocol will differ from the standard regimens used at sites. It may be possible for an agreement to be made for sites to use their own regimen. The premedication regimens specified in the protocol are often for guidance.

The treatment schedule for the trial is clearly stated in the protocol, including details on the method to be used for calculating the drug dose where applicable. The protocol also provides specifications and information on dose adjustments, dose modifications, treatment delays, expected side effects, management of side effects, time points of investigations, response assessment, and discontinuation of protocol treatment.

The protocol for the clinical trial must be strictly adhered to at all times. If this is not done, it is deemed a protocol violation or deviation and may render the patient ineligible for the trial. Whether the patient's treatment is changed or the patient's data are considered ineligible for analysis of the trial will depend on the severity of the protocol violation or deviation. An example would be a patient being given the wrong treatment.

Patients generally are reviewed prior to each course of treatment by the responsible clinician. Prior to treatment, the clinician assesses the patient's current medical condition, taking into consideration any toxicities that have occurred during the previous cycle, to establish whether treatment can be given, and if so, at what dose.

It is common practice in the UK for either a chemotherapy nurse (IV nurse) or research nurse to administer the treatment. Clinicians and research nurses regularly assess patients during the treatment cycle and document in their hospital case notes any side effects or reaction, known as adverse events (AEs), experienced by the patient, regardless of whether they are related to trial treatment.

For the majority of cancer trials in the UK, AEs are graded according to the National Cancer Institute Cancer Therapy Evaluation Program's Common Terminology Criteria for Adverse Events, which can be downloaded from http://ctep.cancer.gov. These provide standard terminology to name and describe the severity (grade) of AEs that occur in the treatment of cancer. The protocol will specify which version is to be used.

Serious adverse events (SAEs) occurring during treatment and up to 30 days from the last administration of the protocol treatment are required to be reported within 24 hours of the site becoming aware of the event. SAEs are reported by fax or telephone, normally by the clinical trial coordinator, data manager, or research nurse, to the pharmacovigilance department of the trial sponsor or the coordinating site. This department is responsible for determining whether the SAE is a suspected unexpected serious adverse reaction (known as a SUSAR). If so, it must be reported to the competent authority, which is MHRA in the UK, and to the ethics committees within the correct timelines. The protocol provides clear guidance on the reporting of SAEs.

Many trials have trial steering committees and data monitoring committees. Trial steering committees are independent bodies that include a majority of members not involved in running the trial. Their role is to monitor and supervise the progress of the trial toward its interim and overall objectives. They regularly review relevant information from other sources and consider recommendations of the data monitoring committee (Medical Research Council, 1998).

Data monitoring committees are independent bodies whose members are not involved in the trial. They generally have a minimum of three members, including one or more clinicians and one or more statisticians with experience in trials. Committee members are the only people to see the data during the trial. They are independent and look at the trial from the point of view of trial participants. The members are responsible for protecting patients from exposure to any excess risk by recommending that the trial stops early if the safety or efficacy results are sufficiently convincing.

Genetics and Genomics

The Human Tissue Authority (HTA) in the UK is a watchdog agency that supports public confidence by licensing organizations that store and use human tissue for purposes such as research, patient treatment, postmortem examination, teaching, and public exhibitions (HTA, n.d.). HTA also gives approval for organ and bone marrow donations from living people. Its aim is to set standards that are clear and reasonable and in which the public and professionals can have confidence.

The Human Tissue Act 2004 covers England, Wales, and Northern Ireland. It established HTA to regulate activities concerning the removal, storage, use, and disposal of human tissue. Consent is the fundamental principle of the legislation and underpins the lawful removal, storage, and use of body parts, organs, and tissue. Different consent requirements apply when dealing with tissue from the deceased and the living. Separate legislation exists in Scotland, the Human Tissue (Scotland) Act 2006. While provisions of the Human Tissue (Scotland) Act 2006 are based on authorization rather than consent, they are essentially both expressions of the same principle. Key points regarding the Human Tissue Act 2004 are as follows.

- The Human Tissue Act 2004 regulates the removal, storage, and use of human tissue. This is defined as material that has come from a human body and consists of, or includes, human cells.
- The Human Tissue Act 2004 created a new offense of DNA "theft." It is unlawful to have human tissue with the intention of its DNA being analyzed, without the consent of the person from whom the tissue came.
- The Human Tissue Act 2004 makes it lawful to take minimum steps to preserve the organs of a deceased person for use in transplantation while steps are taken to determine the wishes of the deceased, or, in the absence of their known wishes, obtaining consent from someone in a qualifying relationship. (HTA, 2010)

The UK Genetic Testing Network advises NHS on genetic testing for inherited disorders. It aims to ensure the provision of high-quality, equitable genetic testing services for all NHS patients across the UK (UK Genetic Testing Network, n.d.). This involves evaluating new tests and making recommendations to commissioners on new NHS services. The network is a collaborative group of genetic testing laboratories, clinicians, and commissioners of NHS genetic services and involves patient support groups.

The Economic and Social Research Council (ESRC) Genomics Network was a major investment by the ESRC from 2002 to 2013. It was dedicated to examining the development and use of the science and technologies of genomics. Network activities spanned the field of genomics, covering areas as diverse as plant and animal genetics, embryonic stem cell research, and associated health applications. The network contributed to many publications, public and policy engagement initiatives, and the involvement of nearly 300 research staff and visiting research fellows (ESRC Genomics Network, n.d.).

Correlative Trials

Correlative or ancillary studies, commonly known as add-on studies, are incorporated into many of the cancer clinical trials in the UK. Examples of these studies are quality-of-life questionnaires, neurologic questionnaires, health economics, translational research, pharmacokinetics, and nursing. The types of correlative studies incorporated are dependent on the trial's protocol and objectives. Patients are fully informed of any additional studies in the patient information sheet for the trial and will often sign an additional consent form for these. Correlative studies often are optional.

Documentation and Data Management

Data Management Tools and Systems

The provision of accurate data in clinical trials is vital, as the data determine the results of a clinical trial. The trial protocol defines the required data and timing of collection. When a site is activated to begin recruitment to the trial, the site is provided with the necessary study materials for conducting the trial, including the CRFs and, where applicable, quality-of-life questionnaires, neurotoxicity questionnaires, patient diary cards, and any other materials. Guidelines that provide step-by-step instructions for the completion of the CRFs are generally provided to sites. During site initiation, time is spent reviewing the data management aspects of the trial.

The clinical trial coordinator/data manager or the clinical research nurse for the trial normally completes the CRF and subsequent queries. Sites involved in clinical trials tend to have methods that they employ to ensure that the required data are collected. Examples of these include creating trial-specific worksheets to ensure the investigations/procedures are carried out at the specified times or adding prompts to patients' case notes to remind the investigator when investigations are required or to be arranged at each patient visit. Copies of the table of investigations from the protocol also may be inserted in patients' case notes, confirming that current versions of study protocols are readily available in treatment areas. The investigator, co-investigator, or research nurse requests the investigations required for the trial.

Various formats of CRFs exist. The most commonly used are paper and electronic. Paper CRFs generally are in the form of ring binders or books. Multiple "no carbon required" papers are used, which allow the study site, sponsor, and coordinating site to each have an original copy of the data.

The electronic CRF format is carried out by data entry to a database on a laptop at sites or via a website. This method is becoming more widely used. The electronic format is beneficial to sponsors because it allows quicker access to the data. The disadvantages of this type of system are that more training is required and the setup costs can be high.

Commercial trials are generally fully monitored. Site monitoring visits are conducted either by a clinical research associate (CRA) from the pharmaceutical company or a CRA from a clinical research organization employed by the company. Source data verification (SDV) is completed at monitoring visits by checking the data recorded on CRFs with patients' case notes to ensure the accuracy of the data recorded. Protocol compliance is checked at monitoring visits, as is the sites' compliance with GCP and necessary regulatory requirements. The level of monitoring required for the trial is determined following initial risk assessment performed for the trial.

Noncommercial trials do not routinely involve full monitoring, mainly because of a lack of resources. Following the implementation of the EU CTD, it has now become more common for noncommercial trials to have some form of monitoring to meet the directive's requirements. In the UK, a risk-based approach generally is taken for noncommercial trials, with the level of monitoring required for the trial determined following the risk assessment performed for the trial.

Trials are required to have quality assurance measures in place to ensure that they meet the requirements for safety, reliability, and completeness. Actions will be taken if the data returned from a site give concerns as to their accuracy, consistency, completeness, or timeliness, or if any serious deficiencies are suspected in SAE reporting. Generally, recruitment will be suspended from the site until a selection of CRFs have been checked against the original patients' case notes.

Information Systems Resources

The World Wide Web provides a great resource for education and information on current clinical research in the UK. Many CTUs, such as the CR-UK Clinical Trials Unit Glasgow, have established their own websites to provide information about their unit and research activities. Larger groups and organizations such as CR-UK, NRES, NCRN, and MHRA have their own websites that will be used regularly by research professionals. Some, such as the NRES and MHRA websites, provide a question-and-answer facility that allows researchers to ask the experts within NRES and MHRA for advice on ethical issues and regulations.

Patients also can access information via these sites. In addition, a number of charities and research groups in the UK provide information for patients, such as CR-UK and Macmillan Cancer Support as discussed previously. Tumor-specific patient support groups also exist, such as Ovacome, Breakthrough Breast Cancer, and Bowel Cancer UK. Websites for patient support organizations in United Kingdom are listed in Figure 62-4.

Quality Assurance

For any clinical trial, the appropriate quality assurance procedures and systems must be in place to ensure the trial is conducted according to the appropriate regulatory standards. It is important that the company, group, and CTU coordinating the clinical trial can be assured of the participants' safety and of producing good quality data that provide the answer to the research question posed.

During the setup phase and the course of the study, version control of study documents is very important. Protocols, patient information sheets, consent forms, and investigator drug brochures should display the version number and date on all pages of the document. When the study undergoes the ethics review, the reviewers will note which version of the documents they have approved, which is the version that should be used and referred to. This is particularly important for the protocol and patient information sheet, as these documents often change during the course of the study. Staff members must be able to easily identify the current version in use.

Site selection is very important to ensure good quality research and timely recruitment to the trial. Participating sites must have the appropriate expertise available to participate in the study, such as clinical, nursing, and research support staff (e.g., data management).

Once the study is underway, a number of different systems are typically initiated to ensure quality, such as the following:

- SDV: The study data are compared and verified with the patients' medical notes to ensure that all the appropriate information has been collected. This can range from 10% SDV to a full 100% check of study data. As discussed previously, the level of monitoring is often determined by the risk assessment of the protocol.
- Checking of patient consent: It is normal practice for the consent forms to be checked for all patients recruited to the study. The monitor will check that form is the correct version and has been signed.

In addition to SDV of patient data, the coordinating site may carry out a number of checks on the quality of data returned by the participating site. Manual and computer-generated checks on the data are produced, and any subsequent data queries will be created and returned to the site. Any sites that continually produce a large amount of queries and poor data quality may be examined more closely, leading to an increase in SDV for that site. A system is also in place to monitor the return of data within the timelines set; any problem sites will be identified and the appropriate action taken.

In addition to the previously described quality checks carried out by the study coordinator, it is common practice for CTUs, companies, and groups to have quality assurance staff in place to internally audit a trial. They will check to ensure that the study coordinator and on-site staff are conducting the trial to per SOPs. This includes ensuring that the data have been confirmed and queried appropriately, that SDV is performed correctly, that the sites have been initiated correctly, and that all of the relevant documentation is in place.

On occasion, the trial sponsor will delegate much of the day-to-day trial tasks to a CTU. In this case, the sponsor may undertake an audit of the study to ensure that the CTU is carrying out its responsibilities as outlined in the CTA. The sponsor may decide to audit participating sites to ensure they are meeting their responsibilities.

Finally, as the licensing and regulatory body of clinical trials in the UK, MHRA may perform an inspection of any specific trials, research units, and sponsor organizations. MHRA may notify sites of a forthcoming inspection at very short notice. The inspections can range from small study-specific inspections to large inspection of the complete setup and practice of a unit or organization.

Professional Development

Within the UK clinical research environment, a number of sources are available for the professional development of research nurses, trial coordinators, and data managers. Most CTUs and hospitals provide ongoing in-house training for staff by making use of the on-site experts in their field, such as oncology and tumor-related education sessions, treatment (chemotherapy and radiation therapy) education sessions, update sessions on current research in various tumor areas, and pathology presentations.

A number of organizations are located throughout UK communities that provide training and development, including the Institute of Clinical Research (ICR), the Royal College of Nursing, and the United Kingdom Oncology Nursing Society (see Figure 62-4). These organizations hold annual general meetings where members can participate and vote on issues, as well as attend a forum for education. Regular training courses are available on topics such as data management, GCP, and presentation skills, to name but a few. ICR sponsors longer-term courses at universities in the UK, including master's degrees in clinical research, postgraduate diplomas, and a certificate in clinical research. NCRN, NCRI, UKCRC, and MHRA offer training courses on issues such as GCP, audit, pharmacovigilance, and SOPs.

Internationally, the European Organisation for Research and Treatment of Cancer organizes training courses for staff involved in cancer clinical research. Conferences such as those held by the American Society for Clinical Oncology and European Society for Medical Clinical Oncology allow staff to stay current with developments in the diagnosis and treatment of cancer.

Summary

Over the past 10–15 years, significant changes and restructuring of the clinical research infrastructure have occurred within the UK, with the aim of making it a desirable location for clinical research activity to take place.

Strategic review by all stakeholders is ongoing, with the goal of streamlining processes and reducing the timelines within which the research is delivered.

Key Points

- The UK has a National Health Service.
- The UK has a strong clinical research heritage and has long been a world leader in medical research. Since the birth of the pharmaceutical industry over a century ago, only the United States has developed more drugs, and British researchers played a central role in many of the revolutionary breakthroughs in scientific understanding and patient care standards (House of Commons Science and Technology Committee, 2013).
- The UK has a well-established research framework for conducting research, particularly in the cancer field.

References

Department of Health. (2012). *Attributing the costs of health and social care research (AcoRD)*. Retrieved from https://www.gov.uk/government/publications/guidance-on-attributing-the-costs-of-health-and-social-care-research

Directive 2001/20/EC of the European Parliament and of the Council of 4 April 2001 on the approximation of the laws, regulations and administrative provisions of the Member States relating to the implementation of good clinical practice in the conduct of clinical trials on medicinal products for human use. Retrieved from http://ec.europa.eu/health/files/eudralex/vol-1/dir_2001_20/dir_2001_20_en.pdf

ESRC Genomics Network. (n.d.). *ESRC Genomics Network (archive)*. Retrieved from http://www.genomicsnetwork.ac.uk

Health and Safety Executive. (n.d.). *Control of substances hazardous to health*. Retrieved from http://www.hse.gov.uk/coshh

House of Commons Science and Technology Committee. (2013, January 1). *Third report of session 2013–14: Clinical trials*. Retrieved from http://www.publications.parliament.uk/pa/cm201314/cmselect/cmsctech/104/10404.htm

Human Tissue Act 2004. Retrieved from http://www.legislation.gov.uk/ukpga/2004/30/contents

Human Tissue Authority. (n.d.). *About us*. Retrieved from https://www.hta.gov.uk/about-us

Human Tissue Authority. (2010, July). *Human Tissue Act 2004*. Retrieved from https://www.hta.gov.uk/human-tissue-act-2004

Human Tissue (Scotland) Act 2006. Retrieved from http://www.legislation.gov.uk/asp/2006/4/contents

International Conference on Harmonisation of Technical Requirements for Registration of Pharmaceuticals for Human Use. (1996). *ICH harmonised tripartite guideline: Guideline for good clinical practice, E6(R1)*. Retrieved from http://www.ich.org/fileadmin/Public_Web_Site/ICH_Products/Guidelines/Efficacy/E6/E6_R1_Guideline.pdf

Medical Research Council. (1998). *MRC guidelines for good clinical practice in clinical trials*. London, England: Author.

UK Genetic Testing Network. (n.d.). *About us*. Retrieved from http://ukgtn.nhs.uk/about-us

World Medical Association. (n.d.). *Declaration of Helsinki: Ethical principles for medical research involving human subjects*. Retrieved from http://www.wma.net/en/30publications/10policies/b3

Appendices

Appendix 1. Terms of the Federalwide Assurance for the Protection of Human Subjects

1. **Human Subjects Research Must Be Guided by a Statement of Principles**
   All of the Institution's human subjects research activities, regardless of whether the research is subject to the U.S. Federal Policy for the Protection of Human Subjects (also known as the Common Rule), will be guided by a statement of principles governing the institution in the discharge of its responsibilities for protecting the rights and welfare of human subjects of research conducted at or sponsored by the institution. This statement of principles may include (a) an appropriate existing code, declaration (such as the World Medical Association's Declaration of Helsinki), or statement of ethical principles (such as the Belmont Report: Ethical Principles and Guidelines for the Protection of Human Subjects of Research of the U.S. National Commission for the Protection of Human Subjects of Biomedical and Behavioral Research), or (b) a statement formulated by the institution itself.

2. **Applicability**
   These terms apply whenever the Institution becomes engaged in human subjects research conducted or supported* by any U.S. federal department or agency that has adopted the Common Rule, unless the research is otherwise exempt from the requirements of the Common Rule or a U.S. federal department or agency conducting or supporting the research determines that the research shall be conducted under a separate assurance. (For guidance on the meaning of "engaged," see OHRP's guidance at http://www.hhs.gov/ohrp/policy/engage08.html.)
   [*For the purposes of the FWA, federally-supported means the U.S. Government providing any funding or other support.]

3. **Compliance with Laws, Regulations, Policies, and Guidelines**
   (a) U.S. Institutions:
   When the Institution becomes engaged in research to which the FWA applies, the Institution and institutional review boards (IRBs) upon which it relies for review of such research will comply with the Common Rule.
   The reference in the U.S. Code of Federal Regulations is shown below for each U.S. federal department and agency which has adopted the Common Rule:
   7 CFR part 1c – Department of Agriculture
   10 CFR part 745 – Department of Energy
   14 CFR part 1230 – National Aeronautics and Space Administration
   15 CFR part 27 – Department of Commerce
   16 CFR part 1028 – Consumer Product Safety Commission
   22 CFR part 225 – Agency for International Development
   24 CFR part 60 – Department of Housing and Urban Development
   28 CFR part 46 – Department of Justice
   32 CFR part 219 – Department of Defense
   34 CFR part 97 – Department of Education
   38 CFR part 16 – Department of Veterans Affairs
   40 CFR part 26 – Environmental Protection Agency
   45 CFR part 46, subpart A – Department of Health and Human Services
   45 CFR part 46, subpart A – Central Intelligence Agency (by Executive Order 12333)
   45 CFR part 46, subpart A – Department of Homeland Security (by federal statute)
   45 CFR part 690 – National Science Foundation
   49 CFR part 11 – Department of Transportation
   (b) Non-U.S. Institutions:
   When the Institution becomes engaged in research to which the FWA applies, the Institution and IRBs upon which it relies for review of such research at a minimum will comply with one or more of the following:
   - The Common Rule;
   - The U.S. Food and Drug Administration regulations at 21 CFR parts 50 and 56;
   - The current International Conference on Harmonization E-6 Guidelines for Good Clinical Practice;
   - The current Council for International Organizations of Medical Sciences International Ethical Guidelines for Biomedical Research Involving Human Subjects;
   - The current Canadian Tri-Council Policy Statement: Ethical Conduct for Research Involving Humans;
   - The current Indian Council of Medical Research Ethical Guidelines for Biomedical Research on Human Subjects; or
   - Other standard(s) for the protection of human subjects recognized by U.S. federal departments and agencies which have adopted the U.S. Federal Policy for the Protection of Human Subjects.

   If a U.S. federal department or agency head determines that the procedures prescribed by the Institution afford protections that are at least equivalent to those provided by the Common Rule, the department or agency head may approve the substitution of the foreign procedures in lieu of the procedural requirements provided above, consistent with the requirements of section 101(h) of the Common Rule.
   (c) U.S. and non-U.S. Institutions:
   For any research to which the FWA applies, the Institution also will comply with any additional applicable human subjects regulations and policies of the U.S. federal department or agency which conducts or supports the research and any other applicable federal, state, local, or institutional laws, regulations, and policies. When the Institution is engaged in non-exempt human subjects research conducted or supported by HHS, the Institution will comply with the requirements of subparts B, C, D, and E of the HHS regulations at Title 45 Code of Federal Regulations part 46, when applicable, for research involving pregnant women, fetuses, and neonates; prisoners; and children, respectively.

(Continued on next page)

Appendix 1. Terms of the Federalwide Assurance for the Protection of Human Subjects *(Continued)*

Human subjects research conducted or supported by each U.S. federal department or agency listed above will be governed by the regulations as implemented by the respective department or agency. The head of the U.S. federal department or agency retains final judgment as to whether a particular activity conducted or supported by the respective department or agency is covered by the Common Rule. If the Institution needs guidance regarding implementation of the Common Rule and/or other applicable U.S. federal regulations, the Institution should contact appropriate officials at the U.S. federal department or agency conducting or supporting the research. For U.S. federally-conducted or –supported research covered by the FWA, the U.S. federal department or agency that conducts or supports the research retains final authority for determining whether the Institution complies with the Terms of Assurance. If HHS receives an allegation or indication of noncompliance related to research to which the FWA applies and that is conducted or supported solely by a U.S. federal department or agency other than HHS, HHS will refer the matter to the other U.S. federal department or agency for review and action as appropriate.

4. **Written Procedures**
   (a) The Institution submitting the FWA has established written procedures for ensuring prompt reporting to the IRB, appropriate institutional officials, the head of any U.S. federal department or agency conducting or supporting the research (or designee), and OHRP of any:
       (1) unanticipated problems involving risks to subjects or others;
       (2) serious or continuing noncompliance with the applicable U.S. federal regulations or the requirements or determinations of the IRB(s); and
       (3) suspension or termination of IRB approval.
   (b) The Institution will ensure that the IRB(s) that reviews research to which the FWA applies has established written procedures for:
       (1) conducting IRB initial and continuing review (not less than once per year), of research, and reporting IRB findings to the investigator and the Institution;
       (2) determining which projects require review more often than annually and which projects need verification from sources other than the investigator that no material changes have occurred since the previous IRB review; and
       (3) ensuring prompt reporting to the IRB of proposed changes in a research activity, and for ensuring that such changes in approved research, during the period for which IRB approval has already been given, may not be initiated without IRB review and approval, except when necessary to eliminate apparent immediate hazards to the subjects.
   (c) Upon request, the Institution will provide a copy of these written procedures to OHRP or any U.S. federal department or agency conducting or supporting research to which the FWA applies.

5. **Institutional Support for the IRB(s)**
   The Institution will ensure that each IRB upon which it relies for review of research to which the FWA applies has meeting space and sufficient staff to support the IRB's review and recordkeeping duties.

6. **Reliance on an External IRB**
   Whenever the Institution relies upon an IRB operated by another institution or organization for review of research to which the FWA applies, the Institution must ensure that this arrangement is documented by a written agreement between the Institution and the other institution or organization operating the IRB that outlines their relationship and includes a commitment that the IRB will adhere to the requirements of the Institution's FWA. OHRP's sample IRB Authorization Agreement may be used for such purpose, or the parties involved may develop their own agreement. This agreement must be kept on file at both institutions/organizations and made available upon request to OHRP or any U.S. federal department or agency conducting or supporting research to which the FWA applies.

7. **Renewal or Update of the Assurance**
   The Institution must renew its FWA every 5 years, even if no changes have occurred, in order to maintain an active FWA.

   The Institution must update its FWA within 90 days after changes occur regarding the legal name of the Institution, the Human Protections Administrator, or the Signatory Official.

   Any renewal or update that is submitted to, and accepted by, OHRP begins a new 5-year effective period.

   Failure to renew or update an FWA appropriately may result in restriction, suspension, or termination of OHRP's approval of the Institution's FWA.

FWA—Federalwide Assurance; HHS—Health and Human Services; OHRP—Office for Human Research Protections

Note. From "Federalwide Assurance (FWA) for the Protection of Human Subjects," by U.S. Department of Health and Human Services Office for Human Research Protections, 2011. Retrieved from http://www.hhs.gov/ohrp/assurances/assurances/filasurt.html.

Appendix 2. Oncology Nursing Society Oncology Clinical Trials Nurse Competencies

The oncology clinical trials nurse demonstrates critical thinking and implementation of the nursing process, thus providing leadership in the conduct of clinical trials, improving outcomes for patients, and enhancing study integrity. This is accomplished through competent practice in the following functional areas.

I. Protocol Compliance
The oncology clinical trials nurse facilitates compliance with the requirements of the research protocol and good clinical research practice while remaining cognizant of the needs of diverse patient populations.
   A. Identifies the requirements of various types and phases of clinical trials, including objectives, sample sizes, and patient care needs.
   B. Identifies sources for and facilitates adherence to current regulations, guidance, and policies that affect research at the institutional, state, federal, and international levels.
   C. Promotes compliance with the varied processes and procedures required by different types of sponsors (e.g., private industry, National Cancer Institute Cancer Therapy Evaluation Program, investigator-initiated).
   D. Protects patient, protocol, and scientific confidentiality by ensuring security of research data and personal health information.
   E. Participates in discussions regarding feasibility of protocol implementation based on knowledge of institutional capabilities and limitations, therapy, or population of interest.
   F. Complies with the International Air Transport Association and institutional policies for shipping and receiving biological specimens, experimental agents, and devices.
   G. Collaborates with the research team to implement procedures for maintaining patient study participation from enrollment through completion.
   H. Identifies the institutional review board (IRB) of record (local, central, or commercial), protocol-related policies of the IRB, and preferred contact method.
   I. Participates in providing timely, informative, and accurate communication to the IRB as required.
   J. Facilitates and participates in the preparation for and implementation of scheduled and unscheduled meetings with external and internal monitors and auditors, including but not limited to the U.S. Food and Drug Administration (FDA), Medicare reviewers, the IRB, and quality assurance.
   K. Ensures validity of research results by ensuring timely, accurate, and complete data documentation, reporting deviations, violations, and serious adverse events.
   L. Collaborates with the principal investigator, pharmacy, and other appropriate personnel to ensure proper use of and accountability for experimental devices or drugs as indicated.

II. Clinical Trials–Related Communication
The oncology clinical trials nurse utilizes multiple communication methods to facilitate the effective conduct of clinical trials.
   A. Ensures ongoing formal and informal communication regarding clinical trials with team members.
   B. Provides general clinical research as well as trial-specific information to research, clinical, and other organizational staff.
   C. Develops relationships with referring physicians, clinical staff, and ancillary departments to facilitate compliance with and accrual to clinical trials.
   D. Participates in study initiation meetings.
   E. Provides education related to clinical trials to patients and their significant others.
   F. Advocates for clinical trials by participating in community outreach efforts to provide general clinical trials education when opportunities arise.
   G. Advocates for the safety and care of clinical trial patients as well as for the promotion and integrity of the clinical trial.

III. Informed Consent Process
The oncology clinical trials nurse demonstrates leadership in ensuring patient comprehension and safety during initial and ongoing clinical trial informed consent discussions.
   A. Ensures the initial and ongoing consent process is performed and documented in compliance with FDA, International Conference on Harmonization Good Clinical Practice (GCP), institutional, sponsor, IRB, and other applicable regulations, guidances, and policies.
   B. Participates in the education of clinical trial patients about their clinical trial and significant new information that is forthcoming during or after the conduct of the trial.
   C. Assesses for barriers to effective informed consent discussions and implements plans to overcome them.

IV. Management of Clinical Trial Patients
The oncology clinical trials nurse uses a variety of resources and strategies to manage the care of patients participating in clinical trials, ensuring compliance with protocol procedures, assessments, and reporting requirements as well as management of symptoms.
   A. Collaborates with the investigator to ascertain study patient eligibility for a clinical trial, including documentation of criteria specified in the protocol.
   B. Ensures adherence to the protocol schedule of events and other requirements.
   C. Ensures scheduling of all procedures required to assess for adverse events and disease response to the study intervention.
   D. Ensures the successful completion of correlative components of the clinical trial (e.g., pharmacokinetic, pharmacoeconomic, and quality-of-life studies).
   E. Assesses patients for trial-related and non–trial-related symptoms and ensures evidence-based symptom management while maintaining trial compliance.
   F. In collaboration with the investigator, assesses patients for adverse events and then documents and reports these findings per the protocol and FDA, sponsor, and IRB policies.

(Continued on next page)

Appendix 2. Oncology Nursing Society Oncology Clinical Trials Nurse Competencies *(Continued)*

G. Utilizes adverse event assessment data and clinical judgment to determine if a dose-limiting toxicity has occurred or if any treatment schedule or drug dose modifications are necessary and communicates findings to the study team and sponsors.
H. During phase I/dose escalation studies, collaborates with the principal investigator to determine when the maximum tolerated dose has been achieved based on adverse event assessment data and clinical judgment.
I. Evaluates disease response results and physical assessment data in conjunction with the principal investigator to determine response per the protocol.
J. Supports and evaluates patient adherence to the protocol by utilizing various methods to assist with documentation, patient education, and study agent return.
K. Identifies vulnerable patients who require increased nursing assessment and management in addition to the clinical trial requirements.

V. Documentation

The oncology clinical trials nurse provides leadership to the research team in ensuring collection of source data and completion of documentation that validate the integrity of the conduct of the clinical trial.

A. Complies with regulations, institutional policies, and sponsor requirements governing source data and documentation.
B. Documents assessment, management, and evaluation in source documents for patients on clinical trials as appropriate to the protocol and role.
C. Educates research and clinical team members regarding appropriate and accurate source documentation for participants in clinical trials.
D. Ensures that relevant data from the source document are abstracted and recorded in the clinical trial case report forms and that every data point can be verified within the source document.
E. Follows appropriate guidelines in making corrections to data entry in clinical records and case report forms as recommended by good clinical practices, standards, or institutional procedures.
F. Ensures that all regulatory documents are processed and maintained per institution, IRB, and GCP regulations.
G. Demonstrates proficiency in the use of clinical and research-related computer programs.

VI. Patient Recruitment

The oncology clinical trials nurse utilizes a variety of strategies to enhance recruitment while being mindful of the needs of diverse patient populations.

A. Assists in implementation of recruitment plans to identify and assess individuals who might be eligible for clinical trials, taking into consideration the study entry criteria, required procedures, and other potential factors.
B. Identifies and develops processes to overcome barriers to recruitment related to patient demographic factors, underserved populations, and healthcare system influences.
C. Identifies institutional or community-based resources or groups that can assist in achieving recruitment goals.

VII. Ethical Issues

The oncology clinical trials nurse demonstrates leadership in ensuring adherence to ethical practices during the conduct of clinical trials in order to protect the rights and well-being of patients and the collection of quality data.

A. Advocates for ethical care of clinical trial patients and the conduct of clinical trials in accordance with standards of nursing practice.
B. Promotes ongoing compliance with key ethical concepts by the research team, including informed consent, documentation, respect for persons, beneficence, and justice.
C. Ensures that members of vulnerable populations enrolled in clinical trials are identified and that their rights are addressed.
D. Identifies and follows institutional procedures to report any falsification of data or scientific misconduct.

VIII. Financial Implications

The oncology clinical trials nurse identifies the financial variables that affect research and supports good financial stewardship in clinical trials.

A. Describes the key components included in study budgets and institutional resources for budget details.
B. Confers with the principal investigator or finance personnel when protocol revisions will affect the costs of protocol management.
C. Identifies routine care versus research-related costs, the financial impact on patients, and any need for financial counseling.
D. Ensures and tracks submission of specified items (e.g., completed case report forms, specimens) to facilitate timely recovery of protocol-related activity costs.
E. Ensures that stipends to patients for protocol-related activities are disclosed to the IRB during approval of the consent form.

IX. Professional Development

The oncology clinical trials nurse takes responsibility for identifying his or her ongoing professional development needs and seeks resources and opportunities to meet those needs, such as through membership in nursing, oncology, or research organizations.

A. Participates in educational opportunities to increase knowledge about clinical trials, regulations and guidance, and the role of the clinical trials nurse.
B. Seeks resources on an ongoing basis that provide oncology treatment and nursing practice updates, such as through professional mentoring and meetings, journals, and Web sites.

Note. From "Oncology Clinical Trials Nurse Competencies" (pp. 11–14), by Oncology Nursing Society, 2010, Pittsburgh, PA: Oncology Nursing Society. Retrieved from https://www.ons.org/sites/default/files/ctncompetencies.pdf. Copyright 2010 by Oncology Nursing Society. Reprinted with permission.

Appendix 3. National Cancer Institute Consent Form Template for Adult Cancer Trials

NOTES FOR CONSENT FORM AUTHORS* (instructions updated 12/13/13):
- This document provides a Template to follow when writing consent forms for the majority of oncology trials. It recognizes the significant differences between various types of trials and provides phase-specific examples of recommended consent form language. This Template is not meant to be fully comprehensive; however, the lay language used and the format of the information should be followed as closely as possible when applying it to a specific study. In all cases, consent form authors should use simple language and be concise.
- Based upon the consensus of an expert, cross-disciplinary panel, the NCI strongly recommends that consent forms not exceed six to nine pages. Suggestions for making the consent form more concise include:
  1. Focus on what makes the study different from the care a patient would typically receive. Instead of trying to cover everything that might happen during the trial, limit the information to the research issues.
  2. Eliminate repetition of information.
  3. Use lay language and explain concepts simply.
  4. Use Times New Roman size 12 font.
- In the Template, instructions to consent form authors are formatted in a box. Placeholders for protocol-specific details, e.g., drug/intervention names and descriptions, are in italics; however, regular font should be used when inserting the details into the suggested consent form language.
- A blank line, "_____", indicates that the local investigator should provide the appropriate information before submitting to the IRB.
- The Template date in the header is for reference to this Template only and should not be included in the consent form distributed to investigators.
- A simplified study schema should be included in the consent form if the study includes randomization, otherwise it is optional.
- Recommendations for use of educational attachments to the consent form may be found on the last page of this Template. For example, while a lay-language, easy-to-read study calendar is a useful tool for study participants, it should not be part of the main consent form but could be included as an optional attachment. IRB review of attachments is required. **For CTEP-sponsored trials**, the ICD and all attachments must be submitted as a **single Word** or **PDF** document.

*These notes for authors are instructional and should not be included in the consent form distributed to investigators.

NOTES FOR LOCAL INVESTIGATORS*:
- The goal of the informed consent process is to provide people with sufficient information for making informed choices about participating in research. The consent form provides a summary of the study, of the individual's rights as a study participant, and documents their willingness to participate. The consent form is, however, only one piece of an ongoing exchange of information between the investigator and study participant. For more information about informed consent, review the "Recommendations for the Development of Informed Consent Documents for Cancer Clinical Trials" prepared by the Comprehensive Working Group on Informed Consent in Cancer Clinical Trials for the National Cancer Institute. The Web site address for this document is http://cancer.gov/clinicaltrials/understanding/simplification-of-informed-consent-docs/
- A blank line, "_____", indicates that the local investigator should provide the appropriate information before submitting to the IRB.

*These notes for investigators are instructional and should not be included in the consent form sent to IRBs.

Consent Form

> Notes to consent form authors about the Study Title:
> 1. **Section length limit: Both titles together should take up no more than one-quarter page.**
> 2. Include two titles:
>   a. The reader-friendly lay title, which is called the "Study Title for Study Participants".
>   b. The official title, which can be used by potential study participants for Internet searches and aids in tracking by study administrative personnel.
> 3. For the lay title:
>   a. Provide a brief (<20 words) title of the study in lay language.
>   b. Use general terms.
>   c. To make title concise, list the usual approach generically; e.g., chemotherapy, radiation therapy, surgery; rather than providing specific names, e.g., docetaxel, IMRT, laparoscopy.
>   d. The study drug should be named.
>   e. Use BOLD font.
> 4. For the official title:
>   a. Insert study ID number, e.g., Protocol 0000, and official study title as provided by the study sponsor.
>   b. Do not use BOLD font.

Study Title for Study Participants: (Insert Lay Title here)

Text Examples for Lay Title:
- **Testing the addition of the antibody, cetuximab, to usual chemotherapy in advanced lung cancer**

  OR
- **Testing the combination of two approved chemotherapy drugs after surgery for early stage lung cancer**

  OR
- **Testing pioglitazone to prevent oral cancer in people with oral leukoplakia**

Official Study Title for Internet Search on http://www.ClinicalTrials.gov: (Insert Official Title here)

(Continued on next page)

Appendix 3. National Cancer Institute Consent Form Template for Adult Cancer Trials *(Continued)*

What is the usual approach to my *(insert type of cancer, precancerous condition, early detection, prevention of cancer, diagnosis, other)*?

Notes to consent form authors:
- **Section length limit: This section should be between five and nine sentences and take up no more than one-quarter page.**
- While there may not be a single, uniformly adopted standard of care in a particular disease, precancerous condition, or high-risk group, clinical trials generally assume a usual approach that the research hopes to improve upon. Providing a brief description of a usual approach, which should not be overly specific or detailed, allows the research to be placed into an appropriate context. Whenever appropriate, include an estimate of the expected outcome if the usual approach is utilized.
- For chemoprevention trials, state the precancerous condition or high-risk status (e.g., current or former smoker, oral leukoplakia) and the usual intervention received if not participating in a study.
- Avoid naming specific drugs as these could change with the availability of new treatments, except where a particular agent is so commonly accepted that it provides the easiest explanation.

Text Examples for Chemoprevention/ Supportive Care Studies:

Text Example: Chemoprevention Studies
You are being asked to take part in this study because you are at increased risk for *(insert type of cancer, e.g., lung)* cancer. People who are at increased risk and choose not to participate in a study are usually followed closely by their doctor to watch for the development of cancer or *(as appropriate)* may receive a hormonal agent *(specify)* that has been approved by the FDA.

Text Example: Screening/Supportive Care/Symptom Management Studies
Treatments for cancer can cause side effects such as nausea and vomiting. People who do not take part in this study will receive standard medications that have been approved by the FDA for nausea and vomiting.

Text Example: Behavioral Study
Treatments for cancer can cause side effects such as fatigue. People who do not take part in this study will receive recommendations, such as encouragement to exercise, and/or ways to adjust their daily activities so they are less tired.

Text Examples for Chemotherapy/Radiation Therapy/Surgery/Biologics/Imaging/Other Studies:

Text Example: Phase 1 First in Human/Novel Route/Combination Studies or Non-randomized Phase 2 Studies
You are being asked to take part in this study because you have *(insert type of cancer, e.g., advanced pancreas)* cancer. You have already been treated with *(insert treatment modality, e.g., chemotherapy)* and your disease is now growing. People who are not in a study are usually treated with *(insert usual treatment modality, e.g., more chemotherapy) (indicate if FDA-approved)*.

Text Example: Phase 2 Single Arm Study of a New Agent
You are being asked to take part in this study because you have *(insert type of cancer, e.g., advanced brain cancer)* which has grown or has recurred. People who are not in a study are usually treated with either surgery, radiation, or with drugs *(indicate if FDA approved)*. Sometimes, combinations of these are used and your doctor can explain which may be best for you. These treatments can reduce symptoms and may stop the tumor from growing for several months or more.

Text Example: Randomized Phase 2/3 Studies in Previously Untreated Patients
You are being asked to take part in this study because you have *(insert type of cancer, e.g., advanced prostate cancer that is sensitive to hormones)*. People who are not in a study are usually treated with hormonal drugs *(indicate if FDA approved)*. Chemotherapy drugs are not usually used until the hormonal drug stops working against your type of cancer. For patients who receive the usual approach for this cancer, about *(insert appropriate number)* out of 100 are free of cancer at five years.

Text Example: Phase 3 Randomized Studies with Multiple Randomizations
You are being asked to take part in this study because you have *(insert type of cancer, e.g., advanced non-small cell lung cancer)*. People who are not in a study are usually treated with surgery, chemotherapy, and radiation therapy. There are several FDA-approved chemotherapy drugs that are commonly used along with the radiation therapy. *(Modify the following sentence to be consistent with the study)* For patients who receive the usual approach for this cancer, about *(insert appropriate number)* out of 100 are free of cancer at five years.

Text Example: Imaging Studies
You are being asked to take part in this study because you have *(insert type of cancer, e.g., advanced lung)* cancer. People who are not in a study are usually diagnosed or have their treatment monitored with a *(insert type of scan, e.g., CT)* scan. These scans use *(insert type of mechanism, e.g., radiation, magnets)* to take pictures of your cancer.

What are my other choices if I do not take part in this study?

Notes to consent form authors:
1. **Section length limit: This section should be no more than one-quarter page.**
2. Additional bullets should include, when appropriate, alternative procedures or interventions.
3. For comparative effectiveness studies in which two approved commercially-available approaches (tests, drugs, surgery, radiation, diagnostics, etc.) are being compared, the option of receiving one of the approaches outside of the trial should be included.

(Continued on next page)

Appendix 3. National Cancer Institute Consent Form Template for Adult Cancer Trials *(Continued)*

Use the following text for all studies:
If you decide not to take part in this study, you have other choices. For example:
- you may choose to have the usual approach described above
- you may choose to take part in a different study, if one is available
- or you may choose not to be treated for cancer *(as appropriate, consider adding)* but you may want to receive comfort care to relieve symptoms.

Why is this study being done?

> <u>Notes to consent form authors:</u>
> 1. **Section length limit: This section should be between five and seven sentences and take up no more than one-quarter page.**
> 2. Provide a brief, phase-specific description of why the study is being done. For single arm phase 2 studies, indicate what is known about the drug/approach and indicate the amount of improvement (e.g., tumor shrinkage by one quarter is expected compared to the tumor's present size). For randomized phase 2 or 3 trials only, indicate the type and amount of improvement (e.g., survival, time to cancer recurrence, decrease in symptoms) that can be observed if the study is positive.
> 3. Insert the names and types of investigational drugs/agents/interventions where indicated.
> 4. Insert the number of people taking part in the study.
> 5. If modifying the Template language is necessary, use simple, concise, lay language.

Text Examples for Chemoprevention/Supportive Care/Other Studies:

Text Example: Phase 1 Dose Escalation Chemoprevention Studies
The purpose of this study is to test the safety of *(insert name of drug or agent)* at different doses to find out what effects, if any, it has on people. There will be about *(insert number)* people taking part in this study.

Text Example: Phase 2 Non-randomized Chemoprevention Studies
The purpose of this study is to test the safety of *(insert name of drug or agent)* and find out what effects, if any, *(insert name of drug or agent)* has on people and their risk of *(insert type)* cancer. *(Indicate if the drug is FDA-approved or not)*. *(Add the following sentence as appropriate)*. The study drug has not been shown to shrink *(specify cancer type)* but it has shrunk several types of cancer in animals. There will be about *(insert number)* people taking part in this study.

Text Example: Phase 2 or 3 Randomized Chemoprevention Studies
The purpose of this study is to compare the safety and effects of *(insert name of drug or agent)* with *(insert name of currently-used drug or placebo)* on people and their risk of *(insert type)* cancer. In this study, you will get either *(insert name of drug/agent)* or placebo, a *(insert appropriate description for the placebo, e.g., pill/liquid)* that looks like the study drug but contains no medication. To be better, the study drug should increase life by 1 year or more compared to the usual approach. There will be about *(insert number)* people taking part in this study.

Text Example: Supportive Care Studies
You have cancer and will be receiving chemotherapy that may cause nausea and vomiting. The purpose of this study is to test whether *(insert name of drug/intervention)* can reduce nausea and vomiting. The effects of *(insert name of drug/intervention)* will be compared to *(a placebo or the usual approach)*. *(If applicable, include the following sentence.)* A placebo is a *(insert appropriate description for the placebo, e.g., pill/liquid)* that looks like the study drug but contains no medication. There will be about *(insert number)* people taking part in this study.

Text Example: Behavioral Study
You have *(insert type)* cancer and will be receiving chemotherapy that will cause fatigue. The purpose of this study is to test whether *(insert intervention, e.g., yoga)* can reduce fatigue. The effects of *(insert intervention)* will be compared to *(describe comparative intervention, e.g., listening to relaxation tapes, or "the usual approach")*.

Text Examples for Chemotherapy/Radiation Therapy/Surgery/Biologics/Imaging/Other Studies:

Text Example: Phase 1 Dose Escalation Studies
The purpose of this study is to test the safety of a study drug called *(insert name of research drug, e.g., TST1234)*. This drug has been tested in animals but not yet in people. This study tests different doses of the drug to see which dose is safer in people. There will be about *(insert number)* people taking part in this study.

Text Example: Phase 1 Novel Route/Combination Studies
This study uses a combination of drugs *(insert names of drugs, e.g., carboplatin and paclitaxel)* that have already been FDA-approved to be given by vein. The purpose of this study is to test whether giving one of the drugs *(insert name of drug, e.g., carboplatin)* through the belly along with the other drug *(insert name of drug, e.g., paclitaxel)* by vein is safe. There will be about *(insert number)* people taking part in this study.

Text Example: Phase 2 Non-randomized Studies
The purpose of this study is to test any good and bad effects of the study drug called *(insert name of drug, e.g., bevacizumab)*. *(Insert name of drug(s) or investigational approach)* could shrink your cancer but it could also cause side effects. Researchers hope to learn if the study drug will shrink the cancer by at least one-quarter compared to its present size. *(The following sentence should be included as appropriate)*. *(Insert name of drug(s))* has already been FDA-approved to treat other cancers. *(The following sentence should be included only if the agent has not shown evidence of activity in humans)*. It has not been tested in *(insert type of cancer, e.g., rectal)* cancer, but has shrunk several types of tumors in animals. There will be about *(insert number)* people taking part in this study.

(Continued on next page)

Appendix 3. National Cancer Institute Consent Form Template for Adult Cancer Trials *(Continued)*

Text Example: Phase 2 or 3 Randomized Studies
The purpose of this study is to compare any good and bad effects of using a *(specific drug, surgery or radiation approach)* along with the usual *chemotherapy*, surgery or radiation therapy to using the usual chemotherapy, surgery or radiation approach alone. The addition of *(insert name of drug(s) or investigational approach)* to the usual *(chemotherapy, surgery or radiation)* could shrink your cancer/prevent it from returning *(as appropriate)* but it could also cause side effects. This study will allow the researchers to know whether this different approach is better, the same, or worse than the usual approach. To be better, the study drug(s)/study approach should increase life by six months or more compared to the usual approach *(select other study primary endpoints as appropriate). (The following sentence should be included if appropriate).* This chemotherapy drug, *(insert name of drug, e.g., docetaxel)*, is already FDA-approved for use in *(insert type of cancer, e.g., prostate)* cancer but is usually not used until *(e.g., hormone drug)* stops working. There will be about *(insert number)* people taking part in this study.

Text Example: Phase 3 Randomized Studies with Multiple Randomizations
The purpose of this study is to test two things:
1. Compare any good and bad effects of using *(e.g., a higher dose [74 Gray] of radiation)* to the usual dose of *(e.g., 60 Gray)*.
2. Compare any good and bad effects of adding *(e.g., an extra antibody drug called cetuximab)* to the usual chemotherapy *(e.g., carboplatin and paclitaxel)* to using the usual chemotherapy alone.

Either of these different approaches could shrink your cancer but could also cause side effects. This study will allow the researchers to know whether this different approach is better, the same, or worse than the usual approach. If better, the new approaches should improve survival by 6 months compared to the usual approach. *(Include the following sentence, if applicable.)* Both the *(insert description of first research intervention, e.g., higher radiation dose)* and *(insert description of second research intervention, e.g., cetuximab)* have already been tested for safety; however, they are not part of the usual approach. There will be about *(insert number)* people taking part in this study.

Text Example: Phase 2 or 3 Study with Integral Biomarker(s)
Another purpose of this study is for researchers to learn if a biomarker test is helpful to decide … *(insert purpose of biomarker test, e.g., decide who should be enrolled in this study or decide which study group you will be in).* An *(insert how biomarker sample will be obtained, e.g., extra tube of blood will be drawn or tissue from your surgery will be used, etc. ...)* for the biomarker test. Researchers do not know if using the biomarker test is better, the same, or worse than if you . . . *(insert purpose of biomarker test, e.g., enrolled in this study or were put in a study group)* without using the biomarker test.

Text Example: Imaging Studies (Diagnostic, staging, or response to therapy)
The purpose of this study is to test *(insert name of research intervention, e.g., PET)* scans, which are a different way to take pictures of your type of cancer. The researchers want to see if *(insert name of intervention, e.g., PET)* scans are better or the same as what is usually used, *(insert name of usual approach, e.g., CT)* scans, at diagnosing or monitoring your type of cancer. There will be about *(insert number)* people taking part in this study.

Text Example: Phase 0/First-in-human Imaging Study
The purpose of this study is to test if *(insert name of research intervention, e.g., F18-Fluoroglutamine)* can be used to take pictures of your type of cancer. This will be the first time that *(insert name of research intervention, e.g., F18-Fluoroglutamine)* is being tried in people. There will be about *(insert number)* people taking part in this study.

Text Example: Phase 2 Non-randomized Imaging Agent Studies (biomarker example)
The purpose of this study is to test if an imaging drug, not approved by the FDA, called *(insert name of drug/agent, e.g., 18F-fluoride)* is useful for evaluating your type of cancer. This drug is used to perform a *(insert type of scan, e.g., PET)* scan. The researchers want to see if the *(insert type of scan, e.g., PET)* scan, using the study drug, can improve upon the usual scans at diagnosing or monitoring your type of cancer. There will be about *(insert number)* people taking part in this study.

What are the study groups?

> Notes to consent form authors:
> 1. **Section length limit: This section should be between seven to ten sentences and take up no more than three-quarters page.**
> 2. Provide a brief, phase-specific description of the study groups.
> 3. Insert the names and types of drugs/agents/interventions as needed.
> 4. For randomized studies, if the assignment is not 1:1, include a brief description of the assignment.
> 5. Clearly identify the investigational arm(s).
> 6. If modifying the Template language is necessary, use simple, concise, lay language.

Text Example: Phase 1 Dose Escalation Studies
Different doses of the study drug *(insert name of research drug)* will be given to several study participants. The first several study participants will receive the lowest dose. If the drug does not cause serious side effects, it will be given to other study participants at a higher dose. The doses will continue to increase for every group of study participants until side effects occur that require the dose to be lowered. Then the study is stopped. You *(insert appropriate information, e.g., will/will not)* be able to receive additional doses of the drug.

Text Example: Phase 2 Non-randomized Studies
All study participants will get the same study intervention. It will include the usual radiation therapy and chemotherapy *(insert usual chemotherapeutics, e.g., 5-fluorouracil or capecitabine)*. All study participants will also get the study drug *(insert name of research drug, e.g., bevacizumab)*.

Appendix 3. National Cancer Institute Consent Form Template for Adult Cancer Trials *(Continued)*

Text Example: Randomized Phase 2 Treatment Studies and Chemoprevention Studies
This study has two study groups. Group 1 will receive the study drug *(insert name of research drug)* and Group 2 will receive a placebo, a *(insert appropriate description for the placebo, e.g., pill/liquid)* that looks like the study drug but contains no medication.

A computer will by chance assign you to treatment groups in the study. This is called randomization. This is done by chance because no one knows if one study group is better or worse than the other.

Text Example: Phase 3 Randomized Studies
This study has two study groups.
- Group 1 will get the usual *(insert description of intervention, e.g., hormone or chemotherapy)* drug used for this type of cancer *(insert name of drug[s])*.
- Group 2 will get the usual *(insert description of intervention, e.g., hormone or chemotherapy)* drug used for this type of cancer *(insert name of drug[s])* plus a study drug called *(insert name of research drug, e.g., docetaxel)*.

A computer will by chance assign you to treatment groups in the study. This is called randomization. This is done by chance because no one knows if one study group is better or worse than the others.
(Note to informed consent authors: Study chart is optional if there is no randomization.) Another way to find out what will happen to you during this study is to read the chart below. Start reading at the left side and read across to the right, following the lines and arrows.

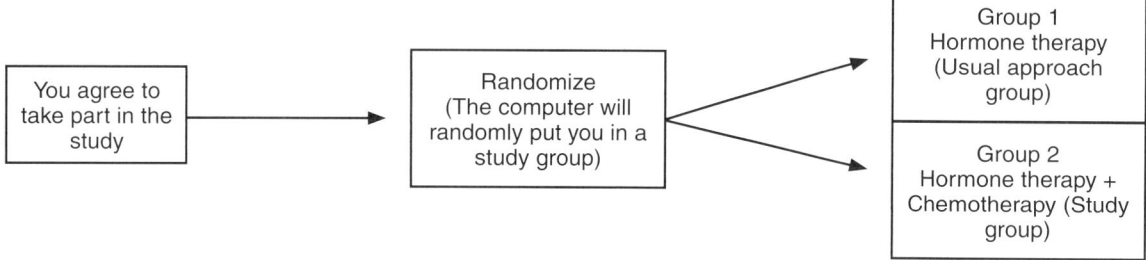

Text Example: Phase 3 Randomized Studies with Multiple Randomizations
All participants in this study will be given chemotherapy and radiation therapy.
- Group 1 will get the usual chemotherapy *(insert names of drugs, e.g., carboplatin and docetaxel)* and the usual radiation dose *(insert dose, e.g., 60 Gray)*.
- Group 2 will get the usual chemotherapy *(insert names of drugs, e.g., carboplatin and docetaxel)* with a higher radiation dose than usual *(insert research dose, e.g., 74 Gray)*.
- Group 3 will get the usual chemotherapy *(insert names of drugs, e.g., carboplatin and docetaxel)* and the usual radiation dose *(insert dose, e.g., 60 Gray)* and a study drug called *(insert name of research drug, e.g., cetuximab)*.
- Group 4 will get the usual chemotherapy plus the higher radiation dose plus the study drug called *(insert name of research drug, e.g., cetuximab)*.

A computer will by chance assign you to treatment groups in the study. This is called randomization. This is done by chance because no one knows if one study group is better or worse than the others. Another way to find out what will happen to you during the study is to read the chart below. Start reading at the left side and read across to the right, following the lines and arrows.

(Insert chart with four Groups, similar to the randomized study chart provided in the Phase 3 example above.)

How long will I be in this study?

> Note to consent form authors:
> 1. **Section length limit: This section should be one or two sentences and take up no more than one-eighth page.**

Use the following text for all studies:
You will receive the *(insert description of intervention, e.g., study drugs)* for *(insert intervention length)*. After you finish *(insert description of intervention)*, your doctor will continue to watch you for side effects and follow your condition for *(insert study follow-up length)*.

What extra tests and procedures will I have if I take part in this study?

> Notes to consent form authors:
> 1. **Section length limit: If the study has extra tests and procedures, this section is required but should be as brief as possible and take up no more than one-half page. If the study includes mandatory specimen collection, five to ten more sentences may be added and the length can be expanded to one page.**
> 2. You **do not** need to list those exams, tests, and procedures that are part of the usual approach. If the only exams, tests, or procedures that are being done are those performed using the usual approach, omit this section.
> 3. Provide a list of research-related exams, tests, and procedures that are not part of the usual approach or that will be done more frequently than usual. Specify the frequency, if applicable.
> 4. Please note: Sample text has been provided below for <u>mandatory</u> specimen collection. Sample text for <u>optional</u> specimen collection is provided in the "…Optional studies…" section located prior to the Signature line.

(Continued on next page)

Appendix 3. National Cancer Institute Consent Form Template for Adult Cancer Trials *(Continued)*

Use the following text for all studies requiring extra exams, tests, and/or procedures:
Most of the exams, tests, and procedures you will have are part of the usual approach for your cancer. However, there are some extra *(insert appropriate word, e.g., exams, tests, and/or procedures)* that you will need to have if you take part in this study.

Before you begin the study:

You will need to have the following extra *(insert appropriate word, e.g., exams, tests, and/or procedures)* to find out if you can be in the study:
List exams, tests, and procedures that either would not be done for the usual approach or are performed more frequently than usual. Use bulleted format. Examples of extra exams, tests and procedures:
- MUGA scan
- Blood tests for studies of drug levels
- CT scan of abdomen
- Bone scan

The following text example is provided for studies which include <u>mandatory</u> *specimen collection:*

[Insert specimen type: Small pieces of cancer tissue removed by surgery, biopsies; A blood sample; A urine sample] will be taken for the study *[state when the sample will be taken, for example, before you begin study drug; after the third dose; etc.]* This sample is required in order for you to take part in this study because the research on the sample is an important part of the study. *[Include brief description of how the specimen will be collected, e.g., "The research biopsy is done in a similar way to biopsies done for diagnosis." Include a brief description of how the specimen will be used.]*

[If applicable, include risks of biopsy or other specimen collection, e.g., "Common side effects of a biopsy are a small amount of bleeding at the time of the procedure, pain at the biopsy site, which can be treated with regular pain medications, and bruising. Rarely, an infection can occur."] [If applicable, include, "You will sign a separate consent form before the biopsy is taken. This will be a standard surgical consent form from the institution where the biopsy procedure takes place."]

[If applicable, include whether any of the specimen left over will be stored for biobanking. If so, indicate that this will be discussed in the section on optional studies.]

[If applicable, describe how the test results will be stored to protect privacy, e.g., "Your privacy is very important and the researchers will make every effort to protect it. Your test results will be identified by a unique code and the list that links the code to your name will be kept separate from your sample and health information." Also include whether or not the results will be available to the study participant or study doctor.]

Neither you nor your health care plan/insurance carrier will be billed for the collection of the *[insert sample type]* that will be used for this study.

Use the following text for all studies requiring extra exams, tests, and/or procedures:

If the exams, tests, and procedures show that you can take part in the study, and you choose to take part, then you will need the following extra *(insert appropriate words, e.g., exams, tests, and/or procedures)*. They are not part of the usual approach for your type of cancer. *(If chemoprevention trial, state, "These are not part of the usual approach for your precancerous condition.")*

During the study:
Examples of exams, tests, and procedures:
- Blood tests every month for 1 year
- CT scan of abdomen every 3 months for 2 years
- Bone scan every 3 months for 2 years
- Bone marrow biopsy immediately after study treatment is completed and 1 year later
- Echocardiogram or MUGA scan to see how your heart is working every 3 months

If study calendar is attached, this statement may be included instead of the bullets: A study calendar that shows how often these *(insert appropriate words, e.g., exams, tests, and/or procedures)* will be done is attached.

What possible risks can I expect from taking part in this study?

> Notes to consent form authors:
> 1. **Section length limit: Limit this section to two to four pages maximum.**

If you choose to take part in this study, there is a risk that:
Note to consent form authors: Select reasonably foreseeable risks and discomforts that are not physical side effects from the bullets below and/or include others, as relevant. Keep bulleted lists to no more than four items, if possible.
- You may lose time at work or home and spend more time in the hospital or doctor's office than usual
- You may be asked sensitive or private questions which you normally do not discuss
- (For randomized studies only) The study drug(s)/study approach may not be better, and could possibly be worse, than the usual approach for your cancer.

(Continued on next page)

Appendix 3. National Cancer Institute Consent Form Template for Adult Cancer Trials *(Continued)*

- *(For studies requiring genetic testing)* There is a risk someone could get access to the personal information in your medical records or other information researchers have kept about you. Someone might be able to trace this information back to you. The researchers believe the chance that someone will identify you is very small, but the risk may change in the future as people come up with new ways of tracing information. In some cases, this information could be used to make it harder for you to get or keep a job. *(For non-U.S. participants, please verify the existence of such laws before including the following sentence.)* There are laws against misuse of genetic information, but they may not give full protection. The researchers believe the chance these things will happen is very small, but cannot promise that they will not occur.
- There can also be a risk in finding out new genetic information about you. New health information about inherited traits that might affect you or your blood relatives could be found during a study.

The *(specify type of study intervention, such as surgery, radiation therapy, drugs, etc.)* used in this study may affect how different parts of your body work such as your liver, kidneys, heart, and blood. The study doctor will be testing your blood and will let you know if changes occur that may affect your health.

There is also a risk that you could have side effects from the study drug(s)/study approach.

Here are important points about side effects:
- The study doctors do not know who will or will not have side effects.
- Some side effects may go away soon, some may last a long time, or some may never go away.
- Some side effects may interfere with your ability to have children.
- Some side effects may be serious and may even result in death.

Here are important points about how you and the study doctor can make side effects less of a problem:
- Tell the study doctor if you notice or feel anything different so they can see if you are having a side effect.
- The study doctor may be able to treat some side effects.
- The study doctor may adjust the study drugs to try to reduce side effects.

The tables below show the most common and the most serious side effects that researchers know about. There might be other side effects that researchers do not yet know about. If important new side effects are found, the study doctor will discuss these with you.

Notes to consent form authors on how to present possible side effects:
1. Side effects of study group(s):
   a. For single-arm studies, list all possible side effects of the study drugs according to the recommendations given in 2-6 below.
   b. For multiple-arm studies with a control, the Table(s) of Possible Side Effects for the control arm should appear first and be followed by the Tables of Possible Side Effects for the drugs/agents used in the experimental arm(s).
   c. If the experimental arm consists of the usual treatment drugs/regimens (the control arm) plus experimental agent(s)/drug(s), the Table of Possible Side Effects for the usual treatment should not be repeated. The following statement should appear before the Table of Possible Side Effects for the investigational drugs/agents: "In addition to side effects outlined above for Group 1 and Group 2, people in this study who are in Group 2 may also experience the possible side effects of (insert name of research drug) listed below."
2. Side effects of procedures:
   a. When describing risks for procedures, describe risks only for procedures that are beyond what would be considered as occurring during the usual treatment approach. The determination of deeming a procedure as part or not part of the usual treatment approach is left to the discretion of the investigator.
   b. Examples of procedures that are not part of the usual treatment approach could include an unusually large amount of blood to be drawn for PK, central line placement to administer the investigational agent, research biopsy, etc.
3. Side effects of supportive drugs named in the consent form:
   a. Non-experimental supportive drugs need not have their side effects listed unless the treatment they support is the research question tested in the study. For example, side effects of Bactrim need not be listed when transplant is part of a study unless transplant is the actual study question in the trial.
4. Side effects of classes of medications:
   a. If general classes of approved medications, such as a hormonal therapy or anti-emetics – where no specific drug is named – are required by the protocol, these do not need to be listed, nor their possible side effects included, in the consent form.
5. Extremely specific possible side effects which are not perceived by the study participant, such as minor changes in lab values, should not be included in the consent form. Lab value changes that could be perceived by the study participant, or could be indicative of harm, should be listed, for example, the phrase "you could have liver damage," would be much more understandable to the study participant than "you could have elevated liver enzymes" or "you could have an elevation in (such-and-such lab value)."
6. Definitions of frequency categories:
   a. "Common, some may be serious" - There is no standard definition of the frequency of risks included in this category however, as a guideline, "Common, some may be serious" can be viewed as occurring in greater than 20% and up to 100% of patients receiving the drug/agent.
   b. "Occasional, some may be serious" - There is no standard definition of the frequency of risks included in this category however, as a guideline, "Occasional, some may be serious" can be viewed as occurring between 4 and 20% of patients.

(Continued on next page)

Appendix 3. National Cancer Institute Consent Form Template for Adult Cancer Trials *(Continued)*

    c. "Rare, and serious" - Side effects that occur in less than 3% of patients do not have to be listed unless they are serious, in which case they should appear in the "Rare, and serious" category. This categorization will need to be modified for prevention studies.

    d. "Serious" is defined as side effects that may require hospitalization or may be irreversible, long-term, or life-threatening.

    e. "Possible, some may be serious" – This is a unique frequency category and may be used, when appropriate, for informing study participants of possible side effects related to IND agents for which the frequency of individual side effects has not yet been determined.

Notes to consent form authors on how to present possible side effects (continued):

7. Note on stating possible side effects for imaging agents: Certain FDA regulations will need to be considered when imaging agents are used depending on the imaging agent (IND vs. commercial) and the protocol. As examples of such guidances, please refer to: FDA's draft guidance for industry standards for clinical trial imaging endpoints, found at http://www.fda.gov/downloads/Drugs/GuidanceComplianceRegulatoryInformation/Guidances/UCM268555.pdf, and FDA's final guidance: "Developing Medical Imaging Drug and Biological Products" found at http://www.fda.gov/Drugs/DevelopmentApprovalProcess/DevelopmentResources/ucm092895.htm. Radiation Safety Committees may also require the mention of certain radiation-related information in the informed consent form.

The following bullets are required for NCI's Cancer Therapy Evaluation Program (CTEP)-sponsored studies. Consent form authors for studies from other sponsors have the option of using them:

1. CTEP is in the process of developing tables of possible side effects for its IND agents as well as for many other drugs commonly used in cancer treatment trials. These Tables should be inserted as illustrated below for the agents/drugs used in the cancer treatment trial. A list of agents/drugs for which tables of possible side effects have been developed, as well as the tables themselves, are available on CTEP's website at the following URL: http://ctep.cancer.gov/protocolDevelopment/#informed_consent
2. If a study uses a drug for which CTEP has not built a table of possible side effects, the same URL can be accessed for the tools and instructions to custom-build a table.
3. For custom-built tables of possible side effects, the same format and frequency categories should be used.

Note to consent form authors:
The following tables of possible side effects for selected drugs and agents have been supplied as examples of what should be included for the regimens or drugs used in the study. Text and tables are examples for a randomized, phase 3 trial in colorectal cancer with Group 1 consisting of FOLFOX or FOLFIRI and Group 2 consisting of FOLFOX or FOLFIRI plus bevacizumab.

Study Group 1 and Group 2 - Possible side effects of FOLFOX or FOLFIRI, either of which is the usual approach for this type of cancer:

Possible Side Effects of FOLFOX

COMMON, SOME MAY BE SERIOUS
In 100 people receiving FOLFOX, more than 20 and up to 100 may have:

- Anemia which may require blood transfusion
- Diarrhea, nausea, vomiting
- Difficulty swallowing
- Tiredness
- Bruising, bleeding
- Numbness and tingling of the arms and legs
- Increased risk of sunburn

(Continued on next page)

Appendix 3. National Cancer Institute Consent Form Template for Adult Cancer Trials *(Continued)*

OCCASIONAL, SOME MAY BE SERIOUS
In 100 people receiving FOLFOX, from 4 to 20 may have:

- Heart attack
- Chest pain
- Abnormal heartbeat which may cause fainting
- Hearing loss
- Swelling and redness of the eye
- Dry eye, mouth, skin
- Problem with eyelid
- Blurred vision with chance of blindness
- Discomfort from light, watering eyes
- Sores in internal organs
- Fluid in the belly
- Internal bleeding which may cause black tarry stool, coughing up blood, or blood in vomit or urine
- Constipation, heartburn, passing gas
- Sores in the throat or mouth
- A tear or hole in internal organs that may require surgery
- Chills, fever
- Difficulty walking, opening mouth, with balance and hearing, smelling, eating, sleeping, talking or emptying the bladder
- Swelling and redness at the site of the medication injection
- Liver damage which may cause yellowing of eyes and skin
- Allergic reaction which may cause rash, low blood pressure, wheezing, shortness of breath, swelling of the face or throat
- Weight gain, weight loss, loss of appetite
- Infection, especially when white blood cell count is low
- Dehydration
- Pain
- Inability to move shoulder or turn head
- Dizziness, headache
- Changes in taste
- Abnormal body movement including the eye and eyelid
- Bleeding from multiple sites including the vagina, testis, or brain
- Stroke which may cause paralysis, weakness
- Muscle weakness
- Seizure
- Worry, confusion, depression
- Increased urination
- Stuffy nose
- Cough, hiccups, sinus problems
- Swelling of the body which may cause shortness of breath
- Scarring of the lungs
- Changes in voice
- Increased sweating
- Hives, hair loss, itching, rash
- Flushing, hot flashes
- High blood pressure
- Low blood pressure which may cause feeling faint
- Blood clot which may cause swelling, pain, shortness of breath
- Damage to organs which may cause shortness of breath

RARE, AND SERIOUS
In 100 people receiving FOLFOX, 3 or fewer may have:

- Kidney damage which may require dialysis
- Redness, pain or peeling of palms and soles

Appendix 3. National Cancer Institute Consent Form Template for Adult Cancer Trials *(Continued)*

Possible Side Effects of FOLFIRI

COMMON, SOME MAY BE SERIOUS
In 100 people receiving FOLFIRI, more than 20 and up to 100 may have:

- Infection, especially when white blood cell count is low
- Anemia which may require blood transfusion
- Constipation, vomiting, nausea, diarrhea
- Sores in mouth
- Difficulty swallowing
- Fever
- Pain
- Weight loss, loss of appetite
- Bruising, bleeding
- Tiredness, dizziness
- Cough
- Hair loss

OCCASIONAL, SOME MAY BE SERIOUS
In 100 people receiving FOLFIRI, from 4 to 20 may have:

- Abnormal heartbeat
- Watering eyes, discomfort from light, blurred vision
- A tear or hole in the stomach which may require surgery
- Allergic reaction which may cause rash, low blood pressure, wheezing, shortness of breath, swelling of the face or throat
- Headache
- Abnormal eye movement
- Difficulty walking
- Shortness of breath
- Rash, itching
- Increased risk of sunburn
- Redness, pain or peeling of palms and soles
- Scarring of the lungs
- Blood clot

RARE, AND SERIOUS
In 100 people receiving FOLFIRI, 3 or fewer may have:

- Damage to the heart which may cause swelling
- Chest pain
- Heart attack which may cause chest pain, shortness of breath

Study Group 2 - In addition to side effects outlined above, people who are in Group 2 may also experience the possible side effects of bevacizumab listed below.

Possible Side Effects of Bevacizumab

COMMON, SOME MAY BE SERIOUS
In 100 people receiving bevacizumab, more than 20 and up to 100 may have:

- Diarrhea, nausea, vomiting
- Tiredness
- Headache
- High blood pressure which may cause blurred vision

(Continued on next page)

Appendix 3. National Cancer Institute Consent Form Template for Adult Cancer Trials *(Continued)*

OCCASIONAL, SOME MAY BE SERIOUS
In 100 people receiving bevacizumab, from 4 to 20 may have:

- Anemia which may require blood transfusion
- Abnormal heartbeat which may cause fainting
- Dizziness, fainting
- Pain
- Constipation, heartburn
- Bleeding from multiple sites including the vagina or nose, or bleeding in the brain which may cause confusion
- Internal bleeding which may cause black, tarry stool, blood in vomit or urine, or coughing up blood
- Sores in mouth which may cause difficulty swallowing
- Allergic reaction which may cause rash, low blood pressure, wheezing, shortness of breath, swelling of the face or throat
- Infection, especially when white blood cell count is low
- Non-healing surgical site
- Weight loss
- Loss of appetite
- In children or adolescents: may interfere with growth
- Kidney damage which may require dialysis
- Cough, hoarseness, stuffy nose, shortness of breath
- Itching, rash, hives
- Blood clot which may cause swelling, pain, shortness of breath

RARE, AND SERIOUS
In 100 people receiving bevacizumab, 3 or fewer may have:

- Heart attack or heart failure which may cause shortness of breath, swelling of ankles, or tiredness
- A tear or hole in internal organs that may require surgery
- Sores in the throat
- Stroke which may cause paralysis, weakness
- Brain damage, Reversible Posterior Leukoencephalopathy Syndrome, which may cause headache, seizure, blindness

Examples of research imaging studies:

Text Example: Radiation Risk for Research Imaging Studies
(Each site may need to modify this section to quote correct dosimetry for the type of study being performed and dosimetry for its own scanners and imaging protocols in accordance with its own institutional policies and procedures. The following text and risk estimate is an example only.)

The *(insert type of scan, e.g., PET, CT)* that you will receive in this study will expose you to low amounts of radiation. Every day, people are naturally exposed to low levels of radiation that come from the sun and the environment. This type of radiation is called "background radiation". No one knows for sure whether exposure to low amounts of radiation is harmful for your body. However, scientists believe that being exposed to too much radiation can cause harmful side effects, including causing a new cancer.

The *(insert type of scan, e.g., PET, CT)* that you will receive in this study will expose you to extra radiation that is equal to about *(insert estimate, e.g., 2 year's worth)* of background radiation. Most of the time, this low amount of extra radiation is not harmful to you. However, scientists believe that if you get extra radiation that is more than about 30 year's worth of background radiation, there is a chance of having a harmful side effect, including causing a new cancer. It is estimated that this could occur in about 1 out of every 1000 people who get a very large amount of extra radiation.

Table example of risk presentation for Radiation Therapy Studies.
Examples should be modified to add possible side effects related to treatment location.

Possible Side Effects of Research Radiation Therapy

COMMON, SOME MAY BE SERIOUS
In 100 people receiving radiation therapy, more than 20 and up to 100 may have:

- Reddening, tanning, or peeling of the skin
- Mild pain
- Hair loss
- Tiredness
- Diarrhea, nausea
- Anemia, which may require transfusion
- Infection, especially when white blood cell count is low

(Continued on next page)

Appendix 3. National Cancer Institute Consent Form Template for Adult Cancer Trials *(Continued)*

OCCASIONAL, SOME MAY BE SERIOUS
In 100 people receiving radiation therapy, from 4 to 20 may have:

- Thickening and numbness of the skin
- Sores or ulcers on the skin or near the cancer location
- Permanent hair loss
- Bleeding from the skin
- Sores in mouth which may cause difficulty swallowing

RARE, AND SERIOUS
In 100 people receiving radiation therapy, 3 or fewer may have:

- Damage to internal organs
- Abnormal opening in internal organs which may cause pain and bleeding

Use the following text for all studies:
Let your study doctor know of any questions you have about possible side effects. You can ask the study doctor questions about side effects at any time.

Reproductive risks: You should not get pregnant, breastfeed, or father a baby while in this study. The *(specify intervention)* used in this study could be very damaging to an unborn baby. Check with the study doctor about what types of birth control, or pregnancy prevention, to use while in this study.

What possible benefits can I expect from taking part in this study?

Notes to consent form authors:
1. **Section length limit: This section should be between two and three sentences and take up no more than one-eighth page.**
2. The statements below are generic and consent form authors should try to make their language specific to the study question when describing the potential research benefit.

Text Example: Phase 1 Studies
This study is unlikely to help you. This study may help us learn things that may help people in the future.

Text Example: Phase 2 Non-randomized Studies
This study has only a small chance of helping you because we do not know if the study drug/study approach is effective. This study may help researchers learn things that may help other people in the future.

Text Example: Phase 2 and 3 Randomized Studies
It is not possible to know at this time if the study drug(s)/study approach is better than the usual approach so this study may or may not help you. This study will help researchers learn things that will help people in the future.

Can I stop taking part in this study?

Notes to consent form authors:
1. **Section length limit: This section should be between five and eight sentences and take up no more than three-eighths page.**

Use the following text for all studies:
Yes. You can decide to stop at any time. If you decide to stop for any reason, it is important to let the study doctor know as soon as possible so you can stop safely. If you stop, you can decide whether or not to let the study doctor continue to provide your medical information to the organization running the study.

The study doctor will tell you about new information or changes in the study that may affect your health or your willingness to continue in the study.

The study doctor may take you out of the study:
- If your health changes and the study is no longer in your best interest
- If new information becomes available
- If you do not follow the study rules
- If the study is stopped by the sponsor, IRB or FDA.

What are my rights in this study?

Notes to consent form authors:
1. **Section length limit: This section should be about four sentences and take up no more than one-eighth page.**

(Continued on next page)

Appendix 3. National Cancer Institute Consent Form Template for Adult Cancer Trials *(Continued)*

Use the following text for all studies:
Taking part in this study is your choice. No matter what decision you make, and even if your decision changes, there will be no penalty to you. You will not lose medical care or any legal rights.

For questions about your rights while in this study, call the _____ *(insert name of center)* Institutional Review Board at _____ *(insert telephone number).* (Note to Local Investigator: Contact information for patient representatives or other individuals at a local institution who are not on the IRB or research team but take calls regarding clinical trial questions can also be listed here.)

What are the costs of taking part in this study?

Notes to consent form authors:
1. **Section length limit: This section should be between four and eight sentences and take up no more than one-quarter page.**
2. If appropriate, state which study agent(s) or procedures are provided free of charge.
3. Indicate if the study participant and/or health plan is likely to be billed for any charges associated with these "free" tests or procedures.
4. Outline any other pertinent financial support.

Use the following text for all studies:
The *(study agent)* will be supplied at no charge while you take part in this study. The cost of getting the *(study agent)* ready and giving it to you *(As appropriate, add: "…is also provided at no charge." Or "…is not paid by the study sponsor so you or your insurance company may have to pay for this.")* It is possible that the *(study agent)* may not continue to be supplied while you are on the study. Although not likely, if this occurs, your study doctor will talk to you about your options.

You and/or your health plan/insurance company will need to pay for all of the other costs of *(As appropriate, add: "caring for" Or "preventing" Or "treating")* your cancer while in this study, including the cost of tests, procedures, or medicines to manage any side effects, unless you are told that certain tests are supplied at no charge. Before you decide to be in the study, you should check with your health plan or insurance company to find out exactly what they will pay for.

You will not be paid for taking part in this study.

(Note to consent form authors and investigators: Insert a description of any compensation for participation or reimbursement for expenses.)

What happens if I am injured or hurt because I took part in this study?

Notes to consent form authors:
1. **Section length limit: This section should be between four and six sentences and take up no more than one-quarter page.**

Use the following text for all studies:
If you are injured or hurt as a result of taking part in this study and need medical treatment, please tell your study doctor. The study sponsors *(will/will not)* offer to pay for medical treatment for injury. Your insurance company may not be willing to pay for study-related injury. If you have no insurance, you would be responsible for any costs.

If you feel this injury was a result of medical error, you keep all your legal rights to receive payment for this even though you are in a study.

Who will see my medical information?

Notes to consent form authors:
1. **Section length limit: This section should be between four to seven sentences and take up no more than one-quarter page.**
2. The NCI has recommended that HIPAA regulations be addressed by the local institution. Language pertaining to HIPAA compliance may or may not be included in the local consent form, depending on local institutional policy.

Use the following text for all studies:
Your privacy is very important to us and the researchers will make every effort to protect it. Your information may be given out if required by law. For example, certain states require doctors to report to health boards if they find a disease like tuberculosis. However, the researchers will do their best to make sure that any information that is released will not identify you. Some of your health information, and/or information about your specimen, from this study will be kept in a central database for research. Your name or contact information will not be put in the database.

There are organizations that may inspect your records. These organizations are required to make sure your information is kept private, unless required by law to provide information. Some of these organizations are:
- The study sponsor and any drug company supporting the study *(Note to consent form authors: Delete drug company reference if not applicable.)*
- The Institutional Review Board, IRB, is a group of people who review the research with the goal of protecting the people who take part in the study.
- The Food and Drug Administration and the National Cancer Institute in the U.S., and similar ones if other countries are involved in the study.

(Continued on next page)

Appendix 3. National Cancer Institute Consent Form Template for Adult Cancer Trials (Continued)

Where can I get more information?

> Notes to consent form authors:
> 1. **Section length limit:** This section should be between six and eight sentences and take up no more than one-quarter page.
> 2. The second paragraph below complies with the new FDA regulation found at 21 CFR 50.25(c) and must be included verbatim in all consent forms for any applicable trial under the regulation. The text in this paragraph cannot be revised.

Use the following text for all studies:
You may visit the NCI Web site at http://cancer.gov/ for more information about studies or general information about cancer. You may also call the NCI Cancer Information Service to get the same information at: 1-800-4-CANCER (1-800-422-6237).

A description of this clinical trial will be available on http://www.ClinicalTrials.gov, as required by U.S. Law. This Web site will not include information that can identify you. At most, the Web site will include a summary of the results. You can search this Web site at any time.

Who can answer my questions about this study?

> Notes to consent form authors:
> 1. **Section length limit:** This section should be between four and six sentences and take up no more than one-eighth page.

Use the following text for all studies:
You can talk to the study doctor about any questions or concerns you have about this study or to report side effects or injuries. Contact the study doctor _____ (insert name of study doctor[s]) at _____ (insert telephone number).

ADDITIONAL STUDIES SECTION: (Indicate clearly to participants that this is a separate section)
This section is about optional studies you can choose to take part in

> Notes to consent form authors:
> 1. **Section length limit:** If the study mandates some of these optional studies be included, the text should be as brief as possible and take up no more than three pages.
> 2. All of the regulatory elements of consent included in the primary consent form must pertain to the embedded optional study. If any do not apply, they must be addressed in the discussion of the optional study.
> 3. Provide yes/no options at each decision point and do not require initials.
> 4. After choosing which optional studies included below pertain to your specific research, delete the studies that do not pertain.
> 5. If modifying the Template language to include other studies is necessary, use simple, concise, lay language.

Use the following text if optional studies are included:
This part of the consent form is about optional studies that you can choose to take part in. You will not get health benefits from any of these studies. The researchers leading this optional study hope the results will help other people with cancer in the future.

The results *(specify: will/ will not)* be added to your medical records and you or your study doctor *(specify: will/will not)* know the results. You will not be billed for these optional studies. You can still take part in the main study even if you say "no" to any or all of these studies. If you sign up for but cannot complete any of the studies for any reason, you can still take part in the main study.

Circle your choice of "yes" or "no" for each of the following studies.

1. **Optional imaging study – extra scan** (Note to consent form authors: This example pertains to an extra scan for research purposes)
   If you choose to take part in this study, you will have an extra *(insert name of standard clinical imaging procedure, e.g., PET scan)*. This scan is already used in medical care but it would be taken at a time point in your treatment that is not usual. Researchers would use this scan to *(briefly describe purpose, e.g., try to learn more about how treatment works on cancer)*.

   If you agree to have this extra scan, it would involve *(briefly describe procedures, e.g., blood draw, contrast agent, time)*. The risks would be *(briefly describe, focusing on risks of extra scan, e.g., additional radiation risk, risk of contrast)*. *(As applicable, insert:* The scan *[may or would]* be used to guide your medical care. *or* The scan would only be used for research and not to guide your medical care.*) If applicable, include the following statement:* There are educational materials available about this type of scan. Ask your study doctor about them, if you would like more information.*)*
   Please circle your answer: I choose to take part in the imaging study and will have the extra *(insert name of procedure, e.g., PET scan)*:
   YES   NO

(Continued on next page)

Appendix 3. National Cancer Institute Consent Form Template for Adult Cancer Trials *(Continued)*

2. **Optional imaging study – research scan or procedure (Note to consent form authors: This example pertains to an investigational scan or procedure.)**

    If you choose to take part in this study, you will have an experimental *(insert descriptor - scan or procedure)* called *(insert name of investigational imaging scan/procedure)*. Researchers hope this kind of *(insert descriptor - scan or procedure)* might one day be used to *(briefly describe purpose, e.g., learn more about cancer and how treatment works on cancer)*. This *(insert descriptor - scan or procedure)* is still being tested and researchers do not know how accurate or useful it is.

    If you agree to have this *(insert descriptor - scan or procedure)*, it would involve *(briefly describe procedures)*. The risks would be *(briefly describe, e.g., risks of investigational contrast agent)*. The *(insert descriptor - scan or procedure)* would only be used for research and not to guide your medical care.

    Please circle your answer: I choose to take part in the imaging study and will have the experimental *(insert name of scan or procedure)*:
        YES   NO

3. **Optional Quality of Life Study**

    If you choose to take part in this study, you will be asked to fill out a form with questions about *(briefly state topic, e.g., your physical and emotional well-being)*. Researchers will use this information to *(briefly describe purpose, e.g., learn more about how cancer and cancer treatment affects people)*.

    You will be asked to fill out this form at *(insert number)* times: *(insert bulleted list of time indicators, e.g., before surgery, after surgery before chemotherapy, and mode, e.g., inpatient, mail, or phone)*. Each form will take about *(insert number)* minutes to complete. The forms will ask about things like *(briefly describe, e.g., fatigue, diarrhea)*. You may feel uncomfortable answering some of the questions, and you can skip any you do not want to answer.

    Please circle your answer: I choose to take part in the Quality of Life study and will fill out these forms:
        YES   NO

4. **Optional Sample Collections for Laboratory Studies and/or Biobanking for Possible Future Studies**

    > Note to consent form authors:
    > 1. Section title and content should be modified as applicable based on whether study has optional collections and/or biobanking.
    > 2. Some content for the biobanking consent has been used with the consent of the author, L.M. Beskow. The citation is as follows: Beskow LM, Friedman JY, Hardy NC, Lin L, Weinfurt KP (2010) Developing a Simplified Consent Form for Biobanking. PloS ONE 5(10):e13302. doi:10.1371/journal/.pone.0013302

Researchers are trying to learn more about cancer, diabetes, and other health problems. Much of this research is done using samples from your tissue, blood, urine, or other fluids. Through these studies, researchers hope to find new ways to prevent, detect, treat, or cure health problems.

Some of these studies may be about genes. Genes carry information about features that are found in you and in people who are related to you. Researchers are interested in the way that genes affect how your body responds to treatment.

Note to consent form authors: The following is a text example for when a defined/known lab study can be described.)
If you choose to take part in this study, the study doctor for the main study would like to collect *(insert specimen to be collected, e.g., blood)* for research on *(briefly describe purpose)*.
(Note to consent form authors: The following is a text example for when a specimen is being collected for future unspecified research.)
If you choose to take part, *(insert specimen to be collected, e.g., a sample of tissue from your previous biopsy)* will be collected. The researchers ask your permission to store and use your samples and related health information (for example, your response to cancer treatment, results of study tests and medicines you are given) for medical research. The research that may be done is unknown at this time. Storing samples for future studies is called "biobanking". The Biobank is being run by *(insert name of clinical trials organization)* and supported by the National Cancer Institute.

WHAT IS INVOLVED?
If you agree to take part, here is what will happen next:
1. *Choose applicable sentence for the trial:* About *(insert number)* tablespoons of blood will be collected from a vein in your arm. *OR* A sample from the tissue that was collected at the time of your surgery will be sent to the Biobank. *OR* A sample of tissue will be collected from the optional extra biopsy. *[Revise as necessary to describe sample and collection. Should be noted if sample is drawn at same time as other draws, is residual material from embedded correlative, or already exists (archived tissue).]*

Appendix 3. National Cancer Institute Consent Form Template for Adult Cancer Trials *(Continued)*

2. *Choose 'a' or 'b' as applicable for the trial:*
   a. Your sample and some related health information will be sent to a researcher for use in the study described above. *(Include the following sentences, if applicable.)* Remaining samples may be stored in the Biobank, along with samples from other people who take part. The samples will be kept until they are used up.
   OR
   b. *For future unspecified research:* Your sample and some related health information may be stored in the Biobank, along with samples and information from other people who take part. The samples will be kept until they are used up. Information from your medical record will be updated from time to time.
3. Qualified researchers can submit a request to use the materials stored in the Biobanks. A science committee at the clinical trials organization, and/or the National Cancer Institute, will review each request. There will also be an ethics review to ensure that the request is necessary and proper. Researchers will not be given your name or any other information that could directly identify you. *(Note to informed consent authors: In specific instances, if this statement is not accurate and information may be given to researchers, please include appropriate notification information.)*
4. Neither you nor your study doctor will be notified when research will be conducted or given reports or other information about any research that is done using your samples. *(Note to informed consent authors: In specific instances, if this statement is not accurate and information may be given to study doctors, please include appropriate notification information.)*
5. Some of your genetic and health information may be placed in central databases that may be public, along with information from many other people. Information that could directly identify you will not be included.

WHAT ARE THE POSSIBLE RISKS?

1. The most common risks related to drawing blood from your arm are brief pain and possibly a bruise. *(Revise as necessary to describe risks from the sample collection.)*
2. There is a risk that someone could get access to the personal information in your medical records or other information researchers have stored about you.
3. There is a risk that someone could trace the information in a central database back to you. Even without your name or other identifiers, your genetic information is unique to you. The researchers believe the chance that someone will identify you is very small, but the risk may change in the future as people come up with new ways of tracing information.
4. In some cases, this information could be used to make it harder for you to get or keep a job or insurance. *(For non-US participants, please verify existence of such laws before including the following text.)* There are laws against the misuse of genetic information, but they may not give full protection. There can also be a risk in knowing genetic information. New health information about inherited traits that might affect you or your blood relatives could be found during a study. The researchers believe the chance these things will happen is very small, but cannot promise that they will not occur.

HOW WILL INFORMATION ABOUT ME BE KEPT PRIVATE?

Your privacy is very important to the researchers and they will make every effort to protect it. Here are just a few of the steps they will take:

1. When your sample(s) is sent to the researchers, no information identifying you (such as your name) will be sent. Samples will be identified by a unique code only. *(Note to consent form authors: If investigators are receiving samples directly from sites without being coded, modify accordingly.)*
2. The list that links the unique code to your name will be kept separate from your sample and health information. Any Biobank and *(insert name of clinical trials organization)* staff with access to the list must sign an agreement to keep your identity confidential.
3. Researchers to whom *(insert name of clinical trials organization)* sends your sample and information will not know who you are. They must also sign an agreement that they will not try to find out who you are.
4. Information that identifies you will not be given to anyone, unless required by law.
5. If research results are published, your name and other personal information will not be used.

WHAT ARE THE POSSIBLE BENEFITS?

You will not benefit from taking part. *(Note to informed consent authors: In specific studies, if this statement is not accurate and information may be given to the study participant's physician for use in their care, please include appropriate notification information.)*

Appendix 3. National Cancer Institute Consent Form Template for Adult Cancer Trials *(Continued)*

(Use the following sentence as applicable, e.g., when diagnosis has not been established: Your samples may be helpful to research whether you do or do not have cancer.*)* The researchers, using the samples from you and others, might make discoveries that could help people in the future.

ARE THERE ANY COSTS OR PAYMENTS?
There are no costs to you or your insurance. You will not be paid for taking part. If any of the research leads to new tests, drugs, or other commercial products, you will not share in any profits.

WHAT IF I CHANGE MY MIND?
If you decide you no longer want your samples to be used, you can call the study doctor, _____, *(insert name of study doctor for main trial)* at _____ *(insert telephone number of study doctor for main trial)* who will let the researchers know. Then, any sample that remains in the bank will no longer be used and related health information will no longer be collected. Samples or related information that have already been given to or used by researchers will not be returned.

WHAT IF I HAVE MORE QUESTIONS?
If you have questions about the use of your samples for research, contact the study doctor, _____, *(insert name of study doctor for main trial)*, at _____ *(insert telephone number of study doctor for main trial)*.

Please circle your answer to show whether or not you would like to take part in each option *(include only applicable questions)*:

SAMPLES FOR THE LABORATORY STUDIES:
    I agree to have my specimen collected and I agree that my specimen sample(s) and related information may be used for the laboratory study(ies) described above.
    YES   NO

    I agree that my study doctor, or their representative, may contact me or my physician to see if I wish to learn about results from this(ese) study(ies).
    YES   NO

SAMPLES FOR FUTURE RESEARCH STUDIES:
    My samples and related information may be kept in a Biobank for use in future health research.
    YES   NO

    I agree that my study doctor, or their representative, may contact me or my physician to see if I wish to participate in other research in the future.
    YES   NO

Use the following text if optional studies have been included:
This is the end of the section about optional studies.

My Signature Agreeing to Take Part in the Main Study

> Notes to consent form authors:
> 1. **Section length limit: This section should be four to five sentences and take up no more than one-quarter page.**

I have read this consent form or had it read to me. I have discussed it with the study doctor and my questions have been answered. I will be given a signed copy of this form. I agree to take part in the main study *and any additional studies where I circled 'yes'*. *(Note to protocol authors – remove italicized text if not applicable. Remove italics, if the text does apply.)*

Participant's signature_____

Date of signature_____

(The following signature and date lines for the person(s) conducting the discussion may be included at the discretion of the study sponsor.)

Signature of person(s) conducting the informed consent discussion_____

Date of signature_____

Appendix 3. National Cancer Institute Consent Form Template for Adult Cancer Trials *(Continued)*

<u>**Note to Consent Form Authors and Investigators:**</u>
 	
Recommendations about Attachments to the Consent Form (CF)
1. Attachments should contain information for the study participant that is considered optional, and is not required for their understanding of the proposed research. Attachments may provide clarification, additional education, or provide information about other facets of overall cancer care.
2. All required information should be contained within the CF itself. If the information is considered mandatory for the participants' understanding of the proposed research, then it should be in the CF.
   a. If a therapy or procedure is truly part of the research design – whether it is drug therapy, surgery, minimally invasive therapy, imaging, etc. – then information describing this therapy/procedure should be part of the CF.
   b. There is a difference between interventions that are part of standard care vs. a new indication of an already marketed intervention when research is being done. Marketed or available interventions (including scans) that are being used for a new indication should be treated as an experimental intervention and their side effects should be in the CF.
3. A study calendar is useful to include as an optional attachment.
   a. Patient advocates have recommended attaching a calendar that is easy for study participants to understand, conveying what has to be done, when, and for how long. It should help the study participant plan his/her life during the study. It should not be formidable-looking or too complicated in format, especially as dates and timing often change during the course of treatment due to unforeseen events.
4. Patient advocates have recommended the use of supportive educational materials that could help study participants better understand research-related information, such as biospecimen banking and treatment-related information for radiation therapy, surgery, chemotherapy, and imaging.
   a. NCI offers educational materials that cover many aspects of cancer, its treatment, and research, for example, the pamphlet, Taking Part in Cancer Treatment Research Studies. This pamphlet, and other materials, may be ordered on the NCI Web site at https://pubs.cancer.gov/ncipl/home.aspx or call 1-800-4- CANCER (1-800-422-6237) to request free copies.
   b. The FAQs about the NIH Certificate of Confidentiality may be found at http://grants.nih.gov/grants/policy/coc/faqs.htm#187. If a study has a Certificate of Confidentiality, the FAQs can be printed and used as an attachment.
5. Since many people do not have access to the Internet, including only web links in an attachment is not considered to be useful.
6. Friendly reminder – attached consent materials to the CF must be reviewed and approved by the IRB.
7. **For CTEP-sponsored trials:** The ICD and all attachments must be submitted to the PIO as a **single Word** or **PDF** document.

Note. From "NCI Consent Form Template for Adult Cancer Trials," by National Cancer Institute, 2013. Retrieved from http://ctep.cancer.gov/protocolDevelopment/docs/Informed_Consent_Template.docx.

Index

The letter f after a page number indicates relevant content appears in a figure; the letter t, in a table.

A

ABCB1 gene, 320
absolute granulocyte count (AGC), 266
absolute neutrophil count (ANC), 266
abstract, 430–432
academic conflict, 206–207
academic programs for professional development, 416
accelerated titration design (ATD), 31
accident compensation scheme in New Zealand, 568
accountability of research study drug, 260–262
 for audit, 409
 in Australia, 450
 in Mexico, 562–563
 in regulatory file, 391t
accreditation of human subject protection programs, 153
accrual. *See also* recruitment
 education and, 220
 estimation of, 176
 screening for, 180
accrual base
 in Australia, 449
 in Germany, 506
 in Japan, 551
AccrualNet, 235
accrual tracking graph, 234, 234f
acknowledgments, 435
act, 58f
active concurrent control, 26t
active treatment
 in Italy, 538
 in Mexico, 562–563
 in United Kingdom, 598–599
Act of Congress, 58f
acute lymphocytic leukemia (ALL), 340
acute myeloid leukemia (AML), 340–341
adaptive design, 27
adherence, 241–246. *See also* retention
 adverse effects and, 243
 assessment for, 243
 associated costs of treatment and, 242–243
 in Australia, 449
 complexity of regimen and, 242
 compliance vs., 241, 241t
 defined, 241–242
 determination of, 244
 factors affecting, 242–243
 in Germany, 506
 and impact of nonadherence, 243
 interventions to promote, 244–245
 in Japan, 551
 organizational tools for, 244–245
 patient characteristics and comorbidities and, 243
 perception of benefit and, 242
 physician/nurse issues for, 245
 provider and system characteristics and, 243
 randomization and, 242
 and reasons for nonadherence, 244
 risk factors for, 244
ADME, 24t
administration of research study drugs, 264–267, 265f
 in Australia, 450
 documentation of, 266, 367–368
 dosing in, 264–265
 guidelines for, 267
 in Ireland, 527
 laboratory studies on, 265–266, 265f
administrative agency, 58f
administrative barriers to recruitment, 229
administrative binder. *See* regulatory file(s)
adult learners, 292–293
adult learning theory, 422–423
advance directive, research, 122
Advanced Medical Service System B (AMSS-B, Japan), 547
adverse device effects, unanticipated, 273t, 281
adverse effects. *See* adverse event(s) (AEs)
adverse event(s) (AEs), 271–289
 and adherence, 243
 assessment of, 271–274
 in Australia, 450
 in Belarus, 469
 in Canada, 479
 in China, 487
 collection of, 278–279, 279f, 280
 common terminology criteria for, 274, 276t
 how to read, 274, 277f, 277t
 patient-reported outcome, 275–276
 Comprehensive Adverse Events and Potential Risks (CAEPR) list for, 284, 286f
 on consent form, 614–620
 defined, 15, 111, 271, 272–273t
 determining attribution of, 276–277, 278f
 documentation of, 279, 367
 in European Union, 492–493
 in France, 499
 in Germany, 507–508
 in Ireland, 527–528
 in Japan, 552
 life-threatening, 272t, 282
 log for, 279, 280f
 in Mexico, 563
 in New Zealand, 569–570
 permissible values for, 375, 376t
 recording of, 279
 in regulatory file, 390t
 reporting of, 279–284
 expedited, 281–284, 283f, 283t, 284
 forms for, 283–284
 to IRB, 280, 281, 281f, 390t
 for NCI-sponsored clinical trials, 284, 285f, 286f
 routine, 280–281, 281f
 voluntary postmarketing, 284
 in Romania, 576–577
 serious, 272t, 281, 282
 in European Union, 492
 in regulatory file, 390t
 as reportable event, 152t
 in United Kingdom, 599
 severity rating scales for, 274, 276t
 suspected, 272t
 terminology for, 271–274, 275f
 and unanticipated problems, 273t, 285–286, 287f
 unexpected, 273t, 281, 282
 in United Kingdom, 598–599
Adverse Event Expedited Reporting System, 284
adverse events list and reporting requirements in protocol, 110–111
adverse reaction, suspected, 272t, 281
advertisements in regulatory file, 389t
affective domain, 423
Affordable Care Act (2010), 8, 18, 60, 177, 212
African Americans
 education of, 225
 recruitment of, 231
 treatment of, 6
Agencia Española de Medicamentos y Productos Sanitarios (AEMPS), 579–580
agreements and contracts, 185–189
 components of, 185–188

confidentiality in, 185
dispute resolution in, 186
financial conflict of interest with, 209–212, 210f, 211f
in Germany, 505
HIPAA and, 187–188
implications for clinical trial nurses of, 188
indemnification in, 185–186
intellectual property in, 186
in Japan, 550
Medicare secondary payer issues in, 187
payments in, 186
in regulatory file, 389t
scope of work in, 186
termination in, 187
AIDS Clinical Trials Information Service (ACTIS), 248–249
Alaska Natives, education of, 225
ALCOA, 366
Alion Human Research Protection Program Accreditation, 153
Allegro CTMS, 167t
alleles, 317, 318
All-Ireland Cancer Consortium, 521–522
All-Ireland Cooperative Oncology Research Group (ICORG), 519–524, 520f, 521f, 530–531
alternative hypothesis, 134–135, 136f
Amberson, J. Burns, 3
amendments to original protocol document, 150–151
American Indians, education of, 225
American Recovery and Reinvestment Act of 2009 (ARRA), 18
analysis plan, 137
analytical cross-sectional study, 36–37
An Bord Altranais, 530
ancillary studies. See correlative trials
Andragogical Model, 423, 423t
anemia, 266
aneuploidy, 317
anti-EGFR monoclonal antibodies in colon cancer, 346
apoptosis, 340
approval with contingencies by IRB, 150
area under the curve (AUC), 359t
arm of study, 23
"arm's length negotiations," 206
article
created from abstract or poster, 432–433
defined, 430
guidelines for reporting research results in, 430, 431f, 431t
publishing of, 430, 430t

types of, 430, 430t
article abstract, 430–431
Association for the Accreditation of Human Research Protection Programs, 153
Association of Clinical Research Professionals, 71t, 417t, 431, 482
assurances, 143, 144f
ATP-binding cassette (ABC), 320
attribution, 276–277, 278f
attrition, 243
audit(s), 403–411
defined, 403f
directed (for-cause), 403f
FDA, 404–405, 405t
financial. See financial audit
in Germany, 509–510
how to prepare for, 408–410, 409f
Human Research Protection Program, 408
internal, 408
in Ireland, 530
in Japan, 550, 556
purpose of, 403, 404f
routine (not-for-cause), 403f
sponsor, 405–406
auditory learning style, 295t
Australasian Health and Research Data Managers Association, 444
Australian clinical trials, 443–453
adverse events in, 450
clinical research team for, 444
clinical trial registries for, 449–450
companion studies with, 451–452
correlative, 451–452
documentation and data management for, 452
eligibility for, 450
ethical review and site-specific assessment for, 447, 448f
financial factors in, 447–449, 448f
fundamental information on, 444–445
genetics and genomics in, 451
government initiatives for, 444
history and foundation of, 443–444
informed consent and patient recruitment for, 445–446
intergroup, 445
legal, regulatory, and legislative issues with, 444–445
participants in, 450–451
patient, family, and staff education for, 450–451
pharmacokinetic studies with, 451
procurement, administration, and accountability of research study drugs in, 450
professional development for, 452

protocol development, review, and approval for, 445–447, 448f
psychosocial distress in, 451
recruitment and retention for, 449–450
sponsoring agencies for, 445
standard operating procedures for, 445
Australian New Zealand Clinical Trials Registry, 449–450
Austrian clinical trials, 455–461
approval processes for, 456–457, 457f
correlative, 458–459
documentation and data management for, 459
financial factors with, 457
fundamental information on, 455–456, 456f
genetics and genomics in, 458, 458f
history and foundation of, 455
professional development for, 460
protocol development, review, and approval for, 456
quality assurance for, 459–460, 459f
recruitment and retention for, 457–458
team for, 458
useful websites on, 456, 456f
authorship, 433–435, 433f, 434f
autonomy, 53
autosomal dominant inheritance, 317, 327
Avery, Oswald, 4

B

background and rationale section of protocol, 110
baseline symptoms, documentation of, 367
basic research in drug development, 14
basic science in drug development, 13–14
basket trials, 27
Bayh-Dole Act (1980), 205
Beecher, Henry, 98
Belarus clinical trials, 463–471
approval and review of, 465, 466f
correlative, 469
documentation and data management for, 469–470
ethics committees for, 464–465
financial factors with, 468
fundamental information on, 463–466, 466–468f
genetics and genomics in, 469
history and foundation of, 463
legislative documents on, 464
multinational multicenter, 465, 467f, 468f

participants of, 469
professional development for, 470
protocol development, review, and approval for, 467–468
quality assurance for, 470
recruitment and retention for, 468–469
regulatory background of, 463
regulatory bodies for, 464
sites for, 465
Belmont Report (1979), 52–53
on ethical principles, 52–53, 53t
on good clinical practice, 67
on informed consent, 113–114
on research vs. practice, 53, 53t
on social and scientific value, 97, 98f
beneficence, 53, 53t, 113
benefits
and adherence, 242
defined, 53
in risk-benefit analysis, 147, 147f
Best Pharmaceuticals for Children Act (2002), 7
bias
and financial conflict of interest, 214–215
publication, 247
selection, 23
billing compliance for Medicare and third-party payers, 177–178
billing grid, 171, 172–174f
bioavailability, 359t
biologic product, defined, 13
biologic samples
correspondence on, 391t
transmittal forms for, 391t
biologic studies in Germany, 508
biomarker(s)
in breast cancer, 344–345
in colon cancer, 346
defined, 343
in lung cancer, 345–346
multigene, 343
predictive, 343–344
prognostic, 343
in prostate cancer, 347
single-gene, 343
biospecimen(s), 351–355
collection of, 130–131, 352–354, 353f, 354f
data sharing on, 353–354
Genetic Information Nondiscrimination Act protection for, 354
implications for clinical trial nurses of, 354
informed consent for, 351–352, 352f
responsibility for research on, 351
storage of, 351–355, 354f
in Canada, 480
in Japan, 554

biotechnology company as sponsor, 47
blinding, 23–25, 24*t*
block randomization, 25*t*
body surface area (BSA)-based dosing, 264–265
Bord Altranais, 530
brand name, 16
Brazil, clinical trials registry in, 251
BRCA1 gene, 328
BRCA2 gene, 328
breast cancer biomarkers, 344–345
budget(s) and budgeting, 171–183
  administrative components of, 171–176
  in Australia, 447–449, 448*f*
  billing compliance for Medicare and third-party payers in, 177–178
  billing grid in, 171, 172–174*f*
  for device trials, 178
  estimating accrual in, 176
  in Germany, 505
  hidden costs in, 181–182
  in Ireland, 524–526
  in Japan, 549–550
  laboratory fees in, 178–179
  Medicare coverage analysis in, 171, 172–174*f*, 177
  nonrefundable fees in, 175, 176–177, 176*f*
  online tools for, 176
  patient care costs in, 178, 179*f*
  pharmacokinetic sampling in, 179
  pharmacy costs in, 177, 179
  rating system in, 171, 175*f*
  scope of, 171
  scope of budget in, 171
  staff effort in, 179–181, 180*f*, 181*f*
  in Thailand, 587
business associate in agreement, 187–188
business model for recruitment, 236–237

C

Canada Health Act (1985), 473
Canadian Association of Nurses in Oncology/Association Canadienne des Infirmières en Oncologie (CANO/ACIO), 482
Canadian clinical trials, 473–484
  adverse events and unanticipated problems in, 479
  correlative, 480
  documentation and data management for, 480–481
  drug development process and, 474
  ethics of, 475–476
  expanded access and, 474

financial factors for, 477–478
fundamental information on, 474–476, 476*f*
genetic testing for, 479–480
good clinical practice and standard operating procedures for, 475
history and foundation of, 473–474, 473*f*, 474*f*
informed consent for, 476–477
investigational agents for, 479
legal, regulatory, and legislative issues for, 475, 476*f*
participants in, 479
patient and family education on, 479
professional development for, 482
protocol development, review, and approval for, 476–477
psychosocial distress in, 479
quality assurance for, 481–482
recruitment and retention for, 478–479, 478*f*, 479*f*
storage of genetic material from, 480
team for, 474–475
Canadian Institutes of Health Research (CIHR), 477
Cancer Australia, 444
Cancer Biology group (Australia), 443
cancer centers, NCI-designated, 45
cancer genetics, 327, 339–340
CancerNet, 249
Cancer Network (Mexico), 564, 565*f*
Cancer Nurses Society of Australia (CNSA), 444
Cancer Research-UK (CR-UK), 595, 595*f*
Cancer Support Community, 308–309
CancerSupportSource, 308–309
Cancer Therapy Evaluation Program (CTEP), 4
  on adverse event reporting, 284, 285*f*
  on budgeting, 176
  monitoring by, 407
  on research team, 79
  on sponsoring agencies, 46–47
Cancer Trials New Zealand (CTNZ), 567
carcinomas, 340
case-control studies, 36*t*, 37
case report, 35, 36*t*
case report forms (CRFs), 365–366, 366*f*
  design of, 374–375, 375*f*
  electronic, 379–380
  in Italy, 539
  in regulatory file, 392*t*
  transmittal forms for, 392*t*
  in United Kingdom, 600
case series studies, 35, 36*t*
case study, 430*t*
  abstract of, 432*t*

category A devices, 178
category B devices, 178
Center for Drug Evaluation and Research, 14–15
Center for Global Health (NCI), 47
Centers for Medicare and Medicaid Services (CMS), on financial conflict of interest, 212–213
CenterWatch, 60
central monitoring in Japan, 556
central pharmacy, dispensing of research drugs by, 262
centromeric banding (C-banding), 339
certificate programs for professional development, 416
certificates of confidentiality (CoCs), 148
certification, specialty, 416–417
certification statements, 388*t*
charging rules with expanded access, 43
check-in of research drugs, 261
chemical name, 16
Chemotherapy and Pharmacy Advisory Service (CPAS, UK), 596
children
  genetic testing of, 334
  informed consent of, 120–121
  patient education for, 294, 296*f*
  treatment of, 7
Children's Oncology Group, 4
Chinese clinical trials, 485–489
  adverse events in, 487
  correlative, 488
  documentation and data management for, 488
  ethics committee for, 486
  financial factors with, 486
  genetics and genomics in, 487–488
  history and foundation of, 485
  human resources at trial sites for, 487
  informed consent for, 486
  investigational product management in, 487
  participants of, 487
  patient compliance in, 487
  procedures for, 485–486
  professional development for, 488
  protocol development, review, and approval for, 486
  quality assurance for, 488
  recruitment and retention for, 486–487
Chinese Food and Drug Administration (CFDA), 485
Chirac, Jacques, 497
chromosomal abnormalities, 317, 340
chromosome banding techniques, 339
chromosomes, 317

chronic lymphocytic leukemia (CLL), 340
chronic myeloid leukemia (CML), 340
citations, 436, 436*f*, 437*f*
Classic Modified Fibonacci Dose Escalation Scheme, 31, 31*t*
clinical article, 430*t*
Clinical Conductor Site CTMS, 168*t*
clinical data management plans, 369–371, 370*f*
clinical data management practices, 369
clinical data management systems (CDMS)
  capabilities of, 377
  vs. clinical trial management systems, 377
  interoperability of, 378
    semantic, 378, 379
  role assignment for, 380, 381*t*
  scalability of, 378
  scope of, 377–378
  security and confidentiality with, 378–379
  using capabilities of, 379–380
clinical data manager, 84–85
clinical equipoise, 98
Clinical Investigator Inspection List, 404, 405*t*
Clinical Oncology Society of Australia (COSA), 443
clinical research, types of, 17–21
clinical research associate, budgeting for, 181
clinical research coordinator (CRC), 84, 85*f*, 157
  core work tasks of, 160, 162*f*
  workload determination for, 158–163
clinical research nurse, 84
clinical research standards, 375, 376*t*
Clinical Studies Groups (CSGs, UK), 592
clinical study report in regulatory file, 393*t*
clinical trial(s)
  as business, 236–237
  phases of, 27–33, 29*t*
    phase 0, 28–30, 29*t*
    phase I, 29*t*, 30–32, 31*f*, 31*t*
    phase II, 29*t*, 32–33
    phase III, 29*t*, 33
    phase IV, 29*t*, 33
clinical trial agreement (CTA), 46–47
  in Mexico, 561
  in regulatory file, 389*t*
  in United Kingdom, 594
Clinical Trial Application (CTA, Canada), 475, 476*f*
Clinical Trial Application-Amendment (CTA-A, Canada), 475
Clinical Trial Awards and Advisory Committee (CTAAC, UK), 595

clinical trial coordinator, 157
clinical trial designs, 25–27
  adaptive, 27
  basket trials as, 27
  blinding/masking in, 23–25, 24t
  control groups in, 24t, 25, 26t
  crossover, 25, 27f
  factorial, 25–27, 28f
  key concepts in, 23–25, 24t, 25t
  parallel, 25, 26f
  randomization in, 23, 25t
  randomized discontinuation, 27, 28f
clinical trials enterprise (CTE), 20–21
Clinical Trial Exemption scheme (Australia), 445
clinical trial management systems (CTMSs), 164, 167–168t
  capabilities of, 377
  vs. clinical data management systems, 377
  interoperability of, 378
    semantic, 378, 379
  scalability of, 378
  scope of, 377–378
  security and confidentiality with, 378–379
  using capabilities of, 379–380, 381t
clinical trial matching services, 252, 252f
clinical trial material (CTM) documentation, 391t
Clinical Trial Notification scheme (Australia), 444–445
clinical trial nurse (CTN), 82–84, 83f
Clinical Trial Nurse Questionnaire (CTNQ), 82
Clinical Trial Nurses Special Interest Group (CTN SIG), 417t
clinical trial registry(ies), 247–255
  AIDS Clinical Trials Information Service (ACTIS) as, 248–249
  in Australia, 449–450
  in Canada, 478, 479f
  CancerNet as, 249
  central access site for, 252–253
  and clinical trial matching services, 252, 252f
  ClinicalTrials.gov as, 249, 249f, 250, 250f
  Clinical Trials Transformation Initiative (CTTI) for, 253
  current trends in, 252–253, 252f
  Declaration of Helsinki on, 250–251
  defined, 247
  disease, 252
  evolution of, 247–251
  of FDA, 249

federal laws on, 250
foreign, 251
in Germany, 506
implications for clinical trial nurses of, 253
in India, 516
International Clinical Trials Registry Platform (ICTRP) for, 250
International Committee of Medical Journal Editors (ICMJE) on, 249
International Federation of Pharmaceutical Manufacturers and Associations (IFPMA) on, 250
in Japan, 551
pharmaceutical, 251
Physician Data Query (PDQ) database as, 248
purpose of, 247
results submission for, 252
standardization of, 252
timeline of, 248t
Trial Registration Data Set (TRDS) for, 250
Clinical Trials Cooperative Group Program, 4–5, 4f, 20, 45–46
Clinical Trials Directive (CTD), 491, 491f
ClinicalTrials.gov, 249, 249f, 250, 250f
clinical trial site information (CTSI), 481
Clinical Trials Monitoring Branch (CTMB), 407
Clinical Trials Monitoring Service (CTMS), 407
Clinical Trials Registry–India (CTRI), 516
Clinical Trials Research Professionals Group (CRPG), 443
Clinical Trials Transformation Initiative (CTTI), 253, 398
clinical trial units
  in Italy, 540, 540f
  NCRI-accredited, 592, 592f
close-out meeting, 410
close-out visit, 407
cloud computing, 416t
coaching, 422
Cockcroft and Gault method, 265–266, 265f
code, 58f
code of ethics, 5–6
Code of Federal Regulations (C.F.R.), 6, 56, 58f, 67, 114
coding of data, 372–373, 373f
codons, 316–317
coercion, 113
cognitive domain, 423
cohort studies, 36t, 37–38, 37f
ColDx assay, 346
collaborative companion studies, 19

Collaborative Institutional Training Initiative (CITI), 482
collection
  of adverse events, 278–279, 279f, 280
  of biospecimens, 130–131, 352–354, 353f, 354f
  data, 371
collect on delivery (COD) shipping, 263
Collins, Francis S., 205, 377
colon cancer biomarkers, 346
ColoPrint assay, 346
Comisión Coordinadora de Instituciones Nacionales de Salud y Hospitales de Alta Especialidad (CCINSHAE), 559
Comisión Federal para la Protección contra Riesgos Sanitarios (COFEPRIS), 560, 561, 562
commercial agents, 284
commercial DNA banking, 335
commercial IND, 14
Commission for the Protection Against Sanitary Risk (Mexico), 560, 561, 562
commitment, conflict of, 206
common data element (CDE), 379
Common Rule, 6, 55–56, 56t, 58f, 67, 98f
Common Terminology Criteria for Adverse Events (CTCAE), 131
  historical timeline for, 274, 276t
  how to read, 274, 277f, 277t
  patient-reported outcome, 275–276
Common Toxicity Criteria (CTC), 274
communication
  in mentorship, 426
  nursing competencies in, 607
Community Clinical Oncology Program, 5
community health organization, expanded access for, 43
community partnership, 222
comorbidities and adherence, 243
companion studies, 19
  in Australia, 451–452
  in Germany, 508
  in Japan, 554
company-sponsored medical research, authorship for, 434–435, 434f
comparative effectiveness research (CER), 17–19
compartmental model, 359–360, 360f, 361f
compassionate use, 41, 42, 264
  in Italy, 536
compensation for accidental injury in India, 516

compensation for participation in India, 515–516
competencies for mentorship, 423–424, 423f, 424f
competent authority in European Union, 491
complete blood count (CBC), 266
complete response in solid tumor response assessment, 133
compliance
  vs. adherence, 241, 241t
  in China, 487
  with regulations and guidelines, 61–64
Comprehensive Adverse Events and Potential Risks (CAEPR) list, 284, 286f
comprehensive feasibility review, 193–194, 193f, 195f
concomitant treatments, documentation of, 367
conditional approval by IRB, 150
conference abstract, 431–432, 432t
Conference on Oncological and Pediatric Oncological Care (Germany), 506
confidentiality, 57–59
  in agreement, 185
  certificates of, 148
  of clinical data management system, 378–379
conflict, in mentorship, 426
conflicting studies within single institution, 206–207
conflict of commitment, 206
conflict of interest (COI), 102–103
  defined, 205–206
  financial. See financial conflict of interest
  in India, 517
  in Italy, 536
  in Spain, 581–582
consensus data element standards, 375, 376t
consent, informed. See informed consent (IC)
consent form (CF). See informed consent (IC) form
consideration, 208
Consolidated Appropriations Act (2008), 59
Consolidated Standards of Reporting Trials (CONSORT), 430
continuing review, 151, 390t
contract(s). See agreements and contracts
contract research organization (CRO), 45
control groups, 24t, 25, 26t
control pharmacy, dispensing of research drugs by, 262
cooperative agreements, financial conflict of interest with, 209–210

Cooperative Group Outreach Program, 5
cooperative research, in Spain, 580
cooperative research and development agreement (CRADA), 46–47
Coordinating Committee for National Health Institutions and High Specialty Hospitals (Mexico), 559
copyrighted material, 436
correlative trials
    in Australia, 451–452
    in Austria, 458–459
    in Belarus, 469
    in Canada, 480
    in China, 488
    in France, 499
    in Germany, 508–509
    in India, 516–517
    in Ireland, 528
    in Italy, 539
    in Japan, 554–555
    in Mexico, 564
    in New Zealand, 570
    in Romania, 577
    in Spain, 583
    in Thailand, 588
    in United Kingdom, 599–600
correspondence with sponsor, 393t
corresponding author, 433
cost(s)
    hidden, 181–182
    and financial risk reduction, 194, 196–197t
    nonstandard procedure, 178, 179f
    patient care, 178, 179f
    of treatment, and adherence, 242–243
cost estimates in resource planning and allocation, 165
Council for International Organizations of Medical Sciences (CIOMS), 98f
covered entities, 59
    in agreement, 187–188
    and electronic data management systems, 378
covered recipients, financial conflict of interest by, 212–213
creatinine clearance (CrCl), 265–266, 265f
credibility and education, 222
criteria for response assessment in protocol, 111
Critical Path Initiative, 5
crossover design, 25, 27f
cross-sectional studies, 35–37, 36t
cultural aspects of Thai clinical trials, 589–590
curation process, 379
curriculum vitae (CV), 388t

CYP2C19 gene, 318
CYP2D6 gene, 317
cytochrome P450 (CYP450) enzymes, 317–318
cytogenetics, 339–342
    and cancer genetics, 339–340
    chromosome alterations in cancers in, 340
    chromosome banding techniques in, 339
    defined, 339
    history of, 339
    in Japan, 553–554
    of leukemia, 340–341, 340t, 341t
    nomenclature for, 340, 340t

D

data, description of, 371
data abstraction, 372
data access, 371
data and safety monitoring board/committee. *See* data monitoring committee (DMC)
data and safety monitoring plans (DSMPs), 397–402
    background of, 397–398
    benefits of, 401
    Clinical Trials Transformation Initiative (CTTI) on, 398
    in Germany, 509
    indications for, 399, 399f
    International Conference on Harmonisation on, 399
    in Japan, 556
    key elements of, 399, 399f
    National Cancer Institute on, 399
    National Institutes of Health on, 399
    overview of, 397
    purpose of, 397
    U.S. Food and Drug Administration on, 398
data coding, 372–373, 373f
data collection, 371
data discrepancies, 372
data element, 379
data exchange, 373
    standards for, 375
data extraction, 372
data format, standards for, 375
data handling guidelines, 372
data handling rules, 371
data management, 369–383
    adherence to regulations for, 371–372
    in Australia, 452
    in Austria, 459
    in Belarus, 469–470
    in Canada, 480–481
    in China, 488
    clinical research standards for, 375, 376f
    in France, 500

future considerations for, 376
in Germany, 509
in India, 517
in Ireland, 529
in Italy, 540
in Japan, 555
in Mexico, 564
in New Zealand, 570
in Romania, 577
in Spain, 583
in Thailand, 588
in United Kingdom, 600
data management associate, budgeting for, 181
data management plans (DMPs), 369–371, 370f
data management practices, 369
data management processes, 371–375
data management system, electronic, 377–380
    capabilities of, 377
    vs. clinical trial management system, 377
    interoperability of, 378
    role assignment for, 380, 381t
    scalability of, 378
    scope of, 377–378
    security and confidentiality with, 378–379
    semantic interoperability of, 378, 379
    using capabilities of, 379–380
data monitoring committee (DMC), 138, 397, 399–401
    historical perspective on, 399–400
    meetings, follow-up, and ongoing business of, 400–401
    reports of, 390t
    responsibilities of, 400
    structure and composition of, 400
    in United Kingdom, 599
data points, 379
data privacy, 374, 374f
data processing, 371, 372
data quality, 374
data security, 374, 374f
data sharing, 371
data storage, 371, 373–374
data transmission, 373
decision modeling, 18
Declaration of Helsinki (1964), 5–6, 52
    and clinical trial registries, 250–251
    on ethics, 98f
    on good clinical practice, 67
decoding procedures, 392t
delegation, 79
delegation log, 80
delegation of authority form, 259
deletions, 317
dementia, informed consent with, 121–122

deoxyribonucleic acid (DNA), 316, 316f
Department of Defense, 54, 55t
Department of Health and Human Services (DHHS), 6, 54, 54f, 114
descriptive cross-sectional study, 36
descriptive statistics, 136–137, 137f
descriptors, 379
destruction of clinical trial material, 391t
Deutsches Register Klinischer Studien (DRKS), 251
deviation as reportable event, 152t
device research, IRB review for, 148149
device trials, budgeting for, 178
diagnostic accuracy studies, reporting guidelines for, 431t
diagnostic trials, hereditary cancer predisposition testing in, 335
diaries, patient, 278–279, 279f
dictionaries, terminology, 371, 373, 373f
dihydropyrimidine dehydrogenase (DPD), 5-fluorouracil (5-FU) and, 318
direct costs in resource planning and allocation, 165
directed audit/review, 403f
directed payment, 213
direct endpoint, 24t
DISCERN tool, 299, 299f
discontinuation of clinical trial, distress related to, 306, 306f
discrepancy documentation, 368
discrete values, 380
discrimination based on genetic information, 333, 334f
disease-free survival as trial endpoint, 132t
disease registries, 252
disease response as trial endpoint, 131–133, 131–134t
dispensing of research drugs, 262, 391t
dispute resolution in agreement, 186
distress. *See* psychosocial distress
Distress Assessment and Response Tool (DART), 479
Distress Thermometer, 307–308, 307f
Division of Cancer Prevention and Control (DCPC), 5
Division of Cancer Treatment and Diagnosis (DCTD), 79, 260
DMET chip, 322
DNA banking, commercial, 335
document(s), essential, 387
    centralization of, 394

documentation, 365–368
    of adverse events, 279, 280f, 367
    ALCOA for, 366
    in Australia, 452
    in Austria, 459
    of baseline symptoms and concomitant treatments, 367
    in Belarus, 469–470
    in Canada, 480–481
    challenges in, 368
    in China, 488
    clinical trial material (CTM), 391t
    discrepancy, 368
    of eligibility confirmation, 366–367
    in France, 500
    in Germany, 509
    in India, 517
    of informed consent, 118–119, 366–367
    in Ireland, 528–529
    in Italy, 539–540
    in Japan, 555
    laboratory, 391–392t
    in medical record, 365–366, 366f
    in Mexico, 564
    in New Zealand, 570
    nursing competencies in, 608
    of off-label use, 367
    of off study, 368
    of off treatment, 368
    of protocol-specific activities, 367
    of research drug administration, 266, 367–368
    in research record, 365, 366f
    research-specific, 366–368
    of returned drugs by patients, 263
    in Romania, 577
    source documents in, 365–366, 366f
    in Spain, 583
    in Thailand, 588
    in United Kingdom, 600
    of unscheduled visits, 367
Dodd, Christopher, 60
dose
    maximum tolerated, 24t, 30–31, 32
    mouse equivalent lethal 10, 24t
    optimal, 32
    recommended phase II, 24t
dose escalation design, 30–31, 31t
dose-limiting toxicity (DLT), 24t, 30–31, 32, 128
dosing, 264–265
double dipping, 63, 177–178
drug(s)
    defined, 13
    naming of, 16
drug clearance, 359t
drug development, 13–16, 16f, 315–316

in Canada, 474
in Germany, 503
in Japan, 545–546
drug metabolism, 317–318, 319t
drug metabolizing genes, 322
drug transporter genes, 320
duplication, 317

E

eClinForce SmartStudy, 167t
Economic and Social Research Council (ESRC, UK), 599
education
    of other nurses, 417–418
    patient and family. See patient and family education
educational material in regulatory file, 389t
efficacy, 33, 68
"Effort Reporting" concept, 206
EGFR mutation in lung cancer, 345
elderly. See older adults
e-learning, 416t
electronic data capture (EDC) system, 380, 381t
    in Japan, 555
electronic data management system, 377–380
    capabilities of, 377
    vs. clinical trial management system, 377
    interoperability of, 378
        semantic, 378, 379
    role assignment for, 380, 381t
    scalability of, 378
    scope of, 377–378
    security and confidentiality with, 378–379
    using capabilities of, 379–380
electronic mailing lists, 416, 417t
electronic records, 365
electronic screening for recruitment, 236
electronic signatures, 365
eligibility confirmation, documentation of, 366–367
eligibility criteria, 110
    in Australia, 450
    explaining importance of, 222–223
    in France, 499
    in Ireland, 526
    in Mexico, 562
    in New Zealand, 569
    in protocol, 128–129
    in Thailand, 587–588
    in United Kingdom, 598
eligibility screening, 231–232
    electronic, 236
elimination half-life, 359t
e-mentoring, 426–427, 427f
emergency use, expanded access for, 42, 264
emergency use IND, 14
emotional distress. See psychosocial distress

emotional readiness to learn, 292
empirical study article, 430t
end of treatment, distress related to, 306, 306f
end point(s), 131–134, 132–135t
    direct, 24t
    safety, 131
    surrogate, 24t
Enhancing the Quality and Transparency of Health Research (EQUATOR), 430
enrollment logs, 392t
enrollment procedures, 110
epigenetics, 334
equipoise, 98
ERCC1 in lung cancer, 345
essential documents, 387
    centralization of, 394
estimate of survival, 344
ethical concerns
    in Canada, 475–476
    with hereditary cancer predisposition testing, 330–331
    nursing competencies in, 608
ethical principles, 5–6, 52–53, 53t
Ethical Principles and Guidelines for the Protection of Human Subjects of Research (1979). *See* Belmont Report (1979)
ethical review board, 143
ethics, 97–105
    and conflict of interest, 102–103
    historical background of, 97, 98f
    informed consent in, 99, 99f
    institutional review boards and, 101
    and research misconduct, 102, 102f
    and scientific integrity, 101–102
    social and scientific value in, 97–99, 98f
    and therapeutic misconception, 99–101, 100f, 101f
ethics committee (EC), 561–562
    in Australia, 447, 448f
    in Austria, 456–457, 457f, 459–460, 459f
    in Belarus, 464–465
    in China, 486
    in European Union, 491, 492, 492f
    in France, 498
    in Germany, 504
    in India, 515
    in Ireland, 523–524
    in Italy, 536
    in Japan, 548
    in New Zealand, 568
    in Romania, 574
    in Spain, 580–581
    in Thailand, 586
    in United Kingdom, 593–594

ethics consultation, 103
EudraCT, 492, 492f
EudraVigilance Clinical Trial Module, 492
euploidy, 317
European Clinical Trials Database (EudraCT), 251
European Medicines Agency, 491
European Oncology Nursing Society (EONS), 493–494
European Organisation for Research and Treatment of Cancer (EORTC), 494
European School of Oncology (ESO), 494
European Union (EU), member states of, 491, 491f
European Union (EU) clinical trials, 491–495
    adverse events in, 492–493
    competent authority in, 491
    directive for, 491, 491f
    ethics committees for, 491, 492, 492f
    EudraCT registration for, 492, 492f
    guidelines for sponsors of, 492
    implementation and practical issues with, 493, 493f
    inspections for, 493
    proposed regulation of, 493
    resources for clinical trial nurses in, 493–494
    sponsor of, 492
European Union (EU) Clinical Trials Directive, 491
European Union (EU) Clinical Trials Register, 251
evidence-based article, 430t
exclusion criteria, 128–129
exculpatory language in informed consent, 115, 115f
exemptions
    to informed consent, 123
    from IRB review, 147
exome, 316
exons, 316
expanded access, 41–44
    in Canada, 474
    charging rules for, 43
    in community health organizations, 43
    criteria for, 41–42, 41f, 42f
    in Germany, 503
    implications for clinical trial nurses of, 44
    for individual patients, 42
    for intermediate-sized patient populations, 42–43, 42t, 43t
    in Japan, 546
    for large populations, 43, 43t
    programs of, 41–42, 41t, 42t
expanded access protocols (EAPs), 41–43t, 41–44
expedited adverse event reporting, 281–284, 283f, 283t, 284

experiential learning theory, 423
experiential readiness to learn, 292
Experimental Cancer Medicines Centres (ECMC) Network (UK), 592–593
experimental devices, 178
experimental group, 25
experimental research, 23–34
   clinical trial designs for, 25–27
      adaptive, 27
      basket trials as, 27
      blinding/masking in, 23–25
      control groups in, 25, 26t
      crossover, 25, 27f
      factorial, 25–27, 28f
      key concepts in, 23–25, 24t, 25t
      parallel, 25, 26f
      randomization in, 23, 25t
      randomized discontinuation, 27, 28f
   on comparative effectiveness, 18
   observational vs., 17
   phases of clinical trials for, 27–33, 29t
      phase 0, 28–30, 29t
      phase I, 29t, 30–32, 31f, 31t
      phase II, 29t, 32–33
      phase III, 29t, 33
      phase IV, 29t, 33
exploratory IND, 14

F

fabrication, 62, 102, 102f
factorial design, 25–27, 28f
failure mode and effects analysis (FMEA), 199, 201, 202–203t, 202f
Fair Access to Clinical Trials (FACT) Act, 60
fair use doctrine, 436
False Claims Act, 63
falsification, 62, 102, 102f
family education. *See* patient and family education
FDA Modernization Act (1997), 59
feasibility review, comprehensive, 193–194, 193f, 195f
federal clinical trial legislation, 60
Federal Information Security Management Act (FISMA), 374
Federal Register, 56, 58f
Federal Technology Transfer Act (1986), 46–47
Federalwide Assurance for the Protection of Human Subjects (FWA), 6
   on institutional review board registration, 143, 144f
   and Office for Human Research Protections, 56

in regulatory file, 389t
   terms of, 605–606
fees
   IRB, 177
   laboratory, 178–179
   nonrefundable, 175, 176–177, 176f
   pharmacy, 177, 179
fetuses, informed consent and protection of, 121
final study report in regulatory file, 390t
financial assistance in India, 515
financial audit, 199–201
   background of, 199–200
   definition of terms for, 199
   documents used in, 200, 200f
   general guidelines for, 200, 200f
   in Japan, 550
   process of, 200–201
   report of, 201, 201f
   staff involved in, 200, 200f
financial conflict of interest (FCOI), 205–216
   academic and institutional, 206–207
   background of, 205–206
   Centers for Medicare and Medicaid on, 212–213
   of commitment, 206
   consequences of noncompliance with, 211–212, 212f, 213–215, 214f
   consideration and, 208
   defined, 205–206, 207–208
   Food and Drug Administration on, 208, 209
   in Germany, 505
   how to manage, 211–212, 212f, 213–215, 214f
   identifying, 206–207
   institutional responsibilities for, 211–212, 211f, 212f
   in Japan, 550
   National Science Foundation on, 208, 209f
   Office of Management and Budget on, 208
   parties affected by, 207–208
   patient advocacy, 206
   personal, 207
   professional, 207
   suggestions for policies and procedures on, 213–214, 214f
   U.S. Public Health Service on, 205, 209–212
      for contracts, 210–212–211f, 212f
      for grants and cooperative agreements, 209–210
financial disclosure statements, 388t
financial factors
   in Australia, 447–449, 448f
   in Austria, 457

   in Belarus, 468
   in Canada, 477
   in China, 486
   in France, 499
   in India, 515–516
   in Ireland, 524–526
   in Italy, 537
   in Japan, 549–550
   in Mexico, 562
   in New Zealand, 568–569
   in Romania, 576
   in Spain, 582, 582f
   in Thailand, 587
   in United Kingdom, 597
financial fraud and abuse, 63
financial implications, nursing competencies in, 608
financial interest, significant, 210, 211
financial management, 200, 200f
financial monitoring, 197
financial reporting, 197
financial risk, areas of potential, 191–192
financial risk assessment, 191–198
   in Germany, 505
   in Japan, 550
financial risk monitoring
   in Germany, 505
   in Japan, 550
financial risk reduction strategies, 192–197
   being aware of hidden costs as, 194, 196–197t
   choosing protocols strategically as, 193, 193f
   identifying invisible institutional barriers as, 194–197
   monitoring research finances as, 197
   partnering with research bases and sponsors that best fit institution's mission as, 192–193
   putting processes and tools in place as, 193–194, 195f
   setting program direction (goals, timelines, and priorities) as, 192
5-fluorouracil (5-FU) and dihydropyrimidine dehydrogenase (DPD), 318
flow chart for resource planning and allocation, 164, 166f
fluorescence in situ hybridization (FISH), 339
follow-up
   in France, 499
   in Ireland, 526–527
   in Mexico, 563
   in New Zealand, 570
   in United Kingdom, 597–598
Fonds de Recherche du Québec-Santé (FRQS), 475
Food and Drug Act (1906), 5
Food and Drug Administration Amendments Act (FDAAA, 2007), 250

Food and Drug Administration Modernization Act (FDAMA, 1997), 249
for-cause audit/review, 403f
foreign registries, 251
frameshift mutation, 317
French clinical trials, 497–501
   adverse events in, 499
   correlative trials and ancillary studies with, 499
   documentation and data management for, 500
   ethics committee review for, 498
   financial factors with, 499
   fundamental information on, 497–499, 498t
   genetics and genomics in, 499
   history and foundation of, 497
   informed consent for, 498–499
   participants of, 499
   professional development for, 500
   protocol review and approval for, 498
   quality assurance for, 500
   recruitment and retention for, 499
   research team for, 498, 498t
   sponsors of, 498
French National Cancer Institute, 497
funding
   in Australia, 447–449, 448f
   budgeting for. *See* budget(s) and budgeting
   in Germany, 505
   in Japan, 549–550
   in New Zealand, 569
   in United Kingdom, 597

G

gastos catastróficos, 562
gene, 316
gene mutation, 317
General Requirements for Informed Consent, 114–115
generic name, 16
Gene Therapy Advisory Committee (GTAC, UK), 594
genetic information, 332
Genetic Information Nondiscrimination Act (GINA, 2008), 59, 331, 333, 334f
genetic material. *See* biospecimen(s)
genetic polymorphism, 317
genetic research
   in Australia, 451
   in Austria, 458, 458f
   in Belarus, 469
   in China, 487–488
   in France, 499

634 Index

in Germany, 508
in India, 516
informed consent for, 332–333, 333f
in Ireland, 528
in Italy, 539
in Japan, 553–554, 553f
in Mexico, 563–564
in New Zealand, 570
in Romania, 577
in Spain, 583
in Thailand, 588
in United Kingdom, 599
genetics
of cancer, 327, 339–340
review of basic, 316–317, 316f
genetic testing, 327–337
in Canada, 479–480
of children, 334
and commercial DNA banking, 335
in Germany, 508
hereditary cancer predisposition testing as, 327–331
additional ethical concerns influencing, 330–331
benefits and limitations of, 330, 330f
in clinical trials, 334–335
clinical vs. research, 328–330
genetics and cancer development in, 327
hereditary cancer syndrome identification and, 328, 328f
history of, 328
indications for, 328–330, 329f
implications for clinical trial nurses of, 335
informed consent for, 122–123
in commercial or nonresearch setting, 331–332
elements of, 331f
in genetic and genomic research setting, 332–333, 333f
in Japan, 553, 553f
protection against discrimination with, 333–334, 334f
genetic variability, 316
genome, 316
genome-wide association studies (GWASs), 322
genomic research
in Australia, 451
in Austria, 458, 458f
in Belarus, 469
in China, 487–488
in France, 499
in Germany, 508
in India, 516
informed consent for, 122–123, 332–333, 333f
in Ireland, 528

in Italy, 539
in Japan, 553–554, 553f
in Mexico, 563–564
in New Zealand, 570
in Romania, 577
in Spain, 583
in Thailand, 588
in United Kingdom, 599
genomics, 330–331
genotyping assays, 320–322
German clinical trials, 503–511
billing in, 505
correlative, 508–509
documentation and data management for, 509
economic questions in, 508
ethics and, 504
financial factors with, 505
fundamental information on, 504
genetics and genomics in, 508
good clinical practice in, 504
history and foundation of, 503–504
informed consent for, 504–506
legal, regulatory, and legislative issues for, 504
participants in, 506–508, 507t
professional development for, 510
protocol development, review, and approval for, 504–505
psychosocial distress in, 508
quality assurance for, 509–510
recruitment and retention for, 506
research team for, 504
standard operating procedures for, 504
types of, 503
workload determination and resource allocation for, 505
German Clinical Trials Register, 251
germ-line mutations, 317, 340
ghostwriting, 435
Giemsa banding (G-banding), 339
gift authorship, 433
gliomas, 340
global economy, good clinical practice in, 68–69, 69f
glomerular filtration rate (GFR), 265
good clinical practice (GCP), 67–76
background of, 67, 68f
in Canada, 475
checklist for, 69, 72–76t
defined, 67, 68, 69
in European Union, 491
FDA, 69, 70t
in Germany, 504
in global economy, 68–69, 69f
ICH, 68–69, 69f, 70t

in Japan, 545, 547
in New Zealand, 568
in practice, 69
recommended resources for, 69, 71t
Good Clinical Practice Program, 69
good clinical practice (GCP) standards, 6
Good Publication Practice guidelines, version 2 (GPP2), 434, 434f
government agencies as sponsors, 45–47, 46f
government initiatives in Australia, 444
Grady, Christian, 97
grants, financial conflict of interest with, 209–210
graphics for resource planning and allocation, 164–168, 165f, 166f, 167–168t, 169f
group education, 221
group purchasing agencies, financial conflict of interest by, 212–213
Grupo de Investigación en Cáncer Ginecológico de México (GICOM), 560
guidance documents, 54, 56, 58f
guidelines, 58f

H

Harmonisation of Multi-centre Ethical Review (HoMER), 447
Health and Safety Executive (HSE, UK), 594–595
Health Canada, 473–474, 473f, 474f, 475
healthcare reform, 8
Health Insurance Portability and Accountability Act (HIPAA), 6
in agreement, 187–188
on genetic testing, 331, 333
on privacy and confidentiality, 57–58
Health Ministry's Screening Committee (HMSC, India), 514
Health Omnibus Programs Extension (HOPE), 248–249
health-related quality of life (HRQOL)
in Ireland, 528
as trial endpoint, 134
health research, reporting guidelines for, 431t
healthy volunteer, 30
hematologic malignancy response assessment as trial end point, 133, 134t
hemoglobin (Hgb) level, 266
hereditary cancer predisposition testing, 327–331

additional ethical concerns influencing, 330–331
in Austria, 458, 458f
benefits and limitations of, 330, 330f
in clinical trials, 334–335
clinical vs. research, 328–330
ethical concerns with, 330–331
genetics and cancer development in, 327
hereditary cancer syndrome identification and, 328, 328f
history of, 328
indications for, 328–330, 329f
hereditary cancer syndrome identification, 328, 328f
hidden costs, 181–182
and financial risk reduction, 194, 196–197t
High Level Group Term (HLGT), 274, 275f
High Level Term (HLT), 274, 275f
High-Priority Clinical Trials Program, 5
high-value study, 97–99, 98f
Hispanics, education of, 225
historical control, 26t
history of oncology clinical trials, 3–10
Clinical Trials Cooperative Group Program in, 4–5, 4f
Cooperative Group Outreach Program in, 5
Critical Path Initiative in, 5
early, 3–5
and evolution of national healthcare reform, 9
growth of international guidelines and U.S. regulations in, 5–6
National Cancer Institute in, 3–5
National Institutes of Health in, 3
NCI Community Oncology Research Program (NCORP) in, 5
NIH Roadmap in, 5
significant events in, 8, 8–9t
treatment of children and older adults in, 7–8
treatment of minorities and women in, 6–7
human genome, 316
Human Genome Project, 327, 328, 330
human research ethics committee (HREC, Australia), 444–445, 446
Human Research Protection Program (HRPP) audits, 408
human subject protection programs, accreditation of, 153
Human Tissue Act (2004, UK), 599

Index 635

Human Tissue Authority (HTA, UK), 599
human tissue repositories, 353, 354*f*
Hygienic Laboratory, 3
hypothesis, 134–135, 136*f*

I

ICH Harmonised Tripartite Guideline: Guideline for Good Clinical Practice, 6
ideal body weight (IBW), 265
The Immortal Life of Henrietta Lacks (Skloot), 7
Improving Access to Clinical Trials Act (2009), 60
inclusion criteria, 128
indels, 588
indemnification in agreement, 185–186
independent data safety monitoring committee (IDMC) in Japan, 556
independent ethics committee (IEC)
　documentation of, 389*t*
　in Spain, 580–581
India
　cancer incidence in, 513–514
　cancer research in, 514
Indian clinical trials, 513–518
　and cancer scenario in India, 513–514
　correlative, 516–517
　documentation and data management for, 517
　ethics committee for, 515
　financial factors for, 515–516
　fundamental information on, 514
　genetics and genomics in, 516
　history and foundation of, 513
　informed consent for, 515
　international collaboration in, 514
　post-trial access with, 516
　professional development for, 517
　protocol development, review, and approval for, 514–515
　quality assurance for, 517
　recruitment and retention in, 516
　regulatory approval for, 515
　selection of special groups as research participants in, 516
indirect costs in resource planning and allocation, 165
indirect payment, 213
individual education, 220–221
Indo-Foreign Cell (IFC), 514
INDOX Cancer Research Network, 514

IND safety reports (ISRs), 15, 282, 283*f*, 283*t*
inducement vs. reimbursement, 149
industry-sponsored clinical trials, 47
inferential statistics, 136
influence and financial conflict of interest, 214–215
INFOCÁNCER, 564
informational materials, 223, 224*f*
information system resources
　in Mexico, 564, 565*f*
　in United Kingdom, 600
informed consent (IC), 113–125
　assessing comprehension and improving readability of, 117–118, 118*f*
　in audit, 409
　in Australia, 445–446
　Belmont Report on, 113–114
　for biospecimens, 351–352, 352*f*
　in Canada, 476–477
　of child, 120–121
　in China, 486
　DHHS on, 114
　documentation of, 118–119, 366–367
　and ethics, 99, 99*f*
　exculpatory language in, 114–115, 115*f*
　exemptions and waivers for, 123
　in France, 498–499
　for genetic testing and genomic research, 122–123
　in commercial or nonresearch setting, 331–332
　elements of, 331*f*
　in genetic and genomic research setting, 332–333, 333*f*
　in Germany, 504–505
　guiding principles for, 113–115
　in India, 515
　investigators' responsibilities for, 114–115, 115*f*
　IRB reviews of, 150
　in Ireland, 526
　in Italy, 537
　in Japan, 548
　with mental disabilities or dementia, 121–122
　in New Zealand, 569
　of non–English speaker, 119–120
　nursing competencies in, 607
　of older adults, 121
　of prisoners, 122
　process of, 115, 116*t*
　and protection of pregnant women, fetuses, and neonates, 121
　for reconsent, 119, 119*f*

　and registry databank, 116–117
　in regulatory file, 389*t*
　role of clinical trial nurses in, 123
　in Romania, 575–576
　source documentation for process of, 120
　of special populations, 120–123
　therapeutic misconception and, 100–101, 100*f*, 101*f*
informed consent (IC) form, 113
　access to more information on, 622
　additional elements of, 117, 118*f*
　additional studies on, 622–623
　adverse events on, 614–620
　attachments to, 626
　benefits on, 620
　costs on, 621
　extra tests and procedures on, 613–614
　injury or hurt on, 621
　length of study on, 613
　medical information access on, 621
　other choices on, 610–611
　reason for study on, 611–612
　required elements of, 115–117
　rights on, 620–621
　risks on, 614–620
　stopping participation in study on, 620
　study groups on, 612–613
　template for, 117, 609–626
　usual approach on, 610
infrastructural barriers to recruitment, 231
initiation visit, 406, 406*f*
innovative medical devices, 178
inspections
　defined, 403*f*
　in European Union, 493
　in Ireland, 530
　U.S. FDA, 404–405, 405*t*
Institute of Medicine (IOM), 20–21
institutional barriers, invisible, 194–197
institutional biosafety committee (IBC), 142, 142*f*
　reporting of adverse events to, 280–281, 282–283
institutional conflict, 206–207
institutional ethics committee (IEC) in India, 515
institutional regulatory file. *See* regulatory file
institutional responsibilities for financial conflict of interest, 211–212, 211*f*, 212*f*
institutional review board(s) (IRBs), 6, 52, 56, 69, 78

　accreditation of human subject protections programs by, 153
　additional oversight requirements of, 152–153
　administrative support for, 146
　approval by, 390*t*
　　conditional, 150
　　with contingencies, 150
　assurances for, 143, 144*f*
　continuing review to, 390*t*
　correspondence of, 389*t*
　and ethics, 101
　external (commercial, independent, central), 145, 145*f*
　Federalwide Assurance on, 606
　fees for, 177
　general functions and operations of, 145
　internal (local), 145, 145*f*
　meetings of, 146, 147, 148*t*
　membership of, 145–146, 389*t*
　in Mexico, 560–561
　records of, 152
　registration of, 143–145, 144*f*
　reporting of adverse events to, 280, 281, 281*f*, 390*t*
　stipulations by, 150
　in Thailand, 586, 587*f*
　types of, 145–146, 145*f*
institutional review board (IRB) reviews, 143–152
　certificates of confidentiality as, 148
　of changes to original protocol document, 150–151
　continuing, 151
　for device research, 148–149
　exemption from, 147
　expedited, 146–147
　full, 146
　of informed consent, 150
　of other reportable events, 151–152, 152*t*
　outcomes of, 150–152
　of payment, 149–150
　of principal investigator qualifications, 152–153
　risk-benefit analysis as, 147–148, 147*f*, 148*t*
　risk for vulnerable populations as, 148, 149*t*
　of site qualifications, 153
　types of, 146–150
　for verification of IND or investigational device exemption, 153
Institut National du Cancer (INCa), 497
Instituto Nacional de Cancerología (INCan), 559–560, 560*f*
insurance in Spain, 582
Integrated Research Application System (IRAS, UK), 593–594

integrity, scientific, 101–102, 207
intellectual property in agreement, 186
IntelliTRIAL, 168*t*
interdisciplinary team, 85–86
    in Canada, 474–475
intergroup trials in Australia, 445
interim analyses, 138
intermediate-sized patient populations, expanded access for, 42, 42*f*, 43*f*
internal audits, 408
internal financial audit. *See* financial audit
International Air Transport Association (IATA), 61
International Association of Clinical Research Nurses, 417*t*
International Clinical Trials Registry Platform (ICTRP), 250
international clinical trials research, 441, 442*f*
    in Australia, 443–453
    in Austria, 455–461
    in Belarus, 463–471
    in Canada, 473–484
    in China, 485–489
    in European Union, 491–495
    in France, 497–501
    in Germany, 503–511
    in India, 513–518
    in Ireland, 519–533
    in Italy, 535–543
    in Japan, 545–558
    in Mexico, 559–566
    in New Zealand, 567–572
    in Romania, 573–578
    in Spain, 579–584
    in Thailand, 585–590
    in United Kingdom, 591–602
International Committee of Medical Journal Editors (ICMJE), 249
International Conference on Harmonisation (ICH) of Technical Requirements for Registration of Pharmaceuticals for Human Use, 6, 57
    on data and safety monitoring plans (DSMPs), 399
    on good clinical practice, 68–69, 69*f*, 70*t*
    on role of investigator, 79
International Federation of Pharmaceutical Manufacturers and Associations (IFPMA), 250
international standards, laws, and guidelines, 57–59
International System for Human Cytogenetic Nomenclature, 317
Internet
    for education about clinical trial, 223, 224*f*
    for patient education, 299, 299*f*, 300*f*
interoperability of clinical data management system, 378
interpreter for informed consent, 120
intervention in protocol, 129–131, 130*f*
IntraLinks for Study Management, 167*t*
intramural research in Spain, 580
intrapatient escalation studies, 31–32
inversions, 317
investigational agent(s)
    accountability of, 260–262
    for audit, 409
    in Australia, 450
    in Mexico, 562–563
    in regulatory file, 391*t*
    administration of, 264–267
    documentation of, 266
    dosing in, 264–265
    guidelines for, 267
    in Ireland, 527
    laboratory studies on, 265–266, 265*f*
    in New Zealand, 569–570
    in Canada, 479
    check-in of, 261
    compassionate use, special exceptions, or emergency use of, 264
    defined, 24*t*
    destruction of, 391*t*
    dispensing of, 262, 391*t*
    expanded access to, 41–43*t*, 41–44
    in France, 499
    in Germany, 507–508
    in Japan, 552
    labeling of, 391*t*
    procurement of, 259–260
    receipt of, 260–261, 391*t*
    return of
        by patient, 263–264
        to supplier, 263
    role of clinical trial nurses with, 267
    storage of, 261–262
    transfer of, 263–264
Investigational Agent Accountability Record, 261
Investigational Agent Transfer Form, 264
investigational device(s), 178
investigational device exemption (IDE), 149
    and budgeting, 178
    verification of, 153
investigational new drug application (IND), 14–15
    and good clinical practice, 67
    verification of, 153
investigational new drug (IND) process in Germany, 503
investigational new drug (IND) safety reports in regulatory file, 390*t*
investigational product management in China, 487
investigator, 77–80, 78*t*
    qualifications of, 152–153
    responsibility for informed consent, 114–115, 115*f*
investigator agreement, 388*t*
investigator binder. *See* regulatory file(s)
investigator-held IND, 14
investigator-initiated clinical trials, 47
investigator meetings, budgeting for, 180
investigator's brochure, 389*t*
investigator's study files. *See* regulatory file(s)
invoiceable costs, 177
iPLEX ADME pharmacogenomics panel, 322
irinotecan and UDP-glucuronosyl transferase, 320
Irish clinical trials, 519–533
    administration of protocol agents in, 527
    adverse events in, 527–528
    correlative, 528
    documentation and data management for, 528–529
    ethics review and approval process for, 523–524
    financial factors and trial site budgets for, 524–526
    fundamental information on, 521–524, 522*t*
    genetics and genomics in, 528
    history and foundation of, 519–521, 520*f*, 521*f*
    industry collaborations in, 531
    informed consent for, 526
    international, 531, 531*f*
    legal and regulatory approval process for, 523
    long-term follow-up after, 526–527
    participants in, 526–528
    patient education for, 527
    patient selective and eligibility for, 526
    professional development for, 530–531, 531*f*
    protocol development, review, and approach for, 524, 525*f*
    quality assurance for, 529–530
    recruitment and retention for, 526
    sponsoring agencies for, 523
Irish Platform for Patients' Organisations, Science and Industry (IPPOSI), 526
Irish Research Nurses Network (IRNN), 531
isotope dilution mass spectrometry (IDMS)-measured serum creatinine, 265
Italian clinical trials, 535–543
    compassionate use in, 536
    conflicts of interest in, 536
    correlative, 539
    documentation and data management for, 539–540, 540*f*
    ethics committee for, 536
    financial factors with, 537
    fundamental information on, 535–536
    genetics and genomics in, 539
    history and background of, 535
    informed consent for, 537
    legal and regulatory issues for, 536–537
    participants in, 538–539
    professional development for, 540–541, 541*f*
    protocol development, review, and approval for, 536–537
    quality assurance for, 540
    recruitment and retention for, 537–538
    research team for, 536

J

Japan Clinical Oncology Group (JCOG), 545
Japanese clinical trials, 545–558
    adverse events and unanticipated problems in, 552
    correlative, 554–555
    documentation and data management for, 555
    drug development process and, 545–546
    ethics for, 548
    expanded access to investigational drugs in, 546
    financial factors with, 549–550
    fundamental information on, 546–548, 547*f*, 548*f*
    genetics and genomics in, 553–554, 553*f*
    good clinical practice for, 545, 547
    history and foundation of, 545–546, 545*f*
    implications for nurses of, 557
    informed consent for, 548
    investigational agents for, 552
    legal, regulatory, and legislative issues with, 547
    participants of, 551–553
    patient and family education on, 552
    professional development for, 556–557
    protocol development, review, and approval process for, 548–549, 548*f*

psychosocial distress in, 552–553
quality assurance for, 556
recruitment and retention for, 550–551
research team for, 546–547, 547f
sponsoring agencies for, 546
staff education for, 551–552
standard operating procedures for, 547–548, 548f
Japan Medical Association Center for Clinical Trials Clinical Trials Registry (JMACCT-CTR), 551
Japan Pharmaceutical Information Center Clinical Trials Information (JAPIC-CTI), 551
journals, recommended, 415, 416f
justice, 53, 53t, 113

K

Kaplan-Meier survival curve, 344
Kefauver-Harris Amendments (1962), 5, 67
kinesthetic learning style, 295t
Konferenz Onkologischer Kranken- und Kinderkrankenpflege (KOK), 506
Koordinierungszentren für Klinische Studien (KKS Network), 506–507, 507t
KRAS oncogene
 in colon cancer, 346
 in lung cancer, 345

L

labels in regulatory file, 391t
lab-only visits, budgeting for, 180–181
laboratory accreditation, 391t
laboratory certification, 391t
laboratory documentation, 391–392t
laboratory fees, 178–179
laboratory studies of research drug administration, 265–266, 265f
Lacks, Henrietta (HeLa), 7
Latin American Cooperative Oncology Group (LACOG), 560
Latinos, education of, 225
law, 58f
lead author, 433
lead generation, 14
lead optimization, 14
Lean Six Sigma principles, 194
learner, domains of, 423
learning assessment, 292, 293t, 293–294
learning needs, 292, 293–294t
learning readiness, 292

learning style, 292, 295t
learning technology for professional development, 415–416, 416t
legal, 58f
regulatory, and legislative issues, 51–65
 in Australia, 444–445
 on basic ethical principles, 52–53, 53t
 in Canada, 475, 476f
 on clinical trials registration and patient open access, 59–60
 on compliance, 61–64, 62t
 on distinction between research and practice, 52, 53t
 federal clinical trial legislation for, 60
 Federalwide Assurance on, 605–606
 on financial fraud and abuse, 63
 in Germany, 504
 implications for clinical trials nurses of, 63–64
 International Conference on Harmonisation for, 57
 international standards, laws, and guidelines on, 57–59
 in Ireland, 523
 in Italy, 536–537
 in Japan, 547
 on negligence, 63
 in New Zealand, 567–568
 on privacy and confidentiality, 57–59
 on research misconduct, 62–63, 62t
 on retention of records, 61, 61f
 selected historical events on, 51–53, 52t
 on shipment of research specimens, 61
 state clinical trial legislation for, 60–61
 in Thailand, 586, 587f
 in United Kingdom, 593, 593f
 U.S. regulatory authority on, 53–57, 54f, 55t, 56t, 57f, 58f
legally authorized representative (LAR), 114, 118, 121–122
legislative documents in Belarus, 464
legislative issues. *See* legal, regulatory, and legislative issues
leukemias, 340–341, 340t, 341t
life-threatening adverse event, 272t, 282
literature review, 430t

abstract of, 432t
reporting guidelines for, 431t
long-term follow-up
 in Ireland, 526–527
 in New Zealand, 570
looks, 138
Lowest Level Term (LLT), 274, 275f
low-income patients, education of, 224–225
lung cancer biomarkers, 345–346
lymphomas, 340

M

Macmillan Cancer Support, 597
mailing lists, electronic, 416, 417t
MammaPrint, 345
Mammostrat, 345
manual of operations, 90
manual of procedures (MOP), 389t
manufacturers, financial conflict of interest by, 212–213
masking, 23–25, 24t
master timeline, 164, 165f
maximum, 137f
maximum drug concentration (Cmax), 359t
maximum time (Tmax), 359t
maximum tolerated dose (MTD), 24t, 30–31, 32
McKusick, Victor, 339
mean, 137f
measurable disease in solid tumor response assessment, 132, 133, 133t
measures of productivity, 160
media campaign, 222
median, 137f
medical device research, IRB review for, 148–149
Medical Dictionary for Regulatory Activities (MedDRA), 271–274, 275f
medical license, 388t
medical record, 365–366, 366f
medical writers, 435
Medicare
 Advantage Plans, 178
 billing compliance for, 177–178
 Clinical Trial Policy of, 8
 and financial audit, 199–200
Medicare coverage analysis (MCA), 171, 172–174f, 177
Medicare secondary payer (MSP) issues, 187
Medicines and Healthcare Products Regulatory Agency (MHRA, UK), 593
MedWatch, 15
mental disabilities, informed consent with, 121–122
mentorship, 421–428
abilities in, 424, 424f

active listening in, 426
background of, 421–422, 421f, 422f
benefits to institutions of, 422, 422f
communication in, 426
competencies for, 423–424, 423f, 424f
defined, 422
via e-mentoring, 426–427, 427f
feedback in, 426
future of, 427
initiation or formation of, 426
in Japan, 556–557
middle or working phase of, 426
redefinition, resolution, or passing the torch in, 426
relationship of, 424–426, 424f, 425f
responsibilities in, 424, 424f
theoretical frameworks for, 422–423, 423t
virtues in, 423–424, 424f
mentorship agreement, 424, 425f
meta-analyses
abstract of, 432t
reporting guidelines for, 431t
metabolism, 359t
metadata, 379
Mexican clinical trials, 559–566
adverse events in, 563
correlative, 564
documentation and data management for, 564
ethics and regulations for, 561–562
financial factors for, 562
fundamental information on, 560
genetics and genomics in, 563–564
history and foundation of, 559–560, 560f
information system resources and patient support for, 564, 565f
off-treatment follow-up in, 563
participants in, 562–563
professional development for, 565
protocol development, review, and approach for, 560–562, 561f
quality assurance for, 564–565
recruitment and retention for, 562
microdose, 24t
microdose IND, 14
minimal risk, 147
minimum, 137f
minor(s). *See* children
minorities
recruitment of, 231
treatment of, 6–7

Minority-Based Community Clinical Oncology Program (MBCCOP), 6–7
misconduct, 62–63, 62*t*
mismatch repair (MMR) status in colon cancer, 346
mission
  and financial risk reduction, 192
  partnering with research bases and sponsors that best fit, 192–193
MLH1 gene, 328
mobile computing, 416*t*
mode, 137*f*
model-based designs, 30
modifications of original protocol document, 150–151
molecular profiling. *See* tumor profiling
monitoring
  in Germany, 509–510
  in India, 517
  in Ireland, 529–530
  in protocol, 111, 137–138
  in regulatory file, 392*t*
  of research finances, 197
monitoring visit, 403*f*
Mosteller equation, 265
motivation for clinical trial participation, 303–305
mouse equivalent lethal dose (MELD) 10, 24*t*
MSH2 gene, 328
multicenter clinical trials
  authorship in, 434
  guidelines for, 111
multicompartment model, 360, 360*f*
multigene biomarkers, 343
multinational multicenter clinical trials (MMCTs) in Belarus, 465, 467*f*, 468*f*
multiple controls, 26*t*
multiple myeloma, 341
mutations, 317, 327, 339–340
myelosuppression, 266

N

naming of drugs, 16
National Agency for Medicines and Medical Devices (ANMDM, Romania), 573, 574
National Cancer Act (1971), 4, 47
National Cancer Control Programme (NCCP, Ireland), 519, 522, 522*t*
National Cancer Cooperative Trials Groups (NCCTG), 443
National Cancer Institute (NCI) and clinical trial registries, 247–248
  on data and safety monitoring plans (DSMPs), 399
  in history of oncology clinical trials, 3–5
  on role of investigator, 79
  as sponsor, 45–47
  as study sponsor, 407–408
National Cancer Institute Act (1937), 3
National Cancer Institute (NCI) Community Oncology Research Program (NCORP), 5, 46
National Cancer Institute of Canada Clinical Trials Group (NCIC CTG), 477–478
National Cancer Institute of Mexico, 559–560, 560*f*
National Cancer Institute (NCI)-sponsored clinical trials, adverse event reporting for, 284, 286*f*, 825*f*
National Cancer Research Institute (NCRI, UK), 591–592
National Cancer Research Network (NCRN, UK), 592
National Cancer Screening Service (Ireland), 522–523
National Commission for the Protection of Human Subjects of Biomedical and Behavioral Research, 6, 52
National Comprehensive Cancer Network (NCCN) on distress, 305–310, 306–309*f*, 307–308
National Coverage Determination (NCD), 177, 199
national healthcare reform, 8
National Health Service (NHS, UK), 591
National Human Genome Research Institute (NHGRI), 327
National Institute for Health Research (NIHR, UK), 591
National Institutes of Health (NIH)
  and clinical trial registries, 249
  on data and safety monitoring plans (DSMPs), 399
  on definition of program director/principal investigator, 207–208
  in history of clinical trials, 3
  in history of legal and regulatory issues, 52
  on recombinant DNA safety review, 142
National Institutes of Health (NIH) Revitalization Act (1993), 7
National Institutes of Health (NIH) Roadmap, 5
National Plan for Radiation Oncology (Ireland), 522, 522*t*
National Provider Identifier (NPI), 213
National Research Act (1974), 6, 52
National Research Ethics Service (NRES, UK), 593
National Science Foundation (NSF) on financial conflict of interest, 208, 209*f*
National Statement on Ethical Conduct in Human Research (NHMRC), 447
negligence, 58*f*, 63
neonates, informed consent and protection of, 121
Network of the Coordinating Centres for Clinical Trials (Germany), 506–507, 507*t*
New Zealand clinical trials, 567–572
  administration of protocol agents and assessments in, 569–570
  adverse events in, 569–570
  ancillary studies with, 570
  documentation and data management systems for, 570
  eligibility and informed consent for, 569
  ethics committees for, 568
  financial factors with, 568–569
  fundamental information on, 567–568
  genetics and genomics in, 570
  good clinical practice for, 568
  history and foundation of, 567
  legal and regulatory issues with, 567–568
  long-term follow-up for, 570
  participants of, 569–570
  patient education in, 570
  professional development for, 571
  protocol development, review, and approval for, 568
  quality assurance for, 570–571
  recruitment for, 569
no action indicated (NAI), 404
nonadherence
  defined, 241–242
  impact of, 245
  primary or intentional, 241–242
  reasons for, 246
  unintentional, 242
noncommercial IND, 14
noncompartmental model, 360–361
non-complete response in solid tumor response assessment, 133
noncompliance
  with financial conflict of interest, 211–212, 212*f*, 213–215, 214*f*
  with regulations and guidelines, 62
non–English speaker, informed consent of, 119–120
nonmeasurable disease in solid tumor response assessment, 132, 133–134, 134*t*
nonprofit organizations, sponsorship by, 47–48, 48*f*
non-progressive disease in solid tumor response assessment, 133
nonrefundable fees, 175, 176–177, 176*f*
non-significant risk (NSR) device, 149
nonstandard procedure costs, 178, 179*f*
nontarget lesions in solid tumor response assessment, 132–133
nontreatment control, 26*t*
normal reference ranges, 391*t*
notes to file, 393*t*
not-for-cause audit/review, 403*f*
nuclear organizing region (NOR) stains, 339
nucleotides, 316
null hypothesis, 134–135, 136*f*
Nuremberg Code (1949), 5, 51–52, 67, 97, 98*f*
nurse, role on research team of, 81–84, 83*f*, 83*t*
Nursing and Midwifery Board of Ireland (NMBI), 530
nursing companion studies. *See* companion studies
nursing competencies, 607–608
nursing registration in Ireland, 530–531

O

obese patient, dosing for, 265
objective response rate as trial end point, 132*t*
objectives in protocol, 110, 127–128
observational research, 35–39
  case-control studies for, 36*t*, 37
  case report/case series studies for, 35, 36*t*
  cohort studies for, 36*t*, 37–38, 37*f*
  on comparative effectiveness, 18
  cross-sectional studies for, 35–37, 36*t*
  experimental vs., 17
  outcomes research as, 36*t*, 38, 38*f*
  purpose and study design for, 35, 36*t*
  reporting guidelines for, 431*t*
Office for Human Research Protections (OHRP), 6, 54–56, 55*t*
  electronic mailing list of, 417*t*
  on informed consent, 114
  on role of investigator, 78
Office of Biotechnology Activities (OBA), 142, 142*f*

reporting of adverse events to, 280–281, 282–283
Office of Cancer Centers, 45
Office of Management and Budget (OMB) on financial conflict of interest, 208
Office of Research on Women's Health, 7
official action indicated (OAI), 404
off-label use, documentation of, 367
off-study criteria in protocol, 111
off-study documentation, 368
off-treatment documentation, 368
off-treatment follow-up
　in Mexico, 563
　in protocol, 131
　in United Kingdom, 597–598
off treatment in Italy, 538–539
older adults
　education of, 224
　informed consent of, 121
　patient education for, 301
　treatment of, 7–8
Oncology Clinical Trials Nurse Competencies, 607–608
Oncology Nursing Certification Corporation (ONCC), 417
Oncology Nursing Society (ONS), 417t
oncology trial endpoints, 131–134, 132–135t
Oncore clinical trial tracking database, 164, 167t
Oncotype DX Breast Cancer Assay, 344–345
Oncotype DX Colon Cancer Assay, 346
Oncotype DX Prostate Cancer Assay, 347
one-compartment model, 360, 360f
Online Mendelian Inheritance in Man, 316
Ontario Cancer Research Ethics Board (OCREB), 476
Ontario Protocol Assessment Level (OPAL), 158–160, 159t, 161t
　in Australia, 447
open access, 59–60
open label, 24
open study, 24
optimal dose, 32
ordering of research study drugs, 259–260
Order of Generalist Medical Nurses, Midwives and Medical Nurses of Romania (OAMGMAMR), 578
Osservatorio Nazionale della Sperimentazione Clinica (OsSC), 535
outcomes research, 36t, 38, 38f
outcome study, 38

Ovarian Cancer Research Group (Mexico), 560
overall survival as trial endpoint, 132t
overall tumor burden in solid tumor response assessment, 132–133

P

Pan-Canadian Oncology Drug Review (pCODR), 474
parallel companion studies, 19
parallel design, 25, 26f
paraphrasing, 436
partial response in solid tumor response assessment, 133
participants, 80
　in Australia, 450–451
　in Belarus, 469
　in Canada, 479
　in China, 487
　in France, 499
　in Ireland, 526–528
　in Italy, 538–539
　in Japan, 551–553
　in Mexico, 562–563
　in New Zealand, 569–570
　in Romania, 576–577, 576f
　in Spain, 582–583
　in Thailand, 587–588
　in United Kingdom, 598–599
participation, motivation for, 303–305
pass-through costs, 177
pathology reports in eligibility, 129
patient advocacy conflict, 206
patient advocates, recruitment by, 238
patient and family education, 291–302
　for adult learners, 292–293
　in Australia, 450–451
　in Canada, 478–479
　with challenges to learning, 301
　defined, 291
　effective messages in, 292–294
　in Germany, 506, 508
　goal of, 291
　in Ireland, 527
　in Japan, 550, 552
　learning needs and, 292, 293–294t
　learning style and, 292, 295t
　methods for effective, 299, 299f, 300f
　model to determine objectives of, 291, 291f
　in New Zealand, 570
　for older adults, 301
　online resources for, 299, 299f, 300f
　for pediatric learners, 294, 296f
　providing clear and effective, 298–301
　readiness to learn and, 292

for recruitment, 219–227
　and accrual, 220
　of African Americans, 225
　of American Indians and Alaska Natives, 225
　in Australia, 449
　clinical trial nurses' role in, 219–220
　community partnership for, 222
　and credibility, 222
　explaining importance of eligibility criteria in, 222–223
　group, 221
　of Hispanics/Latinos, 225
　individual, 220–221
　informational materials for, 223, 224f
　of low-income patients, 224–225
　media campaign for, 222
　of older adults, 224
　opportunities and preparation for speaking to public for, 221–222
　public, 221
　timing of, 221
　of underrepresented populations, 224–225
setting priorities for, 298
specific to study phases, 294–298, 297f
standards for, 291, 291f
tips for, 299–301
what to teach in, 298
patient care costs, 178, 179f
patient care management, nursing competencies in, 607–608
Patient-Centered Outcomes Research Institute (PCORI), 18
patient characteristics and adherence, 243
patient diaries, 278–279, 279f
Patient Distress Management Report, 309
patient eligibility criteria. *See* eligibility criteria
patient factors in motivation for clinical trial participation, 304
patient navigators, recruitment by, 237–238
patient open access, 59–60
patient-oriented research in Germany, 503
Patient Protection and Affordable Care Act (2010), 8, 18, 60, 177, 212
patient-reported outcomes (PROs)
　in Common Terminology Criteria for Adverse Events (CTCAE), 275–276
　as trial endpoint, 134

patient selection
　in Ireland, 526
　in Mexico, 562
　in Spain, 582
patient support in Mexico, 564, 565f
payment(s)
　in agreement, 186
　IRB reviews of, 149–150
pediatric patients. *See* children
peer review, 60, 99
　in United Kingdom, 595
penetrance, 317, 327
peptide bond, 317
performance status in eligibility, 129
permissible values, 375, 376t, 380
personal conflict, 207
Personal Support Care Plan, 308–309
P-glycoprotein, 320
pharmaceutical industry sponsorship, 47
pharmaceutical information in protocol, 110
Pharmaceutical Management Branch (PMB), 79, 259–260
pharmaceutical registries, 251
Pharmaceuticals and Medical Devices Agency (PMDA, Japan), 545–546
pharmacodynamics (PD), 24t, 316
pharmacoeconomic studies
　in Japan, 554
　in Mexico, 564
pharmacogenetics, 315–325
　in Australia, 451
　and basic pharmacogenomics, 317–318, 319t
　and common anticancer drugs, 318–320, 321t
　defined, 315
　drug development process and, 315–316
　in Germany, 508
　goal of, 315
　in Japan, 553
　and review of basic genetics, 316–317, 316f
　role of oncology clinical trial nurses in, 322
pharmacogenetic testing, 320–322
pharmacogenomics, 315, 317–318, 319t
　in Australia, 451
　in Germany, 508
　in Japan, 553
pharmacokinetic (PK) models, 358–361
　compartmental, 359–360, 360f, 361f
　noncompartmental, 360–361
　physiologically based, 361
　population, 361
pharmacokinetic (PK) parameters, 357f, 358, 359t

pharmacokinetics (PK), 24t, 315, 316
pharmacokinetic sampling (PKS), 179
pharmacokinetic (PK) trials, 357–362
  in Australia, 451
  in Japan, 554
  models for, 358–361
    compartmental, 359–360, 360f, 361f
    noncompartmental, 360–361
    physiologically based, 361
    population, 361
  parameters for, 357f, 358, 359t
  role in oncology drug development of, 357–358, 357f
  setting for, 358, 359f
pharmacokinetic (PK) worksheet, 358, 359f
pharmacy costs, 177, 179
phase 0 trials, 28–30, 29t
phase I trials, 29t, 30–32, 31f, 31t
  motivation for participation in, 304–305
  patient education for, 295–296, 297f
phase II trials, 29t, 32–33
  patient education for, 296, 297, 297f
phase III trials, 29t, 33
  patient education for, 297–298, 297f
phase IV trials, 29t, 33
phenotype, 318
phenotyping assays, 320–321
Philadelphia chromosome, 340, 341
Physician Data Query (PDQ) database, 248
physician factors in motivation for clinical trial participation, 304
Physician Payments Sunshine Act (2013), 8, 18, 60, 177, 212
physiologically based pharmacokinetic (PBPK) model, 361
placebo control, 26t, 98–99
plagiarism, 62, 102, 102f, 435–437, 437f
plan of work, 164, 164f
platelet count, 266
polymerase chain reaction (PCR), 322
polypeptides, 316
population pharmacokinetic model, 361
portfolio, professional, 418
poster, 432–433
postmarketing reporting, voluntary, 284
postmarketing surveillance trials, 29t, 33
power, 135–136
power analysis, 98
practice vs. research, 52, 53t, 100, 100f

precepting, 422
preclinical investigations, 13–14
preclinical testing, 315–316
predictive markers, 343–344
Preferred Term (PT), 274, 275f
pregnant women, informed consent and protection of, 121
Pre-Investigational New Drug Application Consultation Program, 15
prestudy qualification visit, 406
prevention trials, hereditary cancer predisposition testing in, 334
primary objectives in protocol, 110, 127–128
primary source, 430
Princess Margaret Hospital Consortium (PMHC), 477
principal investigator(s) (PIs), 77–80, 78t
  budgeting for, 179–180
  defined, 207–208
  multiple, 208
  qualifications of, 152–153
principal investigator (PI) number, 260
Priority-Driven Collaborative Cancer Research Scheme (PDCCRS), 444
prisoners, informed consent of, 122
privacy, 57–59
  data, 374, 374f
Privacy Rule, 57–59
procedural barriers to recruitment, 229–231
procedures
  for patient entry into study, 110
  in protocol, 129–131, 130f
process map, 194
procurement of research study drugs, 259–260
  in Australia, 450
prodrugs, 317
product limit estimate, 344
professional associations and organizations, 416, 417t
professional conflict, 207
professional development, 415–420
  academic and certificate programs for, 416
  in Australia, 452
  in Austria, 450
  in Belarus, 470
  in Canada, 482
  categories of learning technology for, 415–416, 416t
  in China, 488
  educating other nurses for, 417–418
  electronic mailing lists for, 416, 417t
  in France, 500
  general activities for, 415
  in Germany, 510

  in India, 517
  in Ireland, 530–531
  in Italy, 540–541, 541f
  in Japan, 556–557
  in Mexico, 565
  in New Zealand, 571
  nursing competencies in, 608
  professional associations and organizations for, 416, 417t
  recommended journals for, 415, 416f
  in Romania, 578
  in Spain, 583–584, 584f
  specialty certification for, 416–417
  in Thailand, 589
  in United Kingdom, 601
professional development log, 418, 419–420f
professional portfolio, 418
prognostic markers, 343
program direction and financial risk reduction, 192
program directors (PDs), 207–208
progression-free survival as trial endpoint, 132t
progressive disease in solid tumor response assessment, 133
promotion strategies. See also recruitment
  in Australia, 449
  in Germany, 506
  in Japan, 551
  in United Kingdom, 597
proof of concept, 32
prospective cohort studies, 38
prostate cancer biomarkers, 347
protected health information (PHI), 57–59
  in agreement, 187–188
  and data privacy and security, 374, 374f, 378–379
Protection of Human Research Subjects regulations, 52
protocol
  approvals/authorizations of, 391t
  defined, 109
  elements of, 109–111, 109f
  in regulatory file, 389t
  review of changes to original, 150–151
  strategic choice of, 193, 193f
protocol acuity score, 160, 161t
protocol-based timeline, 164, 164f
protocol compliance, nursing competencies in, 607
protocol data elements, 249, 249f
protocol development, 127–140
  analysis plan in, 137
  in Australia, 445–447
  in Austria, 456
  in Belarus, 467–468
  in Canada, 476–477

  in China, 486
  eligibility in, 128–129
  in Germany, 504–505
  in India, 514–515
  in Ireland, 524, 525f
  in Italy, 536–537
  in Japan, 548–549, 548f
  in Mexico, 560–562, 561f
  monitoring in, 137–138
  in New Zealand, 568
  off-treatment follow-up in, 131
  oncology trial end points in, 131–134, 132–135t
  primary and secondary objectives in, 127–128
  in Romania, 575–576
  in Spain, 580–582
  statistical considerations in, 134–137, 136f, 137f
  study design in, 128–129
  study intervention and required procedures in, 129–131, 130f
  in Thailand, 586–587
  in United Kingdom, 595–597, 595f
protocol deviations in regulatory file, 390t
protocol-directed resource planning, 163–164, 163f, 164f
protocol factors in motivation for clinical trial participation, 305
protocol feasibility review, 193–194, 193f, 195f
protocol planning map, 164, 169f
protocol review and approval, 141–154
  in Australia, 445–447
  in Austria, 456
  in Belarus, 465, 466f, 467–468
  in Canada, 477
  in China, 486
  in France, 498
  in Germany, 505
  in India, 514–515
  by IRBs. see institutional review board(s) (IRBs)
  in Ireland, 524, 525f
  in Italy, 536–537
  in Japan, 548–549, 548f
  in Mexico, 560–562, 561f
  in New Zealand, 568
  pre-IRB, 141–143, 142f
  in Romania, 575–576
  safety reviews for, 141–142, 142f
  scientific review for, 141
  in Spain, 580–582
  sponsor approval in, 142–143
  in Thailand, 586–587
  in United Kingdom, 595–597, 595f
protocol-specific activities, documentation of, 367
protocol templates, 109
provider characteristics and adherence, 243

psychomotor domain, 423
psycho-oncology, 303
Psycho-Oncology Cooperative Research Group, 444
psychosocial distress, 303–312
　in Australia, 451
　background of, 303
　in Canada, 479
　characteristics of patients at risk for, 305–306, 306f
　defined, 305
　in Germany, 508
　incidence of, 305
　in Japan, 552–553
　nursing implications of, 309–310, 309f
　overview of, 305–306
　and patient motivation for clinical trial participation, 303–305
　related to clinical trial discontinuation, 306, 306f
　standards of care for, 309–310, 309f
　tools to evaluate, 307–309, 307f, 308f
　treatment of, 308f
publication bias, 247
publication issues in Japan, 557
public domain, 436
public education, 221. See also patient and family education
　in Australia, 449
　in Canada, 478–479
　in Germany, 506
　in Japan, 550
Public Health Service (PHS) on financial conflict of interest, 205, 209–212
　for contracts, 210–212–211f, 212f
　for grants and cooperative agreements, 209–210
public presentations, opportunities and preparation for, 221–222
publishing, 429–437
　of abstract, 430–432, 432t
　acknowledgments in, 435
　of article, 430, 430t, 431f, 431t
　　created from abstract or poster, 432–433
　authorship for, 433–435
　citations in, 436, 436f, 437f
　and guidelines for reporting research results, 430, 431f, 431t
　integrity in, 435–437
　medical writers in, 435
　plagiarism in, 435–437, 437f
　possible topics for, 429, 429f
　of poster, 432
　reasons for, 429
PubMed Central, 59

Q

Q0 procedure code modifier, 178

Q1 procedure code modifier, 178
Qualified Investigator Undertaking, 481
qualifying status for Medicare or third-party payer coverage, 177
qualifying trials for Medicare or third-party payer coverage, 177
quality assurance, 89, 199
　in Austria, 459–460, 459f
　in Belarus, 470
　in Canada, 481–482
　in China, 488
　in France, 500
　in Germany, 509
　in India, 517
　in Ireland, 529–530
　in Italy, 540
　in Japan, 550, 556
　in Mexico, 564–565
　in New Zealand, 570–571
　in Romania, 577–578
　in Spain, 583
　in Thailand, 588–589
　in United Kingdom, 600–601
quality management plan, 89
quality management system (QMS) in Ireland, 529
quality-of-life (QOL) assessment as trial endpoint, 134
quality-of-life (QOL) studies
　in Austria, 459
　hereditary cancer predisposition testing in, 335
　in Japan, 554–555
　in Mexico, 564
　in Romania, 577
　in Thailand, 588
quality system(s)
　benefits of, 89–90
　defined, 199
quality system framework, failure mode and effects analysis as, 201, 202–203f, 202f
quantitative real time PCR (QRT-PCR), 322
quinacrine banding (Q-banding), 339
quorum, 146
quoting, 436–437

R

radiation safety review, 142
randomization, 23, 24t, 25t
　and adherence, 242
　and ethics, 98
　patient education about, 297
randomized controlled trials (RCTs), 17, 18, 23
　abstract of, 432t
　reporting guidelines for, 431t
randomized discontinuation design, 27, 28f
range, 137f

Ransdell Act (1930), 3
rate of absorption, 359t
rating system to estimate budget per patient, 171, 175f
rationale section of protocol, 110
R&D approval in United Kingdom, 594
readiness to learn, 292
ReBEC, 251
receipt of research drugs, 260–261, 391f
Recombinant DNA Advisory Committee (RAC), 142
recombinant DNA safety review, 142
recommended phase II dose (RP2D), 24t
reconsent, 119, 119f
record(s)
　drug accountability, 409
　electronic, 365
　IRB, 152
　medical, 365–366, 366f
　research, 365, 366f
　study participant, 409–410
　subject accountability, 392t
recording of adverse events, 279, 280f
record keeping in protocol, 111
record retention, 61, 61f
recruitment, 229–240
　in Australia, 445–446, 449–450
　in Austria, 457–458
　barriers to, 229–231, 230t
　in Belarus, 468–469
　in Canada, 478, 478f
　in China, 486–487
　and clinical trials as business, 236–237
　considerations for, 229–235
　electronic screening for, 236
　in France, 499
　in Germany, 506
　in India, 516
　in Ireland, 526
　in Italy, 537–538
　in Japan, 550–551
　in Mexico, 562
　of minority and underserved populations, 231
　in New Zealand, 569
　nursing competencies in, 608
　patient advocates in, 238
　patient navigators in, 237–238
　process of, 235
　research team perspectives on, 232–235, 233f, 234f
　in Romania, 576
　via social media, 237
　in Spain, 582
　strategies for, 235–238, 236f
　in Thailand, 587
　trial focus and, 231–232
　by tumor boards, 236
　in United Kingdom, 597, 597f
recruitment material in regulatory file, 389t
Red Contra el Cáncer, 564, 565f

reference citations, 436, 436f, 437f
reference ranges, 391t
regimen complexity and adherence, 242
registration of clinical trials, 59
registry databank, 116–117
regulation, 58f
regulatory agencies, correspondence with, 391t
regulatory approval in India, 515
regulatory background of Belarus, 463
regulatory bodies in Belarus, 464
regulatory compliance, budgeting for, 182
regulatory file(s), 387–395
　in audit, 408–409
　centralizing essential documents in, 394
　contents of, 387, 388–393t
　format for, 393–394, 394t
　in Germany, 509
　in Japan, 555
　maintenance of, 394
　in Canada, 481
　overview of, 387
　terminology for, 387
regulatory issues. See legal, regulatory, and legislative issues
reimbursable costs in agreement, 186
reimbursement fraud, 63
reimbursement of subjects, 149
remission, 298
remote data capture, 377
renal function tests, 265–266, 265f
reportable events, 151–152, 152t
reportable payments, 213
reporting guidelines for writing research articles, 430, 431t
reporting of adverse events, 279–284
　expedited, 281–284, 283f, 283t, 284
　forms for, 283–284
　to IRB, 280, 281, 281f, 390t
　for NCI-sponsored clinical trials, 284, 285f, 286f
　routine, 280–281, 281f
　voluntary postmarketing, 284
reproducibility of endpoints, 131
request for proposals (RFP), 47
required procedures in protocol, 129–131, 130f
research, vs. practice, 52, 53t, 100, 100f
research abstract, 432t
research advance directive, 122
research bases that best fit institution's mission, 192–193
research data, 369
Research Effort Tracking Assessment (RETA), 158–160, 159t, 161t
research ethics board attestation (REBA), 481
research ethics board (REB) in Canada, 475–476

Research Ethics Committees (RECs), 143
  in United Kingdom, 593–594
research governance in Australia, 445
research IND, 14
research misconduct, 62–63, 62t, 102, 102f
research nurse, role of, 81–84, 83f, 83t
research participant, 80
research record, 365, 366f
research results, guidelines for reporting, 430, 431f, 431t
research-specific documentation, 366–368
research study article, 430, 430t, 431f, 431t
research study drugs. *See* investigational agent(s)
research team, 77–87
  attributes needed for success of, 77
  in Australia, 444
  in Austria, 458
  in Canada, 474–475
  in China, 487
  clinical data manager on, 84–85
  clinical research coordinator on, 84, 85f
  delegation log for, 80
  in France, 498, 498t
  in Germany, 504
  interdisciplinary, 85–86
  investigator on, 77–80, 78t
  in Italy, 536
  in Japan, 546–547, 547f
  nurse's role on, 81–84, 83f, 83t
  and recruitment, 232–235, 233f, 234f
  research participant on, 80
  in Romania, 575
  subinvestigator on, 78t, 80
resource allocation, 157–170
  in Australia, 447
  basic algorithm for, 163–164, 163f
  factors affecting, 157–158
  in Germany, 505
  graphics used for, 164–168, 165f, 166f, 167–168t, 169f
  in Japan, 549
  protocol-directed, 163–164, 163f, 164f
resource planning
  graphics used for, 164–168, 165f, 166f, 167–168t, 169f
  protocol-directed, 163–164, 163f, 164f
respect for persons, 53, 53t, 113
response assessment in Australia, 446
Response Evaluation Criteria in Solid Tumors (RECIST), 132
results database, 247

retention, 241–246. *See also* adherence
  in Austria, 457–458
  in Belarus, 468–469
  in Canada, 478
  in China, 486–487
  in France, 499
  in Germany, 506
  in India, 516
  in Ireland, 526
  in Italy, 537–538
  in Japan, 550–551
  in Mexico, 562
  in Romania, 576
  in Spain, 582
  in Thailand, 587
  in United Kingdom, 597, 597f
retrospective cohort studies, 38
Return Investigational Agent Form, 263
return of research drugs
  by patient, 263
  to supplier, 263
reverse banding (R-banding), 339
revisions of original protocol document, 150–151
ribonucleic acid (RNA), 316, 316f
ribonucleotide reductase enzyme (RRM1) in lung cancer, 345–346
risk(s)
  on consent form, 614–620
  defined, 53, 147, 147f
  for vulnerable populations, 148, 149t
risk assessment in United Kingdom, 596
risk-benefit analysis, 147–148, 147f, 148t
risk priority number (RPN), 201
Romanian clinical trials, 573–578
  adverse events in, 576–577
  correlative, 577
  documentation and data management for, 577
  ethics committees for, 574
  financial factors for, 576
  fundamental information on, 574–575, 575f
  genetics and genomics in, 577
  history and foundation of, 573–574
  informed consent for, 575–576
  participants of, 576–577, 576f
  professional development for, 578
  protocol development, review, and approval for, 575–576
  quality assurance for, 577–578
  recruitment and retention for, 576
  research team for, 575
Roosevelt, Franklin D., 3
routine audit/review, 403f
routine monitoring visit, 406–407

rule, 58f
rule-based designs, 30

S

safe handling in United Kingdom, 594–595
safety, in protocol, 137–138
safety endpoints, 131
safety information in regulatory file, 390t
safety reviews, 141–142
sample size, 135–136
sarcomas, 340
satellite institutions, dispensing of research drugs to, 262
satellite pharmacy, dispensing of research drugs by, 262
scalability of clinical data management system, 378
schedule of events table, 130, 130f
schema section of protocol, 110
scientific integrity, 101–102, 207
scientific misconduct, 215
scientific review, 141
scientific value, 97–99, 98f
scope of work in agreement, 186
screen failures, budgeting for, 180
screening for accrual, budgeting for, 180
screening IND, 14
screening trials, hereditary cancer predisposition testing in, 334–335
secondary objectives in protocol, 110, 127–128
secondary payer issues in agreement, 187
security
  of clinical data management system, 378–379
  of data, 374, 374f
seguro popular, 562
selection bias, 23
self-administered study drugs, documentation of, 367–368
semantic data elements, standards for, 375
semantic interoperability of clinical data management system, 378, 379
serious adverse events (SAEs), 272t, 281, 282
  in European Union, 492
  in regulatory file, 390t
  as reportable events, 152t
  in United Kingdom, 599
severity rating scales for adverse events, 274, 276t
Shalala, Donna, 397–398
shipment of research specimens, 61
signature form, 388t
significance level, 136f
significant financial interest, 210, 211

significant risk (SR) device, 149
silent polymorphism, 317
simple randomization, 25t
single-gene markers, 343
single nucleotide polymorphisms (SNPs), 317, 343
site monitoring in Ireland, 529–530
site qualifications, 153
  in Belarus, 465
site-specific assessment in Australia, 447
6-mercaptopurine (6-MP) and thiopurine S-methyltransferase (TPMT), 318–319
Skloot, Rebecca, 7
social media for recruitment, 237
social value, 97–99, 98f
Society of Clinical Research Associates, 417t
solid tumor response assessment as trial endpoint, 131–133, 132t, 133t
somatic mutations, 317, 340
source data, 365–366, 366f
source document(s), 365–366, 366f
source documentation for informed consent process, 120
source document verification (SDV)
  in Japan, 555
  in United Kingdom, 601
Spanish Agency of Medicines and Medical Devices, 579–580
Spanish clinical trials, 579–584
  conflicts of interest in, 581–582
  correlative, 583
  documentation and data management for, 583
  ethics committee for, 580–581
  financial factors in, 582, 582f
  fundamental in formation on, 579–580
  genetics and genomics in, 583
  history and foundation of, 579
  participants of, 582–583
  professional development for, 583, 584f
  protocol development, review, and approval for, 580–582
  quality assurance for, 583
  recruitment and retention for, 582
  types of, 580
Special Access Program (Canada), 474
Special Exceptions, 263, 264
special exemption, 42
Specialized Programs of Research Excellence (SPOREs), 46
specialty certification, 416–417

Specific Protocol Exceptions to Expedited Reporting (SPEER), 284, 286f
specimen(s), shipment of, 61
specimen collection in protocol, 130–131
sponsor(s), 45–48
　in Australia, 445
　correspondence with, 393t
　defined, 45
　in drug development, 13
　in European Union, 492
　in France, 498
　in Germany, 504
　government agencies as, 45–47, 46f
　of investigator-initiated trials, 47
　in Ireland, 523
　in Japan, 546
　National Cancer Institute (NCI) as, 407–408
　nonprofit organizations as, 47–48, 48f
　pharmaceutical industry, 47
　protocol approval by, 142–143
　reporting of adverse events to, 280, 281–282, 390t
　responsibilities of, 45
　that best fit institution's mission, 192–193
sponsor audits, 405–406
sponsor visits, 406–408, 406f
stable disease in solid tumor response assessment, 133
staff education
　in Germany, 506–507
　in Japan, 551–552
staff effort and budgeting, 179–181, 180f, 181f
staff responsibilities, 388t
stage of disease in eligibility, 129
standard(s), 68–69
　clinical research, 375, 376t
　defined, 375
　list of, 371
standard operating procedures (SOPs), 89–95
　in Australia, 445
　benefits of, 89–90
　in Canada, 475
　decision-making and planning matrix for, 92, 93f
　defined, 89
　development of, 90–92
　in Germany, 504
　implementation of, 92
　in Ireland, 529
　items to include in, 92, 94t
　in Japan, 547–548, 548f
　maintaining, 92
　protocol-specific, 90
　and quality management, 89
　resources for, 90, 90f
　table of contents for, 90–91, 91f
　in United Kingdom, 594
　writing of, 92

Standing Committee on Therapeutic Trials (SCOTT, New Zealand), 568
Stark Law, 63
start-up costs, 176–177
State Cancer Legislative Database, 61
state clinical trial legislation, 60–61
statistical considerations
　in protocol, 111
　in protocol development, 134–137, 136f, 137f
statistical power, 135–136
statistical tests, 136
statute, 58f
stipulations by IRB, 150
storage
　of biospecimens, 351–355, 354f
　in Canada, 480
　in Japan, 554
　of research drugs, 261–262
stratification, 24t, 25t
stratified randomization, 24t, 25t
Stroescu, Valentin, 573
structural barriers to recruitment, 231
study binder. See regulatory file(s)
study completion in regulatory file, 390t
study coordinator, budgeting for, 180–181, 180f, 181f
study design, selection of, 128–129
study drug administration. See administration of research study drugs
study intervention in protocol, 129–131, 130f
study parameters in protocol, 111
study participant records, 409–410
study report in regulatory file, 390t
subinvestigator, 78t, 80
subject accountability records, 392t
subject identification code list, 392t
subject screening list, 392t
substudies. See correlative trials
sum, 137f
summarizing, 436
supplier, return of research drugs to, 263
supportive care trials, hereditary cancer predisposition testing in, 335
surrogate endpoint, 24t
survey, 36–37
suspected adverse event, 272t
suspected adverse reaction (SAR), 272t, 281
suspected unexpected serious adverse reactions (SUSAR), in European Union, 492

systematic review, 18
　reporting guidelines for, 431t
Systematized Nomenclature of Medicine Clinical Terms (SNOMED—CT), 271–274
system characteristics and adherence, 243
System Organ Class (SOC), 274, 275f, 277f

T

Taqman Allelic Discrimination Assay, 321–322
target lesions in solid tumor response assessment, 132–133
task time estimates, 160, 161t
team. See research team
temperature log in regulatory file, 391t
termination
　in agreement, 187
　as reportable event, 152t
terminology dictionaries, 371, 373, 373f
test transfer of data, 373
Thai clinical trials, 585–590
　correlative, 588
　cultural aspects of, 589–590
　documentation and data management for, 588
　ethics committees for, 586
　financial factors and budget for, 587
　fundamental information on, 586, 587f
　genetics and genomics in, 588
　history and foundation of, 585
　international, 585–586
　participants of, 587–588
　professional development for, 589
　protocol development, review, and approval for, 586–587
　quality assurance for, 588–589
　recruitment and retention for, 587
　regulatory issues with, 586, 587f
Thailand, incidence of cancer-related deaths in, 585, 586f
Thai Society of Clinical Oncology (TSCO), 585
Therapeutic Goods Administration (Australia), 444
therapeutic index, 24t, 30
therapeutic intent, 30
therapeutic misconception, 99–101
　case study on, 99–100
　and informed consent, 100–101, 100f, 101f
　and motivation for participation in clinical trials, 305

　and patient education, 296
　in phase 0 studies, 30
therapeutic misestimation, 100
therapeutic optimism, 100
Therapeutic Products Directorate (TPD, Canada), 474
thiopurine S-methyltransferase (TPMT), 6-mercaptopurine (6-MP) and, 318–319
third-party payers, billing compliance for, 177–178
3 + 3 design, 30, 31f
3-D virtual spaces, 416t
threshold resources, 164–165
thrombocytopenia, 266
timeline(s)
　and financial risk reduction, 192
　protocol-based, 164, 164f
time points in protocol, 130
time to progression as trial endpoint, 132t
time to treatment failure as trial end point, 132t
Title 21, 54, 56t, 67
Title 45, 54, 56t
title page of protocol, 109–110
TNM system in eligibility, 129
toxicity, dose-limiting, 24t, 30–31, 32, 128
training certificates, 388t
transcription, 316, 316f
transfer of research drugs, 263–264
transfers of value, 213
translation, 316, 316f
translational research
　in Germany, 508
　in New Zealand, 570
Translational Research Program, 46
translocations, 317
Transparency Reports and Reporting of Physician Ownership of Investment Interests, 212
treatment activities, budgeting for, 180
treatment allocation, 392t
treatment completion, patient education for, 298
treatment costs and adherence, 242–243
treatment IND, 14, 43, 43f
treatment plan in protocol, 110
treatment protocol, 43, 43f
Treatment Referral Center (TRC), 43
treatment trials, hereditary cancer predisposition testing in, 334
trial endpoints, 131–134, 132–135t
trial focus and recruitment, 231–232
Trial Registration Data Set (TRDS), 250

trial steering committees in United Kingdom, 599
tumor boards for recruitment, 236
tumor burden in solid tumor response assessment, 132–133
tumor profiling, 343–349
  and biomarkers in specific cancers, 344–347
  in breast cancer, 344–345
  in colon cancer, 346
  defined, 343
  in Japan, 554
  and Kaplan-Meier survival curve, 344
  in lung cancer, 345–346
  in prostate cancer, 347
  techniques for, 343
  uses for, 343
Tuskegee syphilis experiment, 6
type I error, 135, 136f, 138
type II error, 135, 136f

U

UDP-glucuronosyl transferase, irinotecan and, 320
UGT1A1 gene, 320
UK Clinical Research Collaboration (UKCRC), 591
UK Genetic Testing Network, 599
unanticipated adverse device effects (UADEs), 273t, 281
unanticipated problems (UPs), 273t, 285–286, 287f
  in Canada, 479
  in Germany, 507–508
  in Japan, 552
  in regulatory file, 390t
  as reportable events, 152t
unblinded study, 24
underrepresented populations
  education of, 224–225
  recruitment of, 231
undue influence, 113–114
unequivocal progression in solid tumor response assessment, 133
unexpected event, 273t, 281, 282

United Kingdom (UK) clinical trials, 591–602
  active treatment in, 598–599
  adverse events in, 598–599
  correlative, 599–600
  documentation and data management for, 600
  eligibility for, 598
  ethics and regulations for, 593–594
  financial factors with, 597
  fundamental information on, 593–594, 593f
  genetics and genomics in, 599
  history and foundation for, 591–593, 592f
  legal, regulatory, and legislative issues with, 593, 593f
  off-treatment follow-up for, 597–598
  participants of, 598–599
  preparation for, 596–597
  professional development for, 601
  protocol development, review, and approval for, 595–597, 595f
  quality assurance for, 600–601
  recruitment and retention for, 597, 597f
  safe handling and workplace safety in, 594–595
  standard operating procedures for, 594
University Hospital Medical Information Network Clinical Trials Registry (UMIN-CTR, Japan), 551
unscheduled visits, documentation of, 367
updates of original protocol document, 150–151
U.S. Code of Federal Regulations, 54, 56t
useless steps or tasks, 194
U.S. Food and Drug Administration (FDA)
  and clinical trial registries, 249
  Critical Path Initiative of, 5
  on data and safety monitoring plans (DSMPs), 398

  in drug development, 13
  electronic mailing list of, 417t
  on financial conflict of interest, 208, 209
  Form 1572 of, 388t
  on good clinical practice, 69, 70t
  on informed consent, 114
  inspections by, 404–405, 405t
  organizational structure of, 56, 57f
  reporting of adverse events to, 280, 282, 283f, 283t
  review of IND by, 14–15
  on role of investigator, 78–79
  toxicity grading scales of, 276t
  U.S. regulations by, 5, 54, 55t, 56
U.S. National Library of Medicine on reporting guidelines for writing research articles, 431t
U.S. National Research Act (1974), 6, 52
U.S. regulatory authority, 53–57
  based on type of study and sponsor, 54, 55t
  Department of Health and Human Services as, 54, 54f
  Food and Drug Administration as, 56–57, 57f, 58f
  Office for Human Research Protections as, 54–56
  Titles 21 and 45 as, 54, 56t

V

variance, 137f
Velos, 167t
Veracode ADME chip, 322
Virchow, Rudolf, 3
visual learning style, 295t
Vogel, Robert, 377
volume of distribution, 359t
voluntary action indicated (VAI), 404
voluntary postmarketing reporting, 284
vulnerable participants, 99

vulnerable populations, regulations for, 148, 149t

W

waivers for informed consent, 123
websites for education, 223, 224f
white blood cell (WBC) count, 266
Wichita Protocol Assessment Tool (WPAT), 158–160, 160t, 161t
wild-type allele, 318
women, treatment of, 7
workload determination, 157–170
  in Australia, 447
  empirically developed task-based measures for, 158–161, 161t, 162f
  factors affecting, 157–158
  in Germany, 505
  in Japan, 549
  key lessons learned about measurement for, 160–163
  promise of prospective comprehensive tool for, 158–160
  questions about, 157
  selected clinical studies on, 158, 159–160t
workload measurement
  empirically developed task-based, 158–161, 161t, 162f
  key lessons learned about, 160–163
workload tool, promise of prospective new, 158–160, 159–161t, 162f
workplace safety in United Kingdom, 594–595
World Health Organization (WHO)
  and clinical trial registries, 247, 250
  on solid tumor response assessment, 132
World Medical Association, 5–6, 52, 67, 68f, 98f, 251, 516, 605